ANNUAL REVIEW OF PHARMACOLOGY AND TOXICOLOGY

ANNUAL REVIEW OF PHARMACOLOGY AND TOXICOLOGY

HENRY W. ELLIOTT, *Editor*
California College of Medicine, University of California, Irvine

ROBERT GEORGE, *Associate Editor*
University of California School of Medicine, Los Angeles

RONALD OKUN, *Associate Editor*
California College of Medicine, University of California, Irvine

VOLUME 17

1977

ANNUAL REVIEWS INC.   4139 EL CAMINO WAY   PALO ALTO, CALIFORNIA 94306

ANNUAL REVIEWS INC.
Palo Alto, California, USA

International Standard Book Number: 0-8243-0417-9
Library of Congress Catalog Number: 61-5649

Annual Reviews Inc. and the Editors of its publications assume no
responsibility for the statements expressed by the contributors to this Review.

REPRINTS

The conspicuous number aligned in the margin with the title of each article in this
volume is a key for use in ordering reprints. Available reprints are priced at the
uniform rate of $1 each postpaid. The minimum acceptable reprint order is 10
reprints and/or $10.00, prepaid. A quantity discount is available.

PRINTED AND BOUND IN THE UNITED STATES OF AMERICA

Henry W. Elliott
1920–1976

The Editorial Committee dedicates this volume to the memory of Professor Henry W. Elliott in honor of his invaluable contributions to the *Annual Review of Pharmacology and Toxicology*. Dr. Elliott was instrumental in establishing this series, serving as Associate Editor from 1961 to 1965 and as Editor since 1966. His elegant leadership, wisdom, and guidance benefited all who enjoy the *Annual Reviews*.

CONTENTS

A Career or Two, *Karl H. Beyer, Jr.*   1

The Pharmacology of Renal Lithiasis, *Thomas H. Steele*   11

Common Mechanisms of Hormone Secretion, *J. M. Trifaró*   27

Pharmacokinetic Consequences of Aging, *David P. Richey and A. Douglas Bender*   49

Pharmacology of Magnesium, *Shaul G. Massry*   67

Toxicology of Haloalkane Propellants and Fire Extinguishants, *Kenneth C. Back and Ethard W. Van Stee*   83

Enzymes As Drugs, *John S. Holcenberg and Joseph Roberts*   97

Antineoplastic Agents From Plants, *Monroe E. Wall and M. C. Wani*   117

Vitamin Toxicity, *Joseph R. DiPalma and David M. Ritchie*   133

Specific Pharmacology of Calcium in Myocardium, Cardiac Pacemakers, and Vascular Smooth Muscle, *A. Fleckenstein*   149

Fish and Chemicals: The Process of Accumulation, *Jerry L. Hamelink and Anne Spacie*   167

Immunologic Aspects of Cancer Chemotherapy, *Charles M. Haskell*   179

Exposure of Humans to Lead, *Paul B. Hammond*   197

Poison Control Centers: Prospects and Capabilities, *Anthony R. Temple*   215

The Pharmacologic Principles of Regional Pain Relief, *John Adriani and Mohammad Naraghi*   223

Aquatic Invertebrates: Model Systems for Study of Receptor Activation and Evolution of Receptor Proteins, *Howard M. Lenhoff and Wyrta Heagy*   243

Basic Mechanisms of Prostaglandin Action on Autonomic Neurotransmission, *Per Hedqvist*   259

Thymic Hormones: Biochemistry, and Biological and Clinical Activities, *Jean-François Bach*   281

Cardiovascular Drug Interactions, *D. Craig Brater and Howard F. Morrelli*   293

Pharmacological Basis for Combination Therapy of Hypertension, *C. T. Dollery*   311

Histaminergic Mechanisms in Brain, *Jean-Charles Schwartz*   325

Pharmacologic Control of Temperature Regulation, *Barry Cox and Peter Lomax*   341

Pharmacology of Laxatives, *Henry J. Binder*   355

PHARMACOLOGICAL IMPLICATIONS OF BRAIN ACETYLCHOLINE
TURNOVER MEASUREMENTS IN RAT BRAIN NUCLEI,
D. L. Cheney and E. Costa 369

THE PHARMACOLOGY OF EXPERIMENTAL MYOPATHIES, Michael B.
Laskowski and Wolf-D. Dettbarn 387

THE EFFECTS OF PSYCHOPHARMACOLOGICAL AGENTS ON CENTRAL
NERVOUS SYSTEM AMINE METABOLISM IN MAN, James W.
Maas 411

PUTATIVE PEPTIDE NEUROTRANSMITTERS, Masanori Otsuka and
Tomoyuki Takahashi 425

SELECTIVE CYCLIC NUCLEOTIDE PHOSPHODIESTERASE INHIBITORS AS
POTENTIAL THERAPEUTIC AGENTS, Benjamin Weiss and William
N. Hait 441

THE PHARMACOLOGICAL EFFECTS OF HYMENOPTERA VENOMS, Richard
M. Cavagnol 479

THE EFFECT OF HYPOLIPIDEMIC DRUGS ON PLASMA LIPOPROTEINS,
Robert I. Levy 499

CLINICAL PHARMACOLOGY OF SYSTEMIC CORTICOSTEROIDS, James C.
Melby 511

THE CLINICAL APPLICATIONS OF CELL KINETICS IN CANCER THERAPY,
R. B. Livingston and J. S. Hart 529

PSYCHOPHARMACOLOGICAL IMPLICATIONS OF DOPAMINE AND DOPAMINE
ANTAGONISTS: A CRITICAL EVALUATION OF CURRENT
EVIDENCE, Oleh Hornykiewicz 545

PEDIATRIC CLINICAL PHARMACOLOGY AND THE "THERAPEUTIC
ORPHAN," Alan K. Done, Sanford N. Cohen, and Leon Strebel 561

IN VITRO STUDY OF β-ADRENERGIC RECEPTORS, Barry B. Wolfe,
T. Kendall Harden, and Perry B. Molinoff 575

PHARMACOLOGIC CONTROL OF FEEDING, Bartley G. Hoebel 605

PROXIMAL TUBULAR REABSORPTION AND ITS REGULATION, Harry R.
Jacobson and Donald W. Seldin 623

ETHNOPHARMACOLOGY OF SACRED PSYCHOACTIVE PLANTS USED BY THE
INDIANS OF MEXICO, José Luis Díaz 647

REVIEW OF REVIEWS, Chauncey D. Leake 677

INDEXES

AUTHOR INDEX 683

SUBJECT INDEX 721

CUMULATIVE INDEX OF CONTRIBUTING AUTHORS, VOLUMES 13–17 744

CUMULATIVE INDEX OF CHAPTER TITLES, VOLUMES 13–17 746

ANNUAL REVIEWS INC. is a nonprofit corporation established to promote the advancement of the sciences. Beginning in 1932 with the *Annual Review of Biochemistry*, the Company has pursued as its principal function the publication of high quality, reasonably priced Annual Review volumes. The volumes are organized by Editors and Editorial Committees who invite qualified authors to contribute critical articles reviewing significant developments within each major discipline.

Annual Reviews Inc. is administered by a Board of Directors whose members serve without compensation.

Annual Reviews are published in the following sciences: Anthropology, Astronomy and Astrophysics, Biochemistry, Biophysics and Bioengineering, Earth and Planetary Sciences, Ecology and Systematics, Energy, Entomology, Fluid Mechanics, Genetics, Materials Science, Medicine, Microbiology, Nuclear Science, Pharmacology and Toxicology, Physical Chemistry, Physiology, Phytopathology, Plant Physiology, Psychology, and Sociology. The *Annual Review of Neuroscience* will begin publication in 1978. In addition, two special volumes have been published by Annual Reviews Inc.: *History of Entomology* (1973) and *The Excitement and Fascination of Science* (1965).

Ann. Rev. Pharmacol. Toxicol. 1977. 17:1–10

A CAREER OR TWO ❖6663

Karl H. Beyer, Jr.

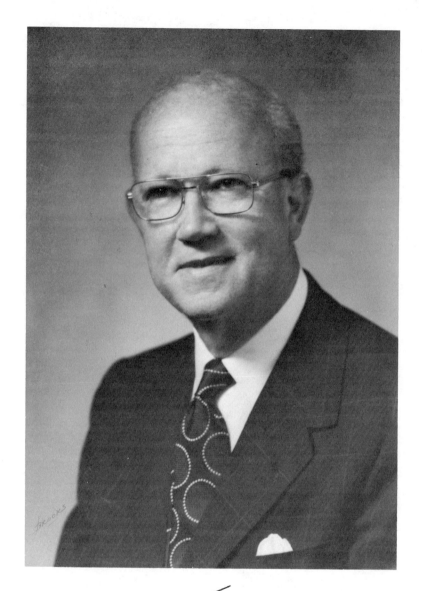

Karl H. Beyer, Jr.

Ann. Rev. Pharmacol. Toxicol. 1977. 17:1–10
Copyright © 1977 by Annual Reviews Inc. All rights reserved

A CAREER OR TWO ♦6663

Karl H. Beyer, Jr.
Department of Pharmacology, The Pennsylvania State University College of Medicine,
Hershey, Pennsylvania 17033 and Department of Pharmacology, The Vanderbilt
University School of Medicine, Nashville, Tennessee 37232

As I stood on the veranda of the little airport terminal at Hershey, Pennsylvania, watching N254-KB hurl itself down runway 26 under the full power and thrust of its engines, I turned to thinking about this prefatory chapter. What of my life would be interesting to those who actually read these bits of memorabilia?

I had touched down at 9:07 EDT. The week before it had been 9:08, which was pretty good reproducibility for a start on still another new chapter in my life. Tom Gelarden, my assistant, was to pick me up at 9:10 for the ten-minute drive across the lovely valley to our laboratory in the Department of Pharmacology of the beautiful new Milton S. Hershey Medical Center, the Pennsylvania State University Medical School. If such a schedule could be sustained, it might be feasible on Wednesdays to breakfast at Stone House (while a Fogarty International Scholar-in-Residence at the National Institutes of Health, Bethesda), put in a reasonable day's work at the Medical School in Hershey, and spend the evening on correspondence at home, near Philadelphia. Wednesday's schedule. In good humor on that lovely morning, August 14, 1974, it occurred to me that such a recitation might be an interesting way to put this prefatory chapter into perspective—prefatory in the sense of anticipating what lay ahead in the next phase of my career as a scientist.

Before my retirement as senior vice president of the Merck Sharp & Dohme Research Laboratories, I had decided that I might accomplish more in the years ahead if I were to build on what I knew rather than start over in an exciting field of research entirely new to me. Thus, as I write I shall look backward to see how my second scientific career is rooted in the past. These reflections will include some highlights of a career that started when I was twelve and had a makeshift lab bench in my room at home, and may shed some light on the direction of my future career as a scientist and teacher.

But first, a few things about my early days that are not likely to be found in such standard references as *American Men and Women of Science*, or *Who's Who*, etc. I was fortunate to have been born (June 19, 1914) to well-regarded residents of a beautiful historic town, Henderson, Kentucky, set high on the banks of the majestic

1

Ohio River and very southern in sentiment. Its lovely main streets were the widest I have known. To me the town, whose economy depended on tobacco, reflected the friendly, leisurely character of substantial people to whom the land had been kind. My two younger sisters and I were reared among people to whom manners seemed more important than means. It was not an industrial town. My father was a capable veterinarian (VMD), hard working and sought after professionally in the surrounding counties. Later, he came to love his own land and animals as a preferred way of life. Mother gave as much of her time as she could to the Methodist Church, in which we all were active. Moderation was taught at home and in the community, and what were considered to be excesses of behavior were dealt with firmly. Those were happy days full of much to learn and do. Time has transformed those wonderful days of learning and doing to years, quite a few of which are behind me, quite a few ahead, I hope.

Even before my high school days, with the encouragement of an excellent and enthusiastic science teacher and friend, Mr. C. P. Rhoads, I discovered a love for chemistry that had to be reconciled with the study of my father's (veterinary) medical textbooks and the dissection of various small animals in my little "laboratory" at home. Even then, it was certain that I should be a medical doctor.

Still another fine teacher and friend, my professor of organic chemistry at Western Kentucky University, Dr. J. T. Skinner, obtained for me from his alma mater a Wisconsin Alumni Research Foundation scholarship in medical physiology (1936). This was exactly what I needed. Dr. Walter J. Meek, my professor and Head of the Department of Physiology at the University of Wisconsin Medical School, made it possible for me to take courses as I pleased and to create my own multifaceted research program as I ranged among the tremendous resources within the university.

Perhaps I should explain that I had taken a double major in chemistry and biology at Western Kentucky. After three years I received my BS degree. I spent an additional year at Western Kentucky taking the graduate courses offered in both zoology and chemistry while teaching in both departments and waiting for such an opportunity as the WARF scholarship afforded.

At Wisconsin, it was possible to work toward the PhD and MD degrees concurrently as one did research and taught. Then, too, some courses, such as Dr. Karl Paul Link's famous Carbohydrate Chemistry (a source of entertainment as well as learning), were given at night. Somehow, one could get to other classes, like Advanced Colloid Chemistry across the street from the medical school in the vast chemistry department, if he was willing to make the effort. Credits and grades had long since become unimportant, and so was the structure of the university when it came to being helpful. If two courses were given at the same time, one got to enough lectures in each to piece together what he wanted to know by additional reading. Sometimes gaining new segments of knowledge was done more expeditiously by bringing specific research problems to the professors. In so doing, one could learn things like diazonium chemistry, which I needed for the colorimetric analysis of sympathomimetic amines; or the physical aspects of organic chemistry, which helped to anticipate structure-activity relationships leading first to metaraminol (that I shall mention again); or the techniques and principles of enzymology, which were reflected in several papers on the metabolism of these compounds. One is tempted to pay tribute to the many people to whom he is indebted for such personal influence, but the list of names would be much too long. Even so, I shall always be grateful for his help to Dr. William B. Youmans who came from Western Kentucky two years before me, who shared his laboratory with me on my arrival, and who succeeded Dr. Meek as chairman of the Department of Physiology.

The purpose of this search for broad academic and research training was straightforward enough. I wanted to be able to synthesize compounds which (by chemical structure–biological activity relationships) seemed interesting, and then to have the capability for evaluating such agents as potential therapy in patients. The advantage of being based in physiology for this training and then moving to pharmacology (as the natural discipline in which to express that ambition) seemed to me that one could acquire the knowledge of the function and the integrative actions of tissues, organs, and systems of organs. One needed this background before trying to modulate such functions during their aberrations, which we call disease, by chemical compounds, which we refer to as drugs. This was to be the marriage of chemistry, which I came to love very early, with medicine, to which I had always been dedicated. This was my way to a career in pharmacology.

Without detailing my research during Wisconsin days, its publication was in journals as diverse as the *Journal of the American Chemical Society,* the *American Journal of Physiology,* or the *Journal of Pharmacology and Experimental Therapeutics,* the *Annals of Internal Medicine,* or *Surgery, Gynecology, and Obstetrics.* Mostly, the work had to do with the actions, metabolism, and elimination of sympathomimetic amines. A gratifying bit of serendipity was that later Dr. Julius Axelrod, by his famous research, successfully and substantially extended my exploratory study of ascorbic acid in the inactivation of sympathomimetic amines (1941),[1] according to personal conversation with him. Seven years at Wisconsin, 18 publications, several advanced degrees (PhM, MD, PhD), and a host of scientist friends later, I was ready for a career that combined these several fascinations in a dedication to the advancement of medicine, of therapeutics. (Later, my friends at Wisconsin added their own distinction, which I cherish, the honorary DSc degree.)

From my structure-activity work that began in 1936 with sympathomimetic amines and carried throughout the Wisconsin days and beyond, I gained a critically important insight that influenced the course of my life. It was the awareness that I would have to team up with capable chemists, biologists, and clinicians if I expected to accomplish as much as I wanted to. For example, the exciting experience of using fuming nitric acid to nitrate β-propiophenone in a physiology laboratory having no exhaust hood was fun and downright hazardous, but not a likely practice

---

[1]Dates in parentheses indicate a date of publication, marketing, etc. They do not indicate dates that concepts or projects were formulated or terminated.

for an extended career! (Actually, I blew some of the fumes out an open window with a cheap home fan.) The logical course then and now for one with my polyvalent inclinations toward research has been within the broad resources of the pharmaceutical industry. I was fortunate in my choice of such associates.

Incidentally, from the structure-activity studies on related chemicals mentioned above, the propiophenone derivative I had decided was worth making and studying (1943) was what we later called metaraminol (Aramine®). A search of the chemical literature revealed that the agent had been synthesized in this country by Dr. Walter H. Hartung, and also in Germany. Its biomedical significance had been overlooked previously, but the compound had the combination of potency and stability that I had anticipated. I called my interest in this agent to the attention of Sharp and Dohme when I joined the company. They marketed the levorotatory form in 1952. Some readers will know metaraminol as a vasopressor agent long used in anesthesiology and the management of hypotension attending shock. Others will recognize it from the literature on false neurotransmitters, a much more recent development to which this compound has contributed. I had synthesized one compound, one drug. A good start, I thought.

There seemed hardly a transition between my graduate and medical school days at Wisconsin and the beginning of research as assistant director of pharmacology at the (then) Sharp and Dohme Research Laboratories, May 1, 1943, except that I had access to more of everything than I knew how to use, at first. The following thirty years and three months, with all their excitement and challenge, never allowed time for looking back or changing course. At the outset of that association, I had intended to return to the academic life several years before I actually did. When I did choose to retire early, it was with immense satisfaction that I could commend to top management those who had worked closely with me in research. These were scientists like Dr. Clement A. Stone, identified with the early work on methyldopa (Aldomet®), and Dr. Ralph F. Hirschmann, who shared honors for the first synthesis of an enzyme, ribonuclease.

My retirement from Merck & Co., Inc. on July 31, 1973, some six weeks after having turned 59, was the termination of a first career. August 1, 1973, marked the beginning of a second.

Indeed, it was at a tremendous retirement party that my second career began to unfold. Dr. Allan D. Bass, long-time friend, chairman of the Department of Pharmacology and acting dean of the Medical School at Vanderbilt, had been asked by my associates to participate in the ceremonies at that affair. It was a surprise to all of us when Dr. Bass presented to me a formal invitation to be a visiting professor of pharmacology at Vanderbilt. I was delighted. On the same occasion, Dr. Elliot S. Vesell, professor and chairman of the Department of Pharmacology at The Milton S. Hershey Medical Center of the Pennsylvania State University, offered me a visiting professorship in his department as well. This seemed too good to be true. I accepted both, for I was familiar with the schools and their excellent faculties. Since Hershey, Pennsylvania, was only 27 minutes by plane into the beautiful foothills of the Appalachian Mountains, it was feasible for me to accept laboratory space for research as well as the teaching responsibilities I had undertaken both there and at Vanderbilt. This has worked out very well.

Teaching at both institutions has been a source of great personal satisfaction— at both the graduate and the medical student level. The experience has not been entirely new, for I have held appointments at four of the Philadelphia medical schools for years. When relating to medical students, I have made it a practice to teach basic pharmacology as a clinical subject, not as molecular biology. The latter is more appropriate to graduate training in research, I think. At the graduate student level, I enjoy teaching the discovery, development, and delivery of new drugs— something about which most graduates in pharmacology know little. Actually, this is the title of a book I hope to finish while I am still intimately familiar with the details of such a complex subject.

Setting up a new laboratory, training personnel, and handling experiments at technical as well as conceptual levels have been as pleasurable in this second time 'round as was learning about such things when a graduate student years ago. Assuming responsibility for ongoing training at the PhD candidate level is new to me and is at least as serious as the responsibility for postdoctoral guidance. In the past, my role in this connection has been to choose from among men and women who have received such advanced training those whom we might help to reach their full potential within a (pharmaceutical) research environment that required the concerted effort and technical ability of many, much of the time. Now, I hope to be so favored by this present effort as to count toward accomplishment the training of useful students, in addition to the contributions to science, knowledge, and therapy with which I have been fortunate to be identified.

Undertaking the renal transport characterization of the quaternary ammonium compound amprolium (Amprol®), since setting up my new laboratory at Hershey, is reminiscent of the earlier days leading to the discovery of probenecid (Benemid®).

When I first joined Sharp and Dohme, I was sent to the laboratory of Dr. James A. Shannon where I learned the conventional renal clearance techniques. I had no prior experience with such concepts and procedures, and so it was fun to see whether I could adapt from a familiarity with sympathomimetic amines to this, for me, new line of research. That was in June and July of 1943. Altogether, about a month was spent in Dr. Shannon's laboratory among bright young men including David P. Earle, Bernard B. Brodie, Julius Axelrod, John E. Baer, Robert W. Berliner, Sidney Udenfriend, and others from that group whom I came to know later. Actually, the work done while at the Goldwater Memorial Hospital laboratories of Dr. Shannon and when I first set up the renal program in our laboratories was on the clearance of sulfonamides. The chemists there, with the guidance of their director, Dr. James M. Sprague, had synthesized sulfamerazine, succinylsulfathiazole, and phthalylsulfathiazole, which the company marketed. This sulfonamide chemistry was to serve us well for many years. The friendship that developed between Jim Sprague and me helped set a standard for personal cooperation between chemists and biologists that I think has contributed to the productivity of these scientists.

At the request of Dr. Homer W. Smith, the leading renal physiologist of his day, the company made available a useful formulation of p-aminohippuric acid (PAH) which he developed as a renal function test at that time, 1943–1944. Perhaps it was providential, at least it was thusly circumstantial, that we should be sensitive to the characteristics of renal tubular secretory mechanisms as set forth for PAH. [In retrospect it does not seem very profound, but not until we began to work with the carinamide (Statacin®) and probenecid analogues did we realize that compounds ultrafiltered at the glomeruli and secreted by the tubules could be reabsorbed by the nephron, actively or by back diffusion. A paper on this three-way pattern of transport was published later by us (1954) that also anticipated the primary renal characteristics of the thiazides.]

To the medical world penicillin was the exciting new chemotherapeutic agent in 1943. Short supply, poor absorption when administered orally, and rapid excretion plagued its early use. Indeed, its national distribution was measured out at that time by the renowned Dr. Chester S. Keefer, professor of medicine at Boston University. In the spring of 1944, by the time we had become used to renal clearance technology, an article that called attention once again to the rapid excretion of penicillin caught my attention at the right time. The availability and lack of toxicity of PAH together with some knowledge of enzymology suggested that PAH might inhibit competitively a transport mechanism for the rapid excretion of penicillin, if that took place by tubular secretion in addition to glomerular ultrafiltration. The practical objective of the project was to increase what we referred to as the physiological economy of the antibiotic agent by decreasing its excretion.

Having first exposed the concept to Dr. A. N. Richards, we took it to Dr. Keefer and procured our first 100,000 units of penicillin-G. The Sharp and Dohme bacteriologists, Dr. Willard F. Verwey, A. Katherine Miller, and Roland Woodward, devised a gadget for collecting urine aseptically from dogs. Their laboratory did the antibiotic assays, we in Pharmacology did the chemical analyses, and the organic chemists soon started synthesizing compounds to inhibit the renal tubular secretion of penicillin. I shall never forget the thrill of seeing those first penicillin clearance calculations. Clearly, the antibiotic was secreted by the renal tubules of the dogs. Just as clearly, PAH coadministered with penicillin depressed its clearance (1944).

A scientist is fortunate if there are even a few such moments of ecstasy in his career. We had applied a basic principle of enzymology to the purposeful advancement of medicine. The two drugs (penicillin-G and PAH) administered intravenously sustained the very high antibiotic plasma concentrations needed to treat effectively the then uniformly lethal subacute bacterial endocarditis. The treatment was about as impractical, though, as the disease was unmanageable otherwise. This deterrent was due to the large amount of PAH needed for its continuous venoclysis with penicillin, neither of which was absorbed very well when administered per os.

Out of this work on competitive inhibition of penicillin secretion came, first, carinamide (1947), then, probenecid (Benemid®, 1951). Probenecid was absorbed well when administered orally, the clinical dosage was practical as predicted from the laboratory data, it inhibited the excretion of other organic acids including uric acid, and it was too late to be a marketing success as a general adjunct to penicillin therapy. Probenecid was the first really useful uricosuric agent for the management of gout. It has gained some popularity combined with penicillin in the one-dose therapy for the "hit-and-run" treatment of gonorrhea. The renal physiologist has found it a tool of many uses. Whereas PAH was first administered at an intravenous dose of some 200 g, the concept that made a practical oral (2 g) daily dose of probenecid seem possible was that the compound should be able to inhibit a definitive component of a transport system for penicillin, yet be refractory to secretion by that mechanism (1947). This concept turned out to lead us toward our objective, only to prove erroneous as a likely explanation of the way probenecid was handled by the kidney. Probenecid secretion was offset by a substantial pH-dependent back diffusion which was sufficient to give, for practical purposes, the same net effect as far as dosage is concerned as was anticipated had the concept been correct.

For all we knew at the time, carinamide, the forerunner of probenecid, inhibited all renal tubular secretion into the lumen—although this seemed unlikely. Therefore, at the First International Physiological Congress after World War II at Oxford in 1947, I was delighted to meet Dr. Ivar Sperber, a young scientist from Uppsala who reported the renal tubular secretion of N-methylnicotinamide by the goat. This was important to us, for if his observation could be generalized to man and other animals, it was evidence for still other secretory mechanisms that might not be affected by our compounds. We reported later that carinamide did not inhibit the renal tubular secretion of N-methylnicotinamide by the dog; neither did probenecid. Over the course of time, we reported the renal tubular secretion of other organic bases, mepiperphenidol (Darstine®), a quaternary anticholinergic agent (1953), and mecamylamine (Inversine®) a tertiary ganglionic blocking antihypertensive amine (1956), from among the therapeutic agents we have brought to the physician. Since retirement from the Merck Sharp & Dohme Research Laboratories, I have returned to this interest as we have undertaken fundamental studies on the transport of basic organic compounds (1974) at our new Hershey Medical Center laboratory.

Even before the probenecid work had been brought to a practical conclusion, we turned to the renal modulation of electrolyte balance. Incidentally, any third-year medical student can recognize gross edema. If he remembers his physiology, the various causes of edema and the forms it takes are comprehensible to him. However, in my student days, the teaching of electrolyte balance was as unconvincing as was respiratory physiology. What was clear, though, was that a good orally active, safe diuretic agent suitable for day-to-day usage would be a godsend. Moreover, if a low salt diet (salt restriction) was useful in the management of hypertension, then what we proposed to call a saluretic agent should be doubly important. It should get rid of excess extravascular fluid, edema. It should lower hypertensive blood pressure also, or so we thought. All this was set forth in a memorandum to management of the company when the program was initiated.

Since the chlorothiazide (Diuril®) story has been made to serve many purposes by many people not intimately associated with its discovery, a few words about this innovation in therapy seems justified in this context. This is my own favorite example of what I like to refer to as *Designed Discovery.* To be sure, the previous probenecid research was (*a*) conceived in terms of sound (enzymological) principles, (*b*) adapted to a hypothetical expression of the nature of (penicillin) tubular secretion, (*c*) reduced to well-defined and controllable laboratory procedures, (*d*) precisely supportive of critical structure-activity studies, and (*e*) directed to an outcome that was translatable to a well-defined clinical objective. Actually, chlorothiazide could be substituted for probenecid in the foregoing resume and only the details would be different. In a way, the sentence is a pattern for Designed Discovery, but it is no guarantee of success. Moreover, the discovery of an interesting compound is only the beginning of product development, of the effort that goes into the tailoring of a new, useful, safe therapeutic agent.

Briefly, the way the research leading to chlorothiazide evolved, as expressed in this five-point formula for discovery, was as follows:

1. It was known, or rather believed at the time, that (*a*) the electrolyte and water content of extravascular-extracellular fluid was essentially the same as plasma; (*b*) the predominant matching of cation and anion in these extracellular fluids that needed to be sustained was sodium and chloride; and (*c*) in the passage of plasma water along the lumen of the proximal portion of the nephron, sodium was actively exchanged and its predominant reabsorption at that site was attended by mostly chloride and water. Thus, an effective diuretic had to inhibit sodium reabsorption and with it predominantly chloride if a proper electrolyte and water balance was to be maintained in the body. Hence, the term *saluretic* was selected to emphasize the importance of these relationships.

2. Theoretically, (*a*) organomercurial diuretic agents worked by inhibiting sulfhydryl-catalyzed enzyme systems involved in the exchange reabsorption of sodium (chloride) and water; (*b*) carbonic anhydrase inhibitors blocked the exchange of sodium for hydrogen from the cells, but at the time this work began the few such compounds that had been studied typically increased bicarbonate excretion along with sodium and water.

3. The conventional renal clearance techniques employed in well-trained dogs gave us precise control of acute changes in specific electrolyte and water balance suitable for quantifying and interpreting the comparative efficacy of even related compounds.

4. The structure-activity studies followed the lines of (*a*) chemistry that mimicked the sulfhydryl binding of mercurials. This led to the phenoxyacetic acid derivatives of which ethacrynic acid (Edecrin®) was a prototype; and (*b*) sulfanilamide analogues that were carbonic anhydrase inhibitors, some of which turned out to increase bicarbonate excretion predominantly, or chloride predominantly, or both bicarbonate and chloride along with sodium (some potassium) and water. For example, the simple substitution of a carboxyl group for the para amino group on sulfanilamide yielded a definite chloruresis (actually a saluretic effect). It was this lead into saluretic sulfonamides that caused the greater initial emphasis and effort by us in this type of chemistry that culminated in chlorothiazide (Diuril).

5. From the laboratory data, it was proposed that one to two grams a day would be an adequate, safe dose of chlorothiazide for an adult man for both diuretic and antihypertensive effects. It was. We marketed chlorothiazide in 1957.

This climaxed an exciting, exacting, cooperative project that will always be a source of the greatest satisfaction to those of us who were a part of it. At the time of the introduction of chlorothiazide, it was more important to recognize and accept the utility of this agent than to know exactly how or where these drugs were thought to act in the kidney. The structure-activity work leading to the thiazides made it clear that the balance of where the compounds acted along the nephron was as important as how they acted, but this was not emphasized at the time.

Likewise, a delicate aspect of the clinical trials was to get our friends in the management of hypertension to recognize that a diuretic, actually a saluretic agent, could be basic antihypertensive therapy. There are some wonderful stories about this. We did not assess the activity of chlorothiazide in hypertensive animals prior to clinical trial. At the time, that methodology seemed even less convincing than the literature on clinical response to dietary salt restriction.

Over the years, there were many who participated in this program to an important extent. Among the chemists, those who come particularly to mind are their director and my counterpart, James M. Sprague; Frederick C. Novello; Everett M. Schultz; Edward J. Cragoe, Jr.; and Carl Ziegler. Among the pharmacologists, Horace F. Russo, who was with me from the outset; John E. Baer; L. Sherman Watson; and George M. Fanelli. This same research team went on from chlorothiazide and hydrochlorothiazide (Hydrodiuril®, 1958) to discover the phenoxyacetic acid ethacrynic acid (Edecrin®) in 1964 which extended the scope of diuretic therapy beyond the capability of the thiazides, and an antikaliuretic agent, amiloride (Colectril®) 1967, used mainly as a potassium-sparing adjunct to saluretic therapy. The latter compound is marketed in the principal countries of the world except the USA. This renal program still makes important advances. Such a new compound (a saluretic-uricosuric indanone) was reported in the Abstracts of the Nephrology Society Meeting in Washington, DC, 1974. As I have moved away from a day-to-day association with the Merck Sharp & Dohme research program and have taken time to think about the more general aspects of transport mechanisms in the kidney and other organs, new questions are beginning to find expression in our research at Hershey.

While a member of the Merck Sharp & Dohme Research Laboratories, it was my privilege to help shepherd a number of interesting compounds to the status of useful drugs in various fields of application. Among these were the antidepressant, amitriptyline (Elavil®); the steroid and nonsteroid anti-inflammatory agents, dexamethasone (Decadron®) and indomethacin (Indocin®), respectively; the antihypertensives, mecamylamine (Inversine®) and methyldopa (Aldomet®); the anthelmintic and the coccidiostat, thiabendazole (Mintezol®) and amprolium (Amprol®), respectively; the unique antiserotonin-antihistamine, cyproheptadine (Periactin®), and a number of less well known drugs not mentioned in this text. Each new drug had its own ups and downs, its own story worth telling. Each brought me into close personal association with different scientists primarily identified with each product, different clinicians both in our laboratory and throughout the world who are better characterized by their publications than is possible here.

In turn, these numerous friends have done me the honor of letting me work for them as their director or counselor, as president of the American Society for Pharmacology and Experimental Therapeutics, as president of the Federation of American Societies for Experimental Biology, as an original member of the National Academy of Sciences Drug Research Board, and in many other ways. My intuition many years ago was right. There is so much more that one can do by working with others.

All our research and the worthwhile therapeutic agents discovered and developed between 1943 and 1973 occurred while my associates and I were members of a pharmaceutical laboratory. It was a natural environment for turning today's theory into tomorrow's therapy. We have been accorded the satisfaction of recognition and respect that should go with reasonable accomplishment. I have been honored by my peers according to their individual expression of recognition throughout the world, and travel to their laboratories has contributed to my education immensely. To mention names and places here would be unseemly. My one regret about such travel is that frequently I have not been able to express my appreciation in the native tongue of my host and his confreres. Still, there are many things I have yet to do. Like the rueful comment of Professor S. V. Anichkov in his delightful 1975 prefatory chapter to the *Annual Review of Pharmacology* about his only trip to London, "I did not even go to the British Museum, putting my visit off to some next time." Having seen what the British left behind in many an exotic land, I have every intention of visiting that museum, some day. It would be pleasant if Professor Anichkov and I met again there!

In bringing this rumination to a close, I return to the basis for the introductory paragraph. When it became generally known that I planned to "retire," Dr. James Shannon—by this time the former "most remarkable" director of the National Institutes of Health and active more recently at The Rockefeller Institute—called to my attention the John E. Fogarty International Center for the Advanced Study of Medical Sciences, an affiliate of the National Institutes of Health. Being a scholar-in-residence on the NIH grounds would help to broaden my awareness of the current status of biomedical sciences while providing opportunity for reading and reflection. I was proposed for and accepted this distinction. On August 1, 1974, Mrs. Beyer and I took up residence at Stone House with the other Fogarty Scholars and their wives from lands abroad, the first stage of a wonderful experience. Having the plane at hand made it possible to take full advantage of this opportunity while supervising the research in my laboratory at Hershey, attending my personal affairs at home, lecturing and participating in the various commitments from which one derives a sense of being helpful.

That August morning flight to Hershey was the beginning of a beautiful and interesting day. I hope I shall be privileged to enjoy many additional productive days. On the other hand, there is a layman's concept of retirement that can wait until research and teaching lose their fascination, if ever. Perhaps then there will be time for things like painting, fishing, sailing, metal working, and music composition that I cannot seem to get to, yet.

One more bit of philosophy that occurs to me as I read these words more times than anyone else ever will—to be a reasonably successful idealist, opportunity needs be met realistically.

Ann. Rev. Pharmacol. Toxicol. 1977. 17:11–25
Copyright © 1977 by Annual Reviews Inc. All rights reserved

THE PHARMACOLOGY OF RENAL LITHIASIS

♦6664

Thomas H. Steele

Department of Medicine, University of Wisconsin, Madison, Wisconsin 53706

Although the history of pharmacologic intervention in patients afflicted with nephrolithiasis is a long one, many of the remedies employed probably have had a more soothing effect upon the conscience of the physician than on the colic of the patient. Striking exceptions have been the efficacy of penicillamine in the treatment of cystinuria and of allopurinol in the treatment of uric acid calculi. In recent years, however, significant advances have occurred in our knowledge regarding the pathogenesis of many (formerly) "idiopathic" cases of calcium stone formation. This, together with improved techniques for diagnosis, has led to several novel pharmacologic approaches to the treatment and prevention of calcium-containing stones. This review is concerned primarily with these newer aspects pertaining to calcium stone disease.

THE PRECIPITATION OF CRYSTALLOIDS

Three interrelated factors contribute importantly to the tendency for crystalloids to precipitate within the urinary tract (1). The first relates to the degree of supersaturation of the urine with respect to the constituents of the particular calculus. The second factor relates to the development of a nucleation site, either of an organic or heterologous inorganic nature, which can then promote the accretion of crystals from supersaturated urine. Finally, because the urine of many normal persons free of calculi is often supersaturated with respect to stone-forming crystalloids, inhibitors of crystallization and crystal aggregation could prevent or reverse a tendency toward stone formation. Although all three factors are important, different investigators usually have concentrated their efforts upon one aspect or the other.

   Because the crystallization process is fundamental to the pathogenesis of any type of nephrolithiasis, a few prefatory remarks related to it are in order. Information regarding the tendency of a given crystalloid in solution to precipitate can be gained by a knowledge of its activity product (Figure 1). The activity product depends on

11

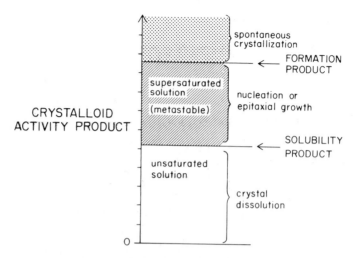

Figure 1   Qualitative representation of the solubility product and formation product, along a hypothetical crystalloid activity product axis (ordinate). Adapted from Pak (1, 23).

the concentrations and electrical charges of the crystalloid constituents, as well as upon the ionic strength of the solution. For example, computation of the activity product for brushite ($CaHPO_4 \cdot 2H_2O$) requires a knowledge of the calcium ion activity and of the monohydrogen phosphate ion activity; these activities are then multiplied to obtain the activity product. Similarly, one needs to know the calcium ion activity and the free oxalate ion activity in order to compute the calcium oxalate activity product. The activity product of monosodium urate is the activity of sodium times the activity of the monohydrogen urate ion. Although, in dilute solution, the activity is similar to the concentration, this does not hold for complex concentrated solutions such as urine. In practice, the activities of various ion species in urine are calculated utilizing computer programs after measuring the concentrations of many urinary constituents (2–4). The methods for computation of absolute ion activities involve the use of certain assumptions that may not be entirely valid. Finally, the computer programs utilize association constant data from various sources, some of which may be incorrect. Fortunately, certain ingenious approaches have permitted the expression of activity products in terms of solubility products, a procedure that cancels out many of the potential errors inherent in the calculation of absolute activities (4, 5). A knowledge of all complexing ion species is necessary, however, as has recently been shown in the case of calcium oxalate where certain soluble charged oxalate-cation species may form (5a).

The calculation of activity products aside, a few generalizations can be made with regard to the tendency of crystalloids to precipitate (1, 6). When the activity product of the crystalloid in question reaches a certain value, nucleation or spontaneous crystallization ensues. The activity product at which precipitation begins to occur is termed the *formation product* (Figure 1). Once this formation product is reached or exceeded and crystallization ensues, the activity product of the crystalloid will diminish as crystal accretion progresses. Finally, equilibrium will be reached between the crystalloid in solution and the solid phase. The activity product at which this equilibrium occurs is termed the *solubility product* (Figure 1). At activity product levels less than the solubility product, the solid crystalline phase will dissolve tending to reestablish equilibrium conditions. As long as the activity product remains less than the solubility product, crystal accretion cannot occur. The formation product, on the other hand, usually is considerably greater than the solubility product (Figure 1). At activity products between the solubility and formation products, the solution is termed *metastable.* In this metastable region, crystallization will not occur spontaneously, but may take place by epitaxial growth if a suitable nucleating site is placed in contact with the supersaturated solution.

CONDITIONS WITH INCREASED URINARY CRYSTALLOID CONSTITUENTS

Hypercalciuria

Hypercalciuria, whatever the cause, predisposes to calcium stone formation—most often oxalate but sometimes apatite, and infrequently, brushite. Because the intestinal absorption of calcium is regulated, the urinary calcium normally should remain relatively stable and reasonably independent of the dietary calcium intake (7, 8). The setting of an upper limit for normal calcium excretion has been problematic (9). Although the excretion of calcium by any one individual is likely to vary from day to day, the upper limit of normal for 24-hr urinary calcium in normal males is frequently set at 300 mg or 4 mg/kg body weight. More restrictive definitions have been proposed. For example, beneficial results have been claimed after decreasing urine calcium in "marginal hypercalciuric" nephrolithiasis patients with 24-hr urinary calcium excretions of 140 mg/square meter of body surface area (10). When hypercalciuria is accompanied by hypercalcemia, the differential diagnosis becomes that of hypercalcemia. Such diagnostic possibilities as primary hyperparathyroidism, sarcoidosis, hyperthyroidism, and neoplasia should be investigated.

The vast majority of patients with calcium-containing stones and increased urinary calcium excretion fall within the broad category of normocalcemic hypercalciuria. Normocalcemic primary hyperparathyroidism accounts for the hypercalciuria in a fraction of these patients (11–13). The diagnosis is best made by finding an elevated serum parathyroid hormone (PTH) concentration or urinary cyclic AMP excretion, which does not return to normal following calcium loading or normalization of the urinary calcium (14, 15). In this condition, a portion of the urinary calcium is derived from bone ("resorptive" hypercalciuria) (16). The treatment of choice is surgical. The syndrome may appear in certain postmenopausal women, probably as a consequence of the lack of estrogen antagonism against the bone-mobilizing action of PTH (17, 18). The signs of hyperparathyroidism in some members of this group (which may include many poor surgical candidates) may be controlled adequately with estrogen replacement (17, 18).

Intestinal hypercalciuria, a consequence of inappropriately increased enteric calcium absorption, may be diagnosed in a substantial percentage of patients with normocalcemic hypercalciuria (14, 19). Several years ago, the Leeds group observed that the urinary calcium varies much more directly with the dietary calcium intake in certain hypercalciuric patients than in comparable normals (7). The cause of the increased calcium absorption in intestinal hypercalciuria is presently unknown. Elevated plasma concentrations of 1,25-dihydroxyvitamin D, together with low plasma PTH values, have been reported in some hypercalciuric stone-formers (20, 21), suggesting that intestinal hyperabsorption may result from the actions of inappropriately elevated amounts of this active vitamin D metabolite. In patients with intestinal hypercalciuria, the serum PTH and urinary cyclic AMP, should be normal or depressed (14, 15, 19). Rational therapy for this condition includes some degree of restriction of the dietary calcium intake in many patients. In addition, cellulose phosphate, a nonabsorbable agent, which prevents calcium absorption by binding it in the intestine, appears to be the treatment of choice (22). The available data indicate that negative calcium balance does not develop during the administration of cellulose phosphate, at least in patients with intestinal hyperabsorption (23). Unfortunately cellulose phosphate currently is unavailable in the United States except as an investigational drug. Therefore, routine treatment is best accomplished by a combination of dietary calcium restriction and thiazide diuretic administration (see below).

Renal hypercalciuria constitutes a third type of normocalcemic hypercalciuria. In this condition, an increased calcium excretion may be ascribed to a defect in the renal tubular reabsorption of calcium (14, 19). The defective calcium reabsorption does not appear to arise from resistance to the renal tubular action of PTH to facilitate calcium reabsorption (24). Interestingly, in this syndrome, parathyroid stimulation occurs during hypercalciuria, and the serum PTH is elevated (19). Presumably the action of PTH to stimulate the renal biosynthesis of 1,25-dihydroxyvitamin D (25) may result in the intestinal absorption of sufficient additional calcium to offset the increment in renal calcium excretion and prevent negative calcium balance. The serum PTH usually returns toward normal upon amelioration of hypercalciuria (19). Thiazide diuretics are the treatment of choice for renal hypercalciuria. Under many types of experimental conditions, thiazides decrease the renal calcium-to-sodium clearance ratio (26, 27). Thus, during chronic thiazide administration, after sodium balance is achieved and the urinary sodium excretion has returned to control levels, calcium excretion is "reset" at a diminished rate. Animal experiments have indicated that this thiazide-induced dissociation between renal calcium and sodium reabsorption occurs within the distal nephron (28) and may be related to the distal delivery of bicarbonate (29). Although it formerly was believed that the presence of PTH is necessary for the hypocalciuric action of thiazides to occur, recent studies have indicated that PTH is not needed (30, 31). Thiazides are capable of normalizing the urinary calcium and decreasing the activity of calculus formation in most hypercalciuric stone-formers. Following the reports of Yendt and collaborators of the clinically beneficial effects of thiazides upon the activity of nephrolithiasis in these patients (32, 33), many other groups have experienced similar results.

The usual side effects of the thiazide diuretics such as electrolyte abnormalities, glucose intolerance, hyperuricemia, metabolic alkalosis, and postural hypotension due to volume depletion may occur. In addition, hypercalcemia has been reported as a consequence of thiazide therapy, although at least a substantial portion of the increase in serum calcium occurred within the protein-bound fraction (34). Rather variable histologic abnormalities of the parathyroid glands have been noted in some patients (35) and in dogs (36) receiving thiazide diuretics for prolonged intervals. Thus, there remains an aura of uncertainty surrounding a putative relationship between thiazides and the parathyroids (37–40). It seems most likely that hypercalciuric patients with occult parathyroid adenomas and relatively nonsuppressible PTH secretion should be optimal candidates to develop thiazide-induced hypercalcemia. Therefore, it is wise to monitor the serum calcium in hypercalciuric patients commencing thiazide therapy.

Hyperoxaluria

At least two types of inherited enzyme abnormalities leading to florid hyperoxaluria secondary to increased oxalate synthesis have been described (41). Clinically the disorders are characterized by calcium oxalate stone formation early in life, followed by renal and systemic oxalosis. The treatment of these patients is particularly vexing, but fortunately the number afflicted is small.

Aside from the "primary hyperoxalurias," stones containing substantial amounts of calcium oxalate constitute about two thirds of the renal calculi in the United States (42). Although it seems surprising that our knowledge of the renal handling of oxalate is not extensive, this void stems largely from difficulties in the measurement of oxalate. Colorimetric procedures require a precipitation step, during which variable quantities of oxalate may be lost. One solution to this problem has been to add ^{14}C-labeled oxalate to urine as an "internal standard." A gas chromatographic technique has been utilized extensively in France (43, 44). Estimates of plasma oxalate concentrations have been obtained by systemically administering ^{14}C-oxalate and allowing sufficient time for its equilibration with the body oxalate pool (45–47). After equilibration the specific activity of labeled oxalate is assumed to be equal in plasma and urine, and oxalate may be measured chemically in the latter. The plasma oxalate values obtained by this method have been exceedingly low— on the order of a few μg/100 ml. An elevated blood oxalate concentration has been reported in a group of patients studied in Spain (47). Limited renal oxalate clearance data have indicated that oxalate may undergo net tubular secretion (45–47), but the details of its renal transport, including possible responsiveness to pharmacologic agents, are not yet well characterized.

A normal 24-hr urinary oxalate excretion appears to be something less than 50 mg. The Leeds group has reported that many calcium oxalate stone-formers have borderline-high urinary oxalate as well as calcium concentrations (3, 48). Presumably, this condition predisposes to intervals of urinary supersaturation, with consequent crystal formation and aggregation (48–51). Similar hyperoxaluric tendencies have been reported in series of nephrolithiasis patients from France (43, 44) and Spain (47). Unfortunately, the pathogenesis of this tendency toward increased urinary oxalate excretion in the usual nephrolithiasis patient is not known at present.

It may derive from an increase in oxalate synthesis or from an increase in the intestinal absorption of dietary oxalate. Oxalate absorption is inversely related to the dietary calcium intake (52, 53). The imposition of a low oxalate diet can result in an increase in the urinary calcium excretion (52). A simple explanation lies in the hypothesis that the calcium and oxalate that form (insoluble) calcium oxalate complexes in the intestine are unavailable for absorption. Thus, changes in the dietary intake of one of these ions will affect the intestinal absorption of the other in a reciprocal fashion.

Intestinal hyperoxaluria is a term applied to a syndrome of calcium oxalate renal lithiasis associated with intestinal disease or resection, chronic diarrhea, or other types of enteric malfunction (54). Daily urinary oxalate excretion in these patients is often greater that 100 mg. Although formerly it was thought that increased oxalate synthesis was responsible for intestinal hyperoxaluria, convincing recent evidence has demonstrated that the dietary oxalate accounts for most if not all of the increment in urinary oxalate excretion (55–57). The explanation for oxalate hyperabsorption probably is related to the concept that, in states of intestinal malfunction, increased amounts of fatty acids are available for complexing with calcium (56). Presumably, this results in decreased intestinal calcium oxalate complex formation, with a resultant increase in the availability of free oxalate for absorption. Therapeutically, dietary oxalate and fat restriction is a rational first step, but this often does not result in normalization of the urinary oxalate excretion. Cholestyramine, a nonabsorbable anion exchange resin, can result in oxalate retention within the intestine and subsequent reduction of the urinary oxalate (54). More recently it has been demonstrated that the feeding of calcium carbonate in patients with intestinal hyperoxaluria can result in a large decrease in urinary oxalate without increasing the urinary calcium (53, 58). By word of caution, it should be remembered that these patients also may have defects in calcium absorption which could explain their failure to develop hypercalciuria. In addition, aluminum hydroxide antacid preparations appear to be effective at binding oxalate within the gut and in reducing oxalate excretion (58). Although aluminum toxicity has been implicated in the pathogenesis of a bizarre neurologic syndrome occurring in patients with end-stage renal disease receiving chronic hemodialysis (59), aluminum has not been convincingly demonstrated as causative to most observers.

Miscellaneous Urinary Solute Alterations

Phosphate-containing stones, brushite, apatite or struvite, may present different types of therapeutic problems. The crystallization of the latter two species is especially pH-dependent. Struvite is often associated with persistent urea-splitting gram-negative urinary tract infections. Aside from antibacterial therapy when appropriate, attempts often are made at urinary acidification. However, acidifying maneuvers which result in metabolic acidosis can elicit an increase in the urinary calcium excretion secondary to an inhibitory effect on the tubular reabsorption of calcium (60). In addition, very large pharmacologic doses of ascorbic acid, sometimes utilized as a urinary acidifying agent, may result in increased oxalate biosynthesis with consequent elevation of the urinary oxalate (61). Preliminary data have indicated that the use of acetohydroxamic acid, a urease inhibitor, may provide a promising therapeutic approach in lithiasis patients with urea-splitting infections (62).

Another program utilized in the treatment of phosphate-containing calculi is essentially that of inducing phosphate depletion. This regimen utilizes oral aluminum hydroxide preparations in order to decrease intestinal phosphate absorption (63). With phosphate depletion, rapid hypophosphaturia occurs as a result of a sharp increase in the renal tubular reabsorption of phosphate (64), but this is accompanied by a reciprocal increase in calcium excretion (65), especially in women (66). A large portion of the increment in urinary calcium is derived from bone (67), and osteomalacia may result from severe phosphate depletion (68). Furthermore, phosphate depletion has other undesirable side effects including diminished phagocytic activity (69) and muscle dysfunction (70). Thus, probably the aluminum hydroxide regimen should be reserved for refractory cases, and then utilized with caution.

DISORDERS OF NUCLEATION INDUCTION

Crystal Nucleation by an Organic Matrix

As already mentioned, the presence of a nucleation site permits the precipitation of crystalloids at activity product values exceeding the solubility product but less than the level at which spontaneous crystallization begins to occur (i.e. the formation product). Work by Boyce and others has demonstrated that urine may contain mucoproteins which provide a nucleating function in urine supersaturated with crystalloids (71). One such substance, designated *matrix substance A*, has been implicated in the pathogenesis of nephrolithiasis in some patients (71). Unfortunately, little is known regarding the processes controlling the formation or excretion of such substances.

Pak's laboratory has demonstrated that collagen can provide the site for epitaxial growth of brushite ($CaHPO_4 \cdot 2H_2O$), a crystalline species which probably is transformed to apatite in alkaline solution (72). In addition, brushite has been implicated as a pathogenetic factor in the formation of other types of calcium-containing stones, as is discussed below (1, 16, 73, 74). The effects of various therapeutic regimens upon brushite activity product ratios have been delineated in detail in Pak's laboratory. For example, corticosteroid administration increases the brushite activity product ratio, whereas cellulose phosphate decreases it (23, 75). Surprisingly, administration of a thiazide diuretic, despite its hypocalciuric action, does not diminish the activity product ratio for brushite because of a concomitant increase in phosphate excretion (23, 76). Likewise, the administration of inorganic phosphate increases the brushite activity product ratio (75, 77).

Nucleation by Heterologous Crystals

It has been proposed that brushite provides a nidus for the epitaxial growth of other calcium-containing crystalline species in urine (1), but this view has been challenged (42). Although direct confirmatory evidence for it is lacking, the hypothesis has many attractive features (1). In addition, many physiologic and pharmacologic influences upon brushite precipitation have been characterized extensively utilizing the assay system devised by Pak (23). For instance, the adequacy of a given type of therapy could be determined by measuring the activity product of brushite and determining its degree of proximity to the formation product. Despite these attractive features, confirmation of the therapeutic efficacy of this approach in a clinical setting is lacking at present. A somewhat similar type of in vitro assay system for calcium oxalate has been utilized in a clinical setting by the Leeds group with reportedly good results (5). A recent observation has been that seed crystals of apatite can induce the epitaxial growth of calcium oxalate monohydrate crystals from supersaturated calcium oxalate solutions (77a).

Many old observations in the renal lithiasis field indicate that stones containing predominantly calcium oxalate may have a central core of uric acid or urate (78). Recent studies, by Coe (79) and Pak (80), have indicated that monosodium urate can act as a nucleator for calcium oxalate. Crystalline monosodium urate, when added to supersaturated calcium oxalate solutions in vitro, initiated calcium oxalate crystallization and increased its rate of precipitation (79, 80).

In a clinical experience with a large group of patients with recurrent calcium-containing stones, Coe & Kavalach found that hyperuricosuria was present in more than one third (81). The etiologies of the hyperuricosuria seemed diverse. Some patients with hyperuricemia and hyperuricosuria probably suffered from urate over-production secondary to increased de novo purine biosynthesis. Others gave a dietary history of excessive purine ingestion. In the remainder, no cause for the hyperuricosuria could be identified. In these patients, the urinary uric acid excretion was shown to be exceptionally responsive to dietary purine loading (81), a type of response which had been noted previously in unilaterally nephrectomized renal transplant donors (82). Although control studies have not been done, preliminary data have indicated that the use of allopurinol in hyperuricosuric oxalate stone-formers affects the activity of the process favorably (10, 81, 83). Coe's laboratory also has found that some patients with recurrent calcium oxalate calculi demonstrate both hyperuricosuria and hypercalciuria. The treatment of those patients with both thiazide diuretics and allopurinol has seemed beneficial (10).

The observation that monosodium urate may act as a nidus for the precipitation of calcium oxalate probably provides an explanation for the old observation that the incidence of calcium-containing kidney stones is increased in patients with gout (84, 85). The fact that crystalline monosodium urate, rather than uric acid, is the offending species is a point of considerable interest and may give rise to some therapeutic dilemmas. Uric acid has usually been considered as the crystalline species which precipitates within and occludes the renal tubules of patients with uric acid nephropathy (86), whereas monosodium urate precipitation occurs within the renal medullary interstitium in gout (86). The solubilities of uric acid and monosodium urate are pH-dependent, but in opposite directions. The solubility of uric acid increases sharply with pH, whereas that of monosodium urate decreases with increasing pH (87–89). Furthermore, an increase in the sodium concentration will decrease the apparent solubility of urate (i.e. by increasing the activity product of monosodium urate) (88, 89). Traditionally, sodium bicarbonate, citrate, or other alkalinizing salts have been utilized to increase the urinary pH in gouty patients with hyperuricosuria and histories of uric acid stones. Such alkalinizing measures in the presence of hyperuricosuria might result in exceeding the formation product of monosodium urate with the resultant formation of a nidus which could promote the deposition and epitaxial growth of calcium oxalate crystals in patients whose urine happened to be supersaturated with respect to the latter crystalloid.

Another potential therapeutic dilemma may arise with the utilization of certain uricosuric natriuretic pharmacologic agents currently being introduced. One such agent, known generically as ticrynafen in the United States and as tienilic acid in Europe, manifests a uricosuric potency exceeding that of probenecid and a natriuretic potency similar to chlorothiazide (90). Whether the use of such an agent would predispose to the formation of calcium oxalate calculi as an indirect consequence of increasing the monosodium urate activity product in urine will have to be determined experimentally (91).

INHIBITORS OF CRYSTAL FORMATION AND GROWTH

Considerable effort has been expended in the identification of organic and inorganic urinary constituents that inhibit the calcification process (92, 92a, 92b). Urinary citrate may diminish somewhat the tendency for calcium stones to form because of its ability to chelate calcium (93). In renal tubular acidosis, the excretion of citrate is diminished because of systemic and probably intracellular acidosis (94), and a diminished urinary citrate has been implicated as a pathogenetic factor in the tendency for some patients with renal tubular acidosis to form calcium-containing stones. The correction of acidosis may ameliorate their tendency toward calcium stone formation (95). However, it is not clear how the administration of alkalinizing salts could correct the stone-forming tendency in patients with *latent* renal tubular acidosis who suffer from nephrolithiasis in the absence of systemic acidosis (95). A diminished urinary citrate probably also partially explains the stone-forming tendencies of patients receiving acetazolamide chronically (96). Stone-forming patients with renal tubular acidosis sometimes are hypercalciuric (95). This may occur because of an inhibitory action of metabolic acidosis upon renal tubular calcium reabsorption (60). In addition, some hypercalciuric patients with renal tubular acidosis have demonstrated intestinal hyperabsorption of calcium (97).

Magnesium oxide has been utilized therapeutically in calcium stone-formers with variable results. Magnesium in high concentration appears to inhibit the crystal growth of calcium oxalate (98, 99). Nevertheless, the diarrhea caused by this and other magnesium-containing compounds sharply curtails their usefulness by forcing limitations on dosage. Methylene blue also has been administered in small doses as a precipitation inhibitor (100, 101). Supplemental ascorbic acid is given in order to avoid the depletion of its body stores. Although patients receiving methylene blue invariably are impressed by the bluish-green color imparted to their urine, a definite salutory effect of methylene blue upon the natural history of stone disease has remained unproved.

Inorganic phosphate has been utilized as a therapeutic agent in patients with calcium-containing stones, with some success at modifying the natural history of the disorder (102, 103). As mentioned earlier, phosphate administration results in an increase in the urinary brushite activity product (23, 75, 77). However, this is offset by the induction of an even greater increase in the formation product for brushite after phosphate administration (75, 77). The salutory effect of phosphate in stone patients has been ascribed to an increase in the urinary pyrophosphate excretion (104, 105). Pyrophosphate has been demonstrated to function as an inhibitor of crystallization and of crystal growth (105). Diarrhea, abdominal cramps, or even constipation are unpleasant side effects of inorganic phosphate administration, but fortunately are short-lived in many patients and often are ameliorated if neutral phosphate is taken in multiple small doses with food. Although phosphate administration does result in an increase in the urinary brushite formation product (75, 77), it probably is unwise to administer phosphate to patients whose calculi contain phosphate as a predominant constituent. The available data indicate that chronic phosphate administration does not elevate the plasma PTH (105a).

Unfortunately, pyrophosphate cannot be administered orally because it is hydrolyzed in the gut. However, the diphosphonates, analogues of pyrophosphate with a carbon atom instead of oxygen bridging the two phosphorus atoms, may be administered orally. The properties of these diphosphonates vary with the nature of the substituents bonded to the carbon bridge. EHDP® (ethane hydroxydiphosphonate) has exhibited a salutory influence on calculus formation in a rat model (106), and also appears to be a highly effective inhibitor of phosphate and oxalate precipitation in crystallization systems in vitro (107–109). EHDP diminishes the renal clearance of phosphate and readily elicits hyperphosphatemia (110). In addition, it interferes with the intrarenal formation of 1,25-dihydroxyvitamin D (111). Finally, EHDP facilitates bone demineralization (111–113). Preliminary studies have suggested a beneficial effect of EHDP on calcium oxalate crystal aggregation in stone-formers (114). Currently, clinical trials of EHDP in nephrolithiasis patients are in progress within the United States but the complete results are not yet generally available (1). Because of its multifactorial toxic potential, it would seem that EHDP is not the ideal agent for the treatment or prevention of renal stones. On the other hand, some other diphosphonate could conceivably provide a better solution for nephrolithiasis patients.

In summary, this review mentions some of the newer (and older) notions regarding the pathogenesis of various types of calcium-containing stones, as well as any currently available or potential pharmacologic interventions which may prove effective. It should be evident that a pharmacologic panacea has yet to be delineated. On the other hand, therapy directed toward decreasing the urinary activity products of crystalloids and eliminating nucleating sites, as well as increasing the concentrations of inhibitors of crystallization in urine, may lead to a more rational and effective pharmacologic assault upon the renal lithiasis problem.

Literature Cited

1. Pak, C. Y. C. 1976. Disorders of stone formation. In *The Kidney*, ed. B. M. Brenner, F. C. Rector, Jr., 1326–54. Philadelphia: Saunders. 28 pp.
2. Robertson, W. G. 1969. Measurement of ionized calcium in biological fluids. *Clin. Chim. Acta* 24:149–57
3. Robertson, W. G., Peacock, M., Nordin, B. E. C. 1968. Activity products in stone-forming and non-stone-forming urine. *Clin. Sci.* 34:579–94
4. Pak, C. Y. C. 1969. Physiochemical basis for the formation of renal stones of calcium phosphate origin: Calculation of the degree of saturation of the urine with respect to brushite. *J. Clin. Invest.* 48:1914–22
5. Robertson, W. G., Peacock, M., Marshall, R. W., Marshall, D. H., Nordin, B. E. C. 1976. Saturation-inhibition index as a measure of the risk of calcium oxalate stone formation in the urinary tract. *N. Engl. J. Med.* 294:249–52
5a. Finlayson, B., Roth, R. 1973. Appraisal of calcium oxalate solubility in sodium chloride and sodium-calcium chloride solutions *Urology* 1:142–44
6. Kallistratos, G. 1974. Physicochemical principles and clinical results concerning the conservative treatment of kidney stones. *Urol. Int.* 29:93–113
7. Peacock, M., Hodgkinson, A., Nordin, B. E. C. 1967. Importance of dietary calcium in the definition of hypercalciuria. *Br. Med. J.* 3:469–71
8. Peacock, M., Knowles, F., Nordin, B. E. C. 1968. Effect of calcium administration and deprivation on serum and urine calcium in stone-forming and control subjects. *Br. Med. J.* 2:729–31
9. Robertson, W. G., Morgan, D. B. 1972. The distribution of urinary calcium excretions in normal persons and stone-formers. *Clin. Chim. Acta* 37:503–8
10. Coe, F. L. 1976. Long term prevention of calcium oxalate nephrolithiasis by chronic thiazide and allopurinol administration. *Clin. Res.* 24:396A (Abstr.)
11. Wills, M. R., Pak, C. Y. C., Hammond, W. G., Bartter, F. C. 1969. Normocalcemic primary hyperparathyroidism. *Am. J. Med.* 47:384–91
12. Muldowney, F. P., Freaney, R., McMullin, J. P., Towers, R. P., Spillane, A., O'Connor, P., O'Donohoe, P., Moloney, M. 1976. Serum ionized calcium and parathyroid hormone in renal stone disease. *Q. J. Med.* 45:75–86

13. Wills, M. R. 1971. Normocalcaemic primary hyperparathyroidism. *Lancet* 1:849–52
14. Pak, C. Y. C., Ohata, M., Lawrence, E. C., Snyder, W. 1974. The hypercalciurias: Causes, parathyroid functions and diagnostic criteria. *J. Clin. Invest.* 54:387–400
15. Pak, C. Y. C., Kaplan, R., Bone, H., Townsend, J., Waters, O. 1975. A simple test for the diagnosis of absorptive, reabsorptive and renal hypercalciurias. *N. Engl. J. Med.* 292:497–501
16. Pak, C. Y. C., East, D. A., Sanzenbacher, L. J., Delea, C., Bartter, F. C. 1972. Gastrointestinal calcium absorption in nephrolithiasis. *J. Clin. Endocrinol. Metab.* 35:261–70
17. Gallagher, J. C., Nordin, B. E. C. 1972. Treatment with oestrogens of primary hyperparathyroidism in post-menopausal women. *Lancet* 1:503–7
18. Gallagher, J. C., Wilkinson, R. 1973. The effect of ethinyloestradiol on calcium and phosphorus metabolism of post-menopausal women with primary hyperparathyroidism. *Clin. Sci. Mol. Med.* 45:785–802
19. Coe, F. L., Canterbury, J. M., Firpo, J. J., Reiss, E. 1973. Evidence for secondary hyperparathyroidism in idiopathic hypercalciuria. *J. Clin. Invest.* 52:134–42
20. Shen, F., Baylink, D., Nielson, R., Hughes, M., Haussler, M. 1975. Increased serum 1,25-dihydroxycholecalciferol in patients with idiopathic hypercalciuria. *Clin. Res.* 23:423A (Abstr.)
21. Shen, F., Baylink, D., Nielsen, R., Sherrard, D., Haussler, M. 1976. A study of the pathogenesis of idiopathic hypercalciuria. *Clin. Res.* 24:460A (Abstr.)
22. Pak, C. Y. C., Delea, C. S., Bartter, F. C. 1974. Successful treatment of recurrent nephrolithiasis (Ca stones) with cellulose phosphate. *N. Engl. J. Med.* 290:175–80
23. Pak, C. Y. C. 1972. Current concepts: Nephrolithiasis (Ca-containing). *Acta Endocrinol. Panam.* 3:45–71
24. Lau, K., Westby, G. R., Bosanac, P., Goldberg, M., Agus, Z. 1976. Idiopathic hypercalciuria: Responsiveness to endogenous PTH. *Clin. Res.* 24:405A (Abstr.)

25. DeLuca, H. F. 1976. Recent advances in our understanding of the vitamin D endocrine system. *J. Lab. Clin. Med.* 87:7–26

26. Costanzo, L. S., Weiner, I. M. 1974. On the hypocalciuric action of chlorothiazide. *J. Clin. Invest.* 54:628–37

27. Costanzo, L. S., Weiner, I. M. 1976. Relationship between clearances of Ca and Na: Effect of distal diuretics and PTH. *Am. J. Physiol.* 230:67–73

28. Edwards, B. R., Baer, P. G., Sutton, R. A. L., Dirks, J. H. 1973. Micropuncture study of diuretic effects on sodium and calcium reabsorption in the dog nephron. *J. Clin. Invest.* 52:2418–27

29. Sutton, R. A. L., Dirks, J. H. 1975. The renal excretion of calcium: A review of micropuncture data. *Can. J. Physiol. Pharmacol.* 53:979–88

30. Quamme, C. A., Wong, N. L. M., Sutton, R. A. L., Dirks, J. H. 1975. The interrelationship of chlorothiazide and parathyroid hormone: A micropuncture study. *Am. J. Physiol.* 229:200–5

31. Costanzo, L. S., Moses, A. M., Rao, K. J., Weiner, I. M. 1975. Dissociation of calcium and sodium clearances in patients with hypoparathyroidism by infusion of chlorothiazide. *Metabolism* 24:1367–73

32. Yendt, E. R., Gagné, R. J. A., Cohanim, M. 1966. The effects of thiazides in idiopathic hypercalciuria. *Am. J. Med. Sci.* 251:449–60

33. Yendt, E. R., Guay, G. F., Garcia, D. A. 1970. The use of thiazides in the prevention of renal calculi. *Can. Med. Assoc. J.* 102:614–20

34. Parfitt, A. M. 1969. Chlorothiazide-induced hypercalcemia in juvenile osteoporosis and primary hyperparathyroidism. *N. Engl. J. Med.* 281:55–59

35. Paloyan, E., Forland, M., Pickleman, J. R. 1969. Hyperparathyroidism coexisting with hypertension and prolonged thiazide administration. *J. Am. Med. Assoc.* 210:1243–45

36. Pickleman, J. R., Strauss, F. G. II, Forland, M., Paloyan, E. 1969. Thiazide-induced parathyroid stimulation. *Metabolism* 18:867–73

37. Koppel, M. H., Massry, S. G., Shinaberger, J. H., Hartenbower, D. L., Coburn, J. W. 1970. Thiazide-induced rise in serum calcium and magnesium in patients on maintenance hemodialysis. *Ann. Intern. Med.* 72:895–901

38. Parfitt, A. M. 1972. Thiazide-induced hypercalcemia in vitamin D-treated hypoparathyroidism. *Ann. Intern. Med.* 77:557–63

39. Stote, R. M., Smith, L. H., Wilson, D. M., Dube, W. J., Goldsmith, R. S., Arnaud, C. D. 1972. Hydrochlorothiazide effects on serum calcium and immunoreactive parathyroid hormone concentrations. *Ann. Intern. Med.* 77:587–91

40. Popovtzer, M. M., Subryan, V. L., Alfrey, A. C., Reeve, E. B., Schrier, R. W. 1975. The acute effect of chlorothiazide on serum ionized calcium. Evidence for a parathyroid hormone-dependent mechanism. *J. Clin. Invest.* 55:1295–1302

41. Williams, H. E., Smith, L. H. Jr. 1972. Primary hyperoxaluria. In *The Metabolic Basis of Inherited Disease*, ed. J. B. Stanbury, J. B. Wyngaarden, D. S. Fredrickson, 196–219. New York: McGraw-Hill. 24 pp. 3rd ed.

42. Williams, H. E. 1974. Nephrolithiasis. *N. Engl. J. Med.* 290:33–38

43. Thomas, J., Melon, J-M., Thomas, E., Steg, A., Desgrez, P., Aboulker, P., 1972. Données recantes sur l'elimination urinaire de l'acide oxalique dans la lithiasis rénale oxalique. *Ann. Urol.* 6:31–33

44. Melon, J-M., Thomas, J. 1973. Le lithiasis rénale oxalique, malade métabolique? *Agressologie* 14:357–65

45. Williams, H. E., Johnson, G. A., Smith, L. H. Jr. 1971. The renal clearance of oxalate in normal subjects and patients with primary hyperoxaluria. *Clin. Sci.* 41:213–18

46. Hodgkinson, A., Wilkinson, R. 1974. Plasma oxalate concentration and renal excretion of oxalate in man. *Clin. Sci. Mol. Med.* 46:61–73

47. Pinto, B., Crespí, G., Solé-Balcells, F., Barcelo, P. 1975. Patterns of oxalate metabolism in recurrent oxalate stone formers. *Kidney Int.* 5:285–91

48. Robertson, W. G., Peacock, M., Nordin, B. E. C. 1971. Calcium oxalate crystalluria and urine saturation in recurrent renal stone formers. *Clin. Sci.* 40:365–74

49. Robertson, W. G., Peacock, M., Nordin, B. E. C. 1969. Calcium crystalluria in recurrent renal stone formers. *Lancet* 2:21–24

50. Robertson, W. G., Peacock, M. 1972. Calcium oxalate crystalluria and inhibitors of crystallization in recurrent renal stone formers. *Clin. Sci.* 43:499–506

51. Hodgkinson, A. 1974. Relations between oxalic acid, calcium, magnesium

and creatinine excretion in normal man and male patients with calcium oxalate kidney stones. *Clin. Sci. Mol. Med.* 46:357–67

52. Marshall, R. W., Cochran, M., Hodgkinson, A. 1972. Relationships between calcium and oxalic acid intake in the diet and their excretion in the urine of normal and renal-stone-forming patients. *Clin. Sci.* 43:91–99

53. Earnest, D. L., Williams, H. E., Admirand, W. H. 1975. A physicochemical basis for the treatment of enteric hyperoxaluria. *Clin. Res.* 23:439A (Abstr.)

54. Smith, L. H., Fromm, H., Hofmann, A. F. 1972. Acquired hyperoxaluria, nephrolithiasis, and intestinal disease. *N. Engl. J. Med.* 286:1371–75

55. Chadwick, V. S., Modha, K., Dowling, R. H. 1973. Mechanism for hyperoxaluria in patients with ileal dysfunction. *N. Engl. J. Med.* 289:172–76

56. Earnest, D. L., Johnson, G., Williams, H. E., Admirand, W. H. 1974. Hyperoxaluria in patients with ileal resection: An abnormality in dietary oxalate absorption. *Gastroenterology* 66:1114–22

57. Smith, L. H., Hofmann, A. F. 1974. Acquired hyperoxaluria, urolithiasis, and intestinal disease: A new digestive disorder? *Gastroenterology* 66:1257–61

58. Earnest, D. L., Gaucher, S., Admirand, W. H. 1976. Treatment of enteric hyperoxaluria with calcium and aluminum. *Gastroenterology* 70:881 (Abstr.)

59. Alfrey, A. C., LeGendre, G. R., Kaehny, W. D. 1976. The dialysis encephalopathy syndrome. Possible aluminum intoxication. *N. Engl. J. Med.* 294:184–88

60. Lemann, J. Jr., Litzow, J. R., Lennon, E. J. 1967. Studies of the mechanism by which chronic metabolic acidosis augments urinary calcium excretion in man. *J. Clin. Invest.* 46:1318–28

61. Hagler, L., Herman, R. H. 1973. Oxalate metabolism. V. *Am. J. Clin. Nutr.* 26:1242–50

62. Musher, D., Templeton, G., Griffith, D. 1976. Further observations on the synergy between acetohydroxamic acid, a urease inhibitor, and methenamine. *Clin. Res.* 24:26A (Abstr.)

63. Larengood, R. W. Jr., Marshall, V. F. 1972. The prevention of renal phosphatic calculi in the presence of infection by the Shorr regimen. *J. Urol.* 108:368–71

64. Steele, T. H., DeLuca, H. F. 1976. Influence of the dietary phosphorus on renal phosphate reabsorption in the para-

thyroidectomized rat. *J. Clin. Invest.* 57:867–74

65. Coburn, J. W., Massry, S. G. 1970. Changes in serum and urinary calcium during phosphate depletion: Studies on mechanisms. *J. Clin. Invest.* 49:1073–87

66. Dominguez, J. H., Gray, R. W., Lemann, J. Jr. 1975. A sex difference in the responses to phosphate deprivation in humans. *Clin. Res.* 23:318A (Abstr.)

67. Bruin, W. J., Baylink, D. J., Wergedal, J. E. 1975. Acute inhibition of mineralization and stimulation of bone resorption mediated by hypophosphatemia. *Endocrinology* 96:394–99

68. Ludwig, G. D., Kyle, G. C., DeBlanco, M. 1967. "Tertiary" hyperparathyroidism induced by osteomalacia resulting from phosphorus depletion. *Am. J. Med.* 43:136–40

69. Craddock, P. R., Yawata, Y., VanSanten, L., Gilberstadt, S., Silvis, S., Jacob, H. S. 1974. Acquired phagocyte dysfunction. A complication of the hypophosphatemia of parenteral hyperalimentation. *J. Engl. J. Med.* 290:1403–7

70. Fuller, T. J., Carter, N. W., Barcenas, C., Knochel, J. P. 1976. Reversible changes of the muscle cell in experimental phosphorus deficiency. *J. Clin. Invest.* 57:1019–24

71. Boyce, W. H. 1968. Organic matrix of human urinary concretions. *Am. J. Med.* 45:673–83

72. Pak, C. Y. C., Ruskin, B. 1970. Calcification of collagen by urine in vitro: Dependence on the degree of saturation of urine with respect to brushite. *J. Clin. Invest.* 49:2353–61

73. Pak, C. Y. C., Eanes, E. D., Ruskin, B. 1971. Spontaneous precipitation of brushite in urine: Evidence that brushite is the nidus of renal stones originating as calcium phosphate. *Proc. Natl. Acad. Sci. USA* 68:1456–60

74. Pak, C. Y. C., Diller, E. C., Smith, G. W. II, Howe, E. S. 1969. Renal stones of calcium phosphate: Physicochemical basis for their formation. *Proc. Soc. Exp. Biol. Med.* 130:753–57

75. Pak, C. Y. C. 1972. Effects of cellulose phosphate and of sodium phosphate on the formation product and activity product of brushite in urine. *Metabolism* 21:447–55

76. Pak, C. Y. C. 1973. Hydrochlorothiazide therapy in nephrolithiasis. Effect on the urinary activity product of

brushite. *Clin. Pharmacol. Ther.* 14: 209–17

77. Pak, C. Y. C., Cox, J. W., Powell, E., Bartter, F. C. 1971. Effect of the oral administration of ammonium chloride, sodium phosphate, cellulose phosphate and parathyroid extract on the activity product of brushite in urine. *Am. J. Med.* 50:67–76

77a. Meyer, J. L., Bergert, J. H., Smith, L. H. 1975. Epitaxial relationships in urolithiasis: The calcium oxalate monohydrate-hydroxyapatite system. *Clin. Sci. Mol. Med.* 49:369–74

78. Prien, E. L., Prien, E. L. Jr. 1968. Composition and structure of urinary stone. *Am. J. Med.* 45:654–72

79. Coe, F. L., Lawton, R. L., Goldstein, R. B., Tembe, V. 1975. Sodium urate accelerates precipitation of calcium oxalate *in vitro. Proc. Soc. Exp. Biol. Med.* 149:926–29

80. Pak, C. Y. C., Arnold, L. 1975. Heterogeneous nucleation of calcium oxalate by seeds of monosodium urate. *Proc. Soc. Exp. Biol. Med.* 149:930–32

81. Coe, F. L., Kavalach, A. G. 1974. Hypercalciuria and hyperuricosuria in patients with calcium nephrolithiasis. *N. Engl. J. Med.* 291:1344–50

82. Shelp, W. D., Rieselbach, R. E. 1968. Increased bidirectional urate transport per nephron following unilateral nephrectomy. *Am. Soc. Nephrol. Abstr.* 2:24 (Abstr.)

83. Coe, F. L., Raisen, L. 1973. Allopurinol treatment of uric acid disorders in calcium stone formers. *Lancet* 1:129–31

84. Gutman, A. B., Yü, T-F. 1968. Uric acid nephrolithiasis. *Am. J. Med.* 45:756–79

85. Yü, T-F., Gutman, A. B. 1967. Uric acid nephrolithiasis in gout. Predisposing factors. *Ann. Intern. Med.* 67: 1133–48

86. Seegmiller, J. E., Frazier, P. D. 1966. Biochemical considerations of the renal damage of gout. *Ann. Rheum. Dis.* 25:668–72

87. Kippen, I., Klinenberg, J. R., Weinberger, A., Wilcox, W. R. 1974. Factors affecting urate solubility *in vitro. Ann. Rheum. Dis.* 33:313–17

88. Weinberger, A., Kippen, I., Klinenberg, J. R. 1972. Solubility of uric acid and monosodium urate. *Med. Biol. Eng.* 10:522–31

89. Klinenberg, J. R., Kippen, I., Bluestone, R. 1975. Hyperuricemic nephropathy: Pathologic features and factors influencing urate deposition. *Nephron* 14:88–98

90. Masbernard, A., Guidicelli, C. 1974. Etude clinique de l'action antihypertensive de l'acide chloro-2,3-(thienyl-2-ceto)-phenoxyacetique en administration prolongee. *Lyon Med.* 232:165–74

91. Reese, O. G. Jr., Steele, T. H. 1976. Renal transport of urate during diuretic-induced hypouricemia. *Am. J. Med.* 60:973–79

92. Howard, J. E., Thomas, W. C. Jr. 1968. Control of crystallization in urine. *Am. J. Med.* 45:693–99

92a. Robertson, W. G., Hambleton, J., Hodgkinson, A. 1969 Peptide inhibitors of calcium phosphate precipitation in the urine of normal and stone-forming men. *Clin. Chim. Acta* 25:247–53

92b. Meyer, J. L., McCall, J. T., Smith, L. H. 1974. Inhibition of calcium phosphate crystallization by nucleoside phosphates. *Calcif. Tiss. Res.* 15: 287–93

93. Harrison, H. E., Harrison, H. C. 1955. Inhibition of urine citrate excretion and production of renal calcinosis in the rat by acetazolamide (Diamox) administration. *J. Clin. Invest.* 34:1662–70

94. Dedmon, R. E., Wrong, O. 1962. The excretion of the organic anion in renal tubular acidosis with particular reference to citrate. *Clin. Sci.* 22:19–22

95. Buckalew, V. M. Jr., Purvis, M. L., Shulman, M. G., Herndon, C. N., Rudman, D. 1974. Hereditary renal tubular acidosis. Report of a 64 member kindred with variable clinical expression including idiopathic hypercalciuria. *Medicine* 53:229–54

96. Parfitt, A. M. 1969. Acetazolamide and sodium bicarbonate induced nephrocalcinosis and nephrolithiasis. *Arch. Intern. Med.* 124:736–40

97. Barzel, U. S., Hart, H. 1973. Studies in calcium absorption: Initial entry of calcium into the gastrointestinal tract in hyperparathyroidism and in a case of renal tubular acidosis. *Nephron* 10: 174–87

98. Melnick, I., Landes, R. R., Hoffman, A. A., Burch, J. F. 1971. Magnesium therapy for recurring calcium oxalate urinary calculi. *J. Urol.* 105:119–22

99. Prien, E. L. Sr., Gershoff, S. F. 1974. Magnesium oxide-pyridoxine therapy for recurrent calcium oxalate calculi. *J. Urol.* 112:509–12

100. Boyce, W. H., McKinney, W. M., Long, T. T., Drach, G. W. 1967. Oral administration of methylene blue to pa-

tients with renal calculi. *J. Urol.*
97:783–89
101. Smith, M. J. V. 1972. Concretions and
methylene blue. *J. Urol.* 107:164–69
102. Bernstein, D. S., Newton, R. 1966.
The effect of oral sodium phosphate
on the formation of renal calculi and
on idiopathic hypercalciuria. *Lancet*
2:1105–7
103. Ettinger, B., Kolb, F. O. 1973. Inorganic phosphate treatment of nephrolithiasis. *Am. J. Med.* 55:32–37
104. Fleisch, H., Bisaz, S., Care, A. D. 1964.
Effect of orthophosphate on urinary
pyrophosphate excretion and the prevention of urolithiasis. *Lancet* 1:
1065–67
105. Russell, R. G. G., Fleisch, H. 1973. Inhibitors of urinary stone disease: Role of
pyrophosphate. *Proc. Int. Symp. Renal
Stone Res.*, Madrid 1972, ed. L. Ci-
fuentes Delatte, A. Rapado, A. Hodgkinson, 307–12. Basel & New York:
Karger
105a. Smith, L. H., Thomas, W. C. Jr., Arnaud, C. D. 1973. Orthophosphate
therapy in calcium renal lithiasis. See
Ref. 105, pp. 188–97
106. Fraser, D., Russell, R. G. G., Pohler,
O., Robertson, W. G., Fleisch, H. 1972.
The influence of disodium ethane-1-
hydroxy-1,1-diphosphonate (EHDP)
on the development of experimentally
induced urinary stones in rats. *Clin. Sci.*
42:197–207
107. Ohata, M., Pak, C. Y. C. 1973. The
effect of diphosphonate on calcium

phosphate crystallization in urine *in vitro. Kidney Int.* 4:401–6
108. Robertson, W. G. 1973. Factors affecting the precipitation of calcium phosphate *in vitro. Calcif. Tiss. Res.* 11:
311–22
109. Pak, C. Y. C., Ohata, M., Holt, K.
1975. Effect of diphosphonate on crystallization of calcium oxalate *in vitro.
Kidney Int.* 7:154–60
110. Recker, R. R., Hassing, G. S., Lau, J.
R., Saville, P. D. 1973. The hyperphos-
phatemic effect of disodium ethane-1-
hydroxy-1,1-diphosphonate (EHDP®):
Renal handling of phosphorus and the
renal response to parathyroid hormone.
J. Lab. Clin. Med. 81:258–66
111. Bonjour, J-P., Trechsel, U., Fleisch, H.,
Schenk, R., DeLuca, H. F., Baxter, L.
A. 1975. Action of 1,25-dihydroxy-
vitamin D_3 and a diphosphonate on
calcium metabolism in rats. *Am. J.
Physiol.* 229:402–8
112. Jowsey, J., Riggs, B. L., Kelly, P. J.,
Hoffman, D. L., Bordier, P. 1971. The
treatment of osteoporosis with disodium ethane-1-hydroxy-1,1-diphos-
phonate. *J. Lab. Clin. Med.* 78:575–84
113. Jowsey, J., Holley, K. 1973. Influence of
diphosphonates on progress of experimentally induced osteoporosis. *J. Lab.
Clin. Med.* 82:567–75
114. Robertson, W. G., Peacock, M., Marshall, R. W., Knowles, F. 1974. The
effect of ethane-1-hydroxy-1,1-diphos-
phonate (EHDP) on calcium oxalate
crystalluria in recurrent renal stone-
formers. *Clin. Sci. Mol. Med.* 47:13–22

Ann. Rev. Pharmacol. Toxicol. 1977. 17:27–47

COMMON MECHANISMS OF HORMONE SECRETION ❖6665

J. M. Trifaró

Department of Pharmacology and Therapeutics, McGill University, Montreal, H3G 1Y6, Quebec, Canada

INTRODUCTION

With the exception of the thyroid gland, which stores hormones extracellularly in the lumen of its follicles, the endocrine tissues store their hormones intracellularly (1). Two main forms of intracellular storage must be recognized: 1. The steroid-secreting glands which store very little amounts of hormone but large quantities of precursor. The adrenal cortex, the ovary, and the testis all belong to this category of endocrine glands in which the presence of secretory granules has not been demonstrated. However, these tissues store large amounts of esterified cholesterol in lipid droplets, and this represents a depot of hormone precursor (1, 2). 2. Endocrine tissues which store large quantities of hormones in membrane-bound organelles, the secretory granules. A similar way of storing secretory products may be observed in exocrine glands (3, 4) and also in nervous tissues which synthesize and release novel transmitter substances (5, 6).

The main concern of this review is with the secretory events which occur in those cells storing hormones in subcellular granules. Among this type of cell are those of the adenohypophysis, the islets of Langerhans of the pancreas, the adrenal medulla, the parathyroid gland, the parafollicular cells of the thyroid, and the neurosecretory cells of the hypothalamus-neurohypophysial system. Because these tissues share the common feature of storing their hormones in granules, it is possible that the cellular and molecular mechanisms of secretion are also similar. Therefore, this article seeks to unify published observations concerning the events involved in the secretory process of these tissues. Because of space limitations, it has been necessary to make an arbitrary selection of references to discuss and illustrate the ideas presented here; in many cases there are other references of equal value which would also support these ideas.

STORAGE OF HORMONES IN GRANULES

Evidence for the storage of hormones in subcellular particles has come to light from results obtained through morphological and biochemical techniques. Centrifugation studies have demonstrated both that the hormone activity in the homogenates of endocrine glands can be sedimented and that the hormone-containing particles of these sediments can be further separated from other subcellular particles by density-gradient centrifugation techniques (1, 7–10). Electron microscopic analysis of the subcellular fractions containing the hormone activity has revealed the presence of membrane-bound granules similar to those observed in intact tissues (7–10). Granule preparations of a quite different degree of purity have been isolated from different encodrine tissues (7–11). Chromaffin granule fractions of a high degree of purity have been isolated from the adrenal medulla (7, 12, 13). The subsequent chemical analysis of these granules (14) has provided a large and valuable body of information on the mechanisms of storage (14, 15) and release of adrenal medullary hormones (14). Therefore it is important that efforts be made to obtain granule preparations of a high degree of purity from other endocrine tissues.

In order to assess the importance of storage granules it is necessary to point out some of the advantages of this type of hormone storage: (a) the hormones may reach very high concentrations within the granules (that is, up to 0.5 M in chromaffin granules); consequently the capacity for hormone storage of these tissues is very high; (b) the hormone is protected from enzyme inactivation or catabolism (that is, monoamine oxidase in the adrenal medulla); (c) since the granules are of approximately the same volume in any given tissue, each granule provides a fixed amount of hormone (quantum) to be released; (d) the granules facilitate the intracellular transport of large quantities of hormones, especially in the case of the granules of the neurohypophysis which contain vasopressin and oxytocin, although it is likely that some kind of mechanism exists in all secretory tissues for the transport of granules from the Golgi apparatus to the cell periphery; and (e) by fusing with the plasma membrane during the release reaction (see below), the granules thus expose their contents directly to the cell exterior.

THE TRANSMEMBRANE POTENTIAL IN SECRETORY CELLS

The transmembrane potentials of the secretory cells are generally much lower than those of the muscle and nerve cells. The published values of resting membrane potentials of the secretory cells under discussion here ranged from –12 to –41 mV (16, 17). The origin of the potential in secretory cells seems to be the same as that in excitable cells, since the intracellular concentration of Na^+ and K^+ are similar to those in nerve and muscle (16, 17). However, secretory cells have higher ratios of membrane permeability of Na^+ to K^+ ($P_{Na}+/P_K+$) than nerve and muscle (16), which would explain the low resting potential observed in secretory cells. The high $P_{Na}+/P_K+$ ratio, together with the large area to volume ratio of secretory cells, is probably responsible for the rapid change in the intracellular concentrations of ions produced in these cells during stimulation (16, 17). Stimulation by raising the extracellular concentration of K^+ depolarizes the endocrine cells, but the potential values always remain negative (18–21). Furthermore, secretory cells have gap junctions which are membrane areas of low resistance (17). For this reason, comparison of membrane resistance in different kinds of secretory cells would be unjustified (17).

IONIC REQUIREMENTS FOR RELEASE

Role of Divalent Cations

In 1928 Houssay & Molinelli first suggested the importance of Ca^{2+} in hormone secretion (22). However, it was W.W. Douglas who conceived of the role of Ca^{2+} in the secretory process as a general one, and who gave the name of *stimulus-secretion coupling* to the events involved in the secretory process because of the similarity to the excitation-contraction coupling in muscle (23). Douglas and co-workers not only established the role of Ca^{2+} in the secretory process of the adrenal medulla (24) but they also extended these observations to the neurosecretory cells of the posterior pituitary (25) and to the submaxillary gland (26). Later on, the requirement of Ca^{2+} for secretion was established in a large variety of secretory systems (27). Thus, the omission of Ca^{2+} from the extracellular environment blocks the release of hormone in response to different secretagogues (25, 28–34). Reintroduction of Ca^{2+} into a Ca^{2+}-free medium produces a sharp increase in hormone release (24, 35, 36). This has been interpreted as arising from a rapid penetration of Ca^{2+} through the plasma membrane, since this divalent cation was added when the plasma membrane was in a state of increased permeability due to the omission of Ca^{2+} (23, 35). It appears, therefore, that stimulation promotes Ca^{2+} entry and this seems to be supported by the results obtained with Mg^{2+}. Increasing the extracellular concentration of Mg^{2+} inhibits hormone release in response to stimulation (28, 35, 37, 38). Replacement of extracellular Ca^{2+} by either Sr^{2+} or Ba^{2+} is effective in maintaining the stimulation-induced release of hormones (35, 38, 42). Furthermore, Ba^{2+} itself is a potent secretagogue, even in the absence of extracellular Ca^{2+} (35, 38–41). The possibility that Ba^{2+} acts by displacing intracellular Ca^{2+} should be considered, since Ba^{2+} interferes with [45]Ca binding by microsomes (43). Therefore, although Ca^{2+} is essential for the release process, different Ca^{2+} pools may be involved, depending upon the secretagogue used (34, 44).

Among the glands storing hormones in secretory granules, the parathyroid gland and the C cells of the thyroid gland seem to be a special case. The parathyroid hormone (PTH) and calcitonin control and maintain the normal levels of Ca^{2+} in plasma (45, 46). One of the most important sites of action responsible for this control is the bone, where PTH stimulates mobilization of Ca^{2+} and calcitonin inhibits this process. Furthermore, the plasma levels of PTH and calcitonin are indirectly and directly, respectively, related to the Ca^{2+} plasma concentration (45). Thus an increase in Ca^{2+} levels triggers calcitonin release whereas the release of PTH is depressed (45, 46). The opposite is true when the concentration of Ca^{2+} in plasma is decreased (45, 46). Therefore, Ca^{2+} ions are the stimulus for calcitonin release. However, it is unknown whether there is an active calcium site in the plasma membrane of the C cell or whether Ca^{2+} can readily penetrate the cell and trigger release (45, 46). In the case of the parathyroid gland, an increase in the extracellular Ca^{2+} does not seem to be responsible for turning off the mechanism of release. On the contrary, a lag of 25–30 min is observed between the increase in Ca^{2+} levels and a 50% decrease in the circulating PTH levels (46). This probably suggests that Ca^{2+} acts on the regulation of the synthesis of the PTH (46, 47). There is, however, not enough available information to understand completely the cellular mechanisms which regulate PTH and calcitonin release.

Effect of Potassium Ions

As discussed above, increasing the concentration of K^+ in the extracellular environment depolarizes the endocrine cell (19–21). This results in an increase in membrane permeability to Na^+ and Ca^{2+} (16, 17). However, only Ca^{2+} is essential in the K^+-induced hormone release reaction. Thus, although the endocrine cell is depolarized by high K^+ in the absence of extracellular Ca^{2+}, hormone release is not triggered (25, 28, 30–35, 48). This effect of K^+ has been observed in many endocrine cells, including the neurosecretory terminals of the neurohypophysis (25, 35).

Sodium-Calcium Interaction, the Late Ca^{2+} Channel, and the Regulation of Intracellular Ca^{2+}

Experiments carried out on the adrenal medulla, the endocrine pancreas, and the neurohypophysis have shown that the omission of Na^+ from the extracellular space produces a sharp increase in hormone output (35, 44, 49). Moreover, after a short exposure to a Na^+-free solution, hormone release in response to stimulation is potentiated (25, 28, 35, 50). Therefore, it is likely that decreasing the extracellular concentration of Na^+ produces an increase in the $[Na^+]_i/[Na^+]_o$ ratio and, perhaps, a concomitant increase in the intracellular Ca^{2+} levels. This Ca^{2+} increase may be due to a decrease in the Na^+-dependent Ca^{2+} efflux mechanism. The existence of a Na^{2+}-dependent Ca^{2+} efflux has been shown in the squid axon and in the cardiac muscle (51). The potentiation of hormone release may also be due to an increased Ca^{2+} entry as a result of the removal of extracellular Na^+ (35, 50). The existence of a Na^+-Ca^{2+} antagonism has also been demonstrated in the squid axon and heart muscle (51). However, it is also possible that decreasing the $[Na^+]_o$ may increase $[Ca^{2+}]_i$ by inhibiting the cellular binding or sequestration of Ca^{2+} (44, 52). Therefore, it seems that conditions which produce an increase in the $[Na^+]_i/[Na^+]_o$ ratio will favor the accumulation of intracellular Ca^{2+} which may be necessary to trigger hormone release. The $[Na^+]_i/[Na^+]_o$ ratio can be increased either by removing extracellular Na^+ (28, 35, 44, 49), or by increasing intracellular Na^+ as a result of blocking the Na^+ pump by either K^+ removal or by ouabain treatment (35, 48, 53). Long exposure to Na^+-deprived solutions produced an opposite effect on hormone release, namely, the inhibition of release upon stimulation (44, 48). This diminished response seems to be due to a progressive fall in the intracellular concentration of Na^+ during exposure to a Na^+-free medium (44). Furthermore, diphenylhydantoin, a drug which reduces the intracellular concentrations of Na^+, inhibits glucose-induced release of insulin (54).

Studies on the movement of Ca^{2+} in the squid axon have shown that the entry of this ion is biphasic: an early phase which seems to use the Na^+ channel and which is blocked by tetrodotoxin (51), and a later phase of Ca^{2+} entry which is tetrodotoxin insensitive and which is blocked by Mg^{2+}, Mn^{2+}, Co^{2+}, La^{3+}, and the Ca^{2+} antagonist methoxyverapamil (51). The Ca^{2+} entry through this channel is blocked by the same ions and substances which block neurotransmitter and hormone release (35, 51, 55, 56). Moreover, one of the characteristics of the late Ca^{2+} channel is its inactivation by prolonged depolarization (51). This type of inactivation seems to be responsible for the decrease in catecholamine output observed during K^+ stimulation (57).

Ca^{2+} is also probably involved in the termination of the release reaction. One or more of the following mechanisms may be responsible for this: (a) inactivation of the late Ca^{2+} channel; (b) extrusion of Ca^{2+} to the cell exterior; (c) cellular binding or sequestration of Ca^{2+}. Sequestration of Ca^{2+} by a Mg^{2+} ATP-dependent mechanism has been demonstrated in microsomal and mitochondrial fractions prepared from adrenal medulla (43). Therefore, these organelles may be responsible not only for the termination of the release reaction, but also for the low $[Ca^{2+}]$ levels present during cellular resting conditions. Furthermore, these organelles may be the site of action of drugs like caffeine or theophylline, which are known to induce release in the absence of extracellular Ca^{2+} (58, 59).

Finally, it is worthwhile to stress that all this ion interplay reflects again a very close similarity between two apparently different processes, namely, contraction and secretion.

EXOCYTOSIS

In earlier studies it was suggested that the mechanisms of hormone release from glands containing secretory granules encompassed holocrine and apocrine secretion (60, 61) as well as other forms of release, for example: (a) extrusion of intact secretory granules into the cell exterior (62); (b) release from a "free hormone pool" (63, 64); (c) release by diffusion of hormones out of the granules into the cytoplasm (64, 65); or (d) release by dissolution of the granule membrane in the cytoplasm (66). The final common path proposed for the last three mechanisms of release was the diffusion across the plasma membrane of the hormones from the cytoplasmic sap into the cell exterior. However, in 1957 another mechanism of secretion was proposed by De Robertis & Vaz Ferreira, which suggested that secretion was by "reverse pinocytosis" (exocytosis), a mechanism whereby the membrane of the secretory granule fuses with the plasmalemma allowing the escape of the content of the granules to the cell exterior (67). Exocytosis seems to be the most logical process of hormone release. If the disadvantages of the other forms of release are considered, it is immediately obvious that exocytosis is the simplest, the most economical, and the most efficient mechanism for releasing not only hormones but also enzymes and transmitter substances from the exocrine glands and nerve terminals respectively. If hormones were released from granules into the cytosol they would diffuse in all directions; large quantities of the hormones would be destroyed by enzymes present in the cytosol and only a fraction of the hormones would reach the cell exterior. Furthermore, the hormones in question would have to cross at least two membranes, those of the granules and that of the cell. Finally, if release were not by exocytosis, since the molecular size of the hormones which are stored in granules varies from very simple molecules like adrenaline to more complex ones like somatotropin or adrenocorticotropin, special transport mechanisms through these membranes, namely, the granule and the plasmalemma, would have to exist. There is now good morphological evidence for exocytosis in the adrenal medulla (67, 68); in the neurohypophysis (69); in the α (70), β (71), and δ (70) cells of the pancreas; and in the pituitary cells, namely, the thyrotroph (72), the corticotroph (73), the somatotroph (74), the mammotroph (75), the melanotroph (76), and even in the gonadotroph (77) where earlier studies failed to show the classical "omega" images of exocytosis (78). Exocytosis seems also to be the mechanism of release in exocrine glands (79), nerve terminals (27), and a variety of secretory tissues (27). Furthermore, biochemical studies carried out in some of these tissues have provided chemical evidence in favor of release by exocytosis. These studies have shown that hormones were released during stimulation along with other soluble granule components. In the adrenal medulla, for example, there is a concomitant release of dopamine-β-hydroxylase, chromogranin A, and ATP along with the catecholamines (44, 80–82). These soluble substances are quantitatively recovered in the effluent escaping from stimulated glands (44, 80–82). Furthermore, subcellular fractionation studies carried out on stimulated medullae have shown that the entire soluble content of the granule is discharged to the cell exterior (83–85), and that exocytosis is an all-or-none release process (86). Further work has demonstrated that, in the neurohypophysis, neurophysins I and II are released along with oxytocin and vasopressin (87, 88) and that stimulation of the pancreas brings about the concomitant release of insulin and the connecting peptide C (89). It has also been demonstrated that in the mast cell, a unicellular gland, the release of histamine is accompanied by a parallel release of heparin and granule protein (90). Biochemical evidence in favor of exocytosis obtained in other secretory tissues has also been published. These secretory tissues are the adrenergic neuron, the polymorphonuclear leucocyte, the platelets, and the basophile leucocytes (27). Other biochemical studies have demonstrated that the membrane components are retained within the cell after exocytosis (83, 85, 91, 92) and that, although large molecules, as for example dopamine β-hydroxylase (mol. wt. 290,000), leave the cell during exocytosis, no cytoplasmic marker enzymes like lactate dehydrogenase (44, 92–94), phenylethanolamine N-methyltransferase (95), and adenylate kinase (93) are detected in the effluents escaping from these stimulated tissues. This indicates that the vital feature of the cell, that is, the membraneous isolation of the cytosol from the extracellular environment, is maintained during exocytosis.

ORIGIN AND FATE OF THE SECRETORY GRANULES

Ultrastructural observations have suggested that secretory granules originate from the Golgi apparatus (75, 77, 96–103). The Golgi complex can be viewed as the membrane-bound compartment of the cell which is believed to be involved in the following functions (104): (a) the synthesis of certain polysaccharides; (b) the synthesis or attachment of carbohydrates side chains of glycoproteins (especially the addition of terminal sugars such as galactose, fucose, and sialic acid); (c) the assembling of secretory materials and formation of membrane-bound granules containing these materials; (d) the assembling of lysosomes. According to some investigators (105) the Golgi apparatus is part of the "endomembrane system" of the cell. This system is formed by the following components: rough endoplasmic reticulum $\longrightarrow$ smooth endoplasmic reticulum $\longrightarrow$ Golgi apparatus $\longrightarrow$ secretory granules. The arrows here indicate the direction of the "membrane flow," a term which has been introduced to describe the process of physical transfer of membranes from one cell compartment to another (105). This process of membrane transfer may or may not be accompanied by the concomitant transfer through this endomembrane system of secretory products, in this particular case, prohormones and hormones. Morphological evidence showing the packing of secretory products into granules in the stacked Golgi cisternae, especially in the maturing phase of the Golgi, has been published. This ultrastructural evidence has been collected from studies on all types of secretory cells of the adenohypophysis (75, 77, 96, 97); the α, β, and δ cells of the pancreas (97–100); the adrenal medulla (101, 102); the neurosecretory cells of the hypothalamus-neurohypophysial system (103); and in many other secretory systems in which secretory products are packed in vesicles (106).

Studies using pulse-labeling methods followed by autoradiography have also provided information on the synthesis, transport, and final packaging of secretory products. These experiments involved the incubation of the secretory tissues "in vitro" and the administration of a short pulse (5 min) of a radioactive amino acid, followed by autoradiography at different intervals of time postpulse. The results indicated that a high proportion of silver grains were always found on the surface of the endoplasmic reticulum at 5–10 min after labeling. The labeled material was then transferred to the Golgi apparatus, where the highest concentration was reached at 20–30 min postpulse. The radioactive material appeared largely concentrated in the secretory granules at 60 min postpulse. This pattern of movement of the label from the endoplasmic reticulum to the secretory granules has been observed in studies on somatotrophs (76), melanotrophs (107), β cells of the pancreas (99), and also in some exocrine cells (108, 109).

Although the results obtained with the use of autoradiography indicate the sequential movement of labeled material from one cell compartment to another, they do not indicate whether this transfer represents the movement of soluble or of membrane-bound protein or of both. Therefore, the results indicate only that some components of the granules are derived from the Golgi. Pulse-labeling procedures combined with biochemical techniques have demonstrated, at least in some cases, that the movement of labeled material represents the synthesis and transport of hormones or their precursors. This seems to be true in the case of the pancreas where the movement of radioactive protein along this endomembrane system represents the synthesis and transport of proinsulin and its conversion to insulin (110). These experiments have suggested that the Golgi is probably the place where the conversion of proinsulin to insulin is initiated and that the transfer of material from the Golgi to the granules is an energy-dependent step (110). The synthesis of a precursor of oxytocin and vasopressin has been also suggested (103, 111). Furthermore, a suggestion has been made in favor of the origin of neurophysin I and oxytocin and of neurophysin II and vasopressin from common precursors respectively (112).

Pulse-labeling experiments followed by subcellular fractionation procedures carried out in perfused adrenal glands showed a similar pattern of endomembrane transport of [^{3}H]-leucine labeled protein, and newly synthesized chromogranins were detected in the perfusates as early as 30 min postpulse (113, 114). These pulse-labeling experiments have also shown the lack of labeled amino acids in the proteins of the membranes of secretory granules during the entire 4 hr of postpulse perfusion, this in spite of the fact that after 4 hr of perfusion the release of radioactive chromogranin could be readily detected (113, 114). These results indicate that the turnover of soluble granule components is more rapid than that of the membrane-bound components, which, in turn, suggests that granule membranes may be reutilized several times during the secretory cycle. This suggestion agrees with an earlier observation showing that the attachment of the granule membranes to the plasmalemma does not involve long-term incorporation (115) and that the granule membranes remain as discrete particles within the cells after catecholamine secretion (83, 116).

It seems, therefore, that the granule membrane proteins are not synthesized simultaneously with the granule content, although the morphological evidence discussed above does seem to indicate that the granules are derived from the Golgi complex. Consequently, it was important to obtain more biochemical information as to the origin of the secretory granules. To this end a method for the isolation of the Golgi complex from the adrenal medulla has been published recently (117). The chemical composition and the immunological properties of the Golgi membranes thus isolated have been compared to those of the chromaffin granule membranes (118). The marked biochemical differences observed between these membranes suggested that, if the secretory granules are derived from the Golgi as the morphological evidence seems to indicate, first, the granule membranes are unlikely to be derived by an unspecific "membrane flow," and second, the membranes must undergo considerable biochemical changes (membrane differentiation). The other possibility is, as suggested above, that after secretion the empty granule membranes return to the Golgi apparatus, fuse with it, and become recharged with newly synthesized hormones. Coated vesicles have been found in the proximity of the Golgi in electron microscopy pictures prepared from the adrenal medulla (119). Coated vesicles can also be seen in published electron micrographs prepared from other endocrine tissues (98, 120, 121). The interpretation given for the presence of coated vesicles in secretory tissues is that these vesicles have been derived from the granule membranes after exocytosis (122, 123). Therefore, a process of endocytosis and membrane retrieval would seem to follow exocytosis (122, 123).

The possible fate of these vesicles must also be considered. One possibility, already discussed above, is that they are reused in the formation of new secretory granules. Alternatively, it has also been suggested that these vesicles are incorporated into and digested by lysosomes. This process of digestion (crinophagy) of not only membranes but also intact secretory granules was first described in mammotrophs by Smith & Farquhar (75). Similar observations have been made in somatotrophs (76, 77), in gonadotrophs (76, 77), in thyrotrophs (76, 77), in α cells of the pancreas during spontaneous or experimental diabetes (124), in the neurohypophysis (125), in the normal adrenal medulla (126), and in pheochromocytomas (127). These autophagic bodies are observed mainly when a strong stimulus is removed or when hormonal secretion is suppressed. Therefore, it seems that this internal mechanism operates primarily when overproduction of secretory products occurs (76, 77, 124, 125, 127). Nevertheless, it is not known whether this is a controlled process or a blind one. It does not, however, seem to be the main factor regulating the fate of the membranes after exocytosis.

MECHANISMS OF RELEASE

Energy Requirement and the Possible Role of ATP

It has been shown that in many secretory tissues the release reaction is an energy-dependent process (128–131). Because secretion is blocked by inhibitors of oxidative phosphorylation and glycolysis (128–131) and because these two processes are important in the generation of ATP, it is possible that the energy requirement for the secretory process is in the form of ATP. However, it is not known whether the energy requirement is necessary to maintain a general cell function or whether it is needed in some of the steps involved in stimulus-secretion coupling.

Although the molecular events involved in the secretory process have not yet been completely elucidated, much information has been obtained by studying the effects of ATP on secretory granules isolated from the adrenal medulla. In the presence of Mg^{2+}, ATP produces structural changes in the chromaffin granules (132) and there is a simultaneous release of catecholamines, endogenous ATP, and soluble proteins (133). When ATP acts on chromaffin granules it is hydrolyzed by enzymes present in granule membranes, and part of the P_i so liberated is transphosphorylated to granule membranes (134). The effects of ATP on chromaffin granules can be blocked at either an early (ATP hydrolysis, transphosphorylation) or at a subsequent (conformational changes) step (135). On the basis of the above and other observations, Poisner & Trifaró proposed a hypothetical model for the molecular events involved in exocytosis (133). In this model the stimulation of the chromaffin cells induces an increase in intracellular Ca^{2+} (this being due either to increased Ca^{2+} entry or to liberation from intracellular sources). Then, Ca^{2+} may form a link between anionic groups (possibly phospholipids) of both granule and plasma membranes (133). It is known that Ca^{2+} can cause the aggregation of chromaffin and other secretory granules (136, 137). Moreover, it has been shown that Ca^{2+} causes the attachment of secretory granules of leucocytes to their membranes (138). ATP, which is released from the plasma membrane upon stimulation (139) and is perhaps also freed from some other places within the cell, acts on chromaffin granules. During this interaction ATP is hydrolyzed by granule membrane enzymes; membrane protein and lipid are phosphorylated; and this is followed by the production of some conformational change (contractile event?) in the granule membrane leading to the release of soluble granule components. This hypothesis involves Ca^{2+} as one of the principal elements in membrane fusion. In connection with this it has been shown that ATP induces the synthesis of diphosphatidyl inositol in granule membranes (85, 140, 141). This lipid has great affinity for Ca^{2+} and, in some membranes, there is a direct correlation between Ca^{2+} binding and diphosphatidyl inositol content (142). It should be remembered that this hypothesis has been formulated on the basis of in vitro observations and although it accommodates all that is known about the release reaction, further work is necessary to see whether this mechanism will operate during release in vivo.

Nevertheless, ATP-induced release from secretory granules has also been demonstrated in other preparations such as zymogen granules (143), cholinergic synaptic vesicles (144), and posterior pituitary granules (145). The results obtained with ATP on granules isolated from the β cell of the pancreas are controversial (146, 147). This is perhaps because the experiments were carried out with "crude granule preparations," that is, fractions that were heavily contaminated with lysosomes, mitochondria, and microsomes (11). Furthermore, granule membrane phosphorylation by ATP has also been demonstrated in granules isolated from the adenohypophysis (148) and in zymogen granules (149). One of the criticisms of the hypothesis discussed above is the lack of effect of Ca^{2+} on chromaffin granules. However, it is possible that a factor which makes the granule ATPase sensitive to Ca^{2+} is lost or inactivated during the isolation of the granules. In this connection it has been shown recently that a protein fraction prepared from the cytosol of adrenal medullary cells sensitizes the granule to Ca^{2+} (150). In the presence of this cytosol factor, Ca^{2+} potentiates the ATP-induced release process (150).

Microtubules

It has been proposed recently that microtubules are involved in the mechanisms of hormone release in a variety of endocrine tissues (151–153). This hypothesis is based on indirect observations that agents which disrupt microtubules, such as colchicine and vinblastine, inhibit the release process. The first observation of this kind was made by Lacy et al (151), who reported that colchicine inhibits glucose-induced release of insulin from the pancreas. Lacy has suggested that secretory granules which are attached to microtubules, in contrast to those that are free in the cytosol of the β cell, are available for immediate release and that Ca^{2+} may trigger contraction or a change in the physical conformation in the microtubule system which results in granule extrusion (154). This hypothesis is subject to criticism for the following reasons. 1. The glucose-induced release of insulin from the pancreas is a biphasic event (155, 156): an immediate and acute release response (phase I) is followed by a late and long-lasting release response (phase II). Puromycin blocks by 50% the release during phase II without affecting phase I (157). Moreover, when pancreatic islets were prelabeled with [3H]-leucine, the insulin released during phase

II was of higher specific activity than that collected during phase I (158). These observations suggest that insulin release during phase II is, at least in part, the result of either the conversion of proinsulin to insulin, or the release of newly synthesized insulin. These two phases of release are observed either when the pancreas is perfused or when pancreatic islets are perifused (155, 156). Colchicine blocks phase II of glucose-induced insulin release without affecting phase I (159). This differential effect of colchicine could not have been detected in the early experiments in which β-cell islets were incubated for 90 min (151). These results suggest that microtubules are not involved in the exocytosis process itself, and that the granules available for immediate release are not attached to microtubules. However, it still may be possible that, in this tissue, microtubules are involved in the intracellular transport of secretory granules from the Golgi (see above) to the periphery of the cell. 2. Lacy's suggestions that Ca^{2+} triggers contraction of microtubules also seems unlikely because Ca^{2+} blocks the polymerization of microtubules (160). In in vitro experiments, this divalent cation seems to be as effective as both colchicine and low temperatures in blocking microtubule polymerization (160). Furthermore, it has been postulated that the levels of free intracellular Ca^{2+} may control microtubule polymerization (161). If this is the case, microtubule polymerization should decrease during the release reaction, a condition in which an increase in free intracellular Ca^{2+} has been assumed (see above).

Therefore, a prerequisite for the study of these agents on the secretory process seems to be an adequate preparation of perfused glands in which exocytosis per se can be temporarily separated from the exocytotic process which follows intracellular transport. This prerequisite has not always been complied with, and many of the studies on hormone release from the adenohypophysis, neurohypophysis, and pancreas have been carried out in pieces or slices of tissues incubated in vitro and exposed to these agents for long periods of time (151, 153, 162–165). Therefore, in the presence of these agents a decrease in the amount of hormone collected during the stimulation was observed in some cases (151, 153, 162, 163); no changes (162, 164, 165) or even a potentiation of release was observed in others (164). Results obtained after long incubation periods in the presence of these agents are also difficult to interpret because of other effects of these drugs on living tissues. These effects are a decrease in production of ATP by colchicine and vincristine (166), the binding of colchicine to cell membranes (167), a drastic inhibition by colchicine and its analogues of nucleoside uptake (168), the tubocurarine-like effects of colchicine and vinblastine (169), and the anticholinergic effects of colchicine and vinblastine (170). This latter effect was observed in an endocrine gland, the adrenal medulla, in experiments in which perfused adrenal glands showed that the exocytotic release of catecholamines in response to either nicotine (152) or acetylcholine (152, 170, 171) was blocked by colchicine and vinblastine. However, catecholamine release induced by depolarizing concentrations of K^+ was unaffected (170, 171). This suggested an anticholinergic effect of these drugs, which was confirmed in experiments with perfused cervical ganglia (170). Furthermore, the lack of effect of colchicine on the histamine release from the mast cell induced by the Ca^{2+} ionophore A23187 suggests that in this tissue, as in the adrenal medulla, microtubules are not involved in exocytosis (172). Therefore, the role of microtubules in the secretory process still remains to be elucidated.

Contractile Proteins

The similarities between the processes of secretion and contraction (23) taken together with the idea that excytosis is a true contractile event (133) raise questions about the presence and possible role of contractile proteins in secretory cells. In this connection the following observations have been made: (a) the presence of an actomyosin-like protein in adrenal medullary cells has been demonstrated (173, 174); (b) neurostenin, a protein which resembles actomyosin, has been isolated from the brain (175); (c) actin-like filaments have been detected by immunofluorescence in the β cell of the pancreas (176); (d) a protein of the same molecular weight and showing a similar finger printing pattern as muscle actin has been detected in the adrenal medulla (177); (e) a protein has also been isolated from this tissue which shows ATPase activity, electrophoretic mobility, molecular weight, amino acid composition, and electron microscopic appearance which closely resembles myosin (178); (f) in vitro interaction between muscle myosin and actin and chromaffin granules has been described recently (179); (g) a calcium-binding protein has been purified from the adrenal medulla (180); (h) actin has been shown in electron micrographs of glycerinated nerve terminals (181); and (i) cytochalasin B, a drug known to interact with microfilaments (182), has been shown to block release in some secretory tissues (163). Although the blocking effect of this drug might be due to its other metabolic inhibitor properties (183, 184), it is worthwhile to point out that the cytochalasin B blocks the polymerization of G actin into F actin (185). In consequence, it is possible that these contractile proteins are involved in one or more of the steps of secretion, for example, in the intracellular transport of secretory granules, in the extrusion of the granule contents, or in the formation of "coated vesicles" during membrane retrieval. The vesicle "coat" is perhaps formed by actin molecules. However, actin and myosin have also been isolated and characterized from a variety of nonmuscle cells (186) and these proteins are thought to be involved in the maintenance of cell shape, in cell motility, and in mitosis (186–188). Therefore, the possibility exists that the presence of actin and myosin in secretory cells is related to cell architecture rather than to the secretory process. Nevertheless, the possible role of myosin and actin in the secretory process should be fully investigated.

Membrane Fusion

Release by exocytosis involves the interaction of both the granule and plasma membranes. The discovery of a large amount of lysolecithin in chromaffin granule membranes (189, 190) has led to the suggestion that, during stimulation, this lipid is involved in the process of membrane fusion (190). Lysolecithin is not formed during stimulation, and it is present in the granule membranes during resting conditions (191, 192). Lysolecithin can cause the fusion of cell membranes (193), but its role in exocytosis has not yet been demonstrated. Furthermore, with the exception of chromaffin granules (189, 190) and the secretory granules of neurohypophysis (194), there is no available information concerning the content of lysolecithin in other hormone storage granules.

As discussed above, Ca^{2+} may be another important factor in membrane fusion. In fact an electrostatic function for Ca^{2+} in exocytosis has been proposed recently (195, 196). The authors of this proposal have suggested that one possible function of Ca^{2+} ions in exocytosis is to reduce the potential at the surfaces of both the granule and cell membranes, thus decreasing the potential energy barrier for granule-membrane interaction (195, 196). This would enable contact or coalition to occur between the two membranes (195, 196). Whereas Ca^{2+} ions may play an important role in membrane fusion, the possible role of ATP and ATPase in this process cannot be ignored. In a review recently published on the mechanism of membrane fusion, a unitary theory of membrane fusion is proposed (197). This theory stresses the role of Ca^{2+}, ATP, and membrane-associated ATPase systems in the regulation of membrane changes responsible for fusion (197).

CONCLUSIONS

This review is an attempt to unify published observations about the secretory process in endocrine glands which store hormones in subcellular granules. One of the most interesting ultrastructural features of these tissues is the presence of secretory granules. Morphological evidence seems to indicate that secretory granules originate in the Golgi apparatus, and biochemical studies suggest that a selective process of membrane flow and differentiation must take place during granule formation. Granule storage not only allows these endocrine tissues to store large amounts of hormones in a relatively small volume, but also protects the hormones from intracellular degradation and provides a very efficient means of transporting and releasing fixed amounts (quantum) of hormones. In these tissues release is by exocytosis and this is an energy-dependent process which requires ionized Ca^{2+}. Therefore, an increase in intracellular Ca^{2+} seems to be a necessary requirement for triggering release. Increase in cytoplasmic Ca^{2+} may be produced by substances which interfere with the Ca^{2+} sequestration by intracellular organelles. However, it is more likely that an increase in Ca^{2+} entry under physiological conditions, through a specific Ca^{2+} channel, would account for this increase in intracellular Ca^{2+}. Where Ca^{2+} is needed still remains to be elucidated. Ca^{2+} may play a role in membrane fusion or it may be involved in some kind of contractile event leading to the release of hormones. Myosin and actin have been found in secretory tissues, but the role of these proteins in secretory cells still remains to be determined. Nevertheless, the close similarities which exist between two apparently different processes, namely, secretion and muscle contraction, suggest that the molecular events involved in secretion may be of similar nature to those involved in muscle contraction.

ACKNOWLEDGMENTS

Original studies in the author's laboratory were supported by grants from the Medical Research Council of Canada.

40   TRIFARÓ

Literature Cited

1. Smith, A. D. 1968. The storage of hormones. *Biochem. J.* 109:17–19
2. Claesson, L. 1954. The intracellular localization of the esterified cholesterol in the living interstitial gland cell of the rabbit ovary. *Acta Physiol. Scand.* 31: Suppl. 113, pp. 53–78
3. Siekevitz, P., Palade, G. E. 1958. A cytochemical study of the pancreas of the guinea pig. I. Isolation and enzymatic activities of cell fractions. *J. Biophys. Biochem. Cytol.* 4:203–18
4. Rothman, S. S., Burwen, S., Liebow, C. 1974. In *Advances in Cytopharmacology*, ed. B. Ceccarelli, J. Meldolesi, F. Clementi, 2:341–48. New York: Raven. 388 pp.
5. Whittaker, V. P. 1974. See Ref. 4, pp. 311–17
6. Bloom, F. E. 1972. In *Handbook of Experimental Pharmacology, Catecholamines*, ed. H. Blaschko, E. Muscholl, 33:46–78. Berlin & New York: Springer-Verlag. 1054 pp.
7. Banks, P. 1965. The adenosine-triphosphatase activity of adrenal chromaffin granules. *Biochem. J.* 95:490–96
8. Bindler, E., Labella, F. S., Sanwal, M. 1967. Isolated nerve endings (neurosecretosomes) from the posterior pituitary. *J. Cell Biol.* 34:185–205
9. Sorenson, R. L., Lindall, A. W., Lazarow, A. 1969. Studies on the isolated goosefish insulin secretion granule. *Diabetes* 18:129–37
10. Hymer, W. C. 1975. In *The Anterior Pituitary*, ed. A. Tixier-Vidal, M. G. Farquhar, 137–80. New York: Academic. 283 pp.
11. Coore, H. G., Hellman, B., Pihl, E., Täljedal, I. B. 1969. Physiochemical characteristics of insulin secretion granules. *Biochem. J.* 111:107–13
12. Smith, A. D., Winkler, H. 1967. A simple method for the isolation of adrenal chromaffin granules on a large scale. *Biochem. J.* 103:480–82
13. Trifaró, J. M., Dworkind, J. 1970. A new and simple method for isolation of adrenal chromaffin granules by means of an isotonic density gradient. *Anal. Biochem.* 34:403–12
14. Winkler, H., Smith, A. D. 1975. *Handb. Physiol., Endocrinology* 6:321–39
15. Pletscher, A., Da Prada, M., Berneis, K. H., Steffen, H., Lütold, B., Weder, H. G. 1974. See Ref. 4, pp. 257–64
16. Williams, J. A. 1970. Origin of transmembrane potentials in non-excitable cells. *J. Theor. Biol.* 28:287–96
17. Matthews, E. K. 1974. In *Secretory Mechanisms of Exocrine Glands*, ed. N. A. Thorn, O. H. Petersen, 185–95. New York: Academic. 645 pp.
18. Douglas, W. W., Kanno, T., Sampson, S. R. 1967. Effects of acetylcholine and other medullary secretagogues and antagonists on the membrane potentials of adrenal chromaffin cells: an analysis employing techniques of tissue culture. *J. Physiol. London* 188:107–20
19. Dean, P. M., Matthews, E. K. 1970. Electrical activity in pancreatic islet cells: effects of ions. *J. Physiol. London* 210:265–75
20. Martin, S., York, D. H., Kraicer, J. 1973. Alterations in transmembrane potential of adenohypophysial cells in elevated potassium and calcium-free media. *Endocrinology* 92:1084–88
21. Douglas, W. W., Kanno, T., Sampson, S. R. 1967. Influence of the ionic environment on the membrane potential of the adrenal chromaffin cells and on the depolarizing effect of acetylcholine. *J. Physiol. London* 191:107–21
22. Houssay, B. A., Molinelli, E. A. 1928. Excitabilité des fibres adrénalinosécrétories du nerf grand splanchnique. Fréquences, seuil et optimum des stimulus. Rôle de l'ion calcium. *C. R. Soc. Biol.* 99:172–74
23. Douglas, W. W. 1968. Stimulus-secretion coupling: the concept and clues from chromaffin and other cells. *Br. J. Pharmacol.* 34:451–74
24. Douglas, W. W., Rubin, R. P. 1961. The role of calcium in the secretory response of the adrenal medulla to acetylcholine. *J. Physiol. London* 159:40–47
25. Douglas, W. W., Poisner, A. M. 1964. Stimulus-secretion coupling in a neurosecretory organ: the role of calcium in the release of vasopressin from the neurohypophysis. *J. Physiol. London* 172:1–18
26. Douglas, W. W., Poisner, A. M. 1963. The influence of calcium on the secretory response of the submaxillary gland to acetylcholine or to noradrenaline. *J. Physiol. London* 165:528–41
27. Smith, A. D. 1971. Summing up: some implications of the neuron as a secretory cell. *Philos. Trans. R. Soc. London Ser. B* 261:423–37
28. Douglas, W. W., Rubin, R. P. 1963. The mechanism of catecholamine release from the adrenal medulla and the role of calcium in stimulus-secretion

coupling. *J. Physiol. London* 167:288–310

29. Douglas, W. W. 1963. A possible mechanism of neurosecretion: release of vasopressin by depolarization and its dependence on calcium. *Nature* 197: 81–82

30. Vale, W., Guillemin, R. 1967. Potassium-induced stimulation of thyrotropin release *in vitro*. Requirement for presence of calcium and inhibition by thyroxine. *Experientia* 23:855–57

31. Samli, M. H., Geschwind, I. I. 1968. Some effects of energy-transfer inhibitors and Ca^{++}-free or K^{+}-enhanced media on the release of luteinizing hormone (LH) from the rat pituitary gland *in vitro*. *Endocrinology* 82:225–31

32. Wakabayashi, K., Kamberi, I. A., McCann, S. M. 1969. In vitro response of the rat pituitary to gonadotrophin-releasing factors and to ions. *Endocrinology* 85:1046–56

33. Parsons, J. A. 1970. Effects of cations on prolactin and growth hormone secretion by rat adenohypophyses *in vitro*. *J. Physiol.* 210:973–87

34. Kraicer, J. 1975. See Ref. 10, p. 21–43

35. Douglas, W. W. 1974. *Handb. Physiol., Endocrinology* 4(Part 1):191–224

36. Devis, G., Somers, G., Malaisse, W. J. 1975. Stimulation of insulin release by calcium. *Biochem. Biophys. Res. Commun.* 67:525–29

37. Grodsky, G. M., Bennett, L. L. 1966. Cation requirements for insulin secretion in the isolated perfused pancreas. *Diabetes* 15:910–13

38. Hales, C. N., Milner, R. D. G. 1968. Cations and the secretion of insulin from rabbit pancreas *in vitro*. *J. Physiol. London* 199:177–87

39. Douglas, W. W., Rubin, R. P. 1964. Stimulant action of barium on the adrenal medulla. *Nature* 203:305–7

40. Buchs, M., Dreifuss, J. J., Grau, J. D., Nordmann, J. J. 1972. Strontium as a substitute for calcium in the process leading to neurohypophyseal hormone secretion. *J. Physiol. London* 222: 168–69

41. Ishida, A. 1968. Stimulus-secretion coupling on the oxytocin release from the isolated posterior pituitary lobe. *Jpn. J. Physiol.* 18:471–80

42. Hales, C. N. 1970. Ion fluxes and membranes function in β-cells and adipocytes. *Acta Diabetol. Lat.* 7: Suppl. 1, pp. 64–75

43. Poisner, A. M., Hava, M. 1970. The role of ATP and ATPase in the release of catecholamines from the adrenal medulla. IV. ATP-activated uptake of calcium by microsomes and mitochondria. *Mol. Pharmacol.* 6:407–15

44. Lastowecka, A., Trifaró, J. M. 1974. The effect of sodium and calcium ions on the release of catecholamines from the adrenal medulla: Sodium deprivation induces release by exocytosis in the absence of extracellular calcium. *J. Physiol. London* 236:681–705

45. Copp, D. H. 1969. Calcitonin and parathyroid hormone. *Ann. Rev. Pharmacol.* 9:327–44

46. Rubin, R. P. 1974. In *Calcium and the Secretory Process*. New York & London: Plenum. 189 pp.

47. Hamilton, J. W., Cohn, D. V. 1969. Studies on the biosynthesis *in vitro* of parathyroid hormone. I. Synthesis of parathyroid hormone by bovine parathyroid gland slices and its control by calcium. *J. Biol. Chem.* 244:5421–29

48. Hales, C. N., Milner, R. D. G. 1968. The role of sodium and potassium in insulin secretion from rabbit pancreas. *J. Physiol. London* 194:725–43

49. Griffey, M. A., Conaway, H. H., Whitney, J. E. 1974. Insulin secretion induced by Na^{+} deprivation. *Endocrinology* 95:1469–72

50. Dreifuss, J. J., Grau, J. D., Bianchi, R. E. 1971. Antagonism between Ca^{2+} and Na^{+} ions at neurohypophyseal nerve terminals. *Experientia* 27:1295–96

51. Baker, P. F., Reuter, H. 1975. In *Calcium Movement in Excitable Cells*. New York: Pergamon. 102 pp.

52. Dransfeld, H., Greeff, K., Schron, A., Ting, B. T. 1969. Calcium uptake in mitochondria and vesicles of heart and skeletal muscle in presence of potassium, sodium, K-strophanthin and pentobarbital. *Biochem. Pharmacol.* 18: 1335–45

53. Banks, P. 1967. The effect of ouabain on the secretion of catecholamines and on the intracellular concentration of potassium. *J. Physiol. London* 193:631–37

54. Levin, S. R., Booker, J., Smith, D. F., Grodsky, G. M. 1970. Inhibition of insulin secretion by diphenylhydantoin in the isolated perfused pancreas. *J. Clin. Endocrinol. Metab.* 30:400–1

55. Russell, J. T., Thorn, N. A. 1974. Calcium and stimulus-secretion coupling in the neurohypophysis. II. Effects of lanthanum, a verapamil analogue (D–600) and prenylamine on 45-calcium transport and vasopressin release in isolated

rat neurohypophyses. *Acta Endocrinol.* 75:471–87

56. Pinto, J. E. B., Trifaró, J. M. 1976. The different effects of D-600 (methoxyverapamil) on the release of adrenal catecholamines induced by acetylcholine, high potassium or sodium deprivation. *Br. J. Pharmacol.* 57:127–32

57. Baker, P. F., Rink, T. J. 1975. Catecholamine release from bovine adrenal medulla in response to maintained depolarization. *J. Physiol. London* 253:593–620

58. Poisner, A. M. 1973. In *Frontiers in Catecholamine Research,* ed. E. Usdin, S. Snyder, 477–82 New York: Pergamon. 1219 pp.

59. Brisson, G. R., Malaisse-Lagae, F., Malaisse, W. J. 1972. The stimulus-secretion coupling of glucose-induced release. *J. Clin. Invest.* 51:232–41

60. Graumann, W. 1956. Beobachtungen uber Bildung and Sekretion perjodatreaktiver Staffe im Nebennierenmark des Gold-hamsters. *Z. Anat. Entwicklungsgesch.* 119:415–30

61. Franzen, D. 1964. Beiträge zur morphologie und chemohistologie des Nebennierenmarks des Goldhamsters (Mesocricetus auratus). *Anat. Anz.* 115:35–38

62. Cramer, W. 1918. Further observations on the thyroid-adrenal apparatus. A histochemical method for the demonstration of the adrenalin granules in the suprarenal gland. *J. Physiol. London* 52:viii–x

63. Hillarp, N. Å. 1960. Different pools of catecholamines stored in the adrenal medulla. *Acta Physiol. Scand.* 50:8–22

64. Thorn, N. A. 1965. Role of calcium in the release of vasopressin and oxytocin from posterior pituitary protein. *Acta Endocrinol.* 50:357–64

65. Blaschko, H., Welch, A. D. 1953. Localization of adrenaline in cytoplasmic particles of the bovine adrenal medulla. *Naunyn-Schmiedebergs Arch. Exp. Pathol. Pharmakol.* 219:17–22

66. Lever, J. D., Findlay, J. A. 1966. Similar structural basis for the storage and release of secretory material in adrenomedullary and β-pancreatic cells. *Z. Zellforsch. Mikrosk. Anat.* 74:317–24

67. De Robertis, E., Vaz Ferreira, A. 1957. Electron microscope study of the secretion of catechol-containing droplets in the adrenal medulla. *Exp. Cell Res.* 12:568–74

68. Diner, O. 1967. L'expulsion des granules de la médulla-surrénale chez le hamster. *C.R. Acad. Sci. Paris* 265:616–19

69. Nagasawa, J., Douglas, W. W., Schulz, R. A. 1970. Ultrastructural evidence of secretion by exocytosis and of "synaptic vesicle" formation in posterior pituitary glands. *Nature* 227:407–9

70. Gómez-Acebo, J., Parrilla, R., Candela, L. R. 1968. Fine structure of the A and D cells of the rabbit endocrine pancreas *in vivo* and incubated *in vitro.* I. Mechanism of secretion of the A cells. *J. Cell Biol.* 36:33–44

71. Lacy, P. E. 1961. Electron microscopy of the beta cell of the pancreas. *Am. J. Med.* 31:851–59

72. Farquhar, M. G. 1969. In *Lysosomes in Biology and Pathology,* ed. J. T. Dingle, H. B. Fell, 2:462–82. Amsterdam: North-Holland. 668 pp.

73. Rennels, E. G., Shiino, M. 1968. Ultrastructural manifestations of pituitary release of ACTH in the rat. *Arch. Anat. Histol. Embryol.* 51:575–90

74. Farquhar, M. G. 1961. Origin and fate of secretory granules in cells of the anterior pituitary gland. *Trans. NY Acad. Sci.* 23:346–51

75. Smith, R. E., Farquhar, M. G. 1966. Lysosome function in the regulation of the secretory process in cells of the anterior pituitary gland. *J. Cell Biol.* 31:319–47

76. Farquhar, M. G., Skutelsky, E. H., Hopkins, E. R. 1975. See Ref. 10, pp. 83–135

77. Farquhar, M. G. 1971. Processing of secretory products by cells of the anterior pituitary gland. *Mem. Soc. Endocrinol.* 19:79–122

78. Pelletier, G., Peillon, F., Vila-Porcile, E. 1971. An ultrastructural study of sites of granule extrusion in the anterior pituitary of the rat. *Z. Zellforsch. Mikrosk. Anat.* 115:501–7

79. Palade, G. E. 1959. In *Subcellular Particles,* ed. T. Hayashi, pp. 64–83. New York: Ronald. 213 pp.

80. Banks, P., Helle, K. 1965. The release of protein from the stimulated adrenal medulla. *Biochem. J.* 97:40C–41C

81. Douglas, W. W., Poisner, A. M., Rubin, R. P. 1965. Efflux of adenine nucleotides from perfused adrenal glands exposed to nicotine and other chromaffin cell stimulants. *J. Physiol. London* 179:130–37

82. Viveros, O. H., Arqueros, L., Kirshner, N. 1968. Release of catecholamines and dopamine β-oxidase from the adrenal medulla. *Life Sci.* 7:609–18

83. Poisner, A. M., Trifaró, J. M., Douglas, W. W. 1967. The fate of the chromaffin granule during catecholamine release from the adrenal medulla. II. Loss of protein and retention of lipid in subcellular fractions. *Biochem. Pharmacol.* 16:2101–8
84. Viveros, O. H., Arqueros, L., Connett, R. J., Kirshner, N. 1969. Mechanism of secretion from the adrenal medulla. 4. The fate of the storage vesicles following insulin and reserpine administration. *Mol. Pharmacol.* 5:69–82
85. Trifaró, J. M. 1973. See Ref. 58, pp. 501–3
86. Viveros, O. H., Arqueros, L., Kirshner, N. 1969. Quantal secretion from adrenal medulla: all or none release of storage vesicle content. *Science* 165:911–13
87. Uttenthal, L. O., Livett, B. G., Hope, D. B. 1971. Release of neurophysin together with vasopressin by a Ca²⁺-dependent mechanism. *Philos. Trans. R. Soc. London Ser. B* 261:379–80
88. Nordmann, J. J., Dreifuss, J. J., Legros, J. J. 1971. A correlation of release of "polypeptide hormones" and of immunoreactive neurophysin from isolated rat neurohypophyses. *Experientia* 27:1344–45
89. Rubenstein, A. H., Clark, J. L., Malani, F., Steiner, D. F. 1969. Secretion of proinsulin C-peptide by pancreatic β cells and its circulation in blood. *Nature* 224:697–99
90. Fillion, G. M. B., Slorach, S. A., Uvnäs, B. 1970. The release of histamine, heparin, and granule protein from rat mast cells treated with compound 48/80 *in vitro. Acta Physiol. Scand.* 78:547–60
91. Trifaró, J. M., Poisner, A. M., Douglas, W. W. 1967. The fate of the chromaffin granule during catecholamine release from the adrenal medulla. I. Unchanged efflux of phospholipid and cholesterol. *Biochem. Pharmacol.* 16:2095–2100
92. Schneider, F. H., Smith, A. D., Winkler, H. 1967. Secretion from the adrenal medulla: biochemical evidence for exocytosis. *Br. J. Pharmacol.* 31:94–104
93. Edwards, B. A., Edwards, M. E., Thorn, N. A. 1973. The release *in vitro* of vasopressin unaccompanied by the axoplasmic enzymes: lactic acid dehydrogenase and adenylate kinase. *Acta Endocrinol.* 72:417–24
94. Matthews, E. K., Legros, J. J., Grau, J. D. Nordmann, J. J., Dreifuss, J. J. 1973. Release of neurohypophysial hormones by exocytosis. *Nature* 241:86–88
95. Kirshner, N., Sage, H. J., Smith, W. J., Kirshner, A. G. 1966. Release of catecholamines and specific protein from adrenal glands. *Science* 154:529–31
96. Tixier-Vidal, A., Picart, R. 1971. Electron microscopic localization of glycoproteins in pituitary cells of duck and quail. *J. Histochem. Cytochem.* 19:775–97
97. Fawcett, D. W., Long, J. A., Jones, A. L. 1969. The ultrastructure of endocrine glands. *Recent Prog. Horm. Res.* 25:315–68
98. Lazarus, S. S., Shapiro, S., Volk, B. W. 1968. Secretory granule formation and release in rabbit pancreatic A-cells. *Diabetes* 17:152–60
99. Howell, S. L., Kostianovsky, M., Lacy, P. E. 1969. Beta granule formation in isolated islets of Langerhans. A study by electron microscopic radioautography. *J. Cell Biol.* 42:695–705
100. Kobayashi, S., Fujita, T. 1969. Fine structure of mammalian and avian pancreatic islets with special reference to D cells and nervous elements. *Z. Zellforsch. Mikrosk. Anat.* 100:340–63
101. De Robertis, E., Sabatini, D. D. 1960. Submicroscopic analysis of the secretory process in the adrenal medulla. *Fed. Proc.* 19:Suppl. 5, pp. 70–78
102. Coupland, R. E. 1972. See Ref. 6, pp. 16–45
103. Sachs, H., Fawcett, P., Takabatake, Y., Portanova, R. 1969. Biosynthesis and release of vasopressin and neurophysin. *Recent Prog. Horm. Res.* 25:447–84
104. Whaley, W. G., Dauwalder, M., Kephart, J. E. 1972. Golgi apparatus: Influence on cell surfaces. *Science* 175:596–99
105. Morré, D. J., Keenan, T. W., Huang, C. M. 1974. See Ref. 4, pp. 107–25
106. Jamieson, J. D., Palade, G. E. 1967. Intracellular transport of secretory proteins in the pancreatic exocrine cell. I. Role of the peripheral elements of Golgi complex. *J. Cell Biol.* 34:577–96
107. Hopkins, C. R. 1972. The biosynthesis, intracellular transport, and packaging of melanocyte-stimulating peptides in the amphibian pars intermedia. *J. Cell Biol.* 53:642–53
108. Caro, L. G., Palade, G. E. 1964. Protein synthesis, storage and discharge in the pancreatic exocrine cell. An autoradiography study. *J. Cell Biol.* 20:473–95
109. Castle, J. D., Jamieson, J. D., Palade, G. E. 1972. Radioautographic analysis of the secretory process in the parotid

44   TRIFARÓ

acinar cell of the rabbit. *J. Cell Biol.* 53:290–311

110. Howell, S. L. 1972. Role of ATP in the intracellular translocation of proinsulin and insulin in the rat pancreatic β cell. *Nature* 235:85–86

111. Sachs, H., Takabatake, Y. 1964. Evidence for a precursor in vasopressin biosynthesis. *Endocrinology* 75:943–48

112. Burford, G. D., Jones, C. W., Pickering, B. T. 1971. Tentative identification of a vasopressin-neurophysin and an oxytocin-neurophysin in the rat. *Biochem. J.* 124:809–13

113. Winkler, H., Hörtnagl, H., Schöpf, J. A. L., Zur Nedden, G. 1971. Bovine adrenal medulla: Synthesis and secretion of radioactively labelled catecholamines and chromogranins. *Naunyn-Schmiedebergs Arch. Pharmakol.* 271: 193–203

114. Winkler, H., Schöpf, J. A. L., Hörtnagl, H., Hörtnagl, H. 1972. Bovine adrenal medulla: Subcellular distribution of newly synthesized catecholamines, nucleotides, and chromogranins. *Naunyn-Schmiedebergs Arch. Pharmacol.* 273: 43–61

115. Malamed, S., Poisner, A. M., Trifaró, J. M., Douglas, W. W. 1968. The fate of the chromaffin granule during catecholamine release from the adrenal medulla. III. Recovery of a purified fraction of electron-translucent structures. *Biochem. Pharmacol.* 17:241–46

116. Viveros, O. H., Arqueros, L., Kirshner, N. 1969. Mechanism of secretion from the adrenal medulla. 5. Retention of storage vesicle membranes following release of adrenaline. *Mol. Pharmacol.* 5:342–49

117. Trifaró, J. M., Duerr, A. C. 1976. Isolation and characterization of a Golgi-rich fraction from the adrenal medulla. *Biochim. Biophys. Acta* 421:153–67

118. Trifaró, J. M., Duerr, A. C., Pinto, J. E. B. 1976. Membranes of the adrenal medulla: A comparison between the membranes of the Golgi apparatus and chromaffin granules. *Mol. Pharmacol.* 12:536–45

119. Benedeczky, I., Smith, A. D. 1972. Ultrastructural studies on the adrenal medulla of golden hamster: origin and fate of secretory granules. *Z. Zellforsch. Mikroskok. Anat.* 124:367–86

120. Baker, B. L. 1974. See Ref. 35, pp. 191–224

121. Pictet, R., Rutter, W. J. 1972. In *Handb. Physiology, Endocrinology* 1: 25–66

122. Douglas, W. W., Nagasawa, J., Schulz, R. A. 1971. Coated microvesicles in neurosecretory terminals of posterior pituitary glands shed their coats to become smooth "synaptic" vesicles. *Nature* 232:340–41

123. Nagasawa, J., Douglas, W. W. 1972. Thorium dioxide uptake into adrenal medullary cells and the problem of recapture of granule membrane following exocytosis. *Brain Res.* 37:141–45

124. Orci, L., Junod, A., Pictet, R., Renold, A. E., Rouiller, C. 1968. Granuloysis in A cells of endocrine pancreas in spontaneous and experimental diabetes in animals. *J. Cell Biol.* 38:462–66

125. Rufener, C. 1973. Autophagy of secretory granules in the rat neurohypophysis. *Neuroendocrinology* 13:314–20

126. Holtzman, E., Dominitz, R. 1968. Cytochemical studies of lysosomes, Golgi apparatus and endoplasmic reticulum in secretion and protein uptake by adrenal medulla cells of the rat. *J. Histochem. Cytochem.* 16:320–36

127. Blaschko, H., Jerrome, D. W., Robb-Smith, A. H. T., Smith, A. D., Winkler, H. 1968. Biochemical and morphological studies on catecholamine storage in human phaeochromocytoma. *Clin. Sci.* 34:453–65

128. Hokin, L. E. 1951. The synthesis and secretion of amylase by pigeon pancreas in vitro. *Biochemistry* 48:320–26

129. Coore, H. G., Randle, P. J. 1964. Regulation of insulin secretion studied with pieces of rabbit pancreas incubated *in vitro. Biochem J.* 93:66–78

130. Douglas, W. W., Ishida, A., Poisner, A. M. 1965. The effect of metabolic inhibitors on the release of vasopressin from the isolated neurohypophysis. *J. Physiol. London* 181:753–59

131. Kirshner, N., Smith, W. J. 1969. Metabolic requirements for secretion from the adrenal medulla. *Life Sci.* 8(part 1): 799–803

132. Trifaró, J. M., Poisner, A. M. 1967. The role of ATP and ATPase in the release of catecholamines from the adrenal medulla. II. ATP-evoked fall in optical density of isolated chromaffin granules. *Mol. Pharmacol.* 3:572–80

133. Poisner, A. M., Trifaró, J. M. 1967. The role of ATP and ATPase in the release of catecholamines from the adrenal medulla. I. ATP-evoked release of catecholamines, ATP, and protein from isolated chromaffin granules. *Mol. Pharmacol.* 3:561–71

134. Trifaró, J. M., Dworkind, J. 1971. Phosphorylation of membrane components of adrenal chromaffin granules by adenosine triphosphate. *Mol. Pharmacol.* 7:52–65
135. Dworkind, J., Trifaró, J. M. 1971. Chromaffin granules: Effects of ions and ATP on catecholamine content, ATPase activity, and membrane phosphorylation. *Experientia* 27:1277–79
136. Banks, P. 1966. An interaction between chromaffin granules and calcium ions. *Biochem. J.* 101:18C–20C
137. Vilhardt, H., Jørgensen, T. 1972. Free flow electrophoresis of isolated secretory granules from bovine neurohypophyses. *Experientia* 28:852–53
138. Woodin, A. M., French, J. E., Marchesi, V. T. 1963. Morphological changes associated with the extrusion of protein induced in the polymorphonuclear leucocyte by staphylococcal leucocidin. *Biochem. J.* 87:567–71
139. Abood, L. G. 1966. Interrelationships between phosphates and calcium in bioelectric phenomena. *Int. Rev. Neurobiol.* 9:223–61
140. Trifaró, J. M. 1972. Solubilization and partial characterization of the phosphorylated component(s) of the membrane of adrenal chromaffin granules. *FEBS Lett.* 23:237–40
141. Trifaró, J. M., Dworkind, J. 1975. Phosphorylation of the membrane components of chromaffin granules: Synthesis of diphosphatidylinositol and presence of phosphatidylinositol kinase in granule membranes. *Can. J. Physiol. Pharmacol.* 53:479–92
142. Buckley, J. T., Hawthorne, J. N. 1972. Erythrocyte membrane polyphosphoinositide metabolism and the regulation of calcium binding. *J. Biol. Chem.* 247:7218–23
143. Yoshida, H., Miki, N., Ishida, H., Yamamoto, T. 1968. Release of amylase from zymogen granules by ATP and a low concentration of Ca^{2+}. *Biochem. Biophys. Acta* 158:489–90
144. Matsuda, T., Hata, F., Yoshida, H. 1968. Stimulatory effect of Na^+ and ATP on the release of acetylcholine from synaptic vesicles. *Biochem. Biophys. Acta* 150:739–41
145. Poisner, A. M., Douglas, W. W. 1968. A possible mechanism of release of posterior pituitary hormones involving adenosine triphosphate and an adenosine triphosphatase in neuro-secretory granules. *Mol. Pharmacol.* 4:531–40

146. Howell, S. L., Young, D. A., Lacy, P. E. 1969. Isolation and properties of secretory granules from rat islets of Langerhans. III. Studies of the stability of isolated Beta granules. *J. Cell Biol.* 41:167–76
147. Hellman, B., Täljedal, I. B. 1970. Solubilizing effect of nucleotides on isolated insulin secretory granules. *J. Cell Biol.* 47:289–93
148. Labrie, F., Lemaire, S., Poirier, G., Pelletier, G., Boucher, R. 1971. Adenohypophyseal secretory granules. I. Their phosphorylation and association with protein kinase. *J. Biol. Chem.* 246:7311–17
149. Lambert, M., Camus, J., Christophe, J. 1974. Phosphorylation of protein components of isolated zymogen granule membranes from the rat pancreas. *FEBS Lett.* 49:228–32
150. Oka, M., Izumi, F., Kashimoto, T. 1972. Effects of cytoplasmic and microsomal fractions on ATP-Mg^{++} stimulated catecholamine release from isolated adrenomedullary granules. *Jpn. J. Pharmacol.* 22:207–14
151. Lacy, P. E., Howell, S. L., Young, D. A., Fink, C. J. 1968. New hypothesis of insulin secretion. *Nature* 219:1177–79
152. Poisner, A. M., Bernstein, J. 1971. A possible role of microtubules in catecholamine release from the adrenal medulla: effect of colchicine, vinca alkaloids and deuterium oxide. *J. Pharmacol. Exp. Ther.* 171:102–8
153. Labrie, F., Gauthier, M., Pelletier, G., Borgeat, P., Lemay, A., Gouge, J. J. 1973. Role of microtubules in basal and stimulated release of growth hormone and prolactin in rat adenohypophysis *in vitro*. *Endocrinology* 93:903–14
154. Lacy, P. E., Greider, M. H. 1972. See Ref. 121, pp. 77–89
155. Grodsky, G. M., Landahl, H., Curry, D., Bennett, L. 1969. In *Structure and Metabolism of the Pancreatic Islets,* ed. S. Falkmer, B. Hellman, I. B. Täljedal, 409–20. Oxford: Pergamon. 568 pp.
156. Hoshi, M., Shreeve, W. W. 1973. Release and production of insulin by isolated, perifused rat pancreatic islets. *Diabetes* 22:16–24
157. Randle, P. J., Hales, C. N. 1972. See Ref. 121, pp. 219–35
158. Pipeleers, D. G., Pipeleers-Marichal, M. A., Kipnis, D. M. 1976. Microtubule assembly and intracellular transport of secretory granules in pancreatic islets. *Science* 191:88–90

159. Lacy, P. E., Walker, M. M., Fink, J. 1972. Perifusion of isolated rat islets *in vitro*. *Diabetes* 21:987–98

160. Weisenberg, R. C. 1972. Microtubule formation *in vitro* in solutions containing low calcium concentrations. *Science* 177:1104–5

161. Shelanski, M. L. 1973. Chemistry of the filaments and tubules of brain. *J. Histochem. Cytochem.* 21:529–39

162. Kraicer, J., Milligan, J. W. 1971. Effect of colchicine on *in vitro* ACTH release induced by high K^+ and by hypothalamus-stalk-median eminence extract. *Endocrinology* 89:408–12

163. Douglas, W. W., Sorimachi, M. 1972. Effects of cytochalasin B and colchicine on secretion of posterior pituitary and adrenal medullary hormones. *Br. J. Pharmacol. Chemother.* 45:143–44

164. Sundberg, D. K., Krulich, L., Fawcett, C. P., Illner, P., McCann, S. M. 1973. The effect of colchicine on the release of rat anterior pituitary hormones *in vitro*. *Proc. Soc. Exp. Biol. Med.* 142:1097–1100

165. Temple, R., Williams, J. A., Wilber, J. F., Wolff, J. 1972. Colchicine and hormone secretion. *Biochem. Biophys. Res. Commun.* 46:1454–61

166. Jamieson, J. D. 1972. Transport and discharge of exportable proteins in pancreatic exocrine cells: *In vitro* studies. *Curr. Top. Membr. Transp.* 3:273–338

167. Stadler, J., Franke, W. W. 1974. Characterization of the colchicine binding of membrane fractions from rat and mouse liver. *J. Cell Biol.* 60:297–303

168. Mizel, S. B., Wilson, L. 1972. Nucleoside transport in mammalian cells. Inhibition by colchicine. *Biochemistry* 11:2573–78

169. Spoor, R. P., Ferguson, F. C. 1965. Colchicine. IV. Neuromuscular transmission in isolated frog and rat tissues. *J. Pharm. Sci.* 54:779–80

170. Trifaró, J. M., Collier, B., Lastowecka, A., Stern, D. 1972. Inhibition by colchicine and by vinblastine of acetylcholine-induced catecholamine release from the adrenal gland: an anticholinergic action, not an effect upon microtubules. *Mol. Pharmacol.* 8:264–67

171. Douglas, W. W., Sorimachi, M. 1972. Colchicine inhibits adrenal medullary secretion evoked by acetylcholine without affecting that evoked by potassium. *Br. J. Pharmacol.* 45:129–32

172. Lagunoff, D., Chi, E. Y. 1975. Effect of colchicine on mast cell secretion stimulated by polymyxin B and A23187. *J. Cell Biol.* 67:230a (Abstr.)

173. Poisner, A. M. 1970. Actomyosin-like protein from the adrenal medulla. *Fed. Proc.* 29:545 (Abstr.)

174. Trifaró, J. M., Ulpian, C. 1975. Actomyosin-like protein isolated from the adrenal medulla. *FEBS Lett.* 57:198–202

175. Berl, S., Puszkin, S., Nicklas, W. J. 1973. Actomyosin-like protein in brain. *Science* 179:441–46

176. Gabbiani, G., Malaisse-Lagae, F., Blondel, B., Orci, L. 1974. Actin in pancreatic islet cells. *Endocrinology* 95:1630–35

177. Phillips, J. H., Slater, A. 1975. Actin in the adrenal medulla. *FEBS Lett.* 56:327–31

178. Ulpian, C., Trifaró, J. M. 1976. Isolation of myosin from the adrenal medulla. *Can. Fed. Biol. Soc. Meet.*, p. 178 (Abstr.)

179. Burridge, K., Slater, J. H. 1975. Association of actin and myosin with secretory granule membranes. *Nature* 254:526–29

180. Brooks, J. C., Siegel, F. L. 1973. Purification of a calcium-binding phosphoprotein from beef adrenal medulla. *J. Biol. Chem.* 248:4189–93

181. LeBeux, Y. J., Willemot, J. 1975. An ultrastructural study of the microfilaments in rat brain by means of E-PTA staining and heavy meromyosin labeling. II. The Synapses. *Cell Tissue Res.* 160:37–68

182. Wessels, N. K., Spooner, B. S., Ash, J. F., Bradley, M. O., Ludueña, M. A., Taylor, E. L., Wrenn, J. T., Yamada, K. M. 1971. Microfilaments in cellular and developmental processes. *Science* 171:135–43

183. Mizel, S. B., Wilson, L. 1972. Inhibition of the transport of several hexoses in mammalian cells by cytochalasin B. *J. Biol. Chem.* 247:4102–5

184. Nakazato, Y., Douglas, W. W. 1973. Cytochalasin blocks sympathetic ganglionic transmission: a presynaptic effect antagonized by pyruvate. *Proc. Natl. Acad. Sci. USA* 70:1730–33

185. Sanger, J. W., Sanger, J. M. 1975. States of actin and cytochalasin-B. *J. Cell Biol.* 67:381a (Abstr.)

186. Pollard, T. D., Weihing, R. R. 1974. Actin and myosin and cell movement. *CRC Crit. Rev. Biochem.* 2:1–65

187. Lazarides, E., Weber, K. 1974. Actin antibody: The specific visualization of actin filaments in non-muscle cells.

Proc. Natl. Acad. Sci. USA 71:2268–72

188. Sanger, I. W. 1975. Changing patterns of actin localization during cell division. *Proc. Natl. Acad. Sci. USA* 72:1913–16

189. Douglas, W. W., Poisner, A. M., Trifaró, J. M. 1966. Lysolecithin and other phospholipids in the adrenal medulla of various species. *Life Sci.* 5:809–15

190. Blaschko, H., Firemark, H., Smith, A. D., Winkler, H. 1967. Lipids of the adrenal medulla: lysolecithin, a characteristic constituent of chromaffin granules. *Biochem. J.* 104:545–49

191. Trifaró, J. M. 1969. Phospholipid metabolism and adrenal medullary activity. I. The effect of acetylcholine on tissue uptake and incorporation of orthophosphate-^{32}P into nucleotides and phospholipids of bovine adrenal medulla. *Mol. Pharmacol.* 5:382–93

192. Trifaró, J. M. 1969. The effect of Ca^{2+} omission in the secretion of catecholamines and the incorporation of orthophosphate-^{32}P into nucleotides and phospholipids of bovine adrenal medulla during acetylcholine stimulation. *Mol. Pharmacol.* 5:420–31

193. Lucy, J. A. 1970. The fusion of biological membranes. *Nature* 227:815–17

194. Koening, H. 1974. See Ref. 4, pp. 273–301

195. Dean, P. M. 1975. Exocytosis modelling: An electrostatic function for calcium in stimulus-secretion coupling. *J. Theor. Biol.* 54:289–308

196. Dean, P. M., Matthews, E. K. 1975. The London–Van der Waals attraction constant of secretory granules and its significance. *J. Theor. Biol.* 54:309–21

197. Poste, G. 1971. Membrane fusion reaction: A theory. *J. Theor. Biol.* 32:165–84

Ann. Rev. Pharmacol. Toxicol. 1977. 17:49–65
Copyright © 1977 by Annual Reviews Inc. All rights reserved

PHARMACOKINETIC CONSEQUENCES OF AGING

❖6666

David P. Richey and A. Douglas Bender
Smith Kline & French Laboratories, Philadelphia, Pennsylvania 19101

INTRODUCTION

For the purpose of this review we have chosen a rather narrow definition of geriatric pharmacology. We deal with the influence of increasing age on the plasma concentration of a drug and the factors that influence the peak concentration and the rate at which the drug leaves the body. We also discuss what changes in tissue sensitivity occur with age that would affect the overall response to a drug at a given blood level concentration. We do not discuss the extensive literature on the safety and utility of drugs in geriatric patients or the effect of increasing age on the incidence of adverse reactions and altered drug utility. Reviews on these have been published (1–5). Not considered as part of this review is one other aspect of geriatric pharmacology, namely, the effect of drugs on the aging process. Information on this aspect of the subject can be found in other reviews (6,7).

We would like to remark on the progress that has been made in our understanding of the effects of age on how a drug is handled by the body and the implications that these changes have on the utility of pharmacological agents in the treatment of diseases of old age. Until recently, most of the work has concerned the use of drugs in the elderly patient to determine their safety and their efficacy. There have been few comparisons with the response in younger populations. Even when such comparisons have been made, however, there have been few attempts to explain the reason for these differences and the basic biological rationale for them. In the last several years, however, greater attention has been focused on the effect of age on mechanisms responsible for drug disposition, and we are gradually laying the foundation for understanding how drugs may be more effectively used in the treatment of diseases of the elderly patient (8–13). It is our hope that the review of this biological rationale, and more specifically the pharmacokinetic aspects of increasing age, will contribute to this understanding.

AGE-RELATED CHANGES IN DRUG HANDLING SYSTEMS

Accepting the general principle that pharmacological effects—as well as side effects and toxic effects—are closely related to the circulating level of an administered drug, it is instructive to consider the physiologic processes which influence that level. Pharmacotherapeutic problems encountered in the elderly are due largely to age-related functional changes in the body's drug-handling machinery.

Absorption

Oral dosage forms must initially undergo dissolution, and although the decrease in stomach acid production which accompanies increasing age has sometimes been cited as a factor mitigating against adequate drug absorption, there is no real evidence for such an effect. It is quite possible that the only clinically important aspect of gastric pH as regards drug absorption is that it affects gastric motility, with higher pH values favoring absorption by hastening the movement of stomach contents to the small intestine. The pharmacologic consequence of abnormal gastric motility may not be simply in the timing of the onset of drug action but rather an alteration in the rate at which the drug enters the circulation so that an excessive and adverse physiologic reaction may occur or so that an inadequate blood level is achieved and thus a limited drug effect is developed. Bianchine et al (14) demonstrated the importance of this factor in treating patients whose parkinsonism was unrelieved by L-DOPA therapy.

The effects of increasing age on the drug absorption process per se have not been carefully or thoroughly studied. An early review of this topic (15) cited the general paucity of such information and concluded that there was an overall suggestion of reduced absorption in the elderly. Age-related decreases in the absorption of glucose and calcium (specifically transported substances unlike most drugs which are passively absorbed) are of uncertain significance, but the decreased absorption of xylose (16) and iron (17) in older subjects may indicate some decrease in the efficiency of drug absorption. A possible basis for decreased drug absorption in the aged has been developed (8) and concerns itself with a decrease in intestinal blood perfusion. While circulation to the coronary and cerebral regions is only slightly changed in the older subjects, intestinal perfusion is decreased by 40–50% (18), and this presents the potential for decreasing transfer of a drug across the serosal membrane.

Metabolism

A limitation on the duration of action of many drugs is established by the rate at which they are metabolized by the hepatic microsomal hydroxylating system and converted to (multi)hydroxylated forms and their conjugates and subsequently excreted. Gorrod (19) has reviewed at length the reports on the effects of age on drug-metabolizing ability. Kato and his co-workers (20) found that after the attainment of sexual maturity, rats steadily lose their capacity for the metabolism of a variety of drugs and that this decrease is mirrored by increases in the serum levels of such drugs and by the intensity or duration of their pharmacologic effects. Good support for the interpretation of this finding was supplied by Kuhlmann et al (21) who found that hexobarbital is metabolized more slowly by older rats and gives a more prolonged effect, whereas barbital (which is not metabolized at all) gave effects of equal duration for old and young rats.

Excretion

The ultimate elimination of a drug or its metabolite(s) from the body is predominantly through the kidneys, mostly by simple glomerular filtration but also by active excretion at the tubule (for organic acids and antibiotic metabolites). This step can limit the pharmacolgic effect for nonmetabolized drugs, and will regulate the elimination of drug metabolites for other drugs. As will be noted in the clinical studies to be described later, renal function is probably the single factor most responsible for altered drug levels in an aging population. The age-related decrease in renal perfusion is estimated at about 1.5% per year after maturity, totaling a decrease of roughly 40–50% from age 25 to age 65. This blood flow decrement is reflected by a 45% drop in both glomerular filtration rate and urea clearance (22) and a corresponding 50% increase in blood urea nitrogen. Even in the absence of any active intrinsic renal disease, creatinine clearance is reduced in the elderly to about half normal (23) and can often be referred to as an index of relative drug clearance capacity. A number of dosage guidelines and nomograms have been developed on the basis of endogenous creatinine clearance (24, 25).

CLINICAL STUDIES

Antibiotics

The earliest studies depicting differences in drug handling by young and geriatric subjects were concerned with antibiotics. Leikola & Vartia (26) reported on the results of a large study of penicillin levels in patients administered penicillin G and procaine penicillin i.m. A young group of subjects (average age 25 years) had a half-time of 0.55 hr for penicillin G while an older group (average age 77 years) had a 1.0 hr half-time. For the procaine form also, younger subjects displayed more rapid elimination with a half-time of about 10 hr compared with 18 hr for the older group. Extrapolation of the serum level curves to zero time indicated that the effectiveness of absorption of penicillin from the intramuscular site was equal for both age groups. The investigators attributed the group differences in half-time to the reduced renal secretion of the antibiotic through active tubular processes known to decrease with age. It is worth mentioning that all of the subjects were hospitalized throughout the study to minimize other influences on drug handling.

Vartia & Leikola (27) extended their work to include dihydrostreptomycin and tetracycline. For dihydrostreptomycin, the serum half-time of a young group (aged 27 years) was 5.2 hr, and this was extended to 8.4 hr for an elderly group (aged 75 years). A similar situation existed for tetracycline, with the same older group having a 4.5 hr half-time vs 3.5 hr for the younger patients. These age-related decreases in half-time are realized as two- to threefold greater serum levels of these two antibiot-

Table 1 Age-related pharmacokinetic results

Drug	Age group (years)	Pharmacokinetic observations	Age-related effect	Reference
Penicillin	Avg. 25	$T_{1/2} = 0.55$ hr (penicillin-G) $T_{1/2} = 10$ hr (procaine penicillin)	Decreased renal function (tubular secretion)	26
	Avg. 77	$T_{1/2} = 1.0$ hr (penicillin-G) $T_{1/2} = 18$ hr (procaine penicillin)		
	Females < 50 Females > 70	$T_{1/2} = 23.7$ min $T_{1/2} = 55.5$ min	Decreased renal function (tubular secretion)	28
	Males < 30 Males > 65	$T_{1/2} = 20.7$ min $T_{1/2} = 39.1$ min		
Dihydrostreptomycin	Avg. 27 Avg. 75	$T_{1/2} = 5.2$ hr $T_{1/2} = 8.4$ hr	Decreased renal function (glomerular filtration)	27
Tetracycline	Avg. 27 Avg. 75	$T_{1/2} = 3.5$ hr $T_{1/2} = 4.5$ hr Elderly have 2–3 × serum level of young	Decreased renal function	27
Kanamycin	20–50 50–70 70–90	$T_{1/2} = 107$ min $T_{1/2} = 149$ min $T_{1/2} = 282$ min Good inverse correlation with creatinine clearance	Decreased renal function	29
Propicillin	20–30 60–80	$V_d = 28.7$ liters $V_d = 19.9$ liters Absorption and elimination constants are similar for both groups, and serum levels are twice as high in the elderly	Decreased distribution volume	30

Table 1 *(Continued)*

Drug	Age/Values	Observations	Consequence	Ref.
Digoxin	Avg. 27 Avg. 27	$T_{1/2} = 51$ hr $T_{1/2} = 73$ hr Blood levels about twice as high in older group. Creatinine clearance = 122 ml/min in young vs 56 ml/min in elderly	Decreased renal function	44
		Plasma level (on equal maintenance dose) increases 2X from age 60 to 80; highly correlated with creatinine clearance values	Decreased renal function	62
		Absorption unaltered with age. Plasma level increased 3X in over 50s compared with young adults Toxic states 3 to 4X greater in over 70s and related to excessive serum creatinine levels	Decreased renal function	63
Antipyrine	Avg. 26 Avg. 78 18–39 40–59 60–92 20–40 65–92	$T_{1/2} = 12$ hr $T_{1/2} = 17.4$ hr $T_{1/2} = 12.7$ hr $T_{1/2} = 13.8$ hr $T_{1/2} = 14.8$ hr $T_{1/2} = 12.5$ hr $T_{1/2} = 16.8$ hr Doubling dose did not alter $T_{1/2}$, so metabolism may be limited not by simple enzymatic capacity, but perhaps by splanchnic circulation	Decreased metabolism	35 36 37

Table 1 *(Continued)*

Drug	Age group (years)	Pharmacokinetic observations	Age-related effect	Reference
Aminopyrine	25–30	$T_{1/2} = 3$ hr		38
	65–85	$T_{1/2} = 10$ hr		
Pethidine/meperidine		Absorption unaltered by age		
		Plasma levels twice as high in over 70s as in the young		39
		Red cell binding of drug is 50% in young vs 20% in elderly		41
		Plasma binding of drug decreased from 75% in young to 35% in elderly		
Phenytoin		Serum level (equal maintenance dose) increased 2× from 20 to 80 year olds	Decreased metabolism	32
	20–43	Phenytoin clearance = 26 ml/kg/hr		31
	67–95	Phenytoin clearance = 42 ml/kg/hr		
		Decrease (18%) in binding by plasma proteins in elderly; binding correlates well with plasma albumin concentration; no affinity change		
		Clearance not affected by induction of hepatic enzymes		
Amylobarbitone	20–40	Urinary metabolite excretion = 14.2%. Plasma drug level = 1.3 µg/ml	Decreased metabolism	34
	> 65	Urinary metabolite excretion = 4.3%. Plasma drug level = 1.0 µg/ml		
Phenobarbital	20–40	$T_{1/2} = 71$ hr		32
	50–60	$T_{1/2} = 77$ hr		
	> 70	$T_{1/2} = 107$ hr		

Table 1 *(Continued)*

Drug	Age	Pharmacokinetic data	Mechanism	Ref.
Lithium	Avg. 25 Avg. 58 Avg. 63	Li clearance = 41.5 ml/min Li clearance = 16.8 ml/min Li clearance = 7.7 ml/min		64
		Dose required to achieve therapeutic plasma level decreases approximately 30% from age 20 to age 80		65
Phenylbutazone	Avg. 26 Avg. 78	$T_{1/2}$ = 81 hr $T_{1/2}$ = 105 hr	Decreased metabolism	35
	Avg. 24 Avg. 81	$T_{1/2}$ = 87 hr $T_{1/2}$ = 110 hr		43
		$T_{1/2}$ correlated (inverse) with plasma albumin concentration		
Propranolol		Plasma level approximately 4× in elderly (avg. age 77) compared to young (avg. age 27) at all time periods after administration (p.o.)	Decreased metabolism (first pass effect)	46
Practolol	Avg. 27 Avg. 80	$T_{1/2}$ = 7.1 hr $T_{1/2}$ = 8.6 hr	Decreased renal function	46
Diazepam		$T_{1/2}$ increased linearly with age, from 20 hr at age 20 to 80 hr at age 70 Distribution volume increased 3× from 20 to 80 yr		47
Ampicillin	21–30 60–76	$T_{1/2}$ = 1.0 hr $T_{1/2}$ = 1.2 hr		66
Doxycycline	20–28 42–55	$T_{1/2}$ = 11.95 hr $T_{1/2}$ = 17.74 hr		67

ics in older subjects. In contrast to penicillin, both dihydrostreptomycin and tetracycline are removed by simple filtration, and the observed decrease in their removal rates in elderly patients is thought to reflect the known decrease in glomerular filtration rate (GFR) which accompanies aging.

A significant observation regarding antibiotic elimination was reported by Hansen et al (28). In their note on the kinetics of penicillin G in different age groups, they found half-time values of 39 and 55 min in older men and women respectively, versus 21 and 24 min for their younger counterparts. Most important, Hansen et al noted that the serum creatinine concentration was of no value in estimating healthy patients' kidney function, while endogenous creatinine clearance measurements were good (inverse) reflections of intrinsic kidney efficiency and correlated very well with half-time measurements for penicillin. This observation pointed up not only that kidney function may be increased by 50% before it is reflected in an increased serum creatinine level, but also that this age-related functional decrement occurs even in the absence of overt renal disease and will greatly decrease the elimination of many drugs in older patients.

Hansen's group (29) provided more support for the above conclusions with their report on kanamycin half-life values in young (20–50 years), intermediate (50–70 years), and elderly (70–90 year) patients. The kanamycin half-time increased from 107 min to 149 min to 282 min with increasing age and was apparently related to a concomitant decrease in creatinine clearance from 94 to 75 to 43 ml per minute. There was no difference in serum creatinine values for the three groups, and the authors cautioned against drug dosage based on serum creatinine data without consideration of urinary creatinine excretion.

A more formalized kind of analysis of drug pharmacokinetics in different age groups was performed by Simon et al (30) with orally administered propicillin. This study used a computer program to generate kinetic constants for drug handling based on serum propicillin levels. Although the older patient group (aged 60–80) had an area-under-curve twice that of the younger group (aged 20–30), both groups had comparable values for the absorption rate and for the drug serum half-life. Nevertheless, peak concentration was twice as high in the older group and the computations indicated a similarly higher initial serum concentration (hypothetical). The investigators concluded that the drugs must be distributed through a smaller circulatory and tissue volume in the older subjects, and this view was supported by calculated distribution volumes of about 29 liters in the younger group and 20 liters in the aged subjects.

Phenytoin and Barbiturates

Hayes et al (31) observed that plasma binding of phenytoin was decreased by about 20% in people over 65 as compared to those under 45. This difference was due not to an altered affinity for the drug but to reduced albumin concentration. Apparently related to this binding difference was an increased phenytoin clearance in the older group presumably reflecting the greater "available" drug circulating in the older subjects. Since Hayes et al did not include serum level data in their report, it is unclear how older subjects' serum phenytoin concentrations compared with the levels in younger subjects. Other clinical results with phenytoin (32) indicate that serum levels are in fact increased in older patients. This increase amounts to approximately a doubling of phenytoin levels over the range 20–80 years. It is possible that the two reports may well be in harmony since more rapid metabolism of phenytoin in younger subjects would lead to both lower serum levels and a lower drug clearance value. Phenytoin is of course extensively metabolized and it is unfortunate that neither of these groups included estimates of this factor in their investigations. It is not possible from the data supplied to determine whether the differences reported are due to age-related alterations in drug binding, renal function, or drug metabolism.

The serum half-life of phenobarbital was found by Traeger et al (33) to increase from 71 hr in a 20–40 age group to 77 hr in 50–60 year olds and to 107 hr in those subjects over 70. Somewhat more information was gathered by Irvine et al (34) who found that oral amylobarbitone gave significantly higher plasma levels in an elderly patient group than in a 20–40 year old group. Furthermore, the older subjects excreted only one third to one half as much of the drug as its primary metabolite, 3-hydroxyamylobarbitone, as did the young group. Irvine et al concluded that an age-related decrease in hepatic drug metabolism was responsible for the higher drug levels in the elderly. Because of the known deficit in renal function in the elderly, one cannot assume that urinary metabolite excretion reflects metabolism accurately. In this instance the conclusion of decreased metabolism is probably correct (especially because none of the subjects had greatly reduced creatinine clearance values), but without plasma metabolite levels or urinary drug estimation to complete the picture, this verdict is uncertain.

Antipyrine and Aminopyrine

Because of its minimal binding by proteins and its clearance from the plasma almost solely by hydroxylation, antipyrine is a favorite for drug metabolism studies. A paper of significant impact on clinical pharmacokinetics is that of O'Malley et al (35) who studied the plasma half-life of antipyrine and phenylbutazone in different age and sex groups. These investigators recorded a substantial increase in the antipyrine plasma half-time for the elderly (average 78 years) group, 17.4 hr, as compared with 12 hr for a group averaging 26 years of age. Some sex differences in metabolism rate were noted for antipyrine, and there were some suggestions of age differences in drug distribution volumes, but these were not impressive or of the importance of the other findings. An elaborate project designed to evaluate the separate and collective effects of age, smoking, caffeine, and alcohol on antipyrine metabolism [Vestal et al (36)] arrived also at a longer plasma half-life for elderly subjects, albeit a modest 16% increment compared to young subjects. The investigators cautioned that smoking habits could account for much of even this small difference, however, and that other factors should be considered when estimating age-related changes in pharmacokinetics. Results similar to those of O'Malley et al were obtained by an Australian group (37). They found that the elderly displayed a 16.8 hr plasma half-life for antipyrine with a 12.5 hr value for younger subjects. The half-time differences were not the result of altered distribution volumes. A similar study by Jori et al (38) led to the same conclusions as the O'Malley group with the plasma half-life of aminopy-rine prolonged from about 3 hr in 25–30 year olds to about 10 hr in a geriatric group aged 65–85.

Analgesics and Anti-Inflammatory Agents

Plasma levels of pethidine were consistently twice as high in a geriatric group as in a younger group (39). While much of this difference seemed to be related to a comparably decreased urinary excretion of pethidine, there was also the strange observation that the elderly excreted larger amounts of pethidine metabolites (40). It was also observed that approximately 50% of any level of pethidine was bound to the red cells of the younger subjects whereas only 20% was bound to the red cells of the geriatric subjects. If the bound drug is protected from metabolism, the elderly of course experience more rapid metabolism and excrete more metabolites than does a younger group. While Mather et al (41) did not find the same age effect as Chan et al on the half-life of pethidine (meperidine), they did find a striking decrease in plasma binding of the drug. A linear decrease in binding occurred with increasing age, proceeding from 75% bound at age 25 to only 35% bound at age 75. It is an interesting contrast to consider that a minimally bound drug such as antipyrine is less metabolized in older than in younger subjects, while highly bound drugs such as pethidine may be more rapidly metabolized if their binding decreases with age.

It has been reported (42) that indomethacin has a slightly greater half-life in the elderly (104 min) than in the young (92 min), but that the difference is not signifi-cant. The data indicated nevertheless that the younger control group excreted much more unchanged drug than did the elderly and that serum levels of indomethacin were higher in the latter. Again, because of incomplete information on comparative metabolite levels and excretion, it is impossible to ascribe the differences to any specific component of the drug-handling apparatus.

Phenylbutazone administered to the O'Malley groups of patients showed a more modest age effect than did antipyrine, but still showed a longer plasma half-time (104.6 hr) in the geriatric group than in the controls (81.2 hr). These values are very similar to those obtained by Triggs et al (43) who reported 110 hr for the elderly versus 87 hr for the young. They calculated this difference to be of little statistical significance. They did report, however, that the half-life of phenylbutazone, which is highly bound by plasma proteins, correlated well (and inversely) with the plasma albumin concentration, suggesting that if the elderly do indeed have reduced albu-min levels they will experience a prolonged half-life for this drug.

Digoxin

Few drugs are as well known to the geriatric practitioner as digoxin. There is a great familiarity with the problem of establishing an effective but nontoxic regimen of digoxin therapy for cardiac patients. Ewy et al (44) showed that a given i.v. dose of digoxin gave rise to higher blood levels and longer blood half-life in the elderly. They established that this was due to reduced renal function as reflected by creati-nine clearance values approximately half those of young patients and that digoxin clearance bore a linear relationship to creatinine clearance. Chamberlain et al (45) extended the pharmacokinetic observations of Ewy et al to show that in patients with good renal function, plasma digoxin levels were roughly proportional to daily dosage and that plasma level was positively correlated with ventricular rate. This latter observation showed that the elderly have in fact essentially the same sensitivity to digoxin as younger patients but need a lower dose to achieve the proper serum level.

Miscellaneous Drugs

Two β-blocker drugs, propanolol and practolol, have been administered orally to elderly and young groups and the plasma levels monitored by Castleden et al (46). Propanolol, which is eliminated almost exclusively by the hepatic route, gave plasma levels approximately five times as great in the elderly as in the younger subjects. Since this included also the peak level, it appears that propanolol's first-pass effect is the primary site of the age-related difference; the sustained constant ratio of serum levels in the decay phase indicates no significant renal influence on this difference. Conversely practolol gave similar plasma levels in both groups until near the peak level, after which the elderly group levels approached levels twice that of the young group, suggesting primarily a difference in renal elimination.

In a concerted study of three drugs—sulphamethizole, paracetamol, and phenyl-butazone—Triggs et al (43) compiled a number of pharmacokinetic measurements on young and geriatric subjects. The phenylbutazone results were mentioned above. Both sulphamethizole clearance and the elimination rate constant for sulphame-thizole were linearly related to creatinine clearance as might be expected for a drug eliminated by renal excretion. Half-lives of 181 min and 105 min were reported for the geriatric and young groups respectively. Similar results were found for paraceta-mol although with a smaller difference in half-time (130 min vs 109 min).

Both of these drugs have relatively short half-lives although paracetamol is elimi-nated predominantly by metabolism. For all three drugs no difference in absorption was noted with age nor was there any age-dependent variation in drug distribution volumes.

The β-phase half-time for diazepam shows a pronounced (and linear) age depen-dence, increasing from about 20 hr at age 20 to 70 hr at age 70. Klotz et al (47) reported that plasma and red cell binding of the drug was independent of age. Computer analysis of their data also implied that there is a linear increase in distribution volume with increasing age.

PLASMA PROTEIN BINDING

Once they enter the circulation, many drugs are bound to circulating plasma pro-teins, and it is for the most part the concentration of the free drug (in equilibrium with the drug that is bound) that determines the drug response interaction with receptor site. Drugs are ordinarily bound to plasma albumin, but other plasma proteins can also bind certain drugs. The binding involves a reversible bonding of the ionic, hydrogen, or van der Vaals type. Not all drugs are equally bound. Some may be bound to a major extent (up to 98% for phenylbutazone) or only very slightly as with barbital, or for all practical purposes not at all as is the case with antipyrine.

Our immediate concern in this review with drug binding is twofold. First, we are concerned with the effect of increasing age per se on the binding of drugs by plasma albumin and the interaction of one drug on the binding of another; and second, on the effect that various diseases have on the binding of drugs.

Plasma Binding and Age

With increasing age there is a decrease in the plasma binding of some drugs, which in some cases can be explained on the basis of lower serum albumin concentrations in the elderly. The character of the binding to plasma protein seems qualitatively the same as in healthy subjects, however. Studies by Bender et al (48) suggest that age per se is not associated with a defect in drug-binding proteins or the presence of endogenous materials that would compete with a drug for binding sites on the albumin molecule. Additionally, Hayes et al (49) have found that the strength of warfarin binding is uninfluenced by age. In a separate study the same investigators have ruled out any change in liver function that might influence the plasma binding of drugs in normal, healthy elderly subjects (31).

Bender et al (48) reported no change with age in the plasma binding of phenytoin, penicillin G, and phenobarbituric acid. In this study the serum albumin for normal, healthy subjects less than 50 years of age was 4.0 g/100 ml and for subjects over 50 years of age the serum albumin concentration was 3.4 g/100 ml. Klotz et al (47) also reported no change in plasma binding of diazepam with age; however, in this study serum albumin levels were not given. In another study, Wallace et al (50) compared drug binding in young and old healthy subjects who had serum albumin levels of 4.2 and 3.6 g/100 ml respectively. In this study they found that the binding of phenylbutazone was significantly reduced in the elderly; however, the binding of sulfadiazine and salicylate was unchanged. The binding of these two drugs was not as dependent on serum albumin levels as was the binding of phenylbutazone. Other authors have reported a consistent decrease in plasma binding with increase in age, and in these studies a large and rather significant drop in the concentration of serum albumin has been reported. For example, Hayes et al (31) found a signifi- cant reduction in plasma binding of phenytoin when data for subjects less than 45 years of age were compared to the binding for patients over 65 years of age. The serum albumin level in the two groups was 4.1 and 2.9 g/100 ml respectively. In this study the decrease in the maximum binding capacity paralleled the decrease in plasma albumin. A similar finding has also been recorded by Hooper et al (51). A decrease in the binding capacity of elderly people for warfarin (49) and carbenoxo- lone (52) has been reported and the decrease correlated with a fall in plasma albumin concentration. A decrease in meperidine binding with age has also been reported (41).

The question of drug-drug interactions with regard to the level and extent of binding of drugs in the elderly has not yet received a great deal of experimental attention. One study concerning this was carried out by Wallace et al (50) who studied the binding of three drugs—salicylate, sulfadiazine, and phenylbutazone—

to plasma protein in young and elderly subjects who previously had not been taking any drugs and in subjects who had received prior drug therapy with one or more drugs. They found that the presence of one or more drugs significantly decreased the binding of salicylate, sulfadiazine, and phenylbutazone to plasma proteins. They found the reduction in plasma binding to be greatest in a group of elderly patients who at the time the study was carried out were receiving one or more drugs. The authors suggest that because of their low albumin levels elderly patients may be more susceptible to the effects of multiple drug therapy on drug binding and that this effect is of particular importance for highly bound drugs like phenylbutazone.

Plasma Binding and Disease

Decreased drug binding has been observed in certain disease states (53), and as opposed to what we have just reviewed as changes occurring in normal elderly subjects, the changes that occur in drug binding in various disease states cannot be explained simply in terms of hypoalbuminemia. It has been postulated from various studies that abnormal or "damaged" albumin and/or the accumulation of endogenous materials apparently contribute to the decrease in drug binding. When considering the use of drugs in the treatment of diseases commonly found in elderly people, the prescribing physician must be alert not only to the potential for decreased drug binding per se because of lowered serum albumin levels and the interaction of one drug on the binding of another but also to the influence that specific disease states will have on the drug-binding capacity of the patient.

To cite the work of a single investigator, Andreasen (54) found in a series of in vitro experiments that the protein binding of acetylsalicylic acid, salicylic acid, phenylbutazone, phenytoin, sulfadiazine, and thiopental was decreased in the plasma of ten surgical patients with acute renal failure. The decreased binding of these drugs could only partly be explained by the lower concentration of serum albumin. In a follow-up study (55) the author conducted a series of experiments using dialyzed plasma samples and concluded that the reduced binding capacity in patients with acute renal failure may be explained only in part by a decrease in the serum albumin level and may be due to a structural change in the plasma protein itself and in part to the accumulation of competitively or noncompetitively bound substances.

CHANGES IN TISSUE RESPONSIVENESS

The response to a drug is a reflection first of the drug's concentration at its site of action, and second the ability of a given amount of drug to affect the receptor and to translate the effect on the receptor to a responsive tissue or tissue system. Decreases in response may occur specifically with an increase in the threshold of a receptor to the effect of a drug, to a decrease or a change in the number of receptor sites, to a decrease in available enzymes that help translate the effect of the drug, to structural changes in the tissue itself which could be rate limiting with respect to the response of a specific tissue, and finally to an alteration in the interrelationship of various organ systems as they change in response to the primary effect of the drug.

A number of changes have been reported to occur in old experimental animals and in elderly human subjects which cannot be explained merely by a change in the plasma concentration of a drug; it has been inferred from these studies that the tissue itself is modified in some way. It is not our intent to review here in exhaustive detail all of these examples but to outline a few as they reflect various possible changes in the status of the receptor site and its behavior.

In rats, amphetamine was on the one hand less effective in increasing spontaneous motor activity in older animals (56) while on the other hand the depressant effect of amphetamine on food intake was enhanced in older animals (57). This response is explained on the basis of a reduced number of cells in the central nervous system, creating a situation where it is more difficult for stimulants to exert an effect but easier for the depressant actions of a drug to be expressed.

A reduction in the number of target cells has also been used to explain the increased activity of alloxan in older rats (58). In this study alloxan administered to young and old rats produced a far larger increase in serum glucose levels in older rats; this was attributed to a decrease in the number of β cells in the pancreas of older rats. An increase in protein and collagen in aortic strips has been cited by Tuttle (59) to explain a decreased response of aortic smooth muscle strips in response to norepinephrine. With increasing age there is a change in the innervation of the heart which is reflected in a decreased response to atropine, suggesting a reduction in the number of receptor sites (60).

In a more recent study, Hewick et al (61) found a difference in the sensitivity to warfarin in young and old rats and humans and stated that the difference appears to be due to a greater depression of hepatic clotting factor synthesis by warfarin in elderly rats and humans.

Table 1 summarizes the clinical results we have presented.

CONCLUSIONS

On balance, the clinical pharmacokinetic studies we have reviewed lead us to these simple generalizations:

1. Changes in absorption with increasing age are not very significant but may be an occasional cause of ineffective therapy in the aged.

2. Drug metabolism changes may be significant in the elderly either because of decreased hepatic enzyme levels or because of reduced hepatic circulation.

3. Plasma binding of drugs is often decreased in the elderly giving rise to higher blood levels.

4. Renal performance is always decreased in the aged and leads frequently to increased blood levels and prolonged drug half-life.

Literature Cited

1. Bender, A. D. 1964. Pharmacologic aspects of aging. A survey of the effect of increasing age on drug activity in adults. *J. Am. Geriatr. Soc.* 12:114–34
2. Bender, A. D. 1969. Geriatric pharmacology—age and its influence on drug action in adults. *Drug Inf. Bull.* 3:153–58
3. Fann, W. E., Maddox, G. L., eds. 1974. *Drug Issues in Geropsychiatry.* Baltimore: Williams & Wilkins. 122 pp.
4. Freeman, J. T. 1974. Some principles of medication in geriatrics. *J. Am. Geriatr. Soc.* 22:289–95
5. Petersen, D. M., Thomas, C. W. 1975. Acute drug reactions among the elderly. *J. Gerontol.* 30:552–56
6. Bender, A. D., Kormendy, C., Powell, R. 1970. Pharmacological control of aging. *Exp. Gerontol.* 5:97–129
7. Kormendy, C., Bender, A. D. 1971. Experimental modification of the chemistry and biology of the aging process. *J. Pharm. Sci.* 60:167–80
8. Richey, D. P., Bender, A. D. 1975. Effects of human aging on drug absorption and metabolism. In *Physiology and Pathology of Human Aging,* ed. R. Goldman, M. Rockstein, 59–93. New York: Academic.
9. Beck, H., Vignalou, J. 1975. Pharmacocinetique des medicaments chez les personnes agees. *Therapie* 30: 331–38
10. Estler, C.-J. 1975. Wirkungsanderungen von pharmaka im alter. *Med. Welt* 26:795–99
11. Vignalou, J. 1974. Generalites sur la therapeutique en geriatrie. *Cah. Med.* 15:573–78
12. Lodola, E. 1973. Farmacocinetica nell-'eta' senile. *Boll. Chim. Farm.* 112: 324–32
13. Triggs, E. J., Nation, R. L. 1975. Pharmacokinetics in the aged: A review. *J. Pharmacokinet. Biopharm.* 3:387–418
14. Bianchine, J. R., Calimlim, L. R., Morgan, J. P., Dujovne, C. A., Lasagna, L. 1971. Metabolism and absorption of L-3,4dihydroxyphenylalanine in patients with Parkinson's disease. *Ann. NY Acad. Sci.* 179:126–39
15. Bender, A. D. 1968. Effect of age on intestinal absorption: Implications for drug absorption in the elderly. *J. Am. Geriatr. Soc.* 16:1131–39
16. Webster, S. G. P., Leeming, J. T. 1974. Assessment of small bowel function in the elderly using a modified xylose tolerance test. *Gut* 16:109–13
17. Dietze, V. F., Kalbe, I., Kranz, D., Bruschke, G., Richter, H. 1971. Geriatrische aspekte der eisenresorption. *Z. Alternsforsch.* 24:229–35
18. Bender, A. D. 1965. The effect of increasing age on the distribution of peripheral blood flow in man. *J. Am. Geriatr. Soc.* 13:192–98
19. Gorrod, J. W. 1974. Absorption, metabolism and excretion of drugs in geriatric subjects. *Gerontol. Clin.* 16:30–42
20. Kato, R., Vassanelli, P., Frontino, G., Chiesara, E. 1964. Variation in the activity of liver microsomal drug-metabolizing enzymes in rats in relation to the age. *Biochem. Pharmacol.* 13: 1037–51
21. Kuhlmann, K., Oduah, M., Coper, H. 1970. Uber die wirkung von barbituraten bei ratten verschiedenen alters. *Naunyn Schmiedebergs Arch. Pharmakol.* 265:310–20
22. Holloway, D. A. 1974. Drug problems in the geriatric patient. *Drug Intell. Clin. Pharm.* 8:632–42
23. Friedman, S. A., Raizner, A. E., Rosen, H., Solomon, N. A., Sy, W. 1972. Functional defects in the aging kidney. *Ann. Intern. Med.* 76:41–45
24. Dettli, L. C. 1976. Drug dosage in renal disease. *Clin. Pharmacokinet.* 1:126–34
25. Christiansen, N. J. B., Kolendorf, K., Siersbaek-Nielsen, K., Hansen, J. M. 1973. Serum digoxin values following a dosage regimen based on body weight, sex, age and renal function. *Acta Med. Scand.* 194:257–59
26. Leikola, E., Vartia, K. O. 1957. On penicillin levels in young and geriatric subjects. *J. Gerontol.* 12:48–52
27. Vartia, K. O., Leikola, E. 1960. Serum levels of antibiotics in young and old subjects following administration of dihydrostreptomycin and tetracycline. *J. Gerontol.* 15:392–94
28. Hansen, J. M., Kampmann, J., Laursen, H. 1970. Renal excretion of drugs in the elderly. *Lancet* I:1170
29. Kristensen, M., Hansen, J. M., Kampmann, J., Lumholtz, B., Siersbaek-Nielsen, K. 1974. Drug elimination and renal function. *J. Clin. Pharmacol.* 14:307–8
30. Simon, C., Malerczyk, V., Muller, U., Muller, G. 1972. Zur pharmakokinetik von propicillin bei geriatrischen patienten im vergleich zu jungeren er-

wachsenen. *Dtsch. Med. Wochenschr.* 97:1999–2003

31. Hayes, M. J., Langman, M. J. S., Short, A. H. 1975. Changes in drug metabolism with increasing age. 2. Phenytoin clearance and protein binding. *Br. J. Clin. Pharmacol.* 2:73–79

32. Houghton, G. W., Richens, A., Leighton, M. 1975. Effect of age, height, weight, and sex on serum phenytoin concentration in epileptic patients. *Br. J. Clin. Pharmacol.* 2:251–56

33. Traeger, A., Kiesewetter, R., Kunze, M. 1974. Zur pharmakokinetik von phenobarbital bei erwachsenen und greisen. *Dtsch. Gesundheitswes.* 29:1040–42

34. Irvine, R. E., Grove, J., Toseland, P. A., Trounce, J. R. 1974. The effect of age on the hydroxylation of amylobarbitone sodium in man. *Br. J. Clin. Pharmacol.* 1:41–43

35. O'Malley, K., Crooks, J., Duke, E., Stevenson, I. H. 1971. Effect of age and sex on human drug metabolism. *Br. Med. J.* 3:607–9

36. Vestal, R. E., Norris, A. H., Tobin, J. D., Cohen, B. H., Shock, N. W., Andres, R. 1975. Antipyrine metabolism in man: Influence of age, alcohol, caffeine, and smoking. *Clin. Pharmacol. Ther.* 18:425–32

37. Liddell, D. E., Williams, F. M., Briant, R. H. 1975. Phenazone (antipyrine) metabolism and distribution in young and elderly adults. *Clin. Exp. Pharmacol. Physiol.* 2:481–87

38. Jori, A., DiSalle, E., Quadri, A. 1972. Rate of aminopyrine disappearance from plasma in young and aged humans. *Pharmacology* 8:273–79

39. Chan, K., Kendall, M. J., Mitchard, M., Wells, W. D. E. 1975. The effect of ageing on plasma pethidine concentration. *Br. J. Clin. Pharmacol.* 2:297–302

40. Chan, K., Kendall, M. J., Wells, W. D. E., Mitchard, M. 1975. Factors influencing the excretion and relative physiological availability of pethidine in man. *J. Pharm. Pharmacol.* 27:235–41

41. Mather, L. E., Tucker, G. T., Pflug, A. E., Lindop, M. J., Wilkerson, C. 1975. Meperidine kinetics in man: Intravenous injection in surgical patients and volunteers. *Clin. Pharmacol. Ther.* 17:21–30

42. Traeger, A., Kunze, M., Stein, G., Ankermann, H. 1973. Zur pharmakokinetik von indomethazin bei alten menschen. *Z. Alternforsch.* 27:151–55

43. Triggs, E. J., Nation, R. L., Long, A., Ashley, J. J. 1975. Pharmacokinetics in the elderly. *Eur. J. Clin. Pharmacol.* 8:55–62

44. Ewy, G. A., Kapadia, G. G., Yao, L., Lullin, M., Marcus, F. I. 1969. Digoxin metabolism in the elderly. *Circulation* 39:449–53

45. Chamberlain, D. A., White, R. J., Howard, M. R., Smith, T. W. 1970. Plasma digoxin concentrations in patients with atrial fibrillation. *Br. Med. J.* 3:429–32

46. Castleden, C. M., Kaye, C. M., Parsons, R. L. 1975. The effect of age on plasma levels of propranolol and practolol in man. *Br. J. Clin. Pharmacol.* 2:303–6

47. Klotz, U., Avant, G. R., Hoyumpa, A., Schenker, S., Wilkinson, G. R. 1975. The effects of age and liver disease on the disposition and elimination of diazepam in adult man. *J. Clin. Invest.* 55:347–59

48. Bender, A. D., Post, A., Meier, J. P., Higson, J. E., Reichard, G. 1975. Plasma protein binding of drugs as a function of age in adult human subjects. *J. Pharm. Sci.* 64:1711–13

49. Hayes, M. J., Langman, M. J. S., Short, A. H. 1975. Changes in drug metabolism with increasing age: 1. Warfarin binding and plasma proteins. *Br. J. Clin. Pharmacol.* 2:69–72

50. Wallace, S., Whiting, B., Runcie, J. 1976. Factors affecting drug binding in plasma of elderly patients. *Br. J. Clin. Pharmacol.* 3:327–30

51. Hooper, W. D., Bochner, F., Eadie, M. J., Tyrer, J. H. 1974. Plasma protein binding of diphenylhydantoin; effects of sex hormones, renal and hepatic disease. *Clin. Pharmacol. Ther.* 15:276–82

52. Hayes, M. J., Langman, M. J. S. 1974. Analysis of carbenoxolone plasma binding and clearance in young and elderly people. In *Symp. Carbenoxolone Proc., 4th,* ed. F. Avery Jones, D. V. Parke, 107–14. London: Butterworth

53. Lindup, W. E. 1975. Drug-albumin binding. *Biochem. Soc. Trans.* 3:635–40

54. Andreasen, F. 1973. Protein binding of drugs in plasma from patients with acute renal failure. *Acta Pharmacol. Toxicol.* 32:417–29

55. Andreasen, F. 1974. The effect of dialysis on the protein binding of drugs in the plasma of patients with acute renal failure. *Acta Pharmacol. Toxicol.* 34:284–94

56. Verzar, F. 1961. The age of the individual as one of the parameters of phar-

macological action. *Acta Physiol. Acad. Sci. Hung.* 19:313–15

57. Farner, D. 1961. Die boeinflussung des appetites durch amphetamin (Benzedrin) und preludin bei ratten verschiedenen alters. *Gerontologia* 5:35–38

58. Bruckmann, G. 1947. The diabetogenic activity of alloxan in old and young rats. *Endocrinology* 41:201–4

59. Tuttle, R. S. 1966. Age-related changes in the sensitivity of rat aortic strips to norepinephrine and associated chemical and structural alterations. *Gerontology* 21:510–13

60. Grollman, A. 1960. *Pharmacology and Therapeutics*, p. 349. Philadelphia:Lea & Febiger. 4th ed.

61. Hewick, D. S., Moreland, T. A., Shepherd, A. M., Stevenson, I. H. 1975. The effect of age on the sensitivity to warfarin sodium. *Br. J. Clin. Pharmacol.* 2:189P–90P

62. Falch, D. 1973. The influence of kidney function, body size and age on plasma concentration and urinary excretion of digoxin. *Acta Med. Scand.* 194:251–56

63. Chavaz, A., Balant, L., Simonin, P., Fabre, J. 1974. Influence de l'age sur la digoxinemie et la digitalisation. *Schweiz. Med. Wochenschr.* 104:1823–25

64. Lehmann, K., Merten, K. 1974. Die elimination von lithium in abhangigkeit vom lebensalter bei gesunden und niereninsuffizienten. *Int. J. Clin. Pharmacol.* 10:292–98

65. Hewick, D. S., Newbury, P. A. 1976. Age: its influence on lithium dosage and plasma levels. *Br. J. Clin. Pharmacol.* 3:354P

66. Simon, C., Malerczyk, V., Zierott, G., Lehmann, K., Thiesen, U. 1975. Blut-, harn-, und gallespiegel von ampicillin bei intravenoser dauerinfuson. *Arzneim. Forsch.* 25:654–56

67. Simon, C., Malerczyk, V., Engelke, H., Preuss, I., Grahmann, H., Schmidt, K. 1975. Die pharmakokinetik von doxycyclin bei niereninsuffizienz und geriatrischen patienten im vergleich zu jungeren erwachsenen. *Schweiz. Med. Wochenschr.* 105:1615–20

Ann. Rev. Pharmacol. Toxicol. 1977. 17:67–82

PHARMACOLOGY OF MAGNESIUM

*6667

Shaul G. Massry

Division of Nephrology and Department of Medicine, University of Southern California
School of Medicine, Los Angeles, California 90033

In recent years, reliable and easy methods for the determination of magnesium in
body fluids became available. This facilitated the investigative efforts on the various
aspects of magnesium metabolism, and a large body of information has been accumulated in this field. However, two areas received greater attention; first, the hormonal and nonhormonal factors controlling the renal handling of magnesium and,
second, the mechanisms of the hypocalcemia of magnesium depletion. The purpose
of this report is to provide a review of the available data on these two aspects of
the pharmacology of magnesium.

RENAL HANDLING OF MAGNESIUM

Each day, approximately 1800 mg of magnesium (Mg) is lost from plasma into the
glomerulus but only 3–5% of filtered Mg is excreted in the urine. This conservation
process is due to an effective tubular reabsorption of Mg. The normal concentration
of Mg in blood is 1.7–2.2 mg/dl and is present in two forms. A diffusible fraction
constitutes ($75\pm9\%$, mean $\pm$ SD) of the total level; this fraction is filtered at the
glomerulus, and a nondiffusible moiety is bound to protein. The relationship between these two forms follows the simple mass action equilibrium.

Characteristics of Renal Tubular Reabsorption of Magnesium

The concentration of Mg in the urine under diuretic conditions is lower than its
concentration in glomerular filtrate, suggesting that Mg is actively transported by
the nephron. However, it is not known whether active reabsorption occurs throughout the nephron. In studies carried out in the dog, the major portion of filtered Mg
is reabsorbed by the proximal tubule and the reabsorption is isotonic or nearly so
(1). A constant tubular fluid/ultrafiltrable (TF/UF) Mg ratio at unity in the proxi-

67

mal tubule could be interpreted to indicate passive Mg reabsorption at this site. This is based on the assumption that the transtubular potential difference is zero. Under such conditions Mg may leave the tubular lumen with the bulk flow of fluid secondary to active sodium reabsorption. If a small negative potential of less than -5 mv exists in the proximal tubule, active reabsorption of Mg cannot be ruled out. Furthermore, the significant fall in TF/UF Mg to a value below 1.0 during saline infusion suggests that active reabsorption of Mg may exist in the proximal tubule. Micropuncture data obtained from nondiuretic rats and from Psammomys indicate that the concentration of Mg in tubular fluid increases along the proximal tubule (2–4); in the Psammomys, for example, the TF/UF Mg in late proximal tubule is 1.52 ± 0.44 (SD). These observations suggest that in the rat and Psammomys, magnesium is less reabsorbable in proximal tubule than in the dog.

Both micropuncture studies (4,5) and stop-flow experiments (6) demonstrate tubular fluid/plasma ratios of Mg which are well below 1.0, despite an electrical potential difference across the tubule which should lead to the appearance of greater concentration of Mg in the urine than in ultrafiltrate of plasma. These observations suggest that a very active transport mechanism for Mg exists in the distal nephron (5).

The fraction of filtered Mg excreted in the urine is significantly higher than that of calcium or sodium. Since, in the dog, the reabsorptions of sodium (7), calcium (8), and Mg (1) are isotonic in the proximal tubule, one must assume that Mg reabsorption in the distal nephron is dissociated from that of calcium or sodium or that Mg is secreted at these distal sites. In the rat, however, the difference in the proximal reabsorption of these ions may also contribute for the higher fraction of filtered Mg excretion.

Available data regarding Mg secretion by the renal tubule are contradictory. There is evidence that magnesium is secreted by the renal tubule of the aglomerular fish (9). Magnesium secretion by the kidney of the rat following prolonged Mg loading was demonstrated by Averill & Heaton (10), but Alfredson & Walser (11) were unable to confirm this observation. Chickens show no evidence for renal Mg secretion following the injection of Mg into the portal circulation (12). In studies carried out in the dog in our laboratory, Mg excretion did not exceed the filtered load during the infusions of large amounts of $MgCl_2$ (13); moreover, even when factors known to decrease tubular Mg reabsorption, such as saline infusion (14), calcium infusion (15), and chronic DOCA treatment (16), were superimposed on Mg loading, the fraction of filtered Mg excreted did not exceed unity (13). In contrast, others found that urinary Mg may reach values which are 10–20% greater than filtered Mg during the concomitant administration of Mg salts, saline, and furosemide to the dog (17). It appears, therefore, that if Mg secretion by the nephron exists, it plays a minor role in the renal handling of magnesium.

Thus, at least in the dog, the higher fractional excretion of Mg relative to that of sodium is not due to Mg secretion but rather to differences in their reabsorption at nephron sites distal to the proximal tubule. The micropuncture data of Wen, Evanson & Dirks (5) suggest that the loop of Henle is the site where the dissociation between the reabsorption of these two ions occur. Apparently Mg is less well reabsorbed at this site. The studies of De Rouffignac et al in the Psammomys indicate that Mg is added to the tubular fluid in the descending limb of the loop of Henle and reabsorbed in the ascending limb and, hence, a medullary recycling exists for Mg (4). Data from micropuncture experiments during acute Mg loading in rats support the existence of such recycling of Mg (18).

Many observations indicate that a limited capacity for tubular reabsorption of Mg exists. Thus, Averill & Heaton assert that Mg reabsorption is maximal in the rat when plasma level is close to normal (10), and observations of Knippers & Hehl in the dog suggest that Mg reabsorption becomes maximal when plasma levels reach 4 times the normal value (19). Our studies in the dog revealed that Mg reabsorption increased two- to threefold to reach a maximum as the filtered load was gradually raised (13). These data demonstrate a maximal tubular reabsorptive capacity for Mg (T_m Mg) in the dog of approximately 140 μg/min/kg body weight (Figure 1). There was a marked degree of splay, and the full capacity for Mg reabsorption was not observed until the filtered load was approximately twice the T_m value, suggesting a wide heterogeneity in the capacity of individual nephrons to reabsorb Mg. Moreover, the T_m Mg was significantly reduced by extracellular volume expansion, produced either by saline infusion or by the chronic administration of DOCA, and following the infusion of calcium (13).

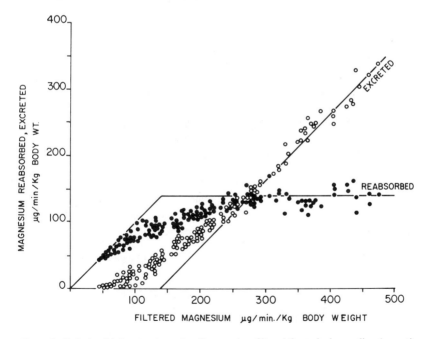

Figure 1   Relationship between quantity of magnesium filtered through glomeruli and quantities reabsorbed by renal tubule and excreted in urine during MgCl$_2$ infusion [Reprinted, by permission, from Massry et al (13)].

Factors Controlling Urinary Excretion of Magnesium

CHANGES IN FILTERED LOAD   An augmentation in the urinary excretion of Mg could occur following an increase in filtered load of these ions, a decrease in its tubular reabsorption, or both. An increase in filtered load of Mg could be produced by a rise in glomerular filtration rate (GFR) and/or an elevation in the concentration of Mg in blood; the effect of such increments in filtered loads on urinary Mg depends on how they are produced. Massry & Kleeman (20) found that a significant augmentation in filtered loads of magnesium induced by acute rise in GFR is associated with small increments in urinary Mg and sodium. These observations are consistent with the existence of glomerular tubular balance for Mg and follows that of sodium. It should be emphasized that a chronic rise in GFR may cause a significant loss of Mg. If the modest increments in the excretion of Mg observed during the acute rise in GFR were to continue over a long period of time, a considerable amount of Mg would be eliminated in the urine. An increase in filtered load of Mg by elevating its concentration in blood results in a marked rise in urinary Mg (13). The absolute quantity of Mg reabsorbed increases during hypermagnesemia, and when T_m Mg is reached, all the excess filtered load of Mg is quantitatively excreted in the urine. Therefore, hypermagnesemia is associated with magnesuria.

CHANGES IN TUBULAR REABSORPTION   There are numerous hormonal and nonhormonal factors that influence the urinary excretion of Mg by altering its tubular reabsorption. These are listed in Table 1.

Extracellular fluid volume expansion   Extracellular fluid volume expansion (ECVE) produced by the infusion of saline increases the excretion of Mg (1, 14). The magnesuria of ECVE occurred despite a significant reduction in its filtered loads, suggesting that ECVE with saline infusion depresses tubular reabsorption of

Table 1   Factors affecting tubular reabsorption of magnesium

Factors that decrease tubular reabsorption
Extracellular fluid volume expansion
Renal vasodilatation
Osmotic diuresis
Diuretic agents
Cardiac glycosides
Hypercalcemia
Alcohol ingestion
High sodium intake
Growth hormone
Thyroid hormone
Calcitonin
Chronic mineralocorticoid effect
Factors that enhance tubular reabsorption
Parathyroid hormone

Mg (14). Indeed, micropuncture studies demonstrated that ECVE inhibits the reabsorption of Mg in the proximal tubule (1).

Renal vasodilatation   Gonda et al (21), Ahumada & Massry (22), and Thompson, Kaufman & DiScala (23) found that renal vasodilatation produced by the infusion of acetylcholine or bradykinin into the renal artery, with and without the intravenous administration of angiotensin, augments the urinary excretion of Mg, probably as a result of a decreased tubular reabsorption. The slope for the relationship between the clearance of Mg and that of sodium was 1.90, a value similar to that of 1.88 seen during saline infusion.

Osmotic diuresis   Osmotic agents such as mannitol, glucose, and urea inhibit the tubular reabsorption of Mg and augment its urinary excretion (24–26). This inhibition is due to the decrease in the concentration of Mg in tubular fluid secondary to the inhibition of water reabsorption in excess of sodium.

Diuretics   The administration of mercurial diuretics, furosemide or ethacrynic acid, causes an increase in the urinary excretion of Mg (26–28). Although these agents may have some action in the proximal tubule, they primarily inhibit tubular transport in the ascending limb of the loop of Henle (29). The acute administration of thiazides to the dog produces either no change (27) or a modest increase in Mg clearance (30). In humans, this drug causes an increase in Mg excretion for one or two days with subsequent return to baseline level (31). In contrast to the hypocalciuria which follows chronic thiazide administration (31–33), hypomagnesuria does not develop. Acetazolamide (Diamox®), a diuretic that augments sodium excretion by inhibiting carbonic anhydrase and reducing sodium reabsorption mediated by Na^+-H^+ exchange, produces either a fall or no change in Mg excretion in humans and in the intact dog (34–36). These observations suggest that sodium reabsorption which is coupled with Na^+-H^+ exchange is not linked with Mg transport. Further support for such a contention is provided by an experiment carried out in our laboratory (36) in which sodium diuresis was produced by the infusion of potassium salts which inhibit Na^+-H^+ exchange by causing intracellular alkalosis. There was no increase in urinary Mg accompanying the natriuresis observed during the potassium infusion.

Diet   The ingestion of glucose or other rapidly metabolizable substances results in an increase in urinary Mg excretion with little or no augmentation in sodium excretion (37, 38). The magnesuria following glucose ingestion is due to a reduction in tubular reabsorption (39). The intake of fat has no effect on urinary Mg (38). The ingestion of 30–45 ml of ethanol produces a prompt increase in urinary Mg with no natriuresis in both normal subjects and chronic alcoholics (40, 41). This effect appears within 20 min after the alcohol ingestion and reaches a maximum in 60–90 min. The mechanism for this response is not clear, but it may represent another example of the effect of ingestion of rapidly metabolizable substrate (38).

A striking relationship exists between Mg intake and the urinary excretion of this ion. The ingestion of a diet deficient in Mg results in the disappearance of this ion from the urine, both in growing and adult animals (42, 43), and in humans (44). Urinary Mg is augmented with high Mg intake (45). Variations in salt intake in humans may be accompanied by concomitant changes in Mg excretion (46). Spontaneous hypercalcemia or that produced by calcium infusion is associated with magnesuria as a result of inhibition of tubular Mg reabsorption (15).

During starvation for periods up to 60 days, there is a continued urinary excretion of substantial amounts of Mg (47). These urinary losses are associated with a reduced content of Mg in muscle but a very small fall in serum Mg. Sodium excretion may average 50–120 meq/day during the first week of fasting and decreases thereafter, to 5–120 meq/day. These observations suggest decreased tubular reabsorption of these two ions, although the site in the nephron where this occurs is not delineated as yet. The administration of small quantities of sodium (40 meq/day) during prolonged fasting causes a marked increase in the urinary excretion of Mg (48). Refeeding with even small amounts of glucose is followed by a rapid reduction in urinary sodium and Mg (47).

Parathyroid hormone   In contrast to the well-established effect of parathyroid hormone (PTH) on renal handling of calcium, the influence of PTH on Mg excretion appears to be less well defined. Heaton (49) reported that administration of PTH increases Mg excretion in rats. However, these animals were hypercalcemic, and hypercalcemia augments urinary Mg independent of PTH (15). In contrast, MacIntyre, Boss & Troughton found a decrease in Mg excretion in rats receiving PTH (50). We have evaluated the influence of PTH on the renal handling of Mg in dogs receiving infusions of Mg (13). In every animal, the intramuscular injection of parathyroid extract decreased fractional Mg excretion. In studies carried out in patients with hypoparathyroidism, Bethune, Turpin & Inoue (51) found a reduction in urinary Mg excretion following the repeated intramuscular injection of parathyroid extract. In humans with hyperparathyroidism, serum Mg levels have been reported to be low with normal or even high urinary Mg excretion (52–54). These observations are not necessarily contradictory in that the hypercalcemia which is present may inhibit the reabsorption of magnesium and overcome the effect of parathyroid hormone.

Adrenal steroids   Urinary Mg may be augmented under the influence of glucocorticoids (46) and urinary Mg losses are increased in patients with Cushing's syndrome. Massry et al (55) reported that the acute administration of methylprednisolone to adrenalectomized dogs does not increase the urinary excretion of Mg. In normal humans, Lemann, Piering & Lennon (56) gave cortisol and found no change in urinary Mg.

The acute administration of mineralocorticoids has no effect on magnesium excretion in dogs or man (55, 56). Thus, the mechanisms for sodium transport, which are stimulated by mineralocorticoids in the distal tubule, are dissociated from the transport of Mg. Certain clinical and experimental data suggest that the excretion of Mg may be affected by long-term action of mineralocorticoids. Thus, Scott & Dobson described an increase in Mg excretion in sheep following prolonged aldosterone administration (57). In primary aldosteronism, hypomagnesemia and a high renal clearance of Mg have been reported (58). These observations suggest that there is a difference between the acute and the long-term action of mineralocorticoids on the renal handling of Mg. Massry et al (16) have studied the effect of long-term administration of DOCA on urinary excretion of Mg in dogs. They found that sodium excretion fell on the first day of DOCA treatment and then returned to baseline values. In contrast, urinary Mg remained unchanged until the second or third day of DOCA administration, when it increased progressively to exceed control levels by two- to fivefold (Figure 2). When similar studies were carried out in dogs fed a sodium-free diet, there were no changes in Mg excretion during the administration of DOCA (Figure 3). Suki and co-workers have reported similar results in rats given mineralocorticoids (59). The initial sodium retention that occurs during prolonged mineralocorticoid administration induces extracellular volume expansion which may lead to escape from the hormonal effect on sodium excretion (60). Extracellular volume expansion produces a decrease in the proximal tubular

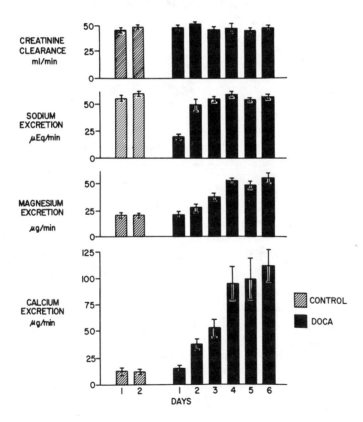

Figure 2 The changes (mean ± SE) in the excretion of sodium, magnesium, and calcium observed in 6 dogs receiving liberal sodium intake and 20 mg of desoxycorticosterone acetate per day over 6 successive days [Reprinted, by permission, from Massry et al (16)].

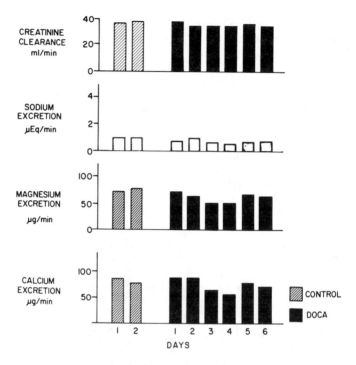

Figure 3   The changes (mean ± SE) in the excretion of sodium, magnesium, and calcium observed in 6 dogs receiving sodium-free diet and 20 mg of desoxycorticosterone acetate per day over 6 successive days.

reabsorption of sodium and Mg, which enhances the delivery of these ions to the distal segment of the nephron where mineralocorticoids may promote sodium reabsorption without a direct effect on Mg transport. The net result would be an increase in the excretion of Mg only. Other data suggest that a decrease in reabsorption in the distal nephron may also contribute to the increase in the excretion of Mg during the escape from the effect of mineralocorticoids (61).

Thyroid hormone   The effect of altered states of thyroid function on Mg metabolism has been studied by Jones and co-workers (62) and Rizek, Dimick, & Wallach (63). They found decreased serum Mg levels and increased urinary excretion of Mg in patients with hyperthyroidism, while those with hypothyroidism had elevated plasma levels and decreased urinary excretion. After treatment of either condition, plasma levels shifted toward normal and urinary excretion of Mg increased in patients with hypoparathyroidism.

Other hormones   The effect of calcitonin on urinary Mg is variable. The administration of this hormone decreased urinary Mg in the rat (64). In humans, Mg excretion either increased (65) or remained unchanged (66). Growth hormone appears to have an effect on the renal handling of Mg, opposite to that of PTH; thus, the administration of growth hormone results in increased urinary excretion of Mg (67).

HYPOCALCEMIA OF MAGNESIUM DEPLETION

Hypocalcemia has been reported with magnesium depletion in a number of species, including chicks (68), rats receiving a low calcium intake (69, 70), sheep (71), pigs (72), calves (73, 74), dogs (75), monkeys (76), and humans (77–81). Although the occurrence of hypocalcemia during magnesium depletion seems well established, the mechanisms underlying this phenomenon are not well understood. Theoretically, several factors should be responsible for the hypocalcemia. These include (a) decreased responsiveness of the skeleton to parathyroid hormone, (b) failure of parathyroid hormone production by the parathyroid glands, (c) inhibition of release of parathyroid hormone from the glands, (d) augmented action or secretion of calcitonin, (e) increased urinary losses of calcium, (f) reduced gastrointestinal absorption of calcium, and (g) altered equilibrium for calcium between bone and extracellular fluid favoring calcium retention or deposition in bone.

Skeletal Resistance to the Calcemic Action of the Parathyroid Hormone

Considerable evidence exists suggesting that magnesium depletion may be associated with unresponsiveness to PTH (69, 77–82), although some investigators did not find such an abnormality (70, 75, 76, 83–87). Estep et al (77), Muldowney and co-workers (79), and Woodward, Webster & Carr (81) found no calcemic response to parathyroid extract administration in patients with hypomagnesemia due to chronic alcoholism, steatorrhea, or severe diarrhea. In most of these patients, the administration of magnesium alone restored the responsiveness to parathyroid extract. Connor et al (80) reported a patient with magnesium depletion secondary to malabsorption; hypocalcemia improved after administration of parathyroid extract but the response was markedly reduced when compared to the effect observed after magnesium repletion. On the other hand, Salet et al (83), Paunier et al (84), and Stromme et al (85) reported an increase in serum calcium after parathyroid extract administration in infants with hypomagnesemia and concluded that there was normal responsiveness to parathyroid extract. Similar observations were reported recently in a child with primary hypomagnesemia (87). These reports led Hahn, Chase & Avioli (70) and Suh et al (87) to suggest that factors other than magnesium depletion might have accounted for unresponsiveness of the skeleton to parathyroid hormone in the patients with alcoholism or malabsorption. Careful evaluation of the data obtained in the hypomagnesemic infants revealed that the response to parathyroid extract was delayed, that seven doses of the extract were required to produce a significant rise in serum calcium in the case of Paunier et al (84), and, that the calcemic response to PTE was markedly reduced in the case of Salet et al (83) when compared with the response after magnesium repletion. Moreover, the patients of Stromme et al had received parenteral magnesium up until a few days before treatment with parathyroid extract, and the serum magnesium was 1.1 mg/100 ml at the time of study (85); it is likely that the degree of magnesium deficiency was mild, accounting for the prompt calcemic response to parathyroid extract.

In the chick, magnesium depletion is associated with marked hypocalcemia which is unresponsive to the administration of parathyroid extract (68). In magnesium-depleted rats, MacManus, Heaton & Lucas reported data from experiments carried out both in vitro and in vivo showing skeletal unresponsiveness to parathyroid extract (69). On the other hand, Hahn and co-workers found similar increments in serum calcium and urinary excretion of hydroxyproline in both normal and magnesium-depleted rats (70). The discrepancies between these results may be related to the degree of magnesium depletion and/or hypomagnesemia; in the studies of MacManus et al (69), the mean value for serum magnesium was 0.46 ± 0.03 (SE) mg/100 ml (29% of control), while the mean serum magnesium was 0.95 ± 0.5 mg/100 ml (58% of control) in the magnesium-depleted rats of Hahn et al (70).

Levi et al (82) found that magnesium depletion is associated with reduced calcemic response to parathyroid extract in adult dogs when this is evaluated after a 7-hr infusion of the exogenous hormone; magnesium repletion completely restored the calcemic response to parathyroid extract (Figure 4). In contrast, Suh, Csima & Fraser evaluated the effect of parathyroid extract on serum calcium in growing puppies with magnesium depletion (75). They found that the changes in serum calcium in magnesium-depleted puppies after 17–48 hours of parathyroid extract infusion were not different from those observed in control animals; they suggested that unresponsiveness of the skeleton to PTH was not responsible for the hypocalcemia in the magnesium-depleted puppies. It is possible that the differences between the results of Suh et al (75) and those of Levi et al (82) are related to the age of the dogs or to the duration of the infusion of the parathyroid extract.

Dunn administered parathyroid extract to monkeys both before and after magnesium depletion and found no significant difference between the changes in serum calcium (76). These results are difficult to reconcile with other reported data; how-

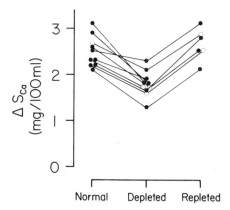

Figure 4   The changes in serum calcium (Δ SCa) induced by the infusion of parathyroid extract in the normal animals, during magnesium-depleted state and after magnesium repletion. *Open circles* represent the mean of two studies in the same animal, and the *lines* connect data in the same dog [Reprinted, by permission, from Levi et al (82)].

ever, there may be species differences in the response to parathyroid extract during magnesium depletion.

Function of Parathyroid Glands

Despite the reduced calcemic response to parathyroid extract in the study of Levi et al (82), serum calcium was either normal or slightly elevated after the infusion of the extract. This finding suggested that the spontaneous hypocalcemia observed in these animals would not have occurred had there been adequate secretion of endogenous parathyroid hormone. It is possible that complete or partial failure of parathyroid hormone secretion during magnesium depletion is an important factor leading to the initial appearance of hypocalcemia. Indeed, Levi et al (82) found that the blood levels of parathyroid hormone were not elevated during magnesium depletion despite the hypocalcemia, suggesting impaired function of the parathyroid glands. Anast and co-workers (86) and Suh et al (87) each found a reduced or undetectable plasma level of immunoreactive parathyroid hormone in separate patients with magnesium depletion. A similar finding was reported by Chase & Slatopolsky (88). In addition, studies by Targovnik, Rodman & Sherwood (89) showed that the release of parathyroid hormone from parathyroid glands in vitro was markedly reduced when magnesium concentration in the media was below 0.70 mg/dl. These findings are not necessarily inconsistent with data showing that acute reduction in the concentration of magnesium in blood perfusing the parathyroid glands causes increased release of parathyroid hormone (90). Chronic hypomagnesemia may have a different effect on parathyroid gland metabolism, and this effect may depend on the degree of hypomagnesemia. There is evidence that parathyroid gland activity may be normal or increased during magnesium deficiency. Thus, Sherwood (91) and Connor et al (80) each reported elevated circulating levels of parathyroid hormone in an individual patient with magnesium depletion, and parathyroid hyperplasia has been reported in calves with magnesium deficiency (74). However, even when the levels of parathyroid hormone are elevated during magnesium depletion, they may not represent an adequate or appropriate response of the parathyroid glands for the degree of hypocalcemia.

Recent observations by Anast and associates (92) and Rude and co-workers (93) indicate that marked magnesium deficiency may inhibit the release of PTH from the parathyroid glands. They found that blood levels of PTH increased markedly within one minute of the administration of magnesium. These observations are consistent with in vitro studies showing that low magnesium concentration in the incubation media diminished the secretion of PTH (89) but not its synthesis (94) by bovine parathyroid glands.

Equilibrium Between Calcium in Extracellular Fluid and Bone

During magnesium depletion, an altered equilibrium may exist between the calcium in extracellular fluid and bone, and such a disturbance may contribute to the hypocalcemia. Neuman & Neuman postulated that magnesium ion may exchange for calcium on the bone surface (95). MacManus & Heaton found that the calcium released from bone, in vitro, by both physicochemical processes and metabolic activity was dependent upon the magnesium concentration in the incubation media (96). Similar observations have been reported by Pak & Diller (97). It is possible that, in the intact animal, magnesium depletion may both reduce the release of calcium from the bone surface and exert an inhibitory effect on normal process of bone resorption; moreover, a defective action of parathyroid hormone on bone may be, at least in part, a consequence of such interrelationships between magnesium and bone. The hypocalcemia, itself, could be a factor preventing a skeletal response to PTE (98,99), possibly as a result of the presence of excess osteoid (99). Indeed, the presence of excess osteoid has been found in magnesium-deficient chicks (68).

Other Factors

Although it is possible that decreased gastrointestinal absorption of calcium, enhanced urinary excretion of calcium, or increased release of calcitonin could be responsible for the hypocalcemia, all available data make these possibilities remote. Thus, during magnesium depletion, calcium absorption is either not impaired or increased (68,100–103), and urinary calcium is low (78,104). An increase in the secretion of calcitonin during magnesium depletion seems unlikely. Elevated levels of magnesium may stimulate the release of calcitonin in the rat (105), although perfusion of the goat thyroid with hypermagnesemic blood did not alter calcitonin secretion (106). Moreover, thyroidectomy and thyroparathyroidectomy failed to alter the hypocalcemia seen with magnesium depletion (75, 76) suggesting that calcitonin is not of importance. Finally, Suh et al (87) did not find an elevation in the blood levels of calcitonin during hypomagnesemia.

SUMMARY

The available data, therefore, indicate that the factors responsible for the hypocalcemia in magnesium deficiency are multiple. Relative or complete failure of the function of parathyroid glands, inhibition of release of parathyroid hormone from the glands, impaired skeletal response to parathyroid hormone, and abnormalities in the equilibrium between bone and extracellular fluid may each or all be operative in various species.

Literature Cited

1. Brunette, M., Wen, S. F., Evanson, R. L., Dirks, J. H. 1969. Micropuncture study of magnesium reabsorption in the proximal tubule of the dog. *Am. J. Physiol.* 216:1510–16
2. LeGrimellec, C., Roinel, N., Morel, F. 1973. Simultaneous Mg, Ca, P, K, Na, and Cl analysis in rat tubular fluid. I. During perfusion of either inulin or ferrocyanide. *Pfluegers Arch.* 340:181–96
3. Morel, F., Roinel, N., LeGrimellec, C. 1969. Electron probe analysis of tubular fluid composition. *Nephron* 6:350–64
4. DeRouffignac, C., Morel, F., Moss, N., Roinel, N. 1973. Micropuncture study of water and electrolyte movements along the loop of Henle in Psammomys with special reference to magnesium, calcium and phosphorus. *Pfluegers Arch.* 344:309–26
5. Wen, S. F., Evanson, R. L., Dirks, J. H. 1970. Micropuncture study of magnesium transport in proximal and distal tubule of the dog. *Am. J. Physiol.* 219:570–76
6. Samiy, A. H. E., Brown, J. L., Globus, D. L., Kessler, R. H., Thompson, D. D. 1960. Interrelations between renal transport system of magnesium and calcium. *Am. J. Physiol.* 189:559–602

7. Bennett, C. M., Clapp, J. R., Berliner, R. W. 1967. Micropuncture study of the proximal and distal tubule in the dog. *Am. J. Physiol.* 213:1254–62

8. Duarte, C. G., Watson, J. F. 1967. Calcium reabsorption in proximal tubule of the dog nephron. *Am. J. Physiol.* 212:1355–60

9. Berglund, F., Forster, R. P. 1958. Renal tubular transport of inorganic divalent ions by the aglomerular marine teleost, Lophius Americanus. *J. Gen. Physiol.* 41:429–40

10. Averill, C. M., Heaton, F. W. 1960. The renal handling of magnesium. *Clin. Sci.* 31:353–60

11. Alfredson, K. S., Walser, M. 1970. Is magnesium secreted by the rat renal tubule? *Nephron* 7:242–47

12. Robinson, R. R., Postwood, R. M. 1962. Mechanism of magnesium excretion by the chick. *Am. J. Physiol.* 202:309–12

13. Massry, S. G., Coburn, J. W., Kleeman, C. R. 1969. Renal handling of magnesium in the dog. *Am. J. Physiol.* 216:1460–67

14. Massry, S. G., Coburn, J. W., Chapman, L. W., Kleeman, C. R. 1967. Effect of NaCl infusion on urinary CA^{++} and Mg^{++} during reduction in their filtered load. *Am. J. Physiol.* 213:1218–24

15. Coburn, J. W., Massry, S. G., Kleeman, C. R. 1970. The effect of calcium infusion on renal handling of magnesium with normal and reduced glomerular filtration rate. *Nephron* 7:131–43

16. Massry, S. G., Coburn, J. W., Chapman, L. W., Kleeman, C. R. 1968. The effect of long-term desoxycorticosterone acetate administration on the renal excretion of calcium and magnesium. *J. Lab. Clin. Med.* 71:212–19

17. Wen, S. F., Wong, N. L., Dirks, J. H. 1971. Evidence for renal magnesium secretion during magnesium infusion in the dog. *Am. J. Physiol.* 220:33–37

18. LeGrimellec, C., Roinel, N., Morel, F. 1973. Simultaneous Mg, Ca, P, K, Na and Cl analysis in rat tubular fluid. II. During acute Mg plasma loading. *Pfluegers Arch.* 340:197–210

19. Knippers, R., Hehl, U. 1965. Die renale Ausscheidung von Magnesium, Calcium, und Kalium nach Erhohung der Magnesium Kenzentration in Plasma des Hundes. *Z. Gesamte Exp. Med.* 139:154–65

20. Massry, S. G., Kleeman, C. R. 1972. Calcium and magnesium excretion during acute rise in glomerular filtration rate. *J. Lab. Clin. Med.* 80:654–64

21. Gonda, A., Wong, N., Seely, J. F., Dirks, J. H. 1969. The role of hemodynamic factors on urinary calcium and magnesium excretion. *Can. J. Physiol. Pharmacol.* 47:619–26

22. Ahumada, J. J., Massry, S. G. 1971. Renal vasodilatation: Effect on renal handling of phosphate. *Clin. Sci.* 41:109–21

23. Thompson, R. B., Kaufman, C. E., DiScala, V. A. 1971. Effect of renal vasodilatation on divalent ion excretion and Tm PAH in anesthetized dogs. *Am. J. Physiol.* 221:1097–1104

24. Better, O. S., Gonick, H. C., Chapman, L. C., Varrady, P. D., Kleeman, C. R. 1966. Effect of urea-saline diuresis on renal clearance of calcium, magnesium, and inorganic phosphate in man. *Proc. Soc. Exp. Biol. Med.* 121:592–96

25. Wesson, L. G. Jr. 1962. Magnesium, calcium and phosphate excretion during osmotic diuresis in the dog. *J. Lab. Clin. Med.* 60:422–33

26. Parfitt, A. M. 1969. The acute effects of mersalyl, chlorothiazide, and mannitol on the renal excretion of calcium and other ions in man. *Clin. Sci.* 36:267–82

27. Eknoyan, G., Suki, W. N., Martinez-Maldonado, M. 1970. Effect of diuretics on urinary excretion of phosphate, calcium, and magnesium in thyroparathyroidectomized dog. *J. Lab. Clin. Med.* 76:257–66

28. Walser, M. 1967. Magnesium metabolism. *Ergeb. Physiol. Biol. Chem. Exp. Pharmakol.* 59:185–296

29. Seldin, D. W., Eknoyan, G., Suki, W. N., Rector, F. C. Jr. 1966. Localization of diuretic action from the pattern of water and electrolyte excretion. *Ann. NY Acad. Sci.* 139:328–43

30. Duarte, C. G., Bland, J. H. 1965. Calcium, phosphorus and uric acid clearances after intravenous administration of chlorothiazide. *Metabolism* 14:211–19

31. Parfitt, A. M. 1972. The interaction of thiazide diuretics with parathyroid hormone and vitamin D. Studies in patients with hypoparathyroidism. *J. Clin. Invest.* 51:1879–88

32. Brickman, A. S., Massry, S. G., Coburn, J. W. 1972. Changes in serum and urinary calcium during treatment with hydrochlorothiazide: Studies on mechanisms. *J. Clin. Invest.* 51:945–54

33. Yendt, E. R., Gagne, R. J. A., Cohanim, M. 1966. The effect of thiazides in

idiopathic hypercalciuria. *Am. J. Med. Sci.* 251:449–60

34. Barker, E. S., Elkinton, J. R., Clark, J. K. 1959. Studies of the renal excretion of magnesium in man. *J. Clin. Invest.* 38:1733–45

35. Heidland, A., Rockel, A., Maidhof, R., Hennemann, H. 1970. Divergenz der Renalen Natrium und Magnesium Excretion nach Trometaniol (Trispuffer), Amerloride HCl, Acetazolemel und Parathormone ein Effekt der Harnalkalisierung? *Klin. Wochenschr.* 48:371–74

36. Massry, S. G., Popovtzer, M. M., Chapman, L. W., Kleeman, C. R. 1968. Effect of potassium infusion and intravenous diamox on the interdependence between the renal handling of sodium, calcium, and magnesium. *Clin. Res.* 16:391 (Abstr.)

37. Hodgkinson, A., Heaton, F. W. 1965. The effect of food ingestion on the urinary excretion of calcium and magnesium. *Clin. Chim. Acta* 11:354–62

38. Lindeman, R. D., Adler, S., Yiengst, M. J., Beard, E. S. 1967. Influence of various nutrients on urinary divalent cation excretion. *J. Lab. Clin. Med.* 70:236–45

39. Lemann, J. Jr., Lennon, E. J., Piering, W. F., Prien, E. L. Jr., Ricanati, E. S. 1970. Evidence that glucose ingestion inhibits net tubular reabsorption of calcium and magnesium in man. *J. Lab. Clin. Med.* 75:578–85

40. McCollister, R. J., Prasad, A. S., Doe, R. P., Flink, E. B. 1958. Normal renal magnesium clearance and the effect of water loading, chlorothiazide and ethanol on magnesium excretion. *J. Lab. Clin. Med.* 52:928

41. Kalbfleisch, J. M., Lindeman, R. D., Ginn, H. E., Smith, W. O. 1963. Effects of ethanol administration on urinary excretion of magnesium and other electrolytes in alcoholic and normal subjects. *J. Clin. Invest.* 42:1471–75

42. Chutkow, J. G. 1965. Studies on the metabolism of magnesium in the magnesium deficient rat. *J. Lab. Clin. Med.* 75:912–26

43. Heaton, F. W. 1969. The kidney and magnesium homeostasis. *Ann. NY Acad. Sci.* 16:775–85

44. Barnes, B. A., Cope, O., Harrison, T. 1950. Magnesium conservation in the human being on low magenesium diet. *J. Clin. Invest.* 37:430–40

45. Heaton, F. W., Parson, F. M. 1961. The metabolic effect of high magnesium intake. *Clin. Sci.* 21:273–84

46. Hills, A. G., Parson, D. W., Webster, G. D. Jr., Rosenthal, O., Conover, H. 1959. Influence of the renal excretion of sodium chloride upon the renal excretion of magnesium and other ions by human subjects. *J. Clin. Endocrinol.* 19:1192–1211

47. Drenick, E. J. 1970. The effects of acute and prolonged fasting and refeeding on water, electrolyte, and acid-base metabolism. In *Clinical Disorders of Fluid and Electrolyte Metabolism,* ed. M. H. Maxwell, C. R. Kleeman, 1117–37. New York: McGraw-Hill

48. Brickman, A. S., Drenick, E. J., Fisher, J., Coburn, J. W. 1970. The effect of sodium supplementation on divalent cation excretion during prolonged fasting. *Clin. Res.* 18:183

49. Heaton, F. W. 1968. The parathyroid glands and magnesium metabolism in the rat. *Clin. Sci.* 28:543–53

50. MacIntyre, I., Boss, S., Troughton, V. A. 1963. Parathyroid hormone and magnesium homeostasis. *Nature* 198:1058–60

51. Bethune, J. E., Turpin, R. A., Inoue, H. 1968. Effect of parathyroid hormone extract on divalent ion excretion in man. *J. Clin. Endocrinol Metab.* 28:673–78

52. Heaton, F. W., Pyrah, L. N. 1963. Magnesium metabolism in patients with parathyroid disorders. *Clin. Sci.* 25:475–85

53. King, R. G., Stanbury, S. W. 1970. Magnesium metabolism in primary hyperparathyroidism. *Clin. Sci.* 39:281–303

54. Hanna, S., North, K. A. K., MacIntyre, I., Fraser, R. 1961. Magnesium metabolism in parathyroid disease. *Br. Med. J.* 2:1253–56

55. Massry, S. G., Coburn, J. W., Chapman, L. W., Kleeman, C. R. 1967. The acute effect of adrenal steroids on the interrelationship between the renal excretion sodium, calcium and magnesium. *J. Lab. Clin. Med.* 70:563–70

56. Lemann, J. Jr., Piering, W. F., Lennon, E. J. 1970. Studies of the acute effects of aldosterone and cortisol on the interrelationship between renal sodium, calcium and magnesium excretion in normal man. *Nephron* 7:117–30

57. Scott, D., Dobson, A. 1965. Aldosterone and the metabolism of magnesium and other minerals in sheep. *Q. J. Exp. Physiol.* 50:42–56

58. Horton, R., Bigliere, E. G. 1962. Effect of aldosterone on the metabolism of

Mg. *J. Clin. Endocrinol Metab.* 22: 1187–92

59. Suki, W. N., Schwettmann, R. S., Rector, F. C. Jr., Seldin, D. W. 1968. Effect of chronic mineralocorticoid administration on calcium excretion in the rat. *Am. J. Physiol.* 215:71–74

60. August, T., Nelson, D. H., Thorn, G. W. 1958. Response of normal subjects to large amounts of aldosterone. *J. Clin. Invest.* 37:1549–55

61. Rasteger, A., Agus, Z. S., Connor, T. B., Goldberg, M. 1972. Renal handling of calcium and phosphate during mineralocorticoid "escape" in man. *Kidney Int.* 2:279–86

62. Jones, J. E., Desser, P. C., Shane, S. R., Flink, E. B. 1966. Magnesium metabolism in hyperthyroidism and hypothyroidism. *J. Clin. Invest.* 45:891–900

63. Rizek, J. E., Dimich, A., Wallach, S. 1965. Plasma and erythrocyte Mg in thyroid disease. *J. Clin. Endocrinol Metab.* 25:350–58

64. Aldred, J. P., Kleszynski, R. R., Basticen, J. W. 1970. Effects of acute administration of porcine and salman calcitonin on urine electrolyte excretion in rats. *Proc. Soc. Exp. Biol. Med.* 134:1175–80

65. Paillard, F., Ardaillou, R., Malendin, H., Fillastre, J. P., Prier, S. 1972. Renal effects of salmon calcitonin in man. *J. Lab. Clin. Med.* 80:200–16

66. Cochran, M., Peacock, M., Sacks, G., Nordin, B. E. C. 1970. Renal effects of calcitonin. *Br. Med. J.* 1:135–37

67. Hanna, S., Harrison, M. T., MacIntyre, I., Fraser, R. 1961. Effects of growth hormone on calcium and magnesium metabolism. *Br. Med. J.* 2:12–15

68. Reddy, C. R., Coburn, J. W., Hartenbower, D. L., Friedler, R. M., Brickman, A. S., Massry, S. G., Jowsey, J. 1973. Studies on mechanisms of hypocalcemia of magnesium depletion. *J. Clin. Invest.* 52:3000–10

69. MacManus, J., Heaton, F. W., Lucas, P. W. 1971. Decreased response to parathyroid hormone in magnesium deficiency. *J. Endocrinol.* 49:253–58

70. Hahn, T. J., Chase, L. R., Avioli, L. V. 1972. Effect of magnesium depletion on responsiveness to parathyroid hormone in parathyroidectomized rats. *J. Clin. Invest.* 51:886–91

71. L'Estrange, J. L., Axford, R. F. E. 1964. A study of magnesium and calcium metabolism in lactating ewes fed a semipurified diet low in magnesium. *J. Agric. Sci.* 63:353–68

72. Miller, E. R., Ullrey, D. E., Zutaut, C. L., Baltzer, B. V., Schmidt, D. A., Hoefer, J. A., Luecke, R. W. 1965. Magnesium requirement of the baby pig. *J. Nutr.* 85:13–20

73. Smith, R. H. 1961. Importance of magnesium in the control of plasma calcium in the calf. *Nature* 191:181–83

74. Larvor, P., Girard, A., Brochart, M. 1964. Experimental magnesium deficiency in the calf. II. Interference of magnesium deficiency with calcium metabolism. *Ann. Biol. Anim. Biochim. Biophys.* 4:371–82

75. Suh, S. M., Csima, A., Fraser, D. 1971. Pathogenesis of hypocalcemia in magnesium depletion. *J. Clin. Invest.* 50:2668–78

76. Dunn, M. J. 1971. Magnesium depletion in rhesus monkey: Induction of magnesium-dependent hypocalcemia. *Clin. Sci.* 41:333–43

77. Estep, H., Shaw, W. A., Watlington, C., Hobe, R., Holland, W., Tucker, S. G. 1969. *J. Clin. Endocrinol.* 29:842–48

78. Shills, M. E. 1969. Experimental human magnesium depletion. *Medicine* 48:61–85

79. Muldowney, F. P., McKenna, T. J., Kyle, L. H., Freaney, R., Swan, M. 1970. Parathormone-like effect of magnesium replenishment in steatorrhea. *N. Engl. J. Med.* 282:61–68

80. Connor, T. B., Toskes, P., Mahaffey, J., Martin, L. G., Williams, J. B., Walser, M. 1972. Parathyroid function during chronic magnesium deficiency. *J. Hopkins Med. J.* 131:100–17

81. Woodward, J. C., Webster, P. D., Carr, A. A. 1972. Primary hypomagnesemia with secondary hypocalcemia, diarrhea and insensitivity to parathyroid hormone. *Dig. Dis.* 17:612

82. Levi, J., Massry, S. G., Coburn, J. W., Llach, F., Kleeman, C. R. 1974. Hypocalcemia in magnesium-depleted dogs: Evidence for reduced responsiveness to parathyroid hormone and relative failure of parathyroid gland function. *Metabolism* 23:323–35

83. Salet, J., Polonovski, C., DeGouyon, F., Pean, G., Melekian, B., Fournet, J. P., Aymard, P., Raynaud, C., Vincent, J. 1966. Tetanie hypocalcemique recidivante par hyomagnesemie congenitale: une maladie metabolique nouvelle. *Arch. Fr. Pediatr.* 23:749–68

84. Paunier, L., Radde, I. C., Kooh, S. W., Conen, P. E., Fraser, D. 1968. Primary hypomagnesemia with secondary hypo-

calcemia in an infant. *Pediatrics* 41:385–402

85. Stromme, J. H., Nesbakken, R., Normann, T., Skjorten, F., Skyberg, D., Johannessen, B. 1969. Familial hypomagnesemia. Biochemical, histological and hereditary aspects studied in two brothers. *Acta Paediatr. Scand.* 58:433–44

86. Anast, C. S., Mohs, J. M., Kaplan, S. L., Burns, T. W. 1972. Evidence for parathyroid failure in magnesium deficiency. *Science* 177:606–7

87. Suh, S. M., Tashjian, A. H. Jr., Matsuo, N., Parkinson, D. K., Fraser, D. 1973. Pathogenesis of hypocalcemia in primary hypomagnesemia: Normal endorgan responsiveness to parathyroid hormone, impaired parathyroid gland function. *J. Clin. Invest.* 52:153–60

88. Chase, L. R., Slatopolsky, E. 1974. Secretion and metabolic efficacy of parathyroid hormone in patients with severe hypomagnesemia. *J. Clin. Endocrinol. Metab.* 38:363–71

89. Targovnik, J. H., Rodman, J. S., Sherwood, L. M. 1971. Regulation of parathyroid hormone secretion in vitro: quantitative aspects of calcium and magnesium ion control. *Endocrinology* 88:1477–82

90. Buckle, R. H., Care, A. D., Cooper, C. W., Gitelman, H. J. 1968. The influence of plasma magnesium concentration on parathyroid hormone secretion. *J. Endocrinol.* 42:529–34

91. Sherwood, L. M. 1970. Magnesium ion and parathyroid function. *N. Engl. J. Med.* 282:752

92. Anast, C. S., Winnacker, J. L., Forte, L. R., Burns, T. W. 1976. Impaired release of parathyroid hormone in magnesium deficiency. *J. Clin. Endocrinol. Metab.* 42:707–17

93. Rude, R. K., Oldham, S. B., Singer, F. R. 1976. Functional hypoparathyroidism and parathyroid hormone endorgan resistance in human magnesium deficiency. *Clin. Endocrinol.* 5: In press

94. Hamilton, J. W., Spierto, F. W., MacGregor, R. R., Cohn, D. V. 1971. Studies on the biosynthesis in vitro of parathyroid hormone. II. The effect of calcium and magnesium on synthesis of parathyroid hormone isolated from bovine parathyroid tissue and incubation media. *J. Biol. Chem.* 246:3224–33

95. Neuman, W. S., Neuman, M. W. 1958. The chemical dynamics of bone mineral. *Univ. Chicago Rep.*, p. 55

96. MacManus, J., Heaton, F. W. 1970. The influence of magnesium on calcium release from bone in vitro. *Biochem. Biophys. Acta* 215:360–67

97. Pak, C. Y. C., Diller, E. C. 1969. Ionic interaction with bone mineral. V. Effect of magnesium, citrate, fluoride and sulfate on the solubility, dissolution and growth of bone mineral. *Calcif. Tissue Res.* 4:69–77

98. Au, W. Y. W., Raisz, L. G. 1967. Restoration of parathyroid responsiveness in vitamin D-deficient rats by parental calcium on dietary lactose. *J. Clin. Invest.* 46:1572–78

99. Jowsey, J. 1972. Calcium release from the skeleton of rachitic puppies. *J. Clin. Invest.* 51:9–15

100. Alcock, N., MacIntyre, I. 1961. Interrelation of calcium and magnesium absorption. *Clin. Sci.* 22:185–93

101. Kessner, D. M., Epstein, F. H. 1966. Effect of magnesium deficiency on gastrointestinal transfer of calcium. *Proc. Soc. Exp. Biol. Med.* 112:721–25

102. Lifshitz, F., Harrison, H. C., Harrison, H. E. 1967. Intestinal transport of calcium and phosphate in experimental magnesium deficiency. *Proc. Soc. Exp. Biol. Med.* 125:19–25

103. Morehead, R. M. Jr., Kessner, D. M. 1969. Effects of Mg deficiency and parathyroidectomy on gastrointestinal Ca transport in the rat. *Am. J. Physiol.* 217:1608–13

104. Dunn, M., Walser, M. 1966. Magnesium depletion in normal man. *Metabolism* 15:884–95

105. Radde, I. C., Wittermann, E. R., Pensuwan, S. 1968. Effect of thyroid and parathyroid on hypocalcemia occurring after a magnesium load. *Endocrinology* 83:1285–92

106. Care, A. D., Duncan, T., Webster, J. 1967. Thyrocalcitonin and its role in calcium homeostasis. *J. Endocrinol.* 37:155–67

Ann. Rev. Pharmacol. Toxicol. 1977. 17:83–95

TOXICOLOGY OF ❖6668
HALOALKANE PROPELLANTS
AND FIRE EXTINGUISHANTS

Kenneth C. Back

6570th Aerospace Medical Research Laboratory, Wright-Patterson Air Force Base, Ohio 45433

Ethard W. Van Stee

National Institute of Environmental Health Sciences, Research Triangle Park, North Carolina 27709

INTRODUCTION

Low molecular weight halogenated alkanes, particularly certain fluoroalkanes, are of toxicological interest because of their industrial use as fire extinguishing agents, refrigerants, and solvents. Some fluoroalkanes also find use as aerosol propellants and are of interest to industrial and public health agencies because of widespread consumer use of pressurized household products and drugs. They also have a potential for abuse, particularly among drug-oriented youth. Another fluoroalkane, halothane, has been in common use in most hospitals since 1954 as an inhalation anesthetic.

Pharmacologically significant exposure of the human organism to these compounds, whether by design or accident, is usually by inhalation. Many compounds have a relatively high vapor pressure at ordinary conditions, so that they readily mix with air in pharmacologically significant concentrations. Fluoroalkanes readily diffuse through cell membranes because of their lipid solubility. Availability to the alveolar membrane, coupled with lipid solubility, results in a potential for quantitatively significant pulmonary absorption of fluoroalkanes.

Fluoroalkanes as a rule are not pulmonary irritants. In low concentrations acute inhalation is not an unpleasant experience, nor does prolonged esposure result in pathological changes in the upper respiratory tract or lungs. In somewhat higher concentrations inspiration may be resisted, but this is likely to be a consequence of the activation of certain reflexes such as the Kratschmer reflex.

A very extensive review of the literature concerning general fluorocarbon toxicity was written by Clayton in 1967 (1). More recently, in 1974, Aviado (2) reviewed

83

the toxicity of the fluorocarbon propellants. The propellant group includes but is not limited to such compounds as trichlorofluoromethane (CCl_3F), dichlorodifluoromethane (CCl_2F_2), trichlorotrifluoroethane ($CCl_2F–CClF_2$), dichlorotetrafluoroethane ($CClF_2–CClF_2$), and chlorodifluoromethane ($CHClF_2$). Fire extinguishing agents include trifluorobromomethane ($CBrF_3$), chlorobromodifluoromethane ($CBrClF_2$), dibromotetrafluoroethane ($CBrF_2–CBrF_2$), dibromotrifluoroethane ($CBrF_2–CHFBr$), and chlorobromomethane (CH_2ClBr). Inasmuch as space does not allow complete discussion of all the compounds used, and as each of the compounds has one or more of the toxicological properties discussed, the general field is reviewed using comparisons where possible.

ACUTE TOXICITY

The popularly accepted indexes of acute toxicity of the compounds listed above have been published by Engibous & Torkelson (3) and Clayton (1). Since the compounds have relatively high vapor pressures and are gases at room temperature, their principal mode of entry is via the respiratory route. The Underwriters Laboratories set up a relatively simplistic method for evaluating their relative toxicities. It involved exposing small numbers of guinea pigs for up to 2 hr and counting survivors. It is evident from this system that the fluoroalkanes are low in the order of toxicity.

Indexes such as median lethal concentration (LC_{50}) and approximate lethal concentrations (ALC) are of some comparative value for CH_2ClBr and $CBrClF_2$ when air was used as the diluent. One of the commonly cited figures for the ALC of $CBrF_3$ in rats is 83%. The report (1) indicated that air was used as the diluent in some of these studies, which would invalidate the results since the 83% $CBrF_3$ mixture in air would contain about 3.5% oxygen and the animals would have been severely hypoxic. Clayton did report, however, a mouse LC_{50} of 84% of $CBrF_3$ and a guinea pig LC_{50} of 88% with the balance of the inspired gas mixture, oxygen (1). Svirbely et al (4) reported an LC_{50} for CH_2ClBr of 2.9% in mice. Engibous & Torkelson (3) reported Army Chemical Center results of the exposure of one (!!) animal to CH_2ClBr and arrived an an ALC of 6.5%

The report by Clayton (1) of the levels of $CBrF_3$ and CH_2ClBr required to produce drowsiness in rats is more illuminating than the Army Chemical Center results. The ratio of 50% $CBrF_3$ to 0.475% CH_2ClBr equals about 105. This is very close to the ratio of a composite of cardiovascular effects found by Van Stee et al (5) in dogs.

NEUROLOGICAL EFFECTS

High brain levels of $CBrF_3$ were achieved in rats exposed to a nominal concentration of 75% $CBrF_3$ in oxygen. The levels were 50% higher than heart and blood levels (6). Aware that the compound reached the brain, Chikos et al (7) studied two basic cortical functions, the primary- and direct-evoked cortical responses. Both were depressed by exposure to $CBrF_3$, indicating cerebrocortical depression. The relative lipid solubilities of the compounds are $CBrF_3 < CBrClF_2 < CH_2ClBr$; therefore $CBrClF_2$ and CH_2ClBr would also be expected to accumulate in brain tissue, and probably to a greater extent than $CBrF_3$. Presence of significant levels of the compounds in the brain would be related to the genesis of central nervous system (CNS) dysfunction.

Carter et al (8) studied the performance of operant-trained monkeys during exposure to $CBrF_3$. Exposure to 20–25% of $CBrF_3$ resulted in performance decrements while exposure to higher concentrations resulted in a complete disintegration of operant behavior. Similar effects would be expected from exposure to $CBrClF_2$ or CH_2ClBr although the precise character of the expected responses is unknown.

Van Stee & Back (9) reported that the electroencephalograms (EEG) of monkeys and dogs exposed to 70% of $CBrF_3$ were synchronized and had increased amplitude. The EEG could still be activated by sensory stimuli, however, and no seizure activity was detected. This is evidence of CNS depression without loss of consciousness. Since no seizure activity was elicited in the dogs that were paralyzed with curare during the recording sessions, the genesis of the convulsions may require a functional somatic motor system.

Hine et al (10), Haskell Laboratory (11), and Call (12) conducted human exposure experiments on $CBrF_3$. Hine et al (10) reported that exposure to 10–15% of $CBrF_3$ decreased the subjects' performance of five of six psychomotor tasks and at 15% caused feelings of impending unconsciousness. The volunteers also reported subjective changes in the sensorium at the lower levels. Call (12) reported only a slight increase in reaction time during 3-min exposure to 4 and 7% of $CBrF_3$. He further reported no significant interaction between the presence of $CBrF_3$ and hypoxia. Light-headedness, paresthesia, and diminished performance during exposure to up to 10% were reported by the Haskell Laboratory (11).

Clark (13) exposed human volunteers to 4 and 5% of $CBrClF_2$. Feelings of light-headedness and paresthesia were reported at 4% which were aggravated at 5%. Exposure to 5% of $CBrClF_2$ caused marked symptoms of CNS depression.

Controlled exposure of human volunteers to CH_2ClBr has not been reported. Rutstein (14) has, however, published three case reports involving accidental human exposures in which the absorbed doses could not be estimated. The subjects initially lost equilibrium and then consciousness. The loss of consciousness is consistent with the observation by Svirbely et al (4) of the anesthetic potency of CH_2ClBr in mice. This has been confirmed in other rodent species in our laboratory as well as in others.

During exposure of $CBrF_3$, monkeys have been observed by Van Stee & Back (15) to go into a trance-like state and Carter et al (8) reported behavioral depression. Dogs, on the other hand, convulsed during exposure to 40–80% $CBrF_3$ (10, 15).

Beck et al (16) reported tremors and convulsions in dogs exposed to 5–8.8% of $CBrClF_2$. The neurologically equivalent responses of dogs to 5–8% of $CBrClF_2$ were roughly equivalent to 40–80% of $CBrF_3$, an approximately 1:10 relationship.

CARDIAC ARRHYTHMIAS

That halogenated alkanes can interact with pressor amines to cause cardiac arrhythmias has been known since Levy and others first made the observation with chloroform and epinephrine at the turn of the century. Since then the concept has become popular that hydrocarbons and halogenated hydrocarbons can "sensitize" the heart to the arrhythmogenic action of epinephrine. Cyclopropane-epinephrine arrhythmias have provided a popular standard for the testing of antiarrhythmic drugs for years. Since the phenomenon was recognized for anesthetics, etc, it was logical to try it out using aerosol propellants as well. It came as no surprise that this interaction with not only epinephrine but also with norepinephrine, metaraminol, ephedrine, phenylephrine, etc, can be demonstrated for a long list of substituted hydrocarbons including the aerosol propellants, fire extinguishing agents, and refrigerants.

Much attention has been directed toward the problem of the genesis of cardiac arrhythmias during exposure to the halogenated alkanes (17). Van Stee & Back (6) demonstrated that in addition to the presence of $CBrF_3$, arrhythmias appearing during exposure to this compound were sensitive to blood pressure, acid-base balance, and pressor amines such as epinephrine and by some mechanism other than their ability to raise blood pressure (see following section).

The interaction between the presence of the halogenated alkanes and epinephrine, the so-called sensitization of the heart to epinephrine, has been thoroughly investigated for $CBrF_3$, $CBrClF_2$, and CCl_2F_2 (18–22). The concern is based on the supposed release of endogenous epinephrine from the adrenal medulla during excitement, fear, or other stressful stimuli. The i.v. infusion of exogenous epinephrine during exposure to the halogenated alkanes does not duplicate the sympathoadrenal activation of the stressful situation. Not only is epinephrine liberated from the adrenal medulla, but also adrenergic neurotransmitter (presumably norepinephrine) is elaborated at the adrenergic terminals of the sympathetic innervation of the heart (as well as other sympathetically innervated structures). Furthermore, the volumes of distribution of endogenous and exogenous catecholamines are not identical.

Hine et al (10) came closest to modeling the physiological situation when they exposed dogs to $CBrF_3$ and then frightened them by means of stroboscopic lights and noise. No dog in this study developed ventricular fibrillation. Van Stee & Back (15) did report the death from ventricular fibrillation of one dog exposed to 40% $CBrF_3$ and not given any additional drugs. Marked excitement accompanied the event.

Beck et al (16) and Clark (13) demonstrated the exogenous epinephrine-$CBrClF_2$ interaction on cardiac arrhythmias in dogs.

Hine et al (10) monitored cardiac electrical activity (EKG) during exposure of human volunteers to nominal concentrations of 5, 10, and 15% of $CBrF_3$. Auriculoventricular (AV) dissociation and premature ventricular contractions were recorded during exposure to the highest concentrations (maximum, 16.9%).

Neither Call (12) nor Smith & Harris (23) detected any cardiac arrhythmias during exposure to $CBrF_3$. Call exposed human volunteers to 4 or 7% of $CBrF_3$ for 3 min in hypobaric chambers. Smith & Harris exposed crews to 5 to 7% for 5 min at pressurized altitudes of 1,000–20,000 feet in aircraft flight tests.

CARDIOVASCULAR PHARMACODYNAMICS

The cardiovascular actions of the fluoroalkanes are considered to represent the most significant hazard incident to their use. Detailed studies of the cardiovascular dynamic and myocardial metabolic effects of exposure to $CBrF_3$, $CBrClF_2$, or CH_2ClBr have been accomplished.

Exposures of anesthetized monkeys to 80% $CBrF_3$ or 12% $CBrClF_2$ cause a marked decrease in mean blood pressure together with a marked increase in left ventricular end diastolic pressure. This indicates that myocardial performance shifted up the Starling curve to a region approaching a state of compensated heart failure which would constitute a decrease in myocardial contractility (24).

The negative inotropic effects of exposure to the halogenated alkanes have been quantified and compared by Van Stee et al (25). The decreases in such indexes as dP/dt_{max} and dP/dt_{max} divided by developed pressure were comparable during exposure to approximately 1% CH_2ClBr, 12–14% $CBrClF_2$, and 75–80% $CBrF_3$.

The arrhythmias, particularly premature ventricular contractions (PVC), are dependent on a number of factors in addition to the level of fluoroalkane (6). Experiments were conducted to evaluate the sensitivity of the arrhythmias to mean blood pressure changes. In monkeys, PVCs appeared when pressure was elevated by expanding circulating blood volume by the infusion of 6% dextran. PVCs appeared and disappeared when mean arterial pressure was raised and lowered by aortic constriction or when the blood pressure was lowered and raised by exsanguination and reinfusion. Further, it was demonstrated that circulating catecholamine levels and acidosis altered the arrhythmia threshold independently of changes in blood pressure.

Exposure to the fluoroalkanes often caused a reversible, concentration-dependent fall in mean arterial blood pressure. Cross-circulation experiments have been performed in which the blood from donor dogs was used to perfuse the hind limbs of recipient dogs. The hind limbs of the recipients were in vascular isolation from the dogs' general circulation but the autonomic innervation remained intact. Through the use of combinations of recipient and donor dog exposures, coupled with the administration of autonomic drugs, the mechanism of hypotensive response to the fluoroalkanes $CBrF_3$ and $CBrClF_2$ was determined to be a decrease of vasoconstrictor tone. The compounds were found not to have any direct vascular smooth muscle action (26).

A series of experiments was conducted to test the hypothesis that the decrease in vasoconstrictor tone was the result, in part, of an impairment of ganglionic transmission. The vagosympathetic trunk was severed in the midcervical region and the cut ends were stimulated electrically. Nictitating membrane tissue tension was measured during stimulation of the central end, and vagal inhibition of the heart was monitored during stimulation of the peripheral end. $CBrF_3$ but not CH_2ClBr was found to cause a partial ganglionic blockade.

Regarding the cardiovascular dynamic effects, the conclusion was reached that the fall in blood pressure seen during exposure to the fluoroalkanes resulted from a combination of cardiodynamic functional impairment and ganglionic blockade. A reduction of cardiodynamic performance also was seen during exposure to CH_2ClBr; however, since the pressoreceptor reflexes remained functional in the absence of ganglionic blockade, their activation resulted in the maintenance of normal or slightly elevated mean arterial blood pressure during exposure.

The cardiac arrhythmias were sensitive to changes in mean arterial blood pressure, which implied that myocardial afterload was a determinant of the arrhythmia threshold as well as the presence of the halogenated alkanes. Tension on the myocardium has been demonstrated to alter both the electrical and mechanical properties of cardiac muscle (27). This concept may be extended to include muscle preload, and the authors suspect that this variable may affect the arrhythmia threshold as well as after-load. This hypothesis has not been tested but assumes some importance because end diastolic pressure (and presumably end diastolic volume) may rise during exposure to the compounds.

Having determined that the hypotensive effect was primarily the consequence of a decrease in vasoconstrictor tone secondary to ganglionic blockade, a group of experiments was conducted to investigate the mechanism of the negative inotropic effect.

A general procedure was established in which dogs were anesthetized and instrumented for acute exposure to different gas mixtures under anesthesia (28). Forty variables were either measured directly or computed from measured variables to provide a basis for an evaluation of cardiovascular dynamics and myocardial metabolism during exposure of anesthetized dogs to the halogenated alkanes. The measurements included arterial and coronary venous blood levels of O_2, glucose, lactate, pyruvate, nonesterified fatty acids, and the acid-base variables. Cardiovascular dynamic variables were monitored and Stewart-Hamilton indicator-dilution studies were performed using indocyanine green.

Some animals were pretreated with amine-depleting doses of reserpine 24 hr prior to examination. The results of these experiments indicated that the cardiovascular dynamic impairment that occurred during exposure to $CBrClF_2$ was independent of the integrity of the aminergic neural mechanisms. We have interpreted this to mean that the negative inotropic effect of the compound is independent of myocardial adrenergic postsynaptic activity (5, 29).

Likewise, the determination was made that the myocardial effects of exposure to the halogenated alkanes was not the consequence of an altered availability to the myocardium of oxygen and oxidizable substrates. Delivery to, and extraction by, the myocardium of nutrients was not altered significantly.

The significant finding in this series of experiments was that, whereas the myocardium was presented with adequate oxygen, animals exposed to $CBrClF_2$ and CH_2ClBr failed to extract a normal amount. A rise in the oxygen content of coronary sinus blood was measured and was correlated with the concentrations of $CBrClF_2$ or CH_2ClBr to which the animals were exposed (29). These elevations in coronary venous PO_2 and O_2 content persisted for 30 min after exposure to $CBrClF_2$ but not to CH_2ClBr.

No significant differences among the acid-base variables were detected for any of the compounds. Exposure to $CBrF_3$ resulted in significant elevations of arterial and coronary venous glucose levels which persisted for at least 30 min postexposure. Lactate extraction by the myocardium and arterial pyruvate decreased significantly during exposure to $CBrClF_2$, and venous pyruvate decreased significantly during exposure to CH_2ClBr. None of these changes persisted after exposure.

Mean transit time was prolonged significantly during exposure to $CBrClF_2$. The dP/dt_{max} and left coronary circumflex arterial blood flow were decreased significantly during exposure to $CBrClF_2$ and the dP/dt_{max} divided by developed pressure was decreased significantly during exposure to CH_2ClBr.

Myocardial oxygen extraction followed demand during exposures to $CBrF_3$ and $CBrClF_2$. The same two variables, on the other hand, were apparently significantly dissociated during the CH_2ClBr exposures. This could have been the consequence of a slowing of mitochondrial respiration. All three haloalkanes were found to slow state three respiration without uncoupling in isolated rat liver mitochondria (29). The effectiveness of the compounds was $CBrF_3 < CBrClF_2 < CH_2BrCl$. In the absence of measurements of mitochondrial levels of the compounds during the in vivo and in vitro experiments only limited inferences may be made concerning the treatment-response relationship. The absence of the measurable O_2 demand myocardial oxygen extraction dissociation during exposure to $CBrF_3$ or $CBrClF_2$ may only have reflected a failure to achieve mitochondrial levels of the compounds sufficient to affect respiration significantly.

Coronary flow was higher than controls for any given oxygen demand during $CBrF_3$ exposure. This was attributable to the mild hypoxemia that accompanied exposure of open-chested dogs to the relatively high levels of the compounds that displaced a significant amount of oxygen from the inspired gas mixture. The failure of $CBrF_3$ to dissociate O_2 demand and myocardial oxygen extraction, as well as the normal response of coronary flow to mild hypoxemia during the exposure, supports the conclusion that $CBrF_3$ had no significant effect on the relationship between myocardial O_2 demand, myocardial oxygen extraction, and coronary flow in these experiments.

Coronary flow was somewhat higher than controls for any given oxygen demand during $CBrClF_2$ exposure. The element of hypoxia was not present in these experiments; therefore, a coronary vasodilation was implied which may have explained the elevated coronary sinus blood oxygen level. Arterial hyperoxemia has been shown normally not to increase coronary venous PO_2 significantly in conscious, unmedicated, chronically instrumented dogs.

Coronary flow was somewhat lower than controls for any given O_2 demand during CH_2BrCl exposure. Myocardial oxygen extraction was profoundly lower, however. These results implied that this compound, in contrast to $CBrClF_2$, caused little or no coronary vasodilation. The elevated coronary sinus oxygen was apparently the consequence of a marked reduction of myocardial oxygen extraction.

In summary, $CBrF_3$ did not affect significantly the responses of either myocardial oxygen extraction or coronary arterial blood flow to oxygen demand. Neither was the coronary sinus blood oxygen level elevated. $CBrClF_2$, on the other hand, elevated coronary flow which resulted in a delivery of oxygen to the myocardium in excess of demand. The excess appeared in coronary sinus effluent. CH_2BrCl impaired oxygen extraction in response to demand without markedly affecting the coronary flow response which resulted in an elevation of coronary sinus blood oxygen. It is obvious, though the exact mechanisms are not known, that exposure to $CBrF_3$, $CBrClF_2$, or CH_2ClBr may result in disturbances of myocardial energy metabolism that are connected to myocardial performance. Based on the concentration to which dogs must be exposed to elicit such responses, $CBrF_3$ was least effective and CH_2ClBr was most effective. The $CBrClF_2$ was intermediate between the two but closer to the CH_2ClBr than to the $CBrF_3$ (5, 29).

GENERAL METABOLISM

Paulet et al (30) reported the results of studies on the effects of CCl_2F_2 and CCl_3F on general metabolism in anesthetized rats and rabbits. Single exposures to CCl_3F for 20 min or 3 hr exposures repeated daily for 15 days produced transitory increases in blood glucose and lactate concentrations that were rapidly reversed following cessation of exposure. CCl_3F also caused a general metabolic depression reflected in decreased O_2 consumption. CCl_2F_2 was without significant effects in these experiments.

Dittmann & Etschenberg (31) compared the ability of a series of halogenated methanes to desensitize pulmonary stretch receptors (endoanesthesia) and to produce narcosis in guinea pigs. The relative effectiveness of CCl_3F and CCl_2F_2 in these experiments was the same as that reported by Paulet et al (30), i.e. $CCl_3F >
CCl_2F_2$.

At least two factors contribute to the relationship of biological activities established in the studies by Paulet et al (30) and Dittman & Etschenberg (31). 1. CCl_3F is nine times as soluble in olive oil and four times as soluble in serum as CCl_2F_2 (32). The expectation that CCl_3F would be absorbed more readily than CCl_2F_2 during inhalation exposure was borne out by the studies of Adir et al (33) who determined that 77% of a given dose of CCl_3F and 55% of CCl_2F_2 was absorbed by conscious men and anesthetized dogs. Furthermore, CCl_3F was retained longer than CCl_2F_2 owing to their relative lipid solubilities. 2. Fluorination usually decreases pharmacologic potency and increases the chemical stability of halogenated alkanes. Increased potency in a homologous series usually is accompanied by increased lipid solubility (34).

Van Stee et al (5) monitored myocardial metabolism in anesthetized dogs exposed to $CBrF_3$ and $CBrClF_2$. Four to 12% $CBrClF_2$ increased coronary venous PO_2 and O_2 content whereas 27–75% $CBrF_3$ did not. The effect of $CBrClF_2$ was partially reversed by 30 min after cessation of 90-min exposures. $CBrClF_2$ is 12 times as soluble in olive oil as $CBrF_3$ (24). The relative potencies of $CBrF_3$ and $CBrClF_2$ bore the same relationship to the degree of fluorination and lipid solubility as the relationship between CCl_2F_2 and CCl_3F.

A possible functional basis for the effects of $CBrF_3$ on myocardial metabolism was revealed by the studies of McNutt et al (35) who reported on exposures of free-roaming guinea pigs to 79% of $CBrF_3$ in O_2. Hearts were rapidly fixed in situ by perfusion with glutaraldehyde. Mitochondrial cristae were in the energized configuration in control animals and in the orthodox configuration in $CBrF_3$-exposed animals. No evidence of mitochondrial hypoxia was observed and the suggestion was made that inner mitochondrial membrane-dependent functions may have been compromised in the presence of $CBrF_3$.

A hyperglycemic action of CCl_3F was noted by Paulet et al (30) and of $CBrF_3$ by Van Stee et al (5). Along similar lines, decreased glucose tolerance during halothane ($CHBrCl-CF_3$) anesthesia has been observed in dogs. This was ascribed to an inhibition of insulin secretion in response to an acute glucose load (36). Gingerich et al (37) supported this conclusion with studies on isolated rat pancreas. A structural basis for the possible activity relationship among this group of compounds is not immediately apparent.

UPTAKE AND DISTRIBUTION

Azar et al (38) measured carotid arterial and jugular venous blood levels of CCl_2F_2 and CCl_3F during 10-min exposures of conscious dogs. Consistent arteriovenous differences reflected general tissue uptake during the exposures. The average arteriovenous levels commonly associated with epinephrine-induced arrhythmogenesis were 35 and 23 $\mu g/ml$, respectively, for CCl_2F_2 and 29 and 20 $\mu g/ml$, respectively, for CCl_3F. The relationships among degree of fluorination, lipid solubility, and pharmacologic potency described in the section on general metabolic effects were preserved for this action (32, 34). In this connection, maximal blood levels of the respective compounds attained by human subjects using pressurized bronchodilator dispersers, were a small fraction of those required to elicit epinephrine-induced cardiac arrhythmias in dogs (39, 40).

Venous blood, whole heart, and whole brain levels of $CBrF_3$ were measured serially during and after 5-min exposures of rats to 75% $CBrF_3$ in O_2. Blood and heart levels were not significantly different and brain levels rose to 50% higher than blood levels. These observations supported the conclusion that venous blood levels provided a reasonable index of myocardial tissue levels and that the compound was preferentially distributed to an organ of high lipid content (41). Exposure of dogs and monkeys to similar concentrations of $CBrF_3$ has been reported to elicit cardiac arrhythmias during intravenous epinephrine infusion (15).

The postexposure decline of blood levels of $CBrF_3$, CCl_2F_2, and CCl_3F was biphasic reflecting a rapid initial washout from the central compartment (blood) followed by transition to a slower phase representing delivery of the compounds from the peripheral compartment (extravascular tissues) to the central compartment. The rapidity of the washout increased with decreasing lipid solubility of the compounds and was essentially complete, even after prolonged exposures, within 2 hr after exposure (5, 33).

Chiou & Hsiao (42) demonstrated that CCl_2F_2, CCl_3F, and $CClF_2-CClF_2$ were preferentially distributed to human and bovine serum albumin in phosphate buffer solution in the same rank order as their lipid solubilities, i.e. (from least to greatest) CCl_2F_2, 51%; CCl_3F, 66–71%; and $CClF_2-CClF_2$, 73–79%.

BIOTRANSFORMATION

Recent reports indicate that a number of systems capable of mediating the enzymatic dehalogenation of low molecular weight halogenated compounds may be present in tissues, particularly in the liver. For example, the reductive dechlorination of CCl_4 to $CHCl_3$ was reported by Paul & Rubinstein (43). The oxidative dechlorination of $CHCl_2-CH_2Cl$ by the mixed-function oxidase (MFO) system was characterized by Van Dyke & Gandolfi (44). Evidence consistent with the notion that the glutathione-S-transferases (45) of the 105,000 X G supernatant fraction of homogenized liver may be involved in the defluorination of methoxyflurane was suggested by Warren et al (46). Kubic et al (47) reported that CH_2Cl_2, CH_2I_2, and CH_2ClBr, respectively, were metabolized to CO by a hepatic system neither stimulated by phenobarbital nor inhibited by SKF 525-A. Several other halogenated methanes including CCl_2F_2 did not yield CO.

Although many potential routes for the dehalogenation of fluorinated alkanes apparently exist, most evidence suggests that the biotransformation of these compounds is of little significance quantitatively to their disposition. On the other hand, as is discussed later in connection with $CHClF_2$ and $CH_2=CCl_2$, limited biotransformation could be of substantial biological significance with respect to manifestations of toxicity.

Jenkins et al (48) exposed rats and guinea pigs continuously for 90 days and intermittently for 8 hr/day, 5 days/wk for six weeks to 100 ppm CCl_3F. Urinary F^- excretion and serum F^- levels did not differ significantly from those of controls. Although no evidence for the defluorination of CCl_3F was presented in that study, the report of Cox et al (49) suggested that caution be exercised before dismissing altogether the possibility and its potential biological significance. They observed Type I binding spectra not unlike those reported for CCl_4 which could represent the first step in an interaction of CCl_3F with the MFO system already known to possess dehalogenation activity.

Studies on the metabolism of $^{14}CCl_3F$ and $^{14}CCl_2F_2$ in man and the dog have been reported (50, 51). Exposures to 1,000–12,000 ppm of the compounds in air for < 20 min resulted in virtually complete recovery of all inspired fluoroalkanes. The possibility that trace amounts of metabolites may have been formed could not be confirmed.

The sum of evidence presented so far indicates that very little, if any, CCl_3F or CCl_2F_2 is defluorinated. Studies of possible dechlorination have not been reported. The apparent lack of biochemical reactivity is, no doubt, the consequence of the stabilization of adjacent carbon–halogen bonds by the successive fluorination of these compounds (34).

There is no doubt that animals are able to metabolize bromine from CH_2ClBr. MacEwen et al (52) exposed rats and dogs to CH_2ClBr for 124 6-hr exposures over a six-month period. The levels of 500 and 1000 ppm produced only a slight depression in rat growth, and lethargy was noted. The most significant finding was blood bromide levels in both species in excess of 95 mg/100 ml blood. This probably accounted for the CNS depression noted.

The matter of quantitatively limited biotransformation and toxicologic response to the presence of trace quantities of metabolites formed is worthy of careful consideration. Speizer et al (53) reported an increased incidence of palpitations and supraventricular arrhythmias among workers preparing frozen sections and exposed to $CHClF_2$. Exposures were to low levels and repeated at intervals over a period of years. The disturbing implication of this report was that the arrhythmogenic propensity appeared to be cumulative, with residual effects suggesting that the proximate arrhythmogen was probably a product of the biotransformation of the $CHClF_2$. This is the first report suggesting long-term residual effects on cardiac rhythm associated with chronic, low level exposure to halogenated alkanes. In this connection, it is of interest to note that pretreatment with phenobarbital, which induces the MFO system, reduced the amount of epinephrine required to trigger cardiac arrhythmias in rats exposed to $CH_2{=}CCl_2$ (54).

CONCLUSIONS

The most important toxicological effects of the haloalkanes are on the central nervous and cardiovascular systems. The neurological effects are manifested as alterations of perception and a reduction in reaction time and the ability to concentrate on complex intellectual tasks. The cardiovascular effects are manifested as changes in cardiovascular dynamics and the electrical activity of the heart.

Clinically important central nervous system effects almost always appear at lower levels of exposure than clinically important cardiovascular effects. Behavioral changes and performance decrements during exposure would undoubtedly have some effect on the interaction of the subject with his environment and such consequences of exposure could be life-threatening. Likewise, certain manifestations of halogenated alkane toxicity, such as the occurrence of cardiac arrhythmias, also constitute readily identifiable hazards.

Literature Cited

1. Clayton, J. W. Jr. 1967. Fluorocarbon toxicity and biological action. *Fluorine Chem. Rev.* 1:197–252
2. Aviado, D. 1974. Toxicity of propellants. *Prog. Drug Res.* 18:365–97
3. Engibous, D. L., Torkelson, T. R. 1960. A study of vaporizable extinguishants. *WADC Tech. Rep. 59–463*, Wright Air Dev. Div., Wright-Patterson AFB, Ohio
4. Svirbely, J. L., Highman, B., Alford, W. C., von Oettingen, W. F. 1947. The toxicity and narcotic action of mono-chloro-mono-bromomethane with special reference to inorganic and volatile bromide in blood, urine and brain. *J. Ind. Hyg. Toxicol.* 29:382–89
5. Van Stee, E. W., Harris, A. M., Horton, M. L., Back, K. C. 1975. The effects of three vaporizable fire extinguishing agents on myocardial metabolism and cardiovascular dynamics in the anesthetized dog. *Toxicol. Appl. Pharmacol.* 34:62–71
6. Van Stee, E. W., Back, K. C. 1971. Brain and heart accumulation of bromotrifluoromethane. *AMRL-TR-70-139,* Aerosp. Med. Res. Lab., Wright-Patterson AFB, Ohio
7. Chikos, P. M., Van Stee, E. W., Back, K. C. 1969. Central nervous system effects of bromotrifluoromethane. *AMRL-TR-69-130,* Aerosp. Med. Res. Lab., Wright-Patterson AFB, Ohio
8. Carter, V. L., Back, K. C., Farrer, D. N. 1970. The effect of bromotrifluoromethane on operant behavior in monkeys. *Toxicol. Appl. Pharmacol.* 17:648–55
9. Van Stee, E. W., Back, K. C., Prynn, R. B. 1970. Alteration of the electroencephalogram during bromotrifluoromethane exposure. *Toxicol. Appl. Pharmacol.* 16:779–85
10. Hine, C. H., Elliott, H. W., Kaufman, J. W., Leung, S., Harrah, M. D. 1968. Clinical toxicologic studies on freon FE 1301. *Proc. Ann. Conf. Atmos. Contam. Confined Spaces, 4th, AMRL-TR-68-175,* Aeros. Med. Res. Lab., Wright-Patterson AFB, Ohio

11. Haskell Lab. Toxicol. Ind. Med. 1967. Human exposures to freon FE 1301. *Tech. Rep., E. I.* DuPont De Nemours, Inc., Wilmington, Delaware

12. Call, D. W. 1973. A study of halon 1301 ($CBrF_3$) toxicity under simulated flight conditions. *Aerosp. Med.* 44:202–4

13. Clark, D. G. 1970. The toxicity of bromochlorodifluoromethane (BCF) to animals and man. *Tech. Rep.,* Imperial Chemical Industries, Ltd., Ind. Hyg. Res. Labs., Alderley Park, Cheshire, England

14. Rutstein, H. R. 1962. Acute chlorobromomethane toxicity. *Arch. Environ. Health* 7:440–44

15. Van Stee, E. W., Back, K. C. 1969. Short-term exposure to bromotrifluoromethane. *Toxicol. Appl. Pharmacol.* 15:164–74

16. Beck, P. S., Clark, D. G., Tinston, D. J. 1973. The pharmacologic actions of bromochlorodifluoromethane (BCF). *Toxicol. Appl. Pharmacol.* 24:20–29

17. Chenoweth, M. B. 1946. Ventricular fibrillation induced by hydrocarbons and epinephrine. *J. Ind. Hyg. Toxicol.* 28:151–58

18. Mullin, L. S., Azar, A., Reinhardt, C. F., Smith, P. E., Fabryka, E. F. 1972. Halogenated hydrocarbon-induced cardiac arrhythmias associated with release of endogenous epinephrine. *Am. Ind. Hyg. Assoc. J.* 33:389–96

19. Reinhardt, C. F., Azar, A., Maxfield, M. E., Smith, P. E., Mullin, L. S. 1971. Cardiac arrhythmias and aerosol "sniffing." *Arch. Environ. Health* 22:265–69

20. Reinhardt, C. F., Mullin, L. S., Maxfield, M. E. 1973. Epinephrine-induced cardiac arrhythmia potential of some common industrial solvents. *J. Occup. Med.* 15:953–55

21. Clark, D. G., Tinston, D. J. 1971. The influence of fluorocarbon propellants on the arrhythmogenic activities of adrenaline and iseprealine. *Proc. Eur. Soc. Study Drug Toxicity Meet., XIII,* Berlin

22. Taylor, G. J., Harris, W. S., Bogdonoff, M. D. 1971. Ventricular arrhythmias induced in monkeys by the inhalation of aerosol propellants. *J. Clin. Invest.* 50:1546–50

23. Smith, D. G., Harris, D. J. 1973. Human exposure to halon 1301 ($CBrF_3$) during simulated aircraft cabin fires. *Aerosp. Med.* 44:198–201

24. Van Stee, E. W. 1974. A review of the toxicology of halogenated fire extinguishing agents. *AMRL-TR-74-143,* Aerosp. Med. Res. Lab., Wright-Patterson AFB, Ohio

25. Van Stee, E. W., Diamond, S. S., Harris, A. M., Horton, M. L., Back, K. C. 1973. The determination of the negative inotropic effect of exposure of dogs to bromotrifluoromethane and bromochlorodifluoromethane. *Toxicol. Appl. Pharmacol.* 26:549–58

26. Van Stee, E. W., Back, K. C. 1972. The mechanism of the peripheral vascular resistance change during exposure of dogs to bromotrifluoromethane. *Toxicol. Appl. Pharmacol.* 23:428–42

27. Penefsky, Z. J., Hoffman, B. F. 1963. Effects of stretch on mechanical and electrical properties of cardiac muscle. *Am. J. Physiol.* 204:433–38

28. Van Stee, E. W., Horton, M. L., Harris, A. M., Back, K. C. 1973. The effect of 90-minute exposure to bromotrifluoromethane on myocardial metabolism in the dog. *Proc. Ann. Conf. Environ. Toxicol., 4th, AMRL-TR-72-125,* Aerosp. Med. Res. Lab., Wright-Patterson AFB, Ohio

29. Van Stee, E. W., Harris, A. M., Horton, M. L., Back, K. C. 1974. Toxic hazards evaluation of new air force extinguishing agents. *Proc. Ann. Conf. Environ. Toxicol., 5th, AMRL-TR-74-125,* Aerosp. Med. Res. Lab., Wright-Patterson AFB, Ohio

30. Paulet, G., Roncin, G., Vidal, E., Toulouse, P., Dassonville, J. 1975. Fluorocarbons and general metabolism in the rat, rabbit, and dog. *Toxicol. Appl. Pharmacol.* 34:197–203

31. Dittmann, E. C., Etschenberg, E. 1973. Endoanesthetic and narcotic activity in halogenated methane derivatives. *Eur. J. Pharmacol.* 24:389–98

32. Morgan, A., Black, A., Walsh, M., Belcher, D. R. 1972. The absorption and retention of inhaled fluorinated hydrocarbon vapours. *J. Appl. Radiat. Isot.* 23:285–91

33. Adir, J., Blake, D. A., Mergner, G. W. 1975. Pharmacokinetics of fluorocarbon 11 and 12 in dogs and humans. *J. Clin. Pharmacol.* 15:760–70

34. Krantz, J. C. Jr., Rudo, F. G. 1966. The fluorinated anesthetics. *Handbook of Experimental Pharmacology,* Part I, *Pharmacology of Fluorides,* ed. F. A. Smith, Chap. 10, pp. 501–64. New York: Springer-Verlag

35. McNutt, N. S., Morris, F., Van Stee, E. W. 1973. Ultrastructure of guinea pig heart after exposure to fluorocarbon 1301. *AMRL-TR-73-125,* Aerosp.

Med. Res. Lab., Wright-Patterson AFB, Ohio

36. Camu, F. 1973. Carbohydrate intolerance during halothane anesthesia in dogs. *Acta Anaesthesiol. Belg.* 24: 180–88

37. Gingerich, R., Wright, P. H., Paradise, R. R. 1974. Inhibition by halothane of glucose-stimulated insulin secretion in isolated pieces of rat pancreas. *Anesthesiology* 40:449–52

38. Azar, A., Trochimowicz, H. J., Terrill, J. B., Mullin, L. S. 1973. Blood levels of fluorocarbon related to cardiac sensitization. *Am. Ind. Hyg. J.* 34:102–9

39. Dollery, C. T., Draffan, G. H., Davies, D. S., Williams, F. M., Conolly, M. E. 1970. Blood concentrations in man of fluorinated hydrocarbons after inhalation of pressurised aerosols. *Lancet* 2:1164–66

40. Paterson, J. W., Sudlow, M. F., Walker, S. R. 1971. Blood-levels of fluorinated hydrocarbons in asthmatic patients after inhalation of pressurized aerosols. *Lancet* 2:565–68

41. Van Stee, E. W., Back, K. C. 1971. Brain and heart accumulation of bromotrifluoromethane. *AMRL-TR-70-139,* Aerosp. Med. Res. Lab., Wright-Patterson AFB, Ohio

42. Chiou, W. L., Hsiao, J. H. 1974. A new simple approach to study the protein binding of volatile and gaseous compounds. I. Fluorocarbon aerosol propellants, halothane and cyclopropane. *Res. Commun. Chem. Pathol. Pharmacol.* 8:273–87

43. Paul, B. B., Rubinstein, D. 1963. Metabolism of CCl$_4$ and CHCl$_3$ by the rat. *J. Pharmacol. Exp. Ther.* 141:141–48

44. Van Dyke, R. A., Gandolfi, A. J. 1975. Characteristics of a microsomal dechlorination system. *Mol. Pharmacol.* 11:809–17

45. Jerina, D. M., Bend, J. R. 1976. Glutathione-S-transferase. In *IUPHAR Sa-*

tell. Symp. Act. Intermed.: Form., Toxicity Inactivation, July 26–27, Turku, Finland

46. Warren, W. A., Baker, F. D., Bellantoni, J. 1976. Enzymatic defluorination of methoxyflurane. *Biochem. Pharmacol.* 25:723–24

47. Kubic, V. L., Anders, M. W., Engel, R. R., Barlow, C. H., Caughey, W. S. 1974. Metabolism of dihalomethanes to carbon monoxide. *Drug Metab. Dispos.* 2:53–57

48. Jenkins, L. J. Jr., Jones, R. A., Coon, R. A., Siegel, J. 1970. Repeated and continuous exposures of laboratory animals to trichlorofluoromethane. *Toxicol. Appl. Pharmacol.* 16:133–42

49. Cox, P. J., King, L. J., Parke, D. V. 1972. A study of the possible metabolism of trichlorofluoromethane. *Proc. Biochem. Soc.* 130:13–14

50. Blake, D. A., Mergner, G. W. 1974. Inhalation studies on the biotransformation and elimination of [^{14}C] trichlorofluoromethane and [^{14}C] dichlorodifluoromethane in beagles. *Toxicol. Appl. Pharmacol.* 30:396–407

51. Mergner, G. W., Blake, D. A., Helrich, M. 1975. Biotransformation and elimination of ^{14}C-trichlorofluoromethane (FC-11) and ^{14}C-dichlorodifluoromethane (FC-12) in man. *Anesthesiology* 42:345–51

52. MacEwen, J. D., McNerney, J. M., Vernot, E. H., Harper, D. T. 1966. Chronic inhalation toxicity of chlorobromomethane. *J. Occup. Med.* 8:251–56

53. Speizer, F. E., Wegman, D. H., Ramirez, A. 1975. Palpitation rates associated with fluorocarbon exposure in a hospital setting. *N. Engl. J. Med.* 292:624–26

54. Siletchnik, L. M., Carlson, G. P. 1974. Cardiac sensitizing effects of 1,1-dichloroethylene: Enhancement by phenobarbital pretreatment. *Arch. Int. Pharmacodyn.* 210:259–364

Ann. Rev. Pharmacol. Toxicol. 1977. 17:97–116
Copyright © 1977 by Annual Reviews Inc. All rights reserved

ENZYMES AS DRUGS ❖6669

John S. Holcenberg
Departments of Pediatrics and Pharmacology, Midwest Childhood Cancer Center,
Medical College of Wisconsin and Milwaukee Children's Hospital, Milwaukee,
Wisconsin 53233

Joseph Roberts
Memorial Sloan-Kettering Cancer Center, New York, New York 10021

"Enzymes far exceed man-made catalysts in their reaction specificity, their catalytic efficiency, and their capacity to operate under mild conditions of temperature and hydrogen-ion concentration" (1). These properties have prompted investigators to use specific enzymes as therapeutic agents since the beginning of this century. Undoubtedly for centuries, proteolytic enzymes were part of mixtures of animal and plant materials used topically.

In pioneering experiments in the 1930s, Avery & Dubos isolated and characterized a bacterial enzyme which degraded the capsular polysaccharide of type III pneumococcus. Parenteral administration of this enzyme protected experimental animals from infection by this type of pneumococcus (2). Subsequently, enzymes have been used to promote fibrinolysis, proteolysis, and food digestion. In recent years, enzymic degradation of amino acids and folic acid derivatives have been used in cancer chemotherapy. An exciting new direction is enzyme replacement therapy in certain genetic diseases.

Enzymes have some unique disadvantages as drugs. For parenteral administration, they must be exhaustively purified to eliminate contaminating toxic materials. Enzymes are generally quite costly to prepare and are degraded in the body. They are large molecules with limited distribution within the host. In addition, the enzymes that are foreign proteins to the host are antigenic. The development of antibodies may prevent the use of the drug for prolonged periods of time as a result of decreased enzyme activity or severe hypersensitivity reactions.

In this review, we concentrate on the practical aspects of enzyme therapy by discussing (*a*) development of new enzymes, (*b*) *in vivo* pharmacology, pharmacokinetics, and therapeutic effects of these agents, and (*c*) experimental attempts to overcome the problems of instability, short half-life, limited distribution, and immunogenicity. These aspects are illustrated mainly from experiments with amino acid–degrading enzymes. We briefly discuss the advances and special problems in the use of enzymes as fibrinolytic agents and as replacement in genetic diseases. A detailed discussion of enzyme therapy can be found in a review by Cooney & Rosenbluth (3). Enzyme therapy of cancer recently has been reviewed by Uren & Handschumacher (4). Asparaginase and glutaminase enzymes as antineoplastic agents have been reviewed in this series in 1970 (5) and elsewhere (6, 7).

DEVELOPMENT OF NEW ENZYMES

Sources and Purification of Therapeutic Enzymes

Microorganisms generally constitute the most practical source for producing large amounts of an enzyme for therapeutic use. Large quantities of a microorganism can be cultured at relatively low cost and in little time. Often the yield of enzyme produced may be greatly increased (10 to 100 fold) by manipulation of culture conditions or by selection of a desirable mutant strain. When bacteria are used to produce enzymes that are suitable for parenteral administration, it is essential that the final product be exhaustively purified to remove endotoxins. Enrichment culture techniques (utilizing the substrate compound as the sole carbon and/or nitrogen source) are utilized for selection of useful organisms and for enzyme induction. Microorganisms are ruptured by sonication or homogenization, and the enzymes are purified through the use of procedures that give high recoveries and can be readily scaled-up. These include precipitation by salts, organic solvents, heat treatment, or pH adjustment, and chromatographic separation with ion exchange, gel filtration, and affinity binding.

Replacement of defective lysosomal enzymes in genetic diseases presents special problems, because these enzymes are glycoproteins with determinants that are responsible for efficient incorporation into the lysosomes (8). Bacterial enzymes may lack these determinants. So far the human placenta has been the major source of these enzymes (9).

Characteristics of Therapeutically Useful Enzymes

Enzymes that degrade selected nutrients or metabolites in circulation should have the following characteristics:

1. High activity and stability at physiological pH.
2. Retention of activity and stability in animal serum and whole blood.
3. High affinity for the substrate (low K_m).
4. Slow clearance from the circulation when injected into animals.
5. No inhibition by its products or other constituents normally found in body fluids.
6. No requirement for exogenous cofactors.
7. Effective irreversibility of the enzymatic reaction under physiologic conditions.
8. Availability from a nonpathogenic organism that contains little endotoxin.

A number of amino acid–degrading enzymes that do not exhibit antitumor activity also fail to meet at least one of these criteria. For instance, *Escherichia coli* glutaminase has a pH optimum of 5 and essentially no activity at physiologic pH. An ineffective form of *E. coli* asparaginase has a K_m over 1 mM. Asparaginase enzymes from a yeast, *Bacillus coagulans,* and *Fusarium tricinctum* all have excessively rapid clearance rates in mice (7).

Clearance rates in mice bearing transplantable tumors may be misleading, since most of these tumors contain the lactate dehydrogenase–elevating virus. Infection by this virus greatly slows the clearance of some enzymes (10). Slow clearance in infected mice does not necessarily correlate with a long half-life in other animals.

The activity of some enzymes is tightly controlled by product inhibition, cooperative substrate kinetics, or other effectors. During treatment of mice with glutaminase-asparaginase, the glutamate level rises over 100-fold and greatly exceeds the glutamine concentrations. A glutaminase inhibited by its products would rapidly lose its effect under these conditions (6). A cysteine-degrading enzyme from *Salmonella typhimurium* shows a sharp fall in activity at cysteine concentrations below 0.1 mM (11). The sigmoid kinetics would greatly decrease its ability to deplete cysteine in circulation. The activity of glutaminase B from *E. coli* is allosterically regulated by carboxylic acids, divalent cations and adenine nucleotides (12). Such an enzyme might have very little activity in vivo.

Both *E. coli* asparaginase and *Acinetobacter* glutaminase-asparaginase are located near the surface of the bacterium, presumably in the periplasmic region between the plasma membrane and cell wall (13, 14). The enzymes have very low K_ms for these amino acids. An intracellular location of similar enzymes would require either their compartmentalization, repression of their synthesis, or some kinetic control of their activity to protect the pools of these amino acids from hydrolysis. Theoretically, enzymes secreted into the media or on the surface of the microorganism would not require these controls of their activity. One can select for these enzymes by searching for strains that demonstrate the activity in suspensions of whole cells or in the culture media.

Several amino acid–degrading enzymes require pyridoxal phosphate or other cofactors for activity. Meadows and his co-workers (15) have recently reported that tyrosine phenol-lyase from *Erwinia herbicola* inhibited growth of established B16 melanoma tumors. These workers, however, found that repeated injections of this enzyme caused only partial lowering of tyrosine in plasma of treated animals. The relatively weak depletion of tyrosine in vivo by this enzyme appears to be largely a result of its requirement for pyridoxal phosphate as a coenzyme. Administered pyridoxal phosphate has a half-life of only a few minutes in mice. Meadows and Elmer (16) have shown that the pyridoxal phosphate is rapidly stripped from the enzyme in vivo. The cofactor is also removed by incubation with albumin, alkaline phosphatase, or membrane preparations from liver. Limited antitumor activity has been noted with two other pyridoxal phosphate–requiring enzymes. Parodi et al (17) tested the therapeutic potential of *E. coli* tryptophanase. These workers reported that injections of very high doses [10,200 international units (IUs) per kilogram] of purified tryptophanase into rodents produced only a 35% reduction in the plasma tryptophan level. Kreis & Hession (18) isolated a methionine-degrading enzyme from *Clostridium sporogenes* which partly inhibited the growth of the Walker 256 carcinosarcoma in rats. In addition to its pyridoxal phosphate requirement, this enzyme has a high K_m for methionine (90 mM). A depot form of this cofactor or covalent binding to the enzyme might greatly increase the activity of this type of enzyme.

Oki et al (19) reported that leucine dehydrogenase from *Bacillus sphaericus* was highly inhibitory to the Ehrlich ascites carcinoma. However, Roberts and his co-workers (20) found that a homogeneous preparation of this enzyme did not lower plasma leucine levels or inhibit tumor growth in mice. The lack of in vivo effectiveness of this enzyme may be explained by several factors. The concentration of its cofactor NAD is negligible in serum. The activity of this leucine dehydrogenase at pH 7.4 is less than 5% of that at its optimal pH of 11. Furthermore, the equilibrium constant of this reversible reaction indicates that very little leucine breakdown can occur at the pH and ammonia concentration of plasma.

Contamination by bacterial endotoxin represents a major problem with some enzymes. Loos et al (21) showed that many commercial preparations of *E. coli* asparaginase contain endotoxin. The Limulus gel test allows for much more rapid screening of preparations than did previously used pyrogen tests. Generally, enzymes from bacteria known to have high concentrations of endotoxin should be avoided.

IN VIVO PROPERTIES OF THERAPEUTIC ENZYMES

Pharmacology and Pharmacokinetics

All the asparaginase and glutaminase-asparaginase enzymes used for enzyme therapy are tetrameric molecules with a molecular weight of about 140,000 g/mole, similar to that of 7S gamma globulin (22). *E. coli* asparaginase has an absorption and distribution similar to that of other macromolecules of this size (23–25). In man and dogs, the volume of distribution of asparaginase is 20–30% greater than the plasma space. In man, intramuscular administration resulted in maximal plasma levels that were only half those observed at the same time after intravenous dosing. In contrast, plasma levels are comparable 24 hr after equal intravenous, intramuscular, and intraperitoneal doses in mice. Detailed studies in dogs showed that the enzyme slowly enters lymph and cerebrospinal fluid reaching a maximum 2–3 hr after an intravenous dose. The concentration in thoracic duct lymph rose to 25% of plasma, while neck and leg lymph did not exceed 5% and cerebrospinal fluid was less than 0.5% of plasma. The concentration in bile reached equilibrium rapidly but was never more than 5% that of plasma. Intra-arterial injections of either histamine or bradykinin caused increases of asparaginase activity in draining lymph.

Studies in patients showed slow appearance of the enzyme in thoracic duct lymph, very low levels in the cerebrospinal fluid, and no activity in the urine. When the enzyme was injected directly into the cerebrospinal fluid of the lateral ventricles, the enzyme was rapidly transferred to the plasma so that by 24 hr no activity remained in the spinal fluid.

Schwartz et al (25) noted that pleural fluid in two patients had only 1–3% of the activity in plasma. Asparaginase, however, may persist within abnormal accumulations of body fluids. High levels of activity persisted for at least two days after injection of the enzyme directly into a pleural effusion. J. S. Holcenberg (unpublished observations) found a slow input and removal of several asparaginase and glutaminase enzymes in the peritoneal fluid of mice bearing the Ehrlich ascites tumor. Enzyme levels increased in this fluid for 24 hr and then decreased at a slower rate than plasma, so that the activity in the peritoneal fluid exceeded that in plasma by two to three days.

Extracts of normal and tumor tissues contain enzyme activity in excess of that in their residual blood content (26). We have measured the relative concentration of four asparaginase and glutaminase enzymes in extracts of subcutaneous EARAD tumors and plasma. The activity in tissue extracts was 10–15% of plasma 24 hr after a single dose of 300–2000 IU asparaginase per kilogram of each enzyme. It is not known whether this activity is only in the extracellular fluid or whether part of it is bound to the tumor cells.

Enzymes with high catalytic activity toward both asparagine and glutamine have less antitumor activity than *E. coli* asparaginase toward asparaginase sensitive subcutaneous tumors (27, 28). J. Roberts has shown that asparagine levels in subcutaneous EARAD tumors are lowered more by *E. coli* asparaginase than the glutaminase-asparaginase enzymes (unpublished results). In tissue culture, the dose of *E. coli* asparaginase needed to kill P5178Y cells is one tenth the dose needed for enzymes with high glutaminase activity. Amino acid levels in the tissue culture media show that asparagine is depleted at a slower rate by the glutaminase-asparaginase enzymes (29). Kinetic models predict this difference since the higher level of glutamine in culture media and body fluids effectively competes with asparagine for hydrolysis by the mixed substrate enzymes, but not with *E. coli* asparaginase.

The disappearance of *E. coli* asparaginase activity in mice infected with LDH-elevating virus and in dogs can be described by a single exponential function with a half-life of 24 and 14 hr, respectively (10, 23). After large doses in man the decay of plasma activity follows a biexponential function with half-lives of about 0.5 and 2.5 days (24, 30). Holcenberg (31) has described a model for asparagine concentration during asparaginase treatment. The plasma asparagine concentration at any time is dependent upon the rates of net input of the amino acid into the plasma and its hydrolysis by the enzyme. Woods & Handschumacher (32) have shown that the liver closely regulates the plasma asparagine concentration in the rat. This type of control can be described by the following equation:

$$\text{net plasma input} = I_{max} \cdot (1 - A/\overline{A}), \qquad\qquad 1.$$

where I_{max} is the maximal rate of asparagine input into the plasma, A is the asparagine concentration, and $\overline{A}$ is the normal controlled concentration of this amino acid. This equation fits the observations that the maximal input of this amino acid occurs when plasma asparagine concentration is low. When plasma asparagine exceeds the controlling concentration $\bar{A}$, plasma input becomes negative, corresponding to the observed uptake of the amino acid by liver (32). The model assumes a constant maximal input rate for asparagine. Actually, synthesis of asparagine increases during periods of asparagine depletion.

L-Asparaginase activity follows Michaelis-Menton kinetics with no product inhibition. Therefore, the decay of enzyme activity in plasma with time can be described by the following equation:

$$\text{enzyme activity} = -A/(K_m + A) \cdot V_{max} \cdot exp(-0.693\, t/T_{1/2}) \qquad 2.$$

where A is the concentration of asparagine, t is time, K_m is the Michaelis-Menton constant for the enzyme, $T_{1/2}$ is the half-life for decay of enzyme activity in the plasma, and V_{max} is the maximal velocity of the enzyme at an initial time. In man, two exponential terms are needed to describe the decay of enzyme activity with time.

The change in asparagine concentration dA/dt, is equal to the sum of the input term (Equation 1) and the enzyme activity term (Equation 2). Asparagine concentration at any time can be calculated by integration of this equation with an iterative process. Since the decay rate of the enzyme in plasma is considerably slower than its catalytic activity or the rate of input of asparagine, the calculation can be simplified by first determining the value for the exponential term at a particular time (Equation 2). Equilibrium is rapidly approached between enzyme activity and asparagine input. Therefore, the asparagine concentration can be calculated without integration by assuming that dA/dt equals zero.

The input rate can be determined experimentally by simultaneous measurement of the plasma asparagine and asparaginase activity. The maximal input rate is equal to the least enzyme activity needed to deplete the asparagine level to zero. Measurements indicate that the maximal asparagine input in mice is 1–5 nmole/min/ml plasma. This value is in the same range as the maximal input of asparagine from rat liver during perfusion studies (32). Using this input rate and the observed half-life of the enzyme, this model predicts closely the asparagine levels observed during treatment of mice and patients. The model may be useful in calculating dosing intervals needed to maintain a specific asparagine concentration and in the comparison of different enzymes. Similar calculations with a glutaminase enzyme indicate that the input rate of glutamine into plasma is approximately five times that of asparagine.

These input rates may also explain the inability of hemodialysis to deplete circulating levels of asparagine despite removal of large amounts of asparagine. An input of 2 nmole/min/ml plasma is equivalent to a total input of about 6 μmole/min in man. The clearance rate of asparagine by currently available dialysis techniques is far below this level.

Very little is known about the site or mechanism of clearance of natural or exogenous proteins (33). Modification of the reticuloendothelial system by zymosan did not change the clearance rate of L-asparaginase in dogs or guinea pigs (23). In mice without LDH-elevating virus infections, the half-life of *Acinetobacter* glutaminase-asparaginase is about 60 min. When the enzyme was labeled with I^{125} and injected into mice, the label did not concentrate in any organ but rapidly appeared in the urine as iodinated tyrosine (A. Montanaro, J. DiGiovanni, and J. Holcenberg, unpublished observations). The clearance of this enzyme was not affected by aggregated albumin which blocks Kupffer's cells pinocytosis or by desialylated α_1 acid glycoprotein which blocks the specific glycopeptide receptors on liver parenchymal cells. Thus, these proteins do not appear to be degraded by a selective process in the liver. A fruitful area of study would be the mechanism by which the LDH-elevating virus slows the clearance of this and other enzymes.

Lysosomal glycoprotein enzymes have a unique distribution and clearance after parenteral administration (8, 34). An intravenous dose of hexoseamidase A, ceramide trihexosidase, or glucocerebrosidase was very rapidly cleared from the blood of patients with genetic defects involving these enzymes. These enzymes appear to be incorporated into lysosomes primarily in the liver, but some activity is retained in the liver for prolonged times after plasma activity falls to control levels (34). Study of fibroblasts from patients with lysosomal enzyme defects indicates that the uptake of replacement enzymes is a highly specific process (35, 36). Further study is needed to define the receptors for this uptake and the characteristics of the enzymes that allow their incorporation into and persistence in lysosomes.

Examples of Therapeutic Uses of Enzymes

THERAPY OF NEOPLASIA BY ENZYMIC DEPRIVATION OF NONESSENTIAL AMINO ACIDS   Depletion of specific nonessential amino acids in body fluids by enzymes offers a potential for cancer therapy with relatively high specificity for the neoplasm. Certain neoplasms are critically dependent on extracellular asparagine for their survival. Because asparagine is synthesized by normal cells and enters the bloodstream, simple dietary deprivation is not effective. For therapeutic effectiveness the amino acid must be continuously degraded in the body fluids by parenteral administration of the enzyme. Asparaginase exploits this specified asparagine requirement of certain neoplastic cells and, thereby, offers a much higher degree of selectivity for the susceptible tumor than conventional chemotherapeutic agents. L-Asparaginase was the first enzyme with antitumor activity to be intensively studied in man. About two thirds of acute lymphocytic leukemia patients when treated with asparaginase achieve complete remission (37, 38), whereas other neoplasms in man are relatively insensitive to asparaginase (39). Recent studies have indicated that asparaginase can rescue normal cells from the toxicity of high-dose methotrexate. Combination therapy with high-dose methotrexate and asparaginase has produced encouraging antitumor effects in human neoplasms (40, 41).

Glutaminase enzymes should have a greater antitumor potential than asparaginase enzymes (42). Glutamine, like asparagine, is a nonessential amino acid in the diet of humans. However, glutamine participates in a wide variety of metabolic reactions in mammalian cells (43). Cells grown in tissue culture require over ten times more glutamine than any other amino acid (44, 45). One of the important functions of glutamine in the metabolism of certain tumors may be as a direct precursor of glutamic acid, which can then furnish the carbon for the partial operation of the citric acid cycle (an important energy source) (46). When compared with other tissues, certain tumor cells appear to operate at a marginal level of glutamine availability as a result of a slow rate of synthesis and a rapid utilization (46, 47). Therefore, glutamine deprivation may have selective toxicity toward certain tumor cells.

In 1964 Greenberg and co-workers reported that a glutaminase-asparaginase preparation with a relatively high K_m (7 mM) for glutamine decreased the initial rate of growth of a number of tumors, including an Ehrlich ascites carcinoma, but caused no significant increase in the survival time of tumor-bearing animals (48). Roberts and co-workers (14, 49) isolated and crystallized glutaminase-asparaginase from an *Acinetobacter* soil organism with the desired kinetic and molecular characteristics for in vivo activity and showed that asparaginase-resistant Ehrlich ascites carcinomas regressed completely following treatment with this enzyme. In tissue culture, *Acinetobacter* glutaminase-asparaginase selectively killed human leukemic leukocytes at about one hundredth the effective concentration of asparaginase (50). Broome & Schenkein reported that a glutaminase-asparaginase preparation derived from a *Pseudomonas* species caused temporary regression in a number of mouse lymphomas which were resistant to asparaginase (27). Bauer et al reported that glutaminase-asparaginase purified from *Pseudomonas aureofaciens* was inhibitory to 9 of 16 tumors in mice and rats (51). An asparaginase-resistant mouse adenocarcinoma was found to be especially sensitive to this enzyme. Hardy et al, however, noted that glutaminase-asparaginase from *Pseudomonas aureofaciens* had severe animal toxicity (52).

Schmid & Roberts (28) studied the toxicity of highly purified *Acinetobacter* glutaminase-asparaginase in C3H/HeJ, CD1, and BDF$_1$ mice. Daily injections of 250 IU/kg in mice infected with the lactate dehydrogenase-elevating virus maintained plasma glutamine and asparagine at undetectable levels while glutamate levels rose to 1700–2800 nmole/ml. To explore the possible toxicity of such high glutamate levels, C3H/HeJ mice were injected i.p. daily for 14 days with various doses of sodium glutamate. None of the injections, including doses of 100 mg per mouse, caused any overt toxicity. During a 90-min i.v. infusion of 100 mg sodium glutamate per mouse, the plasma glutamate level rose from 73 to 1775 nmole/ml and then dropped to normal by 5.5 hr after infusion. Daily treatment with 250 IU/kg glutaminase-asparaginase caused a maximal weight loss of 6 g in C3H/HeJ mice but little weight loss in CD1 and BDF$_1$ mice. Neutrophil counts reached a nadir of 800–1000/mm^3 on day 5 in each strain. Spleen weights and lymphocyte counts also decreased significantly. The hematocrit values in all treated groups decreased less than 20% from the normal values. BDF$_1$ mice tolerated i.p. administration of 500 IU/kg of *Acinetobacter* glutaminase-asparaginase daily for seven days, and three of five mice survived after treatment with 1000 IU/kg/day for seven days. Single doses of up to 6250 IU/kg were tolerated by these mice with only slight transient weight loss.

Holcenberg et al (53) showed that treatment with this enzyme only partially depleted free glutamine concentrations in muscle, spleen, small intestine, and liver. Brain and kidney glutamine concentrations actually rose with treatment. Only kidney showed a substantial increase in free glutamate and glutamyl transferase activity. Ammonia levels rose less than fourfold.

Daily injections of 250–500 IU/kg of *Acinetobacter* glutaminase-asparaginase for 7–14 days resulted in 90–100% reduction of total packed cell volume of the following asparaginase-resistant ascites tumors: Ehrlich carcinoma, Taper liver tumor, and Meth A sarcoma. Median survival time was increased up to twofold in glutaminase-treated mice. Combination with 6-diazo-5-oxo-L-norleucine, azaserine, or L-methionine-DL-sulfoximine enhanced the antitumor effects of glutaminase. The glutamine antagonists did not appear to interfere with in vivo glutamine breakdown by glutaminase since plasma amide levels were unaffected by their presence. The *Acinetobacter* glutaminase-asparaginase was found to have little or no effectiveness against solid tumors (28).

Recently Roberts isolated and crystallized a new glutaminase-asparaginase from a soil isolate organism *Pseudomonas* 7A (54). Although there are similarities between the glutaminase-asparaginase obtained from *Pseudomonas* 7A and other organisms, a comparison of physical, kinetic, and biological properties shows marked differences. The *Pseudomonas* 7A glutaminase-asparaginase possesses properties that make it ideally suited for therapeutic usefulness in larger animals and humans. This enzyme has an unusually long biologic half-life (13 hr in normal mice and 43 hr in mice infected with LDH-elevating virus). Physical studies showed that at high protein concentration, the enzyme polymerizes in the presence of asparagine or glutamine. Perhaps this property contributes to its unusually long half-life (55). In preliminary studies, *Pseudomonas* 7A glutaminase-asparaginase demonstrated substantial antineoplastic effectiveness against a variety of leukemias and solid tumors including L1210, EARAD-1, C1498 myeloid leukemia, B16 melanoma, and Walker 256 carcinosarcoma. The *Acinetobacter* glutaminase-asparaginase showed less or no effectiveness against these tumors (56). The *Pseudomonas* 7A glutaminase-asparaginase lowered free glutamine and asparagine in solid tumor tissue to a much lower level than *Acinetobacter* glutaminase-asparaginase (J. Roberts and J. Holcenberg, unpublished results). *Pseudomonas* 7A glutaminase-asparaginase, thus, appears to be quantitatively and qualitatively a much more potent antitumor agent than *Acinetobacter* glutaminase-asparaginase.

An important characteristic of glutaminase-asparaginase therapy is that tumors do not seem to develop resistance to this enzyme as they do with asparaginase or other antitumor drugs. *Pseudomonas* 7A glutaminase-asparaginase treatment of mice bearing 13 consecutive generations of EARAD-1 leukemia did not select or induce a resistant line. Drug resistance to *E. coli* asparaginase occurred during two treatment generations [(57) and J. Roberts and J. Holcenberg, unpublished results]. Combination therapy with glutaminase-asparaginase substantially delayed development of resistance of L1210 tumors to methotrexate and also lowered host toxicity to the antimetabolite (56).

Spiers & Wade recently reported that a glutaminase-asparaginase with a short half-life has an antileukemic effect against asparaginase-resistant cells in man (58). Preclinical toxicity studies with a long half-life form of *Acinetobacter* glutaminase-asparaginase are being conducted at the Memorial Sloan Kettering Cancer Center.

J. Roberts and co-workers (unpublished results) have isolated a novel histidine-degrading enzyme from a soil organism. This enzyme has a broad pH-activity curve between pH 7.2 and 9, with 75% of maximum activity at pH 7.2. Injections of this enzyme were well tolerated by mice and lowered plasma histidine to undetectable levels. Although this enzyme is being developed primarily as a potential new antineoplastic agent, it may also be ideally suited for treatment of the inborn error of histidine metabolism known as histidinemia.

There is some discord in the literature regarding the usefulness of arginase in tumor growth retardation in vivo (59). Burton reported that in contrast to the reversible inhibition of growth of normal lymphocytes and fibroblasts, a number of mouse and rat tumor cell lines were killed by exposure in tissue culture to arginase for 6 hr (60). The arginase inhibition was reversed with arginine (61). The tumor cells died when the arginine concentration in the medium was less than 8 μM. These studies utilized arginase from mammalian cells. This enzyme possesses unfavorable characteristics for antitumor effectiveness (K_m is 24 mM, and the pH optimum is near 10). Rosenfeld & Roberts have recently purified arginine desimidase from S. lactis and S. faecalis (unpublished results) and arginine decarboxylase from a Pseudomonas soil isolate (62). Preliminary studies showed that the desimidase and decarboxylase enzymes can deplete plasma arginine in mice. These enzymes have much more favorable K_m amd pH optimum values than the mammalian arginase and, therefore, are much better suited for future studies of the antineoplastic potential of arginine deprivation therapy.

Uren & Lazarus (63) reported that cystine- and cysteine-degrading enzymes inhibited leukemic cell growth in vitro. However, their enzymes did not appear to have the desired properties for therapeutic usefulness in vivo. J. Roberts (unpublished results) has isolated a serine dehydratase from a bacterial organism which lowered plasma serine when injected into mice.

THERAPY OF NEOPLASIA BY ENZYMIC DEPRIVATION OF ESSENTIAL AMINO ACIDS   There are conflicting reports in the literature concerning the antineoplastic effects of maintaining tumor-bearing hosts on synthetic diets deficient in selected essential amino acids. Amino acid–deficient diets were first used for tumor control in animals nearly sixty years ago (64). Extensive work along these lines with different essential amino acids followed in a number of laboratories (65). Recently Schmid et al (66) tested the effects on normal and tumor-bearing animals of three synthetic diets lacking the specific amino acids phenylalanine and tyrosine, isoleucine, or threonine. These studies revealed that even after two to three weeks on deficient diets only partial deficiencies of individual amino acids were observed in plasma of mice.

Studies with amino acid–deficient diets on tumor-bearing mice revealed that tumors were able to grow at the expense of carcass weight and there was very little or no increase in survival time. Relatively few studies of this nature have been conducted in humans suffering from malignancies because the synthetic diets were found to be cumbersome, complex, and unpalatable. Administration of specific amino acid–degrading enzymes may circumvent these problems and also effectively block availability to the tumor of an essential amino acid derived from catabolism of normal tissue protein. An important advantage of enzymically depriving tumor cells of an essential amino acid is that the tumor should not develop resistance to deprivation of an essential amino acid.

Prolonged deprivation of an essential amino acid will be toxic to the tumor-bearing host. However, deprivation of essential amino acids for short periods of time may be relatively well tolerated by the host. Selective inhibition of tumors could result if the tumor cells have a greater requirement for the amino acid than normal tissues. Abell et al have reported on in vivo inhibition of murine leukemia L5178Y by *Rhodotorula glutinis* phenylalanine ammonia-lyase (67); however, Roberts and co-workers (68) found that this enzyme only partially lowered free phenylalanine and tyrosine levels in tumor cells and normal tissues, and that treatment with this enzyme did not significantly increase the median survival time or long-term survival in mice bearing murine leukemias L5178Y, EARAD-1, or melanoma B16.

Poor results have been reported with enzymes requiring soluble or easily removed cofactors (see above). It is clear that new enzymes, with more favorable characteristics for in vivo activity, will have to be developed before the potential for treating neoplasms by deprivation of essential amino acids can be properly evaluated.

THERAPY OF NEOPLASIA BY ENZYMIC FOLATE DEPLETION   Dietary deficiencies of folic acid (69), riboflavin (70), or pyridoxine (71) have been shown to inhibit tumor growth. Generally, it takes several weeks or months to deplete body stores of a vitamin when animals are fed vitamin-deficient diets. In some instances concomitant administration of a vitamin analogue can speed up this process. However, the most rapid and effective method of achieving a vitamin deficiency would be to administer a specific vitamin-degrading enzyme to tumor-bearing hosts. Bertino and his co-workers (72) have reported that carboxypeptidase G_1, a folate-hydrolyzing enzyme isolated from *P. stutzeri,* inhibited growth of murine leukemias L5178Y and L1210, the Walker 256 carcinosarcoma, and a human lymphoblastoid line propagated in vitro. Chabner et al (73) have shown that carboxypeptidase G_1 hydrolyzes methotrexate in vitro and in vivo. Lethal toxicity of large single doses of methotrexate in mice was prevented by carboxypeptidase G_1 given 24–48 hr following methotrexate, with no adverse effect on methotrexate antitumor activity.

Albrecht and co-workers (74) have recently isolated a carboxypeptidase from a water bacterium. This enzyme cleaves folic acid and methotrexate in vitro 20 times more rapidly than 5-methyltetrahydrofolate (the plasma folate). When injected into mice, this enzyme efficiently degraded methotrexate at concentrations as low as $1.5 \times 10^{-8}M$ (A. Albrecht, personal communication). Further studies are in progress to ascertain the usefulness of this carboxypeptidase in ameliorating the toxicity of methotrexate, which is associated with the persistence of low plasma levels of the antifolate. Albrecht et al (75) have also isolated a folic acid deaminase from a *Pseudomonas* sp. This enzyme was reported to inhibit the growth of neoplastic cells in tissue culture.

ENZYMES AS FIBRINOLYTIC AND DEFIBRINATING AGENTS   Fibrin clots are dissolved by the proteolytic enzyme plasmin which is formed in vivo from the inactive precurser plasminogen by endogenous activators. Fibrin lysis can be accelerated by administration of plasminogen activators or other proteolytic enzymes capable of cleaving fibrin. The pharmacology, biochemistry, and clinical experience with these agents have been extensively reviewed (76, 77).

Streptokinase and urokinase are the major plasminogen activators. Both are proteins with a single polypeptide chain and molecular weight of about 50,000. They are rapidly cleared from circulation and, therefore, are administered by constant infusion. Urokinase is a natural product isolated from human urine. It is a trypsin-like enzyme which catalyses cleavage of plasminogen. As a normal constituent of urine, urokinase appears to be nonantigenic. Unfortunately its manufacture is quite costly and the drug is not available in commercial quantities. In contrast, streptokinase, a metabolic product of group C streptococci, is readily available in pure form. It does not have enzymatic activity alone, but forms an equimolar complex with plasminogen. Streptokinase probably induces a conformational change in the plasminogen, producing an active center which cleaves an internal peptide bond to produce plasmin (78). Most patients have circulating antibodies from previous streptococcal infections. These antibodies react with streptokinase and block its effect. Consequently, an initial loading dose must be given to overcome this neutralization.

The lysis of clots depends on activation of plasminogen within the fibrin network. Recently Kakkar and co-workers (79) showed improved lysis of deep-vein thromboses by sequential infusions of plasminogen and streptokinase. Clinically, the rate of lysis of pulmonary emboli and deep-vein thromboses is faster and more complete with the plasminogen activators followed by heparin than with heparin alone. Venous valves were better preserved with the combined therapy. The use of these thrombolytic agents is still controversial in myocardial infarction, retinal vessel thromboses, and arterial thrombi. In fact, a randomized, large cooperative study by the National Heart and Lung Institute showed that even though these agents increased the rate of clot lysis they did not improve survival of patients with pulmonary emboli. Their use in deep-vein thromboses depends on a balance of their therapeutic potential with their significant incidence of fever, allergic reactions, and bleeding (77).

The Malayan pit viper and a South American snake are sources of proteolytic enzymes Ancrod® or Arvin®, and Reptilase®, respectively. These enzymes cleave and clot fibrinogen and thereby produce marked hypofibrinogenemia (80). Many more fibrinolytic enzymes are under study from sources as diverse as molds and Brazilian blood-sucking leeches. The therapeutic role of these enzymes will depend on their antigenicity, ease of control, and toxicity.

REPLACEMENT THERAPY FOR INHERITED ENZYME DEFICIENCIES   Lysosomal storage diseases caused by a single enzyme deficiency should be ideal candidates for enzyme replacement therapy. For successful therapy, it has been suggested that the following problems must be solved (81, 82):

1. Adequate amounts of human enzyme must be obtained. Currently, the major sources are placenta and urine. An enzyme must be chosen which is selectively taken up by cells and is stable within lysosomes.

2. The enzyme should be nonimmunogenic. Even human enzymes may invoke an immunologic response. The mutation responsible for the enzyme deficiency may prevent entirely the production of enzyme protein, so that cross-reacting immunological material is absent.

3. The enzyme must reach the tissues in which storage is clinically important. The enzymes studied so far are rapidly taken up by liver. Unfortunately, the major storage problems in some of these diseases is in the heart, kidney, muscle, and central nervous system.

4. The enzyme in the lysosomal particle must fuse with the storage vacuole. In type II glycogenosis, enzyme replacement with purified human acid α-glucosidase resulted in high levels of enzyme in the liver but very little decrease in glycogen content of the liver or in the amount of intravacuolar glycogen (81).

For these reasons, injections of missing enzymes appears to be effective in very few lysosomal storage diseases. Enzyme therapy can cause temporary decreases in circulating levels of storage material in Fabry and adult Gaucher disease, conditions with slow progression and little central nervous system involvement. The prospects for improved therapy may be enchanced by new enzymes, enzyme modification, encapsulation, or entrapment in extracorporeal shunts and perhaps organ transplantation to supply the deficient enzyme (82).

METHODS FOR IMPROVEMENT OF ENZYME THERAPY

Soluble Chemical Modifications

The plasma half-life of *E. coli* and *Erwinia* asparaginases have been increased by deamination, acylation, and carbodiimide reactions with free amino groups (83, 84). Holcenberg et al (85) showed that *Acinetobacter* glutaminase-asparaginase could be modified by succinylation or by conjugation to low molecular weight glycopeptides, yielding enzyme derivatives with a 9- to 15-fold increased half-life in the circulation of mice, rats, and rabbits. Excessive reaction of the amine groups of each of these enzymes decreases the half-life or causes dissociation of the molecules (86). Cross-linking of lysine groups of *E. coli* asparaginase with dimethyl suberimidate decreased activity equally toward asparagine, glutamine, and diazooxonorvaline (87). In contrast, cross-linking by reaction of tyrosine residues with tetranitromethane altered the substrate specificity (88).

We have shown that succinylation of *Acinetobacter* glutaminase-asparaginase greatly decreases its susceptibility to digestion by trypsin (85). Cross-linking of α-galactosidase by hexamethylene diisocyanate stabilized the enzyme to trypsin digestion (89). Breakdown of these proteins in vivo is probably catalyzed by other proteolytic enzymes in the lysosomes. Gregoriadis (90) has shown that invertase cross-linked with glutaraldehyde is more stable in lysosomes. Such modifications which protect enzymes from digestion by lysosomal enzymes might greatly extend their duration of action.

Morell et al (91) have shown that removal of the terminal sialic acid residues of certain circulating glycoproteins causes their rapid uptake by specific galactose receptors on liver parenchymal cells. Rogers & Kornfeld (92) showed that lysozyme and albumin were also selectively taken up by this liver system when coupled to the asialoglycopeptides of fetuin. G. Schmer and J. Holcenberg have bound asialo-glycopeptides to *Pseudomonas* 7A and *Acinetobacter* glutaminase-asparaginase. These derivatives disappear from the blood with a half-life of less than 10 min and are concentrated in the liver. Homogenates of liver retain enzyme activity for about one hour (G. Schmer and J. Holcenberg, unpublished results). Succinylation and coupling of native gluteraldehyde-activated glycopeptides to the *Acinetobacter* enzyme did not change its distribution or effectiveness against solid tumors (85, 93).

Although *E. coli* asparaginase has immunosuppressive properties and retains half of its activity when complexed with antibody, immunologic effects have been shown to interfere with antitumor therapy in patients and experimental animals. Both anaphylactic hypersensitivity reactions and rapid enzyme clearance have been reported (94, 95). G. Schmer and D. Lagunoff (unpublished observations) have studied antibodies produced in rabbits to native *Acinetobacter* glutaminase-asparaginase and its succinylated and glycosylated derivatives. Antibodies to each enzyme preparation are equally effective in neutralizing and precipitating the natural and modified enzymes. Sela (96) has shown that covering the amino groups with polyalanine polymers can reduce the antigenicity of a protein or synthetic polypeptide antigen. Abuchawski et al (97) have reported that reaction of catalase with polyethylene glycol reduced its immunogenicity in mice. These techniques may have applications in the development of therapeutic enzymes.

Microcapsules, Liposomes, and Red Blood Cells

Enzymes have been encapsulated in inert and biodegradable capsules. Inert semi-permeable ultrathin capsules of nylon or polyurea can separate the enzyme from proteolytic enzymes and prevent antibody response. The reaction rate of the encapsulated enzymes depends on diffusion of substrate and products across the confining polymer membrane. Thus, the K_m for L-asparaginase in capsules is 100 times higher than the native one (98). A further disadvantage of these capsules is the foreign body reactions they provoke after intraperitoneal administration. This reaction causes a clumping and sequestration of the capsules so that they are no longer capable of lowering asparagine in vivo (99).

Liposomes are small capsules composed of lipid bilayers alternating with aqueous compartments. The lipid layer is composed of egg lecithin, cholesterol, and a negatively charged lipid. Enzymes and water-soluble drugs can be entrapped in the aqueous phase. These liposomes remain intact in circulation without leakage of the protein. They are rapidly taken up by endocytosis into the liver and spleen. The liposomes then fuse with lysosomes and are eventually catabolized. Preliminary experiments have been carried out with biodegradable capsules loaded with asparaginase and purified lysosomal enzymes (90, 100). Manipulation of the composition of lipid membrane and incorporation of cell specific immunoglobulins or desiallylated glycoproteins offers promise of directing the liposomes to specific cells other than those of the liver and spleen. Gregonadis has shown that while protein entrapment in liposomes does not prevent an immune response, the stratagem may decrease the severity of the hypersensitivity response upon repeated administration (90).

Proteins can be entrapped in erythrocytes by the technique of rapid reversible osmotic shock (101). Ideally, this technique should produce natural enzyme reactors with a prolonged circulation time. Unfortunately, the loading process appears to alter the red cells so that they often have a very short circulation time. Circulation time may be prolonged by modification of the method by including red cell enzymes, organelles, and substrates in the loading mixture, and size fractionation of the resealed ghosts. Thorpe et al (102) have utilized erythrocyte-entrapped β-glucuronidase to improve the treatment of β-glucuronidase-deficient mice. The erythrocyte-entrapped enzyme was retained fourfold longer in circulation, fivefold longer in hepatic tissue and appeared to deliver more enzyme to the lysosomes than the native enzyme. Suggestive evidence was presented that the enzyme-loaded erythrocytes are taken up intact by the liver cells and then slowly digested by the lysosomes. Thus, enzyme-loaded autologous erythrocytes may provide an intracellular depot form of the enzyme for treatment of lysosomal enzyme deficiencies. Nevertheless, the Kupffer's cells are likely to be largely responsible for the uptake of the red cell ghosts in the liver, and the therapeutic usefulness of loading these cells with enzyme is questionable.

Binding to Surfaces

Enzymes can be chemically attached to surfaces, incorporated within the matrix of the gel during polymerization, or bound to the surfaces in microspheres. Immobilized enzymes may be more stable and less likely to produce immune responses if the enzyme does not leach off the surface. Even if antibodies are formed, the complex of antibodies with the immobilized enzyme might still retain activity. Active anaphylaxis should not occur since the enzyme cannot reach sensitized mast cells. The problems associated with immobilized enzymes include changes in enzyme kinetics, leaching of the enzyme from the surface, bioincompatibility of the surface, and coating of the surface with circulating proteins with consequent inactivation of the enzyme reactor.

Allison et al (103) attached asparaginase to nylon tubing with glutaraldehyde. The immobilized enzyme was more stable but its K_m for asparagine was much higher than native enzyme and varied with flow rate. Horvath et al (104) embedded asparaginase within a polycarboxylic gel attached to nylon tubing. Incorporation of the enzyme within the matrix would be expected to prevent leaching from the surface and exposure of the enzyme to proteolytic enzymes and antibodies. In this case enzyme catalysis was also controlled by the rate of diffusion of the substrate into the matrix. Cooney et al (105) showed that asparaginase coupled to a dacron prosthesis by silanization, reduction, and diazotization gradually leached from the surface and brought about an immune response. In addition, accumulation of plasma protein and fibrin deposits on the surface of the graft impaired the catalytic capacity of the graft. This enzyme bound to glass plates by silanization and glutaraldehyde coupling also came off the surface (106).

D. Salley and J. Roberts (unpublished results) using emulsion polymerization prepared enzymically active, spherical (poly)acrylamide particles of controllable size range, and studied the effects of the degree of cross-linking and density of the polymer gel on enzyme retention and catalytic activity in the gels. Therapeutic enzyme was also entrapped in (poly)N-vinyl pyrrolidone, (poly)hydroxyethyl methacrylate, and (poly)dimethyl siloxane (Silastic ®). These were chosen because of their previous use in biological applications. The polymers were prepared in a particle size suitable for i.p. injection. Injection of the (poly)acrylamide, (poly)vinyl pyrrolidone, and (poly)hydroxyethyl methacrylate enzyme polymers in mice caused a reduction in the plasma asparagine but for no longer than was brought about by injecting free enzyme. This finding is in qualitative agreement with that of O'Driscoll et al (107) who studied the antineoplastic effectiveness of *E. coli* asparaginase trapped in (poly)hydroxyethyl methacrylate. Those workers also reported some leakage of enzyme from the gel. Recently D. Salley and J. Roberts (unpublished results) observed that when a single cylinder of (poly)hydroxyethyl methacrylate gel (6 cm $\times$ 0.6 cm) of high asparaginase activity was inserted in the peritoneal cavity of a rat, the reduction in plasma asparagine persisted approximately five times longer than with native enzyme. When plasma asparagine had returned to the normal concentration, the gel cylinder still possessed 60–70% of its original activity. This decrease in activity in vivo could result from impaired diffusion caused by protein coating of the surface of the gel or increased synthesis of asparagine.

Further research is needed to develop better methods for coupling enzymes to matrices. This chemistry must produce biologically stable bonds, no leaching of the enzyme from the matrix, retention of effective enzyme activity, and retention of biocompatibility of the graft.

CONCLUDING REMARKS

Considerable progress has been made in the development and testing of enzymes for parenteral chemotherapy. The biologic obstacles of susceptibility to proteolytic degradation, restricted distribution, and immunogenicity have limited the uses of these highly efficient and specific catalysts. Further advances require the development and selection of enzymes with properties specifically suited for a particular therapeutic use. These enzymes may require chemical modification, encapsulation, or immobilization on biocompatible matrices to improve their stability and decrease the immunogenicity. Directing the enzymes to extrahepatic sites is a much more difficult problem. Tumor-specific antibodies have a limited distribution in the host and therefore may not improve the effect of antitumor enzymes. Certain drugs and hormones with specific high affinity receptors on the target cells may be ideal agents to bind to soluble or immobilized enzymes.

ACKNOWLEDGMENTS

We wish to thank Drs. D. Lagunoff, G. Schmer, and D. C. Teller for their collaborative efforts and many helpful suggestions. This work was supported by NIH grants CA 11881, CA 15860, CA 08748, CA 25976, and CA 15674.

Literature Cited

1. Lehninger, A. L. 1970. The molecular logic of living organisms. In *Biochemistry*, p. 8. New York: Worth. 833 pp.
2. Avery, O. T., Dubos, R. 1931. The protective action of a specific enzyme against type III pneumococcus infection in mice. *J. Exp. Med.* 54:73–89
3. Cooney, D. A., Rosenbluth, R. J. 1974. Enzymes as therapeutic agents. *Adv. Pharmacol. Chemother.* 12:185–289
4. Uren, J. R., Handschumacher, R. E. 1977. Enzyme therapy of cancer. In *Cancer, A Comprehensive Treatise*, ed. F. F. Becker, Vol. 5. New York: Plenum. In preparation
5. Cooney, D. A., Handschumacher, R. E. 1970. L-Asparaginase and L-asparagine metabolism. *Ann. Rev. Pharmacol.* 10:421–40
6. Holcenberg, J. S., Roberts, J., Dolowy, W. C. 1973. Glutaminases as antineoplastic agents. In *The Enzymes of Glutamine Metabolism*, ed. S. Prusiner, E. R. Stadtman, 277–92. New York: Academic. 615 pp.
7. Wriston, J. C. Jr., Yellin, T. O. 1973. L-Asparaginase: A review. *Adv. Enzymol.* 39:185–248
8. Neufeld, E. F., Lim, T. W., Shapiro, L. J. 1975. Inherited disorders of lysosomal metabolism. *Ann. Rev. Biochem.* 44:357–76
9. Pentchev, P. G., Brady, R. O., Hibbert, S. R., Gal, A. E., Shapiro, D. 1973. Isolation and characterization of glucocerobroside from human placental tissue. *J. Biol. Chem.* 248:5256–61
10. Riley, V., Spackman, D. H., Fitzmaurice, M. A. 1970. Critical influence of an enzyme-elevating virus. *Recent Results Cancer Res.* 33:81–101
11. Kredich, N. A., Foote, L. J., Keenan, B. S. 1973. The stoichiometry and kinetics of the inducible cysteine desulfhydrase from *Salmonella typhimurium*. *J. Biol. Chem.* 248:6187–96
12. Prusiner, S. 1973. Glutaminases of *Escherichia coli:* properties, regulation and evolution. See Ref. 6, pp. 293–316
13. Cedar, H., Schwartz, J. H. 1967. Localization of the two L-asparaginases in anaerobically grown *Escherichia coli. J. Biol. Chem.* 242:3753–55
14. Roberts, J., Holcenberg, J. S., Dolowy, W. C. 1972. Isolation, crystallization, and properties of *Achromobacteraceae* glutaminase-asparaginase with antitumor activity. *J. Biol. Chem.* 247:84–90
15. Meadows, G. G., Digiovanni, J., Minor, L., Elmer, G. W. 1976. Some biological properties and an *in vivo* evaluation of tyrosine phenol-lyase on growth of B-16 melanoma. *Cancer Res.* 36:167–71
16. Meadows, G. G. 1976. *Antimelanoma potential of phenylalanine ammonialyase and tyrosine plenol-lyase.* PhD thesis. Univ. Washington, Seattle
17. Parodi, S., Furlani, A., Scarcia, V., Cavanna, M., Brambilla, G. 1973. Studies on the *in vivo* activity of *E. coli* L-tryptophanase. *Pharmacol. Res. Commun.* 5:1–10
18. Kreis, W., Hession, C. 1973. Biological effects of enzymatic deprivation of L-methionine in cell culture and an experimental tumor. *Cancer Res.* 33:1866–69
19. Oki, T., Shirai, M., Ohshima, M., Yamamoto, Y., Soda, K. 1973. Antitumor activities of bacterial leucine dehydrogenase and glutaminase A. *FEBS Lett.* 33:386–88
20. Roberts, J., Schmid, F. A., Takai, K. 1974. The *in vivo* effects of leucine dehydrogenase from *Bacillus sphaericus*. *FEBS Lett.* 43:56–58
21. Loos, M., Vadlamudi, S., Meltzer, M., Shifrin, S., Borsos, T., Goldin, A. 1972. Detection of endotoxin in commercial L-asparaginase preparations by complement fixation and separation by chromatography. *Cancer Res.* 32:2292–96
22. Holcenberg, J. S., Teller, D. C., Roberts, J. 1974. Active enzyme sedimentation of antitumor asparaginase and glutaminase enzymes. *Arch. Biochem. Biophys.* 161:306–12
23. Ho, D. H. W., Carter, C. J. K., Thetford, B., Frei, E. 1971. Distribution and mechanism of clearance of L-asparaginase. *Cancer Chemother. Rep.* 55:539–45
24. Ho, D. H. W., Thetford, B., Carter, C. J. K., Frei, E. 1970. Clinical pharmacologic studies of L-asparaginase. *Clin. Pharmacol. Ther.* 11:408–17
25. Schwartz, M. K., Lash, E. D., Oettgen, H. F., Tamao, F. A. 1970. L-asparaginase activity in plasma and other biological fluids. *Cancer* 25:244–52
26. Pütter, J. 1970. Pharmacokinetic behavior of L-asparaginase in men and in animals. *Recent Results Cancer Res.* 33:64–74
27. Broome, J. D., Schenkein, I. 1971. Further studies on the tumor inhibitory activity of a bacterial glutaminase-asparaginase. *Colloq. Int. C. N. R. S.* 197:95–105

28. Schmid, F. A., Roberts, J. 1974. Antineoplastic and toxic effects of *Acinetobacter* and *Pseudomonas* glutaminase-asparaginases. *Cancer Treat. Rep.* 58:829–40

29. Holcenberg, J. S., Roberts, J., Schmid, F. A., Lu, P. L. 1975. Kinetics of glutaminase-asparaginase treatment. *Pharmacologist* 17:229 (Abstr.)

30. Haskell, C. M., Canellos, G. P., Cooney, D. A., Hardesty, C. T. 1972. Pharmacologic studies in man with crystallized L-asparaginase. *Cancer Chemother. Rep.* 56:611–14

31. Holcenberg, J. S. 1976. Therapeutic model for asparaginase and glutaminase treatment. *Clin. Pharmacol. Ther.* 17:236 (Abstr.)

32. Woods, J. A., Handschumacher, R. E. 1973. Hepatic regulation of plasma L-asparagine. *Am. J. Physiol.* 224:740–45

33. Posen, S. 1970. Turnover of circulating enzymes. *Clin. Chem.* 16:71–84

34. Brady, R. O., Gal, A. E., Pentchev, P. G. 1975. Evolution of enzyme replacement therapy for lipid storage diseases. *Life Sci.* 15:1235–48

35. Lagunoff, D., Nicol, D. M., Pritzl, P. 1973. Uptake of β-glucoronidase by deficient human fibroblasts. *Lab. Invest.* 29:449–53

36. Hickman, S., Shapiro, L. J., Neufeld, E. F. 1974. A recognition marker required for uptake of a lysosomal enzyme by cultured fibroblasts. *Biochem. Biophys. Res. Commun.* 57:55–61

37. Oettgen, H. F., Old, L. J., Boyse, E. A., Campbell, H. A., Philips, F. S., Clarkson, B. D., Tallal, L., Leeper, R. D., Schwartz, M. K., Kim, J. H., 1967. Inhibition of leukemias in man by L-asparaginase. *Cancer Res.* 27:2619–31

38. Hill, J. M., Loeb, E., MacLellan, A., Khan, A., Roberts, J., Shields, W., Hill, N. 1969. Response to highly purified L-asparaginase during therapy of acute leukemia. *Cancer Res.* 29:1574–80

39. Clarkson, B., Krakoff, I., Burchenal, J., Karnofsky, D., Golbey, R., Dowling, M., Oettgen, H., Lipton, A. 1970. Clinical results of treatment with *E. coli* L-asparaginase in adults with leukemia, lymphoma, and solid tumors. *Cancer* 25:279–305

40. Capizzi, R. L. 1975. Improvement in the therapeutic index of methotrexate by L-asparaginase. *Cancer Chemother. Rep.* 6:37–41

41. Rentschler, R., Livingston, R., Mountain, C. 1976. Methotrexate and asparaginase in drug-refactory human tumors. *Proc. Am. Assoc. Cancer Res.* 17:152 (Abstr.)

42. Roberts, J., Holcenberg, J. S., Dolowy, W. C. 1970. Antineoplastic activity of highly purified bacterial glutaminases. *Nature* 227:1136–37

43. Meister, A. 1965. *Biochemistry of the Amino-Acids*, 2:621–28. New York: Academic. 1084 pp. 2nd ed.

44. Eagle, H., Oyama, V. I., Levy, M., Horton, C. L., Fleischman, R. 1956. The growth response of mammalian cells in tissue culture to L-glutamine and L-glutamic acid. *J. Biol. Chem.* 218:607–16

45. Neuman, R. E., McCoy, T. A. 1956. Dual requirement of Walker carcinosarcoma 256 *in vitro* for asparagine and glutamine. *Science* 124:124–25

46. Roberts, E., Simonsen, D. G. 1960. In *Amino Acids, Proteins and Cancer Biochemistry*, ed. J. T. Edsall, 121–45. New York: Academic. 244 pp.

47. Levintow, L. 1954. The glutamyltransferase activity of normal and neoplastic tissues. *J. Natl. Cancer Inst.* 15:347–52

48. Greenberg, D. M., Blumenthal, G., Ramadan, M. E. 1964. Effect of administration of the enzyme glutaminase on the growth of cancer cells. *Cancer Res.* 24:957–63

49. Roberts, J., Holcenberg, J. S., Dolowy, W. C. 1971. Glutaminase induced prolonged regression of established Ehrlich carcinoma. *Life Sci.* 10:251–55

50. Schrek, R., Holcenberg, J. S., Roberts, J., Dolowy, W. C. 1971. *In vitro* cytocidal effect of L-glutaminase on leukaemic lymphocytes. *Nature* 232:265

51. Bauer, K., Bierling, R., Kaufmann, W. 1971. Wirkung von L-glutaminase aus *Pseudomonas aureofaciens* an experimentellen Tumoren. *Naturwissenschaften* 58:526–27

52. Hardy, W., Iritani, C., Schwartz, M. K., Old, L., Oettgen, H. 1972. Therapeutic and toxic effects of L-glutaminase. *Proc. Am. Assoc. Cancer Res.* 13:111 (Abstr.)

53. Holcenberg, J. S., Tang, E., Dolowy, W. C. 1975. Effect of *Acinetobacter* glutaminase-asparaginase treatment on free amino acids in mouse tissues. *Cancer Res.* 35:1320–25

54. Roberts, J. 1976. Purification and properties of a highly potent antitumor glutaminase-asparaginase from *Pseu-*

domonas 7A. *J. Biol. Chem.* 251: 2119–23

55. Holcenberg, J. S., Teller, D. C., Roberts, J. 1976. Physical properties of antitumor glutaminase-asparaginase from *Pseudomonas 7A. J. Biol. Chem.* 251:5375–80

56. Roberts, J., Schmid, F. 1976. Biological and antineoplastic properties of a novel *Pseudomonas* glutaminase-asparaginase with high therapeutic efficacy. *Proc. Am. Assoc. Cancer Res.* 17:26 (Abstr.)

57. Schmid, F., Hutchison, D. J. 1971. Induction and characteristics of resistance to L-asparaginase (NSC–109229) in mouse leukemia L5178Y. *Cancer Chemother. Rep.* 55:115–21

58. Spiers, A. S. D., Wade, H. E. 1976. Bacterial glutaminase in treatment of acute leukemia. *Br. Med. J.* 1:1317–19

59. Bach, S. J., Swaine, D. 1965. The effect of arginase on the retardation of tumor growth. *Br. J. Cancer* 19:379–86

60. Burton, A. F. 1969. Effect of arginase on tumor cells. *Proc. Am. Assoc. Cancer Res.* 10:12 (Abstr.)

61. Storr, J. M., Burton, A. F. 1974. The effects of arginine deficiency on lymphoma cells. *Br. J. Cancer* 30:50–59

62. Rosenfeld, H. J., Roberts, J. 1976. Arginine decarboxylase from a *Pseudomonas* species. *J. Bacteriol.* 125:601–7

63. Uren, J. R., Lazarus, H. 1975. Enzymatic approaches to cyst(e)ine depletion therapy. *Proc. Am. Assoc. Cancer Res.* 16:144 (Abstr.)

64. Drummond, J. C. 1917. A comparative study of tumor and normal tissue growth. *Biochem. J.* 11:325–77

65. Ghadimi, H., Roberts, J. 1975. In *Total Parenteral Nutrition: Premises and Promises,* ed. H. Ghadimi, 615–23. New York: Wiley. 632 pp.

66. Schmid, F., Roberts, J., Old, L. J. 1975. Antineoplastic and toxic effects of diets deficient in selected amino acids. *Proc. Am. Assoc. Cancer Res.* 16:158 (Abstr.)

67. Abell, C. W., Hodgins, D. S., Stith, W. J. 1973. An *in vivo* evaluation of the chemotherapeutic potency of phenylalanine ammonia-lyase. *Cancer Res.* 33:2529–32

68. Roberts, J., Schmid, F. A., Takai, K. 1976. *In vivo* effects of phenylalanine ammonia-lyase. *Cancer Treat. Rep.* 60:261–63

69. Rosen, F., Nichol, C. A. 1962. Inhibition of the growth of an amethopterin-refractory tumor by dietary restriction of folic acid. *Cancer Res.* 22:495–500

70. Bertino, J. R., Nixon, P. F. 1969. Nutritional factors in the design of more selective antitumor agents. *Cancer Res.* 29:2417–21

71. Mihich, E., Nichol, C. A. 1959. The effect of pyridoxine deficiency on mouse sarcoma 180. *Cancer Res.* 19:279–84

72. Bertino, J. R., O'Brien, P., McCullough, J. L. 1971. Inhibition of growth of leukemia cells by enzymic folate depletion. *Science* 172:161–62

73. Chabner, B. A., Johns, D. G., Bertino, J. R. 1972. Prevention of methotrexate toxicity by carboxypeptidase G₁. *Proc. Am. Assoc. Cancer Res.* 13:33 (Abstr.)

74. Albrecht, A. M., Boldizsar, E., Hutchison, D. J. 1976. Folate and antifolate degradation by an *Acinetobacter* enzyme. *Fed. Proc.* 35:787 (Abstr.)

75. Albrecht, A. M., Fenton, J. J., Zanati, E., Hutchison, D. J. 1974. Folic acid deaminase as an inhibitor of growth of neoplastic cells. *Fed. Proc.* 33:715 (Abstr.)

76. Brogden, R. N., Speight, T. M., Avery, G. S. 1973. Streptokinase: A review of its clinical pharmacology, mechanism of action and therapeutic properties. *Drugs* 5:375–445

77. Fratantoni, J. C., Ness, P., Simon, T. L. 1975. Thrombolytic therapy. *N. Engl. J. Med.* 293:1073–77

78. Kosow, D. P. 1975. Kinetic mechanism of the activation of human plasminogen by streptokinase. *Biochemistry* 14: 4459–65

79. Kakkar, V. V., Sagar, S., Lewis, M. 1975. Treatment of deep-vein thrombosis with intermittent streptokinase and plasminogen infusion. *Lancet* 2:674–76

80. Kwaan, H. C. 1973. Use of defibrinating agents Ancrod and Reptilase in the treatment of thromboembolism. *Thromb. Diath. Haemorrh. Suppl.* 56:237–51

81. Rietra, P. J. G. M., Van den Bergh, F. A. J. T. M., Tager, J. M. 1974. Recent developments in enzyme replacement therapy of lysosomal storage disease. In *Enzyme Therapy in Lysosomal Storage Diseases,* ed. J. M. Tager, G. J. M. Hooghwinkel, W. Th. Daems, 53–79. Amsterdam: North-Holland. 308 pp.

82. Desnick, R. J., Thorpe, S. R., Fiddler, M. B. 1976. Toward enzyme therapy for lysosomal storage diseases. *Physiol. Rev.* 56:57–99

83. Wagner, O., Irion, E., Arens, A., Bauer, K. 1969. Partially deaminated L-asparaginase. *Biochem. Biophys. Res. Commun.* 37:383–92

84. Rutter, D. A., Wade, H. E. 1971. The influence of the isoelectric point of L-asparaginase upon its persistence in the blood. *Br. J. Exp. Pathol.* 52: 610–14

85. Holcenberg, J. S., Schmer, G., Teller, D. C., Roberts, J. 1975. Biologic and physical properties of succinylated and glycosylated *Acinetobacter* glutaminase-asparaginase. *J. Biol. Chem.* 250:4165–70

86. Shifrin, S., Grochowski, B. J. 1972. L-asparaginase from *E. coli* B, succinylation and subunit interactions. *J. Biol. Chem.* 247:1048–54

87. Handschumacher, R. E., Gaumond, C. 1972. Modification of L-asparaginase by subunit cross-linking with dimethyl-suberimidate. *Mol. Pharmacol.* 8:59–64

88. Liu, Y. P., Handschumacher, R. E. 1972. Nitroasparaginase. *J. Biol. Chem.* 247:66–69

89. Snyder, P. D., Wold, F., Bernlohr, R. W., Dullum, C., Desnick, R. J., Krivit, W., Condie, R. M. 1974. Purified human αgalactosidase A stabilization to heat and protease degradation by complexing with antibody and by chemical modification. *Biochim. Biophys. Acta* 350:432–36

90. Gregoriadis, G. 1974. Structural requirements for the specific uptake of macromolecules and liposomes by target tissues. See Ref. 81, pp. 131–48

91. Morell, A. G., Gregoriadis, G., Scheinberg, I. H., Hichman, J., Ashwell, G. 1971. The role of sialic acid in determining the survival of glycoproteins in the circulation. *J. Biol. Chem.* 246:1461–67

92. Rogers, J. C., Kornfeld, S. 1971. Hepatic uptake of proteins coupled to fetuin glycopeptide. *Biochem. Biophys. Res. Commun.* 45:622–29

93. Holcenberg, J. S., Roberts, J., Schmid, F., Schmer, G. 1975. Half-life prolongation of *Acinetobacter* glutaminase-asparaginase by succinylation and glycosylation. *Proc. Am. Assoc. Cancer Res.* 16:54 (Abstr.)

94. Peterson, R. G., Handschumacher, R. E., Mitchell, M. S. 1971. Immunological responses to L-asparaginase. *J. Clin. Invest.* 50:1080–90

95. Goldberg, A. I., Cooney, D. A., Glynn, J. P., Homan, E. R., Gaston, M. R., Milman, H. A. 1973. The effects of immunization to L-asparaginase on antitumor and enzymatic activity. *Cancer Res.* 33:256–61

96. Sela, M. 1966. Immunological studies with synthetic polypeptides. *Adv. Immunol.* 5:30–129

97. Abuchowski, A., Van Es, T., Pulczuk, N. C., Davis, F. F. 1974. Preparation and properties of nonimmunogenic catalase. *Fed. Proc.* 33:1317 (Abstr.)

98. Mori, T., Tosa, T., Chibata, I. 1973. Enzymatic properties of microcapsules containing asparaginase. *Biochim. Biophys. Acta* 321:653–61

99. Chong, E. D. S., Chang, T. M. S. 1974. *In vivo* effects of intraperitoneally injected L-asparaginase solution and L-asparaginase immobilized within semipermeable nylon microcapsules with emphasis on blood L-asparaginase, body L-asparaginase and plasma L-asparaginase levels. *Enzyme* 18:218–39

100. Fishman, Y., Citri, N. 1975. L-asparaginase entrapped in liposomes: preparation and properties. *FEBS Lett.* 60:17–20

101. Ihler, G. M., Glew, R. H., Schnure, F. W. 1973. Enzyme loading of erythrocytes. *Proc. Natl. Acad. Sci.* 70:2663–66

102. Thorpe, S. R., Fiddler, M. B., Desnick, R. J. 1975. *In vivo* fate of erythrocyte-entrapped β-glucuronidase in β glucuronidase-deficient mice. *Pediatr. Res.* 9:918–23

103. Allison, J. P., Davidson, L., Gutierrez-Hartman, A., Kitto, G. B. 1972. Insolubilization of L-asparaginase by covalent attachment to nylon tubing. *Biochem. Biophys. Res. Commun.* 47: 66–73

104. Horvath, C., Sardi, A., Woods, J. S. 1973. L-asparaginase tubes: kinetic behavior and application in physiological studies. *J. Appl. Physiol.* 34:181–87

105. Cooney, D. A., Weetall, H. H., Long, E. 1975. Biochemical and pharmacological properties of L-asparaginase bonded to dacron vascular prostheses. *Biochem. Pharmacol.* 24:503–15

106. Sampson, D., Han, T., Hersh, L. S., Murphy, G. P. 1974. Extracorporeal chemotherapy with L-asparaginase in man. *J. Surg. Oncol.* 6:39–48

107. O'Driscoll, K. F., Korus, R. A., Ohnuma, T., Walczack, I. M. 1975. Gel entrapped L-asparaginase: kinetic behavior and antitumor activity. *J. Pharmacol. Exp. Ther.* 195:382–88

Ann. Rev. Pharmacol. Toxicol. 1977. 17:117–32
Copyright © 1977 by Annual Reviews Inc. All rights reserved

ANTINEOPLASTIC AGENTS ❖6670
FROM PLANTS

Monroe E. Wall and M. C. Wani
Chemistry and Life Sciences Division, Research Triangle Institute,
Research Triangle Park, North Carolina 27709

INTRODUCTION

Since at least 1500 BC plants and plant extracts have been recognized as having anticancer activities (1). Surveys by Hartwell (2, 3) listed at least 3000 species so used. However the rational, organized study of plants as sources of potential antineoplastic agents probably commenced with the pioneering studies of Hartwell et al (4–8) during the period 1947–1953 in which for the first time pure plant constituents were isolated, characterized, and associated with the antitumor activity of the crude plant extract.[1]

This review presents a critical appraisal of the current status of plant antineoplastic agents, with particular emphasis on chemical structure and the significant features (where known) that are required for antitumor activity. This review deals only with plant antineoplastic agents of high activity against mouse leukemia and mouse and rat solid tumors as defined by the National Cancer Institute (9). All of the plant antitumor agents covered have excellent antitumor activity in one or more rodent tumor or leukemia systems combined with reasonable therapeutic indices so that the agents are either in clinical testing or scheduled for such studies. As a consequence, many substances with marginal activity or with high toxicity are not included in this review. Material covered in earlier reviews (1, 10) is not discussed unless additional information has become available since the time of the previous review.

[1]We wish to dedicate this review in honor of Dr. Jonathan L. Hartwell, who retired from the National Cancer Institute in January 1975, after more than 30 years of distinguished service during which he not only pioneered in the rational investigative studies of plant antitumor agents but also provided continuous stimulation and support to many other workers in the field.

ALKALOIDS

Camptothecin and Related Alkaloids

Camptothecin I was isolated by Wall et al from the wood and bark of *Camptotheca acuminata,* a tree which is a native of China (11). The alkaloid is biogenetically related to the well-known indole alkaloid group. The compound is highly active in the L-1210 and P-388 mice leukemia systems as well as against a number of experimental rodent tumors, including Walker 256 carcinosarcoma, Lewis Lung carcinoma, and melanotic melanoma B-16. Wani & Wall (12) isolated the 10-hydroxy and 10-methoxy analogues II and III as minor components of *C. acuminata.* The 9-methoxy analogue IV has also been isolated from *Mappia foetida* (13).

VII , RINGS ABCD AS IN I , R_4= ONa
VIII , RING ABCD AS IN I , R_4= NHCH$_3$

I, R = R$_1$ = H ; R$_2$ = C$_2$H$_5$; R$_3$ = OH

II, R = OH ; R$_1$ = H ; R$_2$ = C$_2$H$_5$; R$_3$ = OH

III, R = OCH$_3$; R$_1$= H ; R$_2$= C$_2$H$_5$; R$_3$ = OH

IV, R = H , R$_1$= OCH$_3$, R$_2$ = C$_2$H$_5$, R$_3$= OH

V, R = R$_1$ = H   ; R$_2$= C$_2$H$_5$; R$_3$ = Cl

VI, R = R$_1$ = H   ; R$_2$= C$_2$H$_5$; R$_3$ = H

Wall (14) has shown that the 20-hydroxyl and the lactone moiety found in Ring E of camptothecin are an absolute requirement for antileukemia activity. The 20-chloro and 20-desoxy analogues V and VI were devoid of activity[2] as was the lactol obtained by reduction of the 21-carbonyl. The 20-ethyl substituent is not an absolute requirement for activity. Thus, Sugasawa et al (15) have shown that the ethyl group can be substituted by allyl, propargyl, and several other substituents, with allyl being the most active. Sugasawa et al confirmed the requirement of the α-hydroxy lactone moiety for activity (15). Compounds, which can regenerate ring E on acidification, such as the sodium salt VII, and the methyl amide VIII, are also active although their activity is less than the parent compound I. Oxygenated ring A analogues II, III, and IV are highly active in life prolongation when tested against mice leukemia systems. A large number of synthetic analogues have been prepared, including

[2]Desoxycamptothecin VI was reported by Hartwell & Abbott (1) to be active against L-1210. The data quoted by these workers were obtained from a compound prepared by Wall et al (11) which Wall and Wani (unpublished data) found to have 5% camptothecin as an impurity. A later sample of VI prepared by Wall and Wani that was extremely pure was found to be inactive in L-1210 leukemia. Unfortunately the original observation (1) has been widely quoted and as the individuals responsible for *both* preparations of VI, we wish to clarify the situation.

bicyclic (ring DE) analogues (16, 17) and tricyclic (ring CDE) analogues (17) which contain the vital hydroxy lactone moiety. Schultz (18) and Shamma & St. Georgiev (19) have extensively reviewed the various synthetic methods and compounds. The bicyclic (16) and tricyclic analogues (17) are inactive as antitumor agents, indicating that factors other than the α-hydroxy lactone moiety are involved. In this connection the extensive studies of Horwitz and her collaborators regarding the effect of I and its analogues on nucleic acid synthesis are very important [cf (20) for a review and complete literature citations]. It was found that camptothecin I was a potent inhibitor of nucleic acid synthesis in HeLa cells and in L-1210 cells. Compound I degrades cellular DNA to lower molecular weight species and also inhibits RNA syntheses. Unlike the rather specific structural requirements for antitumor activity, inhibition of RNA synthesis and DNA degradation is brought about by a number of camptothecin analogues. The requirement for activity seems to be rings ABCD as in I, but the α-hydroxy lactone moiety is not an absolute requirement (20).

The antileukemic properties of camptothecin may be due to several features of the structure of this compound. Thus rings ABCD comprise a flat planar structure which may produce an intercalation effect on DNA similar to that found in the case of aromatic planar bacterial inhibitors such as acridine and proflavine [cf (21) pp. 269–75 for an excellent discussion of this subject]. In addition, however, camptothecin possesses an *alkylating moiety*. The lactone ring of camptothecin is facilely attacked by bases under mild conditions, possibly because of the activating effect of the α-hydroxyl group (1, 14). The potent combination of an alkylating moiety combined with a nucleus capable of intercalation with the DNA helix may well account for the total activity of I. Unfortunately, because of its water insolubility, camptothecin has been tested clinically only as the water-soluble sodium salt VII, which recent studies (M. E. Wall and M. C. Wani, unpublished results) have shown to be much less active than I, II, or III.

Dimeric Benzylisoquinoline and Related Alkaloids

The antitumor activity of this group of alkaloids has been established largely as a result of the researches of Kupchan and his co-workers. Thalicarpine IX is a novel dimeric aporphine-benzylisoquinoline alkaloid isolated from *Thalictrum dasycarpum* Fisch. and Lall. (22), and from other Thalictrum species; its structure was elucidated by Tomita et al (23). Tetrandrine X is a dimeric bis(benzylisoquinoline) alkaloid isolated from *Cyclea peltata* Diels (24). Both of these alkaloids showed significant inhibitory activity against the Walker intramuscular carcinosarcoma-256 (1), and after several years of preclinical toxicological studies, these compounds are on clinical trials (25).

Recent studies have defined some of the structural requirements for tumor-inhibitory activity among benzylisoquinoline alkaloids and related compounds (26). The monomeric benzylisoquinolines and aporphines do not show any tumor-inhibitory activity against the W-256 tumor system. Thus, XI and the aporphine alkaloids

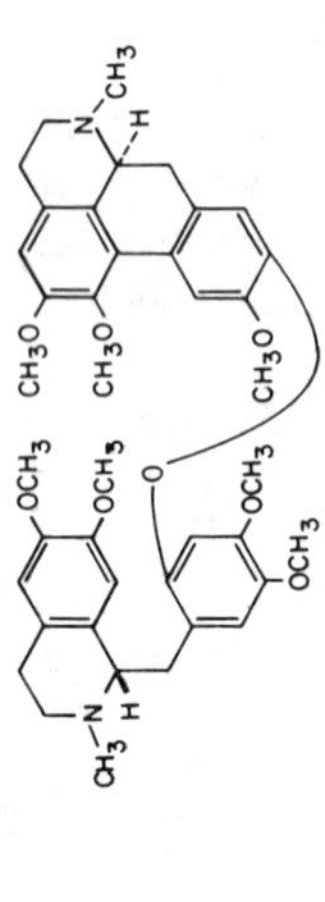

IX

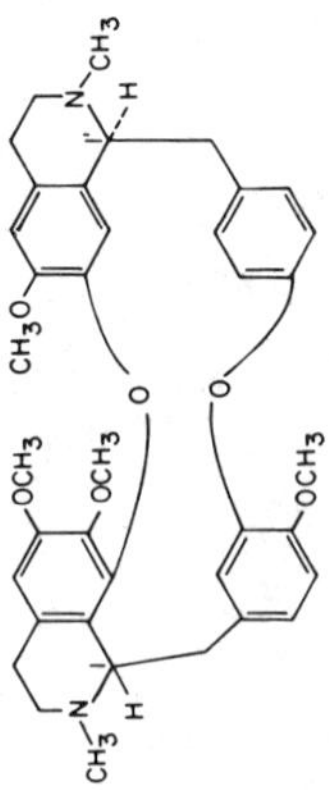

X

XI

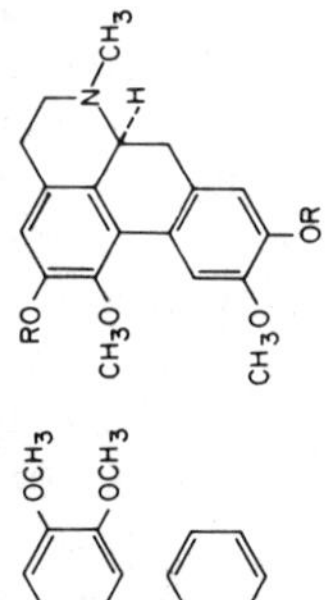

XII, R = CH_3
XIII, R = H

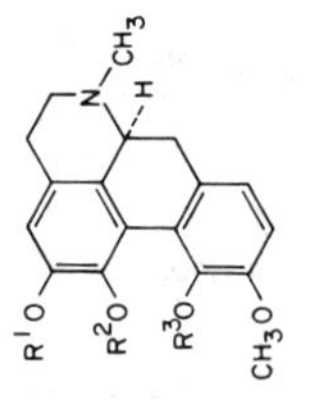

XIV, $R^1 = R^3 = CH_3$; $R^2 = H$
XV, $R^1 = R^2 = CH_3$; $R^3 = H$
XVI, $R^1, R^2 = -CH_2-$; $R^3 = H$

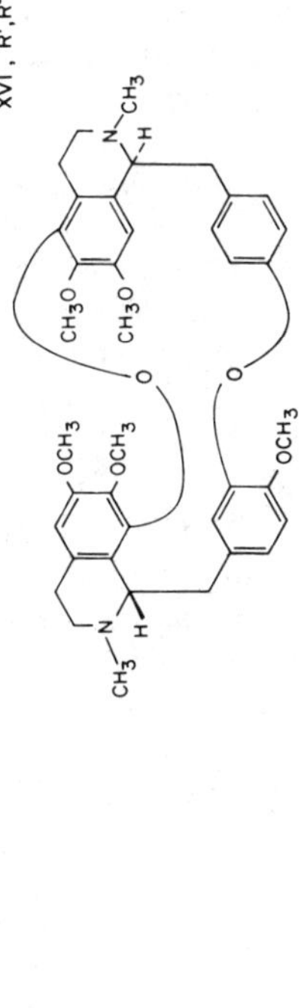

XVII

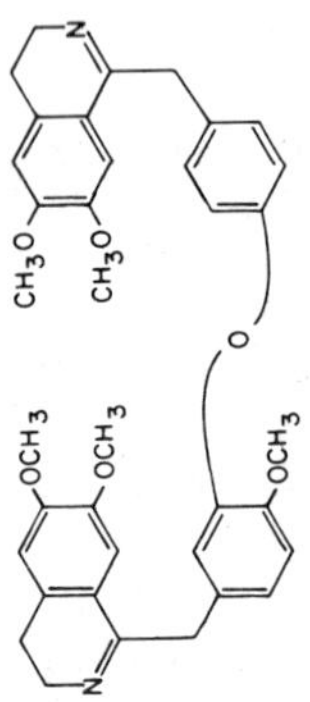

XVIII

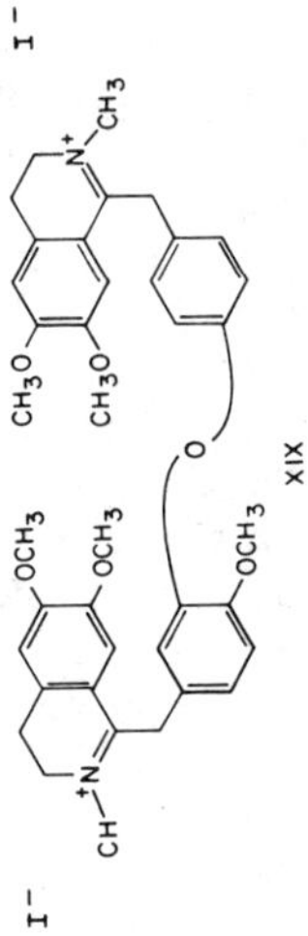

XIX

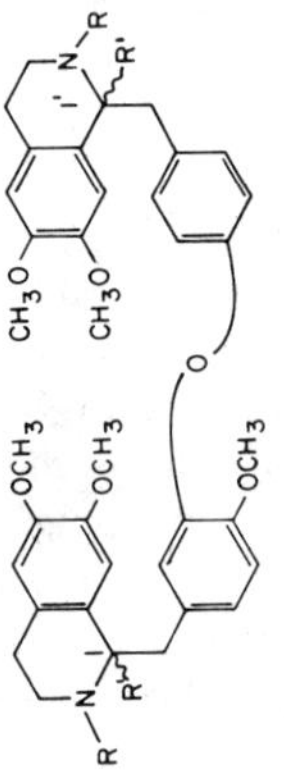

XXa, R = CH_3; R' = H
XXb, R = R' = H
XXc, R = R' = CH_3

glaucine XII, boldine XIII, corydine XIV, isocorydine XV, and bulbocapnine XVI were all inactive. Since both IX and X exhibit equally good activity, it appears that the two components of dimeric alkaloids could be either benzylisoquinoline or aporphine. Thalidaisine XVII is another bisbenzylisoquinoline alkaloid isolated from *Thalictrum dasycarpum* (27). The comparable activities of X and XVII against W-256 suggest that the size of the macrocyclic ring in these alkaloids is not important. In fact, according to Kupchan et al (26), the macrocyclic ring may not be required because *dl*-O-methyldauricine XXa is about as active as X and XVII. An alkyl substituent at the nitrogen atoms is not necessary because XXb and its precursor XVIII are both active. The activity of XVIII also indicates that stereospecificity is not required.

In view of the known sensitivity of the W-256 system toward alkylating agents, it was considered likely that the bis(benzylisoquinoline) alkaloids may exert their tumor-inhibitory activity by bisalkylation of biological nucleophiles (26). This would involve in vivo dehydrogenation to the electrophilic bis(dihydroisoquinolinium) system present in XIX. However, XIX itself was found to be inactive, and XXC which cannot undergo ready transformation to a compound like XIX, was found to be active.

Benzophenanthridine Alkaloids

Nitidine chloride XXIa was first isolated from *Zanthoxylum nitidium* (28) and more recently from *Fagara macrophylla* (29). Both XXIa and a 6-methoxy analogue XXIIa isolated as an artifact during the extraction process (29) are highly active against P-388 leukemia; the latter is also active in the L-1210 leukemia system. A related alkaloid fagaronine XXIb (30, 31) isolated from *F. zanthoxyloides* also shows excellent antitumor activity. On the other hand although sanguinarine XXIIIa and its salt XXIVa are cytotoxic, they are devoid of activity against in vivo tumor systems (J. L. Hartwell, National Cancer Institute, private communication).

In an effort to gain an insight into structure-activity relationships, a number of benzophenanthridine derivatives related to nitidine chloride and sanguinarine have been synthesized and evaluated for antileukemic activity. The antileukemic activity of four analogues of nitidine and the corresponding 6-methoxy-5,6-dihydro derivatives has been reported (32). Allonitidine XXIc and the tetramethoxy analogue XXId are active against P-388 and L-1210 leukemia systems. Zee-Cheng & Cheng (32) report that the antileukemic activity of XXId is slightly greater than that of XXIa which, in turn, shows slightly higher activity than XXIc. The tetrahydroxy analogue XXIe and the tetraacetoxy analogue XXIf are both inactive. The activity of 6-methoxy-5,6-dihydro analogues XXIIa, XXIIc, and XXIId is slightly higher than that of the corresponding salts XXIa, XXIc, and XXId. There is a marked difference between the solubility of the salts and the corresponding 6-methoxy analogues in water. Whether this solubility difference is responsible for the somewhat greater antitumor activity of the latter group of compounds is not clear.

XXI

a, $R_1 + R_2 = CH_2$; $R_3 = R_4 = CH_3$

b, $R_1 = H$; $R_2 = R_3 = R_4 = CH_3$

c, $R_1 = R_2 = CH_3$; $R_3 + R_4 = CH_2$

d, $R_1 = R_2 = R_3 = R_4 = CH_3$

e, $R_1 = R_2 = R_3 = R_4 = H$

f, $R_1 = R_2 = R_3 = R_4 = COCH_3$

XXII

XXIII a, $R_1, R_2 = -CH_2-$; $R_3 = OH$

XXIII b, $R_1, R_2 = -CH_2-$; $R_3 = OCH_3$

XXIII c, $R_1, R_2 = -CH_2-$; $R_3 = OCH_2 CH_3$

XXIII d, $R_1, R_2 = -CH_2-$; $R_3 = OCH_2 CH_2 CH_3$

XXIII e, $R_1, R_2 = -CH_2-$; $R_3 = OCH_2 CH_2 CH_2 CH_3$

XXIII f, $R_1, R_2 = -CH_2-$; $R_3 = CH_2 C(=O) CH_3$

XXIII g, $R_1, R_2 = -CH_2-$; $R_3 = H$

XXV a, $R_1 = R_2 = CH_3$; $R_3 = OH$

XXV b, $R_1 = R_2 = CH_3$; $R_3 = OCH_3$

XXV c, $R_1, R_2 = CH_3$; $R_3 = OCH_2 CH_3$

XXV d, $R_1 = R_2 = CH_3$; $R_3 = OCH_2 CH_2 CH_3$

XXV e, $R_1 = R_2 = CH_3$; $R_3 = OCH_2 CH_2 CH_2 CH_3$

XXV f, $R_1 = R_2 = CH_3$; $R_3 = CH_2 C(=O) CH_3$

XXV g, $R_1 = R_2 = CH_3$; $R_3 = H$

XXIVa, $R_1, R_2 = -CH_2-$

XXIVb, $R_1 = R_2 = CH_3$

Stermitz and collaborators (33) have prepared and tested a series of sanguinarine analogues XXIIIb-XXIIIg, chelerythrine XXVa, and its analogues XXVb-XXVg and XXIVb for cytotoxicity and antileukemic activity (33). These compounds were weakly cytotoxic and failed to show any activity against P-388 and L-1210 leukemia systems. Nitidine chloride XXIa and chelerythrine chloride XXIVb differ from each other only in the position of one methoxyl group in ring A, the former having the 8,9-dimethoxy moiety, the latter the 7,8-dimethoxy moiety. Two possible explanations for the differences in the activity of the above compounds have been offered (33). A common structural feature among many antitumor alkaloids consists of a triangle formed by one nitrogen atom and two oxygen atoms with rather definite interatomic distances (34). The O–O bond distances in all the above derivatives of sanguinarine and chelerythrine fall within the accepted range. However, the N–O bond distances in all cases are shorter than the minimum range found in active compounds (33). The same distances in nitidine and its derivatives do fall within listed values for active antitumor agents. Be this as it may, the mechanism of antitumor activity in this alkaloid series may again be due to a combination of several factors; first a flat, planar structure amenable to intercalation (see section on camptothecin and related alkaloids) and second an alkylation site in the –C–N⁺ region of ring B. In nitidine and analogous substances with 8,9-dimethoxyl substituents in ring A, it has been suggested that there would be no steric hindrance to alkylation of biological nucleophiles (33). In the inactive sanguinarine and chelerythrine series with substitution in the 7,8 position, the substituent at C-7 is in a position to block alkylation sterically at the C-6 position.

Cephalotaxus Alkaloids

This group of active antitumor alkaloids has a structural theme that occurs in a number of other active agents; there is an alcohol (usually a complex, multi-ring structure) that is esterified with a variety of aliphatic acids. Usually both components must be present for retention of activity.

The alkaloids of *Cephalotaxus harringtonia* var. *drupacea* (family Taxaceae) are a group of compounds with an unusual structure. The isolation and partial characterization of the parent alkaloid alcohol cephalotaxine XXVI was first reported by Paudler, Kerley & McKay (35). Subsequently the complete structure of this alkaloid was established by a combination of chemical and physical methods including X-ray crystallography (36–38). The alkaloid esters harringtonine XXVII, isoharringtonine XXVIII, homoharringtonine XXIX, and deoxyharringtonine XXX are minor components of the same plant.

The harringtonines which are esters of cephalotaxine and substituted malic and tartaric acids exhibit significant activity against P-388 lymphocytic leukemia over a wide range of dosage (39, 40). Alkaloids XXVII, XXIX, and XXX show greatest activity at 1–2 mg/kg, XXVII being the most active. In the same system the alkaloid XXVIII has the greatest activity at 7.5 mg/kg. However, against L-1210 lymphocytic leukemia the alkaloids XXVII, XXVIII, and XXIX show only marginal activity. The activity of XXX in this system is not reported. Cephalotaxine XXVI and acetylcephalotaxine XXXI (36) are both inactive in the P-388 leukemia system. The partially synthetic pseudo-deoxyharringtonine XXXII shows only marginal activity at 40 mg/kg. The three esters of cephalotaxine XXXIII, XXXIV, and XXXV (41) and the rearranged ester XXXVI (42) are also inactive, although XXXIII does show marginal activity at 135 mg/kg.

Based on the above results, structure-activity relationships in *Cephalotaxus* alkaloids have been reported (42). The inactivity of XXVI indicates that an ester function at C-6 is necessary for activity. Furthermore, the inactivity or substantially reduced activity of esters XXXI–XXXVI suggests a high degree of structural specificity in the acyl moiety. An α-hydroxyl group and a hindered tertiary carboxyl group in the acyl portion are absolutely required for activity (42) (compare, for example, XXX with XXXV). However, some variations in the acyl side chain are allowed. Insertion of an additional methylene group in the terminal portion of the side chain has little effect on the activity (compare, for example, XXVII with XXIX). Removal of the hydroxyl group from the penultimate carbon atom of the side chain causes a 50% reduction in activity (for example, compare XXVII with XXVIII). Shifting of the ester function from C-6 to C-8 results in an inactive molecule (for example, compare XXVII with XXXVI). It is attractive to propose that the ester function of the biologically active harringtonines not only is involved in processes such as transport or complex formation but also is a part of the electrophilic allylic ester system. The biological nucleophile probably attacks the double bond of the allylic system resulting in the migration of the double bond and elimination of the ester function as the carboxylate anion. Since the ester function is bulky, the latter process should be facilitated by the relief of steric strain. In this connection it is interesting to note that the reaction of cephalotaxine chloride (Cl instead of OH at C-6 in XXVI) with the silver salt of an appropriate half acid results in the formation of the rearranged ester XXXVI (42).

NONALKALOIDS

Groups included here are maytansine and related ansa macrolides, taxol and related diterpenoids, quassinoids and triptolides. Although the first two groups in the above series contain nitrogen, it is in a nonbasic form and hence the compounds are not classified as alkaloids. It will be seen that the maytansine, taxol, and the quassinoids all have ester groups which as in the case of the previously discussed harringtonine alkaloids is a requirement for any activity in some cases or in all cases for normal antitumor activity.

Maytansinoids

Maytansine XXXVII is a novel ansa macrolide isolated from several *Maytenus species* by Kupchan and co-workers (43, 44, 46). It has remarkably potent inhibitory activity against L-1210 and P-388 leukemias and several murine tumors at the level of micrograms per kilogram body weight over a wide dosage range (46). After preclinical toxicological studies, this compound recently has been selected for clinical trials. Maytansine is the first ansa macrolide containing carbinolamide, epoxide, and aryl halide functions. The unusual biological activity of maytansine stimulated interest in the isolation of related maytansinoids.

XXXVII , R = CO.CHCH₃.NCH₃. CO CH₃, R₁ = H

XXXVIII , R = CO.CHCH₃.NCH₃. CO CH₂CH₃, R₁ = H

XXXIX , R = CO.CHCH₃.NCH₃.COCH(CH₃)₂ , R₁= H

XL , R = CO.CHCH₃.NCH₃.COCH(CH₃)₂ , R₁ =OH

XLI , R = CO.CHCH₃.NCH₃.COCH(CH₃)₂ , R₁ =OAC

XLII , R = CO.CHCH₃.NCH₃.COCH₂CH(CH₃)₂ , R₁ = H

XLIII , R = COCH₃, R₁ = H

XLIV , R = R₁ = H

XLV , R = CH₃
XLVI, R = H

XLVII

   Recent studies have resulted in the isolation of ten new maytansinoids. From the antitumor activities of these compounds several deductions can be made concerning structure-activity relationships. Thus, an ester function at C-3 is absolutely necessary for activity. For example maytansine XXXVII, maytanprine XXXVIII (44), maytanbutine XXXIX (44), colubrinol XL (47), colubrinol acetate XLI (47), maytanvaline XLII (45), and maytanacine XLIII (46) exhibit potent antileukemic activity. On the other hand, the parent alcohol maytansinol XLIV (46), maysine XLV (45), normaysine XLVI (45), and maysenine XLVII (45) which lack the ester function have. no antileukemic activity. Kupchan and co-workers have recently shown (46) that an amino acid residue at C₃ is not an absolute requirement and that the simple acetic acid ester XLIII is highly potent. It has been suggested (45) that the ester function in maytansinoids may be involved in the formation of selective molecular complexes with enzymes. The formation of molecular complex may be necessary for the selective alkylation of specific nucleophiles by the carbinol amide and epoxide functions. In support of this hypothesis, maytansine ethyl ether XXXVII (OC_2H_5 instead of OH at C-9) in which the carbinolamide is no longer available for alkylation is devoid of antileukemic activity. Thus we may conclude that the carbinolamide moiety is also absolutely required for activity. The role of the 4,5-epoxide and the 19-chloro substituent remains to be defined. Wani, Taylor & Wall (47) have shown that 15-hydroxy or 15-acetoxy substituents do not affect antineoplastic activity.

Taxane Diterpenoids

Taxol XLVIII, a complex ester isolated from several species of the genus *Taxus* (family Taxaceae) including *T. brevifolia, T. cuspidata,* and *T. baccata,* has been shown to be a taxane derivative containing a rare oxetan ring (48). Taxol shows confirmed activity against L-1210, P-388, and P-1534 leukemia systems, being highly active against the latter two systems. It is also a potent inhibitor of WM-256 carcinosarcoma and shows considerable cytotoxicity in 9KB assay ($ED_{50} = 5.5$ X 10^{-5} μg/ml). Taxol has been selected for advanced preclinical pharmacology by the National Cancer Institute. A mild base-catalyzed methanolysis of taxol gives the methyl ester XLIX and the tetraol L. The latter is also found in the plant (M. E. Wall, M. C. Wani, H. L. Taylor, unpublished results). The cytotoxicities of XLIX and L show that XLIX is inactive and the taxane L to be only one thousandth as active as taxol.

On the basis of limited data, it is interesting to speculate that the activity of taxol is also due to the allylic α-hydroxy ester function. The ester could form molecular complexes and also act as a leaving group developing a positive charge at C-13, thus forming an alkylating center of considerable specificity. Recently the isolation and characterization of a number of oxetan-containing taxane derivatives have been reported (49). Unfortunately, biological data, if any, on these compounds are not available. Therefore, a meaningful structure-activity relationship in this class of compounds is not possible.

Quassinoids

The bitter principles of the simaroubaceae family, which are degraded triterpenoids, are known as the quassinoids. During the last fifteen years, a number of new constituents have been isolated from many genera of this family (50). Most of the quassinoids are fundamentally C_{20}-compounds with basic skeleton A. Some are C_{19}-compounds with basic skeleton B and only two are C_{25}-compounds with basic skeleton C. A number of bitter principles have been known to possess pharmacological activity and in particular antiamoebic activity (51). Recent studies have shown that certain members with basic skeleton A display antitumor activity.

The esters of glaucarubolone such as holacanthone LI (52), glaucarubinone LII (53), 2'-acetylglaucarubinone LIII (53), ailanthinone LIV (53), dehydroailanthinone LV (53), and undulatone LVI (M. E. Wall, M. C. Wani, and H. L. Taylor, unpublished information) are active against P-388 lymphocytic leukemia. However, glaucarubolone LVII, which lacks an ester function at C-15, and glaucarubin LVIII, which has an ester function at C-15 but lacks the conjugated carbonyl in ring A, show a much lower order of activity (M. E. Wall, M. C. Wani, and H. L. Taylor, unpublished information). Saturation of the 3,4 double bond in the quassinoids also resulted in a decrease in cytotoxicity (53).

While the antileukemic activity of the esters of glaucarubolone is not affected significantly by the nature of the ester substituents, that of the esters of bruceolide seems to vary greatly with the ester function (54). Thus, bruceantin LIX and bruceantinol LX containing α,β-unsaturated ester moieties are potent antileukemic agents. Bruceantarin LXI with a benzoate ester is moderately active, whereas bruceine B LXII with a smaller acetate ester and bruceolide LXIII with no ester show only marginal activity. Bruceolide and its congeners differ from glaucarubolone and

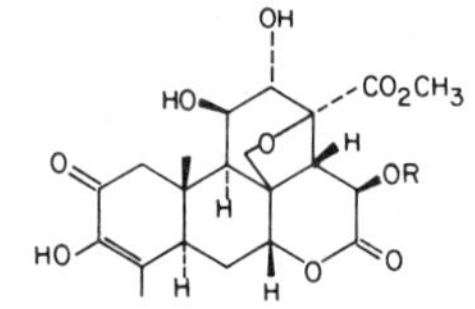

LIX, R = COCH=C—CH(CH₃)₂
              |
              Me

LX, R = COCH=C—C(CH₃)₂
              | |
              Me OH

LXI, R = COC₆H₅

LXII, R = Ac

LXIII, R = H

its congeners in two respects: (a) the hydroxyl group is present at C-3 instead of at C-1; (b) the hydroxymethyl group at C-8 is present as an ether bridge to C-13 instead of a hemiketal bridge to C-11. These structural changes seem to be compatible with biological activity. On the other hand, dehydrobruceantin LXIV and dehydrobruceantarin LXV show only marginal activity suggesting that this modification of ring A destroys activity.

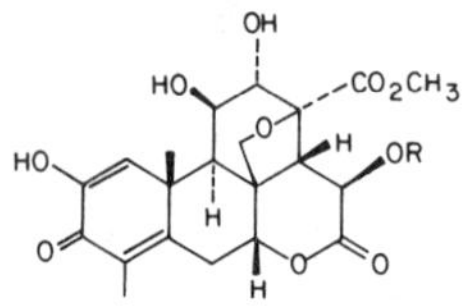

LXIV, R = COCH=C—CH(CH₃)₂
              |
              CH₃

LXV, R = COC₆H₅

The C_{19} quassinoids (50), samaderin C LXVI and cedronine LXVII, both of which lack an ester function, are devoid of activity against P-388 leukemia system (M. E. Wall, M. C. Wani, and H. L. Taylor, unpublished results).

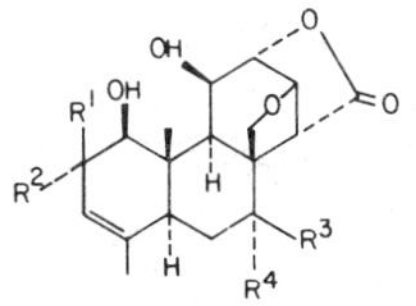

LXVI, R^1=H, R^2=OH, R^3, R^4=O
LXVII, R^1,R^2=O, R^3=H, R^4=OH

Studies regarding the isolation, characterization, and biological activity of quassinoids are continuing in our laboratory. The results obtained to date suggest that (*a*) an ester group adjacent to the lactone carbonyl and (*b*) a conjugated ketone seem absolutely required for antitumor activity in these compounds. As is the case with maytansinoids (cf section on maytansinoids), the ester moiety probably serves as a carrier group in processes such as transport or complex formation (54). The highly electrophilic conjugated ketone is probably involved in the alkylations of biological nucleophiles.

Triptolides

Triptolide LXVIII and tripdiolide LXIX are novel antileukemic diterpenoid triepoxides isolated from *Tripterygium wilfordii* (55). Both of these compounds exhibited very high activity against L-1210 at 0.1 mg/kg. Triptolide LXVIII is currently undergoing advanced pharmacological studies in preparation for clinical trials. The triptonide LXX, which has a carbonyl function at C-14, is inactive. The minor variants epitriptolide LXXI and the thiol adducts LXXII and LXXIII are also inactive (56).

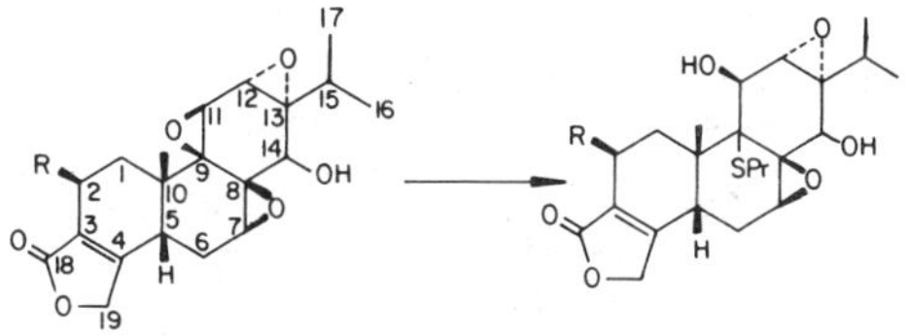

LXVIII, R = H
LXIX, R = OH

LXXII, R = H
LXXIII, R = OH

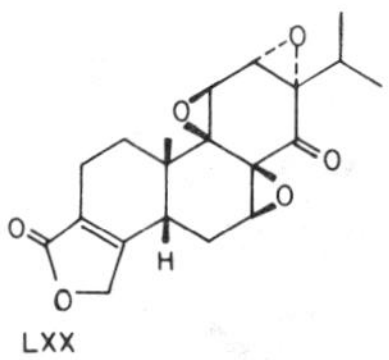

LXX

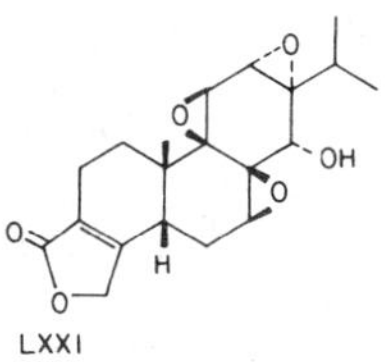

LXXI

All the above triptolides contain electrophilic epoxide and α,β-unsaturated ketone moieties which have been shown to be important for the tumor-inhibiting activity of several classes of terpenoids (57, 58). However, the active triptolides LXVIII and LXIX are the only two that contain a characteristic hydrogen bonded 9,11-epoxy-14-β-hydroxy system. The presence of strong intramolecular hydrogen bonding in LXVIII and LXIX is indicated by NMR spectroscopy. It is proposed that intramolecular catalysis by the 14β-hydroxyl group may assist selective alkylation of biological macromolecules by the 9,11-epoxide (56). In support of this hypothesis, treatment of LXVIII and LXIX with propanethiol resulted in the formation of LXXII and LXXIII respectively by preferential nucleophilic attack at C-9. Similar treatment of the 14-epimeric derivative LXXI gave no reaction.

CONCLUSIONS

The preceding sections cover the structure-activity relationships of a relatively small number of highly active antineoplastic agents of plant origin. In most cases the structural features required for activity have been elucidated. In almost every case a definite alkylation center could be identified. A common theme involved aromatic planar structures which not only could act as intercalation agents but also contained an alkylation site. Another structural feature of frequent occurrence was an ester group (which did not have antineoplastic activity per se) but which was absolutely required for overall activity. Although thousands of plants have been studied, only a small number of the total plants available have been surveyed. Undoubtedly many new agents will be discovered in the future. The current active agents and new compounds as their structures are unraveled will also serve as templates for synthetic modifications which may lead to more active and/or less toxic compounds.

Literature Cited

1. Hartwell, J. L., Abbott, B. J. 1969. Antineoplastic principles in plants: Recent developments in the field. In *Advances in Pharmacology and Chemotherapy*, ed. S. Garrattenie, A. Goldin, F. Hawking, I. J. Kopin, 7:117–209. New York: Academic. 439 pp.
2. Hartwell, J. L. 1967. Plants used against cancer. A survey. *Lloydia* 30:379–436
3. Hartwell, J. L. 1968. Plants used against cancer. A survey. *Lloydia* 31:71–170
4. Hartwell, J. L. 1947. α-Peltatin, a new compound isolated from *Podophyllum peltatum*. *J. Am. Chem. Soc.* 69:2918
5. Hartwell, J. L. 1948. β-Peltatin, a new component of podophyllin. *J. Am. Chem. Soc.* 70:2833
6. Hartwell, J. L., Johnson, J. M., Fitzgerald, D. B., Belkin, M. 1952. Silicicolin, a new compound isolated from *Ju-*
niperus silicicola. *J. Am. Chem. Soc.* 74:4470
7. Hartwell, J. L., Schrecker, A. W., Johnson, J. M. 1953. The structure of silicicolin. *J. Am. Chem. Soc.* 75:2138–40
8. Hartwell, J. L., Johnson, J. M., Fitzgerald, D. B., Belkin, M. 1953. Podophyllotoxin from *Juniperus* species; Savinin. *J. Am. Chem. Soc.* 75:235–36
9. Geran, R. I., Greenberg, N. H., MacDonald, M. M., Schumacher, A. M., Abbott, B. J. 1972. Protocols for screening chemical agents and natural products against animal tumors and other biological systems. *Cancer Chemother. Rep.* 3:1–103
10. Jewers, K., Manchanda, A. H., Rose, H. M. 1973. Naturally-occurring antitumour agents. In *Progress in Medicinal Chemistry*, ed. G. P. Ellis, G. B. West, 9:1–63. New York: Am. Elsevier. 347 pp.

11. Wall, M. E., Wani, M. C., Cook, C. E., Palmer, K. H., McPhail, A. T., Sim, G. A. 1966. Plant antitumor agents. I. The isolation and structure of camptothecin, a novel alkaloidal leukemia and tumor inhibitor from *Camptotheca acuminata*. *J. Am. Chem. Soc.* 88:3888–90

12. Wani, M. C., Wall, M. E. 1969. Plant antitumor agents. II. The structure of two new alkaloids from *Camptotheca acuminata*. *J. Org. Chem.* 34:1364–67

13. Govindachari, T. R., Viswanathan, N. 1972. 9-Methoxy camptothecin. A new alkaloid from *Mappia foetida* Miers. *Ind. J. Chem.* 10:453–54

14. Wall, M. E. 1969. Plant antitumor agents. V. Alkaloids with antitumor activity. Symposiumsberichtes, pp. 77–87. *4th Int. Symp. Biochem. Physiol. Alkaloide*, ed. K. Mothes, K. Schreiber, H. R. Schütte. Berlin: Akad. Verlag

15. Sugasawa, T., Toyoda, T., Uchida, N., Yamaguchi, K. 1976. Experiments on the synthesis of dl camptothecin. IV. Synthesis and antileukemic activity of dl camptothecin analogs. *J. Med. Chem.* 19:675–79

16. Wall, M. E., Campbell, H. F., Wani, M. C., Levine, S. G. 1972. Plant antitumor agents. X. The total synthesis of a ring DE analog of camptothecin. *J. Am. Chem. Soc.* 94:3632–33

17. Plattner, J. J., Gless, R. D., Rapoport, H. 1972. Synthesis of some DE and CDE ring analogs of camptothecin. *J. Am. Chem. Soc.* 94:8613–15

18. Schultz, A. G. 1973. Camptothecin. *Chem. Rev.* 73:385–405

19. Shamma, M., Georgiev, V. S. 1974. Camptothecin. *J. Pharm. Sci.* 63:163–83

20. Horwitz, S. B. 1975. Camptothecin. In *Antibiotics. III. Mechanism of Action of Antimicrobial and Antitumor Agents*, ed. J. W. Corcoran, F. E. Hahn, 48–57, New York: Springer. 742 pp.

21. Albert, A. 1968. *Selective Toxicity.* London: Methuen. 531 pp. 4th ed.

22. Kupchan, S. M., Chakravarti, K. K., Yokoyama, N. 1963. Thalictrum alkaloids. I. Thalicarpine, a new hypotensive alkaloid from *Thalictrum dasycarpum. J. Pharm. Sci.* 52:985–88

23. Tomita, M., Furukawa, H., Lu, S. T., Kupchan, S. M. 1965. The constitution of thalicarpine. *Tetrahedron Lett.,* pp. 4309–16

24. Kupchan, S. M., Yokoyama, N., Thyagarajan, B. S. 1961. Menispermaceae alkaloids. II. The alkaloids of

Cyclea peltata Diels. *J. Pharm. Sci.* 50:164–67

25. Kupchan, S. M. 1974. Novel natural products of biological interest. *Rev. Latinoam. Quim.* 5:133–39

26. Kupchan, S. M., Altland, H. W. 1973. Structural requirements for tumor-inhibitory activity among benzylisoquinoline alkaloids and related synthetic compounds. *J. Med. Chem.* 16:913–17

27. Kupchan, S. M., Yang, T. H., Vasilikiotis, G. S., Barnes, M. H., King, M. L. 1969. Tumor inhibitors. XLII. Thalidasine, a novel bisbenzylisoquinoline alkaloid tumor inhibitor from *Thalictrum dasycarpum. J. Org. Chem.* 34:3884–88

28. Arthur, H. R., Hui, W. H., Ng, Y. L. 1959. An examination of the *Rutaceae* of Hong Kong. II. The alkaloids, nitidine, oxynitidine, from *Zanthoxylum nitidum. J. Chem. Soc.* 1840–45

29. Wall, M. E., Wani, M. C., Taylor, H. L. 1971. Plant antitumor agents. VIII. Isolation and structure of antitumor alkaloids from *Fagara macrophylla.* Presented at 162nd Am. Chem. Soc. Natl. Meet., Washington DC, MEDI–34

30. Messmer, W. M., Tin-Wa, M., Fong, H. H. S., Bevelle, C., Farnsworth, N. R., Abraham, D. J., Trojanek, J. 1972. Fagaronine, a new tumor inhibitor isolated from *Fagara zanthoxyloides* Lam. (Rutaceae). *J. Pharm. Sci.* 61:1858–59

31. Tin-Wa, M., Bell, C. L., Bevelle, C., Fong, H. H. S., Farnsworth, N. R. 1974. Potential anticancer agents. I. Confirming evidence for the structure of fagaronine. *J. Pharm. Sci.* 63:1476–77

32. Zee-Cheng, K. Y., Cheng, C. C. 1975. Preparation and antileukemic activity of some alkoxybenzo[c]phenanthridinium salts and corresponding dihydro derivatives. *J. Med. Chem.* 18:66–71

33. Stermitz, F. R., Larson, K. A., Kim, D. K. 1973. Some structural relationships among cytotoxic and antitumor benzophenanthridine alkaloid derivatives. *J. Med. Chem.* 16:939–40

34. Zee-Cheng, K. Y., Cheng, C. C. 1970. Common receptor-complement feature among some antileukemic compounds. *J. Pharm. Sci.* 59:1630–34

35. Paudler, W. W., Kerley, G. I., McKay, J. 1963. The alkaloids of *Cephalotaxus drupacea* and *Cephalotaxus fortunei. J. Org. Chem.* 28:2194–97

36. Paudler, W. W., McKay, J. 1973. The structures of some of the minor al-

kaloids of *Cephalotaxus fortunei. J. Org. Chem.* 38:2110–12

37. Powell, R. G., Weisleder, D., Smith, C. R. Jr., Wolff, I. A. 1969. Structure of cephalotaxine and related alkaloids. *Tetrahedron Lett.,* pp. 4081–84

38. Arora, S. K., Bates, R. B., Grady, R. A., Germain, G., Declercq, J. P., Powell, R. G. 1976. Crystal and molecular structure of cephalotaxine. *J. Org. Chem.* 41:551–54

39. Mikolajczak, K. L., Powell, R. G., Smith, C. R. Jr. 1972. Deoxyharringtonine, a new antitumor alkaloid from *Cephalotaxus:* structure and synthetic studies. *Tetrahedron,* pp. 1995–2001

40. Powell, R. G., Weisleder, D., Smith, C. R. Jr., 1972. Antitumor alkaloids from *Cephalotaxus harringtonia:* Structure and activity. *J. Pharm. Sci.* 61:1227–30

41. Mikolajczak, K. L., Smith, C. R. Jr., Powell, R. G. 1974. Partial synthesis of harringtonine analogs. *J. Pharm. Sci.* 63:1280–83

42. Mikolajczak, K. L., Powell, R. G., Smith, C. R. Jr. 1975. Preparation and antitumor activity of a rearranged ester of cephalotaxine. *J. Med. Chem.* 18:63–66

43. Kupchan, S. M., Komoda, Y., Court, W. A., Thomas, G. J., Smith, R. M., Karim, A., Gilmore, C. J., Haltiwanger, R. C., Bryan, R. F. 1972. Maytansine, a novel antileukemic ansa macrolide from *Maytenus ovatus. J. Am. Chem. Soc.* 94:1354–56

44. Kupchan, S. M., Komoda, Y., Thomas, G. J., Hintz, H. P. J. 1972. Maytanprine and maytanbutine, new antileukaemic ansa macrolides from *Maytenus buchananii. J. Chem. Soc. D.* 1065

45. Kupchan, S. M., Komoda, Y., Branfman, A. R., Dailey, R. G. Jr., Zimmerly, V. A. 1974. Novel maytansinoids. Structure interrelations and requirements for antileukemic activity. *J. Am. Chem. Soc.* 96:3706–8

46. Kupchan, S. M., Branfman, A. R., Sneden, A. T., Verma, A. K., Dailey, R. G. Jr., Komoda, Y., Nagao, Y. 1975. Novel maytansinoids. Naturally occurring and synthetic antileukemic esters of maytansinol. *J. Am. Chem. Soc.* 97:5294–95

47. Wani, M. C., Taylor, H. L., Wall, M. E. 1973. Plant antitumour agents: colu-brinol acetate and colubrinol, antileukaemic ansa macrolides from *Colubrina texensis. J. Chem. Soc. D.* 390

48. Wani, M. C., Taylor, H. L., Wall, M. E., Coggon, P., McPhail, A. T. 1971. Plant antitumor agents. VI. The isolation and structure of taxol, a novel antileukemic and antitumor agent from *Taxus brevifolia. J. Am. Chem. Soc.* 93:2325–27

49. Della Casa de Marcano, D. P., Halsall, T. G. 1975. Structures of some taxane diterpenoids, baccatins-III, -IV, -VI, and -VII and 1-dehydroxybaccatin-IV, possessing an oxetan ring. *J. Chem. Soc.* 365–66

50. Polonsky, J. 1973. Quassinoid bitter principles. *Fortschr. Chem. Org. Naturst.* 30:101–50

51. Geissman, T. A. 1964. New substances of plant origin. *Ann. Rev. Pharmacol.* 4:305–16

52. Wall, M. E., Wani, M. C. 1970. The isolation and structure of holacanthone, a potent experimental antitumor agent. *7th Int. Symp. Chem. Natl. Prod. IUPAC Riga 614* (Abstr.)

53. Kupchan, S. M., Lacadie, J. A. 1975. Dehydroailanthinone, a new antileukemic quassinoid from *Pierreodendron kerstingii. J. Org. Chem.* 40:654–56

54. Kupchan, S. M., Britton, R. W., Lacadie, J. A., Ziegler, M. F., Sigel, C. W. 1975. The isolation and structural elucidation of bruceantin and bruceantinol, new potent antileukemic quassinoids from *Brucea antidysenterica. J. Org. Chem.* 40:648–54

55. Kupchan, S. M., Court, W. A., Dailey, R. G. Jr., Gilmore, C. J., Bryan, R. F. 1972. Triptolide and tripdiolide, novel antileukemic diterpenoid triepoxides from *Tripterygium wilfordii. J. Am. Chem. Soc.* 94:7194–95

56. Kupchan, S. M., Schubert, R. M. 1974. Selective alkylation: A biomimetic reaction of the antileukemic triptolides. *Science* 185:791–93

57. Herz, W., Subramaniam, P. S., Santhanam, P. S., Aota, K., Hall, A. L. 1970. Structure elucidation of sesquiterpene dilactones from *Mikania scandens* (L.) willd. *J. Org. Chem.* 35:1453–64

58. Kupchan, S. M. 1970. Recent advances in the chemistry of terpenoid tumor inhibitors. *Pure Appl. Chem.* 21:227–46

Ann. Rev. Pharmacol. Toxicol. 1977. 17:133–48
Copyright © 1977 by Annual Reviews Inc. All rights reserved

VITAMIN TOXICITY ❖6671

Joseph R. DiPalma and David M. Ritchie
Department of Pharmacology, The Hahnemann Medical College and Hospital
of Philadelphia, Philadelphia, Pennsylvania 19102

It is the best of times and the worst of times for vitamins. Through the use of modern instrumentation and techniques, research on vitamin functions has provided a mass of accurate data upon which the rational use and avoidance of toxicity should be based (1). Many physicians, however, are lacking in sound knowledge of nutrition and the sensible use of vitamin supplementation. Also, there is a growing therapeutic cult for pharmacological and "megavitamin" doses of vitamins for various diseases (2). A battle rages between legislators and the FDA concerning control of advertising of OTC vitamin preparations (3). The consumption of vitamins increases yearly in the USA and this may be one important factor contributing to the increased incidence of toxicity.

FAT-SOLUBLE VITAMINS

Vitamin A

Extensive articles testify to the toxicity of hypervitaminosis A (4–19). Ever since the curious syndrome of headache, vertigo, and diarrhea following ingestion of bear liver was noted by Arctic explorers in 1857, reports have continued to appear (4). Modern, sophisticated techniques have provided a wealth of detailed data but the exact pathogenesis of toxicity remains obscure.

There is a tendency to associate toxicity with membrane phenomena. Small amounts of vitamin A are essential to maintain stability by providing cross-linking between the lipid and protein of the membrane. Large amounts of vitamin A combine with membrane lipoprotein and then with an exogenous protein to lyse red blood cells (20, 21).

A retinol-binding protein that has an important role in transport has been characterized. It has been suggested that clinical toxicity results in hypervitaminosis A when the amount of retinol binding protein is insufficient to bind and the cell membrane is exposed to unprotected vitamins (22).

This is also true for fibroblastic membranes and for intracellular particles and the degradation of cartilage matrix in vitro (23, 24). The mechanism of increased

133

cerebrospinal fluid pressure so characteristic of vitamin A toxicity remains unresolved but one wonders whether this may not be related to an altered membrane function in the choroid plexus (25, 26). Recent studies in animals have elaborated on this issue (27, 28).

Normally vitamin A is not found in the urine. Yet, in lipoid nephrosis and glomerulonephritis, increased blood levels are found and such patients are intolerant to ordinary doses (29). The mechanism may be related to a carrier and storage disturbance caused by endogenous renal dysfunction. The anorexia, skin dryness, nausea, headache, and other symptoms seen in advanced renal disease may be related to this high serum vitamin A level (30).

Chronic hypervitaminosis A results in a cirrhotic-like liver syndrome including portal hypertension. Liver biopsy shows typical lesions (31). Alcoholic liver cirrhosis may also be associated with vitamin A (32). A detailed study of the microanatomy of the liver in hypervitaminosis A in man and the rat is available (33). Special studies indicate storage of vitamin A in fat storage cells in the perisinusoidal spaces (34).

Cases of hypercalcemia, bony changes, and premature epiphysial closure as a result of hypervitaminosis A continue to be reported (35–39). Older studies linked vitamin A with calcium and phosphorus metabolism although there is some question of contamination of the preparations with vitamin D (39). No clear explanation of the pathogenesis exists.

The tendency to treat acne vulgaris with large doses of vitamin A is attended by much clinical toxicity (18–39). Topical application is safer but still results in erythema and peeling (40, 41). Another therapeutic indication, childhood blindness, seldom produces benefit and contributes to toxicity (42).

There is considerable evidence of the teratogenic effects of vitamin A in the mouse, rat, hamster, and guinea pig. Malformations include cleft palate, fused ribs, spina bifida, meningocele, hydronephrosis, and heart and genitourinary abnormalities (43–46). A human case with congenital renal anomalies resulting in a salt-losing nephritis has been reported (47).

Interaction of vitamin A with vitamin E has been described by several authors (48, 49). A study in normal children showed no greater retention of vitamin A when vitamin E was simultaneously administered (50). On the other hand vitamin E enhances vitamin A utilization in rats. This suggests a degree of protection afforded by vitamin E (48).

Women taking oral contraceptives show an increased serum blood level of vitamin A (51, 52). The suggestion has been made that this could result in fetal abnormalities in women who become pregnant immediately after prolonged oral contraceptive therapy. However, a retrospective study of such women did not reveal increased incidence of birth defects (53).

Vitamin D

Among the fat-soluble vitamins, vitamin D, like A, is a cause of overt toxicity. In the past, therapy of arthritis with large and prolonged doses gave rise to the greatest incidence of overt toxicity, but there are now many such examples in routine nutritional therapy, in infancy, in pregnancy, and in renal disease. All relate to calcium metabolism in all of its intricacies (54–58).

Recent advances in the metabolism of vitamin D and the chemistry and physiology of its metabolites contribute heavily to the understanding of its toxicity (59). There is a growing tendency to regard vitamin D as a hormone rather than as a vitamin. First of all under normal circumstances it is not a dietary requirement. Ultraviolet light converts the "prohormone" 7-dehydrocholesterol in the skin to cholecalciferol (vitamin, D_3). This enters the bloodstream and in the liver vitamin D_3 is metabolized to 25-OH D_3 which then is transported to the kidney where conversion to $1,25(OH)_2$ D_3, $24,25(OH)_2$ D_3, and $1,24,25(OH)_3$ D_3 occurs. Little is known of the function of the latter two metabolites but $1,25(OH)_2$ D_3 proceeds to bone where it influences both deposition and mobilization of calcium and to the intestine where it controls absorption of calcium.

Of interest to toxicologists is the fact that 25-hydroxylation of vitamin D is accomplished by the microsomal fraction of liver homogenates requiring an unidentified cytoplasmic factor (60, 61). Since the reaction is not inhibitied by carbon monoxide, this system is apparently different from the all-inclusive P450 microsomal metabolizing enzyme system of the liver. Suggestive experiments indicate that the rate of this metabolism is inversely related to the blood level of vitamin D_3. This offers some but not complete protection from overdoses. The system responsible for hydroxylation of 25-OH D_3 to $1,25(OH)_2$ D_3 in the kidney is associated with the heavy mitochondrial homogenate fraction. It is dependent on oxygen, Mg^{2+}, and malate and is sensitive to carbon monoxide (62). The most important factor regulating the rate of this conversion is the level of blood calcium. High levels result in greater production of the less active metabolite $24,25(OH)_2$ D_3; conversely, hypocalcemia results in high yields of $1,25(OH)_2$ D_3 (63). A scheme whereby low blood calcium stimulates secretion of parathyroid hormones (PTHs), which in turn is responsible for the increased production of $1,25(OH)_2$ D_3, has been proposed (59). Obviously in turn the higher level of $1,25(OH)_2$ D_3 causes increased absorption of intestinal calcium which provides the inhibiting feedback loop for PTH secretion. Not all investigators accept this explanation (64). Nevertheless, calcium has the pivotal role in the production of the active metabolite.

The above metabolic scheme provides a veritable mecca for drug interaction, for antagonism and stimulation. An earlier observation showed that dactinomycin prevented the in vivo actions of vitamin D. This was presumed to be due to RNA synthesis. (65). It is now believed that the mechanism results from a depressed RNA protein synthesis upon which the rapid turnover rate of the 1-hydroxylase system of the kidney is dependent (66). In rats dactinomycin and cycloheximide inhibit the conversion of 25-OH D_3 to $1,25(OH)_2$ D_3 (67). It might be supposed that vitamin D is necessary for the decalcification of bone by calcitonin. However, no such relationship has been found.

A consistent observation is that adrenal cortical steroids reduce the elevated serum calcium concentration found in hypervitaminosis D, sarcoidosis, and idiopathic hypercalcemia of infancy (69). The mechanism is associated with decreased intestinal calcium absorption. An enigma in this case is that hydrocortisone stimulates vitamin D–dependent intestinal calcium-binding protein (70). In this regard puromycin has been reported to block calcium-binding protein and hence to decrease calcium absorption (71).

Another drug interaction involving intestinal absorption of calcium pertains to the ability of vitamin D_3 to cause increases in brush border alkaline phosphatase (72). The increase is blocked by cycloheximide, suggesting that vitamin D causes de novo synthesis of this enzyme.

Oddly, few drug interactions have been reported for vitamin D despite its tremendous potential in this regard. Hypoparathyroid patients require large doses of vitamin D to maintain plasma calcium concentrations; also, vitamin D–resistant hypoparathyroidism has been reported (73–74). These patients ideally should be treated either with a combination of PTH and vitamin D or with $1,25(OH)_2 \ D_3$.

An older observation is the amelioration of hypervitaminosis D with large doses of vitamin A (75). There does not seem to be a rational explanation for this phenomenon. It has been reported that epileptics on long-term phenytoin therapy have an increased incidence of rickets which is cured by vitamin D (76). Anticonvulsant osteomalacia also shows resistance to low doses of vitamin D_3 (76). More recently in a controlled study the frequency of epileptic seizures was reduced by the addition of vitamin D but not placebo to the usual anticonvulsant drugs (77, 78). The results were not related to serum calcium or magnesium. Another study reports that phenobarbital induces the conversion of vitamin D to more polar metabolites which are more rapidly excreted (79). This appears unlikely, because hydroxylation of vitamin D_3 is accomplished by a different microsomal liver enzyme system than that induced by phenobarbital. This lead needs in vivo work plus identification of the metabolites.

An interesting study relates coronary heart disease and a high blood cholesterol to the high vitamin D diet of a group of farmers (80). A follow-up investigation demonstrated that Vitamin D increases uptake of ^{32}Pi and its incorporation into phospholipids. There was also increase in hepatic cholesterol, total fat, and fatty acid content (81).

Previous studies indicated the propensity of hypervitaminosis D to induce nephrocalcinosis. Recent studies define the histological changes caused by vitamin D in rabbits(82). The exact mechanism remains obscure (83). In jirds, both hypothroidism and hyperthyroidism increased the sensitivity to renal damage to hypervitaminosis D. The pathology differed in the two sets of jirds, suggesting that mitochondria serve as temporary ion buffering systems which are stimulated in the hyperthyroid state (84). A peripheral study related the calcium-mobilizing effect of large doses of vitamin D_3 in anephric rats (85). High doses in rats receiving low calcium, normal vitamin D diets showed no change in serum calcium. On the other hand vitamin D–deficient rats showed variances in serum calcium when challenged with large doses of vitamin D_3. Removal of parathyroids and thyroid did not suppress this effect.

Mobilization of calcium from bone and various degrees of osteoporosis are characteristic features of hypervitaminosis D. Recent studies in mature thyroparathyroidectomized rats show that pharmacological doses of vitamin D produce osteoclastic resorption, pronounced osteoblastic hyperplasia, and proliferation of chondrocytes in the epiphysial plates (68, 86). An ultrastructural evaluation of the effects of pharmacological doses of vitamin D and uremia on bone in the rat characteristically showed increased serum calcium levels, decreased metabolic activity of osteocytes, decreased activity of osteoblasts, and an increased number of osteoclasts (87). In tissue culture, the bone resorptive activity of 25-hydroxydihydrotachysterol (3) is easily demonstrated (88).

Infants are peculiarly susceptible to vitamin D. When the diet of infants is oversupplemented, as occurred in England in World War II, the incidence of infantile hypercalcemia rises. The syndrome consists of cerebral, cardiovascular, and renal damage (89). In particular, supravalvular aortic stenosis is associated with this syndrome (90). An experimental study in pregnant rabbits demonstrated that placental crossing of vitamin D does occur. The offspring showed a high incidence of supravalvular aortic stenosis similar to that seen in man (91).

Vitamin K

Relatively few toxic reactions have been reported for vitamin K in recent years. This is no doubt because it is not available in multivitamin preparations and because no fads have developed for therapeutic use other than specific indications. In addition, vitamin K is seldom administered for prolonged periods; therefore, chronic toxicity is seldom a factor.

The basis of toxicity of vitamin K has been well established as residing mainly in the water-soluble synthetic analogues of which menadione is a prime example. In contrast to phytonadione (vitamin K_1) the water-soluble derivatives act as oxidants in the body, causing red blood cell instability and hemolysis (92). The mechanism is presumed to be similar to that of the oxidant metabolites of primaquine which cause hemolysis in glucose-6-phosphate dehydrogenase–deficient individuals. The effect is more pronounced in the newborn and particularly premature infants (93). Not all agree with the exact mechanism (94). Vitamin K_3 (similar to menadione) oxidizes hemoglobin to methemoglobin in vitro (95).

Toxicity of menadione-like compounds is dose-dependent, especially in infants, and there are now adequate data to provide safe ranges of administration with therapeutic effect and absence of drug-induced hyperbilirubinemia and kernicterus (96). In general, vitamin K_1 is to be preferred in hemorrhagic disease of the newborn (97). However, it is to be noted that intramuscular injection of K_1 into the buttock may cause sciatic nerve paralysis (98).

Vitamin K, especially water-soluble forms, induces radiosensitization. This has been used to amplify the therapeutic effectiveness of X rays (99). Another observation supports the view that vitamin K increases the analgesic effect of opiates and salicylates. This interaction has not resulted in clinical toxicity but has been used therapeutically (100).

Few other drug interactions have been reported. Obviously, vitamin K will antagonize the anticoagulant effects of the coumarins. In this regard vitamin K_1 is used exclusively (101). Too large a dose may wipe out the anticoagulant effect for days. Some have even suggested a thrombotic effect (102).

Experimentally in chicks, actinomycin D antagonized the prothrombin formation induced by vitamin K. The antinomycin D doses used inhibited the synthesis of RNA in the liver. This suggests a genetic action of vitamin K in inducing RNA formation for the synthesis of clotting proteins (103).

An interesting observation demonstrated that vitamin K is a potent inhibitor of choline acetylase (104). If true, chronic administration should result in profound symptoms relative to the functions of acetylcholine. None have been reported. Perhaps this is because reserve stores of acetylcholine are so great that only very large doses for prolonged periods could cause deficiency. It would seem worthwhile to explore this observation further.

Vitamin E

No other vitamin has been as much the target of serious investigators on the one hand and cultists and fadists on the other as α-tocopherol. It continues to be the subject of studies in humans to determine its efficacy for such diverse conditions as heart disease, arteriosclerosis, progressive muscular dystrophy, habitual and threatened abortion, sterility in the male, retrolental fibroplasia, hemolytic disease of the newborn, and many other conditions (105–115). A recent study subjected 28 adults to 100 to 800 international units (IUs) of vitamin E daily for a period of three years. On the average, plasma α-tocopherol was elevated from the control of 650 μg/100 ml to 1340 μg/100 ml under treatment. No apparent toxicity was found but neither were there any objective health improvements. Half of the subjects said they "felt better." Perhaps the only significant finding was a corollary increase in plasma vitamin A level (116).

The difficulty in dealing with vitamin E is that its exact role in metabolism remains conjectural. Most investigators agree that it has antioxidant function but do not understand its role. Many attempts have been made to assign vitamin E as a general protector of structural lipoproteins or of oxidizable lipid components of enzymes. More recently the discovery that selenium is an essential component of glutathione peroxidase, which destroys H_2O_2 and organic hydroperoxides and thus protects against oxidative damage to cell membranes, has implicated vitamin E. In this system the latter is assigned the role of preventing the formation of liquid hydroperoxides (117). In chicks it can be shown that both selenium and vitamin E are essential nutrients for protection against exudative diathesis resulting from increased capillary permeability (118). If this is an important role of vitamin E, how can toxicity be predicted on this basis? Can it be reasonably assumed that an excess presence of an antioxidant ought not to be toxic since it is only protective and is not an actual component of the reaction? It would appear to be so from the lack of toxicity of high doses of vitamin E in many studies (105, 110). On the other hand, in the rat diets high in selenium, vitamin E, and ethyl alcohol showed increased fat deposition in the liver as compared with controls (119).

In man the only significant toxicity seems to be allergy to vitamin E aerosol deodorant (120). In lower animals many toxicities have been reported, but the doses achieved have been much higher. Growth rate, thyroid function, mitochondrial respiration rate, bone calcification, and hematocrit are depressed, and reticulocytosis is increased in the chick (121, 122). Testicular atrophy leading to decreased spermatogenesis but not endocrine functions in the hamster has been reported (123). Secondary sex characteristics are slow to develop in roosters subjected to high doses of vitamin E (124). A teratogenic tendency has been reported in mice (125). Vitamin E or other antioxidants (vitamin C) injected into fertile chicken eggs causes lethality (126).

Among the few drug interactions reported for vitamin E are the increased requirements for vitamins A and D (127). Whether or not this is of clinical significance remains to be confirmed. According to one clinical study the maintenance dose of digitalis should be reduced by 50% in the presence of high doses of vitamin E (128). Oral contraceptives lower the serum level of α-tocopherol and may promote a deficiency (129).

An interesting approach to the reduction of toxicity of the alkyl mercurials is to take advantage of the stabilizing effect of vitamin E on membranes. In tissue culture of rat cerebella DL-α-tocopherol acetate showed considerable protection against the inhibition of development by methylmercuric chloride of nerve fibers, glial cells, and fibroblasts (130). Protection against ozone pulmonary epithelial damage, maintenance of embroynic growth, and enhancement of in vitro immune response are miscellaneous actions of vitamin E recently reported (131–133). It has been known for some time that vitamin E can protect experimentally against carbon tetrachloride hepatotoxicity, but recent studies show that the mechanism is not one of prevention of the perioxidation of this chemical (134).

WATER-SOLUBLE VITAMINS

Thiamin

Aside from hypersensitivity reactions, few instances of toxicity of thiamin have been reported in the recent literature. Numerous reports of thiamin toxicity have appeared in the literature of the forties and fifties primarily showing effects on the cardiovascular system and nervous system. Effects of excess thiamin on the nervous system include nervousness, convulsions, headache, weakness, trembling, and neuromuscular paralysis. Reports of thiamin toxicity on the cardiovascular system include rapid pulse, anaphylactic shock, peripheral vasodilatation, cardiac arrhythmias, and edema (135–141). The decreased use of thiamin, especially parenterally, for various functional disorders appears to have resulted in a reduction of toxic reactions.

Niacin

Reports of niacin toxicity began appearing in the literature coincident with its use in the treatment of schizophrenia, as part of what has become known as the orthomolecular psychiatry therapeutic regimen. Toxic effects of niacin observed in this treatment can be summarized as follows: flushing, pruritus, skin rash, heartburn, nausea, vomiting, diarrhea, ulcer activation, abnormal liver function, hypotension, tachycardia, fainting, and hyperglycemia (142).

The most common serious toxicities reported for niacin are abnormal liver function and jaundice (143–150). Niacin is used physiologically in the formation of the pyridine nucleotides DPN (diphosphopyridine nucleotide or NAD) and TPN (triphosphopyridine nucleotide or NADH). These nucleotides act as coenzymes for a number of dehydrogenase enzymes in oxidation-reduction reactions, which serve to initiate the transfer of reducing equivalents from metabolites to DPN or TPN. Many of the dehydogenases are found in the liver, and alteration of their activity by large amounts of niacin may explain the reports of abnormal liver function.

Niacin has also demonstrated activity on the cardiovascular system. A transient vasodilatory effect, thought to be a direct action on small blood vessels, is a well-known action of nicotinic acid. In examination of its possible use in coronary heart disease, the Coronary Drug Project Research Group conducted a study on the effectiveness of niacin to reduce the incidence of a second myocardial infarction. This study demonstrated very little benefit, but considerable toxicity, showing a greater incidence of atrial fibrillation and other cardiac arrhythmias in the niacin group than in the placebo control (151).

Miscellaneous toxicities of niacin include skin changes with alterations of color and pigmented hyperkeratosis (152, 153).

Riboflavin

Riboflavin has demonstrated very little toxicity. However, in view of the current surge in cancer research, several interactions of riboflavin with other compounds may be of interest. Riboflavin deficiency has been shown to stimulate azo dye carcinogenesis and inhibit tumor growth in man and animals (154, 155). Riboflavin has also been shown to inhibit the uptake of methotrexate into neoplastic cells (154), and to have a slight inhibitory effect in 3,4-benzopyrene-induced skin tumors (156).

Considering the role of riboflavin as a coenzyme in the forms flavin mononucleotide (FMN) and flavin adenine dinucleotide (FAD) and the dependence of folic acid metabolism on a flavin cofactor, there may be an interaction with the flavins and neoplasias yet unknown that may aid in cancer research.

Pyridoxine

Pyridoxine causes convulsive disorders due both to an excess of the vitamin or to a deficiency state (156–158). The problem as to how the convulsant effect of the vitamin is manifested is also demonstrated with the interaction of pyridoxine and the antituberculosis agent isonicotinic acid hydrazide (INH) or isoniazid. One of the side effects of isoniazid therapy is a convulsive disorder, which may or may not be due to pyridoxine deficiency or to the drug itself. It has been generally believed that these convulsive disorders were not due to pyridoxine deficiency; however, some reports have indicated that patients on isoniazid therapy who developed seizures were quickly stabilized by the administration of pyridoxine (159–161). Chemically, it is known that the two agents, pyridoxine and isoniazid, will react together to form a hydrozone which is excreted, eliminating the pyridoxine from the system (162). It is also known that the pyridoxal hydrozones are 10 to 100 times more potent as convulsants than are the parent hydrazides (163, 164). A recent report describes the use of pyridoxine in a case of hydrazine-induced coma (165).

Interactions of pyridoxine with other agents have also been reported. Among these is the ability of pyridoxine to reverse the therapeutic effect of levodopa used in parkinsonism (166). The mechanism of this interaction is apparently due to the increased pyridoxine acting as a stimulator in its coenzyme role in the decarboxylation of dopa to dopamine in the periphery, resulting in less dopa to exert a central nervous system (CNS) effect.

Other toxic effects of pyridoxine have been reported and are adequately described elsewhere (158). Examples of other effects of pyridoxine not covered in this review include the interactions of pyridoxine with oral contraceptives (167), the antagonism of quinidine-induced atrial contractions (168), and the antagonism of penicillamine used in the treatment of Wilson's disease (169).

Folic Acid

Folic acid toxicity has been reported in the CNS and the renal system. Concerning the CNS, folate toxicity deals primarily with epileptic patients and interactions with phenytoin (diphenylhydantoin, DPH). Considerable controversy exists as to whether or not the fit-frequency of epileptics is increased or decreased with the administration of folic acid. Several reports indicate that folic acid therapy causes no change in the fit-frequency of the majority of patients on anticonvulsant drugs (170–175). Others report an increase in the fit-frequency (176–178). A direct convulsant effect of folic acid has also been demonstrated experimentally (179, 180). It seems most likely that the reports showing a decrease in DPH levels and a decrease of DPH effect due to the coadministration of folic acid would favor the reports of increase in fit-frequency with folate (181, 182). Possible explanations of this effect have been proposed. One theory suggests that folic acid alters the metabolism of DPH to an unknown route resulting in rapid inactivation of the anticonvulsant agent (181). Other theories also concern metabolism but suggest an alteration of existing pathways of brain amines causing the convulsant effect (178, 183). Either of these theories could explain the convulsant effect of folic acid.

The other major area of folic acid–induced toxicity is in the area of renal cell hypertrophy. In these studies the effect of large doses of folic acid given to experimental animals caused an immediate increase in DNA synthesis and total protein content along with hypertrophy and hyperplasia of the kidney epithelial cells (184–186). It is suggested that the mechanism for this phenomenon is a regenerative process of the epithelial cells due to folate deposition in the tubule (187–189).

Other miscellaneous toxicities of folic acid have also been controversial. Mental changes, sleep disturbances, gastrointestinal upset, malaise, irritability, and excitability in normal volunteers have been reported (190). In contrast, numerous others have shown no effects of folic acid in normal subjects (191–193).

Ascorbic Acid

Ascorbic acid recently has received considerable exposure in the literature concerning its use as a prophylactic measure against the common cold. The effectiveness of this regimen has yet to be definitively confirmed or disproven (194). There has been very little known concerning the toxicity of ascorbic acid. Recently, it has been demonstrated that large doses of ascorbic acid may cause diarrhea and acidification of the urine causing the precipitation of cystine or oxalate stones in the urinary tract (195). Also, it has been shown that if large doses of ascorbic acid are taken during pregnancy, the infant may develop scurvy when removed from this high ascorbic acid environment by birth (195).

There have been interactions of ascorbic acid with other agents reported. Ascorbic acid has been shown to shorten prothrombin time when the patient is maintained on heparin or warfarin (196). Ascorbic acid has also recently been shown to destroy substantial amounts of vitamin B-12 when it is ingested with food (197, 198). This could develop into a very serious problem since many people use high dose ascorbic acid therapy to prevent the common cold. Should the person continue to destroy vitamin B-12 with this type of self-medication over a period of years the development of megaloblastic anemia may be a potential hazard. Ascorbic acid in a dose of 8.0 g for 3 to 7 days caused sustained uricosuria associated with a fall in uric acid of 1.2–3.1 mg/dl. Possibly, this could cause precipitation of gouty arthritis or renal calculi in susceptible persons (199).

CONCLUSIONS

Excessive and indiscriminate use of vitamins is associated with severe and incapacitating toxicities. This is especially true of vitamins A and D, particularly when used in larger doses, but even in special circumstances when administered in supplemental doses. The water-soluble vitamins have been virtually nontoxic when used in ordinary doses. The advent of medical fadism in the form of "megavitamin" doses has led to serious toxicities in the case of niacin and possibly ascorbic acid. Even folic acid may be toxic in exceptional circumstances. Vitamin E, even though it has been most used in so-called megavitamin doses for a large variety of disorders, has had very little reported toxicity.

There is now advanced and well-documented information of the metabolic role of vitamins in nutrition and in disease. It seems inappropriate that self-medication by the public on the one hand and pharmacological and megavitamin doses of vitamins by the medical profession on the other are allowed to continue indiscriminately without some measure of control.

Literature Cited

1. Sebrell, W. H. Jr., Harris, R. S., eds. 1971. *The Vitamins.* Vols. I–VII. New York & New London: Academic
2. Am. Psychiatr. Assoc. July 1973. *Megavitamin and Orthomolecular Therapy in Psychiatry, Task Force Rep. 7,* Washington DC
3. Drug Res. Rep. February 25, 1976. *"The Blue Sheet."* 19: No. 8
4. Knudson, A. G. Jr., Rothman, P. E. 1953. Hypervitaminosis A. *Am. J. Dis. Child.* 85:316–34
5. Wolf, G. 1969. Symposium on the metabolic function of vitamin A. *Am. J. Clin. Nutr.* 22:897–1138
6. Roels, O. A. 1966. Present knowledge of vitamin A. *Nutr. Rev.* 24:129–32
7. Persson, B., Tunell, R., Ekengren, K. 1965. Chronic vitamin A intoxication during the first half year of life. *Acta Paediatr. Scand.* 54:49–60
8. Bieri, J. G. 1974. Fat soluble vitamins in the eighth revision of the RDA. *J. Am. Diet. Assoc.* 64:171–74
9. Bauernfield, J. C., Newmark, H., Brin, M. 1974. Vitamins A and E nutrition via intramuscular or oral route. *Am. J. Clin. Nutr.* 27:234–53
10. Soler-Bechara, J., Soscia, J. L. 1963. Chronic hypervitaminosis A. *Arch. Int. Med.* 112:462–66
11. Muenter, M. D., Perry, H. O., Ludwig, J. 1971. Chronic vitamin A intoxication in adults. *Am. J. Med.* 50:129–36

12. Mickelsen, O., Yary, M. G. 1968. In *Modern Nutrition in Health and Disease.* ed. M. G. Wohl, R. S. Goodhart, 473–74. Philadelphia: Lea & Febiger
13. Marks, J. 1974. The fat-soluble vitamins in modern medicine. *Vitam. Horm.* NY 32:131–54
14. Jennekens, F. G. I., VanVeelen, C. W. M. 1966. Hypervitaminose A. *Presse Med.* 74:2925–28
15. Goodhart, R. S. 1968. See Ref. 12, pp. 213–27
16. DeLuca, H. F., Suttie, J. W., eds. 1970. *The Fat Soluble Vitamins.* Madison: Univ. Wis. Press
17. Am. Acad. Pediatr. 1974. The use and abuse of vitamin A. *Nutr. Rev.* 32: Suppl., 41–43
18. Berger, S. S., Roels, O. A. 1965. Hypervitaminosis A. *Am. J. Clin. Nutr.* 16:265–69
19. Am. Acad. Pediatr. 1971. The use and abuse of vitamin A. *Pediatrics* 48: 655–56
20. Dingle, J. T., Glauert, A. M., Daniel, M., Lucy, J. A. 1962. Vitamin A and membrane systems. 1. The action of the vitamin on the membranes of cells and intracellular particles. *Biochem. J.* 84:76 pp. (Abstr.)
21. Lucy, J. A., Dingle, J. T. 1962. Vitamin A and membrane systems. 2. Membrane stability and protein–vitamin A–lipid interactions. *Biochem. J.* 84:76 pp. (Abstr.)
22. Smith, F. R., Goodman, D. S. 1976. Vitamin A transport in human vitamin A toxicity. *N. Engl. J. Med.* 294:805–8
23. Fell, H. B., Dingle, J. T. 1963. Studies on the mode of action of excess of vitamin A. *Biochem. J.* 87:403–8
24. Dingle, J. T., Lucy, J. A. 1965. Vitamin A, carotenoids, and cell function. *Biol. Rev.* 40:422–61
25. Maddux, G. W., Foltz, F. M., Nelson, S. R. 1974. Effect of vitamin A on intracranial pressures and brain water in rats. *J. Nutr.* 104:478–82
26. Morrice, G., Havener, W. H., Kapetansky, F. 1960. Vitamin A intoxication as a cause of pseudotumor cerebric. *J. Am. Med. Assoc.* 173:1802–5
27. Eaton, H. D. 1969. Chronic bovine hypo- and hypervitaminosis A and cerebrospinal fluid pressure. *Am. J. Clin. Nutr.* 22:1070–80
28. Frier, H. I., Gorgacz, E. J., Hall, R. C., Gallina, A. M., Rousseau, J. E., Eaton, H. D., Nielsen, S. W. 1974. Formation and absorption of cerebrospinal fluid in adult goats with hypo- and hypervitaminosis A. *Am. J. Vet. Res.* 35:45–55
29. Kagan, B. M., Thomas, E. M., Jordan, D. A., Abt, A. F. 1950. Serum vitamin A and total plasma lipid concentrations as influenced by oral administration of vitamin A to children with nephrotic syndrome. *J. Clin. Invest.* 29:141–45
30. Yatzidis, H., Digenis, P., Fountas, P. 1975. Hypervitaminosis A accompanying advanced chronic renal failure. *Br. Med. J.* 3:352–53
31. Russell, R. M., Boyer, J. L., Bagheri, S. A., Hruban, Z. 1974. Hepatic injury from chronic hypervitaminosis A resulting in portal hypertension and ascites. *N. Engl. J. Med.* 291:435–40
32. Muenter, M. D. 1974. Hypervitaminosis A. *Ann. Intern. Med.* 80:105–6
33. Lane, B. P. 1968. Hepatic microanatomy in hypervitaminosis A in man and rat. *Am. J. Pathol.* 53:591–98
34. Kobayashi, K., Takahasi, Y., Shibusaki, S. 1973. Cytological studies of fat-storing cells in the liver of rats given large doses of vitamin A. *Nature New Biol.* 243:186–88
35. Frame, B., Jackson, C. E., Reynolds, W. A., Umphrey, J. E. 1974. Hypercalcemia and skeletal effects in chronic hypervitaminosis A. *Ann. Intern. Med.* 80:44–48
36. Jowsey, J., Riggs, B. L. 1968. Bone changes in a patient with hypervitaminosis A. *J. Clin. Endocrinol. Metab.* 28:1833–35
37. Fisher, G., Skillern, P. G. 1974. Hypercalcemia due to hypervitaminosis A. *J. Am. Med. Assoc.* 227:1413–14
38. Pease, C. N. 1962. Focal retardation and arrestment of growth of bones due to vitamin A intoxication. *J. Am. Med. Assoc.* 182:980–85
39. Nieman, C., Klein Obbink, H. J. 1954. The biochemistry and pathology of hypervitaminosis A. *Vitam. Horm.* NY 12:69–100
40. Bradford, L. G., Montes, L. F. 1974. Topical application of vitamin A in Acne vulgaris. *South. Med. J.* 67: 683–87
41. Kligman, A. M., Mills, O. H., Leyden, J. J. 1974. Acne vulgaris—a treatable disease. *Postgrad. Med.* 55:99–105
42. Olson, J. A. 1972. The prevention of childhood blindness by the administration of massive doses of vitamin A. *Isr. J. Med. Sci.* 8:1199–1206
43. Murakami, U., Kameyama, Y. 1965. Malformations of the mouse fetus cause by hypervitaminosis A of the mother

during pregnancy. *Arch. Environ. Health* 10:732–41
44. Robens, J. F. 1970. Teratogenic effects of hypervitaminosis A in the hamster and the guinea pig. *Toxicol. Appl. Pharmacol.* 16:88–99
45. Lopes, R. A., Valeri, V., Iucif, S., Azoubel, R., Campos, G. M. 1974. Effect of hypervitaminosis A on the testes of the rat during lactations. *Int. J. Vitam. Nutr. Res.* 44:159–66
46. Nolen, G. A. 1969. Variations in teratogenic response to hypervitaminosis A in three strains of the albino rat. *Food Cosmet. Toxicol.* 7:209–14
47. Bernhardt, I. B., Dorsey, D. J. 1974. Hypervitaminosis A and congential renal anomalies in human infant. *Obstet. Gynecol.* 43:750–55
48. Bieri, J. G. 1973. Effect of excessive vitamins C and E on vitamin A status. *Am. J. Clin. Nutr.* 26:382
49. Bauernfield, J. C., Newmark, H., Brin, M. 1974. Vitamin A and E nutrition via intramuscular and oral route. *Am. J. Clin. Nutr.* 27:234–53
50. Kusin, J. A., Reddy, V., Sivakumar, B. 1974. Vitamin E supplements and the absorption of a massive dose of vitamin A. *Am. J. Clin. Nutr.* 27:774–76
51. Briggs, M., Bennun, M. 1972. Steroid contraceptives and plasma carotenoids. *Contraception* 6:275–80
52. Gal, I., Parkinson, C., Craft, I. 1972. Effects of oral contraceptives on human plasma vitamin A levels. *Br. Med. J.* 2:436–38
53. Wild, J., Schorah, C. J., Smithells, R. W. 1974. Vitamin A, pregnancy, and oral contraceptives. *Br. Med. J.* 1:57–59
54. Comm. Nutrit. Misinf. 1975. Hazards of overuse of vitamin D. *Nutr. Rev.* 33:61–62
55. Mickelsen, O., Yang, M. G. 1968. See Ref. 12, pp. 474–75
56. Yendt, E. R., DeLuca, H. F., Garcia, D. A., Cohanim, M. 1970. See Ref. 16, pp. 125–58
57. Medical Letter. 1974. New developments in pharmacology of vitamin D. *Med. Lett.* 16:15–16
58. Food Nutr. Board, Div. Biol. Sci., Assem. Life Sci., Natl. Res. Counc. 1975. Hazards of overuse of vitamin D. *Am. J. Clin. Nutr.* 28:512–13
59. Omdahl, J. L., DeLuca, H. F. 1973. Regulation of vitamin D metabolism and function. *Physiol. Rev.* 53:327–92
60. Pondron, G., DeLuca, H. F. 1969. Metabolites of vitamin D_3 and their biological activity. *J. Nutr.* 99:157–67

61. Bhattacharyya, M. H., DeLuca, H. F. 1973. The regulation of rat liver calciferol-25-hydroxylase. *J. Biol. Chem.* 248:2969–73
62. Fraser, D. R., Kodicek, E. 1970. Unique biosynthesis by kidney of a biologically active vitamin D metabolite. *Nature* 228:764–66
63. Boyle, I. T., Gray, R. W., DeLuca, H. F. 1971. Regulation of calcium of in vivo synthesis of $1,25.(OH)_2D_3$ and $21,25,(OH)_2 O_3$. *Proc. Natl. Acad. Sci. USA* 68:2131–34
64. Larkins, R. G., Colston, K. W., Galante, L. S., MacAuley, S. J., Evan, I. M. A., MacIntyre, I. 1973. Regulation of vitamin D metabolism without parathyroid hormone. *Lancet* 2:289–91
65. Zull, J. E., Czarnowska-Misztal, E., DeLuca, H. F. 1966. On the relationship between vitamin D action and actinomycin-sensitive processes. *Proc. Natl. Acad. Sci. USA* 55:177–84
66. Tanaka, Y., DeLuca, H. F., Omdahl, J., Holick, M. F. 1971. Mechanism of action of 1,25-dihydroxycholecalciferol on intestinal calcium transport. *Proc. Natl. Acad. Sci. USA* 68:1286–88
67. Gray, R. W., DeLuca, H. F. 1971. Metabolism of 25-hydroxycholecalciferol and its inhibition by actinomycin D and cycloheximide. *Arch. Biochem. Biophys.* 145:276–82
68. Morii, H., DeLuca, H. F. 1967. Relationship between vitamin D deficiency, thyrocalcitonin and parathyroid hormone. *Am. J. Physiol.* 213:358–62
69. Kimberg, D. V., Baerg, R. D., Gershon, E., Graudusius, R. T. 1971. Effect of cortisone treatment on the active transfer of calcium by the small intestine. *J. Clin. Invest.* 50:1309–21
70. Eilon, G., Mor, E., Karaman, H., Menczel, J. 1971. In *Cellular Mechanisms for Calcium Transfer and Homeostasis,* ed. G. Nichols Jr., R. H. Wassemian, 501–2. New York: Academic
71. Bronner, F., Maddaiah, V. T. 1969. In *Symposium on Membrane Proteins,* 134–36. New York: Little, Brown
72. Norman, A. W., Mircheff, A. K., Adams, T. H., Spielvogel, A. 1970. Studies on the mechanism of action of calciferol. *Biochem. Biophys. Acta* 215:348–59
73. Ramussen, H., DeLuca, H., Arnaud, C., Hawker, C., von Stedingk, M. 1963. The relationship between vitamin D and parathyroid hormone. *J. Clin. Invest.* 42:1940–46

74. Pak, C. Y. C., DeLuca, H. F., Chavez de los Rios, J. M., Suda, T., Ruskin, B., Delea, C. S. 1970. Treatment of vitamin D-resistant hypoparathyroidism with 25-hydroxycholecalciferol. *Arch. Intern. Med.* 126:239–47

75. Clark, I., Bassett, C. A. L. 1962. The amelioration of hypervitaminosis D in rats with vitamin A. *J. Exp. Med.* 115:147–55

76. Kruse, R. 1968. Osteopathien bein antiepilepthisches langzeittherapie. *Monatsschr. Kinderheilkd.* 116:378–81

77. Rowe, D. J. F., Stamp, T. C. B. 1974. Anticonvulsant osteomalacia and vitamin D. *Br. Med. J.* 1:392

78. Christiansen, C., Rodbro, P., Sjo, O. 1974. Anticonvulsant action of vitamin D in epileptic patient? A controlled pilot study. *Br. Med. J.* 2:258–59

79. Hahn, T. J., Birge, S. J., Scharp, C. R., Avioli, L. V. 1972. Phenobarbital-induced alterations in vitamin D metabolism. *J. Clin. Invest.* 51:741–48

80. Dalderup, L. M., Stockmann, V. A., Rechsteiner de Vos, H., Slikke, G. T., van der 1965. Survey on coronary heart disease in relation to diet in physically active farmers. *Voeding* 26:245–75

81. Dalderup, L. M. 1968. Vitamin D, cholesterol, and calcium. *Lancet* 1:645

82. Arya, S. N., Das, G. C. 1973. Nephropathy after acute hypervitaminosis D. *J. Indian Med. Assoc.* 61:503–6

83. Avioli, L. V. 1972. Vitamin D, the kidney and calcium homeostasis. *Kidney Int.* 2:241–46

84. Newman, R. J. 1973. The effects of thyroid hormone on vitamin D induced nephrocalcinosis. *J. Pathol.* 111:13–21

85. Pavlovitch, H., Garabedian, M., Balsan, S. 1973. Calcium-mobilizing effect of large doses of 25-hydroxycholecalciferol in anephric rats. *J. Clin. Invest.* 52:2656–59

86. Weisbrode, S. E., Capen, C. C., Nagode, L. A. 1973. Fine structural and enzymatic evaluation of bone in thyroparathyroid-ectomized rats receiving various levels of vitamin D. *Lab. Invest.* 28:29–37

87. Weisbrode, S. E., Capen, C. C., Nagode, L. A. 1974. Ultrastructural evaluation of the effects of vitamin D and uremia on bone in the rat. *Am. J. Pathol.* 76:359–76

88. Trummel, C. L., Raisz, L. G., Hallick, R. B., DeLuca, H. F. 1971. 25-hydroxydihydrotachysterol₃-stimulation of bone resorption in tissue culture. *Biochem. Biophys. Res. Commun.* 44:1096–1101

89. Seelig, M. S. 1969. Vitamin D and cardiovascular, renal and brain damage in infancy and childhood. *Ann. NY Acad. Sci.* 147:537–82

90. Taussig, H. B. 1966. Possible injury to the cardiovascular system from vitamin D. *Ann. Intern. Med.* 65:1195–1200

91. Friedman, W. F., Roberts, W. C. 1966. Vitamin D and the supravalvular aortic stenosis syndrome. *Circulation* 34:77–86

92. Finkel, M. J. 1961. Vitamin K, and the vitamin K analogues. *Clin. Pharmacol. Ther.* 2:794–814

93. Vest, M. 1966. Vitamin K in medical practice: Pediatrics. *Vitam. Horm. NY* 24:649–63

94. Harley, J. D., Robin, H. 1962. Haemolytic activity of vitamin K₃ evidence for a direct effect on cellular enzymes. *Nature* 193:478–80

95. Broberger, O., Ernster, L., Zetterstrom, R. 1960. Oxidation of human hemoglobin by vitamin K₃. *Nature* 188:316–17

96. Owens, C. A. Jr. 1971. In *The Vitamins: Chemistry, Physiology, Pathology, Methods*, ed. W. H. Sebrell, R. S. Harris, 505–10. New York: Academic

97. Shirger, A., Spittell, J. A. Jr., Ragan, P. A. 1959. Small doses of vitamin K₁ for correction of reduced prothrombin activity. *Proc. Staff Meet. Mayo Clin.* 34:453–58

98. Willi, H., Vest, M., Kaser, O. 1959. Das hamatologische verhalten der frühgeborenen unter der einwirkung hoher und niederer dosen von vitamin K₁ (Konakion). *Gynaecologia* 147:481–92

99. Deutsch, E. 1966. Vitamin K in medical practice: adults. *Vitam. Horm. NY* 24:665–80

100. Jurgens, R. 1958. Zur analgetischen wirkung von 1,4,naphthochinonen. *Arzneim. Forsch.* 8:25–28

101. Shoshkes, M., Willner, M., Chiong, R., Palmeri, R. 1962. Oral vitamin K₁ (Phytonadione) as prophylaxis for hypoprothrombinemia in full-term and premature infants. *J. Newark Beth Isr. Hosp.* 13:95–102

102. Geill, T., Ling, E., Darn, H., Sondergaard, E. 1954. Studies on the efficiency of vitamin K₁ in small doses as antidote against anticoagulants of the dicumerol type. *Scand. J. Clin. Lab. Invest.* 6:203–9

103. Olson, R. E. 1964. Vitamin K induced

prothrombin formation: Antagonism by actinomycin D. *Science* 145:926–28

104. Wang, D. H., Koblick, D. C. 1959. Effects of menadione on active sodium transport in isolated frog skin. *Am. J. Physiol.* 196:1112–14

105. Murphy, B. F. 1974. Hypervitaminois E. *J. Am. Med. Assoc.* 227:1381

106. Marks, J. 1962. Critical appraisal of the therapeutic value of αtocopherol. *Vitam. Horm. NY* 20:573–98

107. Briggs, M. H. 1974. Vitamin E in clinical medicine. *Lancet* 1:220

108. Lancet. 1974. Vitamin E in clinical medicine. *Lancet* 1:18–19

109. Berneske, G. M., Butson, A. R. C., Gauld, E. N., Levy, D. 1960. Clinical trial of high dosage vitamin E in human muscular dystrophy. *Can. Med. Assoc. J.* 82:418–21

110. Roels, O. A. 1967. Present knowledge of vitamin E. *Nutr. Rev.* 25:33–37

111. Symp. Vitam. E Metab. 1962. *Vitam. Horm. NY* 20:373–660

112. Anderson, T. W. 1974. Vitamin E in angina pectoris. *Can. Med. Assoc. J.* 110:401–6

113. Weber, H. U. 1973. Hazards of vitamin excess. *Am. J. Clin. Nutr.* 26:1043–44

114. "Therapy" with vitamin E. 1960. *Nutr. Rev.* 18:227–28

115. Olson, R. E. 1973. Vitamin E and its relation to heart disease. *Circulation* 48:179–84

116. Farrell, P. M., Bieri, J. G. 1975. Megavitamin E supplementation in man. *Am. J. Clin. Nutr.* 28:1381–86

117. Holkstra, W. G. 1975. Biochemical function of selenium and its relations to vitamin E. *Fed. Proc.* 34:2083–88

118. Combs, G. F. Jr., Noguchi, T., Scott, M. L. 1975. Mechanisms of action of seleniums and vitamin E in infection of biological membranes. *Fed. Proc.* 34:2090–2100

119. Levander, O. A., Morris, V. C., Higgs, D. J., Varma, R. N. 1973. Nutritional interrelationships among vitamin E, selenium, antioxidants, and ethyl alcohol in the rat. *J. Nutr.* 103:536–42

120. Aeling, J. L., Panagotacos, P. J., Andreozzi, R. J. 1973. Allergic contact dermititis to vitamin E aerosol deodorant. *Arch. Dermatol.* 108:579–80

121. March, B. E., Coates, V., Biely, J. 1968. Reticulocytosis in response to dietary antioxidants. *Science* 164:1398–99

122. March, B. E., Wong, E., Seier, L., Sim, J., Biely, J. 1973. Hypervitaminosis E in the chick. *J. Nutr.* 103:371–77

123. Czyba, J. C. 1960. Effets de l'hypervitaminose E sur le testicule du hamster dore. *C.R. Soc. Biol.* 160:765–68

124. Hill, H., Hamed, M. Y. 1960. Vitamin E metabolism. *Arch. Tierernaehr.* 10:129–41

125. Hook, E. B., Healy, K. M., Niles, A. M., Skalko, R. G. 1974. Vitamin E: Teratogen or anti-teratogen. *Lancet* 1:809

126. Bencze, B., Ugrai, E., Gerloczy, F., Juvancz, I. 1974. The effect of tocopherol on the embryonal development. *Int. J. Vitam. Nutr. Res.* 44:180–83

127. Bieri, J. G. 1975. Vitamin E. *Nutr. Rev.* 33:161–67

128. Vogelsang, A. 1970. Twenty-four years using α tocopherol in degenerative cardiovascular disease. *Angiology* 21:275–79

129. Aftergood, L., Alfin-Slater, R. B. 1974. Oral contraceptive—α tocopherol interrelationships. *Lipids* 9:91–96

130. Kasuya, M. 1975. The effect of vitamin E on the toxicity of alkyl mercurials on nerves tissue in culture. *Toxicol. Appl. Pharmacol.* 32:347–54

131. Warshauer, D., Goldstein, E., Hoeprich, P. D., Lippert, W. 1974. Effect of vitamin E and ozone on the pulmonary antibacterial defense mechanisms. *J. Lab. Clin. Med.* 83:228–39

132. Steele, C. E., Jeffery, E. H., Diplock, A. T. 1974. The effect of vitamin E and synthetic antioxidants on the growth *in vitro* of explanted rat embryos. *J. Reprod. Fertil.* 38:115–23

133. Campbell, P. A., Cooper, H. R., Heinzerling, R. H., Tengerdy, R. P. 1974. Vitamin E enhances in vitro immune response by normal and non-adherent spleen cells. *Proc. Soc. Exp. Biol. Med.* 146:465–69

134. DeFerreya, E. C., Castro, J. A., Diaz Gomez, M. I., D'Acosta, N., Castro, C. R., deFenos, O. M. 1975. Diverse effects of antioxidants on carbon tetrachloride hepatotoxicity. *Toxicol. Appl. Pharmacol.* 32:504–12

135. Stiles, M. H. 1940. Hypersensitivity to thiamin chloride with a note on sensitivity to pyridoxine hydrochloride. *J. Allergy* 12:507–9

136. Effects of excesses of thiamine and pyridoxine. 1960. *Nutr. Rev.* 18:95–96

137. Mills, C. A. 1941. Thiamin overdosage and toxicity. *J. Am. Med. Assoc.* 116:2101

138. DiPalma, J. R., Hitchcock, P. 1958. Neuromuscular and ganglionic block-

ing action of thiamine and its derivatives. *Anesthesiology* 19:762–69

139. Leitner, Z. A. 1943. Untoward effects of vitamin B. *Lancet* 2:474–75

140. Haley, T. J., Flesher, A. M. 1946. A toxicity study of thiamin hydrochloride. *Science* 104:567–68

141. Eisenstadt, W. A. 1942. Hypersensitivity to thiamine hydrochloride. *Minn. Med.* 25:861–63

142. Ban, T. A. 1974. Negative findings with nicotinic acid in the treatment of schizophrenias. *Int. Pharmacopsychiatry* 9:172–87

143. Ananth, J. V., Ban, T. A., Lehmann, H. E. 1973. Potentiation of therapeutic effects of nicotinic acid by pyridoxine in chronic schizophrenics. *Can. Psychiatr. Assoc. J.*

144. Berge, K. G. 1961. Side effect of nicotinic acid in treatment of hypercholesteremia. *Geriatrics* 16:416–22

145. Berge, K. G., Achor, R. W. P., Christensen, N. A., Mason, H. L., Barker, N. W. 1961. Hypercholesteremia and nicotinic acid. *Am. J. Med.* 31:25–36

146. Christensen, N. A., Achor, R. W. P., Berge, K. G., Mason, H. L. 1961. Nicotinic acid treatment of hypercholesteremia. *J. Am. Med. Assoc.* 177:547–50

147. Pardue, W. O. 1961. Severe liver dysfunction during nicotinic acid therapy. *J. Am. Med. Assoc.* 175:137–38

148. Parsons, W. B. 1961. Studies of nicotinic acid use in hypercholesteremia. *Arch. Int. Med.* 107:653–67

149. Sugerman, A. A., Clark, C. G. 1974. Jaundice following the administration of niacin. *J. Am. Med. Assoc.* 228:202

150. Winter, S. L., Boyer, J. L. 1973. Hepatic toxicity from large doses of vitamin B_3 (nicotinamide). *N. Engl. J. Med.* 289:1180–82

151. Coronary Drug Proj. Res. Group 1975. Clofibrate and niacin in coronary heart disease. *J. Am. Med. Assoc.* 231:360–81

152. Wittenborn, J. R., Nenno, R., Rothberg, H., Shelley, W. B. 1974. Pigmented hyperkeratosis among schizophrenic patients treated with nicotinic acid. *Adv. Biochem. Psychopharmacol.* 9:295–300

153. Ruiter, M., Meyler, L. 1960. Skin changes after therapeutic administration of nicotinic acid in large doses. *Dermatologica* 120:139–44

154. Rivlin, R. S. 1973. Riboflavin and cancer: A review. *Cancer Res.* 33:1977–86

155. Roe, F. J. C. 1962. Effect of massive doses of riboflavin and other vitamins of the B group, on skin carcinogenesis in mice. *Br. J. Cancer* 16:252–57

156. Hunt, A. D., Stokes, J., McCrory, W. W., Stroud, H. H. 1954. Pyridoxine dependency: Report of a case of intractable convulsions in an infant controlled by pyridoxine. *Pediatrics* 13:140–45

157. Effects of excesses of thiamine and pyridoxine. 1960. *Nutr. Rev.* 18:95–96

158. Holz, P., Palm, D. 1964. Pharmacological aspects of vitamin B_6. *Pharmacol. Rev.* 16:113–78

159. Parks, R. E., Kidder, G. W., Dewey, V. C. 1952. Thiosemicarbazide toxicity in mice. *Proc. Soc. Exp. Biol. Med.* 79:287–89

160. Jenney, E. H., Smith, R. P., Pfeiffer, C. C. 1953. Pyridoxine as an antidote to semicarbazide seizures. *Fed. Proc.* 12:333

161. T.B. therapy. 1969. *Med. Lett.* 11:10

162. Horton, R. W., Meldrum, B. S. 1973. Seizures induced by allyl-glycine, 3-mercaptopropionic acid, and 4-deoxypyridoxine in mice and photosensitive baboons, and different modes of inhibition of cerebral glutamic acid decarboxylose. *Br. J. Pharmacol.* 49:52–63

163. Dubnick, B., Leeson, G. A., Scott, C. C. 1960. Effect of forms of vitamin B_6 on acute toxicity of hydrazines. *Toxicol. Appl. Pharmacol.* 2:403–9

164. Dixon, R. H., Williams, H. L. 1962. The toxicity of pyradoxal and pyridoxal phosphate hydrazones in mice. *Fed. Proc.* 21:338

165. Kirklin, J. K., Watson, M., Bondoc, C. C., Burke, J. F. 1976. Treatment of thydrazine induced coma with pyridoxine. *N. Engl. J. Med.* 294:938–39

166. Winkelman, A. C., DiPalma, J. R. 1971. Drug treatment of Parkinsonism. *Semin. Drug Treat.* 1:10–62

167. Winston, F. 1973. Oral contraceptives, pyridoxine, and depression. *Am. J. Psychiatry* 130:1217–21

168. Levine, R. R., Smith, E. R., Clark, B. B. 1960. The effect of pyridoxal and other compounds on the mechanical activity and the sodium and potassium content of isolated rabbit atria. *J. Pharmacol. Exp. Ther.* 128:159–67

169. Heddle, J. G., McHenry, E. W., Beaton, G. H. 1963. Penicilliamine and vitamin B_6 interrelationships in the rat. *Can. J. Biochem. Physiol.* 41:1215–22

170. Houben, P. F. M., Hommes, O. R., Knaven, P. J. H. 1971. Anticonvulsant drugs and folic acid in young mentally retarded epileptic patients. *Epilepsia* 12:235–47

171. Gibberd, F. B., Nicholl, A., Dunne, J. F., Chaput de Saintonge, D. M. 1970. Toxicity of folic acid. *Lancet* 1:360–61
172. Mattson, R. H., Gallagher, B. B., Reynolds, E. H., Glass, D. 1973. Folate therapy in epilepsy. *Arch. Neurol.* 29:78–81
173. Norris, J. W. 1970. Folate and vitamin B_{12} in epilepsy. *Br. Med. J.* 4:119
174. Norris, J. W., Pratt, R. F. 1975. A controlled study of folic acid in epilepsy. *Neurology* 21:659–64
175. Ralston, A. J., Snaith, R. P., Hinley, J. B. 1970. Effect of folic acid on fit-frequency and behavior in epileptics on anticonvulsants. *Lancet* 1:867–68
176. Reynolds, E. H. 1967. Effects of folic acid on the mental state and fit-frequency of drug-treated epileptic patients. *Lancet* 1:1086–88
177. Strauss, R. G., Bernstein, R. 1974. Folic acid and dilantin antagonism in pregnancy. *Obstet. Gynecol.* 44:345–48
178. Ch'ien, L. T., Krumdieck, C. L., Scott, C. W. Jr. 1975. Harmful effect of megadoses of vitamins: electroencephalogram abnormalities and seizures induced by intravenous folate in drug-treated epileptics. *Am. J. Clin. Nutr.* 28:51–58
179. Baxter, M. G., Miller, A. A., Webster, R. A. 1973. Some studies on the convulsant action of folic acid. *Br. J. Pharmacol.* 48:350–51
180. Spector, R. G. 1970. Folic acid and convulsions in the rat. *Biochem. Pharmacol.* 20:1730–32
181. Olesen, O. V., Jensen, O. N. 1970. The influence of folic acid on phenytoin (DPH) metabolism and the 24 hours fluctuation in urinary output of 5-(-p-hydroxyphenyl)-5 phenyl hydantoin (HPPH). *Acta Pharmacol. Toxicol.* 28:265–69
182. deWolff, F. A., Hillen, F. C., Sprangers, W. J. J. M., Suijkerbuijk-VanBeek, M. M. A., Noach, E. L. 1971. The influence of folic acid on the action of diphenylhydantoin. *Arch. Int. Pharmacodyn. Ther.* 194:316–17
183. Hunter, R., Barnes, J. 1971.Toxicity of folic acid. *Lancet* 1:755
184. Threlfall, G. 1968. Cell proliferation in the rat kidney induced by folic acid. *Cell Tissue Kinet.* 1:383–92
185. Threlfall, G., Taylor, D. M., Buck, A. T. 1967. Studies of the changes in growth and DNA synthesis in the rat kidney during experimentally induced renal hypertrophy. *Am. J. Pathol.* 50:1–14
186. Searle, C. E., Blair, J. A. 1973. The renal toxicity of folic acid in mice. *Food Cosmet. Toxicol.* 11:277–81
187. Preuss, H. G., Weiss, F. R., Janicki, R. H., Goldin, H. 1972. Studies on the mechanism of folate induced growth in rat kidneys. *J. Pharmacol. Exp. Ther.* 180:754–58
188. Hsueh, W., Rostorfer, H. H. 1973. Chemically induced renal hypertrophy in the rat. *Lab. Invest.* 29:547–55
189. Taylor, D. M., Threlfall, G., Buck, A. T. 1968. Chemically-induced renal hypertrophy in the rat. *Biochem. Pharmacol.* 17:1567–74
190. Hunter, R., Barnes, J., Oakeley, H. F., Matthews, D. M. 1970. Toxicity of folic acid given in pharmacological doses to healthy volunteers. *Lancet* 1:61–63
191. Hellstrom, L. 1971. Lack of toxicity of folic acid given in pharmacological doses to healthy volunteers. *Lancet* 1:59–61
192. Richens, A. 1971. Toxicity of folic acid. *Lancet* 1:912
193. Sheeby, T. W. 1973. Folic acid: lack of toxicity. *Lancet* 1:37
194. Am. Acad. Pediatr. Comm. Drugs. 1974. Vitamin C and the common cold. *Nutr. Rev.* 32:Suppl., 39–40
195. Cochrane, W. A. 1965. Overnutrition in prenatal and neonatal life: A problem? *Can. Med. Assoc. J.* 93:893–99
196. Rosenthal, G. 1971. Interaction of ascorbic acid and warfarin. *J. Am. Med. Assoc.* 215:1671
197. Herbert, V., Jacob, E. 1974. Destruction of vitamin B_{12} by ascorbic acid. *J. Am. Med. Assoc.* 230:241–42
198. Hines, J. D. 1975. Ascorbic acid and vitamin B_{12} deficiency. *J. Am. Med. Assoc.* 234:24
199. Stein, H. B., Hasan, A., Fox, I. R. 1976. Ascorbic acid-induced uricosuria. *Ann. Int. Med.* 84:385–88

Ann. Rev. Pharmacol. Toxicol. 1977. 17:149–66
Copyright © 1977 by Annual Reviews Inc. All rights reserved

SPECIFIC PHARMACOLOGY   ❖6672
OF CALCIUM IN MYOCARDIUM,
CARDIAC PACEMAKERS, AND
VASCULAR SMOOTH MUSCLE

A. Fleckenstein

Physiological Institute, University of Freiburg, D-78 Freiburg,
Federal Republic of Germany

INTRODUCTION

The essential connection of the basic physiological processes of excitation and contraction with transmembrane movements of Na, K, and Ca ions probably originates from an early stage of cellular evolution. Despite innumerable modifications the fundamental processes that developed in the ocean have not undergone major changes during the course of development of higher forms of animal life. Thus in a wide variety of excitable cells the transmembrane exchange of the monovalent marine cations Na and K can be considered the substantial basis of bioelectric membrane activity, whereas Ca ions are required as mediators when, by this superficial process, intracellular reactions such as muscular contraction, glandular secretion, or liberation of transmitter substances are initiated (1, 2). Ca ions can exert this messenger function either in a primitive way, by penetrating into the intracellular space across the depolarized cell membrane or, at a more advanced stage of evolution, by being released from intracellularly located endoplasmic stores.

As to contractile tissues, the development of large endoplasmic Ca pools is most obvious in skeletal muscle, whereas myocardial fibers and, particularly, smooth muscle cells are less specialized in this respect. The natural consequences are as follows:

1. Excitation-contraction coupling of skeletal muscle is practically insensitive to changes in extracellular Ca concentration or transmembrane Ca conductivity since, here, intracellular stores provide sufficient quantities of Ca to guarantee full activation of the contractile system. Probably for this reason excitation-contrac-

tion coupling of skeletal muscle is also rather resistant to pharmacological interventions. Therefore, skeletal muscle is not discussed further in this article.

2. Myocardial and smooth muscle contractility, on the other hand, is much more susceptible to variations in environmental Ca or to pharmacological agents that affect transmembrane Ca supply, because the intracellular Ca stores of myocardial and smooth muscle cells are of rather limited capacity so that they have to be rapidly refilled from extracellular sources during mechanical activity.

3. The sudden inward movement of Ca ions across the excited myocardial or smooth muscle cell membranes is "electrogenic." This means that Ca ions, apart from Na and K, necessarily contribute to the changes in membrane potential during cardiac or smooth muscle activity. Under special conditions Ca ions may even substitute the Na ions as transmembrane charge carriers in the electrogenesis of action potential.

In general, however, there is a clear functional differentiation. For instance, in excited mammalian myocardial fibers the influxes of Na and Ca obviously use separate transmembrane carrier systems, a so-called *fast channel* for Na and a *slow channel* for Ca (3–5). In substantiating these observations it has been shown in our laboratory that, by a selective drug action on one of these two channels, either the particularly Na-dependent excitation phenomena or the strictly Ca-dependent contraction processes can be specifically modified. For instance, some local anesthetics (antiarrhythmic or antifibrillatory drugs such as procaine, procaine amide, lidocaine, or quinidine) predominantly inhibit the Na influx (6, 7). Substances of this type primarily reduce myocardial excitability. On the other hand, it turned out that the new group of organic Ca-antagonists [verapamil = Isoptin®, Iproveratril (8, 9), D 600 (10), nifedipine (11) etc.] first investigated in our laboratory selectively restricts myocardial contractility, because they block the slow channel (7). This article concentrates particularly on these agents. Opposite effects are exerted by sympathetic β-receptor stimulating agents [epinephrine (12), norepinephrine, isoproterenol]. These drugs selectively increase the transmembrane Ca inward current during cardiac excitation, thus augmenting contractile force without major changes in the action potentials (13, 14).

All the facts mentioned indicate that, related to the slow channel, there is indeed a special pharmacology of Ca in heart muscle. The same is true, according to our results, of practically all types of smooth muscle cells. Here the Ca-antagonistic inhibitors of excitation-contraction coupling act as powerful musculotropic relaxants. By this basic action they exert outstanding vasodilator effects in coronary and systemic circulation (15–16) as well as broncholytic and tocolytic activities (17–19). Although Ca-dependent excitation-secretion coupling is out of the scope of this article, it is noteworthy that, here too, the Ca-antagonistic inhibitors of excitation-contraction coupling proved to be surprisingly effective. Thus, in experiments on isolated tissues or perfused organs, suitably high concentrations of verapamil or D 600 specifically block the release of oxytocin and vasopressin from the depolarized neurohypophysis (20, 21) or of insulin from excited B-cells in the islets of Langerhans (22, 23). Extra calcium easily restores the secretory function even in the presence of the inhibitors. Verapamil also interferes specifically with pituitary Ca uptake following in vitro depolarization, and thereby suppresses secretion of ACTH, GH, and TSH (24).

The present article can, of course, not cover more than a small section of this wide field. Therefore, it focuses on only a few important topics: the key-role of Ca ions in the function of heart and vascular smooth muscle, and on the special effects of drugs that antagonize or potentiate these Ca actions.

BASIC INTERACTIONS OF CA AND DRUGS IN CARDIAC ENERGY METABOLISM

The important role of Ca in sustaining myocardial contractility was first appreciated in 1882 by Sidney Ringer (25). He found on isolated frog hearts that Ca-free saline leads to cardiac arrest. As reported later by Mines in 1913, Ca withdrawal primarily impairs mechanical performance, whereas the bioelectric process of ventricular excitation may persist (26). Overwhelming evidence has accumulated in the last two decades that Ca ions are required during excitation to activate the biochemical processes that utilize ATP for contraction. Obviously the rapid rise in free intracellular Ca, resulting from the increased transmembrane Ca influx and a simultaneous liberation of Ca from endoplasmic stores, initiates the splitting of ATP by the Ca-dependent ATPase of the myofibrils so that phosphate-bond energy is transformed into mechanical work. Therefore, contractility is reversibly lost upon Ca withdrawal. As directly shown on isolated frog muscles (27) and beating rabbit auricles (28) the Ca-deficient myocardium exhibits a striking insufficiency in utilizing its high-energy phosphate compounds in the state of excitation. But after addition of Ca, high-energy phosphate consumption is normalized. If, on the other hand, the extracellular Ca concentration is increased above normal, more Ca is taken up by the beating heart so that both splitting of high-energy phosphates and contractility are potentiated. In fact, Ca ions not only trigger the contractile process but also control quantitatively the output of mechanical tension by regulating the amount of ATP that is metabolized during activity (8, 9, 27, 29, 30).

The splitting of ATP will, in turn, give rise to intensified glycolytic and oxidative recovery processes which have to refill, thereafter, the high-energy phosphate stores. This explains that the whole chain of metabolic reactions following contraction is "Ca-sensitive." Thus alterations in the extracellular Ca concentration generally lead to parallel changes in the following three parameters:

(a) the amount of ATP consumed by the contractile system,
(b) the magnitude of mechanical tension developed, and
(c) the extra-uptake of oxygen related to the contractile force generated.
In contrast, the basic respiration rate of the resting myocardium is rather irresponsive to Ca (8, 9, 27, 29).

The determinantal function of Ca in cardiac activity metabolism becomes particularly evident by virtue of the fact that many substances with a positive- or negative-inotropic action on heart muscle exert their influence either by enhancing the Ca effect on utilization of high-energy phosphates, or by interfering with it. This applies, for instance, to β-adrenergic catecholamines (12, 13) and cardiac glycosides (31) which clearly increase, though by different mechanisms, the availability of Ca to the contractile system. In fact, upon administration of these drugs to isolated atria or papillary muscles there is a parallel rise in ATP consumption, contractile force, and oxygen uptake above resting level. Conversely, under the influence of Ca-antagonistic compounds the splitting of ATP, the contractile energy expenditure, and oxygen requirement of the beating heart are lowered (8, 9, 11, 13, 27–29, 32). However, even high doses do not change the basic respiration rate of the arrested myocardium. Hence, the oxygen-saving effects of Ca-antagonistic agents are only due to a restriction of cardiac activity metabolism in which Ca ions play the key role, whereas all other ATP-consuming reactions that are not connected with mechanical activity are insensitive to these drugs.

The restriction of extra-oxygen consumption during activity by the Ca-antagonistic agents listed in Figure 1 is linear to the decrease in isometric peak tension (13, 32, 33). As shown in experiments on isolated myocardial tissue, high concentrations of Ca-antagonistic drugs, just like complete Ca withdrawal, can totally suppress myocardial contractility (9, 13, 30, 33) and lower oxygen consumption even to resting level (13, 32, 33). However, with the relatively small doses applied in human therapy an only moderate reduction of cardiac work and oxygen demand is attainable. Furthermore, on the heart in situ, the cardiodepressant action of Ca-antagonistic compounds is to some extent self-controlled because, each time an unproportionate fall in arterial blood pressure occurs, a reflex release of endogenous sympathetic transmitters is elicited. This can partially neutralize the drug-induced cardiac inhibition because, unlike β-receptor blocking agents, the Ca-antagonistic substances do not abolish the responsiveness of the heart to β-adrenergic catecholamines (13, 29, 30, 34, 35). Thus the new Ca-antagonistic inhibitors of excitation-contraction coupling are safe drugs. They are widely used in Europe for the treatment of patients with a hyperkinetic heart function or coronary heart disease (36–43). Here a certain restriction of cardiac activity metabolism may be helpful to reestablish a suitable balance between the reduced coronary oxygen supply and the actual cardiac oxygen requirement. In this respect the Ca-antagonistic compounds have the same beneficial influence in patients with angina pectoris as the adrenergic β-receptor blocking agents do, even though the mode of action on the myocardial fiber membrane is different.

Ca-antagonistic substances interfere directly with the transmembrane Ca supply, whereas β-blocking agents reduce the transmembrane Ca influx indirectly by neutralizing the promoter effects of β-adrenergic catecholamines on transmembrane Ca uptake. Needless to say, eventually, both Ca-antagonists and β-receptor blocking agents lower Ca-dependent splitting of ATP, contractile tension, and oxygen requirement of heart muscle according to the same basic principle. But only the Ca-antagonistic compounds, by interfering with excitation-contraction coupling of vascular smooth muscle, offer the therapeutic advantage of a concomitant vasodilator action on coronary and systemic circulation comparable to that exerted by nitrites.

The ability of verapamil to reduce the size of experimental myocardial infarction (44, 45) is probably due to both an oxygen-saving effect and to circulatory improvement. Moreover it could be demonstrated in our laboratory that Ca-antagonistic compounds such as verapamil, D 600, or prenylamine are also capable of protecting the heart against noncoronarogenic myocardial necrotization. Since intracellular Ca overload proved to be the decisive factor in the pathogenesis of noncoronarogenic

Prenylamine
(Segontin)

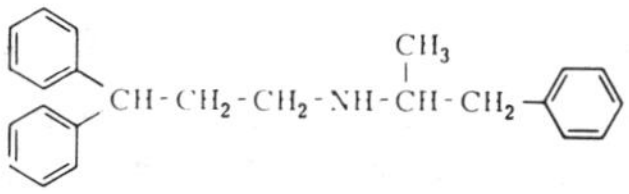

Fendiline
(Sensit)

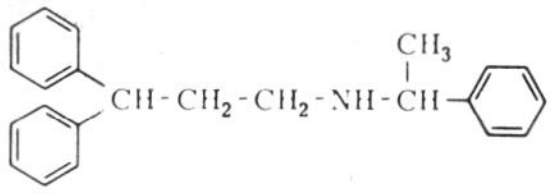

Verapamil
(Isoptin, Iproveratril)

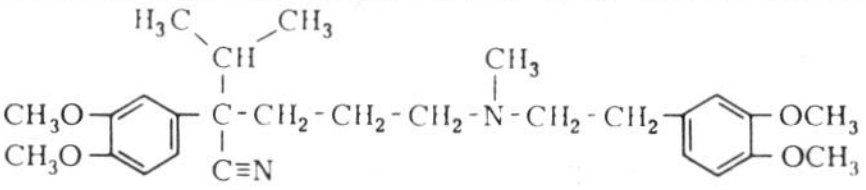

Compound D600

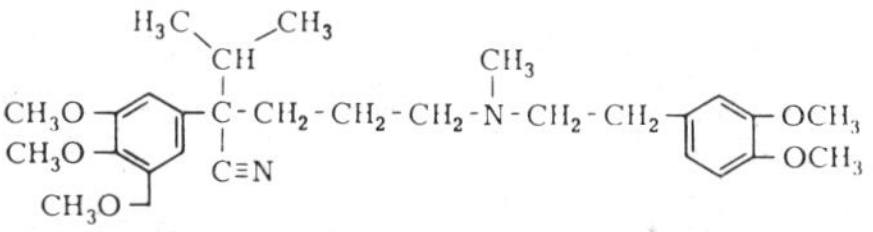

Nifedipine
(Adalat, Bay a1040)

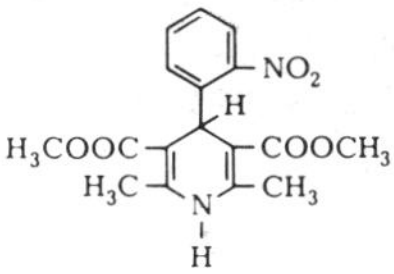

Diltiazem
(Herbesser)

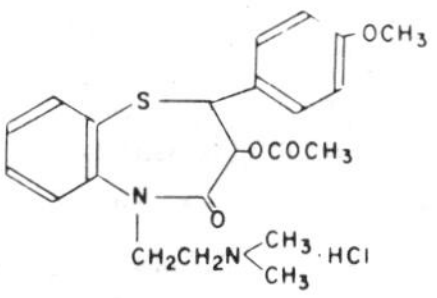

Perhexiline
(Pexid)

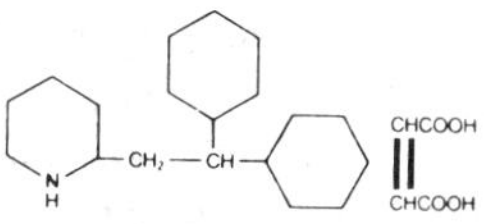

Figure 1 Ca-antagonistic inhibitors of excitation-contraction coupling in mammalian myocardium and vascular smooth muscle.

154   FLECKENSTEIN

myocardial lesions, these Ca-antagonists, by inhibiting excessive Ca uptake, neutralize the cardiotoxic effects of large overdoses of β-adrenergic catecholamines, vitamin D, dihydrotachysterol etc [see (13, 33)]. Similarly, the development of
spontaneous necrotization in cardiomyopathic hamster hearts could be prevented
by long-term treatment with verapamil (46, 47).

BIOPHYSICAL MEMBRANE EFFECTS OF CA-ANTAGONISTIC
AND CA-SYNERGISTIC DRUGS IN HEART MUSCLE

Evidence indicating that excitation-contraction coupling of the mammalian myocardium can be blocked in vitro and in vivo by pharmacological means was first
presented in 1964 by Fleckenstein (8). He reported that two new compounds,
namely Isoptin (= iproveratril, later given the generic name verapamil) and Segon-
tin® (prenylamine) as well as high concentrations of certain adrenergic β-receptor
blocking agents and barbituric acid derivatives mimic the cardiac effects of Ca
withdrawal in that these substances

(a) diminish contractile force without a major change in action potential,
(b) reduce high-energy phosphate utilization of the contractile system,
(c) lower extra-oxygen consumption during activity,
(d) are easily neutralized by administration of additional Ca, β-adrenergic cate-
    cholamines, or cardiac glycosides.

In an extensive search for other Ca-antagonistic inhibitors of this type, a considerable number of substances that also meet these criteria were found in our laboratory.
The Ca-antagonistic compounds can be classified as specific and nonspecific. In the
group of nonspecific inhibitors, Ca-antagonism is merely a side effect which becomes
apparent only if high doses are administered. For instance, the well-known cardiodepressant action of overdoses of barbiturates or, particularly, of certain β-recep-
tor blocking agents such as dichloroisoproterenol, pronethalol, or propranolol is due
to direct interference with Ca-dependent excitation-contraction coupling (9, 29, 30,
33).
    Much more interesting, however, is the family of Ca-antagonistic drugs of the
verapamil type which are capable, according to our observations, of blocking excitation-contraction coupling specifically (see Figure 1). Specificity means that the
Ca-antagonistic action is so predominant that other pharmacodynamic properties,
at least in a reasonable dosage range, are more or less negligible. Apart from
verapamil, compound D 600 [a methoxy-derivative of verapamil (10, 13)], nifedipine
[Bay at 1040, Adalat (11, 13)], and diltiazem (33, 48) proved to be the most specific
and powerful Ca-antagonists. An exemplary experiment is shown in Figure 2. Here,
contractility of an isolated guinea pig papillary muscle was completely abolished by
a large dose of verapamil (30). But resting potential as well as the action potential
parameters such as upstroke velocity and height of the overshoot, indicating the
transmembrane Na influx across the fast channel, remained practically unchanged
(13, 30, 33). Only the plateau of action potential appears to be slightly abbreviated
by verapamil because Ca ions cannot continue to contribute to the maintenance of

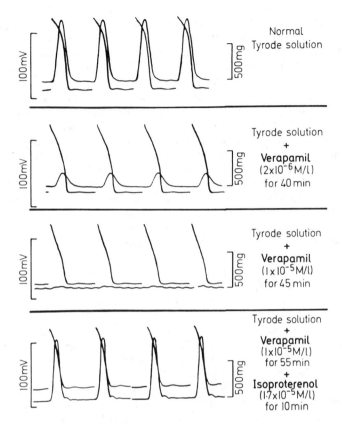

Figure 2 Selective loss of cardiac contractility under the influence of a high overdose of verapamil, and the reversal of this effect by isoproterenol. Experiments on an electrically driven (2 shocks/sec) isolated papillary muscle of a guinea pig [From A. Fleckenstein (30)].

depolarization during the late phase of the plateau when the transmembrane Ca conductivity has been blocked.

The selective inhibition of the slow channel following administration of verapamil and compound D 600 can be directly visualized by separate measurements of the transmembrane Na and Ca currents on ventricular trabeculae of cats with the use of a special voltage clamp technique (7). In fact, verapamil and D 600 produce a drastic reduction in transmembrane Ca conductivity just in the dosage range that suppresses contractile performance, whereas the fast Na current is not altered (7). The inhibitory effects of verapamil on Ca influx and contractile tension can be rapidly overcome by addition of excess Ca or isoproterenol, which is most effective among the β-adrenergic catecholamines tested (8, 9, 33). However, the possibility of controlling contractile force by acting on the Ca channel is lost in skinned myocardial fibers which we have prepared by glycerin water extraction or according to Winegrad's technique (49). In such skinned fibers the Ca-antagonistic compounds produce no inhibition when contraction is directly induced by addition of ATP and Ca. This means that the Ca-antagonistic drugs lose their power if the Ca ions have free access to the myofibrils where ATP is split. Hence there is no direct effect of Ca-antagonistic compounds on myofibrillar ATPase.

Interestingly enough the divalent strontium (Sr) and barium (Ba) ions, which are capable of replacing Ca in excitation-contraction coupling, also use the slow channel when they penetrate into the myocardial fibers (50). This implies that a blockade of the slow channel produced by Ca-antagonistic agents also abolishes the influxes of Sr and Ba provided that the sarcolemma membrane is still intact. Nickel, cobalt, or manganese ions, on the other hand, block the slow channel by themselves because they probably compete with Ca, Sr, and Ba for certain active sites in this particular carrier system (51). Accordingly, nickel and cobalt ions selectively suppress excitation-contraction coupling of mammalian myocardium as found by us in 1965 (52). But again Ni, Co, and Mn have no direct inhibitory effect on the contractile system itself [for more details concerning the basic myocardial effects of Ca-antagonists see (13, 33)].

There is no indication that the Ca-antagonistic inhibitors of excitation-contraction coupling, apart from their well-established action on the slow membrane channel, might also interfere with intracellular Ca movements. For instance, in isolated mitochondria, only an excessive concentration of verapamil, more than 1000 times greater than that required to produce contractile failure, suppresses Ca uptake (53). Similarly in isolated sarcoplasmic reticulum all direct attempts at showing an inhibitory effect of negative inotropic doses of verapamil on accumulation, binding, or exchange of Ca have failed (54–56).

More promising, however, were some recent investigations into the particular action of verapamil on isolated cardiac sarcolemma membranes (54, 57). Here the existence of a membrane-located Ca store was found by Nayler & Szeto (1972) which could be depleted by verapamil (54). The assumption is justified that the Ca ions that enter the cell through the slow channel are derived from this intermediate pool of superficially bound membrane Ca. Thus the principal action of verapamil consists of reducing the Ca-accumulating activity or the Ca-binding capacity of these membrane-located storage sites, so that the availability of Ca to the slow membrane channel is restricted. Conversely, as indicated by observations from our laboratory, the potentiation of transmembrane Ca influx produced by β-adrenergic catecholamines might result from a promoter effect of these agents on sarcolemma Ca binding. Epinephrine and isoproterenol probably increase the affinity of these superficial storage sites to Ca, so that Ca uptake from the environment is intensified. By this action β-adrenergic catecholamines

(a) neutralize the symptoms of Ca deficiency as long as traces of Ca are available (58, 59),

(b) guarantee a sufficient Ca supply to the slow channel even at rather high stimulation rates, and

(c) accelerate the recovery of the transmembrane Ca current considerably when Ca is readmitted to previously Ca-deprived myocardium.

Under all these circumstances verapamil and β-adrenergic catecholamines operate in an exactly opposite sense. Possibly β-adrenergic catecholamines, through formation of cyclic AMP, induce phosphorylation of sarcolemma membrane proteins (60) thus augmenting the number of Ca-accumulating binding sites.

PHARMACOLOGICAL INTERVENTIONS IN CA-DEPENDENT CARDIAC PACEMAKER ACTIVITY

Apart from inhibiting mechanical performance, Ca deficiency impairs cardiac pacemaker activity. Thus the progressive reduction of cardiac work in Ca-free Ringer solution is accompanied by a parallel decrease in heart rate (58). Accordingly, Ca-antagonistic agents such as verapamil, D 600, diltiazem, or nifedipine suppress sinoatrial (SA) or atrioventricular (AV) pacemaker activity of isolated nodal tissue from rabbits, rats, and guinea pigs in the same dosage range that restricts atrial or ventricular contractility (61–64). There is again a recovery of both original heart rate and tension development if appropriate doses of β-adrenergic catecholamines, particularly isoproterenol, are administered (8, 9, 13). Extra Ca is less suitable to restore automaticity. The influence of verapamil on spontaneous pacemaker action potentials obtained from the SA node and the central zone (N-zone) of the AV node was studied by several research groups (63–65) with almost identical results: Verapamil reduces the steepness of the slow diastolic depolarization so that the rate of spontaneous impulse discharge drastically decreases. In addition, the rate of rise and the overshoot of the pacemaker action potential are lowered. Hence, under the influence of verapamil the velocity of impulse propagation within the SA node and especially through the AV node must be considerably diminished. The Ca-antagonistic divalent Co, Ni, and Mn ions too act like verapamil in that they equally suppress cardiac contractility and pacemaker function (64, 66–68). Verapamil, D 600, nifedipine, and Mn ions also block impulse conduction in the perfused AV node of dog hearts in situ (66, 69). Again isoproterenol proved to be an effective antidote.
    The conclusions to be drawn from these observations are as follows:

(a) Impulse production and propagation in cardiac pacemaker tissues require Ca.
(b) Cardiac automaticity is as susceptible to inhibitors (Ca-antagonists) and promoters (β-adrenergic catecholamines) of transmembrane Ca influx as cardiac contractility.
(c) An apparently similar or perhaps identical Ca transport system operates as slow channel in both myocardial fibers and nodal cells.

As to the biophysical characterization of the slow channel it is generally agreed that this carrier mechanism works at a relatively low ventricular membrane potential, whereas the fast Na channel undergoes inactivation if the myocardial fibers are partially depolarized (3–5). Application of tetrodotoxin (TTX) is another means known to abolish fast channel function selectively. Nevertheless, such myocardial fibers are still capable of conducting propagated action potentials. But in this case upstroke and overshoot depend on the slow inward current of Ca which then substitutes, as an auxiliary transmembrane charge carrier, the lacking influx of Na.

The consequence is that upstroke velocity and propagation of Ca-mediated ventricular action potentials are much slower than normal and in addition become highly sensitive to verapamil and other Ca-antagonists (59). Needless to say, in this respect the bioelectric features of Ca-dependent action potentials of partially depolarized myocardial fibers closely resemble those of cardiac pacemakers. Hence it may be argued that this correspondence possibly results from the fact that the nodal cells too operate at a rather low level of membrane potential (70). But whatever the final answer, a decisive involvement of the fast Na channel in normal supraventricular automaticity can be excluded because the SA and AV pacemaker action potentials do not respond to TTX (67, 68). This, however, does not imply that Na is totally inert in pacemaker activity.

There are, indeed, observations indicating that major changes in the extracellular Na concentration also affect upstroke velocity and overshoot of pacemaker action potentials (64). The discrimination between extracellular Ca and Na by the slow channel is probably not so perfect that the influence of large alterations of the transmembrane Na gradient is reduced to zero. A similar finding is that lidocaine, procaine, procaine amide, and quinidine, which according to our voltage clamp studies on cat trabeculae predominantly act as Na-antagonists (7), also restrict SA and AV node automaticity provided that the doses are rather high (61). Nevertheless, the sensitivity of the supraventricular pacemakers to concentration changes in extracellular Ca and to substances that specifically act as slow channel promoters or inhibitors is by far greater. This applies certainly to nomotopic automaticity. But with regard to the successful use of Ca-antagonistic compounds in the treatment of many types of ectopic automaticity it is to be assumed that also in these cases Ca is basically involved.

Verapamil, in particular, has attracted much interest in recent years both pharmacologically (71) and clinically (39, 72–75) because of its pronounced antiarrhythmic and antifibrillatory properties. This is, however, not a peculiarity of verapamil since other Ca-antagonistic drugs listed in Figure 1 share this antiarrhythmic action (43, 76, 77).

INHIBITORS AND PROMOTERS OF CA ACTION IN VASCULAR SMOOTH MUSCLE

Extensive research work on smooth musculature of different origin has revealed that here too Ca ions are required not only for excitation-contraction coupling but also, in analogy to cardiac pacemaker function, for the discharge of propagated action potentials (78–80). Hence smooth muscle relaxation produced by Ca-antagonistic agents may result either directly from inhibition of Ca-dependent contractility or indirectly from suppression of Ca-dependent membrane excitation. For instance, spontaneous impulse discharge in smooth muscle preparations from uterus (18), taenia coli (81), and portal vein (82) is arrested by verapamil, D 600 (and nifedipine) in a concentration range that is considerably lower than that required for the blockade of excitation-contraction coupling. Conversely the latter action is most prominent in vascular smooth muscle from coronary, pulmonal, or brain arteries.

Here, inhibition of excitation-contraction coupling can easily be demonstrated on K-depolarized spiral strips which promptly relax under the influence of Ca-antagonistic drugs, whereas depolarization persists (15, 16, 83, 84). Contractures produced by histamine, serotonin, or pitressin are equally suppressed. Excitation-contraction coupling of coronary smooth muscle is generally three to ten times more sensitive to the Ca-antagonistic agents than that of ordinary myocardial fibers. This explains the high efficacy of Ca-antagonists as coronary vasodilators, even in doses that are insufficient to decrease myocardial contractility (85–90).

Figure 3 represents dose-response curves that indicate the potency of these new Ca-antagonists in neutralizing the K-induced spasm of pig coronary strips. In this study nifedipine proved to be several thousand times stronger than papaverine. However, the vasodilator action of Ca-antagonistic drugs is not confined to coronary circulation because they also lower systemic flow resistance by relaxing basic vascular tone and neutralizing autoregulative vasoconstrictor responses (15, 16, 91). For this reason Ca-antagonists, particularly verapamil and nifedipine, are also used for the treatment of certain types of arterial hypertension (72, 92).

With respect to this dual action on coronary and systemic circulation, the vascular effects of Ca-antagonists resemble those of nitroglycerin and other nitrites. Moreover, as recently found in our laboratory, nitroglycerin and related compounds

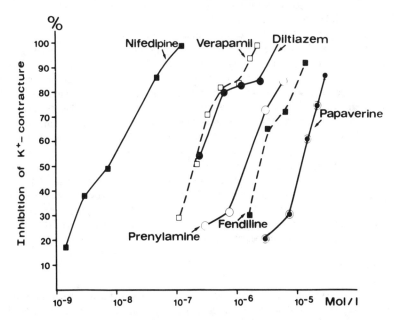

Figure 3 Suppression of K-induced contractures of pig coronary strips by Ca-antagonistic inhibitors of excitation-contraction coupling (From Fleckenstein, Nakayama, Fleckenstein-Grün & Byon. 1976. In *Ionic Actions on Vascular Smooth Muscle,* ed. E. Betz, 117–23. Berlin, Heidelberg & New York: Springer).

also interfere in some way with Ca-dependent excitation-contraction coupling of vascular smooth muscle, even though these drugs have no corresponding action on myocardial fibers (16, 93). However, the kinetics of nitrite-induced vascular relaxation, when thoroughly compared on K-depolarized coronary strips with the action of Ca-antagonists, proved to be rather different. The pecularities of the nitrites are as follows:

(a) The onset of nitrite-induced relaxation is much more rapid, particularly when nitroglycerin or amyl nitrite is applied.

(b) Nitrite-induced relaxation always remains incomplete. Even at high nitrite concentrations a residual contracture of 20–40% persists.

(c) Nitrite-induced relaxation is in most cases transient so that coronary tone tends to recover spontaneously in the presence of the drugs. Extra Ca instantaneously neutralizes the nitrite effects.

The experimental findings on isolated vascular smooth muscle correspond with the old clinical experience that nitroglycerin and amyl nitrite, because of their rapid coronary and systemic action, are most suitable for the interruption of an acute anginal attack. But for the basic long-term treatment of coronary heart disease the Ca-antagonists listed in Figure 1 are more promising. This applies particularly to the prevention of spastic coronary troubles classified as "variant angina" according to Prinzmetal's terminology.

Coronary spasms are facilitated by cardiac glycosides: Because of their interaction with Ca, originally discovered in 1917 by Loewi (94) on frog hearts, cardiac glycosides not only improve myocardial contractility but also increase tension development of coronary smooth muscle (95–98). Furthermore, under the influence of cardiac glycosides a massive sensitization to Ca takes place which again affects both cardiac muscle and coronary arteries (96, 98). Thus, in digitalized hearts, a sudden rise in extracellular Ca concentration not only endangers myocardial function but may also evoke, under certain conditions, coronary vasoconstriction. The same glycoside-induced potentiation of tension development occurs in coronary strips with electric (97, 98) and mechanical stimulation (quick stretch) or with administration of vasoconstrictor agents such as serotonin, histamine, or pitressin (99). However, with the help of Ca-antagonists, all these unpleasant vascular side effects of cardiac glycosides can easily be prevented. The doses of Ca-antagonists required for this purpose are so small that they practically do not impair the desired therapeutic glycoside effects on the myocardium (95).

SUMMARY

During the past decade evidence has been obtained of the existence of a dual membrane carrier system in atrial and ventricular myocardium: a *fast channel* for Na ions that initiate the cardiac fiber action potentials and a separate *slow channel* for Ca ions that activate the contractile machinery. Furthermore, it turned out that transmembrane Ca transport through the slow channel is also involved in nomotopic and ectopic pacemaker activity. Therefore, with the discovery of the new family of highly potent organic Ca-antagonists which are capable of specifically blocking the slow channel, it became possible to limit both cardiac force and automatic impulse discharge to any desired extent. In this respect Ca-antagonists operate in an exactly opposite way than β-adrenergic catecholamines do, since the latter agents exert their positive inotropic and chronotropic effects by acting on the slow channel as promoters of transmembrane Ca influx. In vascular smooth muscle, contractility and tone as well as automaticity also depend on the availability of Ca. This explains the outstanding efficacy of Ca-antagonistic compounds as musculotropic vasodilators in coronary and systemic circulation.

The application of Ca-antagonists as antianginal, antiarrhythmic, antihypertensive, or cardioprotective drugs makes use of these different manifestations of the same basic membrane action. The beneficial influence of Ca-antagonists in coronary disease is probably complex because at least three therapeutically important factors seem to work together: (a) direct reduction of myocardial energy expenditure and, therefore, oxygen demand; (b) indirect decrease in cardiac oxygen requirement by facilitation of heart work at a reduced level of arterial blood pressure, and (c) improvement of myocardial oxygen supply due to vasodilator or spasmolytic effects particularly on extramural coronary vessels (stem arteries, collaterals, anastomoses).

Literature Cited

1. Ebashi, E., Endo, M. 1968. Calcium ions and muscle contraction. *Prog. Biophys. Mol. Biol.* 18:123–83
2. Rubin, R. P. 1970. The role of calcium in the release of neurotransmitter substances and hormones. *Pharmacol. Rev.* 22:389–428
3. Mascher, D., Peper, K. 1969. Two components of inward current in myocardial muscle fibres. *Pfluegers Arch. Gesamte Physiol. Menschen Tiere* 307: 190–203
4. Mascher, D. 1970. Electrical and mechanical responses from ventricular muscle fibres after inactivation of the sodium carrying system. *Pfluegers Arch. Gesamte Physiol. Menschen Tiere* 317:359–72
5. Beeler, G. W., Reuter, H. 1970. Membrane calcium current in ventricular myocardial fibres. *J. Physiol. London* 207:191–209
6. Fleckenstein, A. 1972. Physiologie und Pharmakologie der transmembranären Natrium- , Kalium- und Calcium-Bewegungen. *Arzneim. Forsch.* 22: 2019–28
7. Kohlhardt, M., Bauer, P., Krause, H., Fleckenstein, A. 1972. Differentiation of the transmembrane Na and Ca channel in mammalian cardiac fibres by the use of specific inhibitors. *Pfluegers Arch.*

Gesamte Physiol. Menschen Tiere 335:309–22
8. Fleckenstein, A. 1964. Die Bedeutung der energiereichen Phosphate für Kontraktilität und Tonus des Myokards. *Verh. Dtsch. Ges. Inn. Med.* 70: 81–99
9. Fleckenstein, A., Kammermeier, H., Döring, H. J., Freund, H. J. 1967. Zum Wirkungsmechanismus neuartiger Koronardilatatoren mit gleichzeitig Sauerstoff-einsparenden Myokard-Effekten, Prenylamin und Iproveratril. *Z. Kreislaufforsch.* 56:716–44, 839–53
10. Fleckenstein, A., Tritthart, H., Fleckenstein, B., Herbst, A., Grün G. 1969. A new group of competitive Ca-antagonists (Iproveratril, D 600, Prenylamine) with highly potent inhibitory effects on excitation-contraction coupling in mammalian myocardium. *Pfluegers Arch. Gesamte Physiol. Menschen Tiere* 307:R25
11. Fleckenstein, A., Tritthart, H., Döring, H. J., Byon, Y. K. 1972. Bay a 1040—ein hochaktiver Ca^{++}—antagonistischer Inhibitor der elektro-mechanischen Koppelungsprozesse im Warmblüter-Myokard. *Arzneim. Forsch.* 22: 22–33

12. Reuter, H. 1965. Über die Wirkung von Adrenalin auf den cellulären Ca-Umsatz des Meerschweinchenvorhofs. *Naunyn Schmiedebergs Arch. Exp. Pathol. Pharmakol.* 251:401
13. Fleckenstein, A. 1970/1971. Specific inhibitors and promoters of calcium action in the excitation-contraction coupling of heart muscle and their role in the prevention or production of myocardial lesions. In *Calcium and the Heart,* ed. P. Harris, L. Opie, 135–88. London & New York: Academic
14. Vassort, G., Rougier, O., Garnier, D., Sauviat, M. P., Coraboeuf, E., Gargouil, Y. M. 1969. Effects of adrenaline on membrane inward current during the cardiac action potential. *Pfluegers Arch. Gesamte Menschen Tiere Physiol.* 309:70–81
15. Grün, G., Fleckenstein, A., Byon, Y. K. 1971. Ca-antagonism, a new principle of vasodilation. *Proc. Int. Union Physiol. Sci., XXV Int. Congr., Munich* IX:221
16. Grün, G., Fleckenstein, A. 1972. Die elektromechanische Entkoppelung der glatten Gefäβ-Muskulatur als Grundprinzip der Coronardilatation durch 4-(2'-Nitrophenyl)-2,6-dimethyl-1,4-dihydropyridin-3,5-dicarbonsäure-dimethylester (Bay a 1040, Nifedipine). *Arzneim. Forsch.* 22:334–44
17. Fleckenstein, A., Grün, G. 1969. Reversible Blockierung der elektromechanischen Koppelungsprozesse in der glatten Muskulatur des Ratten-Uterus mittels organischer Ca⁺⁺-Antagonisten (Iproveratril, D 600, Prenylamin). *Pfluegers Arch. Gesamte Physiol. Menschen Tiere* 307:R26
18. Fleckenstein, A., Grün, G., Tritthart, H., Byon, Y. K. 1971. Uterus-Relaxation durch hochaktive Ca⁺⁺-antagonistische Hemmstoffe der elektromechanischen Koppelung wie Isoptin (Verapamil, Iproveratril), Substanz D 600 und Segontin (Prenylamin).—Versuche am isolierten Uterus virgineller Ratten. *Klin. Wocherschr.* 49:32–41
19. Grün, G., Fleckenstein, A., Byon, Y. K. 1971. Hemmung der Motilität isolierter Uterus-Streifen aus gravidem und nicht-gravidem Myometrium durch Ca⁺⁺-Antagonisten und Sympathomimetica. *Arzneim. Forsch.* 21:1585–90
20. Dreifuss, J. J., Grau, J. D., Nordmann, J. J. 1975. Calcium movements related to neurohypophysical hormone secretion. In *Calcium Transport in Contraction and Secretion,* ed. E. Carafoli et al, 271–79. Amsterdam: North-Holland
21. Russell, J. T., Thorn, N. A. 1974. Calcium and stimulus-secretion coupling in the neurohypophysis. II. Effects of lanthanum, a verapamil analogue (D 600) and prenylamine on 45-calcium transport and vasopressin release in isolated rat neurohypophyses. *Acta Endocrinol. Copenhagen* 76:471–487
22. Devis, G., Somers, G., Van Obberghen, E., Malaisse, W. J. 1975. Calcium antagonists and islet function. I. Inhibition of insulin release by Verapamil. *Diabetes* 24:547–51
23. Matthews, E. K., Sakamoto, Y. 1975. Electrical characteristics of pancreatic islet cells. *J. Physiol.* 246:421–37
24. Eto, S., Wood, J. M., Hutchins, M., Fleischer, N. 1974. Pituitary ⁴⁵Ca⁺⁺ uptake and release of ACTH, GH and TSH: effect of verapamil. *Am. J. Physiol.* 226:1315–20
25. Ringer, S. 1882. A further contribution regarding the influence of the different constituents of the blood on the contraction of the heart. *J. Physiol.* 4:29–42
26. Mines, G. R. 1913. On functional analysis by the action of electrolytes. *J. Physiol. London* 46:188
27. Fleckenstein, A. 1963. Metabolic aspects of the excitation-contraction coupling. In *The Cellular Functions of Membrane Transport, Symp. Soc. Gen. Physiol. Woods Hole/Mass., Sept. 4–7,* ed. J. F. Hoffmann, 71–93. Englewood Cliffs, NJ: Prentice-Hall
28. Schildberg, F. W., Fleckenstein, A. 1965. Die Bedeutung der extracellulären Calciumkonzentration für die Spaltung von energiereichem Phosphat in ruhendem und tätigem Myokardgewebe. *Pfluegers Arch. Gesamte Physiol. Menschen Tiere* 283:137–50
29. Fleckenstein, A., Döring, H. J., Kammermeier, H. 1966/1967. Experimental heart failure due to inhibition of utilisation of high-energy phosphates. *Int. Symp. Coronary Circ. Energ. Myocardium,* Milan, 1966, pp. 220–36. Basle & New York: Karger
30. Fleckenstein, A. 1968. Experimental heart failure due to disturbances in high-energy phosphate metabolism. *Proc. Vth Eur. Congr. Cardiol., Athens, Sept. 1968.,* pp. 255–69
31. Lee, K. S., Klaus, W. 1971. The subcellular basis for the mechanism of inotropic action of cardiac glycosides. *Pharmacol. Rev.* 23:193–261
32. Byon, Y. K., Fleckenstein, A. 1969. Parallele Beeinflussung von isometrischer Spannungsentwicklung und O₂-

Verbrauch isolierter Papillarmuskeln unter dem Einfluß von Ca^{++}-Ionen, Adrenalin, Isoproterenol und organischen Ca^{++}-Antagonisten (Iproveratril, D 600, Prenylamin). *Pfluegers Arch. Gesamte Physiol. Menschen Tiere* 312: R8/9

33. Fleckenstein, A., Döring, H. J., Janke, J., Byon, Y. K. 1975. Basic actions of ions and drugs on myocardial high-energy phosphate metabolism and contractility. In *Handbook of Experimental Pharmacology*, ed. G. V. R. Born, O. Eichler, A. Farah, H. Herken, A. D. Welch, J. Schmier, XVI:Part 3, pp. 345–405. Berlin, Heidelberg & New York: Springer

34. Kroneberg, G. 1973. Pharmacology of nifedipine (Adalat). In *1st Int. Nifedipine "Adalat" Symp.*, ed. K. Hashimoto, E. Kimura, T. Kobayashi, 3–10. Tokyo: Univ. Tokyo Press

35. Schümann, H. J., Görlitz, B. D., Wagner, J. 1975. Influence of papaverine, D 600, and nifedipine on the effects of noradrenaline and calcium on the isolated aorta and mesenteric artery of the rabbit. *Naunyn Schmiedebergs Arch. Pharmacol.* 289:409–18

36. Tschirdewahn, B., Klepzig, H. 1963. Klinische Untersuchungen über die Wirkung von Isoptin und Isoptin S bei Patienten mit Koronarinsuffizienz. *Dtsch. Med. Wochenschr.* 88:1702

37. Sandler, G., Clayton, G. A., Thornicroft, S. G. 1968. Clinical evaluation of verapamil in angina pectoris. *Br. Med. J.* 3:224

38. Livesley, B., Catley, P. F., Campbell, R. C., Oram, S. 1973. Double-blind evaluation of verapamil, propranolol and isosorbide dinitrate against placebo in the treatment of angina pectoris. *Br. Med. J.* 1:375–78

39. Krikler, D. 1974. Verapamil in cardiology. *Eur. J. Cardiol.* 2:3–10

40. Winsor, T., Bleifer, K., Cole, S., Goldman, I. R., Karpman, H., Oblath, R., Stone, S. 1971. A double-blind, double crossover trial of prenylamine in angina pectoris. *Am. Heart J.* 82:43

41. Ebner, F. 1973. Survey of the results of world-wide clinical trials with nifedipine (Adalat). In *New Therapie of Ischemic Heart Disease*, See Ref. 34, pp. 282–90

42. Spiel, R., Enenkel, W. 1976. Wirkung von Fendilin auf die Belastungsuntersuchung Koronarkranker. *Wien. Med. Wochenschr.* 126:186–89

43. *Proc. Int. Symp.* R. Soc. Med., London, 3 October, 1972. 1973. *Postgrad. Med. J.* 49:Suppl. 3

44. Smith, H. J., Singh, B. N., Nisbet, H. D., Norris, R. M. 1975. Effects of verapamil on infarct size following experimental coronary occlusion. *Cardiovasc. Res.* 9:569–78

45. Wende, W., Bleifeld, W., Meyer, J., Stühlen, H. W. 1975. Reduction of the size of acute, experimental myocardial infarction by verapamil. *Basic Res. Cardiol.* 70:198–208

46. Lossnitzer, K., Janke, J., Hein, B., Stauch, M., Fleckenstein, A. 1975. Disturbed myocardial calcium metabolism: a possible pathogenetic factor in the hereditary cardiomyopathy of the Syrian hamster. In *Pathophysiology and Morphology of Myocardial Cell Alterations, Vol. 6, Recent Advances in Studies on Cardiac Structure and Metabolism,* 207–17. Baltimore, London & Tokyo: Univ. Park Press

47. Jasmin, G., Bajusz, E. 1975. Prevention of myocardial degeneration in hamsters with hereditary cardiomyopathy. See Ref. 46, pp. 219–29

48. Nakajima, H., Hoshiyama, M., Yamashita, K., Kiyomoto, A. 1975. Effect of diltiazem on electrical and mechanical activity of isolated cardiac ventricular muscle of guinea pig. *Jpn. J. Pharmacol.* 25:383–92

49. Winegrad, S. 1971. Studies of cardiac muscle with a high permeability to calcium produced by treatment with ethylene-diamine-tetraacetic acid. *J. Gen Physiol.* 58:71–93

50. Kohlhardt, M., Haastert, H. P., Krause, H. 1973. Evidence of nonspecificity of the Ca channel in mammalian myocardial fibre membranes. *Pfluegers Arch. Gesamte Physiol. Menschen Tiere* 342:125–36

51. Kohlhardt, M., Bauer, B., Krause, H., Fleckenstein, A. 1973. Selective inhibition of the transmembrane Ca conductivity of mammalian myocardial fibres by Ni, Co and Mn ions. *Pfluegers Arch. Gesamte Physiol. Menschen Tiere* 338:115–23

52. Kaufmann, R., Fleckenstein, A. 1965. Ca^{++}-kompetitive elektro-mechanische Entkoppelung durch Ni^{++}- und Co^{++}-Ionen am Warmblütermyokard. *Pfluegers Arch. Gesamte Physiol. Menschen Tiere* 282:290–97

53. Frey, M., Janke, J. 1975. The effect of organic Ca-antagonists (verapamil, prenylamine) on the calcium transport

system in isolated mitochondria of rat cardiac muscle. *Pfluegers Arch. Gesamte Physiol. Menschen Tiere* 359 (Suppl.):R26

54. Nayler, W. G., Szeto, J. 1972. Effect of verapamil on contractility, oxygen utilization and calcium exchangeability in mammalian heart muscle. *Cardiovasc. Res.* 6:120–28

55. Entman, M. L., Allen, J. C., Bornet, E. P., Gillette, P. C., Wallick, E. T., Schwartz, A. 1972. Mechanisms of calcium accumulation and transport in cardiac relaxing system (sarcoplasmic reticulum membranes): Effects of verapamil, D 600, X537A and A23187. *J. Mol. Cell. Cardiol.* 4:681–87

56. Watanabe, A. M., Besch, H. R. Jr. 1974. Subcellular myocardial effects of verapamil and D 600: comparison with propranolol. *J. Pharmacol. Exp. Ther.* 191:241–51

57. Williamson, J. R., Woodrow, M. L., Scarpa, A. 1975. Calcium binding to cardiac sarcolemma. In *Basic Functions of Cations in Myocardial Activity, Vol. 5, Recent Advances in Studies on Cardiac Structure and Metabolism,* 61–71. Baltimore, London & Tokyo: Univ. Park Press

58. Antoni, H., Engstfeld, G., Fleckenstein, A. 1960. Inotrope Effekte von ATP und Adrenaline am hypodynamen Froschmyokard nach elektro-mechanischer Entkoppelung durch Ca++-Entzug. *Pfluegers Arch. Gesamte Physiol. Menschen Tiere* 272:91–106

59. Tritthart, H., Volkmann, R., Weiss, R., Fleckenstein, A. 1973. Calcium-mediated action potentials in mammalian myocardium: Alterations of membrane response as induced by changes of Ca or by promoters and inhibitors of transmembrane Ca inflow. *Naunyn Schmiedebergs Arch. Pharmacol.* 280: 239–52

60. Langan, T. A. 1973. Protein kinases and protein kinase substrates. In *Advances in Cyclic Nucleotide Research,* ed. P. Greengard, G. A. Robinson, 3:99–153. New York: Raven

61. Haastert, H. P., Fleckenstein, A. 1975. Ca-dependence of supraventricular pacemaker activity and its responsiveness to Ca-antagonistic compounds (verapamil, D 600, nifedipine). *Naunyn Schmiedebergs Arch. Pharmacol.* 287 (Suppl.):R39

62. Refsum, H., Landmark, K. 1975. The effect of a calcium-antagonistic drug, nifedipine, on the mechanical and electrical activity of the isolated rat atrium. *Acta Pharmacol. Toxicol.* 37:369–76

63. Wit, A. L., Cranefield, P. F. 1974. Effect of verapamil on the sinoatrial and atrioventricular nodes of the rabbit and the mechanism by which it arrests reentrant atrioventricular nodal tachycardia. *Circ. Res.* 35:413–25

64. Kohlhardt, M., Figulla, H.-R., Tripathi, O. 1976. The slow membrane channel as the predominant mediator of the excitation process of the sinoatrial pacemaker cell. *Basic Res. Cardiol.* 71: 17–26

65. Tritthart, H., Fleckenstein, B., Fleckenstein, A. 1970. Some fundamental actions of antiarrhythmic drugs on the excitability and the contractility of single myocardial fibers. *Naunyn Schmiedebergs Arch. Pharmacol.* 269:212–19

66. Zipes, D. P., Fischer, J. C. 1974. Effects of agents which inhibit the slow channel on sinus node automaticity and atrioventricular conduction in the dog. *Circ. Res.* 34:184–92

67. Zipes, D. P., Mendez, C. 1973. Action of manganese ions and tetrodotoxin on atrioventricular nodal transmembrane potentials in isolated rabbit hearts. *Circ. Res.* 32:447–54

68. Lenfant, J., Mironneau, J., Gargouil, Y. M., Galand, G. 1968. Analyse de l'activité électrique spontanée du centre de l'automatisme cardiaque de lapin par les inhibiteurs de perméabilitiés membranaires. *C. R. Acad. Sci. Ser. D* 266:901–4

69. Taira, N., Narimatsu, A. 1975. Effects of nifedipine, a potent calcium-antagonistic coronary vasodilator, on atrioventricular conduction and blood flow in the isolated atrioventricular node preparation of the dog. *Naunyn Schmiedebergs Arch. Pharmacol.* 290: 107–12

70. Kreitner, D. 1975. Evidence for the existence of a rapid sodium channel in the membrane of rabbit sinoatrial cells. *J. Mol. Cell. Cardiol.* 7:655–62

71. Singh, B. N., Vaughan-Williams, E. M. 1972. A fourth class of anti-dysrhythmic action? Effect of verapamil on ouabain toxicity, on atrial and ventricular and intracellular potentials and on other features of cardiac function. *Cardiovasc. Res.* 6:109–19

72. Bender, F. 1970. Die Behandlung der tachycarden Arrhythmien und der arteriellen Hypertonie mit Verapamil. *Arzneim. Forsch.* 20:1310–16

73. Schamroth, L., Krikler, D. M., Garrett, C. 1972. Immediate effects of intravenous verapamil in cardiac arrhythmias. *Br. Med. J.* 1:660–62
74. Spurrell, R. A. J., Krikler, D. M., Sowton, E. 1974. Effects of verapamil on electrophysiological properties of anomalous atrioventricular connexion in Wolff-Parkinson-White syndrome. *Br. Heart J.* 36:256–64
75. Härtel, G., Hartikainen, M. 1976. Comparison of verapamil and practolol in paroxysmal supraventricular tachycardia. *Eur. J. Cardiol.* 4:87–90
76. Lindner, E., Kaiser, J. 1975. Die antiarrhythmische Wirkung des Segontin. *Herz Kreisl. Z. Kardiol. Angiol. Klin, Prax.* 7:88–94
77. Refsum, H. 1975. Calcium-antagonistic and anti-arrhythmic effects of nifedipine on the isolated rat atrium. *Acta Pharmacol. Toxicol.* 37:377–86
78. Bohr, D. F. 1964. Electrolytes and smooth muscle contraction. *Pharmacol. Rev.* 16:85–111
79. Somlyo, A. P., Somlyo, A. V. 1970. Vascular smooth muscle, II. Pharmacology of normal and hypertensive vessels. *Pharmacol. Rev.* 22:249–353
80. Rüegg, J. C. 1971. Smooth muscle tone. *Physiol. Rev.* 51:201–48
81. Riemer, J., Dörfler, F., Mayer, C.-J., Ulbrecht, G. 1974. Calcium-antagonistic effects on the spontaneous activity of guinea-pig taenia coli. *Pfluegers Arch. Gesamte Physiol. Menschen Tiere* 351:241–58
82. Golenhofen, K., Hermstein, N. 1975. Differentiation of calcium activation mechanism in vascular smooth muscle by selective suppression with verapamil and D 600. *Blood Vessels* 12:21–37
83. Peiper, U., Schmidt, E. 1972. Relaxation of coronary arteries by electromechanical decoupling or adrenergic stimulation. *Pfluegers Arch. Gesamte Physiol. Menschen Tiere* 337:107–17
84. Haeusler, G. 1972. Differential effect of verapamil on excitation-contraction coupling in smooth muscle and on excitation-secretion coupling in adrenergic nerve terminals. *J. Pharmacol. Exp. Ther.* 180:672–82
85. Lindner, E. 1960. Phenyl-propyl-diphenyl-propyl-amin, eine neue Substanz mit coronargefäßerweiternder Wirkung. *Arzneim. Forsch.* 10:569–73
86. Haas, H., Härtfelder, G. 1962. α-Isopropyl-α-(N-methylhomoveratryl)-γ-aminopropyl)-3,4-dimethoxy-phenylacetonitril, eine Substanz mit coronargefäß

erweiternden Eigenschaften. *Arzneim. Forsch.* 12:549–58
87. Haas, H., Busch, E. 1967. Vergleichende Untersuchungen der Wirkung von α-Isopropyl-α-(N-methyl-N-homoveratryl)-γ-aminopropyl)-3,4-dimethoxy-phenylacetonitril, seiner Derivate sowie einiger anderer Coronardilatatoren und β-Receptor-affiner Substanzen. *Arzneim. Forsch.* 17:257–71
88. Sato, M., Nagao, T., Yamaguchi, I., Nakajima, H., Kiyomoto, A. 1971. Pharmacological studies on a new 1,5-benzothiazepine derivative (CRD-401 = Diltiazem). *Arzneim. Forsch.* 21:1338–43
89. Hudak, W. J., Lewis, R. E., Kuhn, W. L. 1970. Cardiovascular pharmacology of perhexiline. *J. Pharmacol. Exp. Ther.* 173:371
90. Vater, W., Kroneberg, G., Hoffmeister, F., Kaller, H., Meng, K., Oberdorf, A., Puls, W., Schloβmann, K., Stoepel, K. 1972. Zur Pharmakologie von 4-(2'Nitrophenyl)-2,6-dimethyl-1,4-dihydropyridin-3, 5-dicarbonsäuredimethylester (Nifedipin, Bay a 1040). *Arzneim. Forsch.* 22:1–14
91. Ono, H., Kokubun, H., Hashimoto, K. 1974. Abolition by calcium antagonists of the autoregulation of renal blood flow. *Naunyn Schmiedebergs Arch. Pharmacol.* 285:201–7
92. Brittinger, W. D., Schwarzbeck, A., Wittenmeier, K. W., Twittenhoff, W. D., Stegaru, B., Huber, W., Ewald, R. W., von Henning, G. E., Fabricius, M., Strauch, M. 1970. Klinischexperimentelle Untersuchungen über die blutdrucksenkende Wirkung von Verapamil. *Dtsch. Med. Wochenschr.* 95: 1871–77
93. Weder, U., Grün, G. 1973. Ca++-antagonistische elektromechanische Entkoppelung der glatten Gefäßmuskulatur als Wirkungsprinzip vasodilatatorischer Nitroverbindungen. *Naunyn Schmiedebergs Arch. Pharmacol.* 277(Suppl.):R88
94. Loewi, O. 1917. Über den Zusammenhang zwischen Digitalis und Calciumwirkung. *Naunyn Schmiedebergs Arch. Pharmacol.* 82:131–58
95. Fleckenstein, A., Byon, Y. K. 1974. Prevention by Ca-antagonistic compounds (verapamil, D 600) of coronary smooth muscle contractures due to treatment with cardiac glycosides. *Naunyn Schmiedebergs Arch. Pharmacol.* 282(Suppl.):R20

96. Grün, G., Fleckenstein, A., Weder, U. 1974. Changes in coronary smooth muscle tone produced by Ca, cardiac glycosides and Ca-antagonistic compounds (verapamil, D 600, prenylamine etc.). *Pfluegers Arch. Gesamte Physiol. Menschen Tiere* 347(Suppl.):R1

97. Fleckenstein, A., Fleckenstein-Grün, G. 1975. Further studies on the neutralization of glycoside-induced contractures of coronary smooth muscle by Ca-antagonistic compounds (verapamil, D 600, prenylamine, nifedipine, fendiline or nitrites). *Naunyn Schmiedebergs Arch. Pharmacol.* 287 (Suppl.):R38

98. Fleckenstein, A., Nakayama, K., Fleckenstein-Grün, G., Byon, Y. K. 1975. Interactions of vasoactive ions and drugs with Ca-dependent excitation-contraction coupling of vascular smooth muscle. See Ref. 20, pp. 555–66

99. Nakayama, K., Fleckenstein-Grün, G., Byon, Y. K., Fleckenstein, A. 1976. Opposite effects of cardiac glycosides and Ca-antagonistic compounds on vascular smooth muscle contractility under electrical, mechanical and pharmacological stimulation (Observations on helical strips from rabbit coronary and brain arteries). *Pfluegers Arch. Gesamte Physiol. Menschen Tiere* 365(Suppl.):R7

Ann. Rev. Pharmacol. Toxicol. 1977. 17:167–77

FISH AND CHEMICALS: ♦6673
THE PROCESS OF ACCUMULATION[1]

Jerry L. Hamelink
Lilly Research Laboratories, Greenfield, Indiana 46140

Anne Spacie
Department of Forestry and Natural Resources, Purdue University, West Lafayette,
Indiana 47907

INTRODUCTION

After three decades (1, 2) of intensive research, the environmental behavior of DDT
is still almost incomprehensible. Consider for a moment that fish can easily accumulate a million times the concentration of DDT found in the water they inhabit. Yet,
incredible as it may seem, fish are doing that every day with DDT and several other
interesting compounds. At the same time, there are numerous other chemicals they
cannot bioaccumulate with such efficiency. These associations constitute the subject
for this review. Fish and chemicals—how does the one accumulate the other?

The effects of pollutants on fish have been comprehensively reviewed annually
since 1968 (3a–h) in the *Journal of the Water Pollution Control Federation*. Johnson
has published two critical reviews (4, 5) dealing with pesticides and fish that are

[1]Symbols and identities of compounds mentioned in the text (in order of appearance): DDT
(p,p'-DDT), 2,2-bis (*p*-chlorophenyl)-1,1,1-trichloroethane; DDT-R, sum of all isomers and
alteration products of DDT detected in sample; Dieldrin, 1,2,3,4,10,10-hexachloro-6,7-epoxy-
1,4,4a,5,6,7,8,8a-octahydro-1,4-*endo,exo*-5,8-dimethanonaphthalene; Aroclor® 1254, registered trademark of the Monsanto Co., St. Louis, Mo., for a mixture of PCBs; DDD
(p,p'-DDD), 2,2-bis(*p*-chlorophenyl)-1,1-dichloroethane; DDE (p,p'-DDE), 2,2-bis (*p*-chlorophenyl)-1,1-dichloroethylene; PCBs, polychlorobiphenyls (mixtures of chlorinated biphenyl compounds); 2,2',4,4'-tetrachlorobiphenyl, a single isomer of PCB; Endrin, 1,2,3,4,
10, 10-hexachloro-6,7-epoxy-1,4,4a,5,6,7,8,8a-octahydro-1,4-*endo-endo*-5, 8-dimethanonaphthalene; Chlorpyrifos, O,O-Diethyl O-(3,5,6-trichloro-2-phyridyl) phosphorothioate (Dursban); 3,5,6-trichloropyridinol, 3,5,6-trichloro-2-pyridinol (a metabolite of chlorpyrifos);
Hexachlorobenze, hexachlorobenzene; Trifluralin, α,α,α-trifluro-2,6-dinitro,N,N-dipropyl-
p-toluidine; Methyl mercury, methyl mercury.

particularly useful because they summarize the state of the art at two distinct stages of development. In his first review (4), acute toxic effects of various chemicals on many different kinds of fish were emphasized. But he recognized that "major gaps obviously exist in understanding the modes and temporal relationships of pesticide uptake by fishes. . . . " Although considerable progress was made in the next five years (5), many questions and apparent contradictions remained unresolved before chemical residue accumulation by fish could be quantified.

UNIQUE ASPECTS OF THE PROBLEM

Predicting when, where, and to what degree a fish will accumulate a particular chemical has ecologic and economic importance. This need for predictability has many unique aspects foreign to mammalian toxicology. The fish themselves display a vast diversity of anatomical design, represented by over 20,000 species spanning 400 million years of evolution (6). Because they live in a world virtually devoid of oxygen by terrestrial standards, fish are required to satisfy their oxygen demands by extracting volumes of water weighing thousands of times their body weight each day. Osmoregulation is a continuous battle. Freshwater fish must actively absorb salts and excrete copious volumes of dilute urine. Conversely, marine fish drink sea water and actively excrete salts to maintain ionic homeostasis. Water itself undergoes an extremely rapid flux (i.e. the half-life of water in a whole fish is only 0.5–1.5 hr) (7). Furthermore, contrary to the conclusions drawn from some early investigations, certain metabolic detoxication processes, such as conjugation, are important in fish (8, 9). Finally, fish are poikilothermous, so rates of metabolism and chemical uptake are inexorably linked to the temperature of their environment. Thus, we find that the uptake of DDT directly from water by fish increases with temperature in proportion to their oxygen consumption (10, 11).

The residue problem is further complicated by the tremendous size range and indeterminate growth patterns within a single species of fish. For example, adult carp (*Cyprinus carpio*) may weigh a million times more than their newly hatched larvae (12). In addition, the size differences between species are equally great. Yet, for practical reasons, essentially all experimental research on pesticide accumulation has been done on small fish (13), making extrapolations to natural populations difficult. Consequently, while unique aspects such as these have impeded the direct adoption of predictive models designed for mammalian systems, they have fostered many innovative interchanges between a variety of disciplines that may ultimately benefit mammalian studies.

HOW FISH ACQUIRE CHEMICAL RESIDUES

Laboratory Studies

The accumulation of chemical residues by fish was originally attributed to a process defined as biological magnification through the "food-chain" (2, 14–16). The basic assumption underlying this hypothesis is that for each step in the food-chain proportionately more chemical residues are retained than energy (in the form of body weight gain). This process was illustrated by Woodwell (16) who shaded each segment of an ecological pyramid with colored dots to represent DDT. The dots were widely spaced within the broad base of primary producers, more closely spaced in the consumer levels, and crowded in the narrow pinnacle of top carnivores. Accompanied by an illustration of DDT levels in an estuarine food web, it made an artistic and convincing portrayal of the accumulation process. But, direct experimental studies were later to reveal that the factors controlling uptake and retention of chemicals by fish were more complex than originally envisioned.

The growth efficiency (i.e. body weight gained per weight of food consumed) of fish is about 8% (17). Hence, any dietary uptake efficiency of contaminants which is greater than 8% will result in an accumulation of residues. The dietary uptake efficiencies reported for various chlorinated hydrocarbons range from 9 to 68% (18–26). As might be expected, this variability appears to be largely attributable to the length of exposure, dosage level, and the type of food employed. For example, Grezenda et al fed individual goldfish (*Carassius auratus*) artificial diets contaminated with DDT (19) or dieldrin (20). They found that the dietary uptake efficiency of DDT declined as the residue concentrations of DDT-R increased with time (19). Also, the proportion of dieldrin retained was less in fish receiving the higher of two treatment levels (20). Furthermore, dieldrin residue concentrations rose throughout the trial while DDT-R levels reached a steady state. Reinert et al (26) observed that the uptake efficiency for DDT dissolved in corn oil and then mixed into an artificial diet was only about 20%. This is substantially less than the 68% retention of Aroclor® 1254 observed by Lieb et al (21) under similar experimental conditions. However, Lieb et al incorporated the Aroclor with salmon oil, which may improve availibility. Because dietary factors compromise availability, the utility of laboratory data to predict dynamics under natural conditions may be highly arbitrary.

Fish can rapidly take up high concentrations of DDT and other chemicals directly from the water (27–29). Atempting to assess the importance of this source relative to uptake from food by means of laboratory studies is confusing. For example, Macek & Korn (24) demonstrated that brook trout (*Salvelinus fontinalis*) obtained only 10 times more residues from food contaminated with 3 ppm DDT than from water containing 3 pptr DDT. It must be noted that the dose levels were selected to approximate concentrations present in forage organisms and water of Lake Michigan, not to bias the results.

Reinert et al (26) obtained somewhat different results with lake trout (*S. namaycush*) dosed with 6 to 9 pptr of both DDT and dieldrin in the water and/or 2.3 ppm DDT and 1.7 ppm dieldrin in food. After 152 days of exposure the fish obtained progressively higher concentrations of DDT from water alone ($\bar{x} = 352$ ppb), food alone ($\bar{x} = 648$ ppb), and food and water combined ($\bar{x} = 776$ ppb). On the other hand, there was no significant difference between dieldrin levels obtained from water ($\bar{x} = 478$ ppb) or from food ($\bar{x} = 470$ ppb) even though water and food combined still appeared to be additive ($\bar{x} = 670$ ppb). Hence, the actual differences in the concentration of each chemical taken up were relatively slight regardless of the source. Furthermore, they estimated that the efficiency of uptake directly from the

water ranged somewhere between 12 and 59% for DDT and 20 to 102% for
dieldrin, while dietary uptake efficiencies were only 20 and 17%, respectively.
Contrary to these observations, Chadwick & Brocksen (18) and other investigators
(22, 25) demonstrated that natural food and water sources did not appear to be
additive for dieldrin uptake by various species of small-sized fish under a variety of
laboratory conditions. Therefore, we must conclude that uptake from *both* water
and food can be substantial depending on the conditions of exposure, duration, dose
level, and individual fish involved in the process.

Field Studies

Synthetic pollutants do not behave in the same manner as essential nutrients,
notably phosphorus, in aquatic environments. If a single dose of radioactive phosphorus is added to a lake, the concentration in each trophic level rises and falls in
an orderly succession, following the tranfer of the element through the food-chain
(30). By comparison, a single dose of DDT produces a very rapid and simultaneous
concentration increase in all organisms from all trophic levels, yet substantial differences in concentrations between trophic levels still develop (31). Furthermore,
virtually the same concentration differences result whether a complete food-chain
or an artificially interrupted food-chain is used. To explain these results, Hamelink
et al (31) proposed that the processes of absorption onto body surfaces and partition
into lipids control the accumulation of chlorinated hydrocarbons by the various
members of a lake biota. Thus, under this hypothesis, the physical characteristics
of the organisms, such as size and lipid content, become more important factors than
their ecological interactions.

The influence of age, body weight, and lipid content on chemical residue levels
in natural fish populations has been evaluated by many authors (13, 32–39). In fact,
residue concentrations are commonly reported on both a lipid basis and a whole
body basis in fish, which frequently helps reduce variability among samples (32–37).
However, no consistent pattern has emerged, as illustrated by the data for landlocked salmon (*Salmo salar*) from Sebago Lake, Maine (33, 35). DDD and DDE
increased with age and lipid content, dieldrin only increased with lipid content,
while age and lipid content were interdependent on DDT levels found in the salmon
(35). However, one should recognize that residue-lipid content correlations do not
necessarily prove a cause and effect relationship. That is, the presence of more lipids
may not cause greater quantities of residues to be accumulated; rather the factors
that result in lipid deposition may also promote residue storage.

Fish must obviously expend energy in order to acquire and store energy. Because
lipids have a greater caloric content than muscle, a "fat" fish must do more eating,
swimming, and respiring than a "lean" fish of the same weight and age. As a result,
the "fat" salmon from Sebago Lake presumably had more opportunities to take up
residues than "lean" fish. That the "fat" fish did in fact retain greater concentrations
of residues probably just relates to the lipophilic nature of the chemicals. There just
happened to be a convenient place to store the chemicals, but the presence of the
lipids did not cause the compounds to be taken up and stored.

The factors of age and weight cannot be separated because they normally co-vary in fish populations. Residues of DDT-R and PCBs in lake trout (38, 39) show exponential increases with age of fish under uniform conditions of exposure. Since weight also increases exponentially, the data give good correlations between residue concentration and weight as well. For this reason, Eberhardt (13) has recommended that the log of residue concentration be expressed as a function of log body weight to reduce variability among samples. Such correlations in field data again suggest that the mechanism of residue uptake is ultimately linked to the metabolic activities of the fish. Given these realizations, the use of various kinetic and bioenergetic growth models becomes a more plausible means for solving the prediction problem.

PARTITION AND KINETIC MODELS

The exchange-equilibria hypothesis (31), coupled with some uptake and clearance data (19, 23, 28, 29), presumably helped foster interest in using pharmacokinetic models to predict bioaccumulation in fish. Branson et al (40) applied a two-compartment kinetic model to the uptake and clearance of 2,2',4,4'-tetra-chlorobiphenyl by rainbow trout (*Salmo gairdneri*) in the laboratory. The validity of this approach was demonstrated when the projected steady state residue levels based on five days of exposure compared favorably to experimental results obtained during 42 days of exposure. Neely, Branson & Blau used this same technique to develop a regression equation for projected steady state residue concentrations in trout muscle versus calculated n-octanol-water partition coefficients (P) for a variety of synthetic compounds (41). Over a log P range of 2.64 to 7.62 they obtained the regression: log (bioconcentration factor) = 0.542 (log P) + 0.124. This regression was verified by using the P values for endrin (log P = 5.6), chlorpyrifos (log P = 4.82), and 3,5,6-trichloropyrindinol (log P = 1.35) to predict the bioconcentration factors reported for whole mosquito fish (*Gambusia affinis*). Except for the more water-soluble pyridinol, which is a metabolite of chlorpyrifos, very close agreement was obtained between the predicted and observed bioconcentration factors. The predicted values for endrin and chlorpyrifos were log 3.47 ± 0.989 and 2.87 ± 0.963 compared to experimentally observed factors of log 3.17 and 2.67, respectively. The predicted value for the pyridinol on the other hand was 0.88 ± 1.139 verus an observed value of 0.49.

Metcalf and associates (42, 43) derived similar uptake-partition regressions for other organic chemicals and mosquito fish as evaluated in model ecosystems. However, they based their regression on experimentally determined n-octanol-water partition coefficients which were substantially lower than the calculated values used by Neely et al (41). For example, the log P value measured by Lu (43) for hexachlorobenzene was 4.13 compared to a calculated value of 6.18 reported by Neely et al (41). Hence, the upper range log P values reported by Metcalf et al (42) appear to be low, and as a result their equation (log BCF = 1.1587 log P – 0.7504) has a much steeper slope than Neely et al (41) since comparable bioconcentration factors were observed by both groups.

The Neely et al (41) regression also provided a reasonable estimate for the bioconcentration of trifluralin (calculated log $P = 5.33$) measured in several species of large fish from the Wabash River (44). The equation yielded a log value of 3.01 compared to observed mean values of 3.22 in golden redhorse (*Moxostoma erythrurum*), 3.45 in shorthead redhorse (*M.macrolepidotum*), and 3.73 in sauger (*Stizostedion canadense*). Thus, the partition coefficient of a lipophilic compound can often provide a good measure of its bioaccumulation potential in fish and presumably other aquatic organisms.

In reality, predicting bioaccumulation based on partition values alone is risky. Satisfactory results usually can be derived for an analogue series within a family of chemicals for which confirmatory experiments have been conducted on a few representative compounds. Many pitfalls and exceptions exist. For example, compounds with low P values, being more polar, may be more susceptible to biodegradation or excretion (8, 45) such that accumulation may be overestimated. Likewise, the uptake of acidic or basic compounds is strongly affected by the degree of ionization as regulated by the pH (46). Conversely, direct application of a partition coefficient regression appears to underestimate bioaccumulation of compounds having P values something greater than log 6 (41, 47, 48). Compounds in this class often display bioconcentration factors greater than log 5 in whole fish from natural environments (49). Because the amount of time required to reach a steady state is extremely long (40), growth and fat deposition have to be considered in the analysis (48). Consequently, the bioaccumulation of a few "super pollutants" such as DDT and some PCBs require more complex models that incorporate the bioenergetics of the fish (47).

FISH GROWTH AND BIOMASS DYNAMICS

Models for growth have been based either on the biomass (50) or on the energy content (51) of fish as the primary unit of measure. Both methods are complex and require detailed knowledge of the biology of each species, as well as the community they inhabit (52). As a consequence we do not dwell on the specifics involved, but encourage our readers to carefully review the literature we have cited before attempting to employ these more advanced techniques for predicting chemical residue accumulation.

Norstrom et al (53) reasoned that the uptake rate of pollutants by fish should fall within limits set by those factors that control metabolism and growth, as modified by environmental factors such as temperature and food availability. To evaluate this concept, they developed a pollutant accumulation model based on fish bioenergetics (51, 54) combined with some data on pollutant biokinetics. In essence, they devised an equation that stated that pollutant body burden changes with respect to time were equal to the uptake from the water plus uptake from the food minus the depuration rate, wherein each rate was modified by complex body weight–dependent functions. The obvious disadvantage of this approach is the difficulty one encounters in measuring all of the various metabolic rate constants needed for the model. Nevertheless, their detailed analysis did serve to support the log-log transformation, mentioned previously (13), and further demonstrated that for PCBs and mercury in yellow perch (*Perca flavesens*) the entire model could be approximated by

$$dP/dt \doteq AW^{0.7} - k_{cl} \, PW^{-0.58}, \qquad\qquad 1.$$

where A is a constant which combines all the coefficients in the uptake parts of the model, W the body weight, and P the pollutant body burden. Since this is essentially the equation for a simple compartment model, one might expect an equilibrium state to be reached. However, the exponents operating on the changes in body weight prevent an equilibrium from actually being achieved. That is, if the relative value of the exponent terms on body weight are correct, then the uptake factors for methyl mercury and PCBs have increasing "power" over the depuration factors (0.7 > 0.58) as the weight of the aquatic animal increases with time. Thus, it follows that if a compound is persistent, has a high bioconcentration potential, and the animal gains appreciable weight with time, there is more opportunity to "capitalize" on these seemingly small differences and steady state conditions cannot be reached.

Accepting an assumption that a fish's "fill" works faster than its "flush" relative to body weight, is certainly tempting. In fact, an adjustment factor of this sort would undoubtedly account for some of the anomalies observed in residue studies with natural fish populations. However, a physiological reason for this disproportionality still needs to be elucidated.

The equation implies that the surface area or metabolic rate of uptake tissues (e.g. gills and gut) decreases less relative to body weight than that of the excretory tissues (e.g. gills, kidney, and ovaries) as fish gain weight while growing older. How this sort of differentiation would be physiologically possible is a mystery. Alternatively, it may arise as a result of a difference between adsorption and desorption or some other physical-chemical phenomena unique to these "super pollutants." Regardless of the cause, the absolute value of these exponents must vary between species and between various life-stage stanzas for each species.

Thus, one can envision that the kinetic rates and relative importance of body weight would change as the fish grows, matures, spawns, and finally reaches senescence. Furthermore, overlying these physiological changes, their food habits change and seasonal factors (such as temperature), alter food consumption, habitat selection, etc. Each of these factors contributes to the bioenergetics of the fish and its subsequent bioaccumulation of various trace contaminants. Therefore, to be absolutely precise would require a combined biomass-bioenergetics model which incorporated seasonal changes from year to year in the pollutant levels of the environment, plus various subroutines for individual fish stocks that might be further subdivided on the basis of sex and year class.

Achieving this level of refinement would be a truly monumental task! Consider for example that Kitchell et al (50) estimated that over 100 man-years of effort were required just to compile the relatively simple set of data needed to formulate a growth model for bluegills (*Lepomis macrochirus*) in a small lake. Expanding this model to include pollutant kinetics both within a lake and the fish would be staggering, although not impossible. So, we have to ask ourselves: Is this level of refinement really needed? In truth, we have to conclude it would be informative but probably is not necessary at this time. There are just too many other questions pertinent to the environmental behavior of pollutants which need to be resolved before we, as fisheries scientists, need this degree of sophistication.

CONCLUSION

The environmental behavior of pollutants appears to depend more on their chemical-physical properties than on the biological-ecological features of the receiving body. By this statement we do not intend to imply that biology and ecology are not important. They are! It is just that greater insight can probably be achieved more quickly by applying the structure-activity concepts developed by Hansch (55) and others (56) before we try to develop totally comprehensive models for pollutants in aquatic environments.

The environmental fate and effects of chemicals have to relate, ultimately, to the unique properties of each compound. We have discussed how one biological event, that of accumulation, can frequently be related to the parameter of partition. Perhaps then photo-decomposition can be related to metabolism (47) and environmental distribution to surface area and mass ratios via adsorption (57). Thus, what is needed now are more simple, universal approximations which can serve to guide future studies intended to resolve particular issues and unique situations, not more complex solutions to the peculiar problem posed by a few chlorinated hydrocarbons.

We have briefly discussed the concepts of exchange equilibria (31), kinetics (40), and bioenergetics (53). Taken together, these may form the basis for a simpler approach to the problem of quantifying residue accumulation by fish in natural environments. Bioenergetics can define the range of food consumption and respiration that might be expected for a given species under reasonably narrow environmental conditions. Kinetic studies should be able to define quickly the various rate constants for both direct and dietary sources. The concept of exchange equilibria can then be used to delineate the residue concentrations expected for both the water and food sources, provided that total inputs can be quantified. Given this framework it should be relatively easy to derive approximations for residue accumulation which are accurate within an order of magnitude. Considering the latitude associated with most dose-effect relationships, we should then be able to judge whether some definable effect threshold is likely to be exceeded. Thus, by following a rationale of this nature we should be able to streamline our research activities, yet maximize our opportunity for identifying potentially hazardous substances in the environment.

Overall, we are encouraged by the progress made in this field during the past few years. Furthermore, we expect to see even more dramatic results in future years. However, in contrast to the eye-catching headlines generated by studies on fish and chemicals over the past decade, these results will be dramatic for their simplicity and sobriety. As such, they will not be very newsworthy, but for those of us who have muddled through the myriad of environmental toxicology, they will be most welcome.

Literature Cited

1. Surber, E. W. 1948. Chemical control agents and their effects on fish. *Prog. Fish Cult.* 10:125–31
2. Carson, R. 1962. *Silent Spring.* Boston: Mifflin. 368 pp.
3a. Katz, M., Sparks, A. K., Pederson, L., Woelke, C. E., Woodey, J. 1968. Effects of pollution on fish life. *J. Water Pollut. Control Fed.* 40:1007–33
3b. Katz, M., Pederson, L., Yoshinaka, M., Sjolseth, D. 1969. Effects of pollution on fish life. *J. Water Pollut. Control Fed.* 41:994–1016
3c. Katz, M., Sjolseth, D. E., Anderson, D. R., Tyner, L. R. 1970. Effects of pollution on fish life. *J. Water Pollut. Control Fed.* 42:983–1002
3d. Katz, M., Wahtola, C. H., LeGore, R. S., Anderson, D., McConnell, S. 1971. Effects on freshwater fish. *J. Water Pollut. Control Fed.* 43:1334–63
3e. Katz, M., LeGore, R. S., Weitkamp, D., Cummins, J. M., Anderson, D., May, D. R. 1972. Effects on freshwater fish. *J. Water Pollut. Control Fed.* 44:1226–50
3f. McKim, J. M., Christensen, G. M., Tucker, J. H., Lewis, M. J. 1973. Effects of pollution on freshwater fish. *J. Water Pollut. Control Fed.* 45:1370–1407
3g. McKim, J. M., Christensen, G. M., Tucker, J. H., Benoit, D. A., Lewis, M. J. 1974. Effects of pollution on freshwater fish. *J. Water Pollut. Control Fed.* 46:1540–91
3h. McKim, J. M., Benoit, D. A., Biesinger, K. E., Brungs, W. A., Siefert, R. E. 1975. Effects of pollution on freshwater fish. *J. Water Pollut. Control Fed.* 47:1711–68
4. Johnson, D. W. 1968. Pesticides and fishes—a review of selected literature. *Trans. Am. Fish. Soc.* 97:398–424
5. Johnson, D. W. 1973. Pesticide residues in fish. In *Environmental Pollution by Pesticides,* ed. C. A. Edwards, 181–212. New York: Plenum. 542 pp.
6. Marshall, N. B. 1966. *The Life of Fishes.* New York: Universe Books. 402 pp.
7. Motais, R., Isaia, J., Rankin, J., Maetz, J. 1969. Adaptive changes of the water permeability of the teleostean gill epithelium in relation to external salinity. *J. Exp. Biol.* 51: 529–45
8. Forster, R. P., Goldstein, L. 1969. Formation of excretory products. In *Fish Physiology,* ed. W. S. Hoar, D. J. Randall, I:313–50. New York: Academic. 465 pp.
9. Lech, J. J., Statham, C. N. 1975. Role of glucuronide formation in the selective toxicity of 3-trifluoromethyl-4-nitrophenol (TFM) for the sea lamprey: Comparative aspects of TFM uptake and conjugation in sea lamprey and rainbow trout. *Toxicol. Appl. Pharmacol.* 31:150–58
10. Reinert, R. E., Stone, L. J., Willford, W. A. 1974. Effect of temperature on accumulation of methylmercuric chloride and p,p'DDT by rainbow trout (*Salmo gairdneri*). *J. Fish. Res. Board Can.* 31:1649–52
11. Murphy, P. G., Murphy, J. V. 1971. Correlations between respiration and direct uptake of DDT in the mosquitofish (*Gambusia affinis*). *Bull. Environ. Contam. Toxicol.* 6:581–88
12. Nikolsky, G. V. 1963. *The Ecology of Fishes.* New York: Academic. 352 pp.
13. Eberhardt, L. L. 1975. Some methodology for appraising contaminants in aquatic systems. *J. Fish. Res. Board Can.* 32:1852–59
14. Rudd, R. L., Genelly, R. E. 1956. Pesticides: Their use and toxicity in relation to wildlife. *Calif. Fish Game Bull.* 7:1–209
15. Hunt, E. G., Bischoff, A. I. 1960. Inimical effects on wildlife of periodic DDD applications to clear lake. *Calif. Fish Game* 46:91–106
16. Woodwell, G. M. 1967. Toxic substances and ecological cycles. *Sci. Am.* 216:24–31
17. Kevern, N. R. 1966. Feeding rate of carp estimated by a radioisotopic method. *Trans. Am. Fish. Soc.* 95: 363–71
18. Chadwick, G. G., Brocksen, R. W. 1969. Accumulation of dieldrin by fish and selected fish-food organisms. *J. Wildl. Manage.* 33:693–700
19. Grzenda, A. R., Paris, D. F., Taylor, W. J. 1970. The uptake, metabolism, and elimination of chlorinated residues by goldfish (*Carassius auratus*) fed a ¹⁴C-DDT contaminated diet. *Trans. Am. Fish. Soc.* 99:385–96
20. Grzenda, A. R., Taylor, W. J., Paris, D. F. 1971. The uptake and distribution of chlorinated residues by goldfish (*Carassius auratus*) fed a ¹⁴C-dieldrin contaminated diet. *Trans. Am. Fish. Soc.* 100:215–21

176   HAMELINK & SPACIE

21. Lieb, A. J., Bills, D. D., Sinnhuber, R. O. 1974. Accumulation of dietary polychlorinated biphenyls (Aroclor 1254) by rainbow trout (*Salmo gairdneri*). *J. Agric. Food Chem.* 22:638–42
22. Lenon, H. L. 1968. *Translocations and storage equilibria for minnows involving sublethal levels of dieldrin in aquatic ecosystems.* PhD thesis. Michigan State Univ., East Lansing, Michigan. 85 pp.
23. Macek, K. J., Rodgers, C. R., Stalling, D. L., Korn, S. 1970. The uptake, distribution and elimination of dietary ¹⁴C-DDT and ¹⁴C-dieldrin in rainbow trout. *Trans. Am. Fish. Soc.* 99:689–95
24. Macek, K. J., Korn, S. 1970. Significance of the food chain in DDT accumulation by fish. *J. Fish. Res. Board Can.* 27:1496–98
25. Reinert, R. E. 1972. Accumulation of dieldrin in an alga (*Scenedesmus obliquus*), *Daphnia magna,* and the guppy (*Poecilia reticulata*). *J. Fish. Res. Board Can.* 29:1413–18
26. Reinert, R. E., Stone, L. J., Bergman, H. L. 1974. Dieldrin and DDT: Accumulation from water and food by lake trout (*Salvelinus namaycush*) in the laboratory. *Proc. 17th Conf. Great Lakes Res.,* pp. 52–58
27. Allison, D., Kallman, B. J., Cope, O. B., Van Valin, C. 1964. Some chronic effects of DDT on cutthroat trout. *US Bur. Sport Fish. Wildl. Res. Rep. #64.* 30 pp.
28. Gakstatter, J. H., Weiss, C. M. 1967. The elimination of DDT-C¹⁴ dieldrin-C¹⁴ and lindane-C¹⁴ from fish following a single sublethal exposure in aquaria. *Trans. Am. Fish. Soc.* 96:301–7
29. Holden, A. V. 1962. A study of the absorption of ¹⁴C-labelled DDT from water by fish. *Ann. Appl. Biol.* 50:467–77
30. Coffin, C. C., Hayes, F. R., Jodrey, L. H., Whiteway, S. G. 1949. Exchange of materials in a lake as studied by the addition of radioactive phosphorus. *Can. J. Res.* 27:207–22
31. Hamelink, J. L., Waybrant, R. C., Ball, R. C. 1971. A proposal: Exchange equilibria control the degree chlorinated hydrocarbons are biologically magnified in lentic environments. *Trans. Am. Fish. Soc.* 100:207–14
32. Burdick, G. E., Harris, E. J., Dean, H. J., Walker, T. M., Skea, J., Colby, D. 1964. The accumulation of DDT in lake trout and the effect on reproduction. *Trans. Am. Fish. Soc.* 93:127–36
33. Anderson, R. B., Everhart, W. H. 1966. Concentrations of DDT in landlocked

salmon (*Salmo Salar*) at Sebago Lake, Maine. *Trans. Am. Fish. Soc.* 95:160–64
34. Reinert, R. E. 1970. Pesticide concentrations in Great Lakes fish. *Pestic. Monit. J.* 3:233–40
35. Anderson, R. B., Fenderson, O. C. 1970. An analysis of variation of insecticide residues in landlocked Atlantic salmon (*Salmo salar*). *J. Fish. Res. Board Can.* 27:1–11
36. Henderson, C., Inglis, A., Johnson, W. L. 1971. Organochlorine insecticide residues in fish—fall 1969. *Pestic. Monit. J.* 5:1–11
37. Reinert, R. E., Bergman, H. L. 1974. Residues of DDT in lake trout (*Salvelinus namaycush*) and coho salmon (*Oncorhynchus kisutch*) from the Great Lakes. *J. Fish. Res. Board Can.* 31:191–99
38. Bache, C. A., Serum, J. W., Youngs, W. D., Lisk, D. J. 1972. Polychlorinated biphenyl residues: Accumulation in Cayuga lake trout with age. *Science* 177:1191–92
39. Youngs, W. D., Gutenmann, W. H., Lisk, D. J. 1972. Residues of DDT in lake trout as a function of age. *Environ. Sci. Technol.* 6:451–52
40. Branson, D. R., Blau, G. E., Alexander, H. C., Neely, W. B. 1975. Bioconcentration of 2,2′,4,4′-tetrachlorobiphenyl in rainbow trout as measured by an accelerated test. *Trans. Am. Fish. Soc.* 104:785–92
41. Neely, W. B., Branson, D. R., Blau, G. E. 1974. Partition coefficient to measure bioconcentration potential of organic chemicals in fish. *Environ. Sci. Technol.* 8:1113–15
42. Metcalf, R. L., Sanborn, J. R., Lu, P.-Y., Nye, D. 1975. Laboratory model ecosystem studies of the degradation and fate of radiolabeled tri-, tetra-, and pentachlorobiphenyl compared with DDE. *Arch. Environ. Contam. Toxicol.* 3:151–65
43. Lu, P.-Y. 1974. *Model aquatic ecosystem studies of the environmental fate and biodegradability of industrial compounds.* PhD thesis. Univ. Ill., Urbana-Champaign, Ill. 138 pp.
44. Spacie, A. 1975. *The bioconcentration of trifluralin from a manufacturing effluent by fish in the Wabash River.* PhD thesis. Purdue Univ., West Lafayette, Indiana. 136 pp.
45. Kapoor, I. P., Metcalf, R. L., Hirwe, A. S., Coats, J. R., Khalsa, M. S. 1973. Structure activity correlations of biode-

gradability of DDT analogs. *J. Agric. Food Chem.* 21:310–15

46. Hunn, J. B., Allen, J. L. 1974. Movement of drugs across the gills of fishes. *Ann. Rev. Pharmacol.* 14:47–55

47. Crosby, D. G. 1975. The toxicant-wildlife complex. *Pure Appl. Chem.* 42:233–53

48. Hamelink, J. L., Waybrant, R. C., Yant, P. R. 1976. Mechanisms of bioaccumulation of mercury and chlorinated hydrocarbon pesticides by fish in lentic ecosystems. In *Fate of Pollutants in the Air and Water Environments, Adv. Environ. Sci. Technol.* 9: In press

49. Hamelink, J. L., Waybrant, R. C. 1976. DDE and lindane in a large-scale model lentic ecosystem. *Trans. Am. Fish. Soc.* 105:124–34

50. Kitchell, J. F., Koonce, J. F., O'Neill, R. V., Shugart, H. H. Jr., Magnuson, J. J., Booth, R. S. 1974. Model of fish biomass dynamics. *Trans. Am. Fish. Soc.* 103:786–98

51. Kerr, S. R. 1971. Prediction of fish growth efficiency in nature. *J. Fish. Res. Board Can.* 28:809–14

52. Regier, H. A., Henderson, H. F. 1973. Towards a broad ecological model of fish communities and fisheries. *Trans. Am. Fish. Soc.* 102:56–72

53. Norstrom, R. J., McKinnon, A. E., de Freitas, A. S. W. 1976. A bioenergetics-based model for pollutant accumulation by fish. Simulation of PCB and methylmercury residue levels in Ottawa River yellow perch (*Perca flavescens*). *J. Fish. Res. Board Can.* 33:248–67

54. Kerr, S. R. 1971. A simulation model of lake trout growth. *J. Fish. Res. Board. Can.* 28:815–19

55. Gould, R. F., ed. 1972. Biological correlations—the Hansch approach. *Adv. Chem. Ser.* No. 114. 304 pp.

56. Veith, G. D., Konasewich, D. E., eds. 1975. *Structure-activity correlations in studies of toxicity and bioconcentration with aquatic organisms. Proc. Symp., March 11–13, 1975.* Int. Joint Comm., 100 Ouellette Ave., Windsor, Ontario, Canada N9A 6T3. 347 pp.

57. Kenaga, E. E. 1972. Factors related to bioconcentration of pesticides. *Environ. Toxicol. Pestic.* 3:193–228

Ann. Rev. Pharmacol. Toxicol. 1977. 17:179–95

IMMUNOLOGIC ASPECTS OF CANCER CHEMOTHERAPY ❖6674

Charles M. Haskell

Department of Medicine, University of California School of Medicine,
Los Angeles, California 90024

INTRODUCTION

Most human and animal tumors bear antigens which may be classified as tumor specific or as tumor associated (1–4). Many scientists believe that the immune response to these antigens constitutes a critical host defense against cancer, and there are numerous reports in which immune manipulation has been utilized as a treatment for cancer (5–8). Clearly, lymphocytes from animals and human patients cured of tumors may destroy cultivated cells from their respective neoplasms; however, this may also be true when the lymphocyte donors have a growing tumor mass (9–10). Even with sophisticated immunologic testing, the majority of patients with early cancer appear to have normal immunologic function (11). Moreover, in many cases the best treatment for these patients is with drugs that can depress immunologic function, and cure or long-term control is nevertheless possible (12).

Because of these conflicting facts, physicians are faced with a serious question: what is the risk to benefit ratio of cancer chemotherapy as it relates to the immune system? This review focuses on the relationship between cancer chemotherapy and the immune system. Initially, I consider the immune response to cancer and immunologic function in patients with cancer. I then review the immune suppression which can be seen with both single-agent chemotherapy and combination chemotherapy and conclude with a discussion of immunotherapy and chemoimmunotherapy as current approaches to the amelioration of immune defects in patients with cancer. This review does not consider the use of immunosuppressive drugs in human transplantation or as treatment in a wide variety of "autoimmune" diseases.

THE IMMUNE RESPONSE IN CANCER

The normal immune response involves an exceedingly complex interaction between cellular and humoral factors (2, 6, 10, 13, 14). A simplified version of the immune system as it relates to cancer is shown in Figure 1, which distinguishes between

179

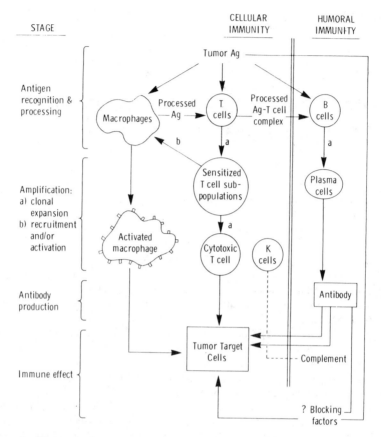

Figure 1 Diagrammatic representation of the immune response to a tumor antigen (Ag). The successive stages of the immune response are depicted on the left side of the diagram. Abbreviations: a, clonal expansion; b, recruitment and/or activation; T cell, thymus-dependent lymphocyte; B cell, bursa or bone marrow—derived lymphocyte; K cell, a lymphocyte population that has neither T- nor B-cell markers.

events involving humoral immunity and those involving cellular immunity. It does not distinguish between the primary and secondary responses to an antigen.

The initial stages of antigen recognition and processing may occur with macrophages, thymus-dependent lymphocytes (T cells), or bursa or bone marrow–dependent lymphocytes (B cells). Interactions between these cell lines are also possible, and subsequent amplification mechanisms follow. Amplification of the immune system may occur by clonal expansion, in which lymphocyte blastogenesis occurs with a proliferation of selected cell populations. Recruitment and/or activation of other cell lines may also occur; for example, it is known that macrophages can be activated by sensitizing T-cell subpopulations through the elaboration of macrophage activating factor (14). The final stage of immune effect involves a complex interaction of one or more of these elements. Activated macrophages are capable of killing tumor cells directly, and cytotoxic T cells can also act independently. A newly described lymphocyte population referred to as K cells (15), which bear neither T nor B lymphocyte surface characteristics, can kill tumor cells in the presence of specific antitumor antibody. Antibody, in the presence of complement, is also capable of killing tumor cells, and recently polymorphonuclear leukocytes in the presence of antibody have been shown to have cytotoxic effects (16).

These components of the immune system are considered critical to the process of killing tumor cells bearing tumor antigens. It is generally assumed that the cellular component of this effect is dominant, with humoral immunity playing a lesser role. Indeed, there is evidence that humoral immunity, through the formation of blocking factors (probable antigen-antibody complexes), may act to abrogate the ability of the cellular immune system to kill these cells (9, 10). Other cellular and humoral immune suppressors and stimulators have also been postulated (6, 17–20).

A diagram such as Figure 1 cannot convey the variety of responses to individual tumors that may occur. Differing levels of immunogenicity (1, 2, 21), changes in immunogenicity developing during the course of tumor dissemination and metastasis (22, 23), nonuniform responses in cell-mediated and humoral immune systems (4, 6, 10), the functional capacity of amplification factors, the importance of host abnormalities in antigen processing such as may occur with inadequate lymphocyte "trapping" in some sites of the body (24), prior antigenic experience, the functional status of the nervous system as it relates to humoral immunity (25), and genetic factors (26) may all serve to individualize the balance within the immune system and between tumor and host.

Many abnormalities in immunologic function have been documented during the course of malignant disease in patients with many different kinds of cancers. There is, however, considerable controversy whether such abnormalities are the result of cancer or represent an important causal factor. Many scientists believe that the immune response is the principal defense against neoplastic cells. This view was formulated by Thomas (27), and subsequently Burnet (28) elaborated on the concept and called it *immunologic surveillance*. They reasoned that the immune response destroyed cancer cells while they were still in the incipient stages of tumor formation, a possible function similar to graft rejection of foreign cells. This theory predicts that impaired immunity would inevitably increase susceptibility to cancer and suggests that immunity against a variety of neoplasms would exist in all normal adults. A tremendous amount of experimental work ensued to define the relationship between oncogenesis and the immunologic status of the host. Results often have been contradictory (29, 30). Many studies demonstrated tumor-specific antigens on human and animal cancer cells, facilitated carcinogenesis by immunosuppression (31), and increased incidence of malignancy in immunosuppressed or immunodeficient patients (14, 32–34). On the other hand, it is clear that some tumors do not seem to be antigenic (29, 30), and other studies failed to demonstrate enhanced carcinogenesis with immunosuppressive treatment (35).

In a critical review of the theory of immunologic surveillance, Schwartz (29) proposed that defective immunity may lead to cancer, not through surveillance against neoplastic cells, but by failure to terminate lymphoproliferation triggered by an antigen. He concluded that it may be unrealistic to expect the enormous complexities of cancer to crystallize within the confines of a single theory. Some neoplasms may well arise as a result of spontaneous mutation, while others may be induced by viruses, chemical carcinogens, X rays, or hormonal stimulation. Some may be eliminated by an immune response, whereas others may actually require an immune response for their development. Clearly, the latter situation has been well documented by Prehn (36), where the initial effect of the immune system on a developing tumor was stimulation of tumor growth at very small tumor cell numbers. A corollary of this is seen in some animal tumors, where manipulation of the immune system has resulted in a marked increase in the rate of tumor growth (37, 38).

Ritts & Neel (4) have provided yet another perspective on the role of the immune system in cancer. Drawing from the work of Voisin (39), they point out that current concepts of the immune system appear to neglect the well-founded physiologic importance of homeostasis. The very vocabulary of immunology with its traditional martial posture of attack versus defense (using such terms as *invader, surveillance, front line of defense, recruitment, escape*) is antithetical to homeostasis. As articulated by Voisin, a posture of dynamic equilibrium is more sensible. In essence, he postulates a dynamic spectrum of immune reaction, which ranges from host rejection to enhancement, allowing one to visualize a finely tuned balance, with both rejection and enhancement utilizing the components of the immune system outlined in Figure 1. This concept considers the facilitation or enhancement of cellular growth equal in importance to the rejection of cells; facilitation represents the necessary counterpart of the rejection reaction to prevent the autodestruction of the individual.

Although immunologic theories of cancer appear to be in a state of crisis, physicians treating patients with cancer must carefully consider both the impact of the tumor on immune function and the impact of treatment on the immunologic status of the host. It may be impossible to prove or disprove the existence of an immune surveillance mechanism (30), but it is possible for us to identify those agents or procedures that appear to increase the probability of neoplastic disease or complications from neoplasms. In terms of cancer chemotherapy, the practical result of these theories is that we should strive for programs of treatment that are minimally immunosuppressive wherever possible (40–42). Even if one believes that the immune system plays no important role in the etiology of cancer, it clearly is an important host defense mechanism for many of the complications that occur during treatment. Specifically, infections commonly lead to the death of patients with advanced cancer, and impaired immunity may contribute to such a death (12, 43). Therefore, while awaiting further studies to define the basic mechanisms involved, we should consider carefully the effect of treatment on the immune system of our patients.

Immune Function in Patients with Cancer

Detailed reviews of immunologic function in patients with cancer are available (3, 4, 11, 40–42, 44), and the techniques of immunologic assessment utilized therein have been reviewed (45). Immunologic studies in patients with cancer commonly utilize tests of delayed cutaneous hypersensitivity, either with recall antigens or with dinitrochlorobenzene (DNCB) to determine cellular immune function (46–49). Humoral immunity is clinically assessed by the level of immunoglobulins (44); however, for research purposes this must be supplemented by additional techniques (45). Considerable controversy surrounds the use of newer techniques of immune evaluation in patients, such as tests of antitumor cellular cytotoxicity (49–51) and T- and B-cell quantitation (52).

Innumerable studies confirm that profound disturbances in immune function may accompany human cancer (11). Patients with early and indolent forms of malignancy are less severely affected than those with rapidly progressive disseminated tumors. Highly sophisticated techniques are required to demonstrate any defects in immune function occurring in very early stages of neoplasia. Leukemias and lymphomas are associated with profound immune defects, as with the well-known anergy which accompanies Hodgkin's disease (11, 44). Cell-mediated immunity is the initial arm of the immune system to be altered in most cases, and disturbances of T-lymphocyte function have been demonstrated by both in vivo and in vitro methods. In late stages of disease, humoral immunity also becomes depressed.

In groups of patients with solid tumors, anergy to DNCB or recall antigens generally signifies a poor prognosis (41, 44, 53). Bolton and colleagues (54) tested the response to DNCB as an indicator of a primary response and the Mantoux reaction as an index of recall responses in patients with colonic cancer, breast cancer, and gastric cancer. Cellular immunity was lost earliest and to the greatest extent in patients with colonic cancer; gastric cancer occupied an intermediate position, and severely depressed immunity was seen in breast cancer only with very advanced disease. A paradoxical result was seen in breast cancer where DNCB responsiveness was excellent in patients with intermediate stages of disease, but was depressed in patients both with early disease and with very advanced disease. This study serves to underline the need to very carefully assess groups of patients by specific type of neoplasm (55–64), with appropriate control groups by stage as well as by age (65, 66), nutritional status (67, 68), and other factors that may influence immunologic function. Unfortunately, this kind of detailed information is not available for most tumors, and statements about the value of DNCB skin testing for populations of patients may not be useful in assessing the prognosis of an individual patient (69).

DRUG-INDUCED IMMUNOSUPPRESSION

Major improvements in cancer chemotherapy have followed a better understanding of the mechanisms of drug action, pharmacology, and cellular biology (12). We now know that one must consider anticancer drug action as a function of the cell cycle (with a distinction between phase specific and phase nonspecific drugs), as well as the fact that tumor cell populations appear to grow by Gomperzian kinetics. It is also known that chemotherapy kills cancer cells by a fractional cell kill mechanism, usually best described as a logarithmic function (log cell kill hypothesis).

We have learned that choosing the proper dose and schedule of drugs is critical, and major improvements in treatment have resulted from combinations of drugs. Combination chemotherapy has been a particularly important factor in improving the treatment of patients with cancer, and several principles underlying combination chemotherapy have emerged. The successful programs of combination chemotherapy utilize only drugs that are active against the cancer in question, have different mechanisms of action, and varying spectra of toxicities so that full doses can be employed. In addition, most successful combination chemotherapy regimens employ intensive pulses of combination drug treatment, followed by a period of rest. This rest period allows for reconstitution of hematopoietic and other cellular functions.

The aforementioned principles have contributed to improvements in cancer chemotherapy over recent years; however, how may we improve these results further and what are the clear-cut deficits of such therapy? The toxicity of these various programs of chemotherapy are fairly well defined as they relate to bone marrow function and the function of other major organ systems. Reasonably extensive studies have defined the immunosuppressive effects of the antineoplastic drugs used as single agents (70). However, most of these studies have been done in animals with the schedule of drug administration chosen to optimize immunosuppression. Much less is known about the immunosuppressive effects in man of cancer chemotherapy used as clinical treatment of cancer (70, 71).

In this review, I do not discuss in detail animal studies of immunosuppression with the clinically useful anticancer drugs. Rather, I summarize the sites of action of the commonly used immunosuppressive agents on the immune response in Table 1, as defined in animal studies. In the sections that follow I briefly describe the results of single-agent chemotherapy and combination chemotherapy on the established immune response in man. It is likely that the major deleterious impact of chemotherapy in man is upon already established immunity, since in all probability the critical event of antitumor immunity occurred before the cancer was diagnosed.

Table 1 Stages of the immune response inhibited by drugs

Antigen recognition and/or processing	Amplification	Antibody production	Immune effect
Alkylating agents (cyclophosphamide)	Alkylating agents (cyclophosphamide)	Alkylating agents (cyclophosphamide)	Corticosteroids
X irradiation	Actinomycin D		Antilymphocyte serum
Actinomycin D	5-Fluorouracil		
Corticosteroids	6-Mercaptopurine		
Antilymphocyte serum	Cytosine arabinoside		
	L-Asparaginase		
	Vinca alkaloids		

Single-Agent Chemotherapy

A recent review details attempts to suppress humoral immunity selectively, while sparing cellular immunity in experimental animals (72). This review and other major ones on immunosuppression (70, 71) clearly illustrate that the commonly used antineoplastic agents rarely suppress previously established immune function.

6-MERCAPTOPURINE   6-Mercaptopurine (6-MP) is one of the most extensively studied immunosuppressive agents (40, 70, 73). Its use in man depresses the primary antibody response; it can retard allograft rejection and prevent the development of new delayed hypersensitivity reactions. It may also induce tolerance with proper scheduling of antigen administration. However, conventional doses of 6-MP used in cancer patients appear to have no important effect on established delayed hypersensitivity (73).

5-FLUOROURACIL   Mitchell & DeConti (74) studied 12 cancer patients undergoing 5-fluorouracil therapy. Eight of 10 patients failed to demonstrate a primary antibody response to Vi-antigen, and a secondary response was completely inhibited in 4 of 9 patients. Five of 6 patients tested failed to achieve a delayed cutaneous hypersensitivity reaction to DNCB. Three of 6 showed reversion to positive of one or more skin tests after therapy. This study suggests that 5-fluorouracil given in clinical doses to man is a potent immunosuppressant, having some effect on established immunity as well as on primary immunity. An additional study of interest is that of Suhrland, Benson & Labelle (75), in which subtherapeutic doses of 5-fluorouracil in mice (1 mg/kg/day) led to an enhanced growth of a transplantable mammary adenocarcinoma, whereas a standard therapeutic dose (15 mg/kg/day) led to marked inhibition of this same tumor. Further studies indicated that the stimulating dose for tumor growth was able to suppress the secondary antibody response to bovine gamma globulin. These findings underline the importance of choosing the proper dose, whether the concern is immunosuppression or antitumor effect.

METHOTREXATE   Methotrexate can suppress humoral antibody formation in man, primarily when given after antigenic stimulation (70, 76). It does not appear to block either the expression of established delayed hypersensitivity or the ability to acquire new delayed hypersensitivity, although it can reduce the intensity of these reactions. It may also inhibit the local inflammatory response in man.

CYTOSINE ARABINOSIDE   Cytosine arabinoside has been intensively studied by Heppner & Calabresi (72) as a potential selective immunosuppressant, based on early studies of its selective ability to inhibit humoral immunity in tumor-bearing mice. Further studies in mice confirmed marked dependency on the schedule of administration of drug and antigen, as well as drug dosage. Mitchell and colleagues (76) have studied schedules of cytosine arabinoside similar to those that are optimal for the treatment of malignancy in patients with cancer. Such schedules partially suppress the primary and secondary antibody response, but established delayed hypersensitivity reactions were unaffected.

CYCLOPHOSPHAMIDE   This drug has been widely studied in animals and man (70, 71, 77–80). Administered as maintenance therapy to patients with lymphomas in an oral dose of 100 mg/day, no interference with the development of normal humoral and cell-mediated immune responses to keyhole limpet hemocyanin was found (71). In vitro lymphocyte blastogenesis after stimulation with phytohemagglutinin was also unaffected. Given in larger doses intravenously (7 mg/kg/day for 7 days), it is capable of blocking the antibody response to Vi antigen. There was, however, no significant reduction in established delayed hypersensitivity. Clearly depending on the timing of administration and dose employed, cyclophosphamide can be a potent immunosuppressant drug. However, I am unaware of any studies demonstrating significant depression of established delayed hypersensitivity reactions.

VINCA ALKALOIDS   Vincristine and prednisone, when combined to treat acute leukemia, inhibit the primary immune response to a variety of antigens (70, 71). Other studies in man are inadequate to make a firm statement about the immunosuppressant qualities of this class of drugs, although most studies suggest that the vinca alkaloids are only weakly immunosuppressant. There are major species differences in the immunosuppressive properties of the vinca alkaloids, and potent immunosuppression has been observed only in the rat (81).

ADRIAMYCIN AND DAUNOMYCIN   I am unaware of any detailed immunologic studies in man with these two drugs. A study comparing the immunosuppressive activity of these drugs on humoral antibody production and tumor allograft rejection has been done in mice (82). It was found that adriamycin induced a greater reduction in the number of antibody-producing cells after primary stimulation with sheep erythrocytes, whereas daunomycin was more suppressive of the secondary response to the same antigen. With a tumor allograft model, daunomycin was significantly more immunosuppressive than was adriamycin administered at equitoxic doses. It was suggested that the greater immunosuppressive effect of daunomycin may account for the superiority of adriamycin in most clinical settings. This interesting hypothesis requires additional study in man, including the effect of drug treatment on established immune function.

IMMUNE SUPPRESSION BY MICROORGANISMS   Schwab (83) has reviewed suppression of the immune response by microorganisms. Of greatest interest has been the suppression of the immune system seen with certain bacterial enzymes, most importantly *l*-asparaginase (84). This appears to inhibit thymus-dependent (T-cell) lymphocytes primarily, although under certain circumstances B cells are also inhibited (85). One fascinating aspect of the toxicity of *l*-asparaginase is the development of allergic reactions to the enzyme. This has been extensively studied in man (86). Prior to treatment, patients are not allergic to this medication and they have no antibody or skin reactivity to the enzyme. After one course of treatment, positive skin test reactivity is observed. Circulating antibodies have also been detected, and patients have, in some cases, developed anaphylactic shock upon repeated exposure.

There are other bacterial products which are immunosuppressive (83), but the important ones (bacillus Calmette-Guérin and *Corynebacterium parvum*) are discussed in the context of immunotherapy in a later section, since these same agents are primarily being employed as immunostimulants.

Combination Chemotherapy

There is a paucity of information on the impact of combination chemotherapy on the immune system. The major studies have taken place in acute leukemia, where a number of investigators have analyzed the impact of various programs of intensive combination chemotherapy on long-term survival and immunologic function (40, 87–91). Leventhal, Cohen & Triem (91) have reviewed the literature on this subject, and concluded that the majority of patients with acute leukemia showed depressed B-cell function during combination chemotherapy. There was also a correlation shown between a poor prognosis and depressed T-cell function during the induction phase of chemotherapy. They postulated that this poor survival was probably due at least in part to an increased incidence of fatal infections. Depressed T-cell function undoubtedly was not a major function of chemotherapy, since it predated the initiation of treatment in most patients.

Of additional interest is the impact of long-term chemotherapy on immunologic function after the conclusion of treatment. Children with acute lymphoblastic leukemia in continuous remission for two and one half to three years treated at St. Jude's Hospital in Tennessee were studied after discontinuation of chemotherapy (87, 88). Children less than five years of age demonstrated a rise in lymphocyte number and increased immunoglobulin and antibody production. This was not seen in the older group of patients. After drugs were discontinued, one fourth of the patients demonstrated a rise in antibody to the Hong Kong influenza virus without evidence of reexposure to the same antigen. Further studies confirmed that lymphocyte function promptly recovered even after three years of antineoplastic therapy, and there were variations from patient to patient in the speed of this form of immunologic rebound. It was suggested that any studies of immunotherapy in this population would have to be carefully controlled, because of the variable rate of immune recovery with immunostimulation.

Several groups have studied the effect of combination chemotherapy on the immune system in patients with solid tumors. The earliest studies were by Hersh and colleagues (40, 70, 92–94), originally performed at the National Cancer Institute and subsequently continued at M. D. Anderson Hospital. One widely quoted study is particularly relevant (12, 42, 94). Patients with solid tumors received five-day courses of intensive combination chemotherapy. The immunological factors included macrophage entry into experimental inflammatory sites (a skin window), antibody response to primary antigenic stimulation, and lymphocyte blastogenic response to phytohemagglutinin. There was a marked decrease in all of these parameters during treatment; however, within two or three days there was complete or nearly complete recovery in immunological response. Indeed, some patients developed an "immunological overshoot" during the recovery period. Thus, when such five-day courses of combination chemotherapy were given every two to four weeks, the patient's immunological function was normal most of the time.

Harris and colleagues (95–97) have extended these results by demonstrating a high correlation of an overshoot response in lymphocyte function in patients with solid tumors who enjoy a substantial reduction in tumor size with combination chemotherapy. Nonresponding patients failed to demonstrate the overshoot, whereas responding patients almost universally demonstrated the phenomenon. This was true for 6 of 13 responding patients who were immunologically hyporeactive before treatment.

Studies are in progress to define further the immunologic effects of combination chemotherapy (98), with attention to the details of patient selection by diagnosis and stage, as well as pretreatment immunologic function. However, while awaiting the results of such studies, it would appear prudent to utilize combination chemotherapy in intermittent regimens wherever possible to take advantage of what appears to be a reduced amount of immunosuppression by such regimens (99).

IMMUNOTHERAPY AND CHEMOIMMUNOTHERAPY

Encouraged primarily by the theory of immunologic surveillance as an explanation for the development of cancer in animals and man, there has been considerable interest in stimulating the immune system as a potential approach to treating or preventing the development of cancer. The subject of immune stimulation has generated a large number of scientific studies and many reviews (4–8, 44, 100).

Immunotherapy can be divided into three areas: passive immunotherapy, adoptive immunotherapy, and active immunotherapy. Passive immunotherapy involves administration to the patient of antibodies produced in other individuals or animals. By definition it does not actively involve the host's resources in the immunotherapeutic process. Adoptive immunotherapy involves the introduction of immunocompetent cells into the cancer patient. These cells may be from related or unrelated individuals, and they may be either immune or nonimmune. Immune cells may be sensitized in vivo or in vitro, either to the patient's tumor, to other tumors, or even to oncogenic viruses. Although both passive and adoptive immunotherapy have been utilized with some success in experimental animals, they have never been proven to be of value in treating human cancer and are not discussed further at this juncture. The remaining form of immunotherapy, active immunotherapy, involves the host playing an active role in the induction or modulation of the immune response. Active immunotherapy can be either specific or nonspecific. A number of agents, including bacillus Calmette Guérin (BCG) (101), methanol-extracted residue (MER) of BCG (102), *Corynebacterium parvum* (103), levamisole (104), and synthetic polynucleosides (105), have been shown to have a nonspecific stimulatory effect. However, as described briefly above, some of these materials may also have immunosuppressive qualities, depending on the dose and route of administration (83).

At the present time, preliminary data suggest that active immunotherapy of a nonspecific type may be useful in the treatment of selected human tumors, primarily adult acute myelogenous leukemia (106–108), metastatic malignant melanoma (7, 109, 110), various skin cancers (111), and possibly Hodgkin's disease (112). However, other human tumors initially thought to be responsive to immune manipulation have failed to respond to such therapy in subsequent trials. This is particularly true of childhood acute lymphocytic leukemia, where initial success (113) failed to be seen in subsequent studies (108, 114). In addition, reports of successful immunotherapy with BCG in malignant melanoma have all utilized retrospective controls, and some of the apparent benefits of BCG in some subsets of patients were not seen in subsequent studies utilizing other strains or doses of BCG (115). These variable results and the inherent risks of BCG in man (116) underline the highly experimental nature of immunotherapy for human malignant diseases. Indeed, given the complexities of the immune system these results should not be a surprise. Lacking a reproducible and consistent record of therapeutic success with immunotherapy, I do not believe that it can be recommended beyond the experimental clinic at the present time.

Programs of chemoimmunotherapy are in a similar state of flux. This form of combined therapy has usually involved single agent or combination agent chemotherapy plus either BCG, *C. parvum,* or levamisole (117). The current status of such studies are reviewed individually by agent.

Bacillus Calmette Guérin

Bacillus Calmette Guérin has been used extensively in malignant melanoma as an immunologic adjunct to chemotherapy with imidazole carboxamide (DIC) (115, 118) or various programs of combination chemotherapy (119, 120). An early study combining DIC with BCG appears to have increased the survival of patients with malignant melanoma involving regional lymph nodes, but it had no effect on survival in patients with lesions involving the trunk (118). In a subsequent study, the Southwest Oncology Group has compared the survival and response of patients with malignant melanoma receiving a program of combination chemotherapy or combination chemotherapy plus BCG. Preliminary analysis of this more recent study has failed to show the dramatic difference which was suggested by the earlier study (120). For malignant melanoma, it remains an open question whether or not the addition of BCG to chemotherapy provides a practical and substantial improvement over the results seen with drug therapy alone. BCG has been combined with 5-fluorouracil in the treatment of patients with potentially cured colon cancer (121), and it has also been used as an adjunct to chemotherapy in advanced breast cancer (122). In both cases, preliminary results suggest that the duration of disease control may be somewhat improved by BCG. These studies require confirmation as well as clarification of some methodological problems (123).

Corynebacterium parvum

C. parvum has been utilized in Europe as an adjunct to chemotherapy (103), primarily in the pioneering studies of Israel and colleagues (124, 125). Israel has shown an increased survival and duration of antitumor response to chemotherapy in patients with lung cancer and breast cancer with the use of subcutaneous *C.*

parvum. Similar studies are currently under way in the United States, using a different preparation of *C. parvum* and different routes of administration. Hopefully, such studies will show a similar improvement in treatment.

Experience at UCLA with *C. parvum*, as well as other available data in the United States, has not been as optimistic (126). In a limited study of patients with breast cancer receiving combination chemotherapy with cyclophosphamide, methotrexate, and 5-fluorouracil, the response rate and duration of response in a small group was similar for those receiving *C. parvum* as for those receiving chemotherapy alone. Bone marrow tolerance to chemotherapy appeared to be reduced by the addition of *C. parvum*, and serious side effects with this agent given intravenously were common. Chills, fever, and changes in blood pressure were not unusual. Therefore, I believe that this drug must be carefully studied in additional patients before its clinical use as an adjunct to chemotherapy can be considered established.

Levamisole

Levamisole is a potent deworming agent which has been shown to stimulate the immune system in immunologically incompetent animals and man (104, 127). It does not appear to stimulate the already intact immune system, and there have been variable results in patients with cancer. Some studies have failed to show a significant immunostimulatory effect with this agent. However, Rojas (128) has shown in a controlled trial a significantly prolonged survival and disease-free interval after radiation therapy for patients with advanced regional breast cancer who received levamisole, in comparison with a control group that did not receive the agent. Similarly, European investigators have found an improved duration of disease-free survival in patients with lung cancer who have received levamisole in a controlled clinical trial (129). Both of these latter studies suggest that levamisole may be a useful agent in improving the survival and outlook for patients with advanced cancer. Further studies are needed to confirm and extend these early observations.

CONCLUSIONS AND PROSPECTS FOR THE FUTURE

Immunologic theories of cancer are clearly in evolution. The immune response has been shown to be extremely complex in patients with cancer, with many interrelated suppressor and stimulator cells or factors. Because of this complexity, it is naive to think that some simple form of immune stimulation will be universally successful in controlling all forms of cancer at all stages of disease in conjunction with all forms of systemic therapy. Indeed, it is likely that immunologic impairment in the majority of cancer patients is a consequence rather than a contributing cause of the illness. Moreover, the suggestion of some workers that one of the reasons for the success of cancer chemotherapy may be due to selective immunosuppression deserves further clarification and study (130–132). An increased effort to define more precisely immunologic function in patients with cancer and the immunologic impact of various forms of local and systemic therapy is needed. In the meantime, cautious and carefully controlled experimental trials of immunotherapy and chemotherapy in patients with cancer appear warranted.

Literature Cited

1. Rowlands, D. T. Jr., Daniele, R. P. 1975. Surface receptors in the immune response. *N. Engl. J. Med.* 293:26–32
2. Smith, R. T. 1968. Tumor-specific immune mechanisms. *N. Engl. J. Med.* 278:1207–14, 1268–75, 1326–31
3. Marx, J. L. 1974. Tumor immunology. I. The host's response to cancer. *Science* 184:552–56
4. Ritts, R. E. Jr., Neel, H. B. III 1974. An overview of cancer immunology. *Mayo Clin. Proc.* 49:118–31
5. Marx, J. L. 1974. Tumor immunology. II. Strategies for cancer therapy. *Science* 184:652–54
6. Fahey, J. L., Brosman, S., Ossorio, R. C., O'Toole, C., Zighelboim, J. 1976. Immunotherapy and human tumor immunology. *Ann. Intern. Med.* 84:454–65
7. Morton, D. L. 1974. Cancer immunotherapy: An overview. *Semin. Oncol.* 1:297–310
8. Bluming, A. Z. 1975. Current status of clinical immunotherapy. *Can. Chemother. Rep.* 59:901–13
9. Baldwin, R. W., Price, M. R. 1976. Tumor antigens and tumor-host relationships. *Ann. Rev. Med.* 27:151–63
10. Hellström, K. E., Hellström, I. 1974. Lymphocyte-mediated cytotoxicity and blocking serum activity to tumor antigens. *Adv. Immunol.* 18:209–77
11. Harris, J., Copeland, D. 1974. Impaired immunoresponsiveness in tumor patients. *Ann. NY Acad. Sci.* 230:56–85
12. Cline, M. J., Haskell, C. M. 1975. *Cancer Chemotherapy.* Philadelphia: Saunders. 324 pp.
13. Craddock, C. G., Longmire, R., McMillan, R. 1971. Lymphocytes and the immune response. *N. Engl. J. Med.* 285:324–31, 378–84
14. Alexander, P. 1976. The functions of the macrophage in malignant disease. *Ann. Rev. Med.* 27:207–24
15. Henney, C. S. 1974. Killer T cells. *N. Engl. J. Med.* 291:1357–58
16. Gale, R. P., Zighelboim, J. 1974. Modulation of polymorphonuclear leukocyte-mediated antibody-dependent cellular cytotoxicity. *J. Immunol.* 113:1793–1800
17. Bach, J-F. 1977. Thymic hormones: Biochemistry, and biological and clinical activities. *Ann. Rev. Pharmacol. Toxicol.* 17: In press
18. Snyderman, R., Pike, M. C. 1976. An inhibitor of macrophage chemotaxis produced by neoplasms. *Science* 192:370–72
19. Mackler, B. F. 1971. Role of soluble lymphocyte mediators in malignant-tumour destruction. *Lancet* 2:297–301
20. Potter, H., Rosenfeld, S., Dressler, D. 1974. Transfer factor. *Ann. Intern. Med.* 81:838–47
21. Jacobs, B. B., Uphoff, D. E. 1974. Immunologic modification: A basic survival mechanism. *Science* 185:582–87
22. Faraci, R. P. 1974. In vitro demonstration of altered antigenicity of metastases from a primary methylcholanthrene-induced sarcoma. *Surgery* 76:469–73
23. Goldman, L. I., Flaxman, B. A., Wernick, G., Zabriskie, J. B. 1974. Immune surveillance and tumor dissemination: In vitro comparison of the B16 melanoma in primary and metastatic form. *Surgery* 76:50–56
24. Frost, P., Lance, E. M. 1973. Abrogation of lymphocyte trapping by ascitic tumours. *Nature* 246:101–3
25. Stein, M., Schiavi, R. C., Camerino, M. 1976. Influence of brain and behavior on the immune system. *Science* 191:435–40
26. Dellon, A. L., Rogentine, G. N. Jr., Chretien, P. B. 1975. Prolonged survival in bronchogenic carcinoma associated with HL-A antigens W-19 and HL-A5: A preliminary report. *J. Natl. Cancer Inst.* 54:1283–86
27. Thomas, L. 1959. Reactions to homologous tissue antigens in relation to hypersensitivity. In *Cellular and Humoral Aspects of the Hypersensitive States*, ed. H. S. Lawrence, 529–32. New York: Hoeber. 667 pp.
28. Burnet, F. M. 1970. The concept of immunological surveillance. *Prog. Exp. Tumor Res.* 13:1–27
29. Schwartz, R. S. 1975. Another look at immunologic surveillance. *N. Engl. J. Med.* 293:181–84
30. Kripke, M. L., Borsos, T. 1974. Immune surveillance revisited. *J. Natl. Cancer Inst.* 52:1393–95
31. Cerilli, J., Hattan, B. A. 1974. Immunosuppression and oncogenesis. *Am. J. Clin. Pathol.* 62:218–23
32. Penn, I., Starzl, T. E. 1972. Malignant tumors arising de novo in immunosuppressed organ transplant recipients. *Transplantation* 14:407–17
33. Brown, R. S., Schiff, M., Mitchell, M. S. 1974. Reticulum-cell sarcoma of host

origin arising in a transplanted kidney. *Ann. Intern. Med.* 80:459–63

34. Waldmann, T. A., Strober, W., Blaese, R. M. 1972. Immunodeficiency disease and malignancy. *Ann. Intern. Med.* 77:605–28

35. Kripke, M. L., Borsos, T. 1974. Immunosuppression and carcinogenesis. *Isr. J. Med. Sci.* 10:888–903

36. Prehn, R. T. 1972. The immune reaction as a stimulator of tumor growth. *Science* 176:170–71

37. Gershon, R. K. 1974. Regulation of concomitant immunity, activation of suppressor cells by tumor excision. *Immunological Parameters of Host-Tumor Relationships,* ed. D. W. Weiss, 3:198–209. New York: Academic. 263 pp.

38. Paranjpe, M. S., Boone, C. W. 1974. Stimulated growth of syngeneic tumors at the site of an ongoing delayed-hypersensitivity reaction to tuberculin in BALB/c mice. *J. Natl. Cancer Inst.* 52:1297–99

39. Voisin, G. A. 1971. Immunity and tolerance: a unified concept. *Cell. Immunol.* 2:670–89

40. Hersh, E. M., Gutterman, J. U., Mavligit, G. M., Reed, R. C. 1975. Immunological aspects of chemotherapy. In *Cancer Chemotherapy—Fundamental Concepts and Recent Advances,* 279–94. Chicago: Yearb. Med. 577 pp.

41. Morton, D. L., Sparks, F. C., Haskell, C. M. 1974. Oncology. In *Principles of Surgery,* ed. S. I. Schwartz, 297–347. New York: McGraw-Hill. 1982 pp.

42. Hersh, E. M. 1973. In *Cancer Medicine,* ed. J. F. Holland, E. Frei III, 681–99. Philadelphia: Lea & Febiger. 2018 pp.

43. Bodey, G. P. 1973. See Ref. 42, pp. 1135–65

44. Hersh, E. M., Gutterman, J. U., Mavligit, G. 1973. In *Immunotherapy of Cancer in Man,* 89–116. Springfield, Ill: Thomas. 141 pp.

45. Mitchell, M. S. 1974. In *Antineoplastic and Immunosuppressive Agents I,* ed. A. C. Sartorelli, D. G. Johns, 555–76. New York: Springer. 762 pp.

46. Catalona, W. J., Taylor, P. T., Rabson, A. S., Chretien, P. B. 1972. A method for dinitrochlorobenzene contact sensitization. *N. Engl. J. Med.* 286:399–402

47. Roth, J. A., Eilber, F. R., Nizze, J. A., Morton, D. L. 1975. Lack of correlation between skin reactivity to dinitrochlorobenzene and croton oil in patients with cancer. *N. Engl. J. Med.* 293:388–89

48. Sokal, J. E. 1975. Measurement of delayed skin-test responses. *N. Engl. J. Med.* 293:501–2

49. Burdick, J. F., Wells, S. A. Jr., Herberman, R. B. 1975. Immunologic evaluation of patients with cancer by delayed hypersensitivity reactions. *Surgery* 141:779–94

50. Heppner, G., Henry, E., Stolbach, L., Cummings, F., McDonough, E., Calabresi, P. 1975. Problems in the clinical use of the microcytotoxicity assay for measuring cell-mediated immunity to tumor cells. *Cancer Res.* 35:1931–37

51. Herberman, R. B., Oldham, R. K. 1975. Problems associated with study of cell-mediated immunity to human tumors by microcytotoxicity assays. *J. Natl. Can. Inst.* 55:749–53

52. Wybran, J., Fudenberg, H. 1974. How clinically useful is T and B cell quantitation? *Ann. Int. Med.* 80:765–67

53. Golub, S. H., O'Connell, T. X., Morton, D. L. 1974. Correlation of in vivo and in vitro assays of immunocompetence in cancer patients. *Cancer Res.* 34:1833–37

54. Bolton, P. M., Mander, A. M., Davidson, J. M., James, S. L., Newcombe, R. G., Hughes, L. E. 1975. Cellular immunity in cancer: Comparison of delayed hypersensitivity skin tests in three common cancers. *Br. Med. J.* 3:18–20

55. Black, M. M. 1973. Human breast cancer a model for cancer immunology. *Isr. J. Med. Sci.* 9:284–99

56. Nemoto, T., Han, T., Minowada, J., Angkur, V., Chamberlain, A., Dao, T. L. 1974. Cell-mediated immune status of breast cancer patients: Evaluation by skin tests, lymphocyte stimulation, and counts of rosette-forming cells. *J. Natl. Cancer Inst.* 53:641–45

57. Daly, J. J., Prout, G. R. Jr., Ahl, C. A., Lin, J. C. 1974. Specificity of cellular immunity to renal cell carcinoma. *J. Urol.* 111:448–52

58. Merrin, C., Han, T. 1974. Immune response in bladder cancer. *J. Urol.* 111:170–72

59. Wolff, J. P., De Oliveira, C. F. 1975. Lymphocytes in patients with ovarian cancer. *Obstet. Gynecol.* 45:656–58

60. Pierce, G. E., DeVald, B. 1975. Microcytotoxicity assays of tumor immunity in patients with bronchogenic carcinoma correlated with clinical status. *Cancer Res.* 35:3577–84

61. Eilber, F. R., Nizze, J. A., Morton, D. L. 1975. Sequential evaluation of general immune competence in cancer pa-

tients: Correlation with clinical course. *Cancer* 35:660–65

62. Gutterman, J. U., Hersh, E. M., McCredie, K. B., Bodey, G. P. Sr., Rodriguez, V., Freireich, E. J. 1972. Lymphocyte blastogenesis to human leukemia cells and their relationship to serum factors, immunocompetence, and prognosis. *Cancer Res.* 32:2524–29

63. Lehane, D. E., Lane, M. 1974. Immunocompetence in advanced cancer patients prior to chemotherapy. *Oncology* 30:458–66

64. Catalona, W. J., Chretien, P. B. 1973. Abnormalities of quantitative dinitrochlorobenzene sensitization in cancer patients: Correlation with tumor stage and histology. *Cancer* 31:353–56

65. Gross, L. 1965. Immunological defect in aged population and its relationship to cancer. *Cancer* 18:201–4

66. Roberts-Thomson, I. C., Whittingham, S., Youngchaiyud, U., Mackay, I. R. 1974. Ageing, immune response, and mortality. *Lancet* 2:368–70

67. Jose, D. G., Good, R. A. 1973. Quantitative effects of nutritional protein and calorie deficiency upon immune responses to tumors in mice. *Cancer Res.* 33:807–12

68. Law, D. K., Dudrick, S. J., Abdou, N. I. 1973. Immunocompetence of patients with protein-calorie malnutrition. *Ann. Intern. Med.* 79:545–50

69. Chakravorty, R. C., Curutchet, H. P., Coppolla, F. S., Park, C. M., Blaylock, W. K., Lawrence, W. Jr. 1973. The delayed hypersensitivity reaction in the cancer patient: Observations on sensitization by DNCB. *Surgery* 73:730–35

70. Hersh, E. M. 1974. Immunosuppressive agents. See Ref. 45, pp. 577–617

71. Harris, J. E. 1970. In *The Immunology of Malignant Disease,* ed. J. E. Harris, J. G. Sinkovics, 176–202. St. Louis: Mosby. 251 pp.

72. Heppner, G. H., Calabresi, P. 1976. Selective suppression of humoral immunity by antineoplastic drugs. *Ann. Rev. Pharmacol.* 16:367–79

73. Levin, R. H., Landy, M., Frei, E. III. 1964. The effect of 6-mercaptopurine on immune response in man. *N. Engl. J. Med.* 271:16–22

74. Mitchell, M. S., DeConti, R. C. 1970. Immunosuppression by 5-fluorouracil. *Cancer* 26:884–89

75. Suhrland, L. G., Benson, J., Labelle, E. 1972. Enhancement of tumor growth and immunosuppression in mice with 5-fluorouracil. *Am. J. Med. Sci.* 263:209–14

76. Mitchell, M. S., Wade, M. E., DeConti, R. C., Bertino, J. R., Calabresi, P. 1969. Immunosuppressive effects of cytosine arabinoside and methotrexate in man. *Ann. Intern. Med.* 70:535–47

77. Santos, G. W., Burke, P. J., Sensenbrenner, L. L., Owens, A. H. Jr. 1970. Rationale for the use of cyclophosphamide as an immunosuppressant for marrow transplants in man. In *Pharmacological Treatment in Organ and Tissue Transplantation,* ed. A. Bertelli, A. P. Monaco, 24–31. Amsterdam: Exerpta Med. 335 pp.

78. Winkelstein, A., Ruben, F. L., Tolchin, S. F., Pollock, B. H. 1974. Mechanisms of immunosuppression: Effect of cyclophosphamide on responses to influenza immunization. *J. Lab. Clin. Med.* 83:504–10

79. Clements, P. J., Yu, D. T. Y., Levy, J., Paulus, H. E., Barnett, E. V. 1974. Effects of cyclophosphamide on B- and T-lymphocytes in rheumatoid arthritis. *Arthritis Rheum.* 17:347–53

80. Hill, D. H. 1975. *A Review of Cyclophosphamide,* 113–71. Springfield, Ill.: Thomas. 340 pp.

81. Aisenberg, A. C., Wilkes, B. 1964. Studies on the suppression of immune responses by the periwinkle alkaloids vincristine and vinblastine. *J. Clin. Invest.* 43:2394–2403

82. Vecchi, A., Mantovani, A., Tagliabue, A., Spreafico, F. 1976. A characterization of the immunosuppressive activity of adriamycin and daunomycin on humoral antibody production and tumor allograft rejection. *Cancer Res.* 36:1222–27

83. Schwab, J. H. 1975. Suppression of the immune response by microorganisms. *Bacteriol. Rev.* 39:121–43

84. Hersh, E. M. 1973. Immunosuppressive enzymes. *Transplant. Proc.* 5:1211–14

85. Gordon, W. C., Mandy, W. J., Prager, M. D. 1976. Differential effect of asparaginase on lymphocyte subpopulations and alleviation of the immunosuppression by lipopolysaccharide. *Cancer Immunol. Immunother.* 1:In press

86. Killander, D., Dohlwitz, A., Engstedt, L., Franzén, S., Gahrton, G., Gullbring, B., Holm, G., Holmgren, A., Höglund, S., Killander, A., Lockner, D., Mellstedt, H., Moe, P. J., Palmblad, J., Reizenstein, P., Skårberg, K-O., Swedberg, B., Udén, A-M., Wadman, B., Wide, L., Åhström, L. 1976. Hypersen-

sitive reactions and antibody formation during l-asparaginase treatment of children and adults with acute leukemia. *Cancer* 37:220–28

87. Borella, L., Green, A. A., Webster, R. G. 1972. Immunologic rebound after cessation of long-term chemotherapy in acute leukemia. *Blood* 40:42–50

88. Green, A. A., Borella, L. 1973. Immunologic rebound after cessation of long-term chemotherapy in acute leukemia. II. In vitro response to phytohemagglutinin and antigens by peripheral blood and bone marrow lymphocytes. *Blood* 42:99–110

89. Greene, W. H., Schimpff, S. C., Wiernik, P. H. 1974. Cell mediated immunity in acute nonlymphocytic leukemia: Relationship to host factors, therapy, and prognosis. *Blood* 43:1–14

90. Jose, D. G., Ekert, H., Colebatch, J., Waters, K., Wilson, F., O'Keefe, D. 1976. Immune function at diagnosis in relation to responses to therapy in acute lymphocytic leukemia of childhood. *Blood* 47:1011–21

91. Leventhal, B. G., Cohen, P., Triem, S. C. 1974. Effect of chemotherapy on the immune response in acute leukemia. *Isr. J. Med. Sci.* 10:866–87

92. Hersh, E. M., Oppenheim, J. J. 1967. Inhibition of in vitro lymphocyte transformation during chemotherapy in man. *Cancer Res.* 27:98–105

93. Cheema, A. R., Hersh, E. M. 1971. Patient survival after chemotherapy and its relationship to in vitro lymphocyte blastogenesis. *Cancer* 28:851–55

94. Frei, E. III 1972. Combination cancer therapy: Presidential address. *Cancer Res.* 32:2593–2607

95. Harris, J. E., Stewart, T. H. M. 1972. *Proc. Leucocyte Culture Conf., 6th*, ed. M. R. Schwarz, 555–80. New York: Academic. 873 pp.

96. Harris, J. E., Bagai, R. C., Stewart, T. H. M. 1973. In *Proc. Leucocyte Culture Conf., 7th*, ed. F. Daguillard, 443–57. New York: Academic. 690 pp.

97. Harris, J., Bagai, R., Stewart, T. 1972. Immunocompetence and response to antitumor treatment. *N. Engl. J. Med.* 286:494

98. Sparks, F. C., Wile, A. G., Ramming, K. P., Morton, D. L. 1976. *Sci. Proc. Am. Soc. Clin. Oncol.* 17:309 (Abstr. C-292)

99. Hersh, E. M., Gutterman, J. U., Mavligit, G., McCredie, K. B., Bodey, G. P., Freireich, E. J., Rossen, R. D., Butler, W. T. 1973. Host defense, chemical im-

munosuppression, and the transplant recipient. Relative effects of intermittent versus continuous immunosuppressive therapy with reference to the objectives of treatment. *Transplant. Proc.* 5:1191–95

100. Fefer, A. 1974. See Ref. 45, pp. 528–54

101. Bast, R. C. Jr., Zbar, B., Borsos, T., Rapp, H. J. 1974. BCG and cancer. *N. Engl. J. Med.* 290:1413–20, 1458–69

102. Weiss, D. W., Stupp, Y., Many, N., Izak, G. 1975. Treatment of acute myelocytic leukemia (AML) patients with the MER tubercle bacillus fraction: A preliminary report. *Transplant. Proc.* 7:545–52

103. Halpern, B., ed. 1975. *Corynebacterium Parvum*. New York: Plenum. 444 pp.

104. Marx, J. L. 1976. Cancer immunotherapy: Focus on the drug levamisole. *Science* 191:57

105. Fourcade, A., Friend, C., Lacour, F., Holland, J. G. 1974. Protective effect of immunization with polyinosinic polycytidylic acid complexed with methylated bovine serum albumin against Friend leukemia virus in mice. *Cancer Res.* 34:1749–51

106. Powles, R. 1974. Immunotherapy for acute myelogenous leukemia using irradiated and unirradiated leukemia cells. *Cancer* 34:1558–62

107. Vogler, W. R., Chan, Y. K. 1974. Prolonging remission in myeloblastic leukaemia by Tice strain Bacillus Calmette Guérin. *Lancet* 2:128–31

108. Gutterman, J. U., Hersh, E. M., Rodriguez, V., McCredie, K. B., Mavligit, G., Reed, R., Burgess, M. A., Smith, T., Gehan, E., Bodey, G. P. Sr., Freireich, E. J. 1974. Chemoimmunotherapy of adult acute leukaemia prolongation of remission in myeloblastic leukaemia with B. C. G. *Lancet* 2:1405–9

109. Gutterman, J. U., Mavligit, G., McBride, C., Frei, E. III, Freireich, E. J., Hersh, E. M. 1973. Active immunotherapy with B. C. G. for recurrent malignant melanoma. *Lancet* 1:1208–12

110. Eilber, F. R., Morton, D. L., Holmes, E. C., Sparks, F. C., Ramming, K. P. 1976. Adjuvant immunotherapy with BCG in treatment of regional-lymph node metastases from malignant melanoma. *N. Engl. J. Med.* 294:237–40

111. Klein, E., Holtermann, O. A., Helm, F., Rosner, D., Milgrom, H., Adler, S., Stoll, H. L. Jr., Case, R. W., Prior, R. L., Murphy, G. P. 1975. Immunologic approaches to the management of pri-

mary and secondary tumors involving the skin and soft tissues: Review of a ten-year program. *Transplant. Proc.* 7:297–315

112. Sokal, J. E., Aungst, C. W., Snyderman, M. 1974. Delay in progression of malignant lymphoma after BCG vaccination. *N. Engl. J. Med.* 291:1226–30

113. Mathé, G., Amiel, J. L., Schwarzenberg, L., Schneider, M., Cattan, A., Schlumberger, J. R., Hayat, M., De Vassal, F. 1969. Active immunotherapy for acute lymphoblastic leukaemia. *Lancet* 1:697–99

114. Heyn, R. M., Joo, P., Karon, M., Nesbit, M., Shore, N., Breslow, N., Weiner, J., Reed, A., Hammond, D. 1975. BCG in the treatment of acute lymphocytic leukemia. *Blood* 46:431–42

115. Gutterman, J. U., Mavligit, G. M., Reed, R. C., Gottlieb, J. A., Burgess, M. A., McBride, C. M., Einhorn, L., Freireich, E. J., Hersh, E. M. 1975. Chemoimmunotherapy for regional and disseminated malignant melanoma. See Ref. 40, pp. 455–82

116. Sparks, F. C., Silverstein, M. J., Hunt, J. S., Haskell, C. M., Pilch, Y. H., Morton, D. L. 1973. Complications of BCG immunotherapy in patients with cancer. *N. Engl. J. Med.* 289:827–30

117. Gutterman, J. U., Mavligit, G. M., Reed, R. C., Hersh, E. M. 1974. Immunochemotherapy of human cancer. *Semin. Oncol.* 1:409–23

118. Gutterman, J. U., Mavligit, G., Gottlieb, J. A., Burgess, M. A., McBride, C. E., Einhorn L., Freireich, E. J., Hersh, E. M. 1974. Chemoimmunotherapy of disseminated malignant melanoma with dimethyl triazeno imidazole carboxamide and bacillus Calmette-Guérin. *N. Engl. J. Med.* 291:592–97

119. Paterson, A. H. G., McPherson, T. A., Katakkar, S., Khaliq, A. 1976. *Sci. Proc. Am. Soc. Clin. Oncol.* 17:310 (Abstr. C-296)

120. Costanzi, J. J. 1976. *Sci. Proc. Am. Soc. Clin. Oncol.* 17:241 (Abstr. C-18)

121. Mavligit, G. M., Gutterman, J. U., Burgess, M. A., Khankhanian, N., Seibert, G. B., Speer, J. F., Jubert, A. V., Martin, R. C., McBride, C. M., Copeland, E. M., Gehan, E. A., Hersh, E. M. 1976. Prolongation of postoperative disease-free interval and survival in human colorectal cancer by BCG or BCG plus 5-fluorouracil. *Lancet* 1:871–76

122. Hortobagyi, G., Gutterman, J., Blumenschein, G., Mavligit, G., Hersh, E. 1976. *Sci. Proc. Am. Soc. Clin. Oncol.* 17:275 (Abstr. C-155)

123. Evans, J. T. 1976. Immunotherapy for colorectal cancer. *Lancet* 1:1248

124. Israel, L. 1975. See Ref. 103, pp. 389–401

125. Israel, L., Edelstein, R. 1975. Immunological control of cancer. *Lancet* 1:979–80

126. Haskell, C. M., Ossorio, R. C., Sarna, G. P., Fahey, J. L. 1976. *Sci. Proc. Am. Soc. Clin. Oncol.* 17:265 (Abstr. C-114)

127. Tripodi, D., Parks, L. C., Brugmans, J. 1973. Drug-induced restoration of cutaneous delayed hypersensitivity in anergic patients with cancer. *N. Engl. J. Med.* 289:354–57

128. Rojas, A. F., Mickiewicz, E., Feierstein, J. N., Glait, H., Olivari, A. J. 1976. Levamisole in advanced human breast cancer. *Lancet* 1:211–16

129. Study Group for Bronchogenic Carcinoma 1975. Immunopotentiation with levamisole in resectable bronchogenic carcinoma: A double-blind controlled trial. *Br. Med. J.* 3:461–64

130. Sadoff, L. 1972. Mechanisms of action of cancer chemotherapy drugs: An alternative hypothesis based on inhibition of immunologic function. *Cancer Chemother. Rep.* 56:559–62

131. Mott, M. G. 1973. Chemotherapeutic suppression of immune enhancement: A primary determinant of successful cancer therapy. *Lancet* 1:1092–94

132. Steele, G., Pierce, G. E. 1974. Effects of cyclophosphamide on immunity against chemically-induced syngeneic murine sarcomas. *Int. J. Cancer* 13:572–78

Ann. Rev. Pharmacol. Toxicol. 1977. 17:197–214
Copyright © 1977 by Annual Reviews Inc. All rights reserved

EXPOSURE OF HUMANS TO LEAD

❖6675

Paul B. Hammond
Department of Environmental Health, University of Cincinnati Medical Center,
Cincinnati, Ohio 45267

INTRODUCTION

Since 1972, several important reviews of lead toxicology have been published (1–3), as well as proceedings of two major conferences (4, 5). One of the reviews (1) was written specifically as a resource document for promulgating air lead standards. In a similar vein, the World Health Organization convened a task force in May 1975 to prepare a document which the member states could use in the establishment of national regulations pertaining to lead. Having participated in the preparation of both of these documents, it seems appropriate that this author should review the recent literature on lead that was most useful in assessing acceptable limits of human exposure.

The focus of this review is on the transfer of lead from the environment into the human organism and on the major consequences thereof. Three target organ systems are generally acknowledged as being of major concern, the heme-hemoprotein system, the kidney, and the nervous system. Although the last-named system may ultimately prove to be the most critical, it is not dealt with in this review, because space is limited and because the subject is in a state of ferment. Hopefully, a separate review of the effects of lead on the central and peripheral nervous system will be published soon.

UPTAKE FROM ENVIRONMENTAL SOURCES

The characteristics of uptake of lead by man from known and suspected environmental sources is a matter of great practical importance, particularly when multiple sources exist or are suspected to exist. Thus, in the general adult population, respiratory intake via ambient air and oral intake via food and beverages are the obvious major sources and routes of entry. But their relative importance has been

197

a matter of considerable uncertainty. It is relatively simple to determine the range of air lead concentrations to which people are exposed and the concentrations of lead in various foods and beverages, but it is more difficult to translate these concentration terms into units of lead inhaled or ingested per unit of time. But the greatest problem of all is determination of the fractional absorption, i.e. the relationship between the internal dose and the external dose.

Uptake from Air

Measurements of the airway deposition and clearance of lead in humans are attended by numerous difficulties. The greatest problem is the nonuniformity of lead aerosols to which people are exposed, both as to chemical composition and as to aerodynamic characteristics. Thus, the aerosols encountered in many industrial exposures consist of lead oxide, which may range from aerodynamic diameters of less than 1 μm to several hundred micrometers. By contrast, the lead aerosol in ambient air attributable to auto exhaust is a complex mixture, mainly of sulfate, carbonate, halides, and oxides (6) which are more uniformly in the respirable range (< 1 μm) than in industrial air (7–9). Experimental studies, conducted mainly in animals but confirmed in man, clearly indicate that great variations occur both in total fractional aerosol deposition and in anatomical distribution patterns, depending on particle size (10, 11). Further, the fraction of deposited lead which ultimately is transferred to the systemic circulation varies greatly, depending on the site of airway deposition and on the solubility and chemical composition of the lead aerosol.

Studies of total airway deposition of lead aerosols in man have been reported (12–14). Results are in general agreement with predictions derived from animal studies (10).

Knowledge of the fate of lead deposited in the airways is virtually nonexistent either in man or in experimental animals. Short-term lung clearance of lead has been studied in man by γ-ray lung scans following inhalation of ^{212}Pb (15). Relevance of this study to the fate of lead aerosols actually inhaled by people in real life is highly questionable because of the artificial nature of Pb-tagged aerosol.

An additional variable relating to lung clearance rates is the possible toxicity of the lead aerosol to the mucociliary-alveolar macrophage clearance mechanism. Lead aerosol exposure, even at concentrations below those commonly inhaled in lead industries, reduces the number of alveolar macrophages in rats (16).

In summary, study of the fate of inhaled lead in man using conventional deposition and clearance measurements has not provided much useful information on the contribution of lead in ambient or industrial air to the internal dose at specified air lead concentrations.

An estimate has been made of the relationship of ambient air lead to total intake by kinetic analysis of the labeling of blood, bone, and excreta following oral administration of the stable isotope ^{204}Pb to two volunteers (17). It was estimated from the data that at an ambient air lead concentration of 2 μg/m^3 about 40% of the total daily internal dose originated from the air. Input from other compartments, e.g. bone, was estimated from very sketchy data. Hence, the conclusions are questionable.

The most common way of estimating relative internal lead exposure in population groups is by analysis of the concentration of lead in the blood, usually expressed as μg Pb/100 g blood, and commonly referred to as PbB. Thus, in industrial populations and in inner city lead screening programs, reliance is placed mainly on PbB as measure of total lead exposure from all sources. The same approach has been used in assessing the specific contribution of ambient air lead to the total internal dose. Air lead exposure has been estimated in a large population of city-dwelling adults using personal air sampling devices. PbB also was determined (18). From analysis of the air Pb vs PbB data it was estimated that the contribution of air lead to PbB was about 1 μg Pb/100 g blood per 1 μg Pb/m^3 of air, within the ambient air lead concentration range encountered by city populations. This estimate was imprecise owing to the large interindividual variability attributable to sources of lead other than air—presumably dietary. Nevertheless, a similar estimate of the contribution of air lead to PbB can be derived from human volunteer studies in which the air lead concentration and dietary lead intake were closely controlled (19).

Absorption from the Gastrointestinal Tract

Even in densely populated cities where the average ambient air lead concentration is of the order of 1–3 μg/m^3, only a small fraction of the internal dose of lead can be attributed to air, since PbBs are of the order of 15–25 μg/100 g — considerably greater than can be accounted for by air sources. Uptake from the gastrointestinal tract probably accounts for most of the PbB found in the general population. The absorption of lead from dietary constituents was established years ago as being about 8% in adults, based on long-term balance studies (12). This estimate has recently been confirmed using ^{204}Pb as a tracer incorporated into the diet (17).

In contrast to the low absorption of lead in adults, the absorption of dietary lead in normal infants and young children has been found to be approximately 50% (20). The accuracy of this estimate is open to question because it was derived from balance studies lasting only three days. Nevertheless, experimental studies in animals using tracer doses of radioactive lead confirm that absorption is much greater in the young than in adults (21, 22).

It has long been known that dietary calcium deficiency enhances lead absorption (23), a fact which was recently reconfirmed (24). It seems unlikely that this interaction involves a competition for an active transport mechanism (25). Other factors have been shown to influence materially the absorption of lead in animals. Thus, milk enhances the absorption of lead (26) while proteins decrease lead absorption (27). It has also been found that lead retention following oral administration is greater in iron-deficient animals (28). But it is not clear whether this interaction involves an increase of lead absorption or an increase in lead retention. Fasting also seems to enhance lead absorption (29).

The availability for absorption of lead in dried paint films is of special interest in view of the importance of lead-based paint as a source of pediatric lead poisoning. Lead chromate and lead naphthenate incorporated into dried paint films are about one half to one third as available for absorption as are lead naphthenate in oil or lead nitrate in aqueous solution (30, 31). Thus, the matrix effect of paint on the availability of lead for absorption is not great.

Absorption from the Skin

Inorganic salts of lead do not readily penetrate the intact skin (32). By contrast, lipid-soluble forms, e.g. tetraethyllead and lead naphthenate, penetrate to a significant degree (32, 33). Such compounds present significant exposure hazards only in special industrially related circumstances.

DISPOSITION OF LEAD

It has long been known that the preponderant site for localization of lead is the calcified matrix of the skeleton. But the major concern has been with the disposition of lead in the other, more toxicologically significant tissues, e.g. brain, kidney, and the hemopoietic system. However, the kinetics of the total system must be considered since exchange of metal occurs among all compartments.

Distribution Among Organs and Systems

Following i.v. administration in rats, the concentration of lead in soft tissues falls rapidly, largely as a result of transfer to the skeleton. An approximate steady state with regard to intercompartmental distribution is attained in about 14 days (34, 35). The pattern of distribution is independent of dose over a wide range and is quite similar for rats and rabbits (35). Probably the best kinetic model for describing the rate of loss of lead from the body is the power function model (34). This, in essence, describes a situation in which the fraction of the body burden which is excreted per unit of time becomes progressively smaller. The fate of single i.p. doses of lead in suckling and mature rats has been compared (36). The rate of loss from the body during the subsequent 8-day period was shown to be much faster in the adults than in the infant animals.

Recent studies of the concentration of lead in human tissues indicate that the total body burden of lead increases throughout life (37, 38). The increase is most pronounced in dense bones. Most soft tissues show no increase after the second decade of life and some, e.g. the kidney, show a progressive decrease. This may be due to replacement of parenchymal cells having a high affinity for lead by connective tissue.

Subcellular Distribution of Lead

The subcellular distribution of lead has been studied in animal systems, mainly by cell fractionation techniques. All such studies must be viewed with a certain amount of suspicion because they are essentially in vitro studies in which redistribution during the preparation of cell fractions is usually not ruled out. Nevertheless, functional and ultrastructural changes are noted following lead exposure, suggesting penetration to the intracellular milieu (39).

Relation Between Exposure and the Blood Lead Concentration

The concentration of lead in peripheral whole blood and blood serum, which probably reflects the concentration in the readily exchangeable pool, does not change systematically with age (40–42). As a matter of fact, the PbB of newborn children and of their mothers differs only slightly, with PbB generally being reported to be slightly lower in the infants (43–45).

The response of PbB to sudden changes in the external lead exposure level has been studied in man. Workers newly introduced into the lead trades show a pronounced rise in PbB which attains a new plateau after about 50–60 days (46). In a more closely controlled study of air lead exposure, the time for attaining an apparent new equilibrium of PbB was about 100 days (19). This is in agreement with studies involving the introduction of ^{204}Pb into the diet on a continuing basis, wherein the labeling of the blood with ^{204}Pb was monitored (17).

The rate at which PbB returns to the normal range following cessation of high exposure seems to be quite variable and probably depends on the duration of prior elevated exposure and possibly on the magnitude of the elevation. Thus, when PbB was somewhat less than doubled as a result of introducing 10.9 μg Pb/m^3 into the air for 19 weeks, about 20 weeks were required for PbB to return to pre-exposure levels with a half-time of about 6 weeks (19). By contrast, the PbB of a group of former lead workers was still abnormally high 15 months following retirement and had fallen only to about 40 μg/100 g from the original level of 64 μg/100 g after 10 months (47). Elevation of PbBs may persist for many years under such circumstances (48). Similarly, a persistence of elevated PbBs has been reported in children with lead poisoning for as long as 5–10 years after exposure (49, 50).

The discrepancy between rate of fall of PbB following short-term vs long-term elevated exposure has not been studied systematically. But it is reasonable to suppose that short-term clearance of lead from the blood involves a greater degree of redistribution to other compartments within the body than does long-term clearance. Following a single dose of ^{210}Pb in dogs, the curve for disappearance from the blood was analyzed as three separate exponents with the last one having a half-time of 103 days (51). The calculations were made on the basis of blood analyses carried out to 280 days. The biological half-life for ^{210}Pb in the body was estimated at 1940 days. Thus, net transfer of lead to other compartments must still have been occurring even at 280 days.

Effects of Chelating Agents

Some investigators have advocated the use of chelating agents for assessing the degree of industrial lead exposure (52). The procedure has also been used as a means of determining whether exposure to lead in early childhood might be involved in renal disease of young and middle-aged adults (53) or in hyperactivity of school children (54). In this procedure the amount of lead mobilized from tissues and excreted in the urine is measured following a standard dose either of calcium disodium ethylenediaminetetraacetate (EDTA) or of D-penicillamine (PCA). In both animals (55) and humans (56), there is a high correlation between pre-treatment PbB and the amount of lead excreted in response to these agents. Contrary to the impression conveyed in some textbooks, most of the metal mobilized in this manner originates from osseous, rather than soft, tissue (35, 37). When given i.v. in comparable doses, EDTA is more effective than PCA (57–59). When given orally the order of effectiveness is reversed (58, 59), probably because of the superior gastrointestinal absorption of PCA. The routine use of these agents for prophylactic and diagnostic purposes is somewhat hazardous. Signs of poisoning in children may be transiently aggravated using EDTA (50), and a nephrotic syndrome has been reported using PCA (60). But the EDTA effect probably occurs only when frank clinical signs are present, and the PCA effect probably occurs only with long-term use at high doses.

The use of lead mobilization by chelating agents as a measure of internal exposure offers no clear advantages over other methods of assessment. Elevated excretion of lead can be obtained by this technique many years after high exposure has terminated, but in such cases PbBs also remain elevated, and the correlation coefficient for the two parameters is about 0.7 (log-log) as calculated from data in the literature (48).

TOXIC EFFECTS VERSUS EXPOSURE

Many organs and systems are affected by lead, with exposure thresholds varying over a wide range for these effects. Some effects, e.g. irritability, weakness, and colic, are subjective. Thresholds of exposure for these are not readily defined and virtually nothing is known regarding why they occur or how they may be measured objectively. Numerous other effects as seen experimentally in animals are measurable but have not been studied in man and may never be. With few exceptions, e.g. studies of nerve conduction velocity, the only target systems to which concepts of dose-response can be applied in man at this time are the heme-hemoprotein and renal systems.

Effects on Heme and Hemoproteins

Certain effects of lead on functions of the erythrocyte and on the heme-synthetic pathway occur even at low levels of lead exposure. Some are readily measured in man. They are of great interest in two respects. First, they may be of toxicological significance. Second, they may provide a more meaningful estimate of the biologically active internal exposure level than PbB, even at exposure levels below those that cause overt signs of toxicity.

The anemia of lead poisoning is probably the most well-known and best-understood effect of lead in man. A decrement in blood hemoglobin appears at relatively low exposure levels. The apparent threshold of exposure is at a PbB of about 40 in children (61, 62) and about 50 in adult males (46). Frank anemia probably only occurs at considerably greater exposure levels, at least in adults (63).

The anemic effects of lead probably are of multiple origins. The vast earlier literature on this subject was reviewed in 1966 (64). At the time of that review, the relative importance of the various demonstrable mechanisms was not clear. An additional ten years of research in many laboratories has clarified the issue to some extent. Thus, earlier studies which suggested a possible shortening of erythrocyte survival have been confirmed using more reliable cell-labeling methodology (65). The subjects were heavily exposed industrial workers with PbBs ranging from 59 to 162. The degree of shortening of cell life span correlated best with reticulocytosis, but also was correlated with PbBs, coproporphyrinuria, and anemia. The mechanism for shortened erythrocyte survival is not well understood, but it is quite moderate in comparison to the shortening observed in hemolytic anemias. Some characteristics of the erythrocyte membrane are altered in lead exposure. Increased resistance to hypoosmotic lysis and increased mechanical fragility have been reported (64, 66). More recently it has been demonstrated that an inhibition of erythrocyte membrane Na^+/K^+-ATPase occurs in people with only moderately elevated lead exposure (67–69). It is not known whether this abnormality plays a role in reduction of the life span of erythrocytes.

Biochemical studies pertaining to the effects of lead on the formation of hemoglobin have dealt mainly with effects on the synthesis of heme. But the possibility exists that effects of significance occur also with reference to globin synthesis. In that connection, inhibition of incorporations of ^3H leucine into α- and β-chain globins of reticulocytes has been observed in two children with clinical lead poisoning (70). This effect, however, seems to occur only secondarily to a deficit in heme production (71).

The lead-induced disturbances in heme synthesis are summarized graphically in Figure 1. Manifestations of these effects are readily quantitated in human blood and urine. As pointed out earlier in this review, alterations in these various parameters are so readily determined and occur at such low levels of lead exposure that they are used as alternatives to PbB in the estimation of internal lead exposure. Two enzymes in the pathway from glycine to heme are clearly sensitive to lead. The first is the cytoplasmic enzyme aminolevulinic acid dehydratase (ALAD), which is responsible for Knorr condensation of two molecules of ALA to form the pyrrole porphobilinogen (PBG) (72). The second enzyme for which there is ample direct evidence for inhibition is heme synthetase, a mitochondrial enzyme that inserts iron into protoporphyrin IX (PROTO) to form heme (64). The significance as to health of lead effects on these enzymes is still uncertain. The concentration of the respective substrates for these two enzymes increases with increasing lead exposure in a dose-related fashion. More specifically, the rate of urinary ALA excretion and the concentration of PROTO in the blood both rise with increasing PbB. But it is not certain whether, over the full range of human lead exposure, these increased substrate concentrations reflect decreased utilization, as distinguished from increased production. Evidence as to the latter possibility is presented later.

Urinary ALA excretion rises above normal limits in a more or less exponential fashion in both adults (73, 74) and children (1) as PbB increases linearly. The threshold for this interaction is at a PbB of about 40 in men and children and somewhat lower in women (75). This effect clearly is prerenal in nature since the elevated ALA excretion is accompanied by elevated plasma ALA concentrations (76, 77). Under conditions of moderate, continuing lead exposure in both man (78) and in animals (79), urinary ALA excretion rises rapidly and returns to normal within a few weeks, suggesting that an adaptive mechanism of some sort has been stimulated.

It is generally assumed that the mechanism for increased ALA levels is inhibition of ALAD with a consequent accumulation of the substrate. The degree of inhibition

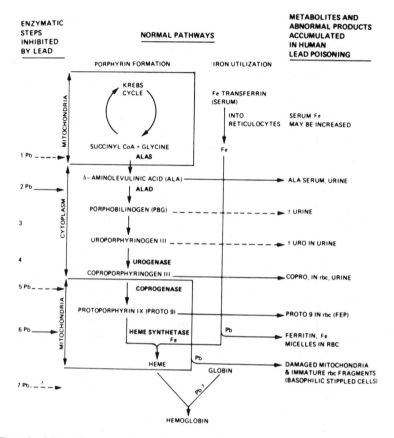

Figure 1   Schematic diagram of hemoglobin synthesis. --→ = weak evidence of Pb-inhibition; —→ = strong evidence of Pb-inhibition (1). (Reproduced with permission of the National Academy of Sciences.)

in peripheral blood correlates very closely with PbB, even within the range of lead exposure found in the general population (80). It occurs very promptly when people are subjected to an increase in lead exposure (46, 80), and enzyme activity returns to normal after termination of exposure at a rate proportional to the return of PbB to the normal range (81, 82). This close correspondence between PbB and enzyme inhibition in erythrocytes has suggested that the effect may be only a test tube phenomenon. This is highly unlikely, however, since the enzyme assay process applied to blood from lead-exposed people does not appear to release free lead ions capable of interacting with additional increments of uninhibited enzyme added to the reaction mixture (83). Furthermore, inhibition caused by in vivo addition of lead can be totally restored by heating the hemolysate for 5 min, whereas no reactivation occurs when lead is added to the erythrocytic enzyme preparation in vitro, suggesting that the inhibition in vivo is of a different nature than in vitro (84, 85). The threshold or no-effect PbB level for ALAD inhibition in erythrocytes is reported to be about 15 in young children (86) and 10–20 in adults (87). Thus, the inhibition in erythrocytes occurs at a lower level of lead exposure than does elevation of plasma or urinary ALA. Since circulating mammalian erythrocytes are largely devoid of the mitochondrial enzymes which participate in heme synthesis, the significance of ALAD inhibition in erythrocytes is of dubious significance. However, roughly equivalent concurrent inhibition of liver ALAD has been reported in man (88) and of liver and brain ALAD in rats (89). The inhibition of the enzyme in the liver is readily reversed by chelation therapy with EDTA in rats, whereas chelation treatment has little effect on the depressed enzyme activity in erythrocytes (90). Since the PbB threshold for elevated ALA in plasma and urine is appreciably higher than for ALAD inhibition, it would appear that the body has a considerable functional enzyme reserve. Indeed, dogs with grossly depressed ALAD activity resulting from lead administration were completely normal in regard to their blood-regenerating capacity following acute hemorrhage (91). In this particular study, excretion of ALA was only marginally elevated, however.

Inhibition of ALAD has been demonstrated with other metals in vitro, e.g. Cu, Hg, and Ag (92). A weak correlation also has been found between urinary Hg excretion and blood inhibition in workers exposed to mercury vapors (93). No interaction could be demonstrated between ALAD inhibition and Cd exposure (94). Aside from Pb and Hg the only other substance that has been shown to inhibit ALAD in vivo in man is ethanol (95).

The toxicological implications of ALAD inhibition are still not adequately known. Attention has been focused mainly on possible effects on hemoproteins, but some attention has been given to the possible toxic effects of ALA per se. Much of this interest actually results from consideration of the neurological manifestations of porphyric diseases, in which the concentration of ALA in tissues and body fluids rises to a considerably greater degree than in lead poisoning. Hyperactivity in mice (96) and vasodepressive effects in rats and rabbits have been observed (97). These observations have been made using high doses of ALA administered acutely. The concentrations of ALA in tissues and body fluids were not determined. The same was true of one study of chronic ALA toxicity in which no toxic effects were noted (98). In one in vitro study it was demonstrated that ALA has an inhibitory effect on erythrocyte and brain Na^+/K^+-ATPase with effects being noted within the range of blood serum ALA concentrations associated with acute neurological manifestations of porphyria (99). The role of porphyrin precursors in the neurological manifestations of porphyria has been reviewed recently (100).

There has been a growing interest in yet another sensitive index of lead exposure, the concentration of protoporphyrin IX (PROTO) in the blood. Recent fluorometric methods have improved the ease and precision with which erythrocytic PROTO can be determined (101–104). Although the substances measured are generally referred to as free erythrocyte porphyrin (FEP), more than 90% of the porphyrin determined is PROTO (104). In both iron deficiency anemia and in excessive lead exposure, FEP is clearly elevated. In adults exposed to lead in industry, there is an increase in FEP which corresponds to the PbB. The FEP increase in women is greater than in men for any given PbB. In these cases, the PbB threshold for effect is approximately 20–30 (105). In effect, the rise in FEP is almost as sensitive an index of lead exposure as is the depression of ALAD activity. There is one significant difference in the two interactions. Depression of ALAD activity occurs very promptly as related to PbB, while the rise in FEB is delayed by about 2 weeks (106). This no doubt reflects the fact that lead acts directly on circulating erythrocytes in producing depression of ALAD activity, whereas the rise in FEP reflects events occurring in the bone marrow. Circulating erythrocytes are devoid of mitochondria. Therefore, the inhibitory effects of lead on mitochondrial enzymes, e.g. heme synthetase, are not expressed in peripheral blood until after erythrocyte maturation and injection into the bloodstream. The delay in FEP response to lead exposure has been confirmed in experimental animals (107).

From all of the studies reported to date, it appears that disturbances in heme synthesis occur at lead exposure levels which are lower than those associated with a decrement in blood hemoglobin levels. It is of particular interest to note that the rises in ALA and FEP occur at roughly equivalent lead exposure levels. These effects occur in spite of maintenance of normal levels of hemoglobin. It is entirely possible that the increased level of these two intermediates of heme synthesis reflects a compensatory derepression of aminolevulinic acid synthetase (ALAS) formation secondary to a marginal reduction of conversion of PROTO to heme by inhibition of heme synthetase. There is some evidence to support this interpretation. Stimulation of ALA formation occurs in the presence of lead in cultured liver cells (108) and in rat liver (109). Further, in one case of human lead poisoning, an increased rate of heme biosynthesis was observed, rather than a decrease (110).

The general assumption that increased PROTO in elevated lead exposure is due to inhibition of heme synthetase may not be correct. The problem may be limitation on the availability of iron for insertion into heme. Lead has been shown to interfere with the transfer of iron from transferrin to human reticulocytes (111) and causes accumulation of iron as ferruginous micelles in developing erythrocytes (112).

Almost all studies of effects of lead on hemoproteins have been concerned with hemoglobin. But some attention has been directed toward possible effects on cytochrome P450. Rates of P450-mediated drug metabolism in adults (113, 114) and children (114) appear to be depressed in some cases of high exposure. Reduction of cytochrome P450 in the liver due to lead has been demonstrated in rats, coincident of a reduction in P450-dependent drug metabolism (115). Cytochrome content of kidney mitochondria also has been shown to be reduced in experimental lead intoxication (116).

In summary, at low levels of lead exposure excessive concentrations of the heme intermediates ALA and PROTO are seen, possibly as a compensatory feedback response to interference with incorporation of iron into PROTO. At higher levels of exposure it is clear that lead causes a reduction in tissue levels of hemoproteins, probably as a result of attainment of a critical uncompensated level of heme synthetase inhibition perhaps combined with other effects, e.g. inhibition of globin synthesis. Dose-response relationships of heme effects as related to PbB in man have been summarized recently (117, 118).

Effects on the Kidney

Studies of the renal effects of lead have been far less extensive than studies of heme effects. Further, studies of renal effects in man have been limited largely to subjects whose lead exposures have been very high. For these reasons and others which will become apparent, dose-response relationships and approximate exposure thresholds have not been defined.

In both adults and children there is extensive evidence for occurrence of two distinctive effects. One is reversible proximal tubular damage. The other is a slow, progressive renal failure involving reduced glomerular function with associated vascular damage and fibrosis.

Tubular damage is manifested in children as Fanconi's syndrome, that is, the triad of glycosuria, hypophosphatemia, and aminoaciduria. Manifestations of proximal tubular damage are inconstant, even among cases of clinical poisoning with PbBs greater than 100 (50), and are readily reversible with chelation therapy (50, 119). Aminoaciduria was described twenty years ago in lead smelter workers (120). More recently, in a study of ten battery factory workers, only one had significant aminoaciduria (121). In another study in which PbBs were markedly elevated, neither aminoaciduria nor glycosuria was observed (122). Thus, as with children, adults seem to experience tubular damage only at very high levels of exposure.

Lead poisoning in adults is sometimes associated with gout, hyperuricemia, and decreased renal urate clearance. These findings are indicative of either an increased tubular reabsorption or a decreased tubular secretion of urate. The condition was first described as a sequela to childhood lead poisoning. Young and middle-aged adults exhibited these abnormalities even though excessive lead exposure had occurred many years earlier in childhood (123–125). A high incidence of gout with extensive morphological evidence of renal tubular degeneration also has been reported in lead poisoning due to long-term drinking of lead-contaminated illicitly distilled whiskey (126). As in the case of gout resulting from earlier childhood exposure, the basic lesion in moonshine whiskey cases appears to be decreased renal urate clearance rather than increased urate production (127). Unlike the case with other tubular lesions due to lead, chronic exposure seems to be a requisite circumstance. Pediatric lead poisoning in the United States does not seem to result in later occurrence of abnormal urate metabolism or other persistent nephropathy in contrast to the situation reported from Australia (128). Similarly, long-term industrial lead exposure has not been reported to cause these disturbances of urate metabolism (129). The special circumstances that lead to gout need clarification.

The cases of gout and associated effects described above occur in conjunction with other renal effects involving a gross reduction of glomerular filtration and progressive renal failure. Histologically, there is evidence of interstitial fibrosis, obliteration of glomeruli, and various lesions of the small renal arteries and arterioles (126). In cases of industrial lead exposure of even moderate intensity and duration, the glomerular filtration rate (GFR) is reduced (122, 129, 130). But tubular function appears to remain essentially normal, at least as to renal PAH extraction (130). Unlike the case with tubular lesions, depression of GFR does not appear to be readily reversible, even with chelation therapy (130).

The level of lead exposure that causes chronic lead nephropathy with the associated glomerular and vascular changes is not known. In view of the progressive nature of the lesions, it does not seem reasonable to ascribe the effects to the PbBs determined only at the time the functional abnormalities happen to be discovered, as was done in one case (131). Rather, it appears from all that is known about this progressive nephropathy that the toxic effects arise as a result of some critical level of exposure maintained for some critical period of time, probably of the order of years. Prolonged administration of lead to rats ultimately results in renal lesions similar to those seen in man (132). Thus, an experimental animal model for chronic lead nephropathy is available. Other renal effects occur, whose significance is obscure. Thus, lead has been shown to decrease activity of the renin-aldosterone system, an effect that would interfere with distal rather than proximal tubular sodium transport (133). Another interesting effect of lead is the appearance in renal proximal tubular cells (and in other tissues as well) of intranuclear inclusion bodies (132, 134). It has been postulated that these serve as a defense mechanism, wherein their formation in response to lead exposure serves to sequester circulating lead. These bodies are composed of protein and lead (133–135). They develop within 6 hr of lead administration, and their formation is dependent upon de novo synthesis of protein (136).

Epidemiological surveys of causes of death among lead workers have been reported on several occasions. In the most recent of these studies it was reported that a marginally significant excess mortality rate occurred in the category of "other hypertensive disease." In 17 out of 20 death certificates in this category there was specific mention of uremia, nephrosclerosis, or other renal disease (137). Many of the workers in this study had been exposed to high levels of lead for more than ten years. PbBs in excess of 80 were common. In a limited recent study of workers exposed to lead at moderate levels, no excess mortalities due to renal diseases were observed (138).

In summary, it appears that the kidney exhibits an array of responses to lead exposure within the range encountered by man as a result of industrial activities and exposure during childhood. The effects involve both the renal tubules and glomerular-vascular apparatus. Dose-response relationships are not clearly definable. Tubular effects appear to be more readily reversible than glomerular effects. Owing to their more pernicious implications, the glomerular effects are of greatest concern at this time.

CONCLUSIONS

In the past few years there has been a great deal of research reported pertaining to toxic effects of lead. Only a small fraction of this research has contributed directly to refinement of dose-response relationships in man. Much of the remaining research not cited in this review may play a role in future refinements of these relationships.

For the present it is concluded that a prolonged lead exposure with PbBs in excess of 40 may be harmful to children. This is based on evidence for a progressive lead-related decrement of hemoglobin concentration as PbBs rise above this level. Below this level of exposure other heme-related biochemical effects are seen. But these seem to be noncritical. Implications for synthesis of other hemoproteins are not adequately known at this time.

Effects of lead on the kidney appear to occur only at exposure levels above those affecting hemoglobin formation. Knowledge as to renal dose-response relationships is even more imperfect than it is in regard to heme-hemoprotein effects. Further work is needed in this area since the renal effects, when they do occur, probably are more pernicious than the heme-hemoprotein effects.

Finally, the reader is cautioned that important effects of lead on the nervous system may prove to occur at relatively low exposure levels. But current information is totally inadequate to assess the situation for man in a dose-time-effect context.

Literature Cited

1. Natl. Acad. Sci.–Natl. Res. Counc. 1972. *Airborne Lead in Perspective.* Washington DC: Natl. Acad. Sci. 330 pp.
2. Goyer, R. A., Rhyne, B. C. 1972. Pathological effects of lead. *Int. Rev. Pathol.* 12:2–78
3. Waldron, H. A., Stöfen, D. 1974. *Subclinical Lead Poisoning.* New York & London: Academic. 224 pp.
4. Comm. Eur. Communities. 1973. *Environmental Health Aspects of Lead. Proc. Symp., Amsterdam, Holland, Oct. 2–6, 1972.* Luxembourg: Comm. Eur. Communities. 1162 pp.
5. Natl. Inst. Environ. Health. Sci., NIH 1974. Perspective on Low Level Lead Toxicity. *Eviron. Health Perspect.* Exp. Issue No. 7, 1–252
6. Ter Haar, G. L., Bayard, M. A. 1971. *Nature* 232:553–54
7. Robinson, E., Ludwig, F. L. 1967. Particle size distribution of urban lead aerosols. *J. Air Pollut. Control Assoc.* 17:664–69
8. Lee, R. E., Patterson, R. K., Wagman, J. 1968. Particle size distribution of metal components in urban air. *Environ. Sci. Technol.* 2:288–90
9. Mueller, P. K. 1970. Discussion (Characterization of particulate lead in vehicle exhaust-experimental techniques.) *Environ. Sci. Technol.* 4:248–51
10. Int. Comm. Radiol. Prot. Deposition and retention models for internal dosimetry of the human respiratory tract. *Health Phys.* 12:173–207
11. Mercer, T. T. 1975. The deposition model of the Task Group on Lung

Dynamics: a comparison with recent experimental data. *Health Phys.* 29:673–80
12. Kehoe, R. A. 1961. The metabolism of lead in man in health and disease. The Harben Lectures. *J. R. Inst. Public Health* 24:101–20, 129–43
13. Nozaki, K. 1966. Method for studies on inhaled particles in human respiratory system and retention of lead fume. *Ind. Health* 4:118–28
14. Mehani, S. 1966. Lead retention by the lungs of lead-exposed workers. *Ann. Occup. Hyg.* 9:165–71
15. Hursh, J. B., Mercer, T. T. 1970. Measurement of ^{212}Pb loss rate from human lungs. *J. Appl. Physiol.* 28:268–74
16. Bingham, E. 1970. Trace amounts of lead in the lung. *Trace Substances in the Environment III.* ed. D. D. Hemphill, 83–90. Columbia, Mo.: Univ. Missouri Press
17. Rabinowitz, M. B. 1974. *Lead contamination of the biosphere by human activity; a stable isotope study.* PhD thesis, Univ. California, Los Angeles. 120 pp.
18. Azar, A., D'Snee, R., Habibi, K. 1973. Relationship of community levels of air lead and indices of lead absorption. See Ref. 4, pp. 581–94
19. Griffin, T. B., Coulston, F., Wills, H., Russell, J. C., Knelson, J. H. 1975. Clinical studies on men continuously exposed to airborne particulate lead. In *Environmental Quality and Safety.* Suppl. Vol. II. Stuttgart:Thieme
20. Alexander, F. W., Delves, H. T., Clayton, B. E. 1973. The uptake and excre-

tion by children of lead and other contaminants. See Ref. 4, pp. 319–30

21. Kostial, K., Simonovic, I., Pisonic, M. 1971. Lead absorption from the intestine of newborn rats. *Nature* 233:564

22. Forbes, G. B., Reina, J. C. 1972. Effect of age on gastrointestinal absorption (Fe, Sr, Pb) in the rat. *J. Nutr.* 102:647–52

23. Sobel, A. E., Wexler, I. B., Petrovsky, D. D., Kramer, B. 1938. Influence of dietary calcium and phosphorus upon action of vitamin D in experimental lead poisoning. *Proc. Soc. Exp. Biol. Med.* 38:435–37

24. Six, K. M., Goyer, R. A. 1970. Experimental enhancement of lead toxicity by low dietary calcium. *J. Lab. Clin. Med.* 76:933–42

25. Gruden, N. 1975. Lead and active calcium transfer through the intestinal wall in rats. *Toxicology* 5:163–66

26. Kello, D., Kostial, K. 1973. The effect of milk on lead metabolism in rats. *Environ. Res.* 6:355–60

27. Barltrop, D., Khoo, H. E. 1975. The influence of nutritional factors on lead absorption. *Postgrad. Med. J.* 51:795–800

28. Six, K. M., Goyer, R. A. 1972. The influence of iron deficiency on tissue content and toxicity of ingested lead in the rat. *J. Lab. Clin. Med.* 79:128–36

29. Garber, B. T., Wei, E. 1974. Influence of dietary factors on the gastrointestinal absorption of lead. *Toxicol. Appl. Pharmacol.* 27:685–91

30. Gage, J. C., Litchfield, M. H. 1968. The migration of lead from polymers in the rat gastro-intestinal tract. *Food Cosmet. Toxicol.* 6:329–38

31. Gage, J. C., Litchfield, M. H. 1969. The migration of lead from paint films in the rat gastro-intestinal tract. *J. Oil Colloid Chem. Assoc.* 52:236–43

32. Lang, E. P., Kunze, F. M. 1948. The penetration of lead through the skin. *J. Ind. Hyg. Toxicol.* 30:256–59

33. Hine, C. H., Cavalli, R. D., Beltran, S. M. 1969. Percutaneous absorption of lead from industrial lubricants. *J. Occup. Med.* 11:568–75

34. Bolanowska, W., Piotrowski, J., Trojanowska, J. 1964. The kinetics of distribution and excretion of lead (Pb[210]) in rats. *Int. Congr. Occup. Health, Proc., 14, Madrid, 16–21 Sept. 1963. Int. Congr. Ser. No. 62*, pp. 420–22. Amsterdam: Excerpta Med. Found.

35. Hammond, P. B. 1971. The effects of chelating agents on the tissue distribu-

tion and excretion of lead. *Toxicol. Appl. Pharmacol.* 18:296–310

36. Momcilovic, B., Kostial, K. 1974. Kinetics of lead retention and distribution in suckling and adult rats. *Environ. Res.* 8:214–20

37. Barry, P. S. I. 1975. A comparison of concentrations of lead in human tissues. *Br. J. Ind. Med.* 32:119–39

38. Gross, S. B., Pfitzer, E. A., Yeager, D. W., Kehoe, R. A. 1975. Lead in human tissues. *Toxicol. Appl. Pharmacol.* 32:638–51

39. Goyer, R. A., Krall, R. 1969. Ultrastructural transformation in mitochondria isolated from kidneys of normal and lead-intoxicated rats. *J. Cell Biol.* 41:393–400

40. US Dep. Health, Educ., Welfare, Public Health Serv. Div. Air Pollut. 1965. Survey of lead in the atmosphere of three urban communities. *Public Health Serv. Publ. 999-AP-12.* Cincinnati: US Public Health Serv. 94 pp.

41. Horiuchi, K., Takada, I. 1954. Studies on the industrial lead poisoning. I. Absorption, transportation, deposition and excretion of lead. 1. Normal limits of lead in the blood, urine and feces among healthy Japanese urban inhabitants. *Osaka City Med. J.* 1:117–25

42. Butt, E. M., Nusbaum, R. E., Gilmour, T. C., Didio, S. L. 1964. Trace metal levels in human serum and blood. *Arch. Environ. Health.* 8:52–57

43. Scanlon, J. 1971. Umbilical cord blood lead concentration. Relationship to urban or suburban residency during gestation. *Am. J. Dis. Child.* 121:325–26

44. Haas, T., Wieck, A. B., Schaller, K. H., Mache, K., Valentin, H. 1972. Die usuelle bleibelastung bei neugeborenen und ihren muttern. *Zentralbl. Bakteriol. Parasitenk. Infektionskr. Hyg. Abt. Orig. Reihe B* 155:341–49

45. Hower, J., Prinz, B., Gono, E., Bohlmann, H. G. 1975. Die bedeutung der blei-immisions belastung fur schwangere und neugeborene im Ruhrgebiet. *Dtsch. Med. Wochenschr.* 100:461–63

46. Tola, S., Hernberg, S., Asp, S., Nikkanen, J. 1973. Parameters indicative of absorption and biological effect in new lead exposure: a prospective study. *Br. J. Ind. Med.* 30:134–41

47. Haeger-Aronsen, B., Abdulla, M., Fristedt, B. I. 1974. Effect of lead on δ-aminolevulinic acid dehydratase activity in red blood cells. *Arch. Environ. Health* 29:150–53

48. Prerovska, I., Teisinger, J. 1970. Excretion of lead and its biological activity several years after termination of exposure. *Br. J. Ind. Med.* 27:352–55

49. Smith, H. D., Baehner, R. L., Carney, T., Majors, W. J. 1963. The sequelae of pica with and without lead poisoning. *Am. J. Dis. Child.* 105:109–16

50. Chisolm, J. J. 1968. The use of chelating agents in the treatment of acute and chronic lead intoxication in childhood. *J. Pediatr.* 73:1–38

51. Hursh, J. B. 1973. Retention of ^{210}Pb in beagle dogs. *Health Phys.* 25:29–35

52. Teisinger, J., Srbova, J. 1959. The value of mobilization of lead by calcium ethylenediaminetetraacetate in the diagnosis of lead poisoning. *Br. J. Ind. Med.* 16:148–52

53. Emmerson, B. T. 1963. Chronic lead nephropathy. The diagnostic use of calcium EDTA and the association with gout. *Aust. Ann. Med.* 12:310–24

54. David, O., Clark, J., Voeller, K. 1972. Lead and hyperactivity. *Lancet* 2:900–3

55. Hammond, P. B., Aronson, A. L. 1960. The mobilization and excretion of lead in cattle: a comparative study of various chelating agents. *Ann. NY Acad. Sci.* 88:498–511

56. Selander, S., Cramer, K., Hallberg, L. 1966. Studies in lead poisoning. *Br. J. Ind. Med.* 23:282–91

57. Hammond, P. B. 1973. The effects of D-pencillamine (PCA) on the tissue distribution and excretion of lead. *Toxicol. Appl. Pharmacol.* 26:241–47

58. Ohlsson, W. T. L. 1962. Penicillamine as lead-chelating substance in man. *Br. Med. J.* 1:1454–56

59. Selander, S. 1967. Treatment of lead poisoning. A comparison between the effects of sodium calcium edetate and penicillamine administered orally and intravenously. *Br. J. Ind. Med.* 24: 272–82

60. Adams, D. A., Goldman, R., Maxwell, M. H., Latta, H. 1964. Nephrotic syndrome associated with penicillamine therapy of Wilson's disease. *Am. J. Med.* 36:330–36

61. Pueschel, S. M., Kopito, L., Schwachman, H. 1972. Children with an increased lead burden. A screening and follow-up study. *J. Am. Med. Assoc.* 222:462–66

62. Betts, P. R., Astley, R., Raine, D. N. 1973. Lead intoxication in children in Birmingham. *Br. Med. J.* 1:402–6

63. Williams, M. K. 1966. Blood lead and haemoglobin in lead absorption. *Br. J. Ind. Med.* 23:105–11

64. Waldron, H. A. 1966. The anaemia of lead poisoning. A review. *Br. J. Ind. Med.* 23:83–100

65. Hernberg, S., Nurminen, M., Hasan, J. 1967. Nonrandom shortening of red cell survival times in men exposed to lead. *Environ. Res.* 1:247–61

66. Hasan, J., Hernberg, S. 1966. Interaction of inorganic lead with human red blood cells. *Work Environ. Health* 2:26–44

67. Hasan, J., Vihko, V., Hernberg, S. 1967. Deficient red cell membrane Na$^+$+K$^+$-ATPase in lead poisoning. *Arch. Environ. Health* 14:313–18

68. Hernberg, S., Vihko, V., Hasan, J. 1967. Red cell membrane ATPase in workers exposed to inorganic lead. *Arch. Environ. Health* 14:319–24

69. Secchi, G., Alessio, L., Cambiaghi, G. 1973. Na$^+$/K$^+$ATPase activity of erythrocyte membranes. *Arch. Environ. Health* 27:399–400

70. White, J. M., Harvey, D. R. 1972. Defective synthesis of α and β globin chains in lead poisoning. *Nature* 236:71–73

71. Piddington, S. K., White, J. M. 1974. The effect of lead on total globin and α and β chain synthesis; *in vitro* and *in vivo*. *Br. J. Haemotol.* 27:415–27

72. Shemin, D. 1970. On the synthesis of heme. *Naturwissenschaften* 57:185–90

73. Selander, S., Cramer, K. 1970. Interrelationships between lead in blood, lead in urine, and ALA in urine during lead work. *Br. J. Ind. Med.* 27:28–39

74. Haeger-Aronsen, B. 1971. An assessment of the laboratory tests used to monitor the exposure of lead workers. *Br. J. Ind. Med.* 28:52–58

75. Roels, H. A., Lauwerys, R. R., Buchet, J. P., Vrelust, M.-T. 1975. Response of free erythrocyte porphyrin and urinary δ-aminolevulinic acid in men and women moderately exposed to lead. *Int. Arch. Arbeitsmed.* 34:97–108

76. Chisolm, J. J. 1968. Determination of δ-aminolevulinic acid in plasma. *Anal. Biochem.* 22:54–64

77. Cramer, K., Goyer, R. A., Jagenburg, R., Wilson, M. H. 1974. Renal ultrastructure, renal function and parameters of lead toxicity in workers with different periods of lead exposure. *Br. J. Ind. Med.* 31:113–27

78. Stuik, E. J. 1974. Biological response of male and female volunteers to inorganic lead. *Int. Arch. Arbeitsmed.* 33:83–97

79. Kao, R. C. L, Forbes, R. M. 1973. Lead and vitamin A effect on heme synthesis in rats. *Arch. Environ. Health* 27:31–35

80. Hernberg, S., Nikkanen, J., Mellin, G., Lilius, H. 1970. δ-Aminolevulinic acid dehydrase as a measure of lead exposure. *Arch. Environ. Health* 21:140–45

81. Tola, S. 1972. Erythrocyte δ-aminolevulinic acid dehydratase activity after termination of lead exposure. *Work Environ. Health* 9:66–70

82. Haeger-Aronsen, B., Abdulla, M., Fristedt, B. I. 1974. Effect of lead on δ-aminolevulinic acid dehydratase activity in red blood cells. II. Regeneration of enzyme after cessation of lead exposure. *Arch. Environ. Health* 29:150–53

83. Roels, H. A., Buchet, J. P., Lauwerys, R. R. 1974. Inhibition of human erythrocyte δ-aminolevulinate dehydratase by lead. In vitro artifact or real phenomenon in vivo? *Int. Arch. Arbeitsmed.* 33:277–84

84. Vergnano, C., Cartasegna, C., Ardoino, V. 1969. Meccanismi di inibizione dell' attivita' δ amino-levulinico deidratasica eritrocitaria nell' intossicasione da piombo umana e sperimentale. *Med. Lav.* 60:505–16

85. Vergnano, C., Cartasegna, C., Bonsignore, D. 1968. Regolazione allosterica della attivita δ-amino-levulinico-deidratasica eritrocitaria. *Bull. Soc. Ital. Biol. Sper.* 64:692–99

86. Granick, J. L., Sassa, S., Granick, S., Levere, R. D., Kappas, A. 1973. Studies in lead poisoning. II. Correlation between the ratio of activated to inactivated δ-aminolevulinic acid dehydratase of whole blood and blood lead level. *Biochem. Med.* 8:149–59

87. Tola, S. 1973. The effect of blood lead concentration, age, sex, and time of exposure upon erythrocyte δ-aminolevulinic acid dehydratase activity. *Work Environ. Health* 10:26–35

88. Secchi, G., Erba, L., Cambiaghi, G. 1974. Delta-aminolevulinic acid dehydratase activity of erythrocytes and liver tissue in man. *Arch. Environ. Health* 28:130–32

89. Millar, J. A., Cumming, R. L. C., Battistini, V., Carswell, F., Goldberg, A. 1970. Lead and δ-aminolevulinic acid dehydratase levels in mentally retarded children and in lead-poisoned suckling rats. *Lancet* 2:695–98

90. Hammond, P. B. 1973. The relationship between inhibition of δ-aminolevulinic acid dehydratase by lead and lead mobilization by ethylenediaminetetraacetate (EDTA). *Toxicol. Appl. Pharmacol.* 26:466–75

91. Maxfield, M. E., Stopps, G. J., Barnes, J. R., Snee, R. D., Azar, A. 1972. Effect of lead on blood regeneration following acute hemorrhage in dogs. *Am. Ind. Hyg. Assoc. J.* 33:326–37

92. Gibson, K. D., Neuberger, A., Scott, J. J. 1955. The purification and properties of δ-aminolevulinic acid dehydrase. *Biochem. J.* 61:618–29

93. Wada, O., Toyokawa, K., Suzuki, T., Suzuki, S., Yano, Y., Nakao, K. 1969. Response to a low concentration of mercury vapor. Relation to human porphyrin metabolism. *Arch. Environ. Health* 19:485–88

94. Lauwerys, R. R., Buchet, J. P., Roels, H. A. 1973. Comparative study of effect of inorganic lead and cadmium on blood δ-aminolevulinate dehydratase in man. *Br. J. Ind. Med.* 30:359–64

95. Moore, M. R., Beattie, A. D., Thompson, G. G., Goldberg, A. 1971. Depression of δ-aminolaevulic acid dehydrase activity by ethanol in man and rat. *Clin. Sci.* 40:81–88

96. McGillion, F. B., Moore, M. R., Goldberg, A. 1973. The effect of δ-aminolaevulinic acid on the spontaneous activity of mice. *Scott. Med. J.* 18:133

97. McGillion, F. B., Moore, M. R., Goldberg, A. 1975. Some pharmacological effects of δ-aminolaevulinic acid on blood pressure in the rat and on rabbit isolated ear arteries. *Clin. Exp. Pharmacol. Physiol.* 2:365–71

98. Kennedy, G. L., Arnold, D. W., Calandra, J. C. 1976. Toxicity studies with δ-aminolaevulinic acid. *Food Cosmet. Toxicol.* 14:45–48

99. Becker, D., Viljoen, D., Kramer, S. 1971. The inhibition of red cell and brain ATPase by δ-aminolaevulinic acid. *Biochim. Biophys. Acta* 225:26–34

100. Kramer, S., Becker, D., Viljoen, D. 1973. Significance of the porphyrin precursors delta-aminolaevulinic acid (ALA) and porphobilinogen in the acute attack of porphyria. *S. Afr. Med. J.* 47:1735–38

101. Granick, S., Sassa, S., Granick, J. L., Levere, R. D., Kappas, A. 1972. Assays for porphyrins, δ-aminolevulinic-acid dehydratase, and porphyrinogen synthetase in microliter samples of whole blood: applications to metabolic defects involving the heme pathway. *Proc. Natl. Acad. Sci. USA* 69:2381–85

102. Piomelli, S. 1973. A micromethod for free erythrocyte protoporphyrins: the

FEP test. *J. Lab. Clin. Med.* 81:932–40
103. Chisolm, J. J., Hastings, C. W., Cheung, D. K. K. 1974. Microfluorometric assay for protoporphyrin in acidified acetone extracts of whole blood. *Biochem. Med.* 9:113–35
104. Lamola, A. A., Joselow, M., Yamane, T. 1975. Zinc protoporphyrin (ZPP): A simple, sensitive fluorometric screening test for lead poisoning. *Clin. Chem.* 21:93–97
105. Roels, H. A., Lauwerys, R. R., Buchet, J. P. 1975. Response of free erythrocyte porphyrin and urinary δ-aminolevulinic acid in men and women moderately exposed to lead. *Int. Arch. Arbeitsmed.* 34:97–108
106. Stuik, E. J. 1974. Biological response of male and female volunteers to inorganic lead. *Int. Arch. Arbeitsmed.* 33:93–94
107. Sassa, S., Granick, J. L., Granick, S., Kappas, A., Levere, R. D. 1973. Studies in lead poisoning. 1. Microanalysis of erythrocyte protoporphyrin levels by spectrophotofluorometry in the detection of chronic lead intoxication in the subclinical range. *Biochem. Med.* 8:135–48
108. Strand, L. J., Manning, J., Marver, H. S. 1972. The induction of δ-aminolevulinic acid synthetase in cultured liver cells. *J. Biol. Chem.* 247:2820–27
109. Suketa, Y., Aoki, M., Yamamoto, T. 1975. Changes in hepatic δ-aminolevulinic acid in lead-intoxicated rats. *J. Toxicol. Environ. Health* 1:127–32
110. Berk, P. D., Tschudy, D. P., Shepley, L., Waggoner, J. G., Berlin, N. I. 1970. Hematologic and biochemical studies in a case of lead poisoning. *Am. J. Med.* 48:137–44
111. Jandl, J. H., Inman, J. K., Simmons, R. L., Allen, D. W. 1959. Transfer of iron from serum iron-binding protein to human reticulocytes. *J. Clin. Invest.* 38:161–85
112. Bessis, M. C., Jensen, W. N. 1965. Sideroblastic anemia, mitochondria and erythroblastic iron. *Br. J. Haematol.* 11:49–51
113. Alvares, A. P., Fischbein, A., Sassa, S., Anderson, K. E., Kappas, A. 1976. Lead intoxication: effects on cytochrome P-450-mediated hepatic oxidations. *Clin. Pharmacol. Ther.* 19:183–90
114. Alvares, A. P., Kapelner, S., Sassa, S., Kappas, A. 1975. Drug metabolism in normal children, lead-poisoned children, and normal adults. *Clin. Pharmacol Ther.* 17:179–83

115. Scoppa, P., Roumengous, M., Penning, W. 1973. Hepatic drug metabolizing activity in lead-poisoned rats. *Experientia* 29:970–72
116. Rhyne, B. C., Goyer, R. A. 1971. Cytochrome content of kidney mitochondria in experimental lead poisoning. *Exp. Mol. Pathol.* 14:386–91
117. Zielhuis, R. L. 1975. Dose-response relationships for inorganic lead. 1. Biochemical and haemotological responses. *Int. Arch. Occup. Health* 35:1–18
118. Chisolm, J. J., Barrett, M. B., Mellits, E. D. 1975. Dose-effect and dose-response relationships for lead in children. *J. Pediatr.* 86:1152–60
119. Chisolm, J. J. 1962. Aminoaciduria as a manifestation of renal tubular injury in lead intoxication and a comparison with patterns of aminoaciduria seen in other diseases. *J. Pediatr.* 60:1–17
120. Clarkson, T. W., Kench, J. E. 1956. Urinary excretion of amino acids by men absorbing heavy metals. *Biochem. J.* 62:361–72
121. Goyer, R. A., Tsuchiya, K., Leonard, D. L., Kahyo, H. 1972. Aminoaciduria in Japanese workers in the lead and cadmium industries. *Am. J. Clin. Pathol.* 57:635–42
122. Cramer, K., Goyer, R. A., Jagenburg, R., Wilson, M. H. 1974. Renal ultrastructure, renal function, and parameters of lead toxicity in workers with different periods of lead exposure. *Br. J. Ind. Med.* 31:113–27
123. Henderson, D. A. 1958. The aetiology of chronic nephritis in Queensland. *Med. J. Aust.* 1:377–86
124. Emmerson, B. T. 1963. Chronic lead nephropathy. The diagnostic use of calcium EDTA and the association with gout. *Australas. Ann. Med.* 12:310–24
125. Emmerson, B. T. 1965. The renal excretion of urate in chronic lead nephropathy. *Australas. Ann. Med.* 14:295–303
126. Morgan, J. M., Hartley, M. W., Miller, R. E. 1966. Nephropathy in chronic lead poisoning. *Arch. Int. Med.* 118:17–29
127. Ball, G. V., Sorensen, L. B. 1969. Pathogenesis of hyperuricemia in saturnine gout. *N. Engl. J. Med.* 280:1199–1202
128. Tepper, L. B. 1963. Renal function subsequent to childhood plumbism. *Arch. Environ. Health* 7:76–85
129. Lilis, R., Gavrilescu, N., Nestorescu, B., Dumitriu, C., Roventa, A. 1968. Nephropathy in chronic lead poisoning. *Br. J. Ind. Med.* 25:196–202

130. Wedeen, R. P., Maesaka, J. K., Weiner, B., Lipat, G. A., Lyons, M. M., Vitale, L. F., Joselow, M. M. 1975. Occupational lead nephropathy. *Am. J. Med.* 59:630–41
131. Vitale, L. F., Joselow, M. M., Wedeen, R. P., Pawlow, M. 1975. Blood lead—an inadequate measure of lead exposure. *J. Occup. Med.* 17:155–56
132. Goyer, R. A., 1971. Lead and the kidney. *Curr. Topics Pathol.* 55:147–76
133. Sandstead, H. H., Michelakis, A. M., Temple, T. E. 1970. Lead intoxication. Its effect on the renin-aldosterone response to sodium deprivation. *Arch. Environ. Health* 20:356–63
134. Richter, G. W., Kress, Y., Cornwall, C. C. 1968. Another look at lead inclusion bodies. *Am. J. Pathol.* 53:189–217
135. Moore, J. F., Goyer, R. A., Wilson, M. 1973. Lead inclusion bodies: solubility, amino acid content, and relationship to residual acidic nuclear proteins. *Lab. Invest.* 29:488–94
136. Choie, D. D., Richter, G. W., Young, L. B. 1975. Biogenesis of intranuclear lead-protein inclusion in mouse kidney. *Beitr. Pathol.* 155:197–203
137. Cooper, W. C., Gaffey, W. R. 1975. Mortality of lead workers. *J. Occup. Med.* 17:100–7
138. Malcolm, D. 1971. Prevention of long-term sequelae following the absorption of lead. *Arch. Environ. Health* 23:292–98

Ann Rev. Pharmacol. Toxicol. 1977. 17:215–22
Copyright © 1977 by Annual Reviews Inc. All rights reserved

POISON CONTROL CENTERS: ❖6676
PROSPECTS AND CAPABILITIES

Anthony R. Temple

Department of Pediatrics, University of Utah, and Intermountain Regional Poison Control
Center, Salt Lake City, Utah 84132

The development of the poison control movement was based on the need to have available a rapid access system to identify the potential danger of an exposure to any of the thousands of chemicals—drugs, household products, industrial chemicals, etc—that are available to man. In that regard, the initial poison control centers were cataloging services providing information to the physician about the contents and toxicity of a product about which he wanted information (1). With the development of newer and better information systems, accumulation of more and better toxicology data, development of new and better poisoning managements, and the development and affiliation with the poison control center movement of clinical or medical toxicologists, the poison control movement has entered a new era.

The poison control concept was initiated in Chicago, Illinois, in 1953. Following the impetus of local health officials, pediatricians, and other interested physicians, a single center for collecting product data was established. The idea soon caught on and numerous other centers were established. In order to provide a coordinating agency for these centers, the then Bureau of Product Safety in the Food and Drug Administration established the National Clearinghouse for Poison Control Centers. This clearinghouse served as a center for collecting and standardizing product toxicology data and for distributing this data in the form of 5" by 8" index cards to recognized poison control centers. State health departments were given the responsibility for identifying poison centers within their states (1). The great interest in poison control eventually resulted in over 580 officially recognized poison control centers and numerous additional nonofficial centers, including drug information services, bringing the total to well over 600 (2). Unfortunately, many poison centers have little if any capability for providing sophisticated information or treatment for poisoning. In fact, some of these recognized poison centers handle as few as one call per week (3).

From the beginning, studies of poison control center operation have shown a wide variability in how services were provided (3–11). For purposes of simplification,

215

poison control services have been defined as poison information centers, poison treatment centers, and poison treatment centers with toxicology laboratory service (12). Poison information centers are services that provide telephone information but do not participate in the treatment of the poisoned patient. An example of this would be the Thomas J. Fleming Poison Information Service at the Children's Hospital of Los Angeles. This center provides information, solely to physicians or health care facilities, for over 30,000 cases annually (C. Ray, personal communication). A poison treatment center is a health care facility that treats poisoning cases and is a referral center for such in addition to providing poison information. The Inter-mountain Regional Poison Control Center at the University of Utah Medical Center is such a center. Poison control services also are variable in that some provide information only to physicians or health care professionals while others provide information to the public or both (3). Staffing of poison control centers likewise is quite variable. The staff of a poison center may consist only of full or part-time clerks or nurses or pharmacists without any direct medical supervision, or they may consist of a full-time M.D. clinical toxicologist-director and specially trained full-time professional staff, such as clinical pharmacists. Other centers may include as staff or consultants pharmacologists, emergency room physicians, ambulatory pediatricians, or other scientifically trained personnel (3, 13).

The current questions facing the poison control center movement two decades following its inception are how best to provide services, how to improve services, how to standardize or monitor services, to whom to provide services, and how to organize such services on a regional or national basis. The question of how to organize these services is still very much open for discussion in poison center circles (3, 4, 11, 13). In the author's view consolidation of manpower and resources into centralized or regional services is crucial. In these centralized or regional centers, information would be provided both to health professionals and to the public. Treatment facilities would be an integral part of the regional poison control center, and the staff, particularly the medical staff, would provide the treatment for poisoning victims. In addition, active supervision and even bedside consultation of poisoning cases admitted to other health care facilities would be provided. The following is a description of what a regional poison control program is and could be.

REGIONAL POISON CONTROL: GENERAL PROGRAM DESCRIPTION

A regional poison control center should be one which, in less densely populated areas, serves a single or multi-state region, or in heavily populated areas serves a portion of a state. Generally, a regional center will be found serving no fewer than one million people, but could serve as many as five to ten million people in areas of high population density. A regional center would provide (a) comprehensive poison information, both to health professionals and consumers, (b) comprehensive poisoning treatment services, (c) a full range of analytical toxicologic services, (d) a toll-free communication system, (e) access to transportation facilities for critically ill patients, (f) professional and public education programs, and (g) collection and dissemination of poisoning experience data. In essence, a regional center must be capable of assuming ultimate responsibility for the provision of poisoning consultations and patient care for all poisonings brought to its attention within its region (13).

Poison Information Services

A regional center's poisoning information capability generally is as comprehensive as is available. The services are available 24 hours a day, every day of the year, and are accessible to both professionals and consumers. These centers have all of the basic toxicology information resources that are available, access to texts and journals related to toxicology, and ready access to a medical library.

In the case of the consumer, information is simplified to meet consumers' needs. Provision of such services is coupled with careful monitoring of consumer understanding, consumer compliance with the suggested recommendations, and assessment of the outcome of such cases. Where appropriate rapport with the consumer is established, it is feasible to manage selected exposures by telephone (14). In order to provide good telephone management, centers obtain as accurate and complete a history of the toxic exposure as possible, make an appropriate assessment of the toxicity, and determine where the victim should be managed.

Poison Treatment Services

Regional centers generally are capable of providing the most sophisticated poisoning treatment available. The medical care facility in which the treatment center is housed is usually a category I comprehensive emergency service and has a fully staffed observation unit and an intensive care unit for both adult and pediatric patients. Comprehensive poisoning treatment services mean that the center is able to provide initial and subsequent treatment of all types of poisonings and to include methods of terminating the exposure, such as gastric lavage, induction of emesis, and irrigation. They have facilities for providing intensive supportive care of the patient, including resuscitation, endotracheal intubation, tracheotomy, cardiac monitoring, monitoring of fluid and electrolyte balance, monitoring of blood gases, and intensive care nursing supervision. They have available all known antidotes. The treatment service generally is staffed with full-time personnel trained specifically in the management of poisoning, including a clinical toxicologist. In addition, they have access to consultant services such as endoscopy, hemodialysis, peritoneal dialysis, exchange transfusions, plasmapheresis, or extracorporeal charcoal hemoperfusion.

Analytical Capabilities

A regional poison control center should have immediate access to appropriate analytical toxicology services. These analytical services provide immediate analysis of blood, urine, and gastric aspirate in terms of an immediate drug screen, and subsequent quantitative analysis for monitoring the patient's progress and assessing the severity of the case.

Communication and Transport

Communication systems are set up by regional centers to provide ready access to the center. Toll-free telephone services generally are established. Outgoing communication is made by telephone or by telecopiers and hard copy information can be transmitted to affiliated hospitals in this way (B. H. Rumack, R. W. Moriarty, personal communication). Regional services also have an established system for referral and transport for patients who are critically ill and provide emergency medical recommendations for the victim prior to transfer to a medical facility in order to facilitate the movement of that victim to medical care. Transportation systems depend upon local geography and circumstances, and in many areas are tied to local emergency medical service systems. In highly populated areas, transportation by specially equipped ambulances or helicopter may be satisfactory. In less densely populated areas with large geographical expanses, more sophisticated air transport has been established (B. H. Rumack, personal communication). These transportation systems usually are used in conjunction with other programs for patient transport, but regional poison centers work with the transport system to see that the transportation equipment includes everything necessary to appropriately manage a poisoned patient during transport.

The regional center additionally services another important role in pulling together the medical care facilities within the region in the management of poisoning cases. Within the region, there may be designated subregional poison treatment centers which provide limited treatment services and which rely on the regional center for backup. In addition, there will be hospital emergency facilities that provide primary emergency management and care of poisoned patients, but are not poison treatment centers. Regional centers ideally develop an administrative posture to encourage adequate communication between themselves and the subregional centers and other primary emergency services. The regional center assumes responsibility for training subregional center personnel and other primary emergency service personnel. While not all cases necessarily are referred to them, either by telephone or in person, these centers maintain adequate liaison with other medical facilities in their region to ensure that appropriate patient care or consultation is given. All in all, regional centers must be willing to assume ultimate responsibility for all consultations regarding poisonings in their region.

POISON CONTROL CENTER STAFFING

As indicated above, staffing of centers is highly variable, but those centers with full-time highly trained individuals have the greatest potential for providing quality information. It has been recommended that each regional center should have a full-time physician who has expertise and skill in the management of poisonings (13). Such a physician would most likely have a background in one of the primary medical care fields—pediatrics, medicine, family practice, or emergency medicine, but also would need to have additional training or experience in the area of clinical toxicology, perferably with certification in that specialty such as is provided by the

American Board of Medical Toxicology of the American Academy of Clinical Toxicology. Unfortunately, very few such individuals are so trained and not all of them are affiliated with poison control programs (15).

Nonmedical staff in poison control centers are drawn from a wide variety of professionals in the health-related field. For daily operation of the information service, pharmacists and nurses with specific clinical training generally are most often used. The background of clinical pharmacists working in regional centers includes basic pharmacy education, special clinical training, and specific experience and/or training in clinical toxicology. In addition to basic nursing training, nurses usually have had additional experience and/or training in emergency care, public health, and occasionally pharmacology and clinical toxicology. While other health professionals may provide poison control information, most do not have a clinical background that would allow them to interact freely with physicians and other health care professionals in providing consultative services, nor do they have the ability to interpret basic toxicology information. We have argued that the physician-pharmacist team, with pharmacologist consultants, is the ideal staffing pattern for poison control (16).

It is neither sufficient nor acceptable that staff in a regional poison control center simply read data as are found in the printed page, so that operational staff must be capable of selecting from various resources appropriate information for specific cases. It is unfortunate but true that information resources may not have accurate data, may lack data entirely, or may have only limited information about a subject. As a result, the ability to interpret literature is a necessity. Management of cases by poison control centers requires a great deal more sophistication than just reading a response from a card file. It is anticipated that soon all operational staff in poison control centers will be certified as to their level of competence through a national certification process.

In addition to the basic operational staff, which provides telephone coverage and consultations, and the administrative staff, a regional poison center will have available an extensive list of consultants who can provide expertise in a wide range of selected fields. These consultants are chosen from various medical fields and fields related to the area of toxicology, and will include such people as an anesthesiologist, endoscopist, ophthalmologist, respiratory care specialist, radiologist, renalogist, pharmacognosist or botanist, analytical chemist, herpetologist, mycologist, pharmacologists, as well as numerous other specialists.

TOXICOLOGY INFORMATION RESOURCES

Accompanying the development of more sophisticated poison centers has been the development of some new, more sophisticated information resources. The most comprehensive resource for listing product names and ingredients in a rapidly accessible manner is Poisindex, a computer-generated microfiche system. Poisindex contains information on over 200,000 separate products, which can be accessed by generic or trade name, manufacturer's name, or selected chemical constituents. This data source lists the product formulation, indexes the major toxic constituents, and provides concise, but thorough, recommendations for the management of exposures or poisonings with the product. The microfiche card file is updated quarterly so that it is extremely current. The managements are written by an editorial board of physicians/toxicologists to ensure the availability of the best possible recommendations (17).

Another new resource is a data bank of information provided by the National Clearinghouse for Poison Control Centers via on-line cathode ray tube (CRT) terminals. Each CRT is on-line to the Food and Drug Administration computer via dedicated telephone lines. Access to the data is as quick as one can type the name of the product or chemical compound. It even has an allowance for phonetic access. Using the well-known poison index card data, the computer-stored data also contains experience data reported to the National Clearinghouse for Poison Control Centers. Because of its cost, the number of terminals made available to regional centers is very limited at the present time.

Numerous other resources also are becoming available. New textbooks in the basic science of poisonings, industrial toxicology, adverse drug effects, and many other topics suggest that for a poison control center to be adequately equipped, dozens of textbooks and access to numerous journals must be maintained. Nonetheless, limitations of information resources is still a major problem.

In most poison control centers, assessment of the toxicity of an agent or exposure must be based on data found in several general rapid retrieval information resources, selected textbooks, and available center-generated files. Ideally the staff of poison centers develop additional expertise in managing cases and learn by experiences how to evaluate discrepancies in the available resources and to fill in the gap of information that is not available, but this may not always be the case. Our personal evaluation of current information resources suggests that unless the staff of a poison control center is capable of evaluation of resources and personally updating them, errors in management can occur. For example, if faced with a case of digoxin poisoning, the information about the types of cardiac manifestations, degree of toxicity, and indication or contraindication of administering potassium are all at variance if one refers to the most commonly used information resources (17–20). It appears that no single information resource at the current time is sufficient to provide comprehensive toxicological data.

ACTIVITIES OF A REGIONAL POISON CONTROL CENTER

Current activities of poison control centers involve the management of large numbers of chemical exposures, but only some of them can be considered actual poisonings. At the Intermountain Regional Poison Control Center, we handled 13,790 calls during July 1974 to June 1975. Of these 11,109 (80.6%) involved actual exposures, the remaining 2681 cases being requests for information only. Of the actual exposures, 8788 (79.1%) were sufficiently minor that they could be managed at home. Of the cases managed at home, most were not considered to be of sufficient potential toxicity that some form of active intervention was initiated. While not all of these cases were followed up in great detail, in a selected group of cases in which ipecac-induced emesis was initiated, careful monitoring of the course of the illness was made (14). In this study, 776 cases were examined that were considered to be of sufficient level of potential toxicity that ipecac emesis at home was warranted but referral to an emergency care facility was not deemed necessary if emesis ensued. Through use of a standardized protocol, 98.8% of the patients vomited successfully. In following these patients we found only 51 (6.7%) had symptoms four hours following ingestion, all of which were minor, and only 11 (1.4%) had symptoms at 24-hour follow-up, again, all of which were minor. In no case did serious symptoms arise. The appearance of some symptoms, even with 98.8% successful emesis, suggests that these ingestions did involve significant exposures, but were not serious and could be managed appropriately as was done in the victims' homes. During this same 12-month period, 1558 (17.7%) cases were either already in emergency rooms or doctors' offices or were referred there. Only 314 (3.6%) of these eventually were admitted to the hospital. Only three (0.03%) were known to result in death. From our experience it would appear that the major efforts of poison control centers are directed toward identifying agent and exposure toxicity, selecting and recommending emergency measures when necessary, while less frequently acting as consultants on serious poisonings. In fact, the principal function of a poison control center still remains that of identifying whether an agent or an exposure is indeed toxic.

LIMITATIONS AND FUTURE NEEDS

As we look at the limitations of the current poison control system, it is apparent that the current principal limitation is that we have not developed more regional programs. In addition, we continue to need more information on product toxicity and human toxicology, and we need to develop better equipped, more highly trained people to service poison control programs.

For many years, the need for regionalization has been stressed (3, 4, 13). This logic is applicable both for information services and treatment services. We must proceed more rapidly at developing regional plans along regional needs and integrating these plans with other regional health care facilities. Centralization of information resources, integration of individual expertise, and coordination of treatment facilities for poisoning should be given high priority.

Just as important a need is the need for increased research in the areas of human toxicology. One of the principal limitations of poison control services is the lack of good information about the real toxicity of a product. Undoubtedly, many patients are undertreated, overtreated, or just mistreated because our knowledge of certain problems is not sufficient. Just how toxic is that cleaning agent? How serious is that industrial exposure? What is the real hazard of eating part of that plant? What is the best way to treat the hepatotoxicity produced by an overdose of that drug? Both basic research and human experience data are vitally needed.

A third limitation is the lack of appropriate manpower. Frequent pleas for more toxicologists are heard, but the need for poison control centers is to develop clinically oriented toxicologists. Programs for training physicians in clinical toxicology are sparse. Programs for training pharmacists or pharmacologists in toxicology are just about as sparse, and clinically oriented programs are rare. Training of nurses in toxicology is nonexistent. As a result, almost all of our manpower development comes as a result of on-the-job experience. While this has proven to be workable in the past, the need for more sophistication in information evaluation and dissemination and in patient management demands the development of training programs. As a minimum, postgraduate fellowships in medical toxicology need to be made available for physicians. In addition, special training programs for poison center staff need to be initiated, hopefully in conjunction with ongoing educational programs such as clinical pharmacy training programs.

Poison control has come of age. Offering sophisticated consultative and patient management services, poison control programs now have the potential for greatly improving the care of poisoning exposures. While limited in number and hampered by limited resources, the development of appropriate regional centers has brought the poison control concept to fruition.

Literature Cited

1. Verhulst, H. L., Crotty, J. J. 1969. Poison control division. *FDA Pap.* March, pp. 11–13
2. Natl. Clgh. Poison Control Cent. July–August 1976. Directory. *Bulletin.* USDHEW, Public Health Serv., FDA, Bethesda, Maryland
3. Lovejoy, F. H., Alpert, J. J. 1970. A future direction for poison centers; a critique. *Pediatr. Clin. North Am.* 17: 747–53
4. Temple, A. R., Done, A. K. 1972. Organization of emergency treatment facilities for the management of acute poisonings. *Emergency Room Care,* ed. W. W. Oaks, S. Spitzer, 107–15. New York: Grune & Stratton. 300 pp.
5. Goulding, R. 1975. Poison control centers—an essay on information and prevention. *Essays Toxicol.* 6:79–100
6. Teitelbaum, D. T. 1968. New directions in poison control. *Clin. Toxicol.* 1:3–13
7. Luckens, M. M. 1972. Developing total service capabilities in poison information centers. *Am. J. Public Health* 62:407–10
8. Matthew, H., Proudfoot, A. T., Brown, S. S., Aitken, R. C. B. 1969. Acute poisoning: organization and work-load of a treatment centre. *Br. Med. J.* 2:489–93
9. Grayson, R. 1962. The poison control movement in the United States. *Ind. Med. Surg.* 31:296–97
10. Adams, W. C. 1963. Poison control centers: their purpose and operation. *Clin. Pharmacol. Ther.* 4:293–96
11. Barry, P. Z. 1974. A workshop on poison control centers. A report of workshop held April 1–2, 1974, Chapel Hill, North Carolina, pursuant to contract no. FDA 74–30
12. Am. Assoc. Poison Control Cent. 1972. Standards
13. Temple, A. R., Veltri, J. C. 1976. A program guide for regional poison control centers. A report prepared for the National Clearinghouse for Poison Control Centers, pursuant to contract no. PHS 223–75–3013
14. Veltri, J. C., Temple, A. R. 1976. Telephone management of poisonings using syrup of ipecac. *Clin. Toxicol.* 9:407–17
15. Diplomates Am. Board Med. Toxicol. 1976. *AACTION* 4:3
16. Temple, A. R. 1972. Role of toxicology education in pharmacy education. *Forum Adv. Toxicol. Newsl.* 5:(4) 4
17. Poisindex, Micromedex, Inc., 2645 South Santa Fe Drive, Denver, Colorado 80223
18. Gosselin, R. E., Hodge, H. C., Smith, R. P., Gleason, M. N. 1976. *Clinical Toxicology of Commercial Products,* III: 124–33. Baltimore: Williams & Wilkins. 1783 pp. 4th ed.
19. Dreisbach, R. H. 1974. *Handbook of Poisoning: Diagnosis & Treatment,* 332–34. Los Altos, Calif: Lange Med. Publ. 517 pp. 8th ed.
20. Poison Index Cards, National Clearinghouse for Poison Control Centers, DHEW-PHS-FDA

Ann. Rev. Pharmacol. Toxicol. 1977. 17:223–42
Copyright © 1977 by Annual Reviews Inc. All rights reserved

THE PHARMACOLOGIC PRINCIPLES OF REGIONAL PAIN RELIEF

❖6677

John Adriani and Mohammad Naraghi
Department of Anesthesiology, Charity Hospital, and Department of Pharmacology,
Louisiana State University, New Orleans, Louisiana 70140

Regional pain relief may be obtained by physical means, such as the application of electric currents to peripheral nerves, the spinal cord, and the brain; the cooling of an extremity; total body cooling; the stimulation of the α, β, and γ of the A fibers by needling (acupuncture); sonic waves; or the application of pressure to nerves. It is more often obtained by the use of drugs that interrupt conduction of impulses when applied directly to peripheral nerves. Drugs that block conduction are of two types: the local anesthetics which provide temporary pain relief and the neurolytic agents that cause destruction of nervous tissues and yield long-lasting relief.

The search for the ideal local anesthetic has continued since Karl Koller introduced local anesthesia into medicine. The search for an ideal neurolytic agent that does not cause neuritis likewise continues. New drugs have been adopted and the older ones discarded, but most of the objections of the old are found with the new. The purpose of this review is to present some of the aspects of clinical pharmacology of local anesthetics and a comparison of the effects of newer drugs with the old. In discussing local anesthetics, emphasis is placed upon the relationship of chemical structure to activity; their presumed mode of action; their absorption, distribution, and mode of elimination; and the relationship of these factors to local and systemic toxicity.

LOCAL VERSUS SYSTEMIC EFFECTS

Local anesthetics behave as such only when placed in direct contact with nervous tissues. The plasma levels during regional block, comparatively speaking, are minute. Undesirable systemic effects occur when local anesthetics gain access to the

223

vascular system in quantities that cause high plasma levels. At certain plasma levels, depression of the inhibitory neurons of the cortex occurs, causing the excitatory neurons to become more active. Convulsions result. As plasma levels increase, the excitatory neurons are affected also, and depression of the central nervous system results. At certain plasma levels there is also a decrease in the electrophysiologic activity of the conductive mechanism of the heart. Increasing the levels further causes a negative inotropic effect on the myocardial tissues and depression of smooth muscle of the vascular tissues. Cardiac output is decreased and hypotension ensues (1–3). Plasma levels attained when these drugs are properly used do not ordinarily exert these effects.

Generally, local anesthetics are applied to somatic nerves, that is, to bundles of axones, and interrupt transmission of stimuli from a nerve cell to a receptor or to another organ. Local anesthetics interfere with this function by causing a temporary, reversible change in the chemical and physical structure of the neuronal membrane. Although they are ordinarily applied to bundles of axones, they are capable of acting anywhere on a neuron. The end result is the same whether they are applied to a cell body, dendrite, axone, or at a synapse.

MOLECULAR CONFIGURATION OF LOCAL ANESTHETICS

Numerous substances are capable of producing the type of blockade referred to as local anesthesia which affords regional pain relief (1–6). Hundreds of compounds that manifest local anesthetic activity have been investigated. Less than several dozen are used clinically. Some were discarded because they were locally destructive to tissue, others because they were too toxic systemically or locally, and others because they were unsatisfactory from the standpoint of potency or effectiveness or duration of action. The majority of the clinically suitable injectable local anesthetics are amines (2). The configuration most consistently associated with the amines is one consisting of an aliphatic chain of two or more carbon atoms, one end of which bears a hydrocarbon nucleus or the other end an amino group. The hydrocarbon nucleus, in the majority of cases, is aromatic although it may be aliphatic or alicyclic. The nitrogen atom is, in most cases, a tertiary amine. Primary amines and secondary amines are unimportant. Thus, an aliphatic chain, sometimes referred to as a pivot, separates a hydrophilic nitrogen atom from a lipophilic carbon residue (1–3).

Local anesthetics possess varying degrees of water and lipid solubility. Lipid solubility is essential for penetration of the drug into the neuronal fiber, since the latter is rich in lipids. The water solubility is essential for the transport of the drug to the neurons by the lymph. A balance between these two solubilities is necessary for local anesthetic activity. A compound of high lipid solubility usually has a correspondingly low water solubility. If the lipid-water partition coefficient has a low numerical value, a compound is usually ineffective because the quantity transported to the fiber or the concentration that penetrates into the neuromembrane is inadequate. The nerve fiber is a lipid-rich metalloprotein surrounded by an aqueous phase. The hydrocarbon residue becomes oriented into the lipid phase and the amino group into the metalloprotein phase of the fiber surrounding the aqueous medium (1–3).

NON-NITROGENOUS LOCAL ANESTHETICS

Presence of the nitrogen atom on a molecule is not mandatory for local anesthetic activity. Certain hydroxy compounds that do not contain nitrogen are used clinically, for surface anesthesia (2). Aliphatic hydroxy compounds possess feeble local anesthetic activity. Derivatives possessing an aromatic nucleus as part of the structure are more effective than aliphatic compounds. The hydroxy compounds are relatively inefficient compared with the nitrogen-containing derivatives. They were used many years ago but have been supplanted by the more effective nitrogenous derivatives. Within the past several years there has been a revival of interest in their efficacy because they are alleged to be the active ingredients in many over-the-counter preparations. The Food and Drug Administration has various advisory panels that are reviewing the efficacy of this type of ingredient in over-the-counter drugs now on sale in order to determine whether or not the claims made in the labeling can be substantiated.

The hydroxyl group probably plays the counterpart of the amino group in the nitrogen-containing compounds and acts as the hydrophilic pole which orients itself into the aqueous phase of the lipid metalloprotein neuronal membrane. The hydrocarbon is lipophilic and orients itself into the lipid phase. Ionization presumably plays no role in pharmacologic activity. The most serviceable compounds of this type which are used clinically are phenol and benzyl alcohol. Benzyl alcohol provides surface anesthesia on the mucous membranes in concentrations ranging from 3–10%. Salicylalcohol (Saligenin®) and monobromosalicyl alcohol (Bromsalizol®) were once used but are no longer in service. Resorcinol and hexylresorcinol are feeble topical local anesthetics.

The hydroxy compounds are locally irritating and may provoke neurolysis when injected perineurally as well as sloughing of soft tissues. Increasing the number of hydroxyl groups in an alcohol causes a decrease in local anesthetic activity (2). Mephenesin, a propane diol, possesses slight local anesthetic activity. Meprobamate, also a diol, possesses some topical anesthetic activity as does glycerol, a triol. The names of the hydroxy compounds usually end with the suffix "ol" in contradistinction to the nitrogen-containing compounds which are designated by appending the suffix "caine" to a descriptive root (4, 7).

ESTERS AND AMIDES

The hydrocarbon nucleus of the amino compounds is usually derived from a carboxylic acid which is joined to the aliphatic pivot by an ester, amide, or ether linkage. The esters are far more numerous than the amides and were once the most widely used drugs. They have now given way to the amides which appear to be superior. Procaine, cocaine, and tetracaine are the most well-known and widely used esters. The amides in current use are lidocaine (Xylocaine®), mepivacaine (Carbocaine®), prilocaine (Citanest®), bupivacaine (Marcaine®), and dibucaine (Nupercaine®).

The amide linkage joins the hydrocarbon to the dimethylene chain or pivot. In lidocaine, mepivacaine, prilocaine, bupivacaine, and dibucaine, the pivot replaces a hydrogen atom of the amide of the acid portion of the molecule. The nitrogen atom carries a positive charge which orients itself to a negative charge on the receptor site, while the electrophilic carbon atom bearing the aromatic nucleus carries a negative charge which becomes oriented to the positive charge on the receptor (1, 2, 4). Optimal activity is noted when the distance between the carbon and nitrogen atom averages 7–9 Å. Some compounds have the nitrogen atom incorporated in a heterocyclic nucleus. The nitrogen atoms when arranged in this manner manifest the attributes of secondary or tertiary amines. Such an arrangement is found in cocaine, piperocaine, diperodon (Diothane®), and various other derivatives. Quaternization of the amino group of a potent local anesthetic nullifies its anesthetic activity. This is explained by the fact that quaternary bases penetrate cellular membranes with difficulty (1, 2). Tertiary amines traverse cellular membranes far more readily.

Exceptions to generalizations are always found. Some compounds possessing the aforementioned general structure of a hydrocarbon residue pivot and amino group may be devoid of local anesthetic activity (2). Some compounds which would appear from their structure to be active local anesthetics are not, while others which do not conform to the generalization are active. The molecular structure of atropine, for example, meets the general specifications of a local anesthetic but possesses only a slight degree of local anesthetic activity (2). The chemical structures of certain narcotics, as for example, ethylmorphine (Dionin®), which is a phenanthrene derivative, certain phenothiazines, various antihistamines, and some barbiturates do not conform to this generalization but manifest varying degrees of local anesthetic activity.

In most cases the hydrocarbon residue is aromatic and is derived from the acid that forms the ester or amide. Derivatives of aminobenzoic acid and benzoic acid were, for many years, the most numerous in clinical use. The aromatic nucleus is most often a single benzine ring which is either a simple phenyl radical or possesses side chains at various positions on the ring. However, a double benzine ring or napthoic nucleus may appear in certain local anesthetics (1). The hydrocarbon nucleus may also be derived from quinoline, a double cyclic structure resulting from a fusion of an aromatic nucleus and pyridine. Dibucaine is the most serviceable amide of the quinoline group. Introducing an additional amino group into the aromatic ring usually increases the local anesthetic activity. The aminobenzoates exemplify this.

Substitutions on the amino group on the ring of aminobenzoates increase potency and toxicity. Tetracaine, for example, has a butyl radical replacing one hydrogen atom of the amino group on the aromatic nucleus. The compound, thus, is both a secondary and tertiary amine. In addition, the ethyl radicals on the alcohol portion of the molecule are shortened to methyl groups. The potency, lipid-water partition coefficient, protein binding capacity, duration of action, and period of latency is increased manyfold over procaine by this alteration in molecular configuration (1, 3).

The amino-acyl amides, of which lidocaine appears to be the most useful, have been studied extensively. Closely allied to these are mepivacaine, prilocaine, bupivacaine, and etidocaine (15). Increasing the molecular weight and substituting into the amino group of the amides likewise increases toxicity, potency, lipid-water partition coefficients, and degree of protein binding. Bupivacaine compared to lidocaine provides longer lasting anesthesia, is more potent and toxic, and manifests a greater degree of protein binding.

Simple esters of aminobenzoic acid series are relatively insoluble (2). Conversion of these esters to amines increases solubility. The conversion of ethyl p-aminobenzoate (benzocaine) to the diethyl amino derivative (procaine) confers additional basic properties to the compound and increases its water and lipid solubility and potency. Benzocaine is one of the most widely used topical analgesics and anesthetics in medications sold over the counter. It manifests practically no degree of systemic toxicity due to its low degree of water solubility (0.5g/liter of water).

BASIC NATURE OF LOCAL ANESTHETICS

All local anesthetics in current use are synthetic, except cocaine which is naturally occurring. Local anesthetics, by virtue of the amino nitrogen groups, are bases that form salts with acids. Aqueous solutions of the free base are alkaline (2). The basicity varies with the molecular configuration, which, in turn, influences solubility and degree of ionization. The pH range of aqueous solutions of the bases, in most cases, is between 7.5 and 9. Compounds that have two amino nitrogen atoms, as for example procaine, are more alkaline than those with single amino groups. The bases are less soluble in water than the salts. The base, which is the active form, is liberated in the tissues and penetrates the axonal membrane. Soluble hydroxides, carbonates, and bicarbonates cause the free base to be precipitated from aqueous solutions of salts. The degree of precipitation depends upon the alkalinity of the resultant solution. The bases are viscous liquids or amorphous solids that, though sparingly soluble in water, easily dissolve in lipid substances and various organic solvents (2). The base is necessary for the preparation of most ointments in petrolatum or fatty bases or for the preparation of oil solutions. Salts are sparingly soluble or insoluble in lipids or organic solvents (2). Salts may be used for preparing ointments in water-soluble bases.

Local anesthetics are dispensed as salts because the salts are more stable than the bases and more soluble in water. The interaction of the base and acid is similar to the union of ammonia with an acid to form an ammonium salt. Most salts are crystalline, water-soluble substances. The pH range of aqueous solutions of salts varies between 4 and 7, depending on the base and the acid used to form the salt. Hydrochloric acid is the most commonly used acid although other acids used are lactic, formic, mucic, sulfuric, etc. Selection of the acid is from the standpoint of solubility, crystal formation, stability, ease in handling the crystals, pH of the resulting aqueous solution, and so on.

The un-ionized base penetrates into the nerve fiber (10, 15). Once it passes into the axone, where the pH is lower than in the membrane, the ionized cation is released and becomes bound to the receptor site. This has been demonstrated by comparing the effect of pH on sheathed and experimentally desheathed nerve fibers. A more effective blockade is obtained in desheathed nerve fibers when solutions of lower pH in which a greater preponderance of ionized base is present than when solutions of higher pH having a more un-ionized base are used (3). Tissue fluids have considerable buffering capacity and, therefore, cause the base to be liberated when solutions of salts and injected into them. The pH of the solution of salts becomes adjusted to that of the tissues (2). Likewise, if an alkaline solution is injected, the pH becomes adjusted to that of the tissues also. The contention that alkalinization of solutions for injection enhances the local anesthetic effect or duration of action is incorrect (2). Enhanced activity does occur when an alkalinized solution is applied topically, because the mucous membranes do not possess the buffering capacity necessary to release the base. Local anesthetics are generally not effective when injected into inflamed areas. Several explanations are offered for this behavior. Absorption from the injection site is increased and the drug is carried away from the tissues because of the hyperemia resulting from the inflammation. Duration of action is thereby shortened (2). The tissues are less alkaline in this area because of the liberation of acid products by the disease process, and the base, which is the effective form of the salt, is not liberated (2).

LIPID SOLUBILITY AND POLAR ASSOCIATION

Both local and general anesthetics are lipid soluble. It was once assumed that local anesthetics followed the Meyer-Overton rule as a result of their lipid solubility and the relative insolubility in water (7, 10, 15). Determining the distribution coefficients of twenty-two local anesthetics of the amino-acyl amide type in oleyl alcohol-water systems indicated that the Meyer-Overton rule, in the true sense, is not valid for local anesthetics (2). Comparisons were made with procaine. No correlation was found between the distribution coefficient and anesthetic potency. Others have since reported similar findings. The Meyer-Overton rule is applicable to inert substances. Inhaled anesthetics are inert when they act to cause anesthesia; local anesthetics are not (2). Local anesthetics have active groups that act by polar association. Isolated nerves are blocked when exposed to ether, chloroform, and other volatile anesthetics. The concentrations of these agents necessary to produce a blockade when applied locally are greater than those that are necessary in the circulating blood to induce general anesthesia. The blockade produced by local anesthetics results from the biochemical changes caused by the drug in the axonal membrane. In the polar association of local anesthetics, the hydrophilic pole becomes oriented into the aqueous phase and the aromatic hydrocarbon residue into the lipid phase as the membrane proper. The indifferent anesthetics, such as ether and chloroform, probably exert their effects by the electronic attraction of forces explained by Van der Waals' concepts (1, 2).

TRANSMISSION OF THE NERVE IMPULSE

Normally a nerve fiber possesses two attributes—the ability to respond to excitation and the ability to conduct. The plasma membrane delineates the cytoplasm of a nerve fiber from the surrounding extracellular fluid. This membrane is composed of a lipid outer and inner phase and a protein layer in between. It is common knowledge that a stimulus applied to a nerve fiber establishes an electrical current, referred to as an action potential, in the plasma membrane in the area of stimulation (3). This action potential is propagated in succession to contiguous areas along the fiber to its point of termination. When the fiber is in the resting state, the plasma membrane is permeable to certain ions, notably potassium and chloride, and impermeable to others, notably ions of sodium, protein, and amino acids (1, 2, 4). The protein ions are, as are those of potassium and sodium, positively charged, since they are derived from the amino group of the amino acids that compose the protein of the nerve. They are unable to diffuse out of the axone into the interstitial fluid. Potassium ions diffuse readily.

As a result of this selective permeability, a difference in ionic concentration develops on either side of the membrane. In a resting fiber, the concentration of potassium ions on the interior of the membrane is greater than on the exterior; the probable ratio is 30 inside to one outside (3). During inactivity, a difference in electrical potential develops between the exterior and the interior of the membrane as a result of this asymmetric ionic distribution. The polarity on the interior of the membrane is negative with reference to the exterior. During the resting phase of a nerve fiber, sodium ions are constantly forced out of the interior, where the concentration is minimal, by a mechanism referred to as the sodium pump.

Energy is necessary to operate the sodium pump, since ions are being extruded outward against a gradient. This energy is provided by the oxidative metabolism of adenosine triphosphate. The potential difference which develops between the two sides of the membrane ranges between 70 to 90 mV. The initiation and transmission of impulses along a nerve fiber are associated with alterations in this membrane potential. Changes in membrane potential are characterized by removal of the polarity, which in turn causes depolarization of the adjacent normal membrane. Thus, a wave of transient depolarization or activity is present along the nerve fiber. When a stimulus is applied, the permeability of the membrane in the area of excitation is altered and the membrane becomes more permeable to sodium. Sodium ions are then able to migrate inward.

Local anesthetics interrupt the propagation of the impulse and prevent its passage at the site of application on the axone. The blockade of a nerve fiber may be accomplished in a number of ways; (a) by alteration of the resting potential of the membrane, (b) by alteration of the threshold potential or "firing" level, (c) by prolonging the rate of depolarization, or (e) by prolonging the rate of repolarization. Most data reveal that local anesthetics alter neither the resting potential nor the threshold potential. Measurements of rate of depolarization and rate of repolarization reveal that there is a marked delay in rate of depolarization (2–4). Rate of repolarization is affected to a minimal degree. Thus, the blockade is due to a delay in the rate of depolarization. This phenomenon is often believed to result from some mechanism which stabilizes the membrane so that changes in permeability to sodium and potassium ions do not occur.

Considerable controversy has existed over the years concerning the mechanism of action of local anesthetics. At one time acetylcholine was believed to be the transmitter substance which caused the membrane to stabilize and inhibit the enlargement of pores that permitted passage of sodium ion inwards. More recent studies implicate the competition of the local anesthetic with calcium ions at the binding site. Calcium ions are believed to play a role in facilitating the migration of sodium ions across the membrane. Thus, development of the action potential is delayed as a result of the decreased concentration of calcium ions and does not attain the "firing" level for complete depolarization. The amplitude of voltage necessary for conduction is not attained and failure of conduction results (3, 6, 7).

IMPORTANCE OF THE MYELIN SHEATH

The myelin sheath which surrounds certain nerve fibers is enclosed by a histologically distinguishable membrane called the neurolemma. The sheath is interrupted at intervals of 1 mm or less into sausage-like segments known to all as the nodes of Ranvier (1–3). At these points myelin is absent and the sheath dips down and makes contact with the nerve fiber. The myelin acts as an insulator for the nerve fiber and increases the efficiency of conduction by conserving energy. Local anesthetics do not penetrate the myelin sheath and can, therefore, pass into the nerve fibers only at the nodes of Ranvier. Seven or eight nodes must be blocked to obtain a complete blockade of a fiber. Local anesthetics penetrate unmyelinated fibers. Anesthesia is established sooner and with less concentrated solutions in such uninsulated fibers.

INFLUENCE OF FIBER SIZE ON THE BLOCKADE

A difference in susceptibility of various types of fibers has been noted both clinically and experimentally. Autonomic and sensory fibers are affected before motor fibers. It is well known now that this behavior is due to fiber size rather than inherent chemical differences of the protoplasm of the axone. The time required for induction of a blockade by a particular drug varies inversely with the concentration of a drug and directly with the square of the radius of the nerve (1–3). Smaller fibers have a greater surface per unit volume than the larger and, therefore, are blocked first. The small, thinly myelinated or the nonmyelinated autonomic fibers are most easily blocked by local anesthetics. Sensory fibers as a rule vary from 1 to 5 μm in diameter. Such fibers conduct temperature and pain impulses and appear to be more resistant to local anesthetics than autonomic fibers. They are more sensitive, however, to local anesthetics than the larger sensory fibers whose diameters vary from 5 to 15 μm. These larger fibers transmit tactile and pressure sensations and vibratory sense. The large myelinated somatic motor fibers are more resistant than the sensory, which are as a rule smaller. A local anesthetic applied in a concentration sufficient to block all fibers in a mixed nerve produces a blockade in this sequence:

the sympathetic and parasympathetic fibers are inactivated first, next the fibers that transmit temperature. The sensation of cold is obtunded before the sensation of warmth. Next to be blocked are somatic motor fibers carrying pin-prick, pain, touch, pressure sense, vibratory sense, and proprioceptive impulses. The recovery of function appears to occur in the reverse order.

EFFECT ON METABOLISM

Normally, there is an increased oxygen uptake by a nerve during transmission of an impulse. This increased uptake appears to be prevented by local anesthetics. The findings concerning the relationship between the local anesthetic effect and the metabolic rate of a nerve fiber are not consistent (1, 2). Depolarization of a nerve with potassium ions, for instance, blocks conduction but causes an increase in oxygen uptake. Decreased oxygen consumption without impairment of conduction has been observed when nonanesthetic substances are applied to a nerve. Cocaine reduces the oxygen consumption when applied in concentrations that block conduction. Chlorobutanol (Chloretone®), on the other hand, has the opposite effect (1, 2).

PENETRATION INTO THE NERVE

The drug requires time for diffusion into the nerve fiber. Relatively speaking, passage into a membrane is quite rapid because of the high external gradient. The rate of entry varies with the chemical nature of the drug, the concentration, and the type and size of the fiber. Thus, a latent period is noted from the moment the drug is applied until a blockade is fully established. After perineural application, as the drug is carried away by the lymph, the concentration gradually falls. When the perineural concentration falls below the intraneural level, the drug begins to pass from the fiber into the lymph. Conduction is reestablished as soon as the concentration falls below the threshold value often referred to as the Cm or minimum effective concentration. The threshold value differs for each drug under a uniform set of experimental conditions. In other words, the blockade is as complete in fibers exposed to a greater than threshold concentration as it is in those exposed to the minimal effective concentration. The blockade continues until the concentration falls below the threshold level and the membrane is restored to its active state. Exceeding the threshold concentration does not increase the intensity of the block, since it is all or none. It may, however, prolong the block somewhat because more time is required to carry the additional quantity from the perineural area. Increase in duration is not proportional to the increase in total quantity applied. For example, doubling the quantity applied does not double the duration of the blockade (2, 3).

BINDING

The passage of the drug into the fiber and its union with receptors in the axonal membrane are often referred to as "fixing" by clinicians. The term is unscientific and should be discarded because it implies that some irreversible chemical union or binding occurs. This term most likely arose because longer-lasting drugs have a slow onset of action or latent period. The interaction, which occurs at the molecular level between protoplasm and local anesthetics, is not clearly understood. The attachment to receptors is reversible. However, the effects of binding to proteins cannot be excluded (8). It has been proposed that certain agents possess chemical affinity for the nerve tissue components which tends to hold the long-acting drugs within the nerve fiber. Correlation between rate of penetration and anesthetic activity is not uniform. Procaine, lidocaine, and propoxycaine have equal rates of penetration but manifest different activity, potency, and duration when compared on the basis of molar concentration (1, 2). Likewise, there is no strict correlation between speed of penetration and duration of action.

The outward diffusion of a local anesthetic from the fiber occurs gradually, the speed, therefore, depending upon the drug, binding power, diffusibility, electric changes in the pores, and so on. Recovery occurs when the intraneural concentration of a drug falls below the threshold level or Cm. Some drug still remains in the fiber even though conduction has been fully restored. The blockade may be reestablished by adding the difference between the amount present and the threshold concentration. If the reapplication is made several hours after recovery, the original threshold concentration is necessary. This is presumptive evidence that none of the drug is present in the fiber at this time (1, 2).

LATENT PERIOD

It has been mentioned that a latent period of several minutes or more elapses from the moment the drug is applied until a blockade is established. Periods of latency increase progressively as the duration of action of a particular drug increases. Thus, dibucaine has a longer latent period than tetracaine, which in turn has a longer latent period than procaine. Lidocaine has a shorter latent period than procaine yet their duration of actions is similar (1, 2). Data concerning time of onset obtained in vitro using isolated nerve preparations differ from those obtained in vivo. In vivo, a number of variable factors are introduced which explain this discrepancy. Clinically the drug is injected into the tissues surrounding the nerve, while experimentally the drug is applied directly to the fibers. Time, concentration, and dosage are fixed in vitro. In vivo, the drug becomes diluted with the perineural tissue fluid. The greater the distance between the point of injection and the nerve, the greater the dilution (7). Then, in addition, some of the drug is carried away by the blood and lymph and does not reach the nerve; therefore, variable results are to be expected in studies in the intact animal or in man, since all conditions are not fixed. In vivo, the concentration of the injected solution must be greater than the threshold concentration necessary to establish an effective block. When isolated nerve preparations are used, data are more precise and present a more realistic picture in regard to the time-dose relationship. The latent period is quite apparent when inducing spinal block (2). When procaine is used, the blockade is established within 1–2 min. When tetracaine is used, sensory changes are apparent within 2–3 min. Hypalgesia appears first, then diminished ability to perceive light touch, pain, and temperature. Ability to perceive pressure and vibratory sense lingers for 5 min or more. Loss of motor function is, in many cases, complete between 5–10 min after application.

The clinical importance of the latent period cannot be emphasized too strongly. Failure to allow sufficient time for establishment of a block conveys the erroneous impression that the dose employed was inadequate and leads to application of unnecessary subsequent doses and uses of quantities that may be lethal. Disastrous results have occurred after the use of excessive quantities of tetracaine and cocaine topically as a result of this misunderstanding (2).

OVERLAPPING OF ACTIONS

Overlapping of actions among drugs is a common finding in pharmacology. Local anesthetics may possess varying degrees of antihistaminic, anticholinergic, myoneural-blocking, narcotic, and vasopressor activity (2). On the other hand, many antihistamines possess varying degrees of local anesthetic, anticholinergic, and central nervous system depressant activity. The local anesthetic activity of antihistaminic drugs has been demonstrated in animals and utilized to a limited extent in man. Tripelennamine (Pyribenzamine®), for example, has been used for topical anesthesia of the mucous membranes of the pharynx, larynx, trachea, and urethra with some degree of success. Considerable local irritation has been reported by some workers. Its virtue as a local anesthetic is in no way comparable to its value as an antihistamine. Anticholinergic drugs also exhibit some local anesthetic as well as antihistaminic activity. Atropine, for example, possesses a feeble local anesthetic action and some antihistaminic activity. The antihistaminic activity, however, is of a low degree and is of little usefulness clinically. It has been estimated to be in the order of one hundredth that of the common antihistamines, such as diphenhydramine (Benadryl®). Procaine manifests some degree of antihistaminic and anticholinergic activity. The anticholinergic activity is less pronounced than the antihistaminic. Usually, when a drug possesses a multitude of actions, one action predominates over all others. This predominant action determines for what purpose a drug will be used. Local anesthetic activity has been ascribed to epinephrine, ephedrine, meperidine, and a host of other substances. Their potency and clinical usefulness in this regard are limited (2).

RATE OF ABSORPTION

Regardless of the site of application of a local anesthetic, ultimately all of it passes into the bloodstream and establishes a plasma level (1, 2, 9–11). The rate of absorption depends to a large extent upon the blood supply to the tissue. Therefore, the absorption, distribution, and elimination of local anesthetics are quite important. Adriani & Campbell (12) studied plasma levels after infiltration and topical application to mucous and cutaneous surfaces and compared them with those after intravenous injection. Their studies were centered about procaine, tetracaine, cocaine, and benzocaine.

Striking differences were noted between blood drug levels that result from a rapid intravenous injection of a particular dose over a period of 1 min and those after the infusion of the same quantity slowly over a 20-min period. Rapid injection results in a marked upsweep of a curve of drug concentration in the blood and a peak level within 2 min. The same quantity infused slowly gives barely detectable blood levels. The basic contours of the drug level curves are the same with use of procaine, tetracaine, and cocaine. The rapid intravenous injection of 6 mg of tetracaine per kilogram of body weight in dogs produced respiratory paralysis. The slow infusion of the same amount causes no significant response. The slow infusion allows time for dilution and storage in various tissues and perhaps hydrolysis or elimination of a portion of the drug. The susceptible cells, therefore, are not suddenly perfused with the high concentration which confronts them after rapid infusion.

Studies on the tissue distribution of local anesthetics in animals indicate that a rapid uptake by all tissues of the body occurs (1, 2, 13, 14). Differences of relative distribution in various tissues do exist between different agents, however. Lidocaine has a greater affinity for fat than procaine. More lidocaine is found in the liver than procaine. A greater amount of prilocaine is found in the lung of rats than lidocaine. Mepivacaine shows a similar distribution pattern to that of lidocaine. A rapid accumulation occurs in liver, kidney, salivary glands, and brain (3, 13).

Curves of drug levels in the blood after topical application simulate those of rapid intravenous injection. Peaks are lower, take longer time to develop, and do not rise as abruptly. However, within 4–6 min the peak is one third to one half that obtained after rapid intravenous injection when an equivalent dose is applied to the pyriform fossae (12).

Plasma erythrocyte distribution (PE) in man reveals higher PE ratios for lidocaine than prilocaine. Values for mepivacaine and lidocaine are similar. There is evidence that there is a correlation between protein binding capacity of the agents and the PE ratio. Bupivacaine shows the highest PE ratio as well as highest protein binding capacity of the amides studied. The muscle mass takes up the greater portion of a local anesthetic, but this is due to redistribution and the fact that the weight of the muscle mass is greater than that of other tissues and not to an affinity of muscle for local anesthetics (3, 13, 15). Thus, a slow infusion continued indefinitely may ultimately cause the plasma level to rise to deleterious levels, with subsequent appearance of symptoms of systemic toxicity.

CAUSE OF SYSTEMIC REACTIONS

Many reactions that occur after the topical use of local anesthetics are caused by the use of excessive quantities at one time (2, 12). Tetracaine levels in the blood are lower when a given dose of the drug is applied to the pyriform fossae in three fractions at 3-min intervals instead of a single dose at one time. Peak levels are approximately one third those obtained after single application. They rise and fall with each application. The contours of the drug level curves are alike for both cocaine and tetracaine when divided doses are used. The levels, even though lower than those resulting with intravenous administration, are measurable and greater than those obtained after infiltration or slow infusion. Thus, it is obvious that blood levels are a function of the total dose and not the concentration of the solution. Plasma levels are similar when a particular total milligram dose of tetracaine is applied over identical areas as a 2 or 4% solution. The same is found to be the case when cocaine was applied as a 4 and 10% solution. The blood levels after infiltration reach a peak of 5–10 min after completion of the injection. With use of comparable doses, the peak level of tetracaine after topical application to the pyriform fossae was 35 μg, while after infiltration the peak was 2 μg. The peak level when slow infusion is used is 3 μg; with rapid infusion 80 μg (12). Thus, it is apparent that application of a local anesthetic to a mucous membrane causes blood levels that simulate those obtained after rapid intravenous injection. Untoward reactions occur far more frequently after topical use than after injection. The pattern of absorption presented by these data strongly suggests that the high plasma levels after topical use are directly responsible for reactions (19).

The rate of absorption varies with the mucous surface. Absorption is more rapid from the trachea than from the pharynx. Instillation of either cocaine or tetracaine into the trachea results in higher peak levels, a steeper slope, and a more rapid buildup than application to the pharynx. Higher levels and steeper curves are obtained when animals were placed in the upright position than prone (2). The solution obviously gravitates into the alveoli, from which it is more rapidly absorbed. Cocaine solutions nebulized into particles of 3 μg or less diameter pass into the alveoli and are rapidly absorbed when inhaled (12).

The absorption from the epithelium of the respiratory tract seems to differ from that of the mucous membranes elsewhere. No significant blood drug levels are noted after instilling cocaine into the stomach of dogs. Adriani & Campbell (12) likewise obtained no detectable drug levels after instilling tetracaine and cocaine into the stomach or esophagus. The most plausible explanation for this type of behavior is the fact that the acid in the stomach forms the salt of the local anesthetic which is highly ionized and poorly absorbed from the gastric mucosa. Massive doses of local anesthetics given orally have been absorbed and have caused death (14).

No blood drug levels can be demonstrated after instillation of either tetracaine or cocaine into the bladder (3). This is a reasonable finding since few drugs pass through the mucous surface of the bladder. Besides, the contents of the bladder are acid. If alkalinized, some absorption of some drugs occurs. Data obtained after urethral instillation are inconclusive. However, reactions are common after urethral instillation in human beings. How many of these reactions are due to absorption from mucosa traumatized by instruments is difficult to say, since this appears as a frequent complicating factor (2, 12).

ABSORPTION FROM THE SKIN

Salts of local anesthetics are not absorbed from the unbroken skin (16–18). They do pass into the blood if the skin is abraded or damaged in other ways. Blood levels are measurable when aqueous solutions of the salts of tetracaine, cocaine, procaine, and ointments of cocaine, tetracaine, and benzocaine in a water-soluble base are applied to the skin over the abdomen, which has been freshly abraded. Peak concentrations of a magnitude obtained after infiltration resulted in 6–10 min (12). Percutaneous absorption of local anesthetics does not occur when the salts are applied but does occur if the base is used. The epithelial barriers permit the passage of unionized, lipid-soluble substances but not those that are ionized. The degree of absorption is related to the lipid-water distribution coefficient. The concentration required for effectiveness is greater than would ordinarily be required on the mucous membranes (16–18).

RETARDING ABSORPTION BY USE OF VASOCONSTRICTORS

Vasoconstrictors are added to solutions of local anesthetics to retard absorption in order to prolong the blockade, decrease the rate of absorption, and reduce systemic toxicity. Their use in highly vascular areas, as for example the scalp, gums, and face is mandatory. The vasoconstrictor also keeps plasma levels minimal and thereby reduces systemic toxicity (1–3).

A host of vasoconstrictor substances has been suggested for the purpose, the majority of which are aromatic amines closely allied to epinephrine (2). It is surprising that, among all these, epinephrine is the most effective. Ephedrine, phenylephrine, nordefrin (Cobefrin®), and other drugs are comparatively less potent and must be used in far greater concentrations than epinephrine. Even then, they are not as effective. Norepinephrine, although as effective as epinephrine, has caused sloughs and for this reason is not used. Anesthesia in intracutaneous wheals using 0.5% procaine with 1:10,000 epinephrine persists for 2 hr compared with the control. Ephedrine (1:100) in 0.5% procaine produced anesthesia for approximately 20 min. This is slightly better than a control using procaine alone. Vasoconstrictors are less effective subcutaneously than intracutaneously because the blood supply is less abundant in intracutaneous structures. The ischemia is, therefore, more transient. Intrathecally, the duration of anesthesia using procaine or lidocaine is increased 60% or more when epinephrine (1.0 mg) (2) is combined with the spinal anesthetic drug. Blood levels of local anesthetics are difficult to measure after intrathecal instillation for spinal anesthesia since only traces appear (2). The circulating blood level is less after epinephrine is combined with the drug, indicating that vasoconstriction retards its passage from the intrathecal space into the blood. The concentration in cerebrospinal fluid persists for a longer period of time when epinephrine is combined with the drug than it does in the control. Interestingly, the systemic effects of the vasopressor are insignificant. Presumably, the quantity of epinephrine absorbed per unit of time is relatively small and undergoes rapid destruction or elimination.

Blood levels after infiltration or perineural injection are less when epinephrine is combined with the agent than they are in the control. On the mucous membranes, however, the situation is different. Neither epinephrine nor norepinephrine remarkably retards absorption of topical anesthetics when mixed with the agent or when sprayed on the surface prior to application of the anesthetic (19, 20). Blood levels do not differ significantly from the control. Clinicians use far more epinephrine for infiltration than is necessary. Effective vasoconstriction is obtained using a dilution of 1:100,000–1:200,000. Absorption of the vasoconstrictor causes pallor, tachycardia, hypertension, and other systemic disturbances. These are mistaken for a "reaction" but such reactions are not difficult to distinguish from the symptoms of overdosage or intolerance to local anesthetics. However, vasoconstrictors never cause convulsions, coma, or respiratory or cardiac failure.

All local anesthetics with the exception of cocaine cause vasodilatation when injected subcutaneously or perineurally. This comes about by a direct action on smooth muscle and by denervation of the blood vessels that supply the area. Cocaine possesses a sympathomimetic action and causes vasoconstriction. The sympathomimetic effects are due to inhibition of binding of norepinephrine at receptor sites and reuptake by monamine oxidase (1). Butethamine (Monocaine®) was alleged to possess some degree of vasoconstrictor activity but not to the degree necessary for clinical effectiveness. Mepivacaine is alleged to possess some vasoconstrictor activity but clear-cut evidence that this is so is lacking (2).

The behavior of cocaine topically on the mucous membranes is interesting. Otolaryngologists use the drug to "shrink" the mucous membranes. The vasoconstrictor effect apparently does not act to retard absorption and reduce blood levels. Ten and 4% cocaine in quantities containing equivalent weights applied over the same surface areas result in similar blood levels. Many clinicians erroneously believe that a 10% solution causes more intense vasoconstriction and retards the absorption to a greater extent, thereby decreasing toxicity (12, 19).

BIOTRANSFORMATION

The importance of the metabolic fate of local anesthetics is obvious. The more slowly and incompletely a drug is detoxified or eliminated, the greater its systemic toxicity. The metabolism of local anesthetics is related to their chemical configuration. Most of the information on detoxification of local anesthetics is from animal studies. Some data are available from studies on man.

The ester type is hydrolyzed by plasma esterases and to a certain extent by the liver. Unmetabolized portions are eliminated unchanged into the urine by the kidney. Detoxification of the amide type is accomplished almost entirely by the liver. Not all esters are metabolized, however. Cocaine is an ester; yet it is eliminated almost unchanged into the urine. Breakdown of some drugs occurs in the kidney. Prilocaine is partially detoxified by kidney slices in vitro (2, 3).

The ester type of compounds is hydrolyzed to its respective acid and amino alcohol (2, 3). Hydrolysis may also be accelerated by enzymes in the liver, in other tissues, and in plasma. The hydrolysis of procaine, for example, is catalyzed by a group of several enzymes, which was once referred to as procaine esterase, into p-aminobenzoic acid with diethylaminoethanol. Procaine esterase was shown to be identical with the pseudocholinesterases. Serum pseudocholinesterases are not specific for procaine, since they aid in the hydrolysis of acetylcholine, tetracaine, chlorprocaine, methylcholine, succinylcholine, and so on. Physostigmine retards the hydrolysis of procaine in vitro. In the intact animal, however, anticholinesterases appear to exert little or no effect on the rate of hydrolysis of local anesthetics (2). The rate of detoxification of a drug depends upon the metabolic state of the individual who receives the drug. Whether or not variations in activity of the enzyme play a role has not been established with certainty. Plasma pseudocholinesterase levels are decreased in certain disease states. Low levels are found in hepatic dysfunction, in toxic goiters, severe anemias, and diseases caused by inadequate nutrition. Detoxification of local anesthetics may be retarded, and symptoms of systemic toxicity may appear in this type of patient (2, 3).

The p-aminobenzoic acid resulting from the breakdown of procaine may be conjugated in the liver with glycine to aminohippuric acid, methylated to p-ethyl aminobenzoic acid, or eliminated unchanged into the urine. The three reactions may occur simultaneously. The conjugated products are also eliminated into the urine (2, 3). Approximately 25% of the alcohol (diethylaminoethanol) is excreted unchanged into the urine. Presumably, the remainder is metabolized in the body. The hydrolysis of procaine occurs rapidly. In the cat, a fatal intravenous dose is hydrolyzed within 20 min. The toxic dose in man is not known. Human plasma hydrolyzes the ester type of compound twenty to forty times faster than plasma of laboratory animals. Halogenation of procaine increases the facility for hydrolysis. Procaine is hydrolyzed at one third the rate of 2-chloroprocaine. This increased facility for hydrolysis is also seen with 2-bromoprocaine, 3,5-dichloroprocaine, and 2-chlorthiocaine. Rapid hydrolysis confers upon a drug the clinical advantage of low systemic toxicity. The majority of benzoic and aminobenzoic acid esters are hydrolyzed partially or completely in the body. Tetracaine is hydrolyzed at one fifth the rate of procaine (2, 3).

The amides are detoxified by amidases and oxidases. Lidocaine is very stable and resists hydrolysis in vitro. In vivo, however, it undergoes rapid metabolic change. The first step appears to be oxidative deethylation to monoethylglycinexylidide and acetaldehyde (22, 26). This is hydrolyzed to xylidine and monoethyl glycine. Less than 10% appears in the urine unchanged. Mepivacaine appears to undergo N-demethylation and some hydroxylation (3, 13). Prilocaine appears to be converted to o-toluidine and L-N-n-propylamine. This occurs in the liver, although the kidney plays a role. Bupivacaine is N-dealkylated to form pipecoloxylidide (11, 22, 26). The metabolites of lidocaine appear to have some convulsive activity and may cause systemic reactions should cumulative effects occur (22, 26). The metabolites of prilocaine, particularly the o-toluidine causes methemoglobinemia (3). Undetoxified portions of local anesthetics are excreted into the urine as are most of the metabolites.

Wide species differences are often noted. In dogs and in man, for example, cocaine is excreted unchanged into the urine, while rabbits detoxify the drug completely by hydrolysis to ecgonine and benzoic acid (2).

DESTRUCTION IN SITU

Little is known about the destruction of the drugs in the nerve and perineural tissues. The general behavior of the drug in the nerve fiber strongly suggests that little or no destruction occurs. Chloroprocaine, for example, is more potent than procaine in regard to its local blocking effect but is hydrolyzed in one third the time in the plasma; yet the block it produces lasts more than 1 hr. The hydrolysis in plasma is complete within 5 min (11).

Drugs that are destroyed or eliminated slowly are, as a rule, more toxic systemically than those that are easily eliminated or detoxified (2, 3). Practically speaking, the safety of most local anesthetics depends upon the balance between the absorption of the drug into the bloodstream and its removal from the blood by destruction, storage, or excretion, into the urine (2).

TOXICITY

Although potency and duration of action are important characteristics, the worthiness of a local anesthetic drug is decided by its toxicity. Toxicity may be either local to the tissues or systemic. Irrespective of the manner by which a drug is administered, whether it be topically, perineurally, or intrathecally, it ultimately passes into the vascular system and then is eliminated. The attainment of a certain blood level, the value of which varies with the drug and the susceptibility of the individual, causes a train of symptoms referred to as a reaction. The type of symptoms that develop, their severity, and their duration depend upon the blood level, the rapidity by which it is attained, and the amount of drug that perfuses the susceptible organs. The organ systems that manifest the most obvious susceptibility are the central nervous system and the cardiovascular system (2, 3, 21, 25).

The more toxic the drug the lower the blood level necessary to precipitate an untoward response. It has been emphasized that blood level depends largely upon the rate of absorption of a drug from the injection site and the rate of clearance from the bloodstream. These two factors are of utmost importance in establishing precautionary measures and in selecting proper drugs for clinical use. The maintenance of a low plasma level depends upon the ease with which destruction of the drug occurs, the rate of clearance by the kidney or detoxification by the liver, and the capability of storage in the tissues (2, 23). After infiltration or nerve-blocking techniques, minute amounts of a local anesthetic drug may be detected in the blood for some time after the injection is completed. A perceptible degree of systemic general analgesia may be detected (2).

Potency and toxicity of local anesthetic drugs do not necessarily parallel each other. A drug may, for example, be ten times more potent than the standard of comparison and fifteen times more toxic on a weight-for-weight basis. On the other hand, the drug could be ten times more potent but only half as toxic. Such a drug, if one could be found, would have a definite clinical advantage over the standard. The potency and toxicity of a drug under study are compared with a standard. Procaine is now used as the standard of comparison for anesthetics intended for infiltration, perineural, and other types of blocking. The effectiveness of drugs intended for surface anesthesia is compared with cocaine, since procaine possesses a feeble topical effect. The principal factors in determining the toxicity of local anesthetic drugs are (a) the rate of inactivation, (b) the rate of diffusion into the tissues, (c) the rate of absorption from the site of injection, (d) the inherent toxicity of the drug, and (e) the susceptibility of the individual to the drug (1, 3).

METHODS OF TESTING

It is virtually impossible to correlate the vast accumulation of data from various laboratories concerning potency and toxicity because of the diversity of the experimental methods employed to obtain the data. Standardized, uniform methods of testing are still nonexistent. Each investigator has his own method or routine for evaluating a new drug. Some authors emphasize the minimal effective concentrations when investigating a drug; others determine the duration of action; others the period of latency. The anesthetic index is used by some in evaluation of a new drug in the laboratory. The anesthetic index takes into consideration toxicity and potency in relationship to a standard of comparison. The index for a particular drug is meaningless unless the method employed and conditions used to determine the index, such as species of animals, status of the animal, environmental room temperature, concentration time, and so on, are stated. Comparisons of indices are valid only when data concerning each drug are obtained under identical experimental conditions. Expressions of potency and anesthetic indices disregard duration of action and period of latency, both of which are important considerations. The more potent drugs not only are longer lasting but also are characterized by slower onset and slower recovery.

The inherent toxicity of a drug is determined by the rapid intravenous administration into several species of animals. The rate of inactivation and diffusion from the site of injection have little influence on the results and, therefore, do not enter to any degree into intravenous studies. Comparisons must be made under identical circumstances to be valid. The rate of injection, concentration of the solution, age, size, and state of nutrition of the animal, body temperature, environmental temperature, temperature of the solution, and so on, must be identical (1–3). Data on toxicity obtained from intravenous administration studies differ from those obtained from subcutaneous or intraperitoneal injection because the rate of absorption and diffusion then enters into the picture. Subcutaneous and intraperitoneal injections are used to study the influence of diffusion and the rate of inactivation. Cumulative effects are studied by observing the responses after intermittent, subcutaneous, or intravenous injection. Delayed and chronic toxicity are studied by repeatedly injecting the drug into animals over a period of weeks or even months. Obviously, information on toxicity of a new local anesthetic can be obtained only from studies in the laboratory of several species of animals. Then cautious clinical use must be resorted to before the drug can be released. Confirmation of the safety and usefulness is obtained only after extensive clinical experience. It is not uncommon for a drug that appears to be ideal in the laboratory to be disappointingly unsuitable clinically.

Clinicians continually seek tables of limits of dosage. It is virtually impossible to provide such information, since so many variable factors are involved in clinical usage of a drug. Qualitatively, species responses are quite similar; quantitatively, they may be quite different. Then, too, variations occur within a species. One variable that cannot be assessed in the clinical use of a local anesthetic is the degree to which tolerance is altered by the pathophysiologic effects of the patient's disease.

PRECAUTIONARY MEASURES

Ordinarily, during various forms of regional anesthesia, blood levels are less than the toxic level for a particular drug and no systemic manifestations develop. Precautionary measures followed to avoid systemic intoxication are (a) limitation of the total quantity of the drug used, (b) use of the minimum quantity of the most dilute effective solution, (c) retardation of absorption by adding vasoconstrictors, and (d) avoidance of inadvertent intravenous injection. When the plasma concentration exceeds the tolerable level, symptoms of overdosage appear. These appear to be directed to either the nervous system or the vascular system (24). Both may be involved simultaneously. Other organ systems may be involved, but the symptoms in these two systems mask effects in other organs. Clinicians refer to reactions as the *vascular type* or the *central nervous system type*. If the drug is one of great potency or if the overdosage is massive, however, both systems may be involved simultaneously. As a rule, when systemic intoxication occurs clinically, the central nervous system is involved more frequently than the vascular system. Central excitation develops when the blood level rises abruptly, as might occur after an inadvertent intravenous administration. The more gradual buildup to the intolerable level usually involves absorption of greater quantities of drug and is characterized by the vascular type of response.

Literature Cited

1. deJong, R. H. 1970. *Physiology and Pharmacology of Local Anesthesia.* Springfield, Ill.: Thomas
2. Adriani, J. 1960. The clinical pharmacology of local anesthetics. *Clin. Pharmacol. Ther.* 1:645–37
3. Corvino, B. G. 1973. Local anesthesia. *N. Engl. J. Med.* 286(18):975–83, 1035–42
4. Corvino, B. G. 1971. Comparative clinical pharmacology of local anesthetic agents. *Anesthesiology* 35:158–167
5. Ritchie, J. M., Ritchie, B., Greengard, P. 1965. The active structure of local anesthetics. *J. Pharmacol. Exp. Ther.* 150:152–59
6. Aceves, J., Machne, X. 1963. The action of calcium and of local anesthetics on nerve cells and their interaction during excitation. *J. Pharmacol. Exp. Ther.* 140:138–48
7. Blaustein, N. P., Goldman, D. E. 1966. Comparative action of calcium and procaine on lobster axone: A study of the mechanism of certain local anesthetics. *J. Gen. Physiol.* 49:1043–63
8. Reynolds, F., Taylor, G. 1970. Maternal and neonatal blood concentrations of bupivacaine: A comparison with lignocaine during continuous extradural analgesia. *Anaethesia* 25:14–23
9. Mazze, R. I., Dunbar, R. W. 1966. Plasma lidocaine concentrations after caudal, lumbar epidural, axillary block, and intravenous regional anesthesia. *Anesthesiology* 27:574–79
10. Moore, D. C., Bridenbaugh, L. D. 1970. Bupivacaine: A review of 2077 cases. *J. Am. Med. Assoc.* 214:713–18
11. Foldes, F. F., Davidson, G. M., Duncalf, D. 1965. The intravenous toxicity of local anesthetic agents in man. *Clin. Pharmacol. Ther.* 6:328–35
12. Adriani, J., Campbell, D. 1956. Fatalities following topical application of local anesthetics to mucous membranes. *J. Am. Med. Assoc.* 162:1527–38
13. Katz, J. 1968. The distribution of C-labelled lidocaine injected intravenously in the rat. *Anesthesiology* 29:249–53
14. Boyes, R. N., Adams, H. J., Duce, B. R. 1970. Oral absorption and disposition kinetic of lidocaine hydrochloride in dogs. *J. Pharmacol. Exp. Ther.* 174:1–8
15. Reynolds, F. 1971. Metabolism and excretion of bupivacaine in man: a comparison with mepivacaine. *Br. J. Anaesth.* 43:33–37
16. Dalili, H., Adriani, J. 1971. Efficacy of local anesthetics in blocking the sensations of itch and pain in normal and

sunburned skin. *Clin. Pharmacol. Ther.* 12:913–19

17. Adriani, J., Dalili, H. 1971. Penetration of local anesthetics through epithelial barriers. *Anesth. Analg. Cleveland* 50: 834–41

18. Monash, S. 1957. Topical anesthesia of the unbroken skin. *Arch. Dermatol.* 76:752–56

19. Adriani, J., Zepernick, R., Arens, J. 1964. The comparative potency and effectiveness of topical anesthetics in man. *Clin. Pharmacol. Ther.* 5:49–62

20. Adriani, J., Zepernick, R. 1964. Clinical effectiveness of drugs used for topical anesthesia. *J. Am. Med. Assoc.* 188: 711–16

21. Strong, J. M., Mayfield, D. E., Atkinson, A. J., Burris, B. C., Raymon, F., Webster, L. T. 1975. Pharmacological activity, metabolism and pharmacokinetics of glycinexylidide. *Clin. Pharmacol. Ther.* 17:184–95

22. Collinsworth, K. A., Strong, J. M., Atkinson, A. J., Winkle, R. A. 1975. Pharmacokinetics and metabolism of lidocaine in patients with renal failure. *Clin. Pharmacol. Ther.* 18:59–64

23. Bonica, J. J., Akamatsu, T. J., Berges, P. U. 1971. Circulatory effects of peridural block: Effects of epinephrine. *Anesthesiology* 34:514–22

24. Bigger, J. T., Mandel, W. J. 1970. Effect of lidocaine on the electrophysiological properties of ventricular muscle and Purkinje fibers. *J. Clin. Invest.* 49:63–77

25. Engel, T. R., Soly, K., Meister, S. G., Frankl, W. S. 1976. Effect of lidocaine on right ventricular muscle refractoriness. *Clin. Pharmacol. Ther.* 19:515–22

26. Halkin, H., Meffin, P., Melmon, K., Rowland, M. 1975. Influence of congestive heart failure on blood levels of lidocaine and its active monodeethylated metabolite. *Clin. Pharmacol. Exp.* 17: 669–76

Ann. Rev. Pharmacol. Toxicol. 1977 17:243–58

AQUATIC INVERTEBRATES: ❖6678
MODEL SYSTEMS FOR STUDY
OF RECEPTOR ACTIVATION
AND EVOLUTION OF
RECEPTOR PROTEINS

Howard M. Lenhoff and Wyrta Heagy

Department of Developmental and Cell Biology and Department of Molecular Biology and Biochemistry, University of California, Irvine, California 92717

INTRODUCTION

A major objective of research in pharmacology, hormone and neurotransmitter action, olfaction, and chemoreception in general, is to understand how specific cellular receptors are activated. Such a concern is evidenced by the large amount of work being carried out on receptors today (see 1–21). Much of the research on receptors deals with molecules of obvious medical importance, such as insulin (1–3), other peptide hormones (2–6), acetylcholine (7–11), other neurotransmitters (12, 13), and opiates (14, 15). The experimental systems used in most of these investigations are as complex as the organisms, usually vertebrates, housing those receptors.

Yet it may be possible to find and use simpler and experimentally more amenable systems if we focus on the primary event common to all receptor systems: the combination of the activator with the receptor. It seems strange, then, that in the study of such a fundamental cellular process as receptor activation, there have not been many systematic searches for organisms free of the complexity of vertebrates. Some recent notable exceptions are the studies on bacterial chemotaxis of Adler (16) and Koshland (17–19). We suggest that lower aquatic organisms might serve as possible fruitful sources of material for research on receptor activation because the chemical senses, relative to other senses, are highly developed in these organisms.

The objective of this review, therefore, is threefold: (*a*) to survey the large spectrum of biological phenomena initiated by activator molecules in lower aquatic organisms that may prove useful in receptor research; (*b*) to present a summary of results obtained with one such system, the glutathione receptor of hydra, that has

243

been used to investigate the activation of cellular receptors; and (c) to present a view which grew out of studies with a large number of lower animals, and which may provide insight into the evolutionary development of receptor proteins.

CHEMICAL ACTIVATION IN LOWER ORGANISMS

Since the turn of the century biologists have been intrigued by aquatic invertebrate behavior in response to chemicals emanating from food, predators, and other environmental sources (22). Within the aquatic environment, chemical cues are often the major stimulus for initiating biological processes.

This interest has led to numerous investigations in which the phenomena activated by chemicals have been defined, and in recent years, the activating substances have been purified, characterized, and, in some cases, identified and synthesized (see 23, 24). Types of activator molecules implicated in stimulating responses include cations, anions, amino acids, polypeptides, proteins, sugars, glycoproteins, lipoproteins, simple alcohols, and steroids (see 23, 25–27).

The phenomena activated by these molecules are diverse (see 23, 25–27). Listed in Table 1 are the classification of the types of activators, the phenomena controlled by the chemicals, and references to major reviews covering these topics in depth. This table does not attempt to be exhaustive but rather it highlights the major types of events activated by chemicals within the aquatic environment. It should be noted that we have not made a distinction between interspecific communication (i.e. between different species as in item V.B. of Table 1) and intraspecific communication (i.e. between members of the same species as in item V.A. of Table 1). Pheromones fit this latter classification.

The common features of interest to the pharmacologist and cellular biologist in all of the examples listed in Table 1 are the binding of a specific activator by cellular receptors and the activation of those receptors to initiate specific coordinated responses. It would seem likely, therefore, that among the wide spectrum of aquatic organisms in which chemical activation of receptors occurs, there exist some in which the receptors are of such a simple and accessible nature that it is possible to investigate this basic phenomenon. We find that the freshwater hydra and related marine cnidarians offer a number of experimental advantages for study of the activation of cellular receptors.

MECHANISM OF ACTION OF THE GLUTATHIONE RECEPTOR OF HYDRA

Research on feeding chemoreceptors in the Cnidaria has reached a high level of sophistication. Not only have specific activators (incitants) been identified in a large number of species, but also it is possible to make reasonable speculations about the evolution of receptors in general, and, with hydra, to study the mechanism by which the receptor is activated.

In this section we focus primarily on the mechanisms by which the tripeptide reduced glutathione (GSH), activates the GSH receptor of hydra to coordinate the

Table 1 Classification of external chemical activators and their functions in aquatic invertebrates

Classification of activator	Function of activator	References
I. Feeding		27–31
A. Attractant	Stimulates orientation toward food	
B. Arrestant	Arrests locomotion toward food	
C. Incitant	Initiates feeding	
D. Suppressant	Inhibits onset of feeding	
E. Stimulant	Promotes ingestion and continuation of feeding	
F. Deterrent	Prevents or interrupts feeding	
II. Symbiosis[a]		32–36
A. Attractant	Orients host-seeking organism toward potential host	
B. Stimulant	Induces and maintains the association after initial contact	
C. Repellent	Repels host-seeking organism	
III. Habitat-niche selection		23, 37, 38
A. Homing attractant	Orients toward habitat by allowing recognition of previous home or territory	
B. Aggregation and schooling attractant	Initiates forming of clusters of organisms belonging to same species	
C. Larval settlement inducer	Initiates settlement of larvae on appropriate substrate	
IV. Development		23, 38
A. Metamorphosis inducer	Initiates change from larval to subsequent developmental stage	
B. Growth inhibitor	Suppresses growth of members of the same species	
V. Avoidance responses		23, 25, 39–41
A. Alarm activator	Initiates response to signal emitted from members of same species	
B. Escape activator	Initiates movement away from predators or in response to environmental factors (pH, salinity)	
C. Defense activator	Initiates specific defense mechanisms	
VI. Reproduction		23, 24
A. Mate attractant	Orients toward opposite sex	
B. Reproductive incitant	Initiates characteristic mating behavior	
C. Spawning inducer	Induces and/or synchronizes release of gametes	
D. Gamete attractant	Orients sperm toward egg	

[a] Includes interactions between different species, such as commensalism, mutualism, and parasitism (see 42).

animal's movements involved in feeding. This system offers a number of experimental advantages for receptor research. For one, the molecule GSH itself is complex enough, though not too large, to allow us to make a sufficient number of analogues for determining the conformation(s) of GSH necessary to activate the receptor.

A second advantage derives from the very nature of hydra itself: (a) it is of simple tissue-level structure (see below), (b) the receptor is on the surface of the outer epithelium, (c) the biological response can be readily quantified, (d) pure clones of the animals can be easily grown in the laboratory in kilogram quantities (wet weight), and (e) the fluid environment ("medium") surrounding the receptor can be accurately controlled within a pH range of about 4 to 8 (see 27).

The animal is shaped like a two-ply hollow tube, about 8 mm by 1 mm when extended, made up of both outer (ectodermal) and inner (endodermal) epithelial layers. At the posterior end of the tube is a basal disc with which the hydra usually attaches to a surface, and at the anterior end is a mouth surrounded by a ring of tentacles. The tentacles are armed with many nematocytes, one of the seven cell types of hydra. The nematocytes contain nematocysts ("stinging capsules") which start the feeding process by piercing the prey with long spear-like tubules.

In nature, the feeding behavior is initiated by trace amounts of GSH which are emitted from wounds in the prey caused by the penetrating nematocyst tubule. The key feature of the behavior is that GSH stimulates the tentacles to writhe and the mouth to open. It is the duration of this mouth opening that can be quantified and used as an accurate and reliable bioassay of GSH activity and the activity of its analogues, and of other factors affecting the feeding behavior.

Evidence for a GSH Surface Receptor

Earlier experiments by Loomis (43) showed that GSH was the substance leaking from the wounded prey that activated feeding in *Hydra littoralis.* To eliminate the possibility of the activity being caused by a contaminant in the GSH preparation, he showed that chemically synthesized GSH was also active (43). Later work by Lenhoff (44), investigating the competitive action of GSH analogues, confirmed that it was the GSH in the prey's fluids that activated the response. Other early experiments (45) showed that the duration of the response was dependent upon the concentration of GSH applied to the hydra and that the response would take place only when GSH remained in the solution. Furthermore, the GSH was neither consumed nor metabolized. These experiments suggested that on the surface of the hydra's outer epithelium, there were receptor sites that would become activated only in the presence of GSH.

A saturable receptor was indicated by analysis of plots of the duration of the feeding response against the concentration of GSH to which the hydra was exposed (45). An analysis of the resultant curve with concepts borrowed from enzymology suggests that there is a receptor which is saturated and gives a maximum response at GSH concentrations of 5×10^{-6} M and greater. A maximum response is considered analogous to the maximum velocity of an enzyme catalyzed reaction; both occur during saturation of an active site.

Determination of the Dissociation Constant

The assumptions made in determining the dissociation constant, K_A, between the activator (A) and the receptor (R) have been reported elsewhere (46, 47). The effect of the activation is signified by ϵ and the maximum effect, by ϵ_M. The equation derived

$$(A)/\epsilon = 1/\epsilon_M \, (A) + K_A/\epsilon_M \qquad\qquad 1.$$

is analogous to the second form of the Lineweaver-Burk (48) plot, the equation developed by Beidler (49) for mammalian taste chemoreception, and, of course, a form of the Langmuir adsorption isotherm. This equation is useful in analyzing chemoreception phenomena because it minimizes deviations in individual animal responses that occur at very low levels of activator.

Previous data (50) show that this equation can be used to interpret the plot of $(A)/\epsilon$ against (A); we obtain straight lines at most glutathione concentrations. From such plots we can determine, for example, at pH 7, a dissociation constant of 10^{-6} M. Such a low K_A is meaningful from at least three viewpoints: (a) the smallness of the constant indicates a high affinity of the receptor for glutathione; (b) concentrations around 10^{-6} M are well within the physiological range to be expected under natural conditions of feeding; (c) this constant provides a means of characterizing the receptor—that is, the glutathione receptor of *H. littoralis* may be said to have a dissociation constant of 10^{-6} M under the given conditions. The constant is a characteristic of the receptor and remains nearly the same no matter what the nutritional state of the hydra (44, 45). Similarly, experiments in which the buffer anion is varied alter the maximum response, but not the dissociation constant (50).

In Vivo Determination of pH Profile of Receptor

Changes in the K_A with pH can be used to determine the pK's of the ionizable groups on glutathione or at the receptor site which are involved in the combination with glutathione. The pK measurements were made by means analogous to those used by enzymologists in determining the pK's of ionizable groups at the active site of enzymes. For our purposes, we needed an equilibrium equation, like Dixon's (51) for enzymes, which would take into account the influence of pH on the dissociation constant. This modified equation (46, 47, 50) involved the assumption that if the activator, receptor site, or activator-receptor complex ionizes, then, in the expression for equilibrium, each component (A, R, AR) equals its concentration multiplied by a term which is a function of pH. For example, if the activator ionized, then the total concentration of free activator, A_t, would be A times the pH function of A, or f_a (pH). The logarithimic form of the equation is:

$$pK_A = pK_A^0 + \log f_{ar} \, (pH) - \log f_r \, (pH) - \log f_a \, (pH). \qquad 2.$$

Here pK_A refers to the negative logarithm of the dissociation constant of AR, while pK_A^0 is the same constant if none of the components has ionic groups; if no component ionizes, then pK_A and pK_A^0 are equal. The derivation of this equation is explained elsewhere (47).

The foregoing equation indicates that a plot of pK_A against pH will consist of a series of straight lines joined by short curved parts, and holds true for the glutathione-hydra system. The results (50) followed almost exactly the predictions from the modified Dixon equations. The following interpretations were made (50): 1. Ionizable groups at the receptor site participated in binding glutathione, because significant variations in pK_A occurred with change in pH. 2. The concave downward inflections at pH's 4.6, 4.8, 6.5, and 7.6 represented pK's of ionizable groups at the receptor site. These pK's probably do not represent ionizable groups of glutathione, which have pK's either below pH 4 (2.1 and 3.5) or above pH 8 (8.7 and 9.6) (52). If the receptor site is protein, then the pK's determined may represent two β-carboxyls of peptide aspartic acid (or γ-carboxyls of peptide glutamic acid), an imidazole group, and a terminal α-amino group, respectively. 3. The horizontal lines indicate pH values that do not affect the combination of glutathione with the receptor site. 4. The quenching of the charges (53) at about pH 4 and 8 indicated that receptor-site groups having pK's of 4.6 and 7.6 may be associated with complementary charged groups of glutathione.

Active Structure of Glutathione

To determine the structure of GSH present at the receptor site, it was necessary to quantify the ability of different structural analogues of GSH either to activate or inhibit a response (54, 55). The aforementioned bioassay experiments were used to determine the effectiveness (K_A and ϵ_M) of synthetic agonists (44, 54, 55). The relative ability of analogues that bind but do not activate, i.e. antagonists, was determined by measuring their ability to inhibit competitively the activity of GSH in eliciting the feeding response (55).

Data from these investigations established that (a) the thiol is not required for activation, because ophthalmic acid (γ-glu-abu-gly), norophthalmic acid (γ-glu-ala-gly), and S-methyl glutathione (S-me-GSH) also activated the response (54, 55); (b) activation of the response requires the intact tripeptide backbone of glutathione, because the just mentioned analogues activated feeding while amino acids, dipeptides, and a number of tripeptide analogues with large and charged substituents at the sulfhydryl group did not activate (44, 55); (c) the receptor has a high affinity for the glutamyl part of the tripeptide because glutamic acid and glutamine were the only amino acids to show competitive inhibition (55) and the tripeptide asparthione (β-asp-cys-gly) did not initiate the response (43, 55); and (d) the α-amino of glutathione is probably required for association of glutathione with the receptor, because glutamic but not α-keto glutaric acid competitively inhibited GSH action (44, 55).

Current research on the specificity of the glutathione receptor of *H. attenuata* agrees with data found using *H. littoralis*. New information was uncovered using tripeptide analogues with substitution of the glycyl residue. For example, when either leucine or tyrosine are substituted for glycine, the resultant tripeptide still activated a response (56).

Currently over 70 analogues are being quantified as to their ability to act as either agonists or antagonists. Both the published and unpublished results indicate that the

GSH receptor of hydra has a unique and rigid specificity for the tripeptide structure of GSH.

Other Factors Influencing the Response

The feeding response of hydra is also influenced by a number of external factors, such as the ionic composition of the medium (46) and certain proteases (57). Environmental cations, for example, affect the response activated by GSH in many ways. Without calcium ions, hydra do not respond to reduced glutathione (58). The requirement for calcium is pH-dependent (H. M. Lenhoff, unpublished), and a concentration of about 10^{-4} M was necessary for a maximum response. Strontium was the only ion that could substitute for calcium, and even it was much less effective (58). The chelating agent ethylenediaminetetraacetic acid (EDTA) also inhibited feeding. This inhibition was completely reversed only by calcium ions, and to some degree by strontium ions (58). Magnesium ions were not required; in high concentrations they inhibited the responses by competing with calcium ions (44, 58). Sodium likewise competed with calcium, but less effectively than magnesium (58).

Potassium ions were found to inhibit the feeding response (46), but, unlike magnesium and sodium ions, they did not act by competing with calcium ions. Concentrations of potassium ions as low as 10^{-4} M could lower the response to glutathione significantly, and this inhibition could be reversed by placing the animals in a potassium-free medium for a few hours (H. M. Lenhoff, unpublished). Since potassium ions play an important role in bioelectric potential, it may be that these ions act by affecting the cellular membrane potential of hydra. More recent work using *H. attenuata* shows that the presence of sodium ions in the environment is an absolute requirement for the glutathione-mediated feeding response (59).

Temperature effects on the feeding response are complex (44), but they do indicate that there is a rate-limiting thermochemical step in the effector system that has an activation energy of about 13,000–14,000 calories (H. M. Lenhoff, unpublished). This step is thought to involve the consumption of some regenerable substance, such as ATP.

A number of nontripeptides can activate a feeding response in some coelenterates in the absence of added GSH (57, 60–62). Of special interest are the proteolytic enzymes papain, ficin, and trypsin (57) because it is now recognized that numerous control mechanisms can be activated by proteases (see 63).

Cyclic Nucleotides

As with higher organisms, cyclic nucleotides are thought to play in lower forms a similar function as second messengers. The first report that cyclic AMP functions in such a fashion in cnidarians is that of Gentleman & Mansour (64) in the sea anemone *Anthopleura elegantissima*. They showed that on the addition of GSH the concentration of cAMP in the oral disc and pharynx tissues increased. Preliminary work with hydra shows that on the addition of GSH there are rapid changes in the levels of both cAMP and cGMP (65).

Summary

In summary, the GSH receptor system of hydra has much in common with the receptor systems of higher organisms now under study. The hydra receptor shows a precise specificity for the activator, the combination of the activator with receptor follows "saturation kinetics," and the cyclic nucleotides appear to be involved as secondary messengers.

The hydra GSH receptor system has a number of advantages that are inherent in the nature of the GSH molecule and in the hydra itself (see above). But perhaps the most unique advantage of this system is that it is possible to investigate in vivo properties of the receptor both while it is carrying out a behavioral response (50) and while measurements are being made on the binding of either activators or competitive inhibitors to the whole animal (65).

ON THE EVOLUTIONARY DEVELOPMENT
OF RECEPTOR PROTEINS

The following view on the evolutionary development of receptor proteins is derived from our analysis of research carried out mostly on feeding activators in lower forms. We propose that the most primitive of cnidarian receptors responded to a range of amino acids and peptides, and that from these general receptors, more specific ones evolved. Furthermore, we propose that receptors in higher forms, such as those involved in chemoreception and in neurotransmitter and hormone action, evolved from similar primitive general receptors which originally functioned in pinocytosis and phagocytosis.

Inspection of Table 2 shows a number of patterns within the Cnidaria which support our hypotheses. The data show that cnidarians tested from every class and most families elicit a feeding response to either one or a few small molecules. The molecules found most commonly to initiate a feeding response are the tripeptide GSH and the imino acid proline. In the Hydrozoa the feeding response of each organism investigated was induced by a single specific molecule (41, 65, 66). Proline is especially prevalent as an activator among the athecate colonial marine hydroids (61, 67–70). For example, all members of these groups thus far tested, i.e. *Cordylophora* (61), *Pennaria* (67), *Tubularia* (69), and *Proboscidactyla* (68), responded only to proline. All hydras tested responded only to GSH (41, 65, 66). The only other hydrozoans tested also responded to GSH (70, 71).

In the Anthozoa we see three trends. In general, although more than one compound may elicit feeding behaviors, the animals exhibit varying ranges of specificity. For example, the most specificity is seen among the sea anemones: *Boloceroides* responds primarily to valine (72), *Anthopleura* to GSH (73), *Haliplanella* to leucine (74), *Actinia* to glutamic acid (75), and *Calliactis* to GSH (76). The specificity broadens when we consider the colonial anemones: whereas *Zoanthus* responds primarily to GSH (77), *Palythoa* responds to relatively high concentrations of either GSH or proline, or to low amounts of these two activators acting synergistically

Table 2 Chemical activation of feeding in the Cnidaria

Type of organism	Activator	References
I. Hydrozoans		
A. Hydroids		
1. Five species of hydra	GSH	43, 65, 66; H. M. Lenhoff, unpublished; W. Heagy, unpublished
2. Four species of colonial marine hydroids (without theca)	Proline	61, 67–69
3. One species of colonial marine hydroid (with theca)	GSH	70
B. Siphonophores		
Two species (including Portuguese man-of-war)	GSH	70, 71
II. Anthozoans		
A. Sea anemones		
1. *Anthopleura*	GSH	73
2. *Boloceroides*	Valine	72
3. *Actinia*	Glutamate	75
4. *Haliplanella*	Leucine	74
5. *Calliactis*	GSH, proline	76
B. Colonial anemones		
1. *Palythoa*	Proline and/or GSH	78
2. *Zoanthus*	GSH	71
C. Corals		
1. Six species	Proline or GSH	66, 79
2. One species	4 amino acids	80
III. Scyphozoa		
One species (large jellyfish)	20 amino acids, GSH, glycylglycine	81

(78). Lastly, corals seem to respond best to proline alone or GSH alone, as well as to numerous other amino acids at relatively higher concentrations (66, 79, 80).

Chrysaora, the only example of the large jellyfishes tested, seems to respond to GSH and to a wide number of amino acids (81). More kinds of these organisms need to be tested before we can make any generalizations about this group.

Do the Glutathione and Proline Receptors Have a Common Origin?

Fulton (61) has suggested that the evolution of a receptor site for glutathione into one for the α-imino acid proline may have proceeded by means of slight structural changes in the receptor site. His postulate was based on the knowledge that one of the possible cyclized forms of glutathione in solution is close in structure to an α-imino acid. Because proline is also present in the fluids released from wounded prey organisms, the change in structure of the receptor site was not disadvantageous to *Cordylophora* but, under some circumstances, advantageous, and so persisted.

In support of Fulton's suggestion (61) are a number of cases reported in Table 2. For example, let us assume that the earliest cnidarians responded to a wider range of amino acids and to GSH, as has been reported for *Chrysaora* (81). Possibly from these early cnidarians there evolved one whose receptor was modified so that it would recognize both GSH and proline. Such a receptor might exist in *Palythoa* (78), although it is also possible that *Palythoa* has two distinct receptors, one for each of those activators. Possibly organisms with this proposed "GSH and proline" receptor might then have evolved into organisms having two distinct receptors, one to GSH and another to proline. Such a situation appears to exist in most of the corals listed in Table 2. And, eventually organisms evolved with only GSH receptors, as seen in hydra and siphonophores, or proline receptors, as found in the athecate colonial hydroids.

A similar argument could be constructed regarding the evolution of receptors to amino acids having apolar side chains. For example, the valine receptor of *Boloceroides* (72) and the leucine receptor of *Haliplanella* (74) may have evolved from a receptor with a specificity for apolar amino acids in general. Possibly receptors for other amino acids may have followed similar pathways from the original primitive cnidarian receptor which responded to many amino acids.

Evolution of Cellular Receptor Sites in General

Among the earliest receptor sites to evolve were probably those associated with the induction of pinocytosis in single cells. In recent years the chemical induction of pinocytosis has been studied in ameba (82, 83) and in white blood cells (84). Both kinds of cells respond to a range of small charged molecules; of the amino acids, aspartate and glutamate are particularly effective (82, 84). In general, it might be said that single cells depend on external chemical cues that stimulate the uptake of nutrients from their environment; hence, these cells may have evolved receptor sites with broad specificity such as might prove useful to guarantee the cell sufficient food to survive.

It thus seems reasonable to suppose that cnidarian cells utilizing pinocytosis to take up nutrients from their gastrovascular cavity also respond to a broad range of molecules. In accord with this supposition is Slautterback's finding that certain amino acids could stimulate the immediate formation of a large network of microvilli at the apical end of the endodermal digestive cells that line the gut of hydra. Among the most active amino acids were the isomers of tyrosine, with *m*-tyrosine the most active. Phenylalanine was ineffective. Other amino acids showing activity were cysteine and glutamate (D. Slautterback, personal communication).

Slautterback's finding that tyrosine stimulates microvilli formation in hydra endoderm cells takes on particular importance in light of the discovery by Blanquet & Lenhoff (85). They showed that hydra have a receptor on the surface of cells lining the gut. When activated by tyrosine, the hydra exhibited a "neck response," i.e. a constriction of the upper third of the body tube. These neck constrictions apparently allow hydra to retain previously ingested food in the gut while swallowing newly captured prey. No other natural amino acid, including phenylalanine, could substitute for tyrosine (85). It is interesting to note, however that m-tyrosine was more active than the other tyrosine isomers in activating both the neck response and in microvilli formation (85).

Recognizing that in response to tyrosine hydra display these two events, a cellular one and an organismic one, we can pose a number of intriguing questions: Is the same receptor site used to trigger both events? If not, did the receptor for neck formation evolve from the receptor for microvilli formation? It would appear simpler for hydra to use an existing receptor for two functions rather than to evolve another.

This reasoning may be stretched even further to postulate that there exists a direct line of evolution of receptor sites from those found on single cells inducing pinocytosis or phagocytosis, to those coordinating feeding responses in such simple "tissue-level" organisms as cnidarians, and finally to the receptors for neurotransmitters and peptide hormones in higher organisms. For example, because dopamine and norepinephrine are formed directly from tyrosine, it seems simpler and more efficient from an evolutionary standpoint for organisms to retain and utilize modifications of a primitive tyrosine receptor to recognize structurally related compounds rather than to evolve new receptor sites for each of these "analogues."

Would not the same argument apply to the evolution of receptors for such neurotransmitters as glutamic acid or glycine? Are there similar evolutionary relationships between the glutathione receptors involved in activating the cnidarian feeding response, and the glutathione site associated with the γ-glutamyl transpeptidase mechanism of amino acid transport (86) (see below)? In any of these cases, it would seem simpler for organisms during evolution to modify existing receptors to control new tasks rather than to develop completely new receptor-effector systems.

Summary and Future Directions

We feel the current information justifies these speculations on the evolution of receptor proteins because such views are analogous to our ideas of the conservative view of the evolution of proteins in general. The difficulty, of course, lies in proving these speculations. Actually, there are a number of ways in which evidence can be obtained. These ways, however, depend upon the development of methods for investigating receptors. One method, for example, would involve the isolation of receptor proteins and the analysis of their amino acid sequence. Based upon the current status of receptor purification, however, such an approach will not be possible for years. A second approach would consist of a search for different kinds of receptors to amino acids and neurotransmitters among members from all the phyla. From such a comparative study it might be possible to determine at which point in evolution the different receptors arose.

We are using a third approach, that of comparing the relative activities of two proteins that might be related to each other, with analogues. In our case, we are interested in proteins that recognize the tripeptide reduced glutathione. Previously we have reported (see 62) that the GSH receptor of hydra is specific for the γ-glutamyl moiety of GSH and can tolerate some changes in the thiol of the cysteinyl moiety. Hydra, for example, can respond to GSH which has its thiol methylated. At that time, no other protein combining with GSH was known to have such an unusual specificity for the molecule. Recent work with the enzyme γ-glutamyl transpeptidase ("GTP"), however, has shown a similar specificity of this enzyme for GSH (87).

We were intrigued by this similar specificity of GTP, especially since this enzyme is implied to act in the transport of amino acids into cells (86). Could it be that the GSH receptor of hydra evolved from the GTP thought to be used in amino acid transport? Could they be the same protein? Next we analyzed hydra for this enzyme (56, 88). We found it present in significant concentrations (see also 89), and its requirement for amino acid acceptors similar to that reported for the same enzyme activity as found elsewhere (56, 88).

To answer the question of whether or not the GSH receptor and the GTP from hydra are the same, we decided to look deeper into their relative specificities for GSH. Using analogues synthesized by our colleagues M. H. Cobb and G. Marshall of Washington University, together with J. Danner we were able to distinguish between the two activities. Whereas both proteins had about the same specificity for the γ-glutamyl-cysteinyl part of GSH, they differed with respect to their activities with analogues having substitutions at the glycine moiety; on one hand the GTP reacted poorly with analogues having amino acids with large side chains substituted for the glycine in GSH, while on the other hand, the GSH receptor of hydra was activated by those same analogues (56).

Such experiments show how those two proteins in hydra have similar and yet different specificities for GSH. Possibly the GSH receptor evolved from a mutation in a repeating unit of a gene controlling the synthesis of GTP.

CONCLUSIONS

The above speculations, like most concerning evolution, are difficult to prove. But they may help to make us aware that unifying concepts, tacitly assumed in the case of enzymes and cell organelles, also may apply to the basic aspects of chemoreception. Specifically, such speculations emphasize that the behavioral responses of lower invertebrates to a peptide or an amino acid may have many fundamental features in common with some hormonal and neurotransmitter responses in higher organisms. By focusing on the primary events of the combination of the activator with the receptor to initiate a series of coordinated activities, we may find new approaches and new insights into universal, yet little understood, chemical control mechanisms.

ACKNOWLEDGMENTS

We thank Dr. David Slautterback for his comments and for allowing us to quote from his unpublished material on microvillus formation. The research discussed was supported by grants from the National Institutes of Health and the National Science Foundation.

Literature Cited

1. Pilkis, S. J., Park, C. R. 1974. Mechanism of action of insulin. *Ann. Rev. Pharmacol.* 14:365–88
2. Cuatrecasas, P., Hollenberg, M. D., Chang, K., Bennett, V. 1975. Hormone receptor complexes and their modulation of membrane function. *Recent Prog. Horm. Res.* 31:37–93
3. Roth, J., Kahn, C. R., Lesniak, M. A., Gorden, P., DeMeyts, P., Megyesi, K., Neville, D. M., Gavin, J. R., Soll, A. H., Freychet, P., Goldfine, I. D., Bar, R. S., Archer, J. A. 1975. Receptors for insulin, NSILA-s, and growth hormone: applications to disease states in man. *Recent Prog. Horm. Res.* 31:95–139
4. Roth, J. 1973. Peptide hormone binding to receptors: a review of direct binding studies *in vitro*. *Metab. Clin. Exp.* 22:1059–73
5. Giorgio, N. A., Johnson, C. B., Blecher, M. 1974. Hormone receptors. III. Properties of glucagon-binding proteins isolated from liver plasma membranes. *J. Biol. Chem.* 249:428–37
6. Marshall, G. R., Bosshard, H. E., Vine, W. H., Glickson, J. D., Needleman, P. 1974. Angiotension II: Conformation and interaction with the receptor. In *Recent Advances in Renal Physiology and Pharmacology,* ed. L. G. Wesson, G. M. Fanelli, 215–55. Baltimore: Univ. Park Press. 388 pp.
7. Cohen, J. B., Changeux, J. P. 1975. The cholinergic receptor protein in its membrane environment. *Ann. Rev. Pharmacol.* 15:83–103
8. McNamee, M. G., Mark, G., Weill, C. L., Karlin, A. 1975. Further characterization of purified acetylcholine receptor and its incorporation into phospholipid vesicles. In *Protein-Ligand Interactions,* ed. H. Sund, G. Blauer, 316–27. Berlin: de Gruyter. 486 pp.
9. Hucho, F., Gordon, A., Sund, H. 1975. Subunit structure and binding sites of the acetylcholine receptor. See Ref. 8, pp. 306–15
10. Sugiyama, H., Popot, J. L., Cohen, J. B., Weber, M., Changeux, J. P. 1975. Binding and functional states of the cholinergic receptor protein from *Torpedo marmorata.* See Ref. 8, pp. 289–305
11. Raftery, M. A., Bode, J., Vandlen, R., Michaelson, D., Deutsch, J., Moody, T., Ross, M. J., Stroud, R. M. 1975. Structural and functional studies of an acetylcholine receptor. See Ref. 8, pp. 328–55
12. Snyder, S. H., Young, A. B., Bennett, J. P., Mulder, A. H. 1973. Synaptic biochemistry of amino acids. *Fed. Proc.* 32:2039–47
13. Roberts, P. J. 1974. Glutamate receptors in the rat central nervous system. *Nature* 252:399–401
14. Dole, V. P. 1970. Biochemistry of addiction. *Ann. Rev. Biochem.* 39:821–40
15. Takemori, A. E. 1974. Biochemistry of drug dependence. *Ann. Rev. Biochem.* 43:15–33
16. Adler, J. 1975. Chemotaxis in bacteria. *Ann. Rev. Biochem.* 44:341–57
17. Lovely, P., Dahlquist, F. W., Macnab, R., Koshland, D. E. Jr. 1974. An instrument for recording the motions of microorganisms in chemical gradients. *Rev. Sci. Instrum.* 45:683–86
18. Taylor, B. L., Koshland, D. E. Jr. 1974. Reversal of flagellar rotation in monotrichous and peritrichous bacteria: generation of changes in direction. *J. Bacteriol.* 119:640–42
19. Strange, P. G., Koshland, D. E. Jr. 1976. Receptor interactions in a signalling system: competition between ribose receptor and galactose receptor in the chemotaxis response. *Proc. Natl. Acad. Sci. USA* 73:762–66
20. Beidler, L. M. 1971. Taste receptor stimulation with salts and acids. In *Handbook of Sensory Physiology,* ed. L. M. Beidler, Vol. 4, Part 2:200–20. New York: Springer. 518 pp.
21. Fischer, R. 1971. Gustatory, behavioral and pharmocological manifestations of chemoreception in man. In *Gustation and Olfaction; Food Science and Technology,* ed. G. Ohloff, A. F. Thomas, 187–235. New York: Academic. 275 pp.
22. Jennings, H. S. 1906. *Behavior of the Lower Organisms.* Republished by Indiana Univ. Press, Bloomington, 1962. 366 pp.
23. Mackie, A. M., Grant, P. T. 1974. Interspecies and intraspecies chemoreception by marine invertebrates. In *Chemoreception in Marine Organisms,* ed. P. T. Grant, A. M. Mackie, 105–33. New York: Academic. 295 pp.
24. Kittredge, J. S. 1974. Comparative biochemistry: Marine biochemistry. In *Experimental Marine Biology,* ed. R. N. Mariscal, 226–55. New York: Academic. 373 pp.

25. Kohn, A. J. 1961. Chemoreception in gastropod molluscs. *Am. Zool.* 1:291–308
26. Barber, S. B. 1961. Chemoreception and thermoreception. In *Physiology of Crustacea*, ed. T. H. Waterman, 2:109–31. New York: Academic. 681 pp.
27. Lenhoff, H. M., Lindstedt, K. J. 1974. Chemoreception in aquatic invertebrates with special emphasis on feeding behavior of Coelenterates. See Ref. 23, pp. 143–72
28. Dethier, V. G., Browne, L., Smith, C. N. 1960. The designation of chemicals in terms of the responses they elicit from insects. *J. Econ. Entomol.* 53:134–36
29. Beck, S. D. 1965. Resistance of plants to insects. *Ann. Rev. Entomol.* 10:207–32
30. Lindstedt, K. J. 1971. Chemical control of feeding behavior. *Comp. Biochem. Physiol.* 39:553–81
31. Laverack, M. S. 1974. The structure and function of chemoreceptor cells. See Ref. 23, pp. 1–41
32. Davenport, D. 1966. The experimental analysis of behavior in symbiosis. In *Symbiosis*, ed. S. M. Henry, 1:381–429. New York: Academic. 478 pp.
33. Cheng, T. O. 1967. Marine molluscs as hosts for symbiosis: with a review of known parasites of commercially important species. In *Advances in Marine Biology*, ed. F. S. Russell, 5:1–424. New York: Academic. 424 pp.
34. McCauley, J. 1969. Marine invertebrates, chemical signals and marine products. *Lloydia* 32:425–37
35. Harris, L. 1971. Nudibranch associations as symbioses. In *Aspects of the Biology of Symbiosis*, ed. T. Cheng, 77–90. Baltimore: Univ. Park Press. 327 pp.
36. Ache, B. W. 1974. The experimental analysis of host location in symbiotic marine invertebrates. In *Symbiosis in the Sea*, ed. W. Vernberg, 45–60. Columbia, SC: Univ. South Carolina Press. 276 pp.
37. Kittredge, J. S. 1971. Marine-fouling organisms: natural attractants and repellents. *U. S. Natl. Tech. Inform. Serv. A.D. Rep. 1971, No. 734106*
38. Crisp, D. J. 1974. Factors influencing the settlement of marine invertebrate larvae. See Ref. 23, pp. 177–253
39. Passano, L. M. 1957. Prey-predator recognition in the invertebrates. In *Recent Advances in Invertebrate Physiology*, ed. B. Y. Scheer, T. H. Bullock,

40. Baylor, E. R., Smith, E. E. 1957. Diurnal migration of plankton crustaceans. See Ref. 39, pp. 21–35
41. Whittaker, R. H., Feeney, P. P. 1971. Allelochemics: chemical interactions between species. *Science* 171:757–70
42. Starr, M. P. 1975. A generalized scheme for classifying organismic associations. In *Symbiosis*, ed. D. H. Jennings, D. L. Lee, 1–20. Cambridge: Cambridge Univ. Press. 633 pp.
43. Loomis, W. F. 1955. Glutathione control of the specific feeding reactions of hydra. *Ann. NY Acad. Sci.* 62:209–28
44. Lenhoff, H. M. 1961. Activation of the feeding reflex in *Hydra littoralis*. In *The Biology of Hydra and of Some Other Coelenterates*, ed. H. M. Lenhoff, W. F. Loomis, 203–32. Coral Gables: Univ. Miami Press. 467 pp.
45. Lenhoff, H. M. 1961. Activation of the feeding reflex in *Hydra littoralis*. I. Role played by reduced glutathione and quantitative assay of the feeding reflex. *J. Gen. Physiol.* 45:331–44
46. Lenhoff, H. M. 1965. Some physicochemical aspects of the microenvironments surrounding hydra during activation of their feeding behavior. *Am. Zool.* 5:515–24
47. Lenhoff, H. M. 1968. Chemical perspectives on the feeding response, digestion and nutrition of selected coelenterates. In *Chemical Zoology*, ed. M. Florkin, B. Scheer, 2:157–221. New York: Academic. 639 pp.
48. Lineweaver, H., Burk, D. 1934. The determination of enzyme dissociation constants. *J. Am. Chem. Soc.* 56:657–66
49. Beidler, L. M. 1954. A theory of taste stimulation. *J. Gen. Physiol.* 38:133–39
50. Lenhoff, H. M. 1969. pH profile of a peptide receptor. *Comp. Biochem. Physiol.* 28:571–86
51. Dixon, M. 1953. The effect of pH on the affinities of enzymes for substrates and inhibitors. *Biochem. J.* 55:161–70
52. Wieland, T. 1954. Chemistry and properties of glutathione. In *Glutathione*, ed. S. Colowick, A. Lazarow, E. Racker, D. R. Schwarz, 45–59. New York: Academic. 341 pp.
53. Dixon, M., Webb, E. C. 1964. *Enzymes*, 154–65. New York: Academic. 950 pp. 2nd ed.
54. Cliffe, E. E., Waley, S. G. 1958. Effect of analogues of glutathione on the feeding reaction of hydra. *Nature* 183:804–5

L. H. Kleinholz, A. W. Martin, 37–47. Eugene: Univ. Oregon Press. 304 pp.

55. Lenhoff, H. M., Bovaird, J. 1961. Action of glutamic acid and glutathione analogues on the hydra glutathione-receptor. *Nature* 189:486–87
56. Danner, J., Lenhoff, H. M., Cobb, M. H., Heagy, W., Marshall, G. R. 1976. *Biochem. Biophys. Res. Commun.* 73: 180–86
57. Lenhoff, H. M., Bovaird, J. 1960. Enzymatic activation of a hormone-like response in hydra by proteases. *Nature* 187:671–73
58. Lenhoff, H. M., Bovaird, J. 1959. Requirement of bound calcium for the action of surface chemoreceptors. *Science* 130:1474–76
59. Asbill, M. 1975. Sodium ion effect on the glutathione induced feeding response of *Hydra attenuata*. *J. Undergrad. Res. Biol. Sci., Univ. Calif., Irvine* 4:210–28
60. Lenhoff, H. M., Zwisler, J. 1963. Zinc activation of a coordinated response in hydra. *Science* 142:1666–68
61. Fulton, C. 1963. Proline control of the feeding reaction of *Cordylophora*. *J. Gen. Physiol.* 46:823–37
62. Lenhoff, H. M. 1974. On the mechanism of action and evolution of receptors associated with feeding and digestion. In *Coelenterate Biology: Reviews and New Perspectives*, ed. L. Muscatine, H. M. Lenhoff, 359–89. New York: Academic. 501 pp.
63. Reich, E., Rifkin, D. B., Shaw, E. eds. 1976. *Proteases and Biological Control*. Cold Spring Harbor, NY: Cold Spring Harbor Lab. 1002 pp.
64. Gentleman, S., Mansour, T. E. 1974. Adenylate cyclase in a sea anemone-implication for chemoreception. *Biochim. Biophys. Acta* 343:469–79
65. Cobb, M. H., Marshall, G. R., Heagy, W., Danner, J., Lenhoff, H. M. 1976. On the mechanism of the glutathione induced feeding response in hydra: hormone-receptor interaction. *Fed. Proc.* 35:1617 (Abstr.)
66. Mariscal, R. N. 1971. The chemical control of the feeding behavior in some Hawaiian corals. In *Experimental Coelenterate Biology*, ed. H. M. Lenhoff, L. Muscatine, V. Davis, 100–18. Honolulu: Univ. of Hawaii Press. 281 pp.
67. Pardy, R. L., Lenhoff, H. M. 1968. The feeding biology of the gymnoblastic hydroid, *Pennaria tiarella*. *J. Exp. Zool.* 168:197–202
68. Spencer, A. N. 1974. Behavior and electrical activity in the hydrozoan *Probos-

cidactyla flavicirrata* (Brandt). *Biol. Bull.* 146:100–15
69. Rushforth, N. B. 1976. Electrophysiological correlates of feeding behavior in the Tubularia. In *Coelenterate Ecology and Behavior*, ed. G. O. Mackie, 729–38. New York: Plenum. 744 pp.
70. Lenhoff, H. M., Schneiderman, H. A. 1959. The chemical control of feeding in the Portuguese man-of-war, *Physalia physalia* L., and its bearing on the evolution of the cnidaria. *Biol. Bull.* 116:452–60
71. Mackie, G. O., Boag, D. A. 1963. Fishing, feeding and digestion in siphonophores. *Publ. Stn. Zool. Napoli* 33: 178–96
72. Lindstedt, K. J., Muscatine, L., Lenhoff, H. M. 1968. Valine activation of feeding in the sea anemone *Boloceroides*. *Comp. Biochem. Physiol.* 26: 567–72
73. Lindstedt, K. J. 1971. Biphasic feeding response in a sea anemone: control by asparagine and glutathione. *Science* 173:333–34
74. Lindstedt, K. J. 1971. Chemical control of feeding behavior. *Comp. Biochem. Physiol.* 39:553–81
75. Steiner, G. 1957. Über die chemische nahrungswahl von *Actinia equina* (L). *Naturwissenschaften* 44:70–71
76. Reimer, A. A. 1973. Feeding behavior in the sea anemone *Calliactis polypus* (Forskal, 1775). *Comp. Biochem. Physiol.* 44:1289–1301
77. Reimer, A. A. 1971. Feeding behavior in the Hawaiian zoanthids *Palythoa* and *Zoanthus*. *Pac. Sci.* 25:512–20
78. Reimer, A. A. 1971. Chemical control of feeding behavior in *Palythoa* (Zoanthidea, Coelenterata). *Comp. Gen. Pharmacol.* 2:383–96
79. Mariscal, R. N, Lenhoff, H. M. 1968. The chemical control of feeding behavior in *Cyphastrea ocella* and some other Hawaiian corals. *J. Exp. Biol.* 49: 689–99
80. Lehman, J. T., Porter, J. W. 1973. Chemical activation of feeding in the Caribbean reef building coral *Montastrea cavernosa*. *Biol. Bull.* 145:140–49
81. Loeb, M., Blanquet, R. S. 1973. Feeding behavior in polyps of the Chesapeake Bay sea nettle, *Chrysaora quinquecirrha* (Desor, 1848). *Biol. Bull.* 145:150–58
82. Chapman-Anderson, C. 1962. Pinocytosis in amoebae. *C. R. Trav. Lab. Carlsberg* 33:73–264
83. Allen, H. J., Ault, C., Winzler, R. J., Danielli, J. 1974. Chemical characteri-

zation of the isolated cell surface of amoebae. *J. Cell. Biol.* 60:26–38

84. Cohn, Z. A. 1967. The regulation of pinocytosis in mouse microphages. II. Factors inducing vesicle formation. *J. Exp. Med.* 125:213–32

85. Blanquet, R. S., Lenhoff, H. M. 1968. Tyrosine enteroreceptor of hydra: its function in eliciting a behavior modification. *Science* 159:633–34

86. Meister, A. 1973. On the enzymology of amino acid transport. *Science* 180: 33–39

87. Tate, S., Meister, A. 1974. Interaction of γ-glutamyl transpeptidase with amino acids, dipeptides, and derivatives and analogs of glutathione. *J. Biol. Chem.* 249:7593–7602

88. Danner, J., Cobb, M. H., Heagy, W., Marshall, G. R. 1976. γ-Glutamyl transpeptidase in hydra. *Fed. Proc.* 35:1529 (Abstr.)

89. Tate, S., Meister, A. 1976. γ-Glutamyl transpeptidase in *Hydra littoralis. Biochem. Biophys. Res. Commun.* 70: 500–5

Ann. Rev. Pharmacol. Toxicol. 1977. 17:259–79
Copyright © 1977 by Annual Reviews Inc. All rights reserved

BASIC MECHANISMS OF ❖6679
PROSTAGLANDIN ACTION ON
AUTONOMIC NEUROTRANSMISSION

Per Hedqvist
Department of Physiology, Karolinska Institutet, S-10401 Stockholm 60, Sweden

INTRODUCTION

More than 40 years ago Euler (1) and Goldblatt (2) independently described the striking pharmacodynamic actions of human seminal plasma and extracts of sheep vesicular gland added to isolated organs or injected into the whole animal. Since the biological effects could not be accounted for by any known naturally occurring compound, the active substance(s) was named prostaglandin (3). Today prostaglandin (PG) is recognized, not as one, but rather a family of fatty acids of almost ubiquitous distribution in the mammalian organism. The principal biosynthetic pathways of the PGs and certain nonprostanoic compounds from their precursor, arachidonic acid, are shown in Figure 1. It should be recalled that PGs are formed from two other precursors as well, the only difference being the number of double bonds in the side chains, as indicated by the subscript numbers of the different PGs.

Although the PG principle has been known for many years, it is only within the last decade that the pharmacology of the PGs has been systematically and extensively investigated. These efforts, greatly aided by the availability of synthetic PGs and potent inhibitors of PG synthesis, have demonstrated that the PGs possess an impressive range of biological activities, which has given rise to many speculations concerning their physiological or pathophysiological significance. Admittedly, the PGs have distinct actions on most mammalian tissues, but few effects seem to be of the same widespread significance as those on autonomic nerves, since the autonomic nervous system is such an essential regulator of the activities of a large number of organs and organ systems.

There is a rapidly growing body of evidence indicating that PGs are released in the vicinity of autonomic neuroeffector junctions, both spontaneously and as a result of physical, chemical, and electrical stimuli; that PGs influence both transmitter release from nerve terminals and the response to the secreted transmitter; and that inhibitors of PG synthesis produce effects opposite to those of the PGs. Taken

259

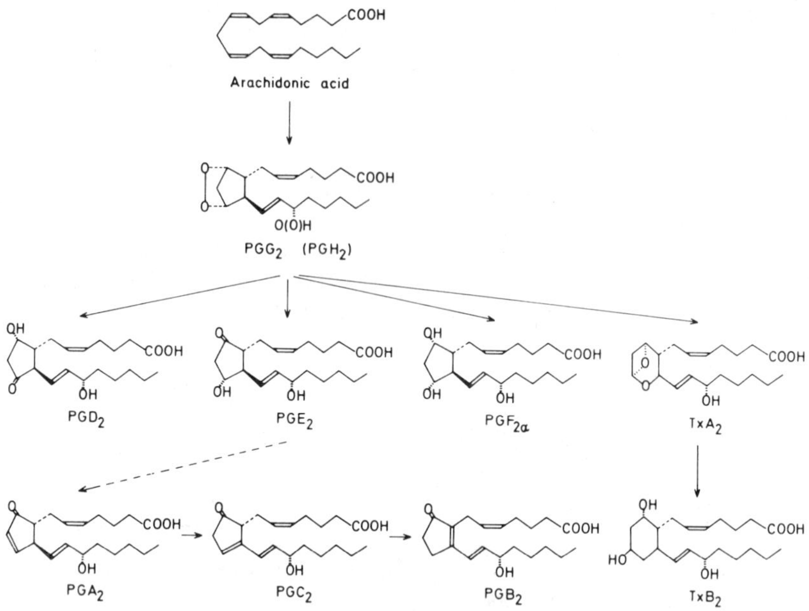

Figure 1   Pathways of biosynthesis of PGs and thromboxanes (Tx) from arachidonic acid.

together, these observations suggest that PGs are important as modulators of the autonomic neuroeffector transmission. In this review special attention is paid to work in which an action on the transmission has been demonstrated directly, rather than implied by the fact that the studied organs or organ systems are autonomically innervated. The presentation focuses on events in the adrenergic neurotransmission, and in particular on the presumed feed-back control mechanism that regulates the release of transmitter in response to forthcoming nerve impulses. Sections on ganglionic and cholinergic transmission are also included, although the available literature on PG actions in these systems is scanty and even controversial. The effects of PGs within the central nervous system are beyond the scope of this presentation.

In order to avoid confusion, contact elements in the neurotransmission are defined. The term *junction* is used when the contacted element is a muscle or a gland cell; *prejunctional* refers to events in the axon terminal membrane or intraaxonally, and *postjunctional* to all events linked to the action of the secreted transmitter on the effector cell membrane. The terms *presynaptic* and *postsynaptic* are used when dealing with ganglionic transmission.

ADRENERGIC NEUROEFFECTOR JUNCTIONS

Action of Prostaglandins of the E Series

Since the discovery of PG in the 1930s much interest has been devoted to its action on the cardiovascular system. Numerous reports have shown that crude PG and synthetic PGEs, although rather modest in their direct action on the heart, are extremely potent as vasodepressors and also reduce the blood pressure–augmenting effect of norepinephrine (NE). These observations are difficult to evaluate in terms of an action on the adrenergic neurotransmission, since the induced vasodilatation alters the geometry of the vascular wall, and, hence the response to pressor agents.

SPLEEN   The first systematic studies were made in 1968 when it was reported that PGE_1 diminished vasoconstrictor responses to nerve stimulation and NE in the feline spleen (without significantly affecting basal perfusion pressure) (4) and that it inhibited the luminal occlusion by nerve stimulation and NE in the rabbit oviduct (5). Although these studies did not permit any conclusion as to a prejunctional inhibitory action on NE release, such an effect was later demonstrated with PGE_1 in the feline spleen (6) and with its congener, PGE_2, in rabbit and human oviduct (7, 8).

In a subsequent study on the feline spleen (9) PGE_2 was shown to inhibit dose dependently and reversibly the release of NE and the splenic contraction response to nerve stimulation. The vascular response was progressively inhibited in the lower dose range, but less so when high doses of PGE_2 were applied. The reason for this escape phenomenon became apparent when nerve stimulation was replaced by intra-arterial injection of NE. NE-induced capsular responses were little affected by PGE_2, while vasoconstrictor responses were inhibited by low PGE_2 doses and markedly enhanced by high doses. It is apparent from these observations that PGE_2 affects adrenergic neurotransmission in the feline spleen in a multifaceted way. It produces prejunctional inhibition of transmitter release and as a consequence also inhibition of the effector response. There are also postjunctional actions which may either further depress or augment the response.

PGE_1 and PGE_2 have little effect on adrenergic neuroeffector transmission in the canine spleen, because reduction in splenic volume (index of capsular contraction) and blood flow induced by nerve stimulation or catecholamines occurred to approximately the same extent before and after administration of PGE, unfortunately given only in one concentration (10). It was also concluded that the PGEs have no effect on induced vasoconstrictor responses. However, the results are difficult to evaluate since the responses were hardly visible even in the control experiments. On the other hand, vascular responses induced by epinephrine in the canine spleen are enhanced after inhibition of local PG synthesis by indomethacin (11). More experiments are needed before the issue can be settled.

HEART   The isolated heart of most laboratory animals is relatively insensitive to the direct action of PGs, and chronotropic effects often observed after intravenous administration of PGEs seem to be mediated largely through reflex sympathetic stimulation as a consequence of decreased arterial blood pressure. On the other hand, chronotropic and inotropic responses to sympathetic nerve stimulation in the isolated rabbit heart are dose dependently and reversibly inhibited by PGE_1 and PGE_2 (12, 13). Positive chronotropic responses to transmural stimulation of the rabbit sinoatrial node preparation are also blocked by PGE_2 in low concentrations (14). Because the PGEs inhibit the overflow of NE in the rabbit heart, at least to the same extent that they depress the effector response to nerve stimulation, and because they have no effect on responses to added NE, the inhibition appears to be solely prejunctional and to consist of reduction of transmitter release from the nerve terminals (12, 13). In agreement with this view is a report that PGE_1 and PGE_2 inhibit the release of NE by nicotine and potassium in the guinea pig heart (15).

VASCULAR BEDS   Besides the spleen PGE_1 and PGE_2 have been tested for actions on adrenergic responses in a great number of vascular beds. In most cases the PGEs have proved inhibitory on responses to sympathetic nerve stimulation, while often causing mixed inhibitory and stimulant effect on responses to NE.

Topical application of PGE_1 to mesenteric and cremasteric vessels in the rat results in a reduced responsiveness to NE which persists long after the direct vasodilating effect has vanished (16, 17). While these observations substantiate a postjunctional inhibitory action, PGE_1 has also been reported to potentiate responses to NE in the rabbit aorta and mesenteric artery in vitro (18, 19), as well as vascular responses to NE in canine uterus in situ (20) and in perfused rat kidney (21).

Vasoconstrictor responses to nerve stimulation are inhibited by PGE_1 and/or PGE_2 in feline and canine hindleg (22–26), and in the kidney of the rabbit, dog, and cat (21–29). Because in most of these cases the responses to NE were less depressed, unchanged, or even enhanced, the PGEs seem to act also by inhibiting the release of transmitter from the adrenergic nerve terminals in vascular tissue. Such an effect has been demonstrated directly in the perfused rabbit kidney and ear (30, 31) and in isolated mesenteric arteries from cat and man (32, 33). An inhibitory action on NE release might be present also in canine subcutaneous adipose tissue, although the effect could be demonstrated only after prior α-adrenoceptor blockade (34). Exceptions may be formed by the canine hindpaw and rat kidney, where PGE_1 and/or PGE_2 enhance the vasoconstrictor responses to nerve stimulation (21, 35). However, at least in the latter case a stimulant postjunctional action might have overshadowed a prejunctional effect which is inhibitory. Admittedly, PGE_1 has been reported to increase the NE overflow response to nerve stimulation in the blood-perfused feline spleen (36). However, extremely high doses were used, exceeding those that are inhibitory by approximately 1000 times. Moreover, the effect could be accounted for by inhibition of platelet thrombus formation and hence improved microcirculation and washout of released NE rather than actual enhancement of the NE release mechanism.

There are at least three ways in which PGEs may affect local blood flow and pressure: 1. PGEs cause vasodilatation in most if not all vascular beds. 2. They depress transmitter release from the nerve terminals, and hence the effector response to nerve impulses. Because this effect has been demonstrated in so many vascular tissues (and nonvascular smooth muscle tissues) from different animal species and from man, it can be concluded that this is an essential and widespread action of the PGEs. Admittedly, the PGEs have been postulated to have the opposite action in some vascular beds, notably the canine hindpaw and the rat kidney. However, this assumption was based only on differential effects of the PGEs on responses to nerve stimulation and NE, and transmitter release, which could have given the proper answer, was not measured. 3. PGEs interact with locally released NE and circulating catecholamines at the level of the effector cell membrane. Both inhibitory effects, probably accentuated by the vasodepressor activity, and stimulant actions have been noted. Although low doses of PGE, which inhibit NE release, often act as postjunctional inhibitors or have no effect at this level, there are several important exceptions to this rule. One can therefore only speculate whether the PGEs, in addition to inhibiting NE release, might serve also another function, that of maintaining the reactivity of the effector cell to catecholamines (37).

MISCELLANEOUS SMOOTH MUSCLE TISSUES   It is well established that PGE_1 and PGE_2 inhibit the twitch response to nerve stimulation and enhance that to NE in the guinea pig vas deferens (38–41), and the same pattern appears to hold true also for the guinea pig seminal vesicle (42). While these observations suggest both prejunctional inhibition and postjunctional enhancement, the results are difficult to evaluate in terms of actions on adrenergic transmission, since, at least in the guinea pig vas deferens, the twitch response behaves as if it were of nonadrenergic origin (43, 44). On the other hand, there is no doubt that the vas deferens is supplied with a heavy adrenergic innervation and that the contraction response to prolonged nerve stimulation bears all the characteristics of being adrenergic. Important contributions to the understanding of PG action on adrenergic transmission have also been obtained in studies on the NE release mechanism in this tissue. These aspects are considered in more detail in a following section. At this stage it is appropriate only to summarize that PGE_1 and PGE_2 produce a dose-dependent, inverse frequency–related, and reversible inhibition of NE release induced by nerve stimulation in the guinea pig vas deferens (45–48).

PGE_1 and PGE_2 inhibit the release of NE from the field stimulated rat and rabbit iris (49, 50). The observation that PGE_1 and PGE_2 counteract or even abolish the inhibition of gut motility resulting from stimulation of periarterial sympathetic nerves, without affecting responses to NE, provides indirect evidence that PGEs inhibit NE release also in this tissue. On the other hand, PGEs do not seem to affect contractions of the feline nictitating membrane induced by transmural or postganglionic nerve stimulation (51, 52).

Action of Other Prostaglandins

Relative to the PGEs, less attention has been paid to the capacity of other PGs to influence the adrenergic neuroeffector transmission. A mainly stimulant effect on neurotransmission in vascular tissue seems to occur with PGs of the F series. In the hindlimb of the dog $PGF_{2\alpha}$ causes vasoconstriction, and this effect is abolished after denervation (53). Similarly, $PGF_{2\alpha}$ enhances reflex vasoconstriction, as well as vasoconstriction induced by direct nerve stimulation in the canine hindpaw (52). In the canine gracilis muscle, vascular responses to nerve stimulation are unchanged by $PGF_{2\alpha}$, and those to NE are actually depressed (52). In the canine spleen and tibial artery $PGF_{2\alpha}$ enhances the response to nerve stimulation, without affecting that to NE (52, 54). While these observations provide circumstantial evidence that

$PGF_{2\alpha}$ facilitates the release of NE, a postjunctional stimulant action has also been demonstrated in several tissues. Thus, $PGF_{2\alpha}$ enhances vasoconstrictor responses to NE in the pulmonary lobar artery and vein (55), and to both nerve stimulation and NE in canine hindlimb superficial veins (56), rabbit and rat kidney (21, 57, 58), and in guinea pig vas deferens (P. Hedqvist, unpublished observations).

PGA_1 and PGA_2 inhibit the vasopressor response to nerve stimulation and NE in the canine hindpaw (25, 26). On the other hand, PGA_1 causes a modest enhancement of canine splenic responses to nerve stimulation (54), and in the rabbit kidney PGA_2 increases vascular responses to both nerve stimulation and NE (58). These observations appear unexpected since deficiency of PGA_2 has been assumed to be a significant etiological factor in essential hypertension (59). It should be recalled, however, that PGA_2 might be enzymatically converted to PGC_2 and subsequently to PGB_2. PGB_2 is a potent vasoconstrictor in canine and human superficial and pulmonary vasculature (60–62). This vasoconstriction produced by PGB_2 is blocked by reserpine pretreatment and by decentralization, as shown in the dog. Moreover, in the canine hindpaw it enhances pressor responses to nerve stimulation, but not to NE. At least some of the above-mentioned effects are consistent with a presynaptic or prejunctional stimulant effect on transmitter release.

$PGF_{2\alpha}$, PGA_2, and PGB_2 have been tested for effects on NE release in several tissues, but in none has a stimulant action been disclosed. In the rabbit heart, $PGF_{2\alpha}$ (in concentrations up to 10^{-6} M) is ineffective in altering the release of NE induced by sympathetic nerve stimulation (12). In both the rabbit kidney and guinea pig vas deferens, $PGF_{2\alpha}$, PGA_2, and PGB_2, in concentrations that enhance the effector response to nerve stimulation, either do not affect NE release or actually decrease it [(57, 58) and unpublished observations]. These observations do not lend any support to a prejunctional stimulant action. Rather they suggest that enhancement of effector responses to adrenergic nerve stimuli by $PGF_{2\alpha}$, PGA_2, or PGB_2 in these and other tissues is mostly, if not wholly, a postjunctional phenomenon.

PGD_2 and the endoperoxides, PGG_2 and PGH_2, are worthy of comment, although so far they have been tested for effects on adrenergic neurotransmission only in the guinea pig vas deferens (57). PGD_2 inhibits the release of NE only in high concentrations, being at least 100 times less active than PGE_2. Moreover, with μg concentrations of this compound, observed effects might be due to the presence of traces of its isomer, PGE_2. Both PGG_2 and PGH_2 inhibit the release of NE induced by nerve stimulation in the guinea pig vas deferens, but they are less than half as potent as PGE_2. One problem when studying the effects of the endoperoxides is that they are nonenzymatically and rapidly ($T_{1/2}$ approximately 5 min in salinic media) degraded mainly into PGE_2. Although attempts were made to minimize this effect by giving the compounds only 30 sec before the stimulation it is conceivable that at least part of the observed effect could be accounted for by newly formed PGE_2.

Mechanism of Prostaglandin-Induced Inhibition of Norepinephrine Release

The demonstration of prejunctional inhibitory action of PGs, in particular the PGEs, in many sympathetically innervated tissues has led to attempts at specifying the target for this effect. Theoretically, the PGEs might reduce the effective outflow of NE from stimulated tissues by promoting its metabolic degradation or uptake. However, observations that PGEs have no effect on monoamine oxidase and catecholamine-O-methyl transferase activities in guinea pig heart (63), that they cause a parallel reduction in the efflux of total tracer and fluorimetrically determined NE induced by nerve stimulation in feline spleen, preloaded with ^{3}H–(–)–NE (6, 9), and that they have no effect on NE uptake in feline spleen and rabbit heart (9, 13) seem to indicate that altered disposition of NE released from the nerve terminals cannot explain the inhibitory effect of the PGEs. Similarly, there is no independent reason to assume that PGEs interfere with the propagation of impulses in the nerve trunk or with the spread of excitation throughout the terminal arborization, because PGE does not affect the compound action potential in splenic nerves (64), and because it readily inhibits the release of NE evoked by potassium in guinea pig heart and vas deferens (15, 65). Rather, the latter observation implies an action on local electrosecretory coupling. In fact, there is a multitude of evidence that indicates that PGEs inhibit NE release by an action on stimulus secretion coupling, and more specifically on the availability of calcium for the release mechanism.

Release of NE by nerve impulses has an absolute requirement for calcium, and upon arrival of a nerve action potential, depolarization is thought to cause an inward movement of membrane calcium which in turn promotes release of NE into the junctional cleft (66–68). It is therefore of particular interest that calcium interacts with the inhibitory effect of PGEs on release of NE from adrenergic nerves. Thus, increasing the ambient calcium concentration counteracts the inhibitory effect of PGE_2 on NE release by nerve stimulation in feline spleen and guinea pig vas deferens (64, 69). On the other hand, NE release by tyramine, which is a calcium-independent process, is not affected by PGE_2, as shown in feline spleen and guinea pig heart (15, 64). Furthermore, in the guinea pig vas deferens the inhibitory effect of PGE_1 and PGE_2 varies inversely with the environmental calcium concentration (45, 70–72), and kinetic analysis of the effect of PGE_2 on the dependence of the release mechanism on calcium has shown that PGE_2 depresses its apparent V_{max} and enhances its K_m, and progressively more so with falling calcium concentration in the medium (72). The inhibitory effect of PGE_2 on NE release by nerve stimulation in the guinea pig vas deferens and rabbit kidney and heart is diminished by increasing the impulse frequency (30, 45, 48, 73). In fact, shortening the pulse interval is considered to leave more residual calcium at the active releasing sites in the axon (74). Evidently, all these observations suggest that PGEs inhibit NE release by interfering with the availability of calcium for the release mechanism, possibly by closure of the calcium gates in the axonal membrane.

Recently it has been shown that prolongation of the nerve action potential, either by lengthening the applied electric pulse or by administering tetraethylammonium or rubidium (75, 76), significantly diminishes the inhibitory effect of PGE_2 on NE release induced by nerve stimulation in the guinea pig vas deferens (77). This observation seems to further link the inhibitory action of PGEs on NE release to interference with calcium availability, since prolongation of the action potential is thought to allow the calcium gates in the axonal membrane to remain open longer, and as a consequence to allow more calcium to enter the axon (68, 78, 79).

As an alternative it has been suggested that PGEs, by analogy with the fact that they may depolarize smooth muscle and cardiac cells (80–83), might similarly depolarize the nerve terminal membrane, and therefore reduce the amplitude of the action potential on arrival of nerve impulses (81). However, it is not known whether PGEs have such an effect on C-terminal fibers; also, the PGE amounts required to produce even a moderate depolarization of muscle cells are high compared with those that forcibly depress transmitter release. Moreover, the observations that PGE_1 and PGE_2 are equipotent on NE release in the heart (12), but that in reasonable concentrations only PGE_2 depolarizes cardiac cells (83, 84), also suggest that PGEs do not inhibit NE release by depolarizing the nerve terminal membrane.

In summary, the inhibitory effect of PGEs on transmitter release from adrenergic nerves is best explained in terms of a direct action on the availability of calcium for the release process. A closely similar mechanism has been proposed for the feedback control NE release by prejunctional α-adrenoceptors (85).

Prostaglandin Release from Adrenergically Innervated Tissues

It is generally accepted that PGs can be extracted from virtually all mammalian tissues. This does not mean that PGs are stored to any appreciable extent in the tissues, but that there is a continuous, and probably very low, PG synthesis and release that can be markedly enhanced by various maneuvers, e.g. extraction procedures.

Increased release of PGs by nerve stimulation and catecholamines readily occurs in a number of adrenergically innervated tissues, such as canine and feline spleen (86–89), rabbit heart and ear (13, 90), canine and rabbit kidney (91, 92), rat and canine adipose tissue (93, 94), and guinea pig and rat vas deferens (95, 96). In most cases the PG predominantly released is PGE_2 followed by $PGF_{2\alpha}$, except in the case of the guinea pig vas deferens, which appears to produce predominantly PGE_1 and PGE_2 and only traces of $PGF_{2\alpha}$. Even though these results have been obtained in perfused tissues, either isolated or kept in situ, they cannot be regarded as artificial. Thus, while the surgical trauma may certainly cause an increased basal PG release, it cannot explain the increased release induced by nerve stimulation. Hence, these PG output figures are relevant and suggest that nerve impulses cause release of PGs in adrenergically innervated organs even under strict in vivo conditions.

The important information provided by these observations is that significant amounts of a PGE are released when adrenergically innervated organs are stimulated by their nerves and the PGEs are particularly well adapted for inhibition of transmitter release in these tissues. In fact, the amounts of PGEs required to produce such an effect are largely of the same order of magnitude as those that can be released by nerve stimulation. On these grounds it may be justified to postulate that locally formed PGEs are able to restrict the release of NE by a negative feedback loop, and hence to act as significant modulators of adrenergic transmission (97). That $PGF_{2\alpha}$, the second principal PG released from adrenergically innervated tissues, should operate by the same mechanism appears less likely, since the concentrations required to produce inhibition of NE release are high compared with the amounts actually released from stimulated tissues. Even though the presence in some tissues of a PGE 9-ketoreductase (98) (which transforms PGE to PGF) might change the pattern into preferential release of $PGF_{2\alpha}$, an inhibitory modulating role is still unlikely since the net effect of $PGF_{2\alpha}$ on adrenergic transmission, if anything, is stimulant.

ORIGIN OF RELEASED PROSTAGLANDINS   Several studies on spleen and kidney have revealed that α-adrenoceptor blockers abolish the release of PGs and the smooth muscle contraction induced by nerve stimulation or catecholamines (86, 88, 89, 99). These observations indicate that contraction of the effector cell, or structural change of its membrane (100), is an essential trigger mechanism for PG synthesis. The finding that PG release in the rabbit heart induced by infusion of NE is inhibited neither by α-adrenoceptor blockers nor by β-adrenoceptor blockers (101) is certainly at variance with this concept, and is difficult to explain.

The observation that the release of PGs from canine spleen and rabbit heart induced by catecholamines is not greatly impaired by surgical or chemical sympathectomy (89, 101) has been regarded as evidence that the source of PGs released by nerve stimulation is strictly extraneuronal. However, none of the studies seems to provide evidence of a complete destruction of all the nerves. Moreover, it is unlikely that destruction of the nerves would significantly alter the total amount of PG overflowing stimulated tissues, because the nerves make up only a fraction of a percent of the total tissue mass. Therefore, possibly a small but nevertheless important fraction of the PGs overflowing from stimulated tissues is neuronal in origin. In fact, PGs have been demonstrated in several different types of nerve tissue (102). The observation that PG synthesis inhibitors enhance NE release by nerve stimulation in the guinea pig vas deferens even in the absence of visible contraction response also seems to support this view (103). On the other hand, it is not contradicted by the finding that α-adrenoceptor blockers abolish the release of PG, since α-adrenoceptors are both pre- and postjunctionally located (104–106). However, more experiments are needed before this issue can be settled.

The inhibitory effect of α-adrenoceptor blockers on PG release may be interesting also from another point of view. α-Adrenoceptor blockers powerfully enhance the release of NE by nerve stimulation (107), and concomitantly fortify the inhibitory effect of exogenous PGEs (8, 42), as would be expected after removal of a significant PGE-mediated feedback control of NE release. However, part of the enhancing effect of α-adrenoceptor blockers on NE release appears to be due to a PG-independent action on prejunctional α-adrenoceptors (45, 47, 108).

Action of Prostaglandin Synthesis Inhibitors

In the search for physiologically relevant functions of the PGs, the experimenter is greatly aided by the availability of specific PG antagonists or of PG synthesis inhibitors. Of these two approaches only the latter has so far proved to be promising.

The literature concerning drugs that inhibit PG biosynthesis has recently been reviewed (109). Principally, two classes of PG synthesis inhibitors have been used. One includes the aspirin-like drugs (110), which, although of diverse chemical structures, all share the analgesic, antipyretic, and anti-inflammatory actions which are characteristic of aspirin. The other consists mainly of substrate analogues, of which only one, the acetylenic derivative of arachidonic acid, 5,8,11,14-eicosatetrayonic acid (ETA) (111), has been tested for effects on adrenergic transmission.

In rabbit heart, feline spleen, and guinea pig vas deferens, ETA blocks the release of PGs and simultaneously enhances the release of NE induced by nerve stimulation (112–114). ETA also has been reported to enhance the release of NE induced by field stimulation in the rabbit iris (50).

Similarly, indomethacin and/or meclofenamic acid, members of the aspirin family, have been shown to increase the release of NE induced by nerve stimulation in the rabbit heart (115), guinea pig vas deferens (47, 116), rabbit kidney (30), and mesenteric arteries from cat and man (32, 33), but not in the feline spleen (117, 118).

The effects of PG synthesis inhibitors on effector responses to nerve stimulation have also been studied in most of the above-mentioned tissues, although the results are somewhat less consistent. The vasoconstrictor responses to nerve stimulation in rabbit kidney are either increased or unchanged by indomethacin (21, 30, 99). In the guinea pig vas deferens, only the initial part of the contraction response to nerve stimulation is markedly affected and enhanced, which is exactly opposite to the effects of exogenous PGEs (39, 96).

Contradictory results have been obtained in the rat kidney, where indomethacin has been reported both to enhance (119) and to inhibit (21) the vascular response to nerve stimulation. However, the results are logical in that exogenous PGEs also caused the opposite effects in the two studies, inhibition when indomethacin was the stimulant and enhancement when indomethacin caused inhibition. There are some inconsistencies in the effects of PG synthesis inhibitors also in the feline spleen. Thus, while ETA produces only enhancement of the vascular response to nerve stimulation, indomethacin or meclofenamic acid causes either enhancement (120, 121) or no effect at all (117, 118). The controversial observations with indomethacin in feline spleen and rat kidney are difficult to explain, although differences in strain, experimental procedure, and drug concentration might have contributed to the different results. In particular the use of indomethacin or meclofenamic acid is worth considering in this context, since they cannot be regarded as specific inhibitors of PG synthetase, but may affect other enzyme systems as well, at least in high concentrations (109).

In addition to the above-mentioned in vitro and in situ experiments, there are several in vivo studies pertaining to the action of PG synthesis inhibitors on adrenergic neurotransmission. Thus, indomethacin has been reported to increase urinary excretion of NE in rats, the animals being either cold-stressed or kept at room temperature (122, 123). There is good reason to believe that this hyperexcretion of NE was initially due to increased NE release from the adrenergic nerves. Only after several days did augmented adrenomedullary secretory activity (as reflected by an increase in urinary epinephrine and a fall in NE content of the adrenal medulla) contribute to the hypersecretion of NE.

Recently, an in vivo effect of indomethacin on adrenergic transmission has been more firmly established (124). Thus, oral administration of indomethacin increases NE turnover rate in a number of rat tissues, such as heart, spleen, submandibular gland, and adipose tissue. Since indomethacin had no effect on monoamine oxidase and catechol-O-methyl transferase activities, or on NE uptake in the different tissues, an action on NE disposition may be excluded. Therefore, the results suggest that indomethacin increased NE turnover, and hence the release of NE per nerve impulse, by blockade of a locally operating feedback inhibition of transmitter release mediated by PGEs. Although forming an important contribution to the concept of PG-mediated control of adrenergic transmission, the results do not exclude the possibility that indomethacin increases also the impulse traffic in the nerves. The significance of such an effect is lessened, however, by the fact that the effect of indomethacin on NE turnover in adipose tissue was low compared with that in heart, spleen, and submandibular gland.

In summary, the bulk of available in vitro and in vivo evidence indicates that inhibitors of PG synthesis increase the release of NE per nerve impulse as a consequence of inhibition of local PGE formation. Admittedly, indomethacin and meclofenamic acid are not exclusive inhibitors of PG synthetase, although the concentrations of these drugs required to inhibit the synthetase are generally much lower than the concentrations that inhibit other enzymes (109). ETA is presumably more specific in its action, but, on the other hand, its metabolic fate is largely unknown (109). However, the finding that members of both classes of PG synthesis inhibitors produce one and the same effect on NE release in several tissues, seems to minimize the possibility that they affect the release of NE by any mechanism other than inhibition of PG synthetase. This view is further supported by observations that PG synthesis inhibitors are unable to enhance NE release when it is sufficiently depressed by administrated PGEs and that the NE release mechanism is hyperreactive to the inhibitory effect of exogeneous PGEs when local PG synthesis is blocked (30, 113, 116). However, conflicting results have been presented and further extensive studies are certainly required before the concept of PG-mediated feedback control can be established as physiologically relevant in adrenergically innervated organs in general, or at least in certain tissues.

GANGLIONIC TRANSMISSION

The information about PG action on ganglionic transmission is sparse and even conflicting. PGE_1 and PGE_2 have been reported to have no effect on postganglionic action potentials elicited by preganglionic stimulation of the feline cervical sympathetic chain (125). On the other hand, the observation that PGE_1 is more prone to inhibit contractile responses to preganglionic than postganglionic nerve stimulation in the guinea pig vas deferens is consistent with PGE_1 interfering with ganglionic transmission (126).

Cardiovascular effects elicited by intracarotid infusion of PGE_1 in intact dogs, or in cross-circulation experiments, are abolished by ganglion blocking drugs (127, 128). At least part of these effects are presumably mediated by the central nervous system, where PGs are capable of either stimulating or inhibiting ganglionic transmission (129–131). Whether or not PGE_1 may have influenced also transmission in peripheral ganglia is not known.

The adrenal medullary cells are homologues to postganglionic nerve cells, and the nerve-effector cell junction may therefore be regarded as a specialized type of ganglionic transmission. It has been shown that PGE_1 and $PGF_{1\alpha}$ do not modify resting outflow or increased secretion of catecholamines induced by acetylcholine, potassium, or splanchnic nerve stimulation in the cat (132). On the other hand, it has been proposed that $PGF_{2\alpha}$ facilitates the adrenal medullary secretion of catecholamines induced by splanchnic nerve stimulation in the dog (52). In this case the venous effluent from the adrenal gland was allowed to perfuse the animal's isolated paw, and variations in perfusion pressure were used as an index of secreted catecholamines. Since $PGF_{2\alpha}$, given in small doses in the left ventricle of the heart, consistently enhanced the vasoconstrictor response to splanchnic nerve stimulation, but not to injected epinephrine, it was concluded that $PGF_{2\alpha}$ actually had facilitated the secretion of catecholamines from the adrenal medulla. Further studies, including direct analysis of catecholamine secretion from the adrenal medulla, are needed to confirm this interesting observation.

CHOLINERGIC NEUROEFFECTOR TRANSMISSION

PGE_1 has been shown to block the negative chronotropic effect of vagal nerve stimulation in the isolated rabbit heart, and in the guinea pig heart in situ (133, 134). In the rabbit study the effect of acetylcholine (ACh) was unaffected by PGE_1, and it was therefore concluded that PGE_1 exerted its effect mainly prejunctionally, that is, on ACh release from the nerve terminals (133). The observation that PGE release from the heart can be induced by vagal nerve stimulation and by ACh (the effect of the latter being blocked by atropine) has subsequently led to the proposal that PGEs might control cholinergic neuroeffector transmission in the heart in a way similar to that proposed for the adrenergic system (13, 135). At least the prejunctional target for such an effect has been questioned, since it has been observed that PGE_1 blocks chronotropic responses to both vagal nerve stimulation and ACh administration in guinea pig atria (136), and that PGE_2 has no effect on negative chronotropic responses (in the presence of propranolol) to electric stimulation of the rabbit sinoatrial node preparation (14). However, the original proposal of a prejunctional action (133) is supported by the recent finding that PGE_1 and PGE_2 inhibit the negative chronotropic responses to vagal nerve stimulation, but not to ACh, in the mouse heart in vivo (137). Further careful characterization of possible prejunctional and postjunctional actions of PGEs in these and other species are needed before this important issue can be settled. In this context it is worth mentioning the inhibitory effect of PGE_1 on gastric secretion induced by vagal nerve stimulation in the rat (138), since besides the heart this appears to be the only case where PGs have been reported to inhibit cholinergic responses. However, the PGs also inhibit the effect of various secretagogues (139), and the effect is presumably postjunctionally located or directly on the secretory cells.

In contrast to the antisecretory property, PGs generally stimulate gastrointestinal smooth muscle, although a few exceptions have been noted (140), and inhibition of

PG synthesis in the intestine is associated with a decrease in muscular tone (141–144). It has been argued that a low continuous PG synthesis may serve the function of maintaining the inherent tone, or that increased PG production might explain the hypermotility that occurs in various pathological conditions in the intestinal tract (141, 142).

Apart from directly affecting gastrointestinal smooth muscle, PGs have also been shown to influence the cholinergic neuroeffector transmission in this region. Thus, PGE_1 and PGE_2 enhance the contraction response to cholinergic nerve stimulation in guinea pig and rabbit ileum (51, 134, 144–146), while the effects on contractions induced by ACh are less clear; both enhanced and unchanged responses have been reported (51, 144). On the other hand, contraction responses to nerve stimulation or administration of angiotensin (a substance which partly acts by releasing ACh) are markedly reduced or almost abolished by indomethacin, and partially or completely restored by subsequent administration of small, subspasmogenic doses of PGE_1 and PGE_2 (134, 144, 147–150). The contraction response to ACh seems to be little affected by indomethacin (144, 151). Taken together, these observations provide evidence that PGEs stimulate cholinergic neuroeffector transmission in the intestinal tract, and imply that part of the stimulant effect is prejunctional on ACh release.

As an alternative to a presumed direct enhancement of ACh release, it has been suggested that PGEs affect ACh secretion indirectly by inhibiting the release of NE from adrenergic nerves (144). The experimental evidence for this assumption is that pretreatment with guanethidine or α-methyl-p-tyrosine (in order to block NE release) prevented the inhibitory effect of indomethacin on the muscular responses to cholinergic nerve stimulation. However, experiments in this laboratory (unpublished) have failed to confirm this observation. Indomethacin was found to be as potent in inhibiting the responses to cholinergic nerve stimulation after guanethidine treatment or degeneration of the adrenergic nerves with 6-hydroxydopamine, which implies that the inhibitory effect of indomethacin does not depend on the functional integrity of the adrenergic nerves.

Several attempts have been made to disclose a prejunctional effect of PGEs and indomethacin (or aspirin) by directly measuring the spontaneous and neurogenically induced release of ACh in the guinea pig ileum (51, 134, 136, 143, 149). However, in none of these studies was there any indication that PGE_1 and PGE_2 enhanced and indomethacin (or aspirin) reduced ACh release induced by nerve stimulation. The spontaneous release of ACh was also unchanged in most cases, although it occasionally decreased in the presence of indomethacin (143). Therefore, the observed effects of PGEs and PG synthesis inhibitors on cholinergic neurotransmission in the gut seem to be mostly, if not wholly, a postjunctional phenomenon.

PGE_1, PGE_2, $PGF_{2\alpha}$, and arachidonic acid all enhance contractions induced by cholinergic nerve stimulation and ACh in the sphincter muscle of the iris (152, 153). The effect of arachidonic acid is blocked by PG synthesis inhibitors, which in addition relax the muscle. PG release, both spontaneous and in response to nerve stimulation, has been noted (154). It is conceivable, therefore, that PGs serve the function of maintaining tone and enhancing motor transmission (presumably post-junctionally) in this muscle. The striking similarities in the actions of PGs and PG synthesis inhibitors in this tissue and the intestinal tract suggests that this might be a principle operating in cholinergically innervated smooth muscle in general.

A mediator role in the cholinergic transmission of salivary glands has been attributed to $PGF_{2\alpha}$ (155–157). This compound, ACh, and stimulation of the corda tympani all induce salivation and increased blood flow in the canine submandibular gland. Tetrodotoxin abolishes the responses to $PGF_{2\alpha}$ and corda tympani stimulation, while those to ACh remain unchanged. Whether or not this means that $PGF_{2\alpha}$ actually facilitates ACh release from the nerve terminals is not clear and can be settled only by direct measurement of ACh release.

CONCLUSION

PGEs are potent inhibitors of neurally induced NE release and effector responses in a great number of tissues. PGEs are also released from adrenergically innervated tissues, and there is considerable in vitro and in vivo evidence that inhibition of local PGE production is associated with increased NE release and effector responses to nerve activity. It is reasonable to assume that NE release from adrenergic terminals is controlled by a local PGE-mediated feedback mechanism, which operates through restriction of availability of calcium for the NE release process, and which seems to be particularly efficient within the "physiological" frequency range of nerve impulses. The fact that even heavy intake of aspirin-like drugs (considered to block almost completely PG synthesis) does not seriously jeopardize the function of adrenergically innervated organs must mean that PGEs are not of vital importance for these organ systems. Rather, the PGEs should be regarded as one of several local inhibitory feed-back control mechanisms that act jointly to regulate adrenergic transmission. PGs other than the PGEs (particularly PGF and PGB) do not appear to take part in this scheme, because their net effect on adrenergic transmission commonly is stimulant, and because they have little or no effect on NE release in concentrations which are of physiological interest. It is conceivable therefore that the spectrum of available PGs influences adrenergic neuroeffector transmission in such a way that, depending on the specialized function of the effector organ and the PG predominantly synthesized (and the level of its synthesis), the overall effect will be either inhibitory or stimulant.

Numerous investigations have dealt with PG action (principally PGE) on cholinergic neuroeffector junctions. On most occasions the effect appears to be stimulant, although vagally induced bradycardia and gastric secretion are inhibited by PGs, and thus seem to form important exceptions. The level of action may be pre- or postjunctional, although most investigations suggest that the latter is principally affected. Release of substantial amounts of PGs occurs from stimulated tissues, and PGs and PG synthesis inhibitors generally produce opposite effects on cholinergic neuroeffector junctions. These observations merit the assumption that this system also is subject to control by locally formed PGs.

Literature Cited

1. Euler, U. S. v. 1934. Zur Kenntnis der pharmakologischen Wirkungen von Nativsekreten und Extrakten männlicher accessorischer Geschlechtsdrüsen. *Naunyn-Schmiedebergs Arch. Exp. Pathol. Pharmakol.* 175:78–84
2. Goldblatt, M. W. 1933. A depressor substance in seminal fluid. *J. Soc. Chem. Ind. London* 52:1056–57
3. Euler, U.S. v. 1935. Über die spezifische blutdrucksenkende Substanz des menschlichen Prostata -und Samenblasensekretes. *Klin. Wochenschr.* 14:1182–83
4. Hedqvist, P. 1968. Reduced effector response to nerve stimulation in the cat spleen after administration of prostaglandin E_1. *Acta Physiol. Scand.* 74:7A
5. Brundin, J. 1968. The effect of prostaglandin E_1 on the response of the rabbit oviduct to hypogastric nerve stimulation. *Acta Physiol. Scand.* 73:54–57
6. Hedqvist, P., Brundin, J. 1969. Inhibition by prostaglandin E_1 of noradrenaline release and of effector response to nerve stimulation in the cat spleen. *Life Sci.* 8(Part 1):389–95
7. Moawad, A., Hedqvist, P., Bygdeman, M. 1975. Noradrenaline release following nerve stimulation and its modification by prostaglandin E_2 in human and rabbit oviduct. *Acta Physiol. Scand.* 95:142–44
8. Hedqvist, P., Moawad, A. 1975. Presynaptic α- and β-adrenoceptor mediated control of noradrenaline release in human oviduct. *Acta Physiol. Scand.* 95:494–96
9. Hedqvist, P. 1970. Control by prostaglandin E_2 of sympathetic neurotransmission in the spleen. *Life Sci.* 9(Part 1):269–78
10. Davies, B. N., Withrington, P. G. 1968. The effects of prostaglandin E_1 and E_2 on the smooth muscle of the dog spleen and on its responses to catecholamines, angiotensin and nerve stimulation. *Br. J. Pharmacol.* 32:136–44
11. Ferreira, S. H., Moncada, S., Vane, J. R. 1971. Indomethacin and aspirin abolish prostaglandin release from the spleen. *Nature New Biol.* 231:237–39
12. Hedqvist, P., Wennmalm, Å. 1971. Comparison of the effects of prostaglandins E_1, E_2 and $F_{2\alpha}$ on the sympathetically stimulated rabbit heart. *Acta Physiol. Scand.* 83:156–62
13. Wennmalm, Å. 1971. Studies on mechanisms controlling the secretion of neurotransmitters in the rabbit heart.

Acta Physiol. Scand. 82:Suppl. 365, pp. 1–36
14. Park, M. K., Dyer, D. C., Vincenzi, F. F. 1973. Prostaglandin E_2 and its antagonists: Effects on autonomic transmission in the isolated sino-atrial node. *Prostaglandins* 4:717–30
15. Westfall, T. C., Brasted, M. 1974. Specificity of blockade of the nicotine-induced release of ^3H-norepinephrine from adrenergic neurons of the guinea-pig heart by various pharmacological agents. *J. Pharmacol. Exp. Ther.* 189: 659–64
16. Weiner, R., Kaley, G. 1969. Influence of prostaglandin E_1 on the terminal vascular bed. *Am. J. Physiol.* 217:563–66
17. Messina, E. J., Weiner, R., Kaley, G. 1974. Microcirculatory effects of prostaglandins E_1, E_2, and A_1 in the rat mesentery and cremaster muscle. *Microvasc. Res.* 8:77–89
18. Strong, C. G., Chandler, J. T. 1972. Interactions of prostaglandin E_1 and catecholamines in isolated vascular smooth muscle. In *Prostaglandins in Cellular Biology*, ed. P. W. Ramwell, B. B. Pharriss, 369–83. New York: Plenum
19. Tobian, L., Viets, J. 1970. Potentiation of in vitro norepinephrine vasoconstriction with prostaglandin E_1. *Fed. Proc.* 29:387
20. Clark, K. E., Ryan, M. J., Brody, M. J. 1973. Effects of prostaglandins E_1 and $F_{2\alpha}$ on uterine hemodynamics and motility. *Adv. Biosci.* 9:779–82
21. Malik, K. U., McGiff, J. C. 1975. Modulation by prostaglandins of adrenergic transmission in the isolated perfused rabbit and rat kidney. *Circ. Res.* 36:599–609
22. Hedqvist, P. 1970. Inhibition by prostaglandin E_1 of vascular response to sympathetic nerve stimulation *in vivo*. *Acta Physiol. Scand.* 80:6A
23. Hedqvist, P. 1972. Prostaglandin-induced inhibition of vascular tone and reactivity in the cat's hindleg in vivo. *Eur. J. Pharmacol.* 17:157–62
24. Hedwall, P. R., Abdel-Sayed, W. A., Schmid, P. G., Mark, A. L., Abboud, F. M. 1971. Vascular responses to prostaglandin E_1 in gracilis muscle and hindpaw of the dog. *Am. J. Physiol.* 221:42–47
25. Kadowitz, P. J., Sweet, C. S., Brody, M. J. 1971. Blockade of adrenergic vasoconstrictor responses in the dog by

prostaglandins E_1 and A_1. *J. Pharmacol. Exp. Ther.* 179:563–72

26. Kadowitz, P. J. 1972. Effect of prostaglandins E_1, E_2 and A_2 on vascular resistance and responses to noradrenaline, nerve stimulation and angiotensin in the dog hindlimb. *Br. J. Pharmacol.* 46:395–400

27. Frame, M. H., Hedqvist, P., Åström, A. 1974. Effect of prostaglandin E_2 on vascular responses of the rabbit kidney to nerve stimulation and noradrenaline, *in vitro* and *in situ*. *Life Sci.* 15:239–44

28. Lonigro, A. J., Terragno, N. A., Malik, K. U., McGiff, J. C. 1973. Differential inhibition by prostaglandins of the renal actions of pressor stimuli. *Prostaglandins* 3:595–606

29. Chapnic, B. M., Paustian, P. W., Klainer, E., Joiner, P. D., Hyman, A. L., Kadowitz, P. J. 1976. Influence of prostaglandins E, A and F on vasoconstrictor responses to norepinephrine, renal nerve stimulation and angiotensin in the feline kidney. *J. Pharmacol. Exp. Ther.* 196:44–52

30. Frame, M. H., Hedqvist, P. 1975. Evidence for prostaglandin mediated prejunctional control of renal vascular sympathetic tone. *Br. J. Pharmacol.* 54:189–96

31. Hadházy, P., Magyar, K., Vizi, E. S., Knoll, J. 1976. Inhibitory effects of prostaglandin E_1 on responses of rabbit ear artery to nerve stimulation and on release of norepinephrine. In *Advances in Prostaglandin and Thromboxane Research*, ed. B. Samuelsson, R. Paoletti, 1,2:365–68. New York: Raven. 1028 pp.

32. Hedqvist, P. 1974. Effect of prostaglandins and prostaglandin synthesis inhibitors on norepinephrine release from vascular tissue. In *Prostaglandin Synthetase Inhibitors*, ed. H. J. Robinson, J. R. Vane, 303–9. New York: Raven. 395 pp.

33. Stjärne, L., Gripe, K. 1973. Prostaglandin-dependent and -independent feedback control of noradrenaline secretion in vasoconstrictor nerves of normotensive human subjects. *Naunyn-Schmiedebergs Arch. Pharmacol.* 280:441–46

34. Fredholm, B. B., Hedqvist, P. 1973. Role of pre- and postjunctional inhibition by prostaglandin E_2 of lipolysis induced by sympathetic nerve stimulation in dog subcutaneous adipose tissue *in situ*. *Br. J. Pharmacol.* 47:711–18

35. Kadowitz, P. J., Sweet, C. S., Brody, M. J. 1971. Differential effects of prosta-

glandins E_1, E_2, $F_{1\alpha}$ and $F_{2\alpha}$ on adrenergic vasoconstriction in the dog hindpaw. *J. Pharmacol. Exp. Ther.* 177:641–49

36. Blakeley, A. G. H., Brown, G. L., Dearnaley, D. P., Woods, R. I. 1968. The use of prostaglandin E_1 in perfusion of the spleen with blood. *J. Physiol. London* 198:31P–32P

37. Horrobin, D. F., Manku, M. S., Karmali, R., Nassar, B. A., Davies, P. A. 1974. Aspirin, indomethacin, catecholamine and prostaglandin interactions on rat arterioles and rabbit hearts. *Nature* 250:425–26

38. Euler, U. S. v., Hedqvist, P. 1969. Inhibitory action of prostaglandins E_1 and E_2 on the neuromuscular transmission in the guinea pig vas deferens. *Acta Physiol. Scand.* 77:510–12

39. Hedqvist, P., Euler, U. S. v. 1972. Prostaglandin-induced neurotransmission failure in the field-stimulated, isolated vas deferens. *Neuropharmacology* 11:177–87

40. Ambache, N., Zar, M. A. 1970. An inhibitory effect of prostaglandin E_2 on neuromuscular transmission in the guinea-pig vas deferens. *J. Physiol. London* 208:30P–32P

41. Baum, T., Shropshire, A. T. 1971. Influence of prostaglandins on autonomic responses. *Am. J. Physiol.* 221:1470–75

42. Hedqvist, P. 1972. Prostaglandin induced inhibition of neurotransmission in the isolated guinea pig seminal vesicle. *Acta Physiol. Scand.* 84:506–11

43. Ambache, N., Zar, M. A. 1971. Evidence against adrenergic motor transmission in the guinea-pig vas deferens. *J. Physiol. London* 216:359–89

44. Euler, U. S. v., Hedqvist, P. 1975. Evidence for an α- and β_2-receptor mediated inhibition of the twitch response in the guinea pig vas deferens by noradrenaline. *Acta Physiol. Scand.* 93:572–73

45. Hedqvist, P. 1973. Aspects of prostaglandin and α-receptor mediated control of transmitter release from adrenergic nerves. In *Frontiers in Catecholamine Research*, ed. E. Usdin, S. Snyder, 583–87. New York: Pergamon. 1219 pp.

46. Hedqvist, P. 1974. Prostaglandin action on noradrenaline release and mechanical responses in the stimulated guinea pig vas deferens. *Acta Physiol. Scand.* 90:86–93

47. Stjärne, L. 1973. Prostaglandin- versus α-adrenoceptor-mediated control of

sympathetic neurotransmitter secretion in guinea-pig isolated vas deferens. *Eur. J. Pharmacol.* 22:233–38

48. Stjärne, L. 1973. Frequency dependence of dual negative feedback control of secretion of sympathetic neurotransmitter in guinea-pig vas deferens. *Br. J. Pharmacol.* 49:358–60

49. Bergström, S., Farnebo, L. O., Fuxe, K. 1973. Effect of prostaglandin E_2 on central and peripheral catecholamine neurons. *Eur. J. Pharmacol.* 21:362–68

50. Neufeld, A. H., Page, E. D. 1975. Regulation of adrenergic neuromuscular transmission in the rabbit iris. *Exp. Eye Res.* 20:549–61

51. Illés, P., Vizi, E. S., Knoll, J. 1974. Adrenergic neuroeffector junctions sensitive and insensitive to the effect of PGE_1. *Pol. J. Pharmacol. Pharm.* 26:127–36

52. Brody, M. J., Kadowitz, P. J. 1974. Prostaglandins as modulators of the autonomic nervous system. *Fed. Proc.* 33:48–60

53. Ducharme, D. W., Weeks, J. R., Montgomery, R. G. 1968. Studies on the mechanism of the hypertensive effect of prostaglandin $F_{2\alpha}$. *J. Pharmacol. Exp. Ther.* 160:1–10

54. Davies, B. N., Withrington, P. G. 1969. Actions of prostaglandins A_1, A_2, E_1, E_2, $F_{1\alpha}$ and $F_{2\alpha}$ on splenic vascular and capsular smooth muscle and their interactions with sympathetic nerve stimulation, catecholamines and angiotensin. In *Prostaglandins, Peptides and Amines,* ed. P. Mantegazza, E. W. Horton, 53–56. London: Academic. 191 pp.

55. Kadowitz, P. J., George, W. J., Joiner, P. D., Hyman, A. L. 1973. Effect of prostaglandins E_1 and $F_{2\alpha}$ on adrenergic responses in the pulmonary circulation. *Adv. Biosci.* 9:501–6

56. Kadowitz, P. J., Sweet, C. S., Brody, M. J. 1971. Potentiation of adrenergic venomotor responses by angiotensin, prostaglandin $F_{2\alpha}$ and cocaine. *J. Pharmacol. Exp. Ther.* 176:167–73

57. Hedqvist, P. 1976. Prostaglandin action on transmitter release at adrenergic neuroeffector junctions. See Ref. 31, pp. 357–63

58. Frame, M. H. 1976. A comparison of the effects of prostaglandins A_2, E_2, and $F_{2\alpha}$ on the sympathetic neuroeffector system of the isolated rabbit kidney. See Ref. 31, pp. 369–73

59. Lee, J. B. 1976. The renal prostaglandins and blood pressure regulation. See Ref. 31, pp. 573–85

60. Greenberg, S., Engelbrecht, J. A., Wilson, W. R. 1974. Prostaglandin B_2-induced cutaneous vasoconstriction of the canine hind paw. *Circ. Res.* 34:491–97

61. Greenberg, S., Howard, L., Wilson, W. R. 1974. Comparative effects of prostaglandins A_2 and B_2 on vascular and airway resistances and adrenergic neurotransmission. *Can. J. Physiol. Pharmacol.* 52:699–705

62. Robinson, B. F., Collier, J. G., Karim, S. M. M., Somers, K. 1973. Effect of prostaglandins A_1, A_2, B_1, E_2 and $F_{2\alpha}$ on forearm arterial bed and superficial hand veins of man. *Clin. Sci.* 44:367–76

63. Bhagat, B., Dhalla, N. S., Ginn, D., La Montagne, A. E., Montier, A. D. 1972. Modification by prostaglandin E_2 (PGE$_2$) of the response of guinea-pig isolated vasa deferentia and atria to adrenergic stimuli. *Br. J. Pharmacol.* 44:689–98

64. Hedqvist, P. 1970. Antagonism by calcium of the inhibitory action of prostaglandin E_2 on sympathetic neurotransmission in the cat spleen. *Acta Physiol. Scand.* 80:269–75

65. Stjärne, L. 1973. Comparison of secretion of sympathetic neurotransmitter induced by nerve stimulation with that evoked by high potassium, as triggers of dual alpha-adrenoceptor mediated negative feed-back control of noradrenaline secretion. *Prostaglandins* 3:421–26

66. Kirpekar, S. M., Misu, Y. 1967. Release of noradrenaline by splenic nerve stimulation and its dependence on calcium. *J. Physiol. London* 188:219–34

67. Simpson, L. L. 1968. The role of calcium in neurohumoral and neurohormonal extrusion processes. *J. Pharm. Pharmacol.* 20:889–910

68. Hubbard, J. I. 1970. Mechanism of transmitter release. *Progr. Biophys. Mol. Biol.* 21:33–124

69. Johnson, D. G., Thoa, N. B., Weinshilboum, R., Axelrod, J., Kopin, I. J. 1971. Enhanced release of dopamine-β-hydoxylase from sympathetic nerves by calcium and phenoxybenzamine and its reversal by prostaglandins. *Proc. Natl. Acad. Sci. USA* 68:2227–30

70. Hedqvist, P. 1974. Interaction between prostaglandins and calcium ions on noradrenaline release from the stimulated guinea pig vas deferens. *Acta Physiol. Scand.* 90:153–57

71. Stjärne, L. 1973. Michaelis-Menten kinetics of secretion of sympathetic neurotransmitter as a function of

external calcium: Effect of graded alpha-adrenoceptor blockade. *Naunyn-Schmiedebergs Arch. Pharmacol.* 278: 323–27

72. Stjärne, L. 1973. Kinetics of secretion of sympathetic neurotransmitter as a function of external calcium: Mechanism of inhibitory effect of prostaglandin E. *Acta. Physiol. Scand.* 87:428–30

73. Junstad, M., Wennmalm, Å. 1973. Prostaglandin mediated inhibition of noradrenaline release at different impulse frequencies. *Acta Physiol. Scand.* 89:544–49

74. Katz, B., Miledi, R. 1968. The role of calcium in neuromuscular facilitation. *J. Physiol. London* 195:481–92

75. Koketsu, K. 1958. Action of tetraethylammonium chloride on neuromuscular transmission in frogs. *Am. J. Physiol.* 193:213–15

76. Baker, P. F., Hodgkin, A. L., Shaw, T. I. 1962. The effect of changes in internal ionic concentrations on the electrical properties of perfused giant axons. *J. Physiol. London* 164:335–74

77. Hedqvist, P. 1976. Further evidence that prostaglandins inhibit the release of noradrenaline from adrenergic nerve terminals by restriction of availability of calcium. *Br. J. Pharmacol.* 58:599–603

78. Katz, B., Miledi, R. 1967. The release of acetylcholine from nerve endings by graded electric pulses. *Proc. R. Soc. London Ser. B.* 167:23–28

79. Katz, B., Miledi, R. 1967. A study of synaptic transmission in the absence of nerve impulses. *J. Physiol. London* 192:407–36

80. Clegg, P. C., Hall, W. J., Pickles, V. R. 1966. The action of ketonic prostaglandins on the guinea-pig myometrium. *J. Physiol. London* 183:123–44

81. Sjöstrand, N. 1972. A note on the dual effect of prostaglandin E_1 on the motor responses of the guinea-pig vas deferens to nerve stimulation. *Experientia* 28: 431–32

82. Taylor, G. S., Einhorn, V. F. 1972. The effect of prostaglandins on junction potentials in the mouse vas deferens. *Eur. J. Pharmacol.* 20:40–45

83. Kecskemeti, V., Kelemen, K., Knoll, J. 1974. Microelectrophysiological analysis of the cardiac effect of prostaglandin E_2. *Pol. J. Pharmacol. Pharm.* 26: 171–76

84. Kecskemeti, V., Kelemen, K., Knoll, J. 1973. Effect of prostaglandin E_1 on the transmembrane potentials of the mammalian heart. *Adv. Biosci.* 9:373–77

85. Stjärne, L. 1973. Inhibitory effect of prostaglandin E_2 on noradrenaline secretion from sympathetic nerves as a function of external calcium. *Prostaglandins* 3:105–9

86. Davies, B. N., Horton, E. W., Withrington, P. G. 1967. The occurrence of prostaglandin E_2 in splenic venous blood of the dog following splenic nerve stimulation. *J. Physiol. London* 188:38P–39P

87. Davies, B. N., Horton, E. W., Withrington, P. G. 1968. The occurrence of prostaglandin E_2 in splenic venous blood of the dog following splenic nerve stimulation. *Br. J. Pharmacol.* 32:127–35

88. Ferreira, S. H., Vane, J. R. 1967. Prostaglandins: Their disappearance from and release into the circulation. *Nature* 216:868–73

89. Gilmore, N., Vane, J. R., Wyllie, J. H. 1968. Prostaglandins released by the spleen. *Nature* 218:1135–40

90. Gryglewski, R. J., Korbut, R. 1973. Prostaglandin feedback mechanism limits vasoconstrictor action of norepinephrine. *Experientia* 31:89–91

91. Dunham, E. W., Zimmermann, B. G. 1970. Release of prostaglandin-like material from dog kidney during renal nerve stimulation. *Am. J. Physiol.* 219:1279–85

92. Davis, H. A., Horton, E. W. 1972. Output of prostaglandins from the rabbit kidney, its increase on renal nerve stimulation and its inhibition by indomethacin. *Br. J. Pharmacol.* 46: 658–75

93. Shaw, J. E., Ramwell, P. W. 1968. Release of prostaglandin from rat epididymal fat pad on nervous and hormonal stimulation. *J. Biol. Chem.* 243:1498–1503

94. Fredholm, B. B., Rosell, S., Strandberg, K. 1970. Release of prostaglandin-like material from canine subcutaneous adipose tissue by nerve stimulation. *Acta Physiol. Scand.* 79:18A–19A

95. Hedqvist, P., Euler, U. S. v. 1972. Prostaglandin controls neuromuscular transmission on guinea-pig vas deferens. *Nature New Biol.* 236:113–15

96. Swedin, G. 1971. Endogenous inhibition of the mechanical response of the isolated rat and guinea-pig vas deferens to pre- and postganglionic nerve stimulation. *Acta Physiol. Scand.* 83:473–85

97. Hedqvist, P. 1970. Studies on the effect of prostaglandins E_1 and E_2 on the sympathetic neuromuscular transmission in some animal tissues. *Acta Physiol. Scand.* 79:Suppl.345, pp. 1–40

98. Lee, S. C., Levine, L. 1974. Prostaglandin metabolism: Cytoplasmic reduced nicotinamide adenine dinucleotide phosphate-dependent and microsomal reduced nicotinamide dinucleotide-dependent prostaglandin E 9-ketoreductase activities in monkey and pigeon tissues. *J. Biol. Chem.* 249:1369–75

99. Needleman, P., Douglas, J. R., Jakschik, B., Stocklein, P. B., Johnson, E. M. 1974. Release of renal prostaglandin by catecholamines: Relationship to renal endocrine function. *J. Pharmacol. Exp. Ther.* 188:453–60

100. Piper, P., Vane, J. 1971. The release of prostaglandins from lung and other tissues. *Ann. NY Acad. Sci.* 180:363–85

101. Junstad, M., Wennmalm, Å. 1973. On the release of prostaglandin E_2 from the rabbit heart following infusion of noradrenaline. *Acta Physiol. Scand.* 87:573–74

102. Karim, S. M. M., Hillier, K., Devlin, J. 1968. Distribution of prostaglandins E_1, E_2, $F_{1\alpha}$ and $F_{2\alpha}$ in some animal tissues. *J. Pharm. Pharmacol.* 20:749–53

103. Stjärne, L. 1972. Prostaglandin E restricting noradrenaline secretion—neural in origin. *Acta Physiol. Scand.* 86:574–76

104. Farnebo, L. O., Malmfors, T. 1971. ^{3}H-noradrenaline release and mechanical response in the field stimulated mouse vas deferens. *Acta Physiol. Scand.* 83:Suppl. 371, pp. 1–18

105. Enero, M. A., Langer, S. Z., Rothlin, R. P., Stefano, F. J. E. 1972. Role of the α-adrenoceptor in regulating noradrenaline overflow by nerve stimulation. *Br. J. Pharmacol.* 44:672–88

106. Starke, K. 1972. Influence of extracellular noradrenaline on the stimulation-evoked secretion of noradrenaline from sympathetic nerves: Evidence for an α-receptor-mediated feed-back inhibition of noradrenaline release. *Naunyn-Schmiedebergs Arch. Pharmacol.* 275:11–23

107. Brown, G. L., Gillespie, J. S. 1957. The output of sympathetic transmitter from the spleen of the cat. *J. Physiol. London* 138:81–102

108. Starke, K., Montel, H. 1973. Sympathomimetic inhibition of noradrenaline release: Mediated by prostaglandins? *Naunyn-Schmiedebergs Arch. Pharmacol.* 278:111–16

109. Flower, R. J. 1974. Drugs which inhibit prostaglandin biosynthesis. *Pharmacol. Rev.* 26:33–67

110. Vane, J. R. 1971. Inhibition of prostaglandin synthesis as a mechanism of action for aspirin-like drugs. *Nature New Biol.* 231:232–35

111. Downing, D. T., Ahern, D. G., Bachta, M. 1970. Enzyme inhibition by acetylenic compounds. *Biochem. Biophys. Res. Commun.* 40:218–23

112. Samuelsson, B., Wennmalm, Å. 1971. Increased nerve stimulation induced release of noradrenaline from the rabbit heart after inhibition of prostaglandin synthesis. *Acta Physiol. Scand.* 83:163–68

113. Hedqvist, P., Stjärne, L., Wennmalm, A. 1971. Facilitation of sympathetic neurotransmission in the cat spleen after inhibition of prostaglandin synthesis. *Acta Physiol. Scand.* 83:430–32

114. Hedqvist, P. 1973. Prostaglandin mediated control of sympathetic neuroeffector transmission. *Adv. Biosci.* 9:461–73

115. Chanh, P. H., Junstad, M., Wennmalm, Å. 1972. Augmented noradrenaline release following nerve stimulation after inhibition of prostaglandin synthesis with indomethacin. *Acta Physiol. Scand.* 86:563–67

116. Fredholm, B., Hedqvist, P. 1973. Increased release of noradrenaline from stimulated guinea pig vas deferens after indomethacin treatment. *Acta Physiol. Scand.* 87:570–72

117. Hoszowska, A., Panczenko, B. 1974. Effects of inhibition of prostaglandin biosynthesis on noradrenaline release from isolated perfused spleen of the cat. *Pol. J. Pharmacol. Pharm.* 26:137–42

118. Dubocovich, M. L., Langer, S. Z. 1975. Evidence against a physiological role of prostaglandins in the regulation of noradrenaline release in the cat spleen. *J. Physiol. London* 251:737–62

119. Needleman, P., Marshall, G. R., Johnson, E. M. 1974. Determinants and modification of adrenergic and vascular resistance in the kidney. *Am. J. Physiol.* 227:665–69

120. Ferreira, S. H., Moncada, S. 1971. Inhibition of prostaglandin synthesis augments the effects of sympathetic nerve stimulation in the cat spleen. *Br. J. Pharmacol.* 43:419P–20P

121. Ferreira, S. H., Moncada, S., Vane, J. R. 1973. Some effects of inhibiting endogenous prostaglandin formation on the responses of the cat spleen. *Br. J. Pharmacol.* 47:48–58

122. Stjärne, L. 1972. Enhancement by indomethacin of cold-induced hyper-

secretion of noradrenaline in the rat *in vivo*—by suppression of PGE mediated feed-back control? *Acta Physiol. Scand.* 86:388–97

123. Junstad, M., Wennmalm, Å. 1972. Increased renal excretion of noradrenaline in rats after treatment with prostaglandin synthesis inhibitor indomethacin. *Acta Physiol. Scand.* 85:573–78

124. Fredholm, B. B., Hedqvist, P. 1975. Indomethacin-induced increase in noradrenaline turnover in some rat organs. *Br. J. Pharmacol.* 54:295–300

125. Kayaalp, S. O., McIsaac, R. J. 1968. Absence of effects of prostaglandins E_1, and E_2 on ganglionic transmission. *Eur. J. Pharmacol.* 4:283–88

126. Swedin, G. 1971. Studies on neurotransmission mechanisms in the rat and guinea-pig vas deferens. *Acta Physiol. Scand.* 83:Suppl. 369, pp. 1–34

127. Carlson, L. A., Orö, L. 1966. Effect of prostaglandin E_1 on blood pressure and heart rate in the dog. *Acta Physiol. Scand.* 67:89–99

128. Kaplan, H. R., Grega, G. J., Sherman, G. P., Buckley, J. P. 1969. Central and reflexogenic cardiovascular actions of prostaglandin E_1. *Int. J. Neuropharmacol.* 8:15–24

129. Duda, P., Horton, E. W., McPherson, A. 1968. The effects of prostaglandins E_1, $F_{1\alpha}$ and $F_{2\alpha}$ on monosynaptic reflexes. *J. Physiol. London* 196:151–62

130. Coceani, F., Dreifuss, J. J., Puglisi, L., Wolfe, L. S. 1969. Prostaglandins and membrane function. See Ref. 54, pp. 73–84

131. Coceani, F., Viti, A. 1973. Actions of prostaglandin E_1 on spinal neurons in the frog. *Adv. Biosci.* 9:481–87

132. Miele, E. 1969. Lack of effect of prostaglandin E_1 and $F_{1\alpha}$ on adreno-medullary catecholamine secretion evoked by various agents. See Ref. 54, pp. 85–93

133. Wennmalm, Å., Hedqvist, P. 1971. Inhibition by prostaglandin E_1 of parasympathetic neurotransmission in the rabbit heart. *Life Sci.* 10(Part I):465–70

134. Hall, W. J., O'Neill, P., Sheehan, J. D. 1975. The role of prostaglandins in cholinergic neurotransmission in the guinea pig. *Eur. J. Pharmacol.* 34:39–47

135. Junstad, M., Wennmalm, Å. 1974. Release of prostaglandin from the rabbit isolated heart following vagal nerve stimulation or acetylcholine infusion. *Br. J. Pharmacol.* 52:375–79

136. Hadházy, P., Illés, P., Knoll, J. 1973. The effects of PGE_1 on responses to cardiac vagus nerve stimulation and acetyl-

choline release. *Eur. J. Pharmacol.* 23:251–55

137. Feniuk, W., Large, B. J. 1975. The effects of prostaglandins E_1, E_2 and $F_{2\alpha}$ on vagal bradycardia in the anaesthetized mouse. *Br. J. Pharmacol.* 55:47–49

138. Shaw, J. E., Ramwell, P. W. 1968. Inhibition of gastric secretion in rats by prostaglandin E_1. In *Prostaglandin Symposium of the Worcester Foundation for Experimental Biology*, ed. P. W. Ramwell, J. E. Shaw, 55–66. New York: Wiley. 402 pp.

139. Robert, A. 1968. Antisecretory property of prostaglandins. See Ref. 138, pp. 47–54

140. Bennett, A. 1972. Effects of prostaglandins on the gastro-intestinal tract. In *The Prostaglandins, Progress in Research*, ed. S. M. M. Karim, 205–21. Oxford: Med. Tech. Publ. 327 pp.

141. Ferreira, S. H., Herman, A., Vane, J. R. 1972. Prostaglandin generation maintains the smooth muscle tone of the rabbit isolated jejunum. *Br. J. Pharmacol.* 44:328P–29P

142. Ferreira, S. H., Herman, A. G., Vane, J. R. 1976. Prostaglandin production by rabbit isolated jejunum and its relationship to the inherent tone of the preparation. *Br. J. Pharmacol.* 56:469–77

143. Botting, J. H., Salzmann, R. 1974. The effect of indomethacin on the release of prostaglandin E_2 and acetylcholine from guinea-pig isolated ileum at rest and during field stimulation. *Br. J. Pharmacol.* 50:119–24

144. Kadlec, O., Masek, K., Šeferna, I. 1974. A modulating role of prostaglandins in contractions of the guinea-pig ileum. *Br. J. Pharmacol.* 51:565–70

145. Harry, J. D. 1968. The action of prostaglandin E_1 on the guinea-pig isolated intestine. *Br. J. Pharmacol.* 33:213P–14P

146. Hedqvist, P., Persson, N. Å. 1975. Prostaglandin action on adrenergic and cholinergic responses in the rabbit and guinea pig intestine. In *Chemical Tools in Catecholamine Research*, ed. O. Almgren, A. Carlsson, J. Engel, 2:211–18. Amsterdam: North-Holland. 310 pp.

147. Chong, E. K. S., Downing, O. A. 1974. Reversal by prostaglandin E_2 of the inhibitory effect of indomethacin on contractions of the guinea-pig ileum induced by angiotensin. *J. Pharm. Pharmacol.* 26:729–30

148. Ehrenpreis, S., Greenberg, J., Belman, S. 1973. Prostaglandins reverse inhibiton of electrically-induced contractions of guinea pig ileum by morphine, indomethacin and acetylsalicylic acid. *Nature New Biol.* 245:280–82

149. Hazra, J. 1975. Evidence against prostaglandin E having a physiological role in acetylcholine liberation from Auerbach's plexus of guinea-pig ileum. *Experientia* 31:565–66

150. Bennett, A., Eley, K. G., Stockley, H. L. 1975. Modulation by prostaglandins of contractions in guinea-pig ileum. *Prostaglandins* 9:377–84

151. Chong, E. K. S., Downing, O. A. 1973. Selective inhibition of angiotensin-induced contractions of smooth muscle by indomethacin. *J. Pharm. Pharmacol.* 25:170–71

152. Gustafsson, L., Hedqvist, P., Lagercrantz, H. 1975. Potentiation by prostaglandins E_1, E_2 and $F_{2\alpha}$ of the contraction response to transmural stimulation in the bovine iris sphincter muscle. *Acta Physiol. Scand.* 95:26–33

153. Gustafsson, L., Hedqvist, P. 1975. Prostaglandin formation participates in the control of tone and contractility in the iris sphincter muscle. *Acta Physiol. Scand.* 95:56A

154. Posner, J. 1973. Prostaglandin E_2 and the bovine sphincter pupillae. *Br. J. Pharmacol.* 49:415–27

155. Hahn, R. A., Patil, P. N. 1972. Salivation induced by prostaglandin $F_{2\alpha}$ and modification of the response by atropine and physostigmine. *Br. J. Pharmacol.* 44:527–33

156. Hahn, R. A., Patil, P. N. 1974. Further observations on the interaction of prostaglandin $F_{2\alpha}$ with cholinergic mechanisms in canine salivary glands. *Eur. J. Pharmacol.* 25:279–86

157. Taira, N., Satoh, S. 1973. Prostaglandin $F_{2\alpha}$ as a potent excitant of the parasympathetic postganglionic neurons of the dog salivary gland. *Life Sci.* 13:501–6

Ann. Rev. Pharmacol. Toxicol. 1977. 17:281–91

THYMIC HORMONES: ❖6680
BIOCHEMISTRY, AND BIOLOGICAL
AND CLINICAL ACTIVITIES[1]

Jean-François Bach
Inserm U 25, Hôpital Necker, 75730 Paris, France

It is now well demonstrated that the thymus plays a central role in the immune system. Thymus-derived cells (or T cells) mediate delayed hypersensitivity reactions and the rejection of allografts and certain tumors. In addition, they regulate antibody production by bone marrow–derived cells (B cells) either positively as helper cells or negatively as suppressor cells. Abnormalities in their function are considered to be at the origin of many pathological situations including some immunodeficiency syndromes, autoimmune diseases, and numerous acute or chronic infections. It is obvious that any means of manipulating T-cell production by the thymus could be of great help to the clinician.

The mode of action of the thymus in the manufacture of T-cells is still incompletely known. There is, however, increasing evidence that the thymus gland produces humoral factors capable of modifying various functions of thymocytes. Many of these factors, which are secreted by the thymic epithelium, are involved in T-cell diffentiation even if they do not represent the exclusive mode of action of the thymus (the role of direct contact of T-cell precursors with the thymic microenvironment cannot be excluded) (1–3).

Several groups have characterized thymic factors (generally from calf thymus glands) and have provided various data on their biochemical nature and their biological activities. Some preliminary clinical trials have been performed. We review these data, on a pharmacological basis, rather than discuss the indirect ap-

---

[1]The following abbreviations are used in this review: ARFC, autologous rosette-forming cell; ATS, antithymocyte serum; BM, bonemarrow; BSA, bovine serum albumin; B/W, black/white; DNP, dinitrophenol; GVH, graft versus host; MLC, mixed lymphocyte culture; MSV, Moloney sarcoma virus; NZB, New Zealand black; PBS, phosphate balanced solution; SDS, sodium dodecyl sulfate; SLE, systemic lupus erythematosus; SRBC, sheep red blood cells; TF, thymic factor; and THF, thymic humoral factor.

proaches of the thymic hormone concept and the site of thymic hormone action in T-cell differentiation (see 1–3).

PREPARATION, ASSAY, AND BIOCHEMISTRY OF THYMIC FACTORS

As mentioned above, several groups of investigators have reported biological activities of thymic extracts or of circulating thymic factors. It is difficult to compare these data because the original source of material varies and especially because the assays utilized are very different. Also, the data presented in this section do not necessarily apply to products used in the biological assays presented in the next section, since functional studies were often performed with relatively crude extracts even if the same authors have reported on more refined and sophisticated preparations. In other words, there is a possibility that many of the biological effects described with thymic extracts are not due to the purified and well-characterized entity present in the crude extract and identified on the basis of another assay.

A. L. Goldstein and White's "Thymosin"

BIOASSAY   The bioassay utilized by Goldstein, Slater & White until 1971 was a "lymphocyte poietic" assay consisting of measuring DNA synthesis by lymph nodes after in vivo injection of the tested extract (4). More recently, these authors have used in vitro rosette assays (5) and an MLC assay (6).

ISOLATION   Calf thymic tissue is homogenized in 0.15 M NaCl and centrifuged at 14,000 g. The supernatant is heated at 80°C and precipitated by acetone. The precipitate is removed by centrifugation and the supernatant is added with ammonium sulfate. The precipitate is collected and dissolved in Tris Cl buffer before being desalted on Sephadex® G-25. This material (called *fraction 5*) has been routinely used in most studies dealing with biological thymosin activities. Further purification has been performed in some studies using DEAE cellulose, Sephadex G-50, and polyacrylamide gel electrophoresis (7).

BIOCHEMICAL CHARACTERISTICS   The purity of the last *fraction* has been assessed by analytical polyacrylamide gel filtration: one single band is visible at pH 8.3 or pH 2.9. Estimates of molecular weight have been done on polyacrylamide gels containing 0.1% SDS. By comparison with several markers it was assumed that thymosin (*fraction 8*) has a molecular weight of approximately 12,000. Amino acid analysis revealed that the molecule was rich in acidic residues, contained not unusual amino acids, and only one tyrosyl residue. The terminal amino acid is blocked (7).

N. Trainin's Thymic Humoral Factor

BIOASSAY   Bioassay is an in vitro model of graft versus host reaction primitively developed to study the immunocompetence of isolated lymphoid cell populations: competent T cells normally induce in vitro an increase in an allogeneic spleen explant whereas spleen cells from neonatally thymectomized mice do not achieve it except if they are previously incubated with thymic extracts (8, 26).

ISOLATION   Thymus glands are cleaned of blood vessels and connective tissues, homogenized in a Virtis® blender in PBS, and centrifuged for 20 min at 2,500 g. The supernatant is strained through gauze and centrifuged again at 100,000 g for 5 hr. The supernatant collected after this ultracentifugation step is then passed through Millipore® filters of 0.45 μm porosity. The last dialysis purification step is based upon the fact that the active material is of low molecular weight and therefore passes through cellophane dialysis bags. Further purification has been achieved for THF biochemical characterization, using Sephadex G-25 and DEAE-Sephadex A-25 chromatography (9, 10, 26).

BIOCHEMICAL CHARACTERISTICS   Purity of the material obtained has been analyzed by isoelectric focusing on polyacrilamide gel. It is probably a polypeptide since it is destroyed by proteolytic enzymes and not by ribonuclease or deoxyribonu-clease. The amino acid analysis reveals the presence of Asp, Ser, Glu, and Gly in large amounts. The pH is acidic (between 5.7 and 5.9). Its molecular weight is certainly less than 10,000 from dialysis data and close to 3,000 from G-25 data. However Sephadex G-25 does not provide precise evaluation of molecular weight and it is not possible from present data to differentiate between THF with a reported molecular weight of close to 3000 and a circulating thymic factor (see section on the circulating thymic factor) (9).

G. Goldstein's Thymopoietins I and II

BIOASSAY   Patients with myasthenia gravis show symptoms of motor weakness as a result of a partial failure of neuromuscular transmission. The association with thymic pathological abnormalities (germinal centers, thymomas, or thymic hyper-plasia) has long been known, and thymectomy has been found empirically to im-prove the status of a large proportion of patients. Hence the idea of characterizing thymic extracts by injecting them into test mice and studying neuromuscular trans-mission electromyographically (11).

ISOLATION   Calf thymus is homogenized and heated at 70°C for 30 min. The material is then centrifuged and the supernatant is concentrated on Amicon® mem-branes before being chromatographed on Sephadex G-50 columns and on hydroxy-apatite (11, 12).

BIOCHEMICAL CHARACTERISTICS   The purity of the two thymopoietins has been assessed by polyacrylamide disc electrophoresis at pH 8.9. With 200 μg of thymopoietin I and II per gel, there was a single major band stained with Coomassie blue ingels run at pH 8.9 and 4.3. Analysis of the terminal amino acids provided further evidence for purity since no residue could be identified. Thymopoietins I and II are related entities, as shown by peptide mapping and by the existence of immuno-logical cross-reactions (12).

The amino acid sequence of thymopoietin II was established using an automated sequenator (13). The peptide contains 49 amino acids. The precise molecular weight is 5562. There is microheterogeneity at the C terminal with approximately two thirds of the molecules lacking the C terminal arginine found on the remaining molecules. It is interesting to note that a randomly selected peptide corresponding to residues 29–41 was synthesized and shown to have a selectivity of action comparable to thymopoietin (14).

The Circulating Thymic Factor

BIOASSAY   The principle of the assay consists in the induction of θ antigen on θ negative T-cell precursors after incubation with the thymic hormone. θ conversion is studied on θ negative rosette-forming cells (toward sheep erythrocytes) in normal bone marrow or adult thymectomized mouse spleen (15, 16).

ISOLATION   Isolation of the polypeptide has been achieved by six successive operations: (a) defibrination, (b) dialysis, (c) concentration on UM2 Amicon membrane, (d) Sephadex G-25 filtration, (e) CM cellulose chromatography, and (f) Sephadex G-25 filtration in acetic acid (15).

BIOCHEMICAL CHARACTERISTICS   The purity of G-25 acetic acid–eluted fractions is assessed (a) by the observation of a single spot in five thin layer chromatographies using different solvents, (b) by the absence of detectable amino acid by dansylation after treatment of protein quantities (1 nM) largely superior to the threshold of the dansyl technique, and (c) by the reproducibility of amino acid analysis with a satisfactory stoichiometry (15).

The molecular weight of the circulating thymic factor has been evaluated by G-25 chromatography in phosphate buffer 0.2 M, pH 7.3, by comparison to several markers, as well as by calibrated dialysis (in a standardized system with 1 m² area). Both evaluations provided a molecular weight which is compatible with the amino acid stoichiometry (15).

The circulating thymic factor loses its biological activity after trypsin, chymotrypsin, or pronase treatment. Its pH is close to 7.5. It contains a lysine but no aromatic amino acids. Absence of detectable amino-terminal, as shown by dansylation studies indicate that the amino-terminal is blocked (likely under the form of pyrroglutamic acid) (our unpublished results). The amino acid sequence of the circulating thymic factor has recently been determined in the pig (52): Gln-Ala-Lys-Ser-Gln-Gly-Gly-Ser-Asn.

Other Preparations

Factors other than the four just described have also been reported. They have been isolated on the basis of various and sometimes unexpected bioassays. The most important are: (a) Luckey's lymphocyte-stimulating hormones, two proteins with molecular weights of 17,000 and 80,000, respectively, evaluated by their action on lymphocytosis and increase in antibody synthesis of newborn mice (17); (b) Comsa's homeostatic thymus hormone, a heat-labile glycopeptide of 1800–2500 mol. wt.

showing antagonistic effects against ACTH, TSH, thyroxine, gonadotropins, and synergy with growth hormone as well as a chemotactic influence on lymphocytes (18); (c) and Mizutani's thymic hypocalcemic factors (T1 and T2) inducing hypocalcemia and lymphocytosis (19).

It should be made clear that the factors mentioned here have often been isolated on the basis of assays not directly related to immunology. This is unfortunate since several of these thymic factors have been fairly well defined biochemically.

Conclusions: One or Several Thymic Hormones?

It is difficult to draw conclusions from the present state of knowledge. The main question is to determine whether the various thymic polypeptidic factors isolated by the groups quoted in the preceding pages are related. There are differences in the molecular weights but this cannot be considered a conclusive argument since the same product could exist under different molecular forms. It could thus be possible that thymosin is a precursor or contains precursors of the circulating TF. A relationship is made unlikely between thymopoietins and circulating TF after examination of the thymopoietin sequence and TF amino acid analysis. In contrast, there are very few differences between THF and circulating TF; it is very possible that they are identical.

BIOLOGICAL ACTIVITIES

Several in vitro and in vivo biological activities of thymic extracts have been demonstrated in the mouse. It should, however, be stressed that none of the biological effects detected in these tests are specific to thymic products. Indeed several pharmacological substances, in particular cyclic AMP, can induce similar or sometimes more dramatic effects. This underlines the need for critical interpretation of the biological significance of these in vitro assays and indicates that in vivo restoration experiments are still highly relevant, all the more so since purified extracts are now available which prevent heavy protein overloading. Finally, the convergence of data from both in vivo and in vitro experiments provides the most convincing arguments for the role of thymic hormones.

Induction of T-Cell Markers on T-Cell Precursors

We reported in 1971 that thymic extracts induce the appearance of the Θ antigen on Θ-negative normal bone marrow rosette forming cells (RFC) or on spleen RFC from adult thymectomized (ATx) mice (5). This induction, which occurs within 60 min at 37°C, was confirmed in 1973 by Komuro & Boyse, who showed that incubation of thymic extracts with normal spleen cells previously fractionated on a BSA gradient rendered a significant proportion of Θ-negative cells Θ-positive (20). In both experiments the minority of precursor cells were separated from the whole population by rosette formation or BSA fractionation. Similar results were also obtained with unfractionated nude mouse spleen cells (21).

The significance of the changes induced by thymic extracts is still open to speculation, particularly with regard to its relevance to T-cell differentiation. One may think that the appearance of T-cell markers is the first step of the irreversible differentiation of precursor cells in the direction of mature T cells. On the other hand, one may speculate that the changes in question are in fact associated with reversible membrane changes. The fact that in vivo Θ induction in ATx mice by thymic extracts (22) or cyclic AMP (23, 24) is reversible within 24–48 hr is compatible with this hypothesis. Such reversible changes could probably better fit with membrane rearrangement than with gene activation and would imply that Θ induction is not equivalent to true T-cell differentiation. However, it might very well be that these changes put the precursor cells in a particular metabolic state, which is a prerequisite for the cell to proceed in the differentiation process (according to its own program, independently of any further thymic stimulus). Consequently, one should not accept definitively the concept of thymic hormone (considered as a thymus substitute) for a given product before other in vitro and especially in vivo activities of the factor have been demonstrated as has been the case for several products (15, 25, 26).

Mitogen and MLC Responses

Several groups of authors have reported thymic factor–induced increase in mitogen responsiveness in thymectomized mice (27) and unexpectedly in normal spleen cells (28, 29, 30) either in vivo or in vitro. The increment in responses, however, remained generally modest and the overall interpretation of these data is not totally convincing. The same comments apply to MLC assays (6, 31).

Homograft and GVH Responses

One of the most salient manifestations of newborn thymectomy is a severe impairment of cell-mediated responses. Many studies have been undertaken in order to try to restore such responses by the administration of thymic extracts. Two models mainly have been investigated: the homograft response directed against either skin or tumor H-2 incompatible grafts and the capacity of inducing GVH reaction in an allogeneic host.

Cytotoxic T lymphocytes are generated and can be easily detected in the course of an immune reaction against histocompatibility antigens. However, the activity of such effector T cells is almost nonexistent in newborn Tx mice. Ikhehara et al have recently reported that thymus-deprived mice treated with a thymosin-like extract developed the capacity to reject an allogeneic sarcoma (27). The repair of T-cell function was also manifested by the presence in the spleen of these animals of specifically committed killer T cells, which could be inhibited by an anti-Θ serum. It had been previously shown by Trainin's group that THF restored the capacity of T cells from Tx donors to become educated after in vivo transfer into an H-2 incompatible irradiated host and to differentiate into cytotoxic cells (32). Lastly, M. A. Bach has recently shown that the decreased capacity of ATx C57Bl/6 mice to generate cytotoxic cells against DBA/2 mastocytoma cells could be returned to normal levels by in vivo treatment with purified circulating TF (33).

In contrast with the above experiments which required in vivo thymic factor administration during several weeks, a series of experiments was reported indicating that a short in vitro incubation (1 to 2 hr) with a thymic extract rendered bone marrow cells immunocompetent in a GVH assay. Goldstein et al showed that bone marrow cells incubated in vitro with thymosin induced splenomegaly after injection into lethally irradiated hosts (34). Trainin et al were unable to obtain with THF such direct conferment of immunocompetence upon BM cells. The THF-treated cells required an additional in vivo or in vitro contact with splenic tissue before acquiring the capacity to induce an in vitro GVH reaction (35).

Anti-Tumor Responses

Zissblatt et al have shown that the administration of thymosin to newborn mice accelerated their ability to reject an MSV-induced sarcoma (36). Thymosin could also delay to a certain extent the death by tumor growth of adult mice immunologically impaired by ATS or thymectomy plus irradiation (37). We have reported similar findings with purified circulating TF: whereas Tx-irradiated mice had no regression of tumor growth, similar mice treated with TF showed a 85% incidence of regression. However, in contrast with normal animals, regression was only transient and tumors reappeared after the treatment was stopped (15).

Antibody Responses

Most data presented above deal with T-cell–mediated response. One may wonder whether thymic hormones can as well influence antibody responses, either positively (by acting on helper T cells) or negatively (by acting on suppressor T cells). Trainin has shown that thymus-deprived mice treated repeatedly with THF had an improved response towards SRBC as compared with nontreated Tx controls (38). However, the degree of restoration was rather modest, especially when compared with that achieved in cell-mediated responses with the same thymic extract. Experiments with nude mice have been recently reported by two groups (27, 39), suggesting that thymic factors can induce the differentiation of prethymic cells into T helper cells. Ikhehara et al injected a thymosin-like extract into nude mice for more than 60 days, and then challenged the animals with SRBC. A low but significant number of plaque-forming cells were found in the spleen of these mice after stimulation with SRBC (27). Katz & Armerding tested the effect of a thymic preparation in Mishell & Dutton's in vitro system of primary antibody response (39). Spleen cells were primed against SRBC or against a DNP protein conjugate with or without thymosin. The presence of thymosin increased the amount of plaque-forming cells. Recently the action of circulating TF on the effect of suppressor T cells on antipolyvinylpyrrolidone antibody production has been described (40).

Control of Autoimmunity

INTRODUCTION   Increasing evidence indicates that a T-cell deficiency could be a major etiological factor in the development of several autoimmune conditions; also, the question of the origin of such T-cell deficiency has been raised. The serum level of the circulating thymus factor (assessed by the rosette assay mentioned above) has been tested in several experimental autoimmune conditions (41, 42).

NZB and B/W mice have a normal T-cell level at birth, but it decreases prematurely between the third and sixth week of life. At two months NZB and B/W mice have no significant thymus factor (TF), whereas TF is still at birth level in control mouse strains and remains at this level until the fourth to the sixth month. The influence of thymic factors on autoreactivity has been demonstrated in two experimental models.

IN VITRO AUTOSENSITIZATION   Cohen & Wekerle have shown that normal lymphoid cells cultured for 5 days on syngeneic fibroblast monolayers differentiate into specifically sensitized T cells able to mediate specific cytotoxicity against syngeneic (43) or H-2–compatible target cells (44) and to induce a GVH-like reaction of splenomegaly or of lymph node enlargement after in vivo transfer into a syngeneic host (45).

This experimental system has been used by Trainin's group to investigate the effects of a calf thymus extract on autoreactivity (46). It has been found that addition of such an extract to the culture medium during the sensitization phase inhibited the generation of effector cells as measured by cell-mediated cytotoxicity or by an in vitro GVH-like assay on syngeneic spleen fragments (47). Normal syngeneic serum also blocked the reaction. However, syngeneic serum from newborn Tx donors did not show any blocking activity. It was therefore assumed that the blocking factor present in normal serum was a humoral substance secreted by the thymus and disappearing from the blood stream after Tx.

AUTOLOGOUS ROSETTES   Further evidence for the role of the thymus in the control of autoreactivity is derived from the study of autologous rosettes (ARFC) formed between lymphocytes and autologous or syngeneic erythrocytes. Thymectomy in adult mice increases more than 10 times the incidence of ARFC in the spleen (48). A high number of RFC are also found in the spleen of athymic nude mice and aging mice. It is likely that ARFC formation expresses a true recognition event of self-antigenic determinants (J. F. Bach, unpublished results). The high number of rosettes found in the spleen of adult Tx animals is reduced to normal values after a single injection of purified TF, which adds support to the concept of a control exerted by the thymus upon ARFC which are probably immature T cells.

CLINICAL ACTIVITIES

All the above data argue in favor of the indication of thymic factors in the treatment of patients with immune deficiency, SLE, and related diseases. A few prelimary clinical trials, mainly in immunodeficiency syndromes, have been made recently in various centers, using A. L. Goldstein's thymosin (49, 50) and Trainin's THF (51). It is too early to interpret the preliminary clinical results. The most clear-cut effects deal with in vivo correction of low E rosette values, reminiscent of what has been shown in in vitro experiments, especially in immunodeficiency and SLE. It will probably take some time before conclusive results are obtained with randomized trials using standardized preparations with well-defined half-lives (delay preparations will be necessary as for most peptidic hormones). In addition, it will perhaps be necessary to select patients who do not have too advanced a disease since, for example in the NZB model, old mice appear to be no longer responsive. Potential clinical applications of thymic hormones raise the problem of their relationship to transfer factor. Transfer factor is a dialyzable leukocyte extract which confers specific delayed hypersensitivity to anergic subjects. Little is known in fact of its biochemical nature because of the lack, until recently, of available in vitro assays. The fact that transfer factor is antigen specific suggests that it is different in nature from thymic factors. However, this specificity is not absolute; thus, the possibility that transfer factor preparations contain thymic hormone-like products especially with small molecular weights cannot be ruled out.

Literature Cited

1. Bach, J. F., Carnaud C. 1976. Thymic factors. *Prog. Allergy* 21:342
2. Friedman, M., ed. 1975. Thymus factors in immunity. *Ann. NY Acad. Sci.* 249
3. Van Bekkum, D. W. 1975. The biological activity of thymic hormones. In *The Biological Activity of Thymic Hormones,* ed. D. W. Van Bekkum. Rotterdam: Kooyker Sci. Publ.
4. Goldstein, A. L., Slater, F. D., White, A. 1966. Preparation, assay and partial purification of a thymic lymphocytopoietic factor (thymosin). *Proc. Natl. Acad. Sci. USA* 56:1010
5. Bach, J. F., Dardenne, M., Goldstein, A., Guha, A., White, A. 1971. Appearance of T-cell markers in bone marrow after incubation with purified thymosin, a thymic hormone. *Proc. Natl. Acad. Sci. USA* 68:2734
6. Cohen, G. H., Hooper J. A., Goldstein, A. L. 1975. Thymosin induced differentiation of murine thymocytes in allogeneic mixed lymphocyte cultures. *Ann. NY Acad. Sci.* 249:145
7. Hooper, J. A., McDaniel, M. C., Thurman, G. B., Cohen G. H., Schulof, R. S., Goldstein, A. L. 1975. Purification and properties of bovine thymosin. *Annals NY Acad. Sci.* 249:125
8. Trainin, N., Small, M., Globerson, A. 1969. Immunocompetence of spleen cells from neonatally thymectomized mice, conferred in vitro by a syngeneic thymus extracts. *J. Exp. Med.* 130:765
9. Kook, A. I., Yakir, Y., Trainin, N. 1975. Isolation and partial chemical characterization of THF, a thymus hormone involved in immune maturation of lymphoid cells. *Cell. Immunol.* 19:151
10. Trainin, N., Small, M. 1970. Studies on some physicochemical properties of a thymus humoral factor conferring immunocompetence on lymphoid cells. *J. Exp. Med.* 132:885
11. Goldstein, G. 1974. Isolation of bovine thymin: a polypeptide hormone of the thymus. *Nature* 247:11
12. Goldstein, G. 1975. The isolation of thymopoietin (thymin). *Ann. NY Acad. Sci.* 72:11
13. Schlesinger, D. H., Goldstein G. 1975. The aminoacid sequence of thymopoietin II. *Cell* 5:361
14. Schlesinger, D. H., Goldstein, G., Scheid, M. P., Boyse E. A. 1975. Chemical synthesis of a peptide fragment of thymopoietin II that induces selective T cell differentiation. *Cell* 5:367
15. Bach, J. F., Dardenne, M., Pleau, J. M., Bach, M. A. 1975. Isolation, biochemical characteristics and biological activity of a circulating thymic hormone in the mouse and in the human. *Ann. NY Acad. Sci.* 249:186
16. Dardenne, M., Bach, J. F., 1975. The sheep cell rosette assay for the evaluation of thymic hormones. See Ref. 3, p. 235
17. Luckey, T. D., Venugopal, B. 1975. Isolation and quantification of LSH and the evaluation of related serum basic proteins in normal adults and cancer patients. *Ann. NY Acad. Sci.* 249:166
18. Comsa, J. 1975. Extraction, fractionation and testing of homogeneous thymic hormone preparation. *Ann. NY Acad. Sci.* 249:402
19. Mizutani, A., Shimizu, M., Suzuki, I., Mizutani, T., Hayase, S. 1975. A hypocalcemic and lymphocyte stimulating substance isolated from thymus extracts

and its physicochemical properties. *Ann. NY Acad. Sci.* 249:220

20. Komuro, K., Boyse, E. A. 1973. Induction of T lymphocytes from precursor cells in vitro by a product of the thymus. *J. Exp. Med.* 138:479

21. Scheid, M. P., Goldstein, G., Boyse, E. A. 1975. Differentiation of T cells in Nude mice. *Science* 190:1211

22. Dardenne, M., Bach, J. F. 1973. Studies on thymus products. I. Modification of rosette forming cells by thymic extracts. Determination of the target RFC subpopulation. *Immunology* 25:425

23. Bach, M. A., Founier, C., Bach, J. F. 1975. Regulation of theta antigen expression by agents altering cyclic AMP level and by thymic factor. *Ann. NY Acad. Sci.* 249:316

24. Bach, M. A., Bach, J. F. 1973. Studies on thymus products. VI. The effects of cyclic nucleotides and prostaglandins on rosette forming cells. Interactions with thymic factor. *Eur. J. Immunol.* 3:778

25. Goldstein, A. L., Guha, A., Zatz, M. M., Hardy, M. A., White, A. 1972. Purification and biological properties of thymosin, a hormone of the thymus gland. *Proc. Natl. Acad. Sci. USA* 69:1800

26. Trainin, N., Small, M., Zipori, D., Umiel, T., Kook, A. I., Rotter, V. 1975. Characteristics of THF, a thymic hormone. See Ref. 3, p. 117

27. Ikehara, S., Hamashima, Y., Masuda, T. 1975. Immunological restoration of both thymectomized and athymic nude mice by a thymus factor. *Nature* 258:335

28. Rotter, V., Trainin, N. 1975. Increased mitogenic reactivity of normal spleen cells to T lectins induced by thymus humoral factor (THF). *Cell. Immunol.* 16:413

29. Basch, R. S., Goldstein, G., 1975. Thymopoietin-induced acquisition of responsiveness to T cell mitogens. *Cell. Immunol.* 20:218

30. Thurman, G. B., Ahmed, A., Strong, D. M., Gershwin, M. E., Steinberg, A. D., Goldstein, A. L. 1975. Thymosin-induced increase in mitogenic responsiveness of lymphocytes of C57Bl/6, NZB/W and Nude mice. *Transpl. Proc.* 7: Suppl. 1, p. 299

31. Umiel, T., Trainin, N. 1975. Increased reactivity of responding cells in the mixed lymphocyte reaction by a thymic humoral factor. *Eur. J. Immunol.* 5:85

32. Lonai, P., Mogilner, B., Rotter, V., Trainin, N. 1973. Studies on the effect of a thymic humoral factor on differentiation of thymus derived lymphocytes. *Eur. J. Immunol.* 3:21

33. Bach, M. A. 1976. Cyclic AMP and T-cell differentiation. *Ann. Immunol. Paris.* 127c:967

34. Goldstein, A. L., Guha, A., Howe, M. L., White, A. 1971. Ontogenesis of cell mediated immunity and its acceleration by thymosin, a thymic hormone. *J. Immunol.* 106:773

35. Small, M., Trainin, N. 1971. Contribution of a thymic humoral factor to the development of an immunologically competent population from cells of mouse bone marrow. *J. Exp. Med.* 134:786

36. Zisblatt, M. A., Goldstein, A. L., Lilly, F., White, A. 1970. Acceleration by thymosin of the development of resistance to murine sarcoma virus-induced tumors in mice. *Proc. Natl. Acad. Sci. USA* 66:1170

37. Hardy, M. A., Zisblatt, M., Levine, N., Goldstein, A. L., Lilly, F., White, A. 1971. Reversal by thymosin of increased susceptibility of immuno suppressed mice to Moloney sarcoma virus. *Transpl. Proc.* 3:926

38. Small, M., Trainin, N. 1967. Increase in antibody forming cells of neonatally thymectomized mice receiving calf thymus extract. *Nature* 216:377

39. Armerding, G., Katz, D. H. 1975. Activation of T and B lymphocytes in vitro. IV. Regulatory influence on specific T cell functions by a thymus extract factor. *J. Immunol.* 114:1248

40. Bach, M. A., Niaudet, P. 1976 Thymic function in NZB mice. II. Regulatory influence of a circulating thymic factor on antibody production against polyvinylpyrrolidone in NZB mice. *J. Immunol.* 117:76

41. Bach, J. F., Dardenne, M., Salomon, J. C. 1973. Studies on thymus products. IV. Absence of serum "thymic activity" in adult NZB and (NZB X NZW)F1 mice. *Clin. Exp. Immunol.* 14:247

42. Dardenne, M., Monier, J. F., Biozzi, G., Bach, J. F. 1974. Studies on thymus product. V. Influence of genetic selection based on antibody production on thymus hormone production. *Clin. Exp. Immunol.* 17:339

43. Cohen, I. R., Wekerle, H. 1973. Regulation of autosensitization. The immune activation and specific inhibition of self

recognizing lymphocytes. *J. Exp. Med.* 137:224

44. Ilfield, D., Carnaud, C., Klein E. 1975. Cytotoxicity of autosensitized lymphocytes restricted to the H-2K end of identical targets. *Immunogenetics* 2:231

45. Cohen, I. R. 1973. Difference between the lymph node response to injection of autosensitized T lymphocytes and that in a graft versus host reaction. *Eur. J. Immunol.* 3:829

46. Trainin, N., Carnaud C., Ilfeld, D. 1973. Inhibition of in vitro autosensitization by a thymic humoral factor. *Nature New Biol.* 245:253

47. Small, M., Trainin, N. 1975. Control of autoreactivity by a humoral factor of the thymus (THF). *Cell. Immunol.* 20:2

48. Charreire, J., Bach, J. F. 1975. Binding of autologous erythrocytes to immature T-cells. *Proc. Natl. Acad. Sci. USA* 71:3201

49. Goldstein, A. L., Wara, D. W., Ammann, A. J., Sakai, H., Harris, N. S., Thurman, G. B., Hooper, J. A., Cohen, G. H., Goldman, A. S., Costanzi, J. J., McDaniel, M. C. 1975. First clinical trial with thymosin: reconstitution of T cells in patients with cellular immunodeficiency diseases. *Transpl. Proc.* 7:681

50. Wara, D. W., Goldstein, A. L., Doyle, N. E., Ammann, A. J. 1975. Thymosin activity in patients with cellular immunodeficiency. *N. Engl. J. Med.* 292:70

51. Handzel, Z. T., Levin, S., Hahn, T., Altman, Y., Ashkenazi, A., Trainin, N., Schechter, B. 1975. Infantile partial thymic deficiency: correction of some in vitro T functions by thymus humoral factor. *Isr. J. Med. Sci.* 11:1391

52. Bach, J. F., Dardenne, M., Pleau, J. M., Rosa, J. 1976. Caractérisation biochimique du facteur thymique circulant. *C. R. Acad. Sci.* 283:1605

Ann. Rev. Pharmacol. Toxicol. 1977. 17:293–309

CARDIOVASCULAR DRUG INTERACTIONS

❖6681

D. Craig Brater and Howard F. Morrelli[1]

Division of Clinical Pharmacology and the Departments of Medicine and Pharmacology, University of California School of Medicine, San Francisco, California 94143

INTRODUCTION

Among the clinically important drug interactions, those involving cardiovascular agents are probably preeminent. Drug interactions change the expected relation between the dose administered and the drug's effect, whether that change is due to the amount of drug available at its site of action (pharmacokinetic), or to a change in "sensitivity" at its receptor (pharmacodynamic). Interactions that decrease a drug's effect leave the patient susceptible to the morbidity and mortality of his primary disease. Interactions that increase a drug's effect may cause toxicity. The narrow benefit:risk ratio of many of the cardiovascular agents increases the importance of drug interactions involving them, for interactions can result in subtherapeutic or toxic responses from doses that would ordinarily be therapeutic.

Though the sequelae of cardiovascular drug interactions are often serious, they often are not recognized (1–5). Many patients with cardiovascular diseases are desperately ill, and the manifestations of drug toxicity may be difficult to distinguish from those of the primary disease. For example, arrhythmias due to digitalis toxicity may be impossible to differentiate from those that are disease induced (6–9). Similarly, arrhythmias may be a toxic manifestation of antiarrhythmic drugs, and may be misinterpreted as lack of efficacy of the drug (10–14). Avoidance of and appropriate response to drug interactions requires understanding of the pharmacology of the drugs and the pathophysiology of the diseases in which they are used. We categorize drug interactions in pharmacokinetic terms and by types of drug. The breadth of this topic and editorial limitations on manuscript length allow us only to use broad outlines here. The references listed will help those who wish to pursue topics in more detail.

[1]During preparation of this report, the authors were supported in part by National Institutes of Health Grants GM-01791, GM-00001, and GM-16496.

293

PHARMACOKINETIC DRUG INTERACTIONS

Drug interactions can affect the absorption of a drug, its distribution to tissues, its elimination by metabolism and excretion, and the relationship between the amount of drug at its site of action and its effect.

Absorption

Drug interactions affecting absorption can change the rate and extent of absorption of a drug, each or both of which may be important. The rate of absorption determines the peak level of drug attained in blood and the rapidity at which the drug reaches its site of action; the extent of absorption determines the total amount of drug that is systemically available and, hence, the level of drug attained at steady state (15, 16).

Interactions affecting rates of absorption are of minor clinical importance. When a rapid onset of action is desired, as in treating arrhythmias, the agent is administered intravenously. Changes in extent of absorption, or bioavailability, however, are often clinically important, for such alterations affect the level of drug maintained at steady state.

There are a number of mechanisms by which changes in absorption can occur. Whether the drug is given as a solution, suspension, tablet, or capsule can importantly affect both the rate and the extent of absorption. In addition, the method of a tablet's formulation can change its dissolution rate and its availability for absorption, as has been observed with various preparations of digoxin (17–28).

Drug interactions of a direct physical or chemical nature are also seen. Complexing of drugs with antacids, with exchange resins, etc occurs with a variety of drugs. The in vitro dissolution of digoxin tablets is drastically decreased by antacids containing magnesium trisilicate (29). Whether these antacids impair the bioavailability of digoxin in vivo has not been reported. By interrupting the enterohepatic circulation of digitoxin, cholestyramine and colestipol enhance its elimination rate, and these resins have been advocated for treatment of digitoxin intoxication (30–32). Cholestyramine similarly increases the elimination of warfarin (33). Antacids appear not to alter the kinetics of warfarin importantly, and cholestyramine does not influence the elimination of digoxin (34, 35). Activated charcoal, on the other hand, may impair digoxin's absorption (36).

Many drugs are weak acids or weak bases. The pH of their milieu, their pK_a, and their lipid solubility determine their ability to cross cell membranes. Theoretically, therefore, a gastrointestinal (GI) pH favoring non-ionized drug facilitates absorption. For weak bases, such as procainamide, quinidine, and mecamylamine, an alkaline pH increases the amount of non-ionized drug; for weak acids, such as salicylate or phenobarbital, an acid pH increases the amount of non-ionized drug. Studies in animals verify that the acidic gastric pH facilitates movement of weak acids from the gastric lumen to blood and promotes movement of weak bases in the opposite direction (37, 38). Gastric luminal pH effects, however, are not as important as might be expected; these pH changes affect the rate of absorption of some noncardiovascular agents to a minor degree, but no important quantitative effects have been reported on the extent of drug absorption, perhaps, because a large intestinal surface area is available for absorption, or the mucosa is "leaky," or there are other unidentified factors important for facilitating complete absorption of drugs (39–40).

The greatest amount of drug absorption occurs in the duodenum or proximal jejunum. Consequently, the rate of gastric emptying influences the time from drug administration to absorption. Drugs that delay gastric emptying, such as morphine, atropine, or meperidine can significantly decrease the rate of absorption of other drugs. Rapid gastric emptying would cause an earlier and higher peak level of drug.

Changes in GI motility can affect the extent of absorption of slowly absorbed drugs such as digoxin, guanethidine, and bishydroxycoumarin. Decreased motility provides more time for and increases the extent of absorption; increased motility has the opposite effect. With a slowly dissolving brand of digoxin, concomitant administration of metaclopramide, which increases GI motility, decreased steady state serum digoxin concentrations by one third. Propantheline, which slows GI motility, increased the steady state serum digoxin concentrations by one third (41). This effect of GI motility on the extent of absorption of digoxin was not observed when a rapidly dissolving formulation of digoxin was used (42).

Congestive heart failure or shock, release of catecholamines or vasoactive peptides, and administration of vasoactive drugs may change perfusion of the intestine or muscle, causing unpredictable absorption. In many settings in which cardiovascular agents are used, perfusion to tissue changes with time; the only certain way to know how much drug is systemically available is to administer it intravenously.

Before reaching peripheral sites, orally administered drugs pass through the intestine and the liver. Metabolism of the drug may occur in either organ and decrease the amount systemically available; this process is called the "first pass" effect. A first pass effect occurs with propranolol, alprenolol, lidocaine, reserpine, dopamine, and other sympathomimetics. This effect is clinically unimportant with reserpine; lidocaine and sympathomimetics are administered parenterally because the first pass effect is so great that insufficient levels of drug are reached systemically after oral dosing. The first pass effect on the absorption of propranolol is partly responsible for the wide variation in plasma levels of this drug that occur among patients given similar oral doses.

Changes in the liver's capacity to metabolize drugs would be expected to change the magnitude of the first pass effect importantly. By decreasing hepatic blood flow, congestive heart failure or propranolol decrease the clearance of lidocaine and other drugs (43–46).

Interference with GI muscosal function does not appear to be important with most cardiovascular agents, although diminished absorption by this mechanism may explain how heptobarbital decreases the absorption of bishydroxycoumarin (47).

Distribution

Interactions involving distribution of drugs to tissue sites of action include effects on serum protein binding and pH-dependent effects on distribution.

Drugs bound to albumin are in equilibrium with free drug in plasma. Only the free drug is available to its site of action; consequently, changes between amounts of bound and free drug may significantly influence a drug's effect. The ability of one drug to displace another depends on the relative concentrations of each drug and their affinities for binding. The clinical significance of displacement of a drug depends on the drug's therapeutic index and its degree of protein binding. Only with drugs that are highly bound will displacement cause significantly increased amounts of free drug. Consequently, clinically important interactions have been observed only with concomitant use of highly bound drugs that have a low therapeutic index (48).

Cardiovascular agents highly bound to protein include warfarin, bishydroxy-coumarin, digitoxin, phenytoin, diazoxide, clofibrate, hydralazine, and quinidine. Other highly bound drugs able to cause displacement interactions include pyrazolone derivatives, salicylates, indomethacin, chloral hydrate's metabolite, and sulfonamides. Theoretically, clinically significant serum protein displacement interactions could occur with concomitant use of any of the drugs mentioned. However, important interactions thus far have been observed only when coumarin anticoagulants are displaced from proteins by clofibrate, pyrazolones, or chloral hydrate (49–52). Displacement of coumarin anticoagulants sufficient to potentiate the anticoagulant effect has been observed in animals or in vitro with administration of diazoxide, ethacrynic acid, indomethacin, sulfinpyrazone, sulfadimethoxine, sulfaphenazole, and tolbutamide (53–56). A study in normal volunteers, however, has shown no clinically important interaction between coumarin and indomethacin (57). Pyrazolones displace digitoxin and diazoxide displaces phenytoin, but the transient increase in levels of free drug is not clinically important (58–60).

Interactions among the other drugs may not be important because changes in free levels are minor, or because the increase of the free level is short-lived and not detected. All protein displacement interactions are transient. Because the described drugs obey first order elimination kinetics, the temporarily increased free drug is eliminated more quickly, causing a new steady state in which the total drug in serum is decreased, but the amount of free drug is the same as before. The duration of the displacement interaction depends on the time necessary to reach the new steady state; this time period is a function of the intrinsic elimination rate of the displaced drug (61, 62). Many drug interactions previously believed to occur by protein displacement mechanisms are now felt to occur through changes in metabolism of one drug induced by another (63). These interactions would persist throughout the concomitant use of the interacting drugs, while protein displacement interactions are clearly short-lived. Concomitant administration of highly bound drugs, therefore, requires dose adjustment and close following of endpoints of drug effect only until the new steady state is reached. These interactions are clinically most important when using coumarin anticoagulants, requiring frequent determinations of the prothrombin time when starting or discontinuing other drugs.

Changes in systemic pH can affect distribution of drugs to tissues. A pH favoring the non-ionized congener of drugs that are weak acids or weak bases would facilitate its diffusion into tissues. The converse is also true. Acidemia increases the hypotensive effect of mecamylamine by increasing its distribution to its extracellular site of action (64). A number of other cardiovascular agents including quinidine and procainamide are weak bases. Changes in systemic pH induced by other drugs might affect their distribution to sites of action, but this phenomenon has not been described.

Metabolism

Significant interactions among cardiovascular drugs occur with induction or inhibition of hepatic metabolism of drugs and from inhibition of monoamine oxidase (MAO). A number of different drugs can affect the hepatic microsomal enzyme system that is responsible for metabolism of various drugs. There is a great deal of interindividual variation in the capacity of this system and the degree to which it may be induced or inhibited (65, 66). This knowledge, plus the realization that many of the potential inducers and inhibitors have been studied only in animals, makes tenuous any prediction of the extent of an interaction in any individual.

Clinically important interactions due to induction of hepatic microsomal enzymes that have been observed with cardiovascular agents occur with the coumarin anticoagulants, phenytoin, and quinidine. Phenobarbital and carbamazepine can significantly increase the metabolism of phenytoin in some patients (67–70). The decreases in phenytoin levels have not resulted in increased seizure activity, presumably because of the seizure inhibiting activity of the inducing agent. A similar interaction when phenytoin is used as an antiarrhythmic could result in subtherapeutic levels of the drug. Phenytoin and phenobarbital increase the clearance of quinidine probably by metabolic induction. Both drugs decreased the half-life of quinidine in normal subjects by approximately 50%, and in two patients decreased quinidine to subtherapeutic levels (71).

Inhibition of metabolism is also important with these same drugs. Inhibition of hepatic metabolism of phenytoin, probably by noncompetitive inhibition of parahydroxylation, occurs with concomitant use of bishydroxycoumarin, disulfiram, antituberculous drugs, phenylbutazone, oxyphenbutazone, chloramphenicol, phenyramidol, sulfaphenazole, sulfamethizole, sulthiame, and methylphenidate (72–76). "Epidemics" of phenytoin toxicity have been reported when isoniazid was administered to a group of patients (77). Phenyramidol, sulthiame, and chloramphenicol doubled the serum half-life of phenytoin in studies of normal subjects (78–80).

A number of drug interactions due to inhibition of MAO are well known (81). Their significance is only lessened by the appropriately infrequent use of these agents. However, procarbazine, a drug used in treating Hodgkin's disease, has MAO inhibitory activity (82). Concomitant use of sympathomimetic agents requires awareness of this potential effect of procarbazine. MAO metabolizes sympathetic neurotransmitters at the synaptic cleft. During inhibition of this enzyme, administration of catecholamines or agents that release catecholamines such as tyramine, ephedrine, amphetamines, and some antihypertensive agents like reserpine and guanethidine can cause fatal hypertensive crises. Conversely, the effects of some antihypertensive agents such as diuretics may be potentiated and prolonged (81).

Inhibitors and inducers of the metabolism of coumarin derivatives are presented in the section on anticoagulants.

Excretion

The kidney excretes many drugs. A drug that changes the glomerular filtration rate might alter excretion of another drug, but changes of sufficient magnitude to be important have not been reported. Active secretion of a variety of drugs occurs at the pars recta of proximal tubules. There appear to be two nonspecific transport systems, one for organic acids and one for bases; any of the secreted drugs can compete for transport with another drug within its group (83–85). Cardiovascular agents for which this effect might be important, but which have not been reported, include the bases, procainamide and quinidine, and the organic acids, thiazides or thiazide derivatives. Spironolactone decreases the renal excretion of digoxin by competing for active secretion. This probably occurs at a site in the distal tubule, and concomitant administration can significantly increase the serum level of digoxin (86).

Passive renal tubular transport of drugs is related to urine flow rate and pH (87). High rates of urine flow induced by diuretics or fluid loading increase excretion of phenobarbital, but this effect has not been observed with cardiovascular agents. Carbonic anhydrase inhibitors or bicarbonate administration causing an alkaline urine, and ammonium chloride, potassium depletion from diuretics etc, inducing acid urine can affect passive transport of weak acids and bases. Alkaline urine decreases excretion of weak bases like amphetamine while acid urine decreases excretion of weak acids like salicylate by increasing the amount of non-ionized drug that can be reabsorbed from the tubular lumen (88). Procainamide, a weak base, follows urine pH-dependent excretion in dogs, but not in man (89, 90). A case of quinidine toxicity has been reported in a patient with renal tubular acidosis receiving "normal" doses of quinidine and has been attributed to accumulation due to a persistently alkaline urine (91). However, the increment of change in quinidine excretion that occurs with changes in urine pH is not of a magnitude that should be clinically important.

PHARMACODYNAMIC INTERACTIONS

Relationship Between Drug Amount and its Effect

Drugs and disease states can alter the effect seen from a known amount of drug; that is, they change the dose-response relationship. Systemic acidemia decreases the expected response to catecholamines (92). Potassium depletion increases the toxicity of digitalis glycosides. This interaction is particularly easy to overlook because substantial decreases in intracellular potassium can occur with normokalemia. Use of digitalis with guanethidine or propranolol can result in profound bradycardia as a result of the "vagal" activity of digitalis during sympathetic blockade (93). In addition, disease states can also affect the relation between drug dose and effect. A pharmacology or clinical pharmacology text, or the *Index Medicus,* should be referred to when unusual responses to a drug are observed.

Drug Interactions at the Receptor Site

Clinically important drug interactions at the receptor site include those involving drugs that have direct and indirect effects on the autonomic nervous system. Interactions among drugs primarily used for their effects on the autonomic nervous system are well known and include blockade of the β-agonist effects of isoproterenol and epinephrine by propranolol, or of the α-agonist effects of norepinephrine by phentolamine or phenoxybenzamine. Less commonly anticipated interactions are those occurring with concomitant administration of drugs that have secondary effects on the autonomic nervous system. For example, phenothiazines, tricyclic antidepressants, and butyrophenones are α-sympathetic antagonists, accounting for the enhanced activity of other α-blockers used concomitantly and the rationale for the use of directly acting α-sympathomimetics to reverse the α blockade of phenothiazines.

Tricyclic antidepressants and guanethidine block neuronal uptake of catecholamines at the synaptic cleft. Because reuptake of catecholamines is a major mechanism of attenuation of their effect, exogenously administered catecholamines may have an increased effect if used with them. In studies of normal subjects who had taken imipramine (25 mg TID) for five days, there was potentiation of the pressor effects of phenylephrine by two to three times, norepinephrine by four to eight times, and epinephrine by two to four times (94). In a similar study in subjects administered debrisoquin, an antihypertensive agent that also blocks the catecholamine reuptake system, the circulatory effects of phenylephrine were markedly potentiated and prolonged (95). Indirectly acting sympathomimetics would not be expected to have an enhanced effect with guanethidine-like drugs, and would more likely have a decreased effect, since guanethidine, debrisoquin, and bethanidine deplete endogenous catecholamines.

Another set of important cardiovascular drug interactions involving the catecholamine reuptake mechanism is that occurring between quanethidine, bethanidine, and debrisoquin and a number of psychoactive agents. The former drugs are taken into the synaptosomes by the catecholamine reuptake system. They then cause release and depletion of endogenous catecholamine stores. A reversal of their effect by tricyclic antidepressants is predictable since the tricyclics would inhibit their uptake to this site of action (96–103). A similar reversal of effect that probably occurs by inhibition of uptake or displacement from the site of action occurs with amphetamine, ephedrine, methylphenidate, doxepin, phenothiazines, butyrophenones, thiothixene, and possibly reserpine (103–109). This interaction has also been seen with use of a nasal decongestant containing chlorpheniramine, isopropamide, and phenylpropanolamine (110). This last interaction is probably not clinically important in most patients, but use of over-the-counter "cold" remedies should probably be avoided in patients on guanethidine-like drugs.

Reversal of the antihypertensive effect of clonidine by desipramine is well documented (111, 112). The site of action of clonidine appears to be central. This observed interaction may imply uptake of clonidine into CNS neurons as integral to its mechanism of action. This interaction requires caution in using other tricyclic antidepressants and psychoactive drugs in patients receiving clonidine.

Drugs, like reserpine, or diseases, like congestive heart failure, that deplete endogenous catecholamine stores can blunt the response to metaraminol and ephedrine, whose major effect depends on release of catecholamines at the nerve ending (113, 114).

Unanticipated but predictable interactions may occur with use of agents that have multiple effects. For example, epinephrine is both an α- and β-sympathetic receptor agonist; the α effect predominates in most instances, causing arteriolar vasoconstriction. However, concomitant use of an α-receptor antagonist not only will attenuate the vasoconstriction, but also may unveil the vasodilation caused by the β effect. Similarly, the use of propranolol for the treatment of hypertension rarely exacerbates the hypertension by blocking β-induced vasodilation and potentiating preexisting α-mediated vasoconstriction, especially in patients with a pheochromocytoma (115–118).

A number of drugs affect the parasympathetic limb of the autonomic nervous system. These agents may unexpectedly antagonize or potentiate the effects of cardiovascular agents used to affect the parasympathetics. Phenothiazines, antihistamines, and tricyclic antidepressants have clinically significant parasympathoplegic effects (119, 120).

Another type of drug interaction that is less clearly defined, but which we categorize as occurring at the receptor, is effects of psychotherapeutic agents on the myocardium. Phenothiazines and tricyclic antidepressants have quinidine-like effects on conductivity and automaticity (121–123). These effects can be manifested as QRS widening, QT prolongation, and arrhythmias. Because of the mechanism of these cardiac effects, concomitant use of quinidine and procainamide may have additive effects. Similarly, treatment of arrhythmias due to this effect of phenothiazines or tricyclic antidepressants requires agents that would not further depress conduction; these include lidocaine, phenytoin, and sympathomimetics. Some arrhythmias caused by these psychoactive agents are due to this quinidine-like effect rather than the parasympathoplegic effect (124). Inappropriate use of physostigmine for arrhythmias due to the quinidine-like effect can result in worsening of the arrhythmias and death.

CARDIOVASCULAR AGENTS

In this section, we discuss drug interactions involving specific types of cardiovascular agents.

Digitalis Glycosides

The effects on absorption of digitalis preparations by tablet formulation, changes in intestinal motility, and possible physiochemical interactions have been discussed. Digitoxin is metabolized by the liver, while the other glycosides are excreted by the kidney. Phenobarbital, phenytoin, phenylbutazone, and spironolactone enhance the metabolism of digitoxin, but this effect is of a clinically important magnitude only with phenobarbital with which the serum half-life of digitoxin is halved (58, 59, 125, 126). Digitoxin is highly bound to serum proteins and is displaced by phenylbutazone, but this interaction does not appear to be clinically important (59). Inhibition by spironolactone of digoxin's secretion by the renal tubule has been mentioned.

The most frequent interactions involving cardiac glycosides are those due to effects of other drugs on electrolyte balance. Increased sensitivity to the toxicity of digitalis occurs with potassium depletion, hypomagnesemia, and hypercalcemia, all of which may be secondary to diuretic therapy. Coadministration of sympathomimetic drugs also appears to increase the sensitivity to the toxic effects of digitalis.

Antiarrhythmic Agents

The different antiarrhythmic agents can have additive or antagonistic effects toward each other (10–14). Their effects on conductivity and the relative refractory period may differ (Table 1). Drugs with opposite effects on these electrophysiologic parameters can antagonize each other; drugs with similar effects can be additive. For example, phenytoin may antagonize the effects on conduction of quinidine, while procainamide predictably potentiates those effects. Understanding the diverse electrophysiologic effects of the different antiarrhythmic drugs increases the potential for their rational use as single agents or in combination.

Table 1 Effects of antiarrhythmic agents on the transmembrane action potential of isolated cardiac tissue[a,b]

Agent	Type of tissue[c]	Resting potential	Amplitude	dv/dt	Membrane responsiveness	Conduction velocity	Duration	Refractory period	Automaticity
Quinidine	Canine PF	0	↓	↓	↓	↓	↑	↑	↓
Procainamide	Canine PF	0	↓	↓	↓	↓	↑	↑	↓
Lidocaine	Canine PF	0	↓	↓	↓	↓	↓	↓	↓
Propranolol	Canine PF	0	↓	↓	↓	↓	↓	↓	↓
Phenytoin	Canine PF	0	0	0, ↓[d]	↓[d], 0, ↑[e]	0, ↓[f]	↓	↓	↓
Phenytoin	Rabbit AM and VM	0	0	↓	↓	↓	0	?	↓
Disopyramide	Canine PF	0	0	↓	↓	↓	↑	↑	↓
Ajmaline	Canine PF, AM, and VM	0	↓	↓	↓	↓	↑[f], ↓[g]	?	↓
Mexiletine	Rabbit AM and VM	0	⸮	↓	↓	↓	0	↑	0
Aprindine	Canine PF	⸮	↓	↓	↓	↓	↓	↑	↓
Verapamil	Canine PF	0	0	0	0, ↓	?	0, ↑[d]	0, ↑[d]	↓
Amiodarone[h]	Rabbit AM and VM	0	0	0	0	0	↑	↑	↓
Dimethyl quaternary propranolol[i]	Canine PF	0	↓	↓	↓	↓	↓	↓	↓
Bretylium	Rat AM and VM	0	↓	↓	↓	?	↑	↑	?

[a] Reprinted with permission from Morgan, P. H., Mathison, I. W. 1976. Arrhythmias and antiarrhythmic drugs: mechanism of action and structure–activity relationships I. *J. Pharm. Sci.* 65:468–82.

[b] 0 = no effect, ? = not reported, ↓ = decrease, ↑ = increase, and ⸮ = questionable or slight effect.

[c] PF = Purkinje fiber, AM = atrial muscle, and VM = ventricular muscle.

[d] At high concentration only.

[e] In acutely depressed fibers.

[f] Atrial muscle and ventricular muscle.

[g] Purkinje fiber.

[h] After 6 weeks of treatment of whole animal.

[i] UM–272.

Antihypertensive Agents

Interactions involving antihypertensive agents that occur at the receptor have been discussed. The most important interactions with these agents, however, are those used therapeutically for rational use of combinations of drugs in the treatment of hypertension. Blood pressure has a number of physiologic components as schematized in Figure 1. Successful treatment of hypertension often requires use of different drugs to treat the different physiologic components. For example, a patient treated with therapeutic doses of vasodilators to reduce peripheral vascular resistance, β-blockers to decrease heart rate, and ganglionic blockers to decrease venous return may still have hypertension if the patient's blood volume is expanded. Combination therapy for hypertension should use drugs acting on the different physiologic determinants of blood pressure. The various antihypertensive agents in Figure 1 are listed according to their dominant cardiovascular effects.

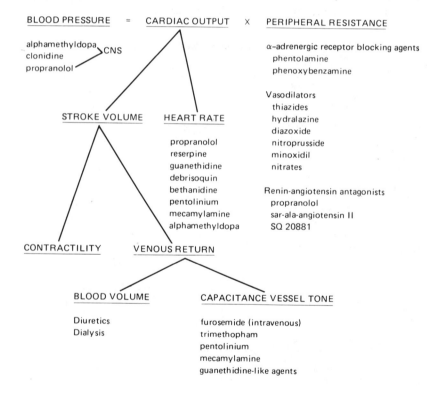

Figure 1   Antihypertensive agents as they affect the physiologic determinants of blood pressure.

Diuretics

Rational therapy with combinations of diuretics requires knowledge of the physiology of sodium, chloride, and water reabsorption by the kidney. Different diuretics affect different segments of renal tubules, and various agents or combinations of diuretics will cause different, but usually predictable effects on extent of volume and electrolyte loss. For example, by avidly reabsorbing chloride, the loop of Henle reclaims more sodium than does the distal tubule; agents acting at the loop are predictably potent. Sodium and potassium are both reabsorbed proximally, while potassium is secreted as sodium is reabsorbed distally. Consequently, the effects on excretion of different electrolytes of drugs used singly or in combination often can be predicted by knowing the tubule segments affected and the pathophysiology of the patient's disease at a given time. The sites of action of the different diuretics are shown in Table 2. Salicylates have been reported to attenuate the diuretic effects of spironolactone (127).

Anticoagulants

Interactions affecting anticoagulants have been partly presented; those affecting coumarin derivatives are summarized in Table 3. Excellent, current reviews of the coumarin anticoagulants are available (128, 129). Effects on coagulation from interactions with other components of the clotting pathway are also clinically important. Acetylsalicylic acid, phenylbutazone, sulfinpyrazone, indomethacin, dipyridamole, and other drugs interfere with platelet function by poorly defined

Table 2 Site of action of commonly used diuretics

Diuretic	Site of action
Carbonic anhydrase (CA) inhibitors:	Proximal tubule by inhibiting CA-mediated $NaHCO_3$ reabsorption
acetazolamide benzolamide	Minor effect more distally
Osmotic agents: mannitol glycerol glucose urea	Main effect at the loop of Henle; also blocks Na^+ and H_2O reabsorption proximally
"Loop" diuretics: furosemide ethacrynic acid	Block active reabsorption of Cl^- in the ascending limb of the loop of Henle—both cortical and medullary portions
Thiazides	Inhibit Na^+ reabsorption at the cortical segment of the ascending limb of the loop of Henle
Spironolaetone	Competitive inhibition of aldosterone-mediated Na^+ reabsorption in the distal tubule
Triamterene, amiloride	Noncompetitive inhibition of Na^+ reabsorption in the distal tubule

Table 3   Interactions affecting the coumarin anticoagulants[a]

Drug	Mechanism
Inhibition of the hypoprothrombinemic action of coumarins	
Barbiturates	Acceleration of coumarin metabolism
Carbamazepine	Acceleration of coumarin metabolism
Cholestyramine	Inhibition of coumarin absorption
Diphenylhydantoin	Acceleration of coumarin metabolism
Ethchlorvynol	Acceleration of coumarin metabolism?
Glutethimide	Acceleration of coumarin metabolism
Griseofulvin	Inhibition of coumarin absorption?
	Acceleration of coumarin metabolism?
Oral contraceptives	Increase of clotting factor synthesis
Rifampin	Acceleration of coumarin metabolism?
Vitamin K	Increase of clotting factor synthesis
Enhancement of the hypoprothrombinemic action of coumarins	
Allopurinol	Inhibition of coumarin metabolism
Anabolic steroids	Decrease in circulating vitamin K?
	Direct depression of clotting factor synthesis?
	Increase in clotting factor catabolism?
Chloral hydrate	Decrease in coumarin albumin binding
Chloramphenicol	Inhibition of coumarin metabolism
Clofibrate	Decrease in circulating vitamin K?
	Decrease in coumarin ablumin binding?
	Inhibition of coumarin metabolism?
Dextrothyroxine	Decrease in circulating vitamin K?
	Increase in clotting factor catabolism?
Diazoxide	Decrease in coumarin albumin binding
Disulfiram	Inhibition of coumarin metabolism
Ethacrynic acid	Decrease in coumarin albumin binding
Glucagon	Decrease in clotting factor synthesis?
Nalidixic acid	Decrease in coumarin albumin binding
Neomycin	Decrease in vitamin K absorption?
Nortriptyline	Inhibition of coumarin metabolism
Phenylbutazone	Decrease in coumarin albumin binding
Quinidine	Direct depression of clotting factor synthesis?
Salicylate	Direct depression of clotting factor synthesis?
Sulfonamides, long-acting	Decrease in coumarin albumin binding
Thyroid drugs	Increase in clotting factor catabolism
Tolbutamide	Decrease in coumarin albumin binding
Triclofos	Decrease in coumarin albumin binding

[a] Reprinted with permission from Koch-Weser, J. 1975. Drug interactions in cardiovascular therapy. *Am. Heart J.* 90:93–116.

mechanisms manifested as decreased secondary release by platelets of ADP (130, 131). Combined platelet inhibition and impairment of the vitamin K–dependent clotting pathways or intrinsic but latent genetic coagulation defects can contribute to a bleeding diathesis.

In summary, there are a wide variety of mechanisms responsible for a large number of clinically relevant drug interactions. Importantly, these interactions are often predictable; if the primary, secondary, or even tertiary effects of the drugs are known and considered, these interactions can be categorized in a way that makes them easier to conceptualize and remember.

Literature Cited

1. Melmon, K. L. 1971. Preventable drug reactions—causes and cures. *N. Engl. J. Med.* 284:1361–68
2. Karch, F. E., Lasagna, L. 1974. Adverse drug reactions in the United States—an analysis of the scope of the problem and recommendations for future approaches. Washington DC: Med. Public Interest. 28 pp.
3. Cluff, L. E., Caranasos, G. J., Stewart, R. B. 1975. Clinical problems with drugs. *Major Problems in Internal Medicine,* V. Philadelphia: Saunders. 308 pp.
4. Karch, F. E., Lasagna, L. 1975. Adverse drug reactions. A critical review. *J. Am. Med. Assoc.* 234:1236–41
5. Karch, F. E., Smith, C. L., Kerzner, B., Mazzullo, M., Weintraub, M., Lasagna, L. 1976. Adverse drug reactions—a matter of opinion. *Clin. Pharmacol. Ther.* 19:489–92
6. Shrager, M. W. 1957. Digitalis intoxication. A review and report of forty cases, with emphasis on etiology. *Arch. Intern. Med.* 100:881–93
7. Rodensky, P. L., Wasserman, F. 1961. Observations on digitalis intoxication. *Arch. Intern. Med.* 108:61–78
8. Chung, E. K. 1970. Digitalis-induced cardiac arrhythmias. *Am. Heart J.* 79:845–48
9. Fisch, C. 1971. Digitalis intoxication. *J. Am. Med. Assoc.* 216:1770–73
10. Mason, D. T. 1970. The clinical pharmacology and therapeutic applications of the antiarrhythmic drugs. *Clin. Pharmacol. Ther.* 11:460–80
11. Bassett, A. L., Hoffman, B. F. 1971. Antiarrhythmic drugs: electrophysiological actions. *Ann. Rev. Pharmacol.* 11:143–70
12. Rosen, M. R., Hoffman, B. F. 1973. Mechanisms of action of antiarrhythmic drugs. *Circ. Res.* 32:1–8
13. Arnsdorf, M. F. 1976. Electrophysiologic properties of antidysrhythmic drugs as a rational basis for therapy. *Med. Clin. North Am.* 60:213–32
14. Morgan, P. H., Mathison, I. W. 1976. Arrhythmias and antiarrhythmic drugs: mechanism of action and structure-activity relationships. I and II. *J. Pharm. Sci.* 65:467–82, 635–48
15. Rowland, M. 1972. Drug administration and regimens. In *Clinical Pharmacology. Basic Principles in Therapeutics,* ed. K. Melmon, H. Morrelli. New York: Macmillan
16. Koch-Weser, J. 1974. Bioavailability of drugs. *N. Engl. J. Med.* 291:233–37, 503–6
17. Manninen, V., Melin, J., Härtel, G. 1971. Serum digoxin concentration during treatment with different preparations. *Lancet* 2:934–35
18. Lindenbaum, J., Mellow, M. H., Blackstone, M. O., Butler, V. P. 1971. Variation in biologic availability of digoxin from four preparations. *N. Engl. J. Med.* 285:1344–47
19. Shaw, T. R. D., Howard, M. R., Hamer, J. 1972. Variation in the biological availability of digoxin. *Lancet* 2:303–7
20. Falch, D., Teien, A., Bjerkelund, C. J. 1973. Comparative study of the absorption, plasma levels, and urinary excretion of the "new" and the "old" Lanoxin. *Br. Med. J.* 1:695–97
21. Johnson, B. F., Fowle, A. S. E., Lader, S., Fox, J., Munro-Faure, A. D. 1973. Biological availability of digoxin from Lanoxin produced in the United Kingdom. *Br. Med. J.* 4:323–26
22. Huffman, D. H., Azarnoff, D. L. 1972. Absorption of orally given digoxin preparations. *J. Am. Med. Assoc.* 222:957–60
23. Sanchez, N., Sheiner, L. B., Halkin, H., Melmon, K. L. 1973. Pharmacokinetics

of digoxin: interpreting bioavailability. *Br. Med. J.* 4:132–34
24. Sorby, D. L., Tozer, T. N. 1973. On the evaluation of biologic availability of digoxin from tablets. *Drug Intell. Clin. Pharm.* 7:78–83
25. Wagner, J. G., Christensen, M., Sakmar, E., Blair, D., Yates, J. D., Willis, P. W., Sedman, A. J., Stoll, R. G. 1973. Equivalence lack in digoxin plasma levels. *J. Am. Med. Assoc.* 224:199–204
26. Greenblatt, D. J., Duhme, D. W., Koch-Weser, J., Smith, T. W. 1973. Evaluation of digoxin bioavailability in single-dose studies. *N. Engl. J. Med.* 289:651–54
27. Beveridge, T., Kalberer, E., Nüesch, E., Schmidt, R. 1975. Bioavailability studies with digoxin-Sandoz and Lanoxin. *Eur. J. Clin. Pharmacol.* 8:371–76
28. Shaw, T. R. D., Raymond, K., Howard, M. R., Hamer, J. 1973. Therapeutic non-equivalence of digoxin tablets in the United Kingdom: Correlation with tablet dissolution rate. *Br. Med. J.* 4:763–66
29. Khalil, S. A. H. 1974. Bioavailability of digoxin in the presence of antacids. *J. Pharm. Sci.* 63:1641–42 (Letter)
30. Caldwell, J. H., Greenberger, N. J. 1971. Interruption of the enterohepatic circulation of digitoxin by cholestyramine. I. Protection against lethal digitoxin intoxication. *J. Clin. Invest.* 50:2626–37
31. Gallo, D. G., Bailey, K. R., Sheffner, A. L. 1965. The interaction between cholestyramine and drugs. *Proc. Soc. Exp. Biol. Med.* 120:60–65
32. Bazzano, G., Bazzano, G. S. 1972. Digitalis intoxication: Treatment with a new steroid-ending resin. *J. Am. Med. Assoc.* 220:828–30
33. Robinson, D. S., Benjamin, D. M., McCormack, J. J. 1971. Interaction of warfarin and nonsystemic gastrointestinal drugs. *Clin. Pharmacol. Ther.* 12:491–95
34. Ambre, J. J., Fisher, L. J. 1973. Effect of coadministration of aluminum and magnesium hydroxides on absorption of anticoagulants in man. *Clin. Pharmacol. Ther.* 14:231–38
35. Bockbrader, H. N., Caldwell, J. L., Reuning, R. H., Lewis, R. P., Goodenow, J. S. 1976. Failure of cholestyramine to enhance digoxin elimination. *Clin. Res.* 24:225 (Abstr.)
36. Zajtchuk, R., Corby, D. G., Miller, J. G. 1975. Treatment of digoxin toxicity with activated charcoal. *Am. J. Cardiol.* 35:178 (Abstr.)
37. Shore, P. A., Brodie, B. B., Hogben, C. A. M. 1957. The gastric secretion of drugs: A pH partition hypothesis. *J. Pharmacol. Exp. Ther.* 119:361–69
38. Milne, M. D. 1965. Influence of acid-base balance on efficacy and toxicity of drugs. *Proc. R. Soc. Med.* 58:961–63
39. Benet, L. Z. 1973. *Drug Des.* 4:24–32
40. Levine, R. R. 1970. Factors affecting gastrointestinal absorption of drugs. *Digest. Dis.* 15:171–88
41. Manninen, V., Melin, J., Apajalahti, A., Karesoja, M. 1973. Altered absorption of digoxin in patients given propantheline and metoclopramide. *Lancet* 1:398–400
42. Manninen, V., Apajalahti, A., Simonen, H., Reissell, P. 1973. Effect of propantheline and metoclopramide on absorption of digoxin. *Lancet* 1:1118–19 (Letter)
43. Stenson, R. E., Constantino, R. T., Harrison, D. C. 1971. Interrelationships of hepatic blood flow, cardiac output, and blood levels of lidocaine in man. *Circulation* 43:205–11
44. Thomson, P. D., Melmon, K. L., Richardson, J. A., Cohn, K., Steinbrunn, W., Cudihee, R., Rowland, M. 1973. Lidocaine pharmacokinetics in advanced heart failure, liver disease, and renal failure in humans. *Ann. Intern. Med.* 78:499–508
45. Branch, R. A., Shand, D. G., Wilkinson, G. R., Nies, A. S. 1973. The reduction of lidocaine clearance by dl-propranolol: An example of hemodynamic drug interaction. *J. Pharmacol. Exp. Ther.* 184:515–19
46. Halkin, H., Meffin, P., Melmon, K. L., Rowland, M. 1975. Influence of congestive heart failure on blood levels of lidocaine and its active monodeethylated metabolite. *Clin. Pharmacol. Ther.* 17:669–76
47. O'Reilly, R. A., Aggeler, P. M. 1969. Effect of barbiturates on oral anticoagulants in man. *Clin. Res.* 17:153 (Abstr.)
48. Koch-Weser, J., Sellers, E. M. 1976. Binding of drugs to serum albumin. *N. Engl. J. Med.* 294:311–16, 526–31
49. Schrogie, J. J., Solomon, H. M. 1967. The anticoagulant response to bishydroxycoumarin. II. The effect of D-thyroxin, clofibrate, and norethandrolone. *Clin. Pharmacol. Ther.* 8:70–77
50. Aggeler, P. M., O'Reilly, R. A., Leong, L. 1967. Potentiation of anticoagulant

effect of warfarin by phenylbutazone. *N. Engl. J. Med.* 276:496–501

51. Hobbs, C. B., Miller, A. L., Thornley, J. H. 1965. Potentiation of anticoagulant therapy by oxyphenylbutazone (a probable case). *Postgrad. Med. J.* 41:563–65

52. Sellers, E. M., Koch-Weser, J. 1970. Potentiation of warfarin-induced hypoprothombinemia by chloral hydrate. *N. Engl. J. Med.* 283:827–31

53. Sellers, E. M., Koch-Weser, J. 1970. Displacement of warfarin from human albumin by diazoxide and ethacrynic, mefenamic, and nalidixic acids. *Clin. Pharmacol. Ther.* 11:524–29

54. Solomon, H. M., Schrogie, J. J., Williams, D. 1967. The displacement of phenylbutazone-^{14}C and warfarin-^{14}C from human albumin by various drugs and fatty acids. *Biochem. Pharmacol.* 17:143–51

55. Seiler, K., Duckert, F. 1968. Properties of 3-(1-phenylpropyl)-4-oxy-coumarin (Marcoumar®) in the plasma when tested in normal cases and under the influence of drugs. *Thromb. Diath. Haemorrh.* 19:389–96

56. Solomon, H. M., Schrogie, J. J. 1967. The effect of various drugs on the binding of warfarin-^{14}C to human albumin. *Biochem. Pharmacol.* 16:1219–26

57. Vesell, E. S., Passananti, G. T., Johnson, A. O. 1975. Failure of indomethacin and warfarin to interact in normal human volunteers. *J. Clin. Pharmacol.* 15:486–95

58. Solomon, H. M., Reich, S., Spirt, N., Abrams, W. B. 1971. Interactions between digitoxin and other drugs in vitro and in vivo. *Ann. NY Acad. Sci* 179:362–70

59. Solomon, H. M., Abrams, W. B. 1972. Interactions between digitoxin and other drugs in man. *Am. Heart J.* 83:277–80

60. Roe, T. F., Podosin, R. L., Blaskovics, M. E. 1975. Drug interaction: diazoxide and diphenylhydantoin. *J. Pediatr.* 87:480–84

61. Brodie, B. B. 1965. Displacement of one drug by another from carrier or receptor sites. *Proc. R. Soc. Med.* 58:946–55

62. Sellers, E. M., Koch-Weser, J. 1971. Kinetics and clinical importance of displacement of warfarin from albumin by acidic drugs. *Ann. NY Acad. Sci.* 179:213–25

63. Wardell, W. M. 1974. Redistributional drug interactions: A critical examination of putative clinical examples. In *Drug Interactions,* ed. P. L. Morselli, S. Garattini, S. N. Cohen. New York: Raven. 406 pp.

64. Payne, J. P., Rowe, G. G. 1957. The effects of mecamylamine in the cat as modified by the administration of carbon dioxide. *Br. J. Pharmacol.* 12:457–60

65. Burns, J. J., Conney, A. H. 1965. Enzyme stimulation and inhibition in the metabolism of drugs. *Proc. R. Soc. Med.* 58:955–60

66. Gelehrter, T. D. 1976. Enzyme induction. *N. Engl. J. Med.* 294:522–26, 589–95, 646–51

67. Cucinell, S. A., Conney, A. H., Sansur, M., Burns, J. J. 1965. Drug interactions in man. I. Lowering effect of phenobarbital on plasma levels of bishydroxycoumarin (Dicumarol) and diphenylhydantoin (Dilantin). *Clin. Pharmacol. Ther.* 6:420–29

68. Buchanan, R. A., Heffelfinger, J. C., Weiss, C. F. 1969. The effect of phenobarbital on diphenylhydantoin metabolism in children. *Pediatrics* 43:114–16

69. Kutt, H., Haynes, J., Verebely, K., McDowell, F. 1969. The effect of phenobarbital on plasma diphenylhydantoin level and metabolism in man and in rat liver microsomes. *Neurology* 19:611–16

70. Hansen, J. M., Siersbaek-Nielsen, K., Skovsted, L. 1971. Carbamazepine-induced acceleration of diphenylhydantoin and warfarin metabolism in man. *Clin. Pharmacol. Ther.* 12:539–43

71. Data, J. L., Wilkinson, G. R., Nies, A. S. 1976. Interaction of quinidine with anticonvulsant drugs. *N. Engl. J. Med.* 294:699–702

72. Kiørboe, E. 1966. Phenytoin intoxication during treatment with Antabuse® (Disulfiram). *Epilepsia* 7:246–49

73. Kutt, H., Verebely, K., McDowell, F. 1968. Inhibition of diphenylhydantoin metabolism in rats and in rat liver microsomes by antitubercular drugs. *Neurology* 18:706–10

74. Garrettson, L. K., Perel, J. M., Dayton, P. G. 1969. Methylphenidate interaction with both anticonvulsants and ethyl biscoumacetate. *J. Am. Med. Assoc.* 207:2053–56

75. Soda, D. M., Levy, G. 1975. Inhibition of drug metabolism by hydroxylated metabolites: Cross-inhibition and specificity. *J. Pharm. Sci.* 64:1928–31

76. Lumholtz, B., Siersbaek-Nielsen, K., Skovsted, L., Kampmann, J., Moelholm-Hansen, J. 1975. Sulfamethizole-

induced inhibition of diphenylhydantoin, tolbutamide, and warfarin metabolism. *Clin. Pharmacol. Ther.* 17:731–34

77. Murray, F. J. 1962. Outbreak of unexpected reactions among epileptics taking isoniazid. *Am. Rev. Respir. Dis.* 86:729–32

78. Solomon, H. M., Schrogie, J. J. 1967. The effect of phenyramidol on the metabolism of diphenylhydantoin. *Clin. Pharmacol. Ther.* 8:554–56

79. Hansen, J. M., Kristensen, M., Skovsted, L. 1968. Sulthiame (Opsollot®) as inhibitor of diphenylhydantoin metabolism. *Epilepsia* 9:17—22

80. Christensen, L. K., Skovsted, L. 1969. Inhibition of drug metabolism by chloramphenicol. *Lancet* 2:1397–99

81. Sjoqvist, F. 1965. Psychotropic drugs (2). Interaction between monoamine oxidase (MAO) inhibitors and other substances. *Proc. R. Soc. Med.* 58:967–77

82. DeVita, V. T., Hahn, M. A., Oliverio, V. T. 1965. Monoamine oxidase inhibition by a new carcinostatic agent, N-isopropyl-A-(2-methyl-hydrazino)-p-toluamide (MIH). *Proc. Soc. Exp. Biol. Med.* 120:561–65

83. Weiner, I. M., Mudge, G. J. 1964. Renal tubular mechanisms for excretion of organic acids and bases. *Am. J. Med.* 36:743–62

84. Rennick, B. R. 1972. Renal excretion of drugs: Tubular transport and metabolism. *Ann. Rev. Pharmacol.* 12:141–56

85. Prescott, L. F. 1972. Mechanisms of renal excretion of drugs. *Br. J. Anaesth.* 44:246–51

86. Steiness, E. 1974. Renal tubular secretion of digoxin. *Circulation* 50:103–7

87. Milne, M. D., Scribner, B. H., Crawford, M. A. 1958. Non-ionic diffusion and the excretion of weak acids and bases. *Am. J. Med.* 24:709–29

88. Beckett, A. H., Rowland, M. 1965. Urinary excretion kinetics of amphetamines in man. *J. Pharm. Pharmacol.* 17:628–39

89. Weily, H. S., Genton, E. 1972. Pharmacokinetics of procainamide. *Arch. Intern. Med.* 130:366–69

90. Galeazzi, R. L., Sheiner, L. B., Lockwood, T., Benet, L. Z. 1976. The renal elimination of procainamide. *Clin. Pharmacol. Ther.* 19:55–62

91. Gerhardt, R. E., Knouss, R. F., Thyrum, P. T., Luchi, R. J., Morris, J. J. 1969. Quinidine excretion in aciduria and alkaluria. *Ann. Intern. Med.* 71:927–33

92. Nash, C. W., Heath, C. 1961. Vascular responses to catecholamines during respiratory changes in pH. *Am. J. Physiol.* 200:755–82

93. Roberts, J., Ito, R., Reilly, J., Carioli, V. J. 1963. Influence of reserpine and beta TM 10 on digitalis induced ventricular arrhythmia. *Circ. Res.* 13:149–58

94. Boakes, A. J., Laurence, D. R., Teoh, P. C., Barar, F. S. K., Benedikter, L. T., Prichard, B. N. C. 1973. Interactions between sympathomimetic amines and antidepressant agents in man. *Br. Med. J.* 1:311–15

95. Allum, W., Aminu, J., Bloomfield, T. H., Davies, C., Scales, A. H., Vere, D. W. 1974. Interaction between debrisoquin and phenylephrine in man. *Br. J. Clin. Pharmacol.* 1:51–57

96. Leishman, A. W. D., Matthews, H. L., Smith, A. J. 1963. Antagonism of guanethidine by imipramine. *Lancet* 1:112

97. Stone, C. A., Porter, C. C., Stavorski, J. M., Ludden, C. T., Totaro, J. A. 1964. Antagonism of catecholamine-depleting agents by antidepressant and related drugs. *J. Pharmacol.* 144:196–204

98. Gokhale, S. D., Gulati, O. D., Udwadia, B. P. 1966. Antagonism of the adrenergic neurone blocking action of guanethidine by certain antidepressant and antihistamine drugs. *Arch. Int. Pharmacodyn.* 160:321–29

99. Mitchell, J. R., Arias, L., Oates, J. A. 1967. Antagonism of the antihypertensive action of guanethidine sulfate by desipramine hydrochloride. *J. Am. Med. Assoc.* 202:973–76

100. Hanahoe, T. H. P., Ireson, J. D., Large, B. J. 1969. Interactions between guanethidine and inhibitors of noradrenaline uptake. *Arch. Int. Pharmacodyn.* 182:349–53

101. Skinner, C., Coull, D. C., Johnston, A. W., 1969. Antagonism of the hypotensive action of bethanidine and debrisoquin by tricyclic antidepressants. *Lancet* 2:564–60

102. Mitchell, J. R., Cavanaugh, J. H., Arias, L., Oates, J. A. 1970. Guanethidine and related agents. III. Antagonism by drugs which inhibit the norepinephrine pump in man. *J. Clin. Invest.* 49:1596–1604

103. Boullin, D. J. 1975. The action of antidepressants on the effects of other drugs. *Primary Care* 2:669–88

104. Day, M. D. 1962. Effect of sympathomimetic amines on the blocking ac-

tion of guanethidine, bretylium, xylo-choline. *Br. J. Pharmacol.* 18:421–39
105. Day, M. D., Rand, M. J. 1962. Antagonism of guanethidine by dexamphetamine and other related sympathomimetic amines. *J. Pharm. Sci.* 14:541–49
106. Day, M. D., Rand, M. J. 1963. Evidence for a competitive antagonism of guanethidine by dexamphetamine. *Br. J. Pharmacol.* 20:17–28
107. Chang, C. C., Costa, E., Brodie, B. B. 1964. Reserpine-induced release of drugs from sympathetic nerve endings. *Life Sci.* 3:839–44
108. Fann, W. E., Cavanaugh, J. H., Kaufmann, J. S. 1972. Doxepin: Effects on transport of biogenic amines in man. *Psychopharmacologia* 22:111–25
109. Janowsky, D. S., El-Yousef, M. K., Davis, J. M., Fann, W. E. 1973. Antagonism of guanethidine by chlorpromazine. *Am. J. Psychiatry* 130:808–12
110. Misage, J. R., McDonald, R. H. 1970. Antagonism of hypotensive action of bethanidine by "common cold" remedy. *Br. Med. J.* 4:347–49
111. Hoobler, S. W., Sagastume, E. 1971. Clonidine hydrochloride in the treatment of hypertension. *Am. J. Cardiol.* 28:67–83
112. Briant, R. H., Reid, J. L., Dollery, C. T. 1973. Interaction between clonidine and desipramine in man. *Br. Med. J.* 1:522–23
113. Burn, J. H., Rand, M. J. 1958. The action of sympathomimetic amines in animals treated with reserpine. *J. Physiol.* 144:314–36
114. Boura, A. L. A., Green, A. F. 1963. Adrenergic neurone blockade and other acute effects caused by N-benzyl-N'-N"-dimethylguanidine and its orthochloro derivative. *Br. J. Pharmacol.* 20:36–55
115. Prichard, B. N. C., Ross, E. J. 1966. Use of propranolol in conjunction with alpha receptor blocking drugs in pheochromocytoma. *Am. J. Cardiol.* 18:394–98
116. Nies, A. S., Shand, D. G. 1973. Hypertensive response to propranolol in a patient treated with methyl dopa—a proposed mechanism. *Clin. Pharmacol. Ther.* 14:823–26
117. McMurtry, R. J. 1974. Propranolol, hypoglycemia, and hypertensive crisis. *Ann. Intern. Med.* 80:669–70
118. Blum, I., Atsmon, A., Steiner, M., Wysenbeeck, H. 1975. Paradoxical rise in blood pressure during propranolol treatment. *Br. Med. J.* 4:623
119. Noble, J., Matthew, H. 1969. Acute poisoning by antidepressants: Clinical features and management of 100 patients. *Clin. Toxicol.* 2:403–21
120. Newton, R. W. 1974. Physostigmine salicylate in the treatment of tricyclic antidepressant overdosage. *J. Am. Med. Assoc.* 231:941–44
121. Davis, J. M., Bartlett, E., Termini, B. S. 1968. Overdosage of psychotropic drugs. A review. *Dis. Nerv. Syst.* 29:157–64, 246–56
122. Williams, R. B. Jr., Sherter, C. 1971. Cardiac complications of tricyclic antidepressant therapy. *Ann. Intern. Med.* 74:395–98
123. Arita, M., Surawicz, B. 1973. Electrophysiologic effects of phenothiazines on canine cardiac fibers. *J. Pharmacol. Exp. Ther.* 184:619–30
124. Fowler, N. O., McCall, D., Chou, T., Holmes, J. C., Hanenson, I. B. 1976. Electrocardiographic changes and cardiac arrhythmias in patients receiving psychotropic drugs. *Am. J. Cardiol.* 37:223–30
125. Solymoss, B., Toth, S., Varga, S., Selye, H. 1971. Protection by spironolactone and oxandrolone against chronic digitoxin or indomethacin intoxication. *Toxicol. Appl. Pharmacol.* 18:586–92
126. Taylor, S. A., Rawlins, M. D., Smith, S. E. 1972. Spironolactone—a weak enzyme inducer in man. *J. Pharm. Pharmacol.* 24:578–79
127. Tweedale, M. G., Ogilvie, R. I. 1973. Antagonism of spironolactone-induced natriuresis by aspirin in man. *N. Engl. J. Med.* 289:198–200
128. Koch-Weser, J., Sellers, E. M. 1971. Drug interactions with coumarin anticoagulants. *N. Engl. J. Med.* 285:487–98, 547–58
129. Koch-Weser, J. 1975. Drug interactions in cardiovascular therapy. *Am. Heart J.* 90:93–116
130. Mustard, J. F., Packham, M. A. 1970. Factors influencing platelet function: Adhesion, release, and aggregation. *Pharmacol. Rev.* 22:97–187
131. Genton, E., Gent, M., Hirsh, J., Harker, L. A. 1975. Platelet-inhibiting drugs in the prevention of clinical thrombotic disease. *N. Engl. J. Med.* 293:1174–78, 1236–40, 1296–1300

Ann. Rev. Pharmacol. Toxicol. 1977. 17:311–23

PHARMACOLOGICAL BASIS FOR COMBINATION THERAPY OF HYPERTENSION

❖6682

C. T. Dollery

Department of Clinical Pharmacology, Royal Postgraduate Medical School,
London W12 OHS England

COMBINATION THERAPY OF HYPERTENSION

One of the basic concepts of modern therapeutics is that drugs should be used only for specific purposes and that blunderbuss therapy should be discouraged. Many clinical scientists are outraged when they learn that patients with severe hypertension often receive treatment with three, four, or even five drugs at the same time, not one of which is directed at an identified etiological factor or specific deviant physiological mechanism. Their concern is justified, but multidrug therapy of hypertension does have a rationale although few of the many combinations in use have had their efficacy, safety, and side effects defined in comparison with possible alternatives.

Originally antihypertensive drugs were combined out of desperation to try to save the lives of patients with accelerated hypertension whose pressure control was inadequate. The hope was to find drugs with a synergistic effect, but what was demonstrated was usually some degree of additive effect.

As the number of effective drugs has increased it has become rare to be confronted with a patient whose blood pressure cannot be reduced with one of the available drugs. The emphasis has shifted to finding means of minimizing the unwanted effects of therapy or producing a more favorable profile of hemodynamic effects (1, 2).

Investigation of Drug Combinations

Demonstration of synergy between two or more antihypertensive drugs in man is no easy matter. In animals, where the number of experiments is not a limiting factor, the normal method is to construct dose-response curves of one drug at one or more dose levels of the second. From these families of dose-response curves the dose ratio can be calculated as a convenient measure of potentiation.

In man it is rarely possible to examine the whole of a dose-response curve because of the risk of excessive hypotension or side effects. The number of subjects and

311

measurement points is also likely to be less than ideal for reaching a precise conclusion.

The usual method for studying drug combinations in man is to add a fixed or variable dose of one drug to a constant dose of another. It is important that the experiment should be double-blind and placebo controlled. Both bias and digit preference are important problems in blood pressure recording and they can be avoided by using a sphygmomanometer that prevents bias (3) or automatic equipment such as the arteriosonde. Placebo responses can confuse the interpretation of results unless a control period on the placebo is included. In the British MRC trial through the use of either bendrofluazide or propranolol in mild hypertension the fall in pressure in the actively treated groups averaged about 24/12 mm Hg but the fall on placebo was about half of this so that the response due to the drug was only about 12/6 mm Hg.

Another problem of clinical trial design lies in the recording of drug side effects. As the choice between drugs often rests upon a claimed lesser incidence of side effects, this is a matter of great importance. The most reliable method is to use a printed questionnaire which is completed by the patient at intervals during the trial; reliance upon symptoms recorded in case notes or checklists is much less satisfactory (4, 5).

Prediction of Response to Antihypertensive Drugs

Efforts to define a specific cause for most cases of human hypertension have not succeeded. In the absence of a known cause, efforts to identify pathophysiological factors that influence the response to particular drugs have also failed, the sole exception being the relationship between renin status and response to β-blocking drugs and diuretics.

Hypertensive patients who maintain a low plasma renin on a low sodium diet do not respond to low doses of propranolol with a fall in pressure (6, 7). However, there may be a dual mechanism of response to propranolol, and the blood pressure of low renin patients can be reduced by higher doses of propranolol (8). Furthermore a combination of a diuretic and a β-blocker may have an additive effect in lowering the blood pressure irrespective of the renin status (9).

Although the pretreatment renin may be of some value in predicting the patients who will respond to propranolol or, in the case of low renin patients, to diuretics there is a poor correlation between the magnitude of the fall in renin with β-blockers and the fall in blood pressure (10). It appears that renin release can be blocked by lower doses of propranolol than are needed to produce a maximal fall in the blood pressure (11).

Thus the specificity of response to β-blockers and diuretics in relation to renin status does not invalidate the concept of using these drugs in combination.

REGULATION OF BLOOD PRESSURE

"Arterial pressure is not regulated by a single pressure controlling system but instead by several interrelated systems that perform specific functions" (12). The level of blood pressure is set by the output of the heart and the level of the systemic vascular resistance, but both output and resistance are under the control of more than one system.

The rapidly acting control systems rely upon the baroreflex and the release of hormones such as norepinephrine, epinephrine, angiotensin, and vasopressin. Of these the baroreflex is the most important for buffering short-term changes of blood pressure but it is probably unimportant in the long term because the baroreceptors reset to a new level of pressure over 24–48 hr. Release of norepinephrine and epinephrine from the adrenal is a useful supplement to the sympathetic innervation of blood vessels in emergency situations, but it is not clear whether these hormones circulate in sufficient concentrations in normal circumstances to play a significant role in maintaining blood pressure. Both the renin-angiotensin system and vasopressin are activated in low pressure states in man and animals, and they play a role in the restoration of blood pressure in an emergency. It is unlikely that angiotensin plays a role in normal pressure regulation because the competitive antagonist saralasin does not lower blood pressure if infused into a normal person on a normal sodium intake (13). Longer-term regulation of blood pressure appears to rely upon other mechanisms. Reduction of blood pressure disturbs the Starling equilibrium of hydrostatic forces in the capillary and brings about a movement of fluid from the tissues into the vascular compartment. However, a much more important mechanism is the kidney's role in changing the output of salt and water in accordance with the level of blood pressure. Guyton has suggested that the relationship between blood pressure and salt and water output by the kidney is fixed and that this system has infinite gain. This would accord a dominant role to this system in all circumstances, but there is some evidence that the relationship is not completely fixed and that adaptive changes take place which alter the renal pressure threshold for sodium excretion. Another important long-term adaptive mechanism is hypertrophy of the vascular smooth muscle in response to pressure elevation (14). Smooth muscle hypertrophy makes the artery better able to withstand a high vascular pressure, moves the high and low autoregulatory breakpoints upwards, and enhances the pressor response to a given degree of fiber shortening in the smooth muscle because of the greater thickness of the wall (15). Guyton assigns an important role to vascular autoregulation in the determination of the long-term level of pressure. If the kidney retains salt and water, the cardiac output will rise because the filling pressure of the heart will increase. Increased perfusion of the tissues will ultimately bring about an increase in vascular resistance as a tissue autoregulatory response to excessive flow. This is the mechanism of the rise in pressure in animals or man without kidneys and explains the excessive sensitivity to fluid overload in the "renoprival" state.

The pharmacological activity of hypotensive agents must be interpreted against this background. Diuretics that increase salt and water output at a given level of blood pressure would be expected to lower blood pressure—perhaps to be more effective than they have proved to be. Reduction of cardiac output by inhibition of the sympathetic innervation of the heart should lower the blood pressure, after the baroreflex has fatigued, by an autoregulatory mechanism. Disabling vascular regulation by sympathetic inhibition or direct dilatation of vascular smooth muscle should also be an effective means of lowering the blood pressure.

However, all these systems are interrelated. A sudden fall in blood pressure activates all of them. The baroreflex fires, sympathetic nerves discharge, the adrenal gland releases catecholamines, the kidney secretes renin, the pituitary, vasopressin. Capillary pressure falls and fluid begins to pass from tissues into the vascular compartment. Renal output of salt and water is restricted or, if the pressure fall is severe, it ceases. All these restorative mechanisms come into play to try to minimize the fall in blood pressure. It is surprising that single antihypertensive drugs are effective in some patients with hypertension. It might be anticipated that these mechanisms would be able to overcome the action of a drug that had disabled only one control system. The rationale of combined drug therapy is that by disabling more than one control system simultaneously these feedback loops are inhibited and there is a greater pressure fall for a given degree of inhibition of a particular control system. As the physiological consequences of disabling any one control system completely may be undesirable, e.g. postural hypotension, such a line of reasoning provides a logical reason for partial inhibition of several systems at the same time.

THE RATIONALE FOR COMBINED USE OF DRUGS IN HYPERTENSION

If two drugs when coadministered have a greater effect than either alone in lowering the blood pressure there may be a case for using them together in a therapeutic regime. However, if this is all they do the advantage would be small and it might be simpler to use a larger dose of one of the drugs by itself. In practice the advantages that are looked for are either a more favorable profile of circulatory effects or a reduction of side effects or toxicity.

The main problem of using sympathetic inhibitory drugs to treat high blood pressure is that these agents interfere with normal circulatory reflexes and lead to a greater fall in blood pressure on standing or after exercise. If addition of a second drug to the first achieved a proportional increase in the fall in blood pressure in recumbency and on standing it would have no therapeutic advantage. For this reason, drugs that have a postural effect upon blood pressure are rarely coadministered (16). However, if the second drug has a different type of action it may be possible to achieve a fall in recumbent pressure without exaggeration of the postural fall. This is why diuretics are combined with many other antihypertensive drugs, particularly sympathetic inhibitors.

An additional reason for administering two or more drugs together is to reduce unwanted effects of some members of the combination while retaining an adequate hypotensive effect. At its simplest this may involve no more than using smaller doses of two drugs together to reduce the side effects of each while retaining the desired effect. Alternatively the properties of one drug may be used to overcome unwanted actions of another. Examples are: (a) use of a potassium-retaining diuretic such as amiloride, triamterene, or spironolactone with a potassium-losing one such as a benzothiadiazine (17); (b) use of a β-receptor–blocking drug with a vasodilator to minimize the tachycardia and palpitations that would otherwise result from stimulation of the baroreflex (18); (c) use of a diuretic with a vasodilator or other hypotensive agent that is liable to cause salt and water retention to prevent this (19).

A convenient way of subdividing the combinations to be discussed is by the number of drug components in the combination, two, three, or four.

Drug Pairs

DIURETIC COMBINATIONS WITH OTHER SINGLE DRUGS   Benzothiadiazine diuretics and related structures are among the most widely used antihypertensive drugs, and it has become almost universal practice to start treatment with them and to add other drugs as required. One of the advantages of diuretics is that they have a flat dose-response curve (20) with a nonpostural effect and thus can be prescribed in a fixed dose.

The mechanism of the hypotensive action of diuretics has not been completely explained but there is little doubt that it is due to depletion of salt and water. Early suggestions that the effect was brought about by a fall in plasma volume were disputed on the grounds that the effect was transitory. However, some long-term contraction of plasma volume persists and this may be one mechanism of the hypotensive action (21). Combination of diuretics with other hypotensive agents increases the magnitude of the fall of pressure obtained with either drug alone. This point has been established with almost all antihypertensive drugs in use.

Diuretics with β-adrenoceptor–blocking agents   Richardson et al (22) studied the effect of a placebo, propranolol, 120 mg daily; chlorthalidone, 50 mg daily; and of propranolol with chlorthalidone in the same doses. The blood pressures were placebo, 172.0/106.7; propranolol, 162.8/98.7; chlorthalidone, 148.6/97.7; combination, 138.7/92.1 mm Hg. Angervall & Bystedt (23) demonstrated that this type of effect was synergistic. They established that alprenolol in a dose of 700 mg was equihypotensive to chlorthalidone in a dose of 50 mg. If the effect was additive it might be expected that half the dose of each would be needed to achieve the same effect, but it turned out that one quarter of the dose of each drug combined was sufficient to match the effect of either alone.

The potentiation of the hypotensive action by combining β-receptor–blocking drugs and diuretics has been established for a great many individual compounds (24–26).

Diuretics with centrally acting drugs   Smith et al (27) showed that a fall of recumbent blood pressure of 17.5/13.7 mm Hg on 1.5 g/day of methyldopa was increased to 23.3/14.9 mm Hg when 500 mg/day of chlorothiazide was added. Other authors have obtained similar results (28, 29). Rosenman (30) observed a blood pressure of 163/99 mm Hg in patients treated with 50 mg/day of chlorthalidone which fell to 142/83 mm Hg when an average of 0.37 mg/day of clonidine was added to the treatment.

Diuretics with reserpine   Fixed ratio drug combinations containing reserpine and a diuretic are among the most popular hypotensive drugs. Their use was called into question in 1974 when several papers were published (31, 32) suggesting an association between the ingestion of reserpine and an increased incidence of breast cancer in middle-aged women. Later work has not confirmed the earlier findings which were critically dependent upon the methods used to choose controls (33, 34). However, the argument still rumbles on and the last word has not yet been written (35). While doubt remains, the tendency to switch to combinations including β-blockers rather than reserpine is likely to continue. The combination of chlorothiazide and reserpine is undoubtedly effective, and in one study it reduced the mean arterial pressure by 20 mm Hg in over two thirds of patients (36).

Diuretics with adrenergic neurone–blocking drugs   Many published reports have demonstrated that the hypotensive effect of adrenergic neurone–blocking drugs is increased to a modest extent by addition of a diuretic (37, 38).

Diuretics with hydralazine   At one time this was also a popular combination (39), but it is used less often now because the triple combination including a β-receptor-blocking drug is preferred.

DIURETICS AND THE PREVENTION OF FLUID RETENTION BY OTHER DRUGS
Most antihypertensive agents apart from the diuretics have been reported to cause salt and water retention in a proportion of patients. Guyton's hypothesis (12) can be invoked to explain this phenomenon. If this pressure threshold is not reset downwards, salt and water retention would be a normal regulatory response whose aim would be to restore the previous level of pressure.

Dustan et al (40) studied changes in plasma volume in 16 patients treated long-term with antihypertensive drugs. Plasma volume was normal or high, and there was a correlation between plasma volume as percentage of normal and the blood pressure. Intensive diuretic therapy lowered the plasma volume below normal and reduced the arterial pressure. Finnerty and his colleagues (19, 41) demonstrated that resistance to diazoxide, hydralazine, or reserpine that developed in the course of treatment was associated with fluid retention. In a group of patients treated with intravenous diazoxide for ten days there was an average increase in weight of 3.1 kg and a rise in extracellular fluid volume of 3.3 liters. Ronnov-Jessen & Hansen (42) showed a rise in exchangeable sodium of 210 meq after 8–14 days treatment with guanethidine with a rise in blood volume of 382 ml. Diuretic treatment returned these values to normal. Fluid retention appears to be especially prominent with powerful vasodilators such as minoxidil. Wilburn et al (43) reported that the average dose of furosemide required to prevent fluid retention was 578 mg/day and some patients require 1200 mg/day.

Thus one justification for using a diuretic as a basic component of the treatment regime is to prevent this fluid retention and thus to avoid the development of resistance in some patients.

THE CASE AGAINST ROUTINE USE OF DIURETICS AS A COMPONENT OF ANTIHYPERTENSIVE COMBINATIONS   There has been some controversy concerning the routine use of diuretics as the first component of antihypertensive regimes.

The argument has never been clearly formulated in public but some of the strands in it are as follows:

1. Diuretics elevate the plasma renin and renin may be a factor responsible for vascular damage (44). There are two main weaknesses to this argument, first, that most subsequent work does not support the assertion that renin does damage blood vessels (45, 46), and, second, that the elevation of plasma renin during prolonged diuretic treatment is modest (21, 47).

2. Diuretics have undesirable metabolic effects such as hypokalemia, hyperuricemia, hyperglycemia, and retention of calcium. This statement is true but the evidence that diuretics cause harm is wanting. A mild degree of hypokalemia does not appear to cause either symptoms or adverse effects upon long-term kidney function (48). Hyperuricemia caused by thiazides rarely appears to cause gout. There may be more room for concern about the long-term effect of thiazides upon glucose tolerance but further evidence is needed before any conclusion can be reached about its clinical significance (49). The mild elevation of serum calcium caused by thiazides appears unimportant unless there is also some other reason for hypercalcemia.

3. Use of diuretics confuses the interpretation of the serum potassium concentration and makes it more difficult to detect primary hyperaldosteronism and to investigate renin mechanisms. These arguments may be important to an investigator whose center of work is renin and aldosterone, but they need not be taken too seriously in therapeutics.

Against these arguments is the important consideration that thiazides are cheap, effective, and easy to use. If the thiazides were not available, the treatment of hypertension would be appreciably more difficult.

OTHER DRUG PAIRS

Vasodilators and sympathetic inhibitors   Vasodilators are one of the most important groups of antihypertensive drugs although only hydralazine has been widely used over long periods. The combination of hydralazine with a ganglion-blocking drug, hexamethonium, was tried as early as 1955 (50). Combinations of reserpine and hydralazine have been thoroughly studied and extensively used. In one study of 426 patients given reserpine 0.5 mg daily and hydralazine 200 mg daily, the changes in pressure were placebo +3.7/+2.0 mm Hg; reserpine alone −3.0/−5.1 mm Hg; and reserpine plus hydralazine −4.9/−10.5 mm Hg (51).

More recently, hydralazine has often been combined with a β-receptor–blocking drug (52–56). It is of interest that there has been some disagreement concerning the effect of combining a β-blocking–drug and hydralazine in animals (57, 58).

Several new and powerful vasodilators have been introduced, including diazoxide, prazosin, and minoxidil. One of the reasons for the revival of interest in vasodilators has been the availability of β-receptor–blocking drugs and diuretics which can be used to overcome the tachycardia and fluid retention which commonly occur when they are used alone (59). A further advantage of combining a vasodilator and a β-blocker is that this prevents the rise in plasma renin caused by the vasodilator (60, 61).

Adrenergic neurone blocking drugs, centrally acting drugs, and β-blockers   Day & Prichard (62) reported an additional fall of blood pressure of 20 mm Hg when propranolol was added to patients under treatment with bethanidine and 12 mm Hg when it was added to treatment with methyldopa. Pearson et al (63) demonstrated a fall in blood pressure averaging 5.7/10.9 mm Hg in patients treated with a mean dose of 27 mg of guanethidine. When oxprenolol 240 mg daily was added, the fall in pressure increased 21.8/17.4 mm Hg. Oxprenolol alone caused a fall in pressure of 17.2/12.2 mm Hg, so the fall on the combined treatment was almost exactly the sum of the individual effects.

Breckenridge & Dollery (64) demonstrated an additive hypotensive effect when bethanidine was added to treatment with methyldopa.

Triple Combinations

Various triple combinations are possible but those that have been most extensively studied have involved the use of a diuretic, vasodilator, and sympathetic inhibitor. Most often the diuretic has been a thiazide, the vasodilator has been hydralazine, and the sympathetic inhibitor reserpine or a β-receptor–blocking drug.

DIURETIC-HYDRALAZINE-RESERPINE   The most significant clinical trials of antihypertensive agents on outcome which have so far been completed were those arranged by the Veterans Administration in the United States (65). These trials used a combination of hydrochlorothiazide (100 mg), hydralazine (75–150 mg), and reserpine (0.2 mg) daily as the therapeutic regime. A particularly instructive study of this combination was conducted by Clark & Troop (66). They treated 114 patients who had previously been on other drugs with a tablet containing reserpine (0.1 mg), hydralazine (25 mg), and hydrochlorothiazide (15 mg) (Ser-Ap-Es) as the sole treatment. The patients had an average pretreatment diastolic pressure of 126 mm Hg, and the average fall in diastolic pressure on the triple combination tablet was 19 mm Hg compared with previous therapy with individual drugs in separate tablets.

DIURETIC–HYDRALAZINE–β-BLOCKING DRUGS   This combination is becoming a very popular one in therapeutics. One of the most convincing studies was that of Zacest and his colleagues (55). They used a regime consisting of hydrochlorothiazide (100 mg), hydralazine (average dose 225 mg/day), and propranolol (average dose 143 mg/day). The recumbent blood pressures of the group of patients were 188/118 on the diuretic alone, 162/102 mm Hg on diuretic plus propranolol, and 142/88 mm Hg on the triple combination. This study provides good evidence to support the contention that each component is making a useful contribution to the end result.

Gottlieb and co-workers (56) reported a fall from 191/128 mm Hg to 169/108 mm Hg when hydralazine was added to a regime that already included a thiazide diuretic and propranolol.

It has proved possible to use the triple combination safely in patients with angina pectoris in whom hydralazine alone would have been contraindicated because of the risk of worsening the angina. Plasma renin values on the triple combination were not significantly different from pretreatment values.

DIURETIC–MINOXIDIL–β-BLOCKING DRUGS   Minoxidil is the most effective of the currently available vasodilatory agents and several studies attest to its effectiveness in treating patients who have proved relatively unresponsive to large doses of other drugs (43, 56, 67). Gottlieb et al compared the efficacy of adding hydralazine or minoxidil to a treatment regime that already included a diuretic and propranolol. Minoxidil proved more effective and reduced the average recumbent pressure to 142/92 compared with 169/108 with hydralazine. This regime has also been used successfully in patients who had angina without worsening their condition (43). The addition of propranolol to treatment with minoxidil produces a further fall in blood pressure, prevents the rise in heart rate which otherwise occurs, and reduces the rise in plasma renin activity caused by minoxidil, although not to control values (60).

There has been less interest in triple combinations which include a centrally acting drug such as methyldopa or clonidine, or an adrenergic neurone–blocking drug. Probably the future of such combinations lies with the β-receptor–blocking agents because of their effectiveness in blocking low rates of traffic such as may be the case in recumbency. Adrenergic neurone–blocking drugs are more effective in blocking higher rates of traffic and thus more likely to cause postural hypotension.

PRACTICAL PROBLEMS

The real world of therapeutics is very different from the pharmacology laboratory or the ward of a university hospital. Things that succeed in the ivory tower sometimes fail outside it. Problems with compliance and the consequent return to respectability of the fixed ratio drug combination illustrate these problems in respect of combined drug treatment of hypertension.

Compliance

Patients often do not take their medicines as prescribed (68). In the Veterans Administration trial of antihypertensive therapy, half the patients were rejected as unreliable pill takers during a run-in period. Urine tests on patients taking para-amino salicylic acid for tuberculosis showed that, on average, only half the patients were taking the medicine at the time of the random tests (69). Children with bacteriologically proven streptococcal sore throats were even less reliable. On the ninth day of treatment only 8% had penicillin in their urine (70).

Factors such as social status, educational attainment, and seriousness of the disease process have not proved to be accurate predictors of which patients will take their medicines regularly (71). The problems of treatment dropout and poor compliance are so serious that they threaten the basis of long-term treatment of symptomless conditions (72).

Both the complexity of the therapeutic regime and the severity of drug side effects appear to contribute to noncompliance. Patients who receive more attention comply better than those given routine care (73). It might be expected that a fixed ratio combination drug might have advantages over the same drugs given as individual tablets, but this is yet to be established conclusively (74).

Compliance problems are a powerful argument against multidrug, multitablet regimes unless the patient is in great danger and there is no effective alternative.

Fixed Ratio Drug Combinations

If the treatment of hypertension could be reduced to one tablet once a day it would be much more convenient for the patient and compliance would probably improve. The only candidates for such a combination are various types of three drug combination in a fixed ratio in the same tablet. Some physicians and pharmacologists object that such a product is irrational, confusing, does not permit individualization of treatment, and is illogical in pharmacokinetic terms because of the differing half-lives of the components. Each argument must be taken seriously. Evidence already presented shows that there is a rational justification for simultaneous moderate inhibition of different blood pressure control loops. The product could be confusing if it were marketed under a snappy uninformative name. But it is possible to use a name to convey the nature of the mixture, e.g. Ser-Ap-Es. The fixed ratio does not permit individual adjustment of the components, but if the ratio is near optimal for a large fraction of the patients this is not a matter of great importance. The pharmacokinetic objection is not insuperable because the amount of each constituent and the dosage interval can be adjusted to the requirements of the shortest acting component.

It is probable that in the future most patients with mild to moderate hypertension will be treated with a fixed ratio combination product although it will be necessary to demonstrate by clinical trials that each exerts a biologically significant effect at the chosen dose in the combination.

CONCLUSION

It would be preferable if the theoretical and experimental basis for the use of drug combinations in the treatment of hypertension were better established. At present, the generalization that all hypotensive agents given to man in submaximal doses are likely to have additive effects with all other hypotensive agents which have a different mode of action appears to be true. The value of combinations rests upon their efficacy in relation to side effects and toxicity, and the number of studies that permit a firm conclusion on all of these points is few. However, a very large clinical experience attests to the value of drug combinations in the treatment of hypertension and it is probable that their use will continue to increase.

ACKNOWLEDGMENTS

I am most grateful to Miss E. M. Reid, Librarian of the Royal Postgraduate Medical School, for her help with MEDLARS II literature searches for this review.

Literature Cited

1. Simpson F. O. 1971. Combination antihypertensive therapy. *Cardiovasc. Clin.* 2:37–54
2. Gifford, R. W. 1974. Drug combinations as rational antihypertensive therapy. *Arch. Intern. Med.* 133:1053–57
3. Rose, G. A., Holland, W. W., Crowley, E. A. 1964. A sphygmomanometer for epidemiologists. *Lancet* i:296
4. Bulpitt, C. J., Dollery, C. T. 1973. Side effects of hypotensive agents evaluated by a self-administered questionnaire. *Br. Med. J.* iii:485–90
5. Bulpitt, C. J., Dollery, C. T., Carne, S. J. 1976. Changes in symptoms of hypertensive patients after referral to hospital clinic. *Br. Heart J.* 38:121–28
6. McGregor, G. A., Dawes, P. H. 1976. Antihypertensive effect of propranolol and spironolactone in relation to plasma angiotensin II. *Clin. Sci. Mol. Med.* 50:18P
7. Buhler, F. R., Laragh, J. H., Baer, L., Vaughan, E. D., Brunner, H. R. 1972. Propranolol inhibition of renin secretion. *N. Engl. J. Med.* 287:1209–16
8. Shand, D. G., Frisk-Holmberg, M., McDevitt, D., Sherman, K., Hollifield, J. 1975. A dual antihypertensive mechanism for propranolol based on plasma level/response relationships. In *Pathophysiology and Management of Arterial Hypertension*, ed. G. Berglund, L. Hansson, L. Werko, 17–82. Molndel, Sweden: Lindgren & Sohn
9. Karlberg, B. E., Kagedal, B., Tegler, L., Tolagen, K. 1976. Renin concentrations and effects of propranolol and spironolactone in patients with hypertension. *Br. Med. J.* 1:251–54
10. Bravo, E. L., Tarazi, R. C., Dustan, H. P. 1975. Beta-adrenergic blockade in diuretic-treated patients with essential hypertension. *N. Engl. J. Med.* 292:66–70
11. Michelakis, A. M., McAllister, R. G. 1972. The effect of chronic adrenergic receptor blockade on plasma renin activity in man. *J. Clin. Endocrinol.* 34:386–94
12. Guton, A. C. 1976. *Textbook of Medical Physiology*, 265–94. London: Saunders
13. Streeten, D. H. P., Anderson, G. H., Freiberg, J. M., Dalakos, T. G. 1975. Angiotensin antagonist in diagnosing angiotensinogenic hypertension. *N. Engl. J. Med.* 292:657–61
14. Folkow, B., Hallback, M., Lundgren, Y., Weiss, L. 1971. The effect of intense treatment with hypotensive drugs on structural design of the resistance vessels in spontaneously hypertensive rats. *Acta Physiol. Scand.* 83:280–82
15. Strandgaard, S., Olesen, J., Skinhoj, E., Lassen, N. A. 1973. Autoregulation of brain circulation in severe arterial hypertension. *Br. Med. J.* i:507–10
16. Dollery, C. T., Harington, M. 1961. Interactions of alpha-methyldopa, guanethidine and pentolinium. In *Hypertension—Recent Advances*, ed. A. N. Brest, A. N. Moyer, 464. Philadelphia: Lea & Febiger.
17. George, C. F., Breckenridge, A. M., Dollery, C. T. 1973. Comparison of the potassium retaining effects of amiloride and spironolactone in hypertensive patients with thiazide-induced hypokalaemia. *Lancet* 2:1288—91
18. Gilmore, E., Weil, J., Chidsey, C. 1970. Treatment of essential hypertension with a new vasodilator in combination with beta-adrenergic blockade. *N. Engl. J. Med.* 282:521–27
19. Finnerty, F. A., Davidov, M., Mroczek, W. J., Gavrilovich, L. 1970. Influence of extracellular fluid volume on response to antihypertensive drugs. *Circ. Res.* 27:Suppl. 1, pp. 71–80
20. Cranston, W. I., Juel-Jensen, B. E., Semmence, A. M., Handfield-Jones, R. P. C., Forbes, J. A., Mutch, L. M. M. 1963. Effect of oral diuretics on raised arterial pressure. *Lancet* ii:966
21. Tarazi, R. C., Frohlich, E. D., Dustan, H. P. 1969. Chronic thiazide therapy in hypertension. Evidence for persistent contraction of plasma volume and increased plasma renin activity. *Circulation* 39–40:Suppl., pp.111–201
22. Richardson, D. W., Freund, J., Gear, A. S., Mauck, H. P., Preston, L. W. 1968. Effect of propranolol on elevated arterial pressure. *Circulation* 37:534–42
23. Angervall, G., Bystedt, U. 1974. Effect of alprenolol and alprenol in combination with saluretics in hypertension. *Acta Med. Scand.* 554:39–45
24. Petrie, J. C., Galloway, D. B., Webster, J., Simpson, W. T., Lewis, J. A. 1975. Atenolol and bendrofluazide in hypertension. *Br. Med. J.* 4:133–35
25. Mitchell, I., Lodge, R., Lawson, A. A. 1972. Adjuvant effect of bendrofluazide on propranolol in hypertension. *Scott. Med. J.* 17:326–29
26. O'Brien, E. T., MacKinnon, J. 1972. Propranolol and polythiazide in treat-

ment of hypertension. *Br. Heart J.* 34:1042–44

27. Smith, W. M., Bachman, B., Galante, J. G., Hanowell, E. G., Johnson, W. P., Koch, C. E., Korfmacher, S. D., Thurm, R. H., Bromer, L. 1966. Co-operative clinical trial of alpha-methyl-dopa. 3. Double-blind control comparison of alpha-methyldopa and chlorothiazide and rauwolfia. *Ann. Intern. Med.* 65:657–71

28. Leonard, J. W., Gifford, R. W., Humphrey, D. C. 1965. Treatment of hypertension with methyldopa alone or combined with diuretics and/or guanethidine. *Am. Heart J.* 69:610–18

29. McMahon, P. C. 1975. Efficacy of antihypertensive agents. Comparison of methyldopa and hydrochlorothiazide in combination and singly. *J. Am. Med. Assoc.* 231:155–58

30. Rosenman, R. H. 1975. Combined clonidine-chlorthalidone therapy in hypertension. Two years experience in 30 patients. *Arch. Intern. Med.* 135:1236–39

31. Editorial 1974. Rauwolfia derivatives and cancer. *Lancet* 2:701–2

32. Boston Collab. Drug Surveillance Program 1974. Reserpine and breast cancer. *Lancet* ii:669–71

33. O'Fallon, W. M., Labarthe, D. R., Kurland, L. T. 1975. Rauwolfia derivatives and breast cancer. *Lancet* ii:292–95

34. Laska, E. M., Siegel, C., Meisner, M., Fischer, S., Wanderling, J. 1975. Matched-pairs of reserpine use and breast cancer. *Lancet* ii:296–99

35. Armstrong, B., Skegg, D., White, G., Doll, R. 1976. Rauwolfia derivatives and breast cancer in women. *Lancet* ii:8–11

36. Smith, W. M., Damato, A. N., Galluzzi, N. J., Garfield, C. F., Hanowell, E. G., Stimson, W. H., Thurm, R. H., Walsh, J. J., Bromer, L. 1964. The evaluation of antihypertensive therapy, cooperative clinical trial method. 1. Double-blind control comparison of chlorothiazide, Rauwolfia serpentina and hydralazine. *Ann. Int. Med.* 61:829–46

37. Page, I. H., Hurley, R. E., Dustan, H. P. 1961. The prolonged treatment of hypertension with guanethidine. *J. Am. Med. Assoc.* 175:543–49

38. Brest, A. N., Moyer, J. H. 1961. Therapeutic use of guanethidine. In *Hypertension Recent Advances,* ed. A. N. Brest, J. H. Moyer, p. 449. Philadelphia: Lea & Febiger

39. Veterans Adm. Co-op. Study Antihypertensive Agents 1962. Double blind control study of antihypertensive agents. III. Chlorothiazide alone and in combination with other agents. *Arch. Intern. Med.* 110:230–36

40. Dustan, H. P., Tarazi, R. C., Bravo, E. L. 1972. Dependence of arterial pressure on intravascular volume in treated hypertensive patients. *N. Engl. J. Med.* 286:861–66

41. Finnerty, F. A. 1971. Relationship of extracellular fluid volume to the development of drug resistance in the hypertensive patient. *Am. Heart J.* 81:563–65

42. Ronnov-Jessen, V., Hansen, J. 1969. Blood volume and exchangeable sodium during treatment of hypertension with guanethidine and hydrochlorothiazide. *Acta Med. Scand.* 186:255–63

43. Wilburn, R. L., Blaufuss, A., Bennett, C. M. 1975. Long-term treatment of severe hypertension with minoxidil, propranolol and furosemide. *Circulation* 52:706–13

44. Laragh, J. H., Baer, L., Brunner, H. R., Buhler, F. R., Sealey, J. E., Vaughan, E. D. 1972. Renin, angiotensin and aldosterone system in pathogenesis and management of hypertensive vascular disease. *Am. J. Med.* 52:633–52

45. Doyle, A. E., Jerks, J., Johnston, C. I., Louis, W. J. 1973. Plasma renin and vascular complications in hypertension. *Br. Med. J.* 2:206–7

46. Mroczek, W. J., Finnerty, F. A., Catt, K. H. 1973. Lack of association between plasma-renin and history of heart attack or stroke in patients with essential hypertension. *Lancet* ii:464–68

47. Bourgoignie, J. J., Catanzaro, F. J., Perry, H. M. Jr. 1968. Renin-angiotensin-aldosterone system during chronic thiazide therapy of benign hypertension. *Circulation* 37:27–35

48. Bulpitt, C. J. 1974. Blood urea changes in hypertensive patients according to therapy given, blood pressure control and serum potassium levels. *Br. Heart J.* 36:383–86

49. Lewis, P. J., Kohner, E. M., Petrie, A., Dollery, C. T. 1976. Deterioration of glucose tolerance in hypertensive patients on prolonged diuretic treatment. *Lancet* i:564–66

50. Stein, D. H., Hecht, H. H. 1955. Cardiovascular and renal responses to the combination of hexamethonium and l-hydrazinophthalazine (Apresoline) in

hypertensive subjects. *J. Clin. Invest.* 34:867

51. Veterans Adm. Co-op. Study Antihypertensive Agents 1962. Double-blind control study of antihypertensive agents. *Arch. Int. Med.* 110:222–29

52. Pape, J. 1974. The effect of alprenolol in combination with hydralazine in essential hypertension. A double-blind, crossover study and a long-term follow-up study. *Acta Med. Scand. Suppl.* 554:55

53. Sannerstedt, R., Stenberg, J., Johnsson, G., Werko, L. 1971. Hemodynamic interference of alprenolol with dihydralazine in normal and hypertensive man. *Am. J. Cardiol.* 28:316–20

54. Hansson, L., Olander, R., Aberg, H., Malmcrona, R., Westerland, A. 1971. Treatment of hypertension with propranolol and hydralazine. *Acta Med. Scand.* 190:531–34

55. Zacest, R., Gilmore, E., Koch-Weser, J. 1972. Treatment of essential hypertension with combined vasodilatation and beta-adrenergic blockade. *New Engl. J. Med.* 286:617–22

56. Gottlieb, T. B., Katz, F. H., Chidsey, C. A. 1972. Combined therapy with vasodilator drugs and beta adrenergic blockade in hypertension. A comparative study of minoxidil and hydralazine. *Circulation* 45:571–82

57. Brunner, H., Hedwall, P. R., Meier, M. 1967. Influence of adrenergic beta-receptor blockade on the acute cardiovascular effects of hydralazine. *Br. J. Pharmacol. Chemother.* 30:122–33

58. Scriabine, A., Ludden, C. T., Bohidar, N. R. 1974. Potentiation of the antihypertensive action of hydralazine by timolol in spontaneously hypertensive rats. *Proc. Soc. Exp. Biol. Med.* 146:509–12

59. Chidsey, C. A., Gottlieb, T. B. 1974. The pharmacologic basis of antihypertensive therapy: The role of vasodilator drugs. *Prog. Cardiovasc. Dis.* 17:99–113

60. O'Malley, K., Velasco, M., Wells, J., McNay, J. L. 1975. Control plasma renin activity and changes in sympathetic tone as determinants of minoxidil-induced increase in plasma renin activity. *J. Clin. Invest* 55:230–35

61. Pedersen, E. B., Kornerup, H. J. 1975. Effect of alprenolol and hydralazine on plasma renin concentration in patients with arterial hypertension. *Acta Med. Scand.* 198:579–83

62. Day, G. M., Prichard, B. N. C. 1971. Hypotensive action from a combination of propranolol and other hypotensive drugs. *Br. J. Pharmacol.* 41:408P

63. Pearson, R. M., Bending, M. R., Bulpitt, C. J., George, C. F., Hole, D. R., Williams, F. M., Breckenridge, A. M. 1976. Trial of combination of guanethidine and oxprenolol in hypertension. *Br. Med. J.* 1:933–36

64. Breckenridge, A., Dollery, C. T. 1966. Combined action of methyldopa and bethanidine. Evidence for a synergistic effect. *Lancet* i:1074–76

65. Veterans Adm. Co-op. Study Group Antihypertensive agents 1970. Effect of treatment on morbidity in hypertension. II. Results in patients with diastolic blood pressure averaging 90 through 114 mm Hg. *J. Am. Med. Assoc.* 213:1143

66. Clark, G. M., Troop, R. C. 1972. One-tablet combination drug therapy in the treatment of hypertension. *J. Chronic Dis.* 25:57–64

67. Limas, C. J., Freis, E. D. 1973. Minoxidil in severe hypertension with renal failure. Effective of its addition to conventional antihypertensive drugs. *Am. J. Cardiol.* 31:355–61

68. Sackett, D. L., Haynes, R. B., Gibson, E. S., Hackett, B. C., Taylor, D. W., Roberts, R. S., Johnson, A. L. 1975. Randomised clinical trial of strategies for improving medication compliance in primary hypertension. *Lancet* i:1205–7

69. Dixon, W. M., Stradlin, P., Wootton, I. D. P. 1957. Outpatient P. A. S. therapy. *Lancet* ii:871

70. Bergman, A. B., Werner, R. J. 1963. Failure of children to receive penicillin by mouth. *N. Engl. J. Med.* 268:1334–38

71. Blackwell, B. 1972. The drug defaulter. *Clin. Pharmacol. Ther.* 13:841–48

72. Stamler, R., Gosch, F. C., Stamler, J., Ticho, S., Civinelli, J., Restivo, B., Pritchard, D., Fine, D. 1975. Adherence and blood pressure response to hypertension treatment. *Lancet* ii:1227–30

73. Haynes, R. B., Sackett, D. L., Gibson, E. S., Taylor, D. W., Hackett, B., Roberts, R. S., Johnson, A. L. 1976. Improvement of medication compliance in uncontrolled hypertension. *Lancet* i:1256–68

74. David, N. A., Welborn, S., Pierce, H. I. 1975. Comparison of multiple and combination tablet drug therapy in hypertension. *Curr. Ther. Res. Clin. Exp.* 18:741–54

Ann. Rev. Pharmacol. Toxicol. 1977. 17:325–39
Copyright © 1977 by Annual Reviews Inc. All rights reserved

HISTAMINERGIC MECHANISMS IN BRAIN ♦6683

Jean-Charles Schwartz
Unité de Neurobiologie, Centre Paul Broca de l'INSERM, 2tr, rue d'Alésia, 75014 Paris, France

Since the initial findings by Sir Henry Dale at the beginning of this century that the imidazoleethylamine histamine (HA) was a potent agonist on a variety of biological systems as well as a normal constituent of many tissues, it was hypothesized that the amine acts as a messenger between the cells in which it is stored and those responding to its application. To characterize precisely the messages delivered by a candidate transmitter substance, i.e. to attribute to it a precise physiological role, requires that the cells from which this substance emanates should be identified and that its actions on the target cells as well as the circumstances of its release should be known. During recent years, significant progress has been made in this direction and HA has been identified as one of a dozen of probable neurotransmitters in the brain. As expected, this evidence has been derived from two kinds of complementary studies that are reviewed here: the first concerns HA localization and metabolism ("HA in the brain") while the second concerns its action on various target systems ("HA on the brain"). Several reviews (1–5) and a symposium (6) have recently been devoted to this matter.

HISTAMINE IN THE BRAIN: LOCALIZATION AND METABOLISM

Occurrence and Distribution

In 1943, Kwiatowski (7) found with a bioassay procedure that HA was present in mammalian brain, more in gray than in white matter. The same procedure was used by Adam (8) to establish in detail the distribution of HA between regions of the dog brain. Large regional differences in amine levels were reported and later confirmed in other species like the cat (9), the rat (10, 11), the mouse (12, 13), the monkey (14), or man (15).

In these studies HA was assayed either with fluorometry following purification by ion-exchange chromatography (16) or with the more sensitive radioenzymatic assay (11), both procedures yielding similar results. The mean cerebral level of HA in most species is around 50 ng/g, about one tenth of noradrenaline or serotonin

325

levels, but its relative distribution is more or less parallel to that of these monoamines: the highest concentration is in the hypothalamus while the lowest is in the cerebellum or in the medulla-pons, and the intermediate levels are in the mesencephalon and telencephalon.

Recently the biochemical mapping of HA in discrete nuclei of rat hypothalamus (17, 18) or rat mesencephalon (19) has confirmed that HA is unevenly distributed even within brain regions. Such observations are compatible with the view that different densities of putative histaminergic neurons occur in various parts of the CNS. However, before interpreting these data in such a way, one must consider that the amine is probably also stored in non-neuronal cells.

Biosynthesis

Labeled HA does not diffuse readily from blood to brain (20–22, 25), indicating that the cerebral stores depend on local biosynthesis. White (24, 25) showed that this was the case in cat brain but did not characterize the enzyme responsible for the decarboxylation of ^{14}C-histidine. In 1970 Schwartz et al (26) studied the kinetics of the enzyme in homogenates from rat hypothalamus and the effects of selective inhibitors and concluded that the "specific" L-histidine decarboxylase (EC 4.1.1.22) was involved rather than the aromatic L-amino acid decarboxylase (EC 4.1.1.26), suggesting that HA synthesis does not take place in catecholaminergic or serotoninergic neurons containing the latter enzyme. Indeed, after chemical degeneration of monoaminergic neurons elicited by 6-hydroxydopamine or 5,7-dihydroxytryptamine, brain L-histidine decarboxylase (HD) is left unaltered (27). The inhibition of HA synthesis in brain slices (28) as well as in vivo (29, 30) by compounds like α-hydrazinohistidine, but not by α-methyldopa, an inhibitor of aromatic-L-amino acid decarboxylase, confirms that the latter enzyme is not involved.

The regional distribution of HD activity in the brains of rats (26, 31) or mice (30, 12) grossly parallels that of HA. However this does not always hold true: in the median eminence of rat hypothalamus an extremely high HA level is associated with an almost undetectable HD activity (18). In fact, the ratio of HA level/HD activity (which is expressed in units of time) appears well correlated with the half-life of the amine in various regions of mouse brain (12, 32).

Subcellular fractionation of homogenates from rat cortex shows that a major portion of HD activity is associated with synaptosomes from which it can be released in soluble form by osmotic shock, indicating that HD is, like other enzymes, responsible for the synthesis of putative transmitters present in the cytoplasm of nerve endings (33). This view is confirmed by the observation that, in vivo, synthesis of ^{3}H-HA from its ^{3}H-precursor takes place predominantly in the nerve-ending fraction (34). In rat hypothalamus, the picture is not so clear because HD activity appears associated to a lesser extent with synaptosomes from which it is only partially releasable in soluble form (35), but this relative discrepancy might be due to technical differences in homogenization or fractionation.

The developmental pattern of HD activity in rat brain is comparable to that of enzymes responsible for the synthesis of other putative neurotransmitters: at birth, when synapses are still few, HD activity is low and predominantly found in the supernatant fraction of homogenates; then its activity increases several fold during synaptogenesis while its subcellular localization is progressively shifted into the fraction rich in nerve endings (23, 36).

Although the rate of ^{3}H-HA synthesis can be rapidly modified, the biochemical mechanisms by which such changes occur are not entirely clear. While HD activity does not appear to be regulated by a feedback mechanism, the rate-limiting step might be the availability of the precursor amino acid (28). In fact the apparent K_m of HD is about 3.10^{-4}M (26, 28), whereas the mean concentrations of L-histidine (L-His) in plasma and brain tissues ($\sim 6.10^{-5}$M) are not sufficient to normally saturate the enzyme. Thus brain HA is increased when the levels of L-His in plasma are elevated either following administration of loads of the amino acid (29, 30, 37) or as a consequence of a genetic defect in histidase (38). Conversely, cerebral HA rapidly decreases when L-His uptake is diminished in a competitive manner in mice loaded with other amino acids (39).

Storage

In peripheral tissues, mast cells constitute a major site of storage of HA in which it is held in large granules also containing heparin (40). The importance of these cells in brain has been overlooked for a long time because they were only rarely encountered upon histological examination (1). However mast cells have been recently identified in different brain regions of various animal species (41–44), even at the electron microscopic level (45). Moreover, in a preliminary report Rönnberg et al (46) have been able to reveal HA in mast cells from rat brain after its condensation with o-phtalaldehyde into a fluorescent product. However, using the same procedure, El-Ackad & Brody (47) did not reach a clear-cut conclusion in this respect. Although particularly abundant in the meninges, mast cells are also encountered in the brain parenchyma and are, in all cases, closely associated with blood vessels. Their number and morphology vary during brain maturation (44, 45).

No suitable histochemical method is available to visualize HA-containing neurons, but the subcellular fractionation approach used in several laboratories (35, 48–51) strongly indicates that such neurons occur in mammalian brain. Although in some studies there was evidence for a bimodal distribution of HA-storing particles, in all cases it was reported that a significant percentage of the amine is recovered in fractions containing synaptosomes. Furthermore, when synaptosomes are subjected to an hypoosmotic treatment, a substantial fraction of HA is recovered attached to synaptic vesicles (49, 51). This finding, together with the observation that HD is highly localized in the cytoplasm of nerve endings, suggests that both synthesis and storage of neuronal HA takes place in the same subcellular structures as other putative neurotransmitters.

Recently, the respective sizes of the neuronal and non-neuronal compartments, the latter probably corresponding to mast cells, have been evaluated in the cerebral cortex of rat (27) and cat (52) by combining data from deafferentation and subcellular studies. Approximately 50% of HA (but almost all HD activity) in cortex appears to be neuronal, while this percentage might be higher in other regions like rat hippocampus (53).

In the neonatal rat brain, i.e. before formation of most synapses, a paradoxically high level of HA (10, 23, 36, 54, 55), predominantly found in the crude nuclear fraction (36, 55), contrasts with a low HD activity (23, 36). These observations, previously attributed to a nuclear localization of HA (55), have been explained by Martres et al (36) on the assumption that mast-cell granules constitute the major store for HA during this period. This latter interpretation is confirmed by the observations that a large number of mast cells occur in the neonatal rat brain (44) and that, upon subfractionation of the crude nuclear pellet, HA-storing particles sediment like mast-cell granules but differently from nuclei (56).

Release

HA has not yet been reported to be released from any brain area following stimulation of corresponding afferent fibers. However, the axotomy of HA-containing pathways afferent to the cortex (27) or the hippocampus (53) is immediately followed by a strong but transient elevation of the amine content in these structures, which precedes the degeneration processes and could be attributed to a diminished release from nerve endings in which the impulse flow is interrupted. In vitro endogenous HA (57, 58), as well as endogenously synthesized ^{3}H-Ha (28) and exogenous ^{3}H-HA (59), is released from brain slices by K^+-evoked depolarization, and the efflux is both temperature- and calcium-dependent. The released amine appears to emanate predominantly from a rapidly turning-over compartment and because this release is accompanied by increased uptake of ^{3}H-L-His and increased ^{3}H-HA formation, there is evidence for a compensatory mechanism adjusting the rate of synthesis to the rate of release (28).

Reserpine releases both endogenous HA and endogenously synthesized ^{3}H-HA from hypothalamic slices (58, 60) and, in vivo, accelerates the disappearance of ^{3}H-HA from rat brain (61). However, there is no extensive depletion, as in the case of monoamines, in the content of endogenous HA in the brain of treated animals (62), except perhaps in cat hypothalamus (9).

Compound 48/80, a mast-cell degranulator, elicits an increased release of HA from slices from neonatal (36) and adult (28) rat brain, but the amine emanates from a slowly turning-over compartment. After systemic injection, this drug elicits a 40% depletion of HA from rat median eminence without affecting other hypothalamic structures inside the blood-brain barrier (18); significant depletion of whole brain HA also follows the intracerebral administration of compound 48/80 to newborn rats (63).

Hence, the data on HA release by various agents are also consistent with the view that the brain amine is stored both in a neuronal and in a mast-cell compartment.

Inactivation

There is apparently no high affinity uptake process to terminate rapidly the actions of HA in brain (2, 59, 64). The catabolism of HA in peripheral organs (65) involves two pathways: (*a*) direct oxidative deamination catalyzed by diamine oxidase and resulting in the formation of imidazoleacetic acid, (*b*) N-methylation into 3-methylhistamine (MHA) which is then converted by monoamine oxidase (MAO) into 3-methylimidazoleacetic acid. The first pathway is not operating in mammalian brain since diamine oxidase is absent (66) and, in contradiction with earlier reports (11, 67) labeled imidazoleacetic acid could not be detected after intracerebral administration of labeled HA (31, 68). On the contrary, high levels of labeled MHA appear soon after the administration of labeled HA (24, 31, 68, 69) or labeled L-His (31, 34, 70), especially in the brain of animals treated with MAO inhibitors. Indeed, methylation is an inactivation process since MHA lacks the characteristic activities of HA on brain tissues (71, 72). Methylation probably follows HA release since this conversion is reduced when the turnover of HA is reduced by anesthesia (34, 73). Minor quantities of MHA might also be formed by decarboxylation of the natural amino acid L-3-methylhistidine (39).

The enzyme responsible for this transformation, histamine-N-methyltransferase, is found in high activity in all regions of mammalian brain (69, 74, 75). It utilizes the methyl-donor S-adenosylmethionine which is, then, converted into S-adenosylhomocysteine, a potent competitive inhibitor of the reaction (76). This mechanism accounts for the interrelationships between the reactions of transmethylation of several amines in brain (69). The enzyme is evenly distributed in neurons and glial cells as indicated by its presence in clones derived from glioma or neuroblastoma (77) as well as by regional (75), subcellular (51), and developmental (36) studies.

Peptido amines are formed when HA and various amino acids are incubated with brain homogenates, but the function of these compounds is as yet obscure (78).

Turnover

Pollard et al (34) and Dismukes et al (70) have determined the turnover of HA in rat brain by examining the fluctuations with time of the specific activity of the amine in relationships with that of ^{3}H-L-His, after intraventricular administration of the latter. While the analytical data were in good agreement in both studies, because of the utilization of different mathematical models, the values for the half-life of cerebral HA were 46 min (34) and 30 sec (70), respectively.

A similar approach used in mice receiving ^{3}H-L-His by i.v. infusion (12, 13, 32) indicated that the half-life of HA in a rapidly turning-over compartment in brain, i.e. about 20 min, was much shorter than in any peripheral organ. Derived from kinetic data, there was also evidence for a second, slowly turning-over compartment (probably held in mast cells), a finding that might account for the partial, although rapid depletion of cerebral HA in animals treated with HD inhibitors (29, 30, 79). In the neonatal rat brain, the half-life of HA is, like in typical mast cells, in the order of several days (36).

The turnover of HA was reported to be accelerated and its endogenous level decreased in the brain of rats stressed by restraint (79) but this result could not be duplicated (80). Actually, in mice, restraint elicits an almost instantaneous decrease in turnover which is not secondary to adrenal stimulation (13). The turnover of HA is also decreased immediately after anesthesia (34, 73) and is higher during periods of arousal of a 24-hr cycle (81–84). Hence, a fraction of HA in brain turns over at a rapid rate which can be modified almost instantaneously, as could be expected for a neurotransmitter.

Anatomical Disposition of Histaminergic Neuron Pathways

In the absence of a suitable histochemical technique, the anatomical disposition of histaminergic neurons in brain has been investigated by following the neurochemical changes elicited by specific lesions. The first attempts were not successful probably because HA level (and not HD activity) was selected as the marker for degenerative changes (85, 86).

In 1974, starting from the similar regional distribution of HA and the monoamines, Garbarg et al (87) lesioned the medial forebrain bundle (MFB) unilaterally in the hypothalamus and presented evidence for an ascending histaminergic pathway in rat brain: after 1 week HD activity is lowered ipsilaterally by 30–50% in all telencephalic areas, while caudal regions are unaffected. The time for half-decline of HD, i.e. 2 days, is consistent with anterograde degeneration of nerve tracts. Shortly after the lesion, i.e. in the period preceding degenerative changes, the reduced ^{3}H-HA synthesis and the progressive enhancement of endogenous HA in cortex indicates that the turnover of HA depends on impulse traffic in terminals of this tract (27). That HD in telencephalic areas is contained in terminals from extrinsic neurons is confirmed by the almost complete disappearance of enzyme activity after surgical isolation of an area of cat cortex (52) or complete deafferentation of rat hippocampus (53). In addition, selective lesions of afferents to the hippocampus demonstrate that histaminergic neurons enter this region, like the monoaminergic ones (88), partly through a dorsal route comprising the fornix and partly via fibers emanating from the amygdaloid area (53). After the various kinds of lesions, the decreases in HA levels, although significant, were less pronounced than those of HD, an observation consistent with the presence of the amine in non-neuronal cells, whereas the enzyme should be almost entirely confined to neurons.

Recently the existence of these histaminergic fibers has received strong support from the electrophysiological work of Haas et al (89) showing that inhibitions recorded in cortex after stimulation of the MFB, or on hippocampal pyramidal cells after stimulation of the fornix, are not only mimicked by HA but also prevented by metiamide, an HA antagonist.

While the precise localization of HA cell bodies remains to be established, recent lesion studies suggest that the ascending fibers emanate from the posterior hypothalamus or upper midbrain (32). There is also evidence for a descending system innervating the brain stem, especially the periventricular gray (19), a feature constituting an additional similarity with the anatomical disposition of noradrenergic and serotoninergic systems.

HISTAMINE ON THE BRAIN: ACTIONS ON TARGET SYSTEMS

The actions of HA have been studied either at the cellular level, i.e. on electrophysiological and biochemical parameters, or on behavior. While the former studies are obviously easier to interpret, the latter might be more informative about the functions in which putative HA neurons are implicated.

Histamine and cAMP

The original finding by Kakiuchi & Rall (90) that HA was one of the most powerful agents in increasing the cyclic adenosine 3',5'-monophosphate (cAMP) level in slices from rabbit cerebellum has been repeatedly confirmed in a variety of regions and species like the chick (91), rabbit (90, 92, 93), guinea pig (72, 94–96), pig (97), rat (98), mouse (98, 99) and man (100). In addition, HA stimulates cAMP accumulation in cultured glioma cells (101). As in the case of other systems, there is no apparent correlation between the HA content of brain regions and their responsiveness: for instance, the hippocampus, which contains a low density of HA nerve endings, is the most responsive structure in the guinea pig (95). The action of HA appears mediated by receptors distinct from those mediating the responses to catecholamines, as indicated by large differences in responsiveness to the two classes of biogenic amines during brain maturation (92) or in various brain regions and, finally, by the lack of effect of adrenergic receptor blockers (95).

The discovery by Black et al (102) of specific agonists and antagonists of the two classes of HA receptors, i.e. H_1 and H_2, has allowed the identification of those mediating the cAMP response in brain. Baudry et al (96) demonstrated that, on slices of guinea pig cortex, HA stimulation is partially inhibited by either a H_1-antagonist (mepyramine) or a H_2-antagonist (metiamide) and totally blocked in the presence of both agents. While these data were essentially confirmed on slices from hippocampus (103), Hegstrand et al (104) found evidence for H_2-receptors only on homogenates from the same region, but the latter result is difficult to interpret since the responsiveness to HA is largely lost upon homogenization of the tissue. In chick brain the stimulation of cAMP formation is exclusively mediated by H_2-receptors (91).

Clonidine, an imidazoline derivative, is a relatively potent agonist of H_2-receptors on slices from guinea pig hippocampus (105) while its hypotensive action is blocked by intraventricular metiamide (106).

The cellular localization and functional roles of the two kinds of HA receptors mediating the stimulation of cAMP synthesis remains to be established. However, the observations that HA acts on isolated nerve endings (107) and that HA and cAMP exert similar actions when iontophoretically applied (71) are consistent with a possible role of the nucleotide as "second messenger" in histaminergic neurotransmission, as postulated in the case of noradrenergic synapses (108).

Electrophysiological Actions

Although few systematic studies have been undertaken, it appears that the actions of HA applied by iontophoresis on individual brain neurons result from the activation of specific receptors since they are generally not affected by antagonists of other putative CNS transmitters. HA elicits variable actions depending on the brain area where it is applied. On most neurons from the cerebral cortex of anesthetized cats or rats (109–111) HA has, like catecholamines and indoleamines, a weak depressant action evidenced by a reduction of spontaneous or glutamate- and acetylcholine-induced firing, without depression of spike amplitude. Excitation is recorded only on a few cortical neurons and might be produced by higher doses of HA.

In contrast, Haas et al (75, 112, 113) have recently demonstrated that HA increased the discharge frequency of a great proportion of hypothalamic neurons including identified neurosecretory cells in the supraoptic nucleus. HA also excites neurons in the ventromedial hypothalamic nucleus (114).

Scarcer are the data on other brain regions. While excitatory actions are observed on neurons from the thalamus and the central gray of midbrain (71) depression is more frequent in the medulla oblongata (115), on neurons of the reticular formation of the brain stem, on the cerebellar Purkinje cells (116), on cells from cuneate nucleus (117), or on the spinal motoneurons (118). The ionic mechanisms responsible for both of the actions of HA on mammalian brain are not known but, in Aplysia, excitation results from an increase in Na^+ conductance while an increase in K^+ conductance might cause slow hyperpolarization (119).

It is tempting to hypothesize that the two opposite actions of HA are mediated by distinct receptors, i.e. excitation by H_1-receptors and inhibition by H_2-receptors. Indeed, this appears to be the case for the opposite actions of HA both on cerebral ganglia of the Aplysia (119) and on the superior cervical ganglion of the rabbit (120). In mammalian brain also, the depressant effects of HA on cerebral cortex, hippocampus, midbrain, or hypothalamus are reduced or blocked by metiamide, while this H_2-receptor antagonist has no specific effect on excitations. The important observation that inhibitions elicited by stimulations of the MFB or the fornix can be selectively reduced by metiamide (89) suggests that H_2-receptors might also be involved in the postsynaptic actions of the endogenous transmitter released from these fiber systems.

However, it must be stressed that these identifications of receptors mediating the various electrophysiological actions of HA remain to be confirmed, inasmuch as they lie mainly on the effects of H_2-antagonists. The actions of specific H_1- and H_2-agonists have not yet been reported and the data derived from the use of H_1-antagonists (the classical antihistamines) are doubtful in view of the nonspecific membrane stabilization elicited by these compounds.

Effects on Vegetative Functions and Behaviors

Intraventricular HA elicits a tachycardia and a rise in blood pressure via stimulation of sympathetic centers, which appears to involve H_1-receptors (121–124). On the other hand, the hypotensive activity of clonidine, a H_2-receptor agonist (105), was reported to be blocked by metiamide (106); however, the finding could not be confirmed by others (H. Schmitt, personal communication).

Intraventricular (125) or intrahypothalamic (126) administration of HA elicits a dose-related hypothermia which appears to involve both H_1- and H_2-receptors (127–129).

Emesis is observed in dogs receiving HA either systemically or intracerebrally (130) and results from a stimulation both of H_1- and H_2-receptors, at the level of the area postrema (131).

The effects of HA in the control of water metabolism have received relatively large attention. Intraventricular HA elicits an increase in water intake in satiated rats (132), an effect which is blocked by H_1-antagonists, and can be reproduced by microinjections of the amine into restricted hypothalamic areas known to be involved in the control of body water homeostasis (133). Following intraventricular HA, there is also a marked antidiuresis (134–136) which is accompanied by a rise in blood ADH (131) and prevented by lesioning the median eminence (136). That this action probably involves a stimulation of neurosecretory cells in the supraoptic nucleus is confirmed by the observation that the firing of these cells is increased by iontophoretically applied HA (113). Since this effect of HA is independent of cholinergic receptors and since both the supraoptic and the paraventricular nuclei of the hypothalamus contain rather high levels of HA and HD activity (17, 18), the hypothesis that histaminergic neurons in the hypothalamus might participate in the control of ADH release deserves consideration.

The actions of HA on complex behaviors is, as yet, poorly substantiated. Increased levels of brain HA elicited by L-His loads do not result in dramatic behavioral changes, except a slight motor depression (37) but this kind of experiment might be misleading in view of the direct pharmacological actions of the amino acid or of imidazoleacetic acid, its main metabolite. Intrahypothalamic administration of HA or L-His causes a dose-related elevation of self-stimulation thresholds, an effect prevented by prior treatment with H_1-receptor antagonists (137).

Desynchronization of electroencephalogram (EEG) patterns is recorded after the intraventricular administration of HA (138). Although this effect might be due to nonspecific (for instance vascular) actions of HA, it might also indicate that histaminergic neurons are involved in the control of arousal mechanisms. This idea is supported by several kinds of observations, i.e. by the anatomical disposition of the ascending pathway diffusely projecting in the whole telencephalon, by the effects of hypnotics on HA turnover (73), by the well-known sedative properties of H_1-receptor antagonists, and by the circadian fluctuations in brain HA levels (82–84) and in rates of HA synthesis (M. Verdière, C. Rose, and J. C. Schwartz, in preparation).

CONCLUSION

When the data concerning the localization and the metabolism of HA in the brain are considered together with those concerning its actions on brain tissues, it appears likely that the amine functions as a messenger in cell-to-cell communications in the CNS.

One of the main difficulties currently encountered in identifying the HA-mediated communications lies in the duality of the histaminergic cells in mammalian brain.

Mast cells have been characterized histologically but, in view of the probably very low turnover of the amine therein, it is doubtful that mast-cell HA participates in physiological regulations under normal conditions. Nevertheless, the close association of cerebral mast cells with blood vessels suggests that HA might be involved in vascular control, at least in the course of immune or inflammatory reactions.

On the other hand, while due to technical shortcomings characterization and localization of histaminergic neurons have been restricted to indirect approaches (mainly neurochemical and not histochemical), there is little reasonable doubt about their occurrence in mammalian brain. Indeed a fraction of brain HA appears to be synthesized at a rapid rate in a distinct population of neurons, to be released in conjunction with nerve activity, to affect selectively the firing of other neurons, possibly through cAMP formation, and then to be enzymatically inactivated.

At this time, the functions of these putative histaminergic neurons are not entirely clear, in spite of preliminary indications that they might be implicated in the control of water metabolism, of wakefulness, or of emotional behaviors. While the functional roles of other aminergic systems in brain has been better unraveled during the recent years, it appears that such a delay in the case of HA rests on a lack of several investigative tools. Undoubtedly, the discovery of a sensitive histochemical method to map out precisely the histaminergic neurons, as well as the development of chemical agents to modify selectively the metabolism and the actions of HA, will lead us in the coming years to a better understanding of the messages that the imidazoleamine delivers in our brain.

ACKNOWLEDGMENT

It is my pleasure to thank Pr. J. P. Green, who kindly reviewed the manuscript.

Literature Cited

1. Green, J. P. 1970. Histamine. In *Handbook of Neurochemistry*, ed. A. Lajtha, 4:221–50. New York: Plenum
2. Snyder, S. H., Taylor, K. M. 1972. Histamine in the brain: A neurotransmitter? In *Perspectives in Neuropharmacology. A Tribute to Julius Axelrod*, ed. S. H. Snyder, 43–73. New York: Oxford Univ. Press
3. Boissier, J. R. 1971. Histamine et cerveau. *Actual. Pharmacol.* 24:51–93
4. Schwartz, J. C. 1975. Histamine as a neurotransmitter in brain. *Life Sci.* 17:503–18
5. Calcutt, C. R. 1976. The role of histamine in the brain. *Gen. Pharmacol.* 7:15–25
6. Boissier, J. R., Hippius, H., Pichot, P. 1975. Histamine in the brain. 549–606. *Neuropsychopharmacology*, ed. J. R. Bossier, H. Hippius, P. Pichot. Amsterdam: Excerpta Med.
7. Kwiatowski, H. 1943. Histamine in nervous tissue. *J. Physiol. London* 102: 32–41
8. Adam, H. M. 1961. Histamine in the central nervous system and hypophysis of the dog. In *Regional Neurochemistry*, ed. S. S. Kety, J. Elkes, 293–306. London: Pergamon
9. Adam, H. M., Hye, H. K. A. 1966. Concentration of histamine in different parts of the brain and hypophysis of the rat and its modification by drugs. *Br. J. Pharmacol.* 28:135–52
10. Ronnberg, A. L., Schwartz, J. C. 1969. Répartition régionale de l'histamine dans le cerveau de rat. *C. R. Acad. Sci.* 268:2376–79
11. Taylor, K. M., Snyder, S. H. 1971. Histamine in rat brain: sensitive assay of endogenous levels; formation in vivo and lowering by inhibitors of histidine decarboxylase. *J. Pharmacol. Exp. Ther.* 173:619–33
12. Schwartz, J. C., Barbin, G., Bischoff, S., Garbarg, M., Pollard, H., Rose, C., Verdiere, M. 1975. Histamine in as ascending pathway in the brain: Localization, turnover and effects of psychopharmacological agents. See Ref. 6, pp. 575–83 ed. J. R. Boissier, H. Hippius, P. Pichot, pp. 575–83, Amsterdam: Excerpta Med.
13. Verdiere, M., Rose, C., Schwartz, J. C. 1977. Turnover of cerebral histamine in a stressful situation. *Brain Res.* In press
14. Taylor, K. M., Gfeller, E., Snyder, S. H. 1972. Regional localization of histamine and histidine decarboxylase in the

brain of the rhesus monkey. *Brain Res.* 41:171–79

15. Lipinski, J. F., Schaumburg, H. H., Baldessarini, R. J. 1973. Regional distribution of histamine in the human brain. *Brain Res.* 52:403–8

16. Medina, M., Shore, P. A. 1966. Increased sensitivity in a specific fluorometric method for brain histamine. *Biochem. Pharmacol.* 15:1627–29

17. Brownstein, M. J., Saavedra, J. M., Palkovits, M., Axelrod, J. 1974. Histamine content of hypothalamic of the rat. *Brain Res.* 77:151–56

18. Pollard, H., Bischoff, S., Llorens-Cortes, C., Schwartz, J. C. 1976. Histamine and histidine decarboxylase in discrete nuclei of rat hypothalamus and the evidence for mast-cells in the median eminence. *Brain Res.* 118:509–13

19. Pollard, H., Barbin, G., Bischoff, S., Garbarg, M., Llorens-Cortes, C., Schwartz, J. C. 1977. Topographical distribution of histamine and histidine decarboxylase activity in hypothalamus and brain stem: modifications by lesions. *Agents Actions.* In press

20. Schwartz, J-C., Lampart, C., Rose, C., Rehault, M. C., Bischoff, S., Pollard, H. 1970. *J. Physiol. Paris* 62: Suppl. 3, p. 447

21. Snyder, S. H., Axelrod, J., Bauer, H. 1964. The fate of C^{14}-histamine in animal tissues. *J. Pharmacol. Exp. Ther.* 144:373–79

22. Schayer, R. W., Reilly, M. A. 1970. In vivo formation and catabolism of ^{14}C-histamine in mouse brain. *J. Neurochem.* 17:1649–55

23. Schwartz, J. C., Lampart, C., Rose, C., Rehault, M. C., Bischoff, S., Pollard, H. 1971. Histamine formation in rat brain during development. *J. Neurochem.* 18:1787–89

24. White, T. 1959. Formation and catabolism of histamine in brain tissue in vitro. *J. Physiol. London* 149:34–42

25. White, T. 1960. Formation and catabolism of histamine in cat brain in vivo. *J. Physiol. London* 152:299–308

26. Schwartz, J. C., Lampart, C., Rose, C. 1970. Properties and regional distribution of histidine decarboxylase in rat brain. *J. Neurochem.* 17:1527–34

27. Garbarg, M., Barbin, G., Bischoff, S., Pollard, H., Schwartz, J. C. 1976. Dual localization of histamine in an ascending neuronal pathway and in non-neuronal cell evidenced by lesions in the lateral hypothalamic area. *Brain Res.* 106:333–48

28. Verdiere, M., Rose, C., Schwartz, J. C. 1975. Synthesis and release of histamine on slices from rat hypothalamus. *Eur. J. Pharmacol.* 34:157–68

29. Schwartz, J. C., Lampart, C., Rose, C. 1972. Histamine formation in rat brain in vivo: Effects of histidine loads. *J. Neurochem.* 19:801–10

30. Taylor, K. M., Snyder, S. H. 1972. Dynamics of the regulation of histamine levels in mouse brain. *J. Neurochem.* 19:341–54

31. Schayer, R. W., Reilly, M. A. 1973. Formation and fate of histamine in rat and mouse brain. *J. Pharmacol. Exp. Ther.* 184:33–40

32. Schwartz, J. C., Barbin, G., Baudry, M., Garbarg, M., Martres, M. P., Pollard, H., Verdiere, M. 1977. Metabolism and functions of histamine in the brain. In *Current Developments in Psychopharmacology*, ed. W. B. Essman, L. Valzelli. New York: Spectrum. In press

33. Baudry, M., Martres, M. P., Schwartz, J. C. 1973. The subcellular localization of histidine decarboxylase in various regions of rat brain. *J. Neurochem.* 21:1301–9

34. Pollard, H., Bischoff, S., Schwartz, J. C. 1974. Turnover of histamine in rat brain and its decrease under barbiturate anaesthesia. *J. Pharmacol. Exp. Ther.* 190:88–99

35. Snyder, S. H., Brown, B., Kuhar, M. J. 1974. The subsynaptosomal localization of histamine, histidine decarboxylase and histamine methyltransferase in rat hypothalamus. *J. Neurochem.* 23:37–45

36. Martres, M. P., Baudry, M., Schwartz, J. C. 1975. Histamine synthesis in the developing rat brain: Evidence for a multiple compartmentation. *Brain Res.* 83:261–75

37. Costentin, J., Schwartz, J. C., Boulu, R. 1974. Histamine et comportements: Effects de surcharges en L-histidine. *J. Pharmacol. Paris* 5:195–208

38. Bulfield, G., Kacser, H. 1975. Histamine and histidine levels in the brain of the histidinaemic mouse. *J. Neurochem.* 24:403–5

39. Schwartz, J. C., Rose, C., Caillens, H. 1973. Metabolism of methylhistamine formed through a new pathway: Decarboxylation of L-3-methylhistidine. *J. Pharmacol. Exp. Ther.* 184:766–79

40. Selye, H. 1965. *The Mast-Cells.* London: Butterworth

41. Cammermeyer, J. 1973. Mast-cells and postnatal topographic anomalies in mammalian subfornical body and su-

41. praoptic crest. *Z. Anat. Entwicklungsgesch.* 140:245–69
42. Dropp, J. J. 1972. Mast-cells in the central nervous system of several rodents. *Anat. Rec.* 174:227–38
43. Kruger, P. G. 1970. Mast-cells in the brain of the hedgehog. Distribution and seasonal variations. *Acta Zool.* 51:85–93
44. Kruger, P. G. 1974. Demonstration of mast-cells in the albino rat brain. *Experientia* 30:810–11
45. Ibrahim, M. Z. M. 1974. The mast-cells in the mammalian central nervous system. Part I: morphology, distribution and histochemistry. *J. Neurol. Sci.* 21:431–78
46. Rönnberg, A. L., Edvinsson, L., Larsson, L. I., Nielsen, K. C., Owman, C. 1973. Regional variations in the presence of mast-cells in the mammalian brain. *Agents Actions* 3:191
47. El-Ackad, T. M., Brody, M. J. 1975. Fluorescence histochemical localization of non-mast-cell histamine. See Ref. 6, pp. 551–59
48. Carlini, E. A., Green, J. P. 1963. The subcellular distribution of histamine, slow-reacting substance and 5-hydroxytryptamine in the brain of the rat. *Br. J. Pharmacol.* 20:264–77
49. Kataoka, K., De Robertis, E. 1967. Histamine in isolated small nerve-endings and synaptic vesicles of rat brain cortex. *J. Pharmacol. Exp. Ther.* 156:114–25
50. Michaelson, I. A., Coffman, P. Z. 1967. The subcellular localization of histamine in guinea-pig brain. *Biochem. Pharmacol.* 16:2085–90
51. Kuhar, M. J., Taylor, K. M., Snyder, S. H. 1971. The subcellar localization of histamine and histamine methyltransferase in rat brain. *J. Neurochem.* 18:1515–27
52. Barbin, G., Hirsch, J. C., Garbarg, M., Schwartz, J. C. 1975. Decrease in histamine content and decarboxylase activities in an isolated area of the cerebral cortex of the cat. *Brain Res.* 92:170–74
53. Barbin, G., Garbarg, M., Schwartz, J. C., Storm-Mathisen, J. 1976. Histamine synthesizing afferents to the hippocampal region. *J. Neurochem.* 26:259–63
54. Pearce, L. A., Schanberg, S. M. 1969. Histamine and spermidine content in rat brain during development. *Science* 166:1301–3
55. Young, A. B., Pert, C. D., Brown, D. G., Taylor, K. M., Snyder, S. H. 1971. Nuclear localization of histamine in neonatal rat brain. *Science* 13:247–48
56. Picatoste, F., Palacois, J. M., Blanco, I. 1977. Subcellular localization of histamine in neonatal rat brain. *Agents Actions.* In press
57. Atack, C., Carlsson, A. 1972. In vitro release of endogenous histamine together with noradrenaline, serotonine from slices of mouse cerebral hemispheres. *J. Pharm. Pharmacol.* 24:990–92
58. Taylor, K. M., Snyder, S. H. 1973. The release of histamine from tissue slices of rat hypothalamus. *J. Neurochem.* 21:1215–23
59. Subramanian, N., Mulder, A. H. 1976. Potassium-induced release of tritiated histamine from rat brain tissue slices. *Eur. J. Pharmacol.* 35:203–6
60. Verdiere, M., Rose, C., Schwartz, J. C. 1974. Synthesis and release of ³H-histamine in slices from rat brain. *Agents Actions* 4:184–85
61. Pollard, H., Bischoff, S., Schwartz, J. C. 1973. Increased synthesis and release of ³H-histamine in rat brain by reserpine. *Eur. J. Pharmacol.* 24:399–401
62. Green, H., Erickson, R. W. 1964. Effects of some drugs upon rat brain histamine content. *Int. J. Neuropharmacol.* 3:315–20
63. Blanco, I., Rodergas, E., Picatoste, F. 1977. In vivo liberation of brain histamine induced by Compound 48/80. *Agents Actions.* In press
64. Tuomisto, L., Tuomisto, J., Walaszek, E. J. 1975. Uptake of histamine by rabbit hypothalamic slices. *Med. Biol.* 53:40–46
65. Schayer, R. W. 1959. Catabolism of physiological quantities of histamine in vivo. *Physiol. Rev.* 39:116–20
66. Burkard, W. P., Géy, K. F., Pletscher, R. 1963. Diamine oxidase in the brain of vertebrates. *J. Neurochem.* 10:183–86
67. Snyder, S. H., Glowinski, J., Axelrod, J. 1966. The physiologic disposition of ³H-histamine in the rat brain. *J. Pharmacol. Exp. Ther.* 153:8–14
68. Schwartz, J. C., Pollard, H., Bischoff, S., Rehault, M. C., Verdiere-Sahuque, M. 1971. Catabolism of ³H-histamine in the rat brain after intracisternal administration. *Eur. J. Pharmacol.* 16:326–35
69. Schwartz, J. C., Baudry, M., Chast, F., Pollard, H., Bischoff, S., Krishnamoorthy, M. S. 1973. Histamine in the brain: Importance of transmethylation process and their regulation. In *Metabolic Regulation and Functional*

Activity in the Central Nervous System, ed. E. Genazzani, H. Herken. Amsterdam: Springer

70. Dismukes, K., Snyder, S. H. 1974. Histamine turnover in rat brain. *Brain Res.* 78:467–81

71. Haas, H. L., Hosli, L., Anderson, E. G., Wolf, P. 1975. Action of histamine and metabolites on single neurones of the mammalian central nervous system. See Ref. 6, pp. 589–96

72. Huang, M., Daly, J. W. 1972. Accumulation of cyclic adenosine monophosphate in incubated slices of brain tissue. 1. Structure-activity-relationship of agonists and antagonists of biogenic amines and of tricyclic tranquilizers and antidepressants. *J. Med. Chem.* 15:458–62

73. Pollard, H., Bischoff, S., Schwartz, J. C. 1973. Decreased histamine synthesis in the rat brain by hypnotics and anaesthetics. *J. Pharm. Pharmacol.* 25: 920–21

74. Brown, D. D., Tomchick, R., Axelrod, J. 1959. The distribution and properties of a histamine-methylating enzyme. *J. Biol. Chem.* 234:2948–50

75. Axelrod, J., MacLean, P. D., Waynes-Albers, R. W., Weissbach, H. 1961. Regional distribution of methyltransferase enzymes in the nervous system and glandular tissues. In *Regional Neurochemistry,* ed. S. S. Kety, J. Elkes, 307–11. London:Pergamon

76. Baudry, M., Chast, F., Schwartz, J. C. 1973. Studies on S-adenosyl-homocysteine inhibition of histamine transmethylation in brain. *J. Neurochem.* 20:13–21

77. Garbarg, M., Baudry, M., Brenda, P., Schwartz, J. C. 1975. Simultaneous presence of histamine-N-methyltransferase and catechol-O-methyltransferase in neuronal and glial cells in culture. *Brain Res.* 83:583–41

78. Kvamme, E., Reichelt, K. L., Edminson, P. D., Sinichkin, A., Sterri, S., Svenneb, G. 1975. N-substituted peptides in brain. In *Proc. FEBS Meet. 10th,* ed. J. Montreuil, P. Mandel, 41: 127–36. Amsterdam: North-Holland

79. Taylor, K. M., Snyder, S. H. 1971. Brain histamine: Rapid apparent turnover altered by restraint and cold stress. *Science* 172:1037–39

80. Kobayashi, R. M., Kopin, I. 1974. The effect of stress and environmental lighting on histamine in the rat brain. *Brain Res.* 74:356–59

81. Schwartz, J. C., Barbin, G., Garbarg, M., Pollard, H., Rose, C., Verdiere, M.

1976. Neurochemical evidence for histamine acting as a transmitter in mammalian brain. First and second messengers in nervous tissues. *Adv. Biochem. Psychopharmacol.* 15:111–26

82. Orr, E., Quay, W. B. 1975. Hypothalamic 24-hour rhythm in histamine, histidine decarboxylase and histamine-N-methyltransferase. *Endocrinology* 96:941–45

83. Orr, E., Quay, W. B. 1975. The effects of castration on histamine levels and 24-hour rhythm in the male rat hypothalamus. *Endocrinology* 97:481–84

84. Schwartz, J. C. 1975. Histamine as a transmitter in mammalian brain. *Proc. Int. Cong. Pharmacol., 6th,* ed. J. Tuomisto, M. K. Paasonen, 2:71–80. New York: Pergamon

85. Garbarg, M., Krishnamoorthy, M. S., Feger, J., Schwartz, J. C. 1973. Effects of mesencephalic and hypothalamic lesions on histamine levels in rat brain. *Brain Res.* 50:361–67

86. Dismukes, K., Kuhar, M. J., Snyder, S. H. 1974. Brain histamine alterations after hypothalamic isolation. *Brain Res.* 78:144–51

87. Garbarg, M., Barbin, G., Feger, J., Schwartz, J. C. 1974. Histaminergic pathways in rat brain evidenced by lesions of the MFB. *Science* 186: 833–35

88. Storm-Mathisen, J., Guldberg, H. C. 1974. 5-hydroxytryptamine and noradrenaline in the hippocampal region: effect of transection of afferent pathways on endogenous levels, high affinity uptake and some transmitter-related enzymes. *J. Neurochem.* 22:793–803

89. Haas, H. L., Wolf, P. 1976. Central actions of histamine: Microelectrophoretic studies. *Brain Res.* In press

90. Kakiuchi, S., Rall, T. W. 1968. The influence of chemical agents on the accumulation of adenosine 3'-5'phosphate in slices from rabbit cerebellum. *Mol. Pharmacol.* 4:367–78

91. Nahorski, S. R., Rogers, K. J., Smith, B. M. 1974. Histamine H_2-receptors and cyclic AMP in brain. *Life Sci.* 15: 1887–94

92. Palmer, G. C., Schmidt, M. J., Robison, G. A. 1972. Development and characteristics of the histamine-induced accumulation of cycle AMP in the rabbit cerebral cortex. *J. Neurochem.* 19: 2251–56

93. Shimizu, H., Creveling, C. R., Daly, J. W. 1970. The effect of histamine and other compounds on the formation of adenosine 3'-5'-monophosphate in slices

from cerebral cortex. *J. Neurochem.* 17:441–44

94. Chasin, M., Rivkin, I., Mamrak, F., Samaniego, S. G., Hess, S. M. 1971. Alpha- and beta-adrenergic receptors as mediators of accumulation of cycle adenosine 3'-5'-monophosphate in specific areas of guinea-pig brain. *J. Biol. Chem.* 246:3037–41

95. Chasin, M., Mamrak, F., Samaniego, S. G., Hess, S. M. 1973. Characteristics of the catecholamine and histamine receptor sites mediating accumulation of cyclic adenosine 3'-5'-monophosphate in guinea-pig brain. *J. Neurochem.* 21: 1415–27

96. Baudry, M., Martres, M. P., Schwartz, J. C. 1975. H_1- and H_2-receptors in the histamine induced accumulation of cycle AMP in guinea-pig brain slices. *Nature* 253:362–63

97. Sato, A., Onaya, T., Kotani, M., Harada, A., Yamada, T. 1974. Effects of biogenic amines on the formation of adenosine 3'-5'-monophosphate in porcine cerebral cortex, hypothalamus and anterior pituitary slices. *Endocrinology* 94:1311–17

98. Schultz, J., Daly, J. W. 1973. Accumulation of cyclic adenosine 3'-5'-monophosphate in cerebral cortical slices from rat and mouse: Stimulation effect of alpha- and beta-adrenergic agents and adenosine. *J. Neurochem.* 21: 1319–26

99. Skolnick, P., Daly, J. W. 1974. The accumulation of adenosine 3'-5'-monophosphate in cerebral cortical slices of the quaking mouse, a neurologic mutant. *Brain Res.* 73:513–25

100. Kodama, T., Matsukado, Y., Shimizu, H. 1973. The cyclic AMP system of human brain. *Brain Res.* 50:135–146

101. Clark, R. B., Perkins, J. P. 1971. Regulation of adenosine 3'-5'-monophosphate concentration in cultured human astrocytoma cells by catecholamines and histamine. *Proc. Natl. Acad. Sci. USA* 68:2757–60

102. Black, J. W., Duncan, W. A. M., Durant, C. J., Ganellin, C. R., Parsons, M. E. 1972. Definition and antagonism of histamine H_2-receptors. *Nature* 236: 385–90

103. Dismukes, K., Rogers, M., Daly, J. W. 1976. Cyclic adenosine 3'-5'-monophosphate formation in guinea-pig brain slices: Effect of H-$_1$- and H_2-histaminergic agonists. *J. Neurochem.* 26:785–90

104. Hegstrand, L. R., Kanof, P. D., Greengard, P. 1976. Histamine-sensitive adenylate cyclase in mammalian brain. *Nature* 260:163–65

105. Audigier, Y., Virion, A., Schwartz, J. C. 1976. Stimulation of cerebral histamine H_2-receptors by clonidine. *Nature* 262:307–8

106. Karppanen, H., Paakari, I., Paakari, P., Huotari, R., Orma, A. L. 1976. Possible involvement of central histamine H_2-receptors in the hypotensive effect of clonidine. *Nature* 259:587–88

107. Von Hungen, K., Roberts, S. 1973. Adenylate-cyclase receptors for adrenergic neurotransmitters in rat cerebral cortex. *Eur. J. Biochem.* 36:391–401

108. Bloom, F. E., Hoffer, B. J., Siggins, G. R. 1972. Norepinephrine mediated cerebellar synapses: a model system for neuropsychopharmacology. *Biol. Psychiatry* 4:157–77

109. Phillis, J. W., Tebecis, A. K., York, D. H. 1968. Histamine and some antihistamines: action on cerebral cortical neurones. *Br. J. Pharmacol. Chemother.* 33:426–40

110. Phillis, J. W., Limacher, J. J. 1974. Effects of some metallic cations on cerebral cortical neurones and their interactions with biogenic amines. *Can. J. Physiol. Pharmacol.* 52:566–74

111. Haas, H. L., Bucher, U. M. 1975. Histamine H_2-receptors on single central neurones. *Nature* 255:634–35

112. Haas, H. L. 1974. Histamine: Action on single hypothalamic neurones. *Brain Res.* 76:363–66

113. Haas, H. L., Wolf, P., Nussbaumer, J. C. 1975. Histamine: Action on supraoptic and other hypothalamic neurones of the cat. *Brain Res.* 88:166–69

114. Renaud, L. P. 1975. Response of identified ventromedial hypothalamic nucleus neurones to putative neurotransmitters applied by microiontophoresis. *Br. J. Pharmacol.* 55:277P–78P

115. Haas, H. L., Anderson, E. G., Hosli, L. 1973. Histamine and metabolites: Their effects and interactions with convulsants on brainstem neurones. *Brain Res.* 51:269–78

116. Siggins, G. R., Hoffer, B. J., Bloom, F. E. 1971. Studies on norepinephrine containing afferents to Purkinje cells of rat cerebellum. III. Evidence for mediation of norepinephrine effects by cyclic 3'-5'-adenosine monophosphate. *Brain Res.* 25:535–53

117. Galindo, A., Krnjevic, K., Schwartz, S. 1967. Micro-iontophoretic studies on neurones in the cuneate nucleus. *J. Physiol. London* 192:105–18

118. Phillis, J. W., Tebecis, A. K., York, D. H. 1968. Depression of spinal motoneurones by noradrenaline, 5-hydroxytryptamine and histamine. *Eur. J. Pharmacol.* 4:471-75

119. Carpenter, D. O., Gaubatz, G. L. 1975. H_1- and H_2-histamine receptors on aplysia neurones. *Nature* 254:343-44

120. Brimble, M. J., Wallis, D. I. 1973. Histamine H_1- and H_2-receptors at ganglionic synapse. *Nature* 246:156-58

121. White, T. 1965. Peripheral vacular effects of histamine administered into the cerebral ventricles of anaesthetized cats. *Experientia* 21:132-33

122. Sinha, J. N., Gupta, M. L., Bhargava, K. P. 1969. Effect of histamine and antihistaminics on central vasomotor loci. *Eur. J. Pharmacol.* 5:235-38

123. Brezenoff, H. E., Jenden, D. J. 1969. Modification of arterial blood pressure in rats following microinjections of drugs into the posterior hypothalamus. *Int. J. Neuropharmacol.* 8:593-600

124. Finch, L., Hicks, P. E. 1976. Central hypertensive action of histamine in conscious normotensive cats. *Eur. J. Pharmacol.* 36:263-66

125. Shaw, G. G. 1971. Hypothermia produced in mice by histamine acting on the central nervous system. *Br. J. Pharmacol.* 42:205-14

126. Brezenoff, H. E., Lomax, P. 1970. Temperature changes following microinjection of histamine into the thermoregulatory centers of the cat. *Experientia* 26:51-52

127. Brimblecombe, R. W., Calcutt, C. R. 1974. The involvement of H_1- and H_2-histamine receptors in the hypothermic response to intracerebroventricularly-injected histamine and related drugs. *J. Pharmacol. Paris* 5: Suppl. 2, p. 11

128. Costentin, J., Boulu, P., Schwartz, J. C. 1973. Pharmacological studies on the role of histamine in thermoregulation. *Agents Actions* 3:177

129. Green, M. D., Cox, B., Lomax, P. 1976. Histamine H_1- and H_2-receptors in the central thermoregulatory pathways of the rat. *J. Neurosci. Res.* 1:353-59

130. Bhargava, K. P., Dixit, K. S. 1968. Role of chemoreceptor trigger zone in histamine-induced emesis. *Br. J. Pharmacol.* 34:508-13

131. Bhargava, K. P. 1975. Some neuropharmocological studies with histamine. See Ref. 6, pp. 597-604

132. Gerald, M. C., Maickel, R. P. 1972. Studies on the possible role of brain histamine in behavior. *Br. J. Pharmacol.* 44:462-71

133. Leibowitz, S. F. 1973. Histamine: A stimulatory effect on drinking behavior in the rat. *Brain Res.* 63:440-44

134. Bhargava, K. P., Kulshrestha, V. K., Santhakumri, G., Srivastava, Y. P. 1973. Mechanism of histamine-induced antidiuretic response. *Br. J. Pharmacol.* 47:700-6

135. Tuomisto, L., Eriksson, L. 1974. Central antidiuretic effect of histamine in the unanesthetized goat: Effects of H_1- and H_2-antagonists. *J. Pharmacol. Paris* 5: Suppl. 2, p. 101

136. Bennett, C. T., Pert, A. 1974. Antidiuresis produced by injections of histamine into the cat supraoptic nucleus. *Brain Res.* 78:151-56

137. Cohn, C. K., Ball, G. G., Hirsch, J. 1973. Histamine: Effects on self-stimulation. *Science* 180:757-58

138. Monnier, M., Sauer, R., Hatt, A. M. 1970. The activating effect of histamine on the central nervous system. *Int. Rev. Neurobiol.* 12:265-305

Ann. Rev. Pharmacol. Toxicol. 1977. 17:341–53
Copyright © 1977 by Annual Reviews Inc. All rights reserved

PHARMACOLOGIC CONTROL ❖6684
OF TEMPERATURE REGULATION

Barry Cox
Department of Pharmacology, The University of Manchester,
Manchester M13 9PT, England

Peter Lomax
Department of Pharmacology, School of Medicine, and the Brain Research Institute,
University of California, Los Angeles, California 90024

INTRODUCTION

During the past two decades the physiology and pharmacology of thermoregulation have been the subjects of a considerable volume of research and numerous books and reviews. The physiologic aspects have been reviewed in detail most recently by Cabanac (1). The effects of drugs on temperature regulation have been discussed at two symposia, which resulted in books containing the proceedings (2, 3), and a third symposium in this series was held in Banff in September 1976. In reviewing this prodigious development of knowledge of the subject, any demarcation of these reports into "pharmacologic" is somewhat arbitrary since in many cases drugs have been used as tools to elucidate physiologic mechanisms.

With respect to the actions of drugs on central thermoregulatory mechanisms, many of the compounds studied affect the CNS by modifying the activity of the several neuronal pathways that impinge on the central thermostats or that mediate the effector responses controlling body temperature. The role of the putative neurotransmitters involved constitutes perhaps the most debatable topic in thermoregulation (4). Because there has been no recent exhaustive review of this subject we restrict the present discussion to the role of these neuroamines and the effects of drugs on their activity in the CNS.

A convenient model on which to base a discussion of the role of amines in thermoregulation is the neural net described by Carlson (5). He divided the system into afferent, central, and efferent components. Of these three components there is little or no evidence for a role of amines in the afferent sensory division. Conversely there is good evidence for a role of amines in the peripheral effector part of the neural net; its pharmacology is easy to analyze and is well understood. The central component is, perhaps predictably, not well understood and it is in this area that apparent inconsistencies exist and controversy abounds.

There are seven distinct efferent pathways in the neural net, of which six involve aminergic mechanisms and the seventh hormonal mechanisms. Of the aminergic systems four were described as sympathetic (5)—those to the skin blood vessels, sweat glands, adipose tissue (nonshivering thermogenesis), and adrenal medulla. The other two involve the somatic nervous system for the production of shivering and changes in respiration.

Pharmacologic manipulation of the effectors produces predictable thermoregulatory effects. For example, sympathomimetic drugs causing vasoconstriction will reduce heat loss, while drugs causing vasodilation (sympatholytics or cholinomimetics) will increase heat loss. Manipulation of these peripheral effectors can modify thermoregulatory behavior and affect heat loss or heat gain systems as well. The effects of a quaternary diphenhydramine derivative, which has ganglion blocking properties and does not pass the blood-brain barrier (6) will serve as an example. This drug, injected into rats, produced a fall in core temperature. However, if the rat was allowed access to a radiant heat source it used this source to maintain its temperature at the original set point (7). In the opposite situation, in which the rat had an elevated core temperature as a result of a 2-hr pretreatment with thyroxine, the rat avoided the heat source in an attempt to keep its temperature near the original set point.

Thus, the effect of drugs acting exclusively via the peripheral effectors are relatively easy to investigate and their actions can often be explained in terms of interactions with known neurotransmitter systems. When the central component of the neural net is considered, the situation is less clear and much of the experimental evidence is conflicting.

A number of models has been devised to explain the role of amines in the central component of the neural net. Problems in constructing such a model arise because of the wide species variations (8) and because of the differences in measured responses that occur after central monoamine injection depending on the route used and the ambient temperature of the study (9).

Typical models for the control of body temperature (10, 11) usually place the central thermostat in the preoptic anterior hypothalamus. This site receives information from peripheral cold and warm receptors. Stimulation of cold receptors is postulated to release 5-hydroxytryptamine (5-HT) in the preoptic anterior hypothalamus, which in turn activates a cholinergic pathway in the caudal hypothalamus to bring about heat conservation. Stimulation of warm receptors is thought to cause preoptic release of norepinephrine, which acts via caudal hypothalamic cholinergic mechanisms to activate heat loss processes. The validity and universality of this model have been subjected to a good deal of experimental study; this review summarizes some of the findings and discusses some of the apparent anomalies.

ACETYLCHOLINE

Central cholinergic mechanisms have been reported to mediate both hypo- and hyperthermic responses; this cannot be explained simply on the basis of either species differences or the duality of the role proposed for acetylcholine in the model. Thus, intraventricular injection of cholinomimetics such as acetylcholine (alone or in combination with a cholinesterase inhibitor) or carbachol have been reported to increase the core temperature of primates (12) and rats (13). Systemic injection of the centrally active muscarinic agonist, oxotremorine, caused a fall in core temperature of rats (14), which occurred even when peripheral muscarinic receptors were blocked. One possible explanation for these divergent results was that different central sites were being activated by the different routes of injection. However, further experiments involving injection into brain tissue have not resolved the problem. When oxotremorine was injected directly into the rostral hypothalamus of the rat a hypothermia was reported (14). Injection into the surrounding tissue was without effect. In contrast, injection of carbachol into the preoptic anterior hypothalamus has been reported to produce a dose-dependent hyperthermia (15, 16). Support for a central hypothermic effect of cholinomimetics came from the work of Beckman & Carlisle (17) who noted that intrahypothalamic injection of acetylcholine led to an immediate fall in brain temperature accompanied by decreases in behavioral responses for heat gain. One reservation about comparing their results with others is that the experiments were carried out at –5°C. Other workers have observed falls in core temperature in rats after a variety of muscarinic agonists (oxotremorine, pilocarpine, nicotine, and acetylcholine) were injected centrally at normal ambient temperatures (15, 18, 19, 20).

In an interesting experiment in which a variety of variables were recorded simultaneously, Crawshaw (21) attempted to resolve the apparent anomalies. He measured hypothalamic and cutaneous tail temperature in lightly restrained rats and made bilateral injections of acetylcholine into the preoptic/anterior hypothalamic region. A coordinated set of heat loss responses occurred almost immediately after injection, which included postural changes and vasodilation. Crawshaw also noted that locomotor activity could prevent the hypothermia and suggested that the hyperthermia reported by other workers (13, 14, 16) was either related to an increase in locomotor activity or to measurements being made at a time (15 to 30 min) when a compensatory rise in temperature was taking place. An alternative view was put forward by Myers (22), who suggested that low doses of cholinomimetics produced hyperthermia and that high doses caused a "swamping of local receptors sites" and hypothermia, presumably as a result of depolarizing blockade. Work in the cat supported this hypothesis, where low doses of cholinomimetics injected into the rostral hypothalamus produced hyperthermia but where increasing the dose at the same site resulted in a hypothermia (23). However, a similar experiment in rats was reported to give exactly the opposite results (24). Which, if either, of these findings is correct remains to be resolved. Another possible view is that the differences are due to the activation of two subsets of cholinergic receptors (muscarinic and nicotinic?), but there are as yet insufficient data to allow analysis of such a suggestion.

Other approaches to the problem have involved the use of anticholinesterase or antimuscarinic drugs. Meeter & Wolthuis (25) found that systemic injection of tertiary nitrogen anticholinesterases lowered core temperature in rats, and in a similar experiment in mice, at least two thirds of the response to the anticholinesterases was shown to be due to an action in the CNS (R. Chitty and B. Cox, unpublished). More recent studies have shown that intraventricular injection of the anticholinesterases caused hypothermia which was blocked by atropine (24). However, once again an alternative view has been presented: studies in the cat have shown that either intraventricular or intrahypothalamic injection of anticholinesterases can result in a hyperthermia (26).

In a detailed study of the effects of atropine on core temperature in the rat (27), systemic injection produced hypothermia but intrahypothalamic injection caused hyperthermia. Confirmation of these earlier studies have come recently from an investigation of cholinergic mechanisms in PGE_1 hyperthermia when central injection of atropine alone caused hyperthermia in the rat (28). Thus, the central injection of atropine gave results consistent with a hypothermia mediated by central cholinergic sites.

Clearly no unitary concept for a role of acetylcholine in thermoregulation can yet be advanced and it is only possible to echo the sentiments of Brimblecombe (29) who in 1973 said, "In view of the conflicting results it is remarkable that, in comparison with the monoamines, so little work has been done to elucidate the role of acetylcholine in central thermoregulation. This is clearly a fruitful field for further research."

NOREPINEPHRINE

The presence of norepinephrine in the hypothalamus, coupled with the known homeostatic function of this area, led in 1957 to a suggestion of a possible thermoregulatory role for this amine (30). Direct evidence of such a role came when it was shown that either intraventricular or intrahypothalamic injections of norepinephrine caused a fall in core temperature of the conscious cat (31, 32). Subsequently a great deal has been published concerning a thermoregulatory role for norepinephrine, but interpretation of these data is difficult. First, there is an apparently wide species variation (33). Second, in many studies, the precise site of injection is not well defined. Third, there are in the literature a number of reports of biphasic effects, which are particularly evident when the intraventricular route of injection is used (34, 35).

In the rat, the species most widely studied, low doses of norepinephrine injected into the hypothalamus are usually reported to increase core temperature (36–38), whereas high doses are reported to produce a fall (16, 36, 37, 39, 40). When the intraventricular route is used, the picture is less clear; in addition to the biphasic effect (35), there are also reports of hypo- or hyperthermia (13, 41, 42), which cannot be explained on the difference in dosage used. Satinoff & Cantor (43) attempted to resolve this problem by studying the effect of intraventricular norepinephrine on thermoregulatory behavior (the rats were trained to press a bar to obtain heat) and brain temperature. They recorded a fall in brain temperature accompanied by an increase in the animals' response to obtain heat. It was concluded that intraventricular injection of norepinephrine activated central heat loss pathways for which the rat attempted to compensate by behavioral responses for heat gain. The earlier investigations of Beckman (38) showed that intrahypothalamic norepinephrine also caused behavioral responses for heat gain but that these were associated with a rising core temperature. The hypothesis resulting from these two findings was that low doses of norepinephrine injected directly into the hypothalamus caused a rise of the set point and an increase in temperature, while higher doses diffused out of the hypothalamus and activated more distant heat loss effectors. This latter site of action would be expected to override the former. Injection into the cerebral ventricles appears preferentially to act on these heat loss effectors, whose precise location is not yet defined. One possible location is in the ventrobasal thalamus, which has been suggested to be involved in behavioral thermoregulation (44).

Bruinvels (45) has also suggested that the hyper- and hypothermic responses in the rat result from activation of different thermosensitive sites in the brain. However, he could not demonstrate a hypothermic effect of high doses of norepinephrine and attributed the fall in core temperature reported by other workers to restraint of the animals. Another finding was that phentolamine, an α-adrenoceptor blocking drug, could modify the temperature changes. This work in the rat supports findings in other species (cats, rabbits, and mice) that the action of norepinephrine in thermoregulation is mediated via α-adrenoceptors (46–50). Recently, norepinephrine has been reported to produce hypothermia in various avian species including the chicken (51, 52) and the pigeon (53). The fall in core temperature in the pigeon was also blocked by phentolamine, but not propranolol, again confirming a role for α-adrenoreceptors. In the cat both norepinephrine and its α-methyl derivative produced hypothermia blocked by phentolamine (33). However, it was noted that although norepinephrine and α-methylnorepinephrine were almost equipotent in their central actions, norepinephrine was eight times more potent on peripheral α-adrenoceptors. Therefore it was concluded that although central thermoregulatory receptors for norepinephrine have some properties in common with α-adrenoceptors, they may not be identical. Further support for an involvement of central α-adrenoceptors came from studies with the drug clonidine (54), which is a centrally acting α-adrenoceptor agonist. This drug produced effects identical with those of norepinephrine when injected intraventricularly in sheep.

The use of other drugs has led to speculation that endogenous norepinephrine is indeed involved in thermoregulation. Imipramine, which prevents inactivation of endogenous norepinephrine by inhibiting neuronal uptake, produced changes analogous to those of injected norepinephrine (55). This finding held whether the response was hyperthermia (rabbit) or hypothermia (rat). Acute injection of 6-hydroxydopamine, which causes release of norepinephrine, has also been reported to produce hypothermia in the rat (56–58). More direct evidence for a role of endogenous norepinephrine comes from the work of Myers & Chinn (59). They showed that at raised ambient temperatures norepinephrine caused a decrease in core temperature of the monkey and that under these conditions there was selective increase in norepinephrine release from the rostral hypothalamus.

Finally, the effect of norepinephrine on electrical activity in the CNS needs to be considered to determine whether any neurophysiological correlates exist for norepinephrine and temperature control. The widespread distribution of thermosensitive cells in the CNS and the limited number of studies made allow few firm conclusions. The effects of norepinephrine on unit activity in the preoptic/anterior hypothalamic area have been studied in rats (60), rabbits (61), and cats (62). In the rat and rabbit there was a correspondence of effects; norepinephrine decreased the rate of warm-sensitive neurons and increased the rate of cold-sensitive ones.

In conclusion, some tentative explanations have been advanced to explain the apparent anomalies in the thermoregulatory effects of norepinephrine, but the total picture is confused and more experiments under controlled conditions are required.

5-HYDROXYTRYPTAMINE

As with norepinephrine, the initial impetus for research into a possible role for 5-HT in temperature control came from the observations of Feldberg & Myers in 1964 (31), who noted that intraventricular injection of 5-HT in the cat increased core temperature. There is once more an apparent wide species variation. Initial reports showed that intraventricular 5-HT caused increased core temperature in the cat and dog (31, 63) and the opposite effect in the rabbit, sheep, rat, and mouse (35, 50, 64, 65). However, a later report of the effect of intrahypothalamic 5-HT in the rat claimed that hyperthermia rather than hypothermia occurred, particularly when low doses were employed (37, 66). 5-HT has also been implicated in the hyperthermia (which occurs in man, rabbit, and mouse) (67), resulting from injection of meperidine and a monoamineoxidase inhibitor. A possible solution to this problem of a hypo- or hyperthermic response has been presented with the finding that 5-hydroxytryptophol, a 5-HT metabolite, was hypothermic (68). It was postulated that 5-HT itself was hyperthermic, but that its metabolite was hypothermic. Some support for this idea came from the observation that monoamineoxidase inhibition, which prevented metabolite production, also prevented 5-hydroxytryptophan (5-HTP)-induced hypothermia. Further support for a hyperthermic role of 5-HT was the finding that stimulation of the midbrain raphe, which is the origin of most central 5-HT neurons, caused an increase in core temperature in the rat (69).

The role of 5-HT in the rabbit is also unclear in contrast to the hypothermia noted above (64); 5-HT has been suggested to mediate drug induced hyperthermia (70). To add to the confusion a biphasic effect has also been suggested, low doses decreasing and high doses increasing core temperature (71). Brimblecombe (72) has looked at 36 different tryptamine derivatives in the rabbit and found a hyperthermic response; in all cases the hyperthermia correlated with another measure of CNS activity.

Work in avian species has noted hyperthermia in the hen (52) and little or no effect in the pigeon (53). Therefore its role in this species requires elucidation.

Iontophoretic studies with 5-HT in the rat and rabbit (60, 61) have supported the original concept of Feldberg & Myers (31) for an opposite action of 5-HT and norepinephrine in these species. However, experiments in the cat, the species in which the hypothesis was first advanced, gave an equivocal result (62). In a more recent study (73) it was reported that 5-HT did not shift the sensitivity of medio-preoptic brain structures in the rat to thermal stimuli. Thus, although support for a neurotransmitter role has been published, the conflicting evidence makes a precise statement about its function impossible. More evidence is likely to accrue from the use of drugs, analogous to 6-hydroxydopamine, which selectively destroy 5-HT neurons. Such a drug, 5,6-dihydroxytryptamine, has been injected into monkey hypothalamus. Acutely it acted like 5-HT to increase core temperature. Chronically the monkeys demonstrated a thermoregulatory deficit to a cold challenge, which supports the hypothesis of a 5-HT link in the pathway carrying information from cold receptors (74).

DOPAMINE

Compared to the other biogenic amines, dopamine was rather late in being considered for a role in thermoregulation. Before 1971, only slight or inconsistent hypothermic effects had been reported after intraventricular or intracisternal injection (13, 41, 50, 57). However, the use and introduction of two pharmacological tools significantly affected the work in this field. The first was apomorphine, a specific dopamine receptor agonist (75) and the specific antagonist, pimozide (76).

In the rat, intraventricular injection of apomorphine, amphetamine, or dopamine has been shown to produce hypothermia (77). Similar findings have been noted for the cat and the baboon (78, 79). In all cases the hypothermia was blocked by pimozide or other dopamine antagonists. The hypothermia in the cat was shown not only to be pimozide sensitive, but also to be located in the preoptic/anterior hypothalamic region (80) and not in the caudal hypothalamus (81). A wide variety of drugs which have in common an ability to stimulate central dopamine receptors consistently have been shown to produce hypothermia in commonly used laboratory animals (82–84). As with norepinephrine, however, the findings are not unanimous. Low doses (10 μg) of dopamine administered intraventricularly have been claimed to increase core temperature in the rat (85). Further studies are required to see whether an explanation similar to that advanced by Satinoff & Cantor (43) for norepinephrine applies in this case. An alternative hypothesis is that the hyperthermia results from the conversion of dopamine to norepinephrine (85). Barnett & Taber (86) postulated a differential role for brain dopamine in temperature control in mice based on experiments with diethyldithiocarbamic acid, which inhibits dopamine-β-oxidase, and l-dopa. They suggested that while dopamine was hypothermic in control mice, it would elevate core temperature in mice pretreated with reserpine. These experiments were subsequently confirmed and extended using a variety of dopamine agonists (82). This study also showed that for complete reserpine reversal a small, but significant, noradrenergic contribution was required.

The rabbit appears to be the only commonly used laboratory species in which injection of dopamine agonists consistently produces a rise in core temperature (87, 88) which is pimozide sensitive. More recent studies have indicated a 5-HT link in the hyperthermia (70); this may apply also to the fall in core temperature in the rat (89).

Evidence for a role of endogenous dopamine in temperature control comes mainly from indirect sources. Bilateral lesioning of the striatum in mice has been reported to prevent apomorphine hypothermia (90), as did injections of scopolamine. This led the authors to postulate a role for dopamine receptors in the striatum, acting through cholinergic mechanisms in the hypothalamus. Other indirect evidence has suggested a role for endogenous dopamine in the rostral hypothalamus. Thus, morphine withdrawal hypothermia was blocked by injection of pimozide into the preoptic/anterior hypothalamic nuclei (91), which suggested that the hypothermia was mediated via endogenous dopamine at this site. Further studies, measuring thermoregulatory behavior in rats undergoing withdrawal, indicated that the effect of this dopamine was to lower the setting of the central thermostats (92).

In general there appears to be less controversy over the thermoregulatory actions of dopamine than for the other amines. However, it is quite possible that this merely reflects its late arrival on the scene.

HISTAMINE

As in the case of dopamine, histamine is a relative latecomer to the field of central control of temperature regulation. It has long been known that systemic administration of histamine can cause changes in body temperature in several species (see 93) but, since the amine does not readily penetrate the blood-brain barrier, these responses must be mediated peripherally. In 1970 Brezenoff & Lomax (94) reported a dose-dependent fall in core temperature after injection of histamine (1–5 μg) into the rostral hypothalamus of rats. This response was prevented by pretreatment of the animals with a histamine H_1-receptor antagonist (chlorcyclazine). Histamine also caused a fall in temperature when injected into the cerebral ventricles of mice but here the effect was not blocked by either systemic or intraventricular injection of chlorcyclazine (95).

An alternative to intracranial injection in the study of histamine as a neurotransmitter has been to increase central histamine concentrations by systemic loading with its precursor L-histidine (96, 97). Such systemic administration causes a fall in temperature of the rat maintained at an environmental temperature of 18°C (93). That this fall is indeed due to the enhancement of central histaminergic activity has been established (98, 99). Histamine H_1-receptor antagonists, injected systemically or centrally, had no effect on the histidine-induced hypothermia, whereas the response was blocked by H_2-receptor antagonists injected into the third ventricle (100).

The above data suggested at least two sites at which histamine affects the central thermoregulatory pathways: H_1-receptors in the rostral hypothalamic thermoregulatory centers and H_2-receptors in the pathways coursing close to the wall of the third ventricle. The responses evoked at these effectors were analyzed further using behavioral responses (7). These studies revealed that activation of H_1-receptors in the rostral hypothalamus lowers the set point of the thermostats causing heat loss mechanisms to be brought into play to lower the body temperature to the new set level. On the other hand, stimulation of the H_2-receptors activates the efferent heat loss pathways directly (101) and the set point is unchanged. A similar lowering of the set point mediated by H_1-receptors has been reported in the cat (102). The data indicating that H_2-receptor stimulation activates heat loss mechanisms directly are supported by studies with 4-methylhistamine, a predominantly H_2-receptor agonist (103).

Whether or not the histamine H_1- and H_2-receptors in the thermoregulator pathways are on the same neuronal chain remains to be determined. However, using oxotremorine, which lowers the set point of the central thermostats after systemic injection (7), the fall in temperature was significantly reduced by an H_2-antagonist (cimetidine) injected into the third ventricle of the rat (unpublished data, M. D. Green and P. Lomax). Possibly, certain heat loss pathways contain this H_2-histaminergic link, and these are activated by any changes involving a lowering of the set temperature. The universality of histaminergic transmission in central temperature regulation has recently been illustrated by evidence that thermal environmental selection in fish can be modulated by histamine and H_1-antagonists (104).

CONCLUSIONS

Although it is not possible to establish rigorously all of the criteria necessary to implicate a specific transmitter function to any central neuroamines, the evidence is certainly compelling in the cases discussed above. The inherent difficulties in investigating neuronal pathways in the central nervous system do not allow, as yet, definitive statements as to the precise sites of action of these several transmitters; nor can one confidently predict whether the neurons involved represent long afferent or efferent pathways or short interneurons.

However, of the several neuroamines discussed it might be concluded that there is strong evidence for assigning a role in central thermoregulation to norepinephrine, 5-HT, and acetylcholine while dopamine and histamine, in the words of Feldberg (105) "although not yet admitted to the club, are knocking at the door." How many of the drug effects on thermoregulation will eventually be explained as due to modification of transmitter function remains the topic of some future review.

Literature Cited

1. Cabanac, M. 1975. Temperature regulation. *Ann. Rev. Physiol.* 37:415–39
2. Schönbaum, E., Lomax, P., eds. 1973. *The Pharmacology of Thermoregulation.* Basel: Karger. 583 pp.
3. Lomax, P., Schönbaum, E., Jacob, J., eds. 1975. *Temperature Regulation and Drug Action.* Basel: Karger. 405 pp.
4. Lomax, P., Green, M. D. 1975. Neurotransmitters and temperature regulation. *Prog. Brain Res.* 42:251–61
5. Carlson, L. D. 1973. Central and peripheral mechanisms in temperature regulation. See Ref. 2, pp. 7–21
6. Lomax, P., Knox, G. V. 1973. The sites and mechanisms of action of drugs affecting thermoregulation. See Ref. 2, pp. 146–54

7. Cox, B., Green, M. D., Lomax, P. 1975. Behavioural thermoregulation in the study of drugs affecting body temperature. *Pharmacol. Biochem. Behav.* 3: 1051–54
8. Veale, W. L., Cooper, K. E. 1973. Species differences in the pharmacology of temperature regulation. See Ref. 2, pp. 289–301
9. Baumann, I. R., Bligh, J. 1975. The influence of ambient temperature on drug induced disturbances of body temperature. See Ref. 3, pp. 241–51
10. Maskrey, M., Bligh, J. 1971. Interactions between the thermoregulatory responses to injection into a lateral cerebral ventricle of the Welsh Mountain sheep of putative neurotransmitter substances and of local changes in anterior

hypothalamic temperature. *Int. J. Biometeorol.* 15:129–33

11. Myers, R. D. 1975. An integrative model of monoamine and ionic mechanisms in the hypothalamic control of body temperature. See Ref. 3, pp. 32–42

12. Myers, R. D., Yaksh, T. L. 1969. Control of body temperature in the unanaesthetized monkey by cholinergic and aminergic systems in the hypothalamus. *J. Physiol. London* 202:483–500

13. Myers, R. D., Yaksh, T. L. 1968. Feeding and temperature responses in the unrestrained rat after injections of cholinergic and aminergic substances into the cerebral ventricles. *Physiol. Behav.* 3:917–28

14. Lomax, P., Jenden, D. J. 1966. Hypothermia following systemic and intracerebral injection of oxotremorine in the rat. *Int. J. Neuropharmacol.* 5:353–59

15. Avery, D. D. 1970. Hyperthermia induced by direct injections of carbachol in the anterior hypothalamus. *Neuropharmacology* 9:175–78

16. Avery, D. D. 1971. Intrahypothalamic adrenergic and cholinergic injection effects on temperature and ingestive behaviour in the rat. *Neuropharmacology* 10:753–63

17. Beckman, A. L., Carlisle, H. J. 1969. Effect of intrahypothalamic infusion of acetylcholine on behavioural and physiological thermoregulation in the rat. *Nature London* 221:561–62

18. Kirkpatrick, W. E., Lomax, P., Jenden, D. J. 1967. The effect of muscarinic agents on the thermoregulatory centers in the rat. *Proc. West. Pharmacol. Soc.* 10:51–55

19. Lomax, P., Foster, R. S., Kirkpatrick, W. E. 1968. Thermoregulation in the rat: interactions of cholinergic and adrenergic agents in the hypothalamus. *Proc. West. Pharmacol Soc.* 15:48–51

20. Knox, G. V., Lomax, P. 1972. The effect of nicotine on thermosensitive units in the rostral hypothalamus. *Proc. West. Pharmacol. Soc.* 15:179–83

21. Crawshaw, L. I. 1973. Effect of intracranial acetylcholine injection on thermoregulatory responses in the rat. *J. Comp. Physiol. Psychol.* 83:32–35

22. Myers, R. D. 1974. *Chemical Stimulation of the Brain.* New York: Van Nostrand–Reinhold. 759 pp.

23. Rudy, T. A., Wolf, H. H. 1972. Effect of intracerebral injections of carbamylcholine and acetylcholine on tempera-

ture regulation in the cat. *Brain Res.* 38:117–30

24. Meeter, E. 1973. Cholinergic factors in central thermoregulation. See Ref. 2, pp. 490–92

25. Meeter, E., Wolthuis, O. L. 1968. The effects of cholinesterase inhibitors on the body temperature of the rat. *Eur. J. Pharmacol.* 4:18–24

26. Metcalf, G., Myers, R. D., Redgrave, P. C. 1975. Temperature and behavioural responses induced in the unanaesthetized cat by central administration of RX72601 a new anticholinesterase. *Br. J. Pharmacol.* 55:9–15

27. Kirkpatrick, W. E., Lomax, P. 1967. The effect of atropine on the body temperature of the rat following systemic and intracerebral injection. *Life Sci.* 6:2273–78

28. Rudy, T. A., Viswanthan, C. T. 1975. Effect of central cholinergic blockade on the hyperthermia evoked by prostaglandin E_1 injected into the rostral hypothalamus of the rat. *Can. J. Physiol.* 53:321–24

29. Brimblecombe, R. W. 1973. Effects of cholinomimetic and cholinolytic drugs on body temperature. See Ref. 2, pp. 182–93

30. Brodie, B. B., Shore, P. A. 1957. A concept for a role of serotonin and norepinephrine as chemical mediators in the brain. *Ann. NY Acad. Sci.* 66:631–42

31. Feldberg, W., Myers, R. D. 1964. Effects on temperature of amines injected into the lateral cerebral ventricles. *J. Physiol. London* 173:226–37

32. Feldberg, W., Myers, R. D. 1965. Changes in temperature produced by microinjections of amines into the anterior hypothalamus of cats. *J. Physiol. London* 177:239–50

33. Lewis, P. J., Rawlins, M. D., Reid, J. L. 1975. Studies on central noradrenergic pathways in the control of body temperature. See Ref. 3, pp. 111–18

34. Hellon, R. 1972. Central transmitters and thermoregulation. In *Essays on Temperature Regulation,* ed. J. Bligh, R. Moore, 71–86. Amsterdam: North-Holland. 436 pp.

35. Feldberg, W., Lotti, V. J. 1967. Temperature responses to monoamines and an inhibitor of MAO injected into the cerebral ventricles of rats. *Br. J. Pharmacol.* 31:152–61

36. Lomax, P., Foster, R. S., Kirkpatrick, W. E. 1969. Cholinergic and adrenergic interactions in the thermoregulatory centres of the rat. *Brain Res.* 15:431–38

37. Rewerski, W., Kubikowski, P. 1969. Influence of biogenic amines on the central regulation of body temperature in rats. *Acta Physiol. Pol.* 6:777–79

38. Beckman, A. L. 1970. Effects of intrahypothalamic norepinephrine on thermoregulatory responses in the rat. *Am. J. Physiol.* 218:1596–1604

39. Avery, D. D. 1972. Thermoregulatory effects of intrahypothalamic injections of adrenergic and cholinergic substances at different environmental temperatures. *J. Physiol. London* 220:257–66

40. Avery, D. D., Penn, P. E. 1973. Effects of intrahypothalamic injections of adrenergic and cholinergic substances on behavioural thermoregulation and associated skin temperature levels in rats. *Pharmacol. Biochem. Behav.* 1:159–65

41. Bruinvels, J. 1970. Effect of noradrenaline, dopamine and 5-hydroxytryptamine on body temperature in the rat after intracisternal administration. *Neuropharmacology* 9:277–82

42. Bruinvels, J. 1973. Effects of intracisternal administration of metaraminol and noradrenaline on body temperature in the rat. See Ref. 2, pp. 194–201

43. Satinoff, E., Cantor, A. 1975. Intraventricular norepinephrine and thermoregulation in rats. See Ref. 3, pp. 103–10

44. Hayward, J. N. 1975. The thalamus and thermoregulation. See Ref. 3, pp. 22–31

45. Bruinvels, J. 1975. Temperature responses to noradrenaline administered by different routes in rats. See Ref. 3, pp. 95–102

46. Burks, T. F. 1970. Central alpha-adrenergic mediation of norepinephrine hypothermia in cats. *Fed. Proc.* 29:417

47. Burks, T. F. 1972. Central alpha-adrenergic receptors in thermoregulation. *Neuropharmacology* 11:615–24

48. Rudy, T. A., Wolf, H. H. 1971. The effect of intrahypothalamically injected sympathomimetic amines on temperature regulation in the cat. *J. Pharmacol. Exp. Ther.* 179:218–35

49. Dhawan, B. N., Dua, P. P. 1971. Evidence for the presence of alpha-adrenoceptors in the central thermoregulatory mechanism of rabbits. *Br. J. Pharmacol.* 43:495–503

50. Brittain, R. T., Handley, S. L. 1967. Temperature changes produced by the injection of catecholamines and 5-hydroxytryptamine into the cerebral

51. ventricles of the conscious mouse. *J. Physiol. London* 192:805–13

51. Marley, E., Stephenson, J. D. 1970. Effects of catecholamines infused into the brains of young chickens. *Br. J. Pharmacol.* 40:639–58

52. Scott, N. R., Van Tienhoven, A. 1974. Biogenic amines and body temperature in the hen *Gallus domesticus. Am. J. Physiol.* 227:1399–1405

53. Hissa, R., Rautenberg, W. 1975. Thermoregulatory effects of intrahypothalamic injections of neurotransmitters and their inhibitors in the pigeon. *Comp. Biochem. Physiol.* 51:319–26

54. Maskrey, M., Vogt, M., Bligh, J. 1970. Central effects of clonidine upon thermoregulation in the sheep and goat. *Eur. J. Pharmacol.* 12:297–302

55. Cranston, W. I., Hellon, R. F., Luff, R. M., Rawlins, M. D. 1972. Hypothalamic endogenous noradrenaline and thermoregulation in the cat and rabbit. *J. Physiol. London* 223:59–68

56. Simmonds, M. A., Uretsky, N. J. 1970. Central effects of 6-hydroxydopamine on the body temperature of the rat. *Br. J. Pharmacol.* 40:630–38

57. Nakamura, K., Thoenen, H. 1971. Hypothermia induced by intraventricular administration of 6-hydroxydopamine in rats. *Eur. J. Pharmacol.* 16:46–54

58. Breese, G. R., Moore, R. A., Howard, J. L. 1972. Central actions of 6-hydroxydopamine and other phenylethylamine derivatives on body temperature in the rat. *J. Pharmacol. Exp. Ther.* 180:591–602

59. Myers, R. D., Chinn, C. 1973. Evoked release of hypothalamic norepinephrine during thermoregulation in the cat. *Am. J. Physiol.* 224:230–36

60. Murakami, N. 1973. Effects of iontophoretic application of 5-hydroxytryptamine, noradrenaline and acetylcholine upon hypothalamic temperature-sensitive neurones in rats. *Jpn. J. Physiol.* 23:435–46

61. Hori, T., Nakayama, T. 1973. Effects of biogenic amines on central thermoresponsive neurones in the rabbit. *J. Physiol. London* 232:71–85

62. Jell, R. M. 1973. Responses of hypothalamic neurones to local temperature and to acetylcholine, noradrenaline and 5-hydroxytryptamine. *Brain Res.* 55:123–24

63. Feldberg, W., Hellon, R. F., Myers, R. D. 1966. Effects on temperature of monoamines injected into the cerebral

ventricles of anaesthetized dogs. *J. Physiol. London* 186:416–23

64. Cooper, K. E., Cranston, W. I., Honour, A. J. 1965. Effects of intraventricular and intrahypothalamic injection of noradrenaline and 5-hydroxytryptamine on body temperature in conscious rabbits. *J. Physiol. London* 181:852–64

65. Bligh, J. 1966. Effects on temperature of monoamines injected into the lateral ventricles of sheep. *J. Physiol. London* 185:46–47P

66. Crawshaw, L. I. 1972. Effects of intracerebral 5-hydroxytryptamine injection on thermoregulation in the rat. *Physiol. Behav.* 9:133–40

67. Gessner, P. K. 1973. Body temperature correlates of the interaction between monoamineoxidase inhibitors and meperidine. See Ref. 2, pp. 473–81

68. Barofsky, I., Feldstein, A. 1970. Serotonin and its metabolites. Their respective roles in the production of hypothermia in the mouse. *Experientia* 26:990–91

69. Sheard, M. H., Aghajanian, G. K. 1967. Neural release of brain serotonin and body temperature. *Nature London* 216:495–96

70. Horita, A., Quock, R. M. 1975. Dopaminergic mechanisms in drug induced temperature effects. See Ref. 3, pp. 75–84

71. Jacob, J., Peindaries, R. 1973. Central effects of monoamines on the temperature of the conscious rabbit. See Ref. 2, pp. 202–16

72. Brimblecombe, R. W. 1967. Hyperthermic effects of some tryptamine derivatives in relation to their behavioural activity. *Int. J. Neuropharmacol.* 6:423–29

73. Gorynia, I., Bartsch, P. 1975. Der Einfluss mediopraoptischer reizung auf die Temperatureregulation der Ratte vor und nach Serotoningabe. *Acta Biol. Med. Ger.* 34:67–68

74. Waller, M. B., Myers, R. D., Martin, G. E. 1976. Thermoregulatory deficits in the monkey produced by 5,6-dihydroxytryptamine injected into the hypothalamus. *Neuropharmacology* 15:61–68

75. Ernst, A. M. 1967. Mode of action of apomorphine and dexamphetamine on gnawing compulsion in rats. *Psychopharmacologia* 10:316–23

76. Andén, N-E., Butcher, S. G., Corrodi, H., Fuxe, K. 1970. Receptor activity and turnover of dopamine and noradrenaline after neuroleptics. *Eur. J. Pharmacol.* 11:303–14

77. Kruk, Z. L. 1972. The effect of drugs acting on dopamine receptors on the body temperature of the rat. *Life Sci.* 11:845–50

78. Kennedy, M. S., Burks, T. F. 1974. Dopamine receptors in the central thermoregulatory mechanism of the cat. *Neuropharmacology* 13:119–28

79. Toivola, P., Gale, C. C. 1970. Effect on temperature of biogenic amine infusion into hypothalamus of baboon. *Neuroendocrinology* 6:210–19

80. Quock, R. M., Gale, C. C. 1974. Hypothermia-mediating receptors in the preoptic anterior hypothalamus of the cat. *Naunyn-Schmiedebergs Arch. Pharmacol.* 285:297–300

81. Saxena, P. N. 1973. Mechanism of hypothermic action of catecholamines in the cat. *Ind. J. Pharmacol.* 5:374–77

82. Cox, B., Tha, S. J. 1975. The role of dopamine and noradrenaline in temperature control of normal and reserpine pretreated mice. *J. Pharm. Pharmacol.* 27:242–47

83. Davies, J. A., Redfern, P. H. 1973. A note on the effect of amantadine on body temperature in mice. *J. Pharm. Pharmacol.* 25:705–7

84. Calne, D. B., Claveria, L. E., Reid, J. L. 1975. Hypothermic action of bromocriptine. *Br. J. Pharmacol.* 54:123–24

85. Przewlocka, B., Kaluza, J. 1973. The effect of intraventricularly administered noradrenaline and dopamine on body temperature of the rat. *Pol. J. Pharmacol. Pharm.* 25:2345–55

86. Barnett, A., Taber, R. I. 1968. The effects of diethyldithiocarbamate and L-dopa on body temperature in mice. *J. Pharm. Pharmacol.* 20:600–4

87. Hill, H. F., Horita, A. 1971. Inhibition of D-amphetamine hyperthermia by blockade of dopamine receptors. *J. Pharm. Pharmacol.* 23:715–17

88. Hill, H. F., Horita, A. 1972. A pimozide sensitive effect of apomorphine on body temperature of the rabbit. *J. Pharm. Pharmacol.* 24:490–91

89. Grabowska, M., Michaluk, J., Antkiewicz, L. 1973. Possible involvement of brain serotonin in apomorphine induced hypothermia. *Eur. J. Pharmacol.* 23:82–89

90. Glick, S. D., Marsanico, R. G. 1974. Apomorphine induced and pilocarpine induced hypothermia in mice: drug interactions and changes in drug sensitivity after caudate nucleus lesions. *Br. J. Pharmacol.* 51:353–57

91. Cox, B., Ary, M., Lomax, P. 1975. Dopaminergic mechanisms in withdrawal hypothermia in morphine dependent rats. *Life Sci.* 17:41–42

92. Cox, B., Ary, M., Lomax, P. 1976. Dopaminergic involvement in withdrawal hypothermia and thermoregulatory behaviour in morphine dependent rats. *Pharmacol. Biochem. Behav.* 4:259–62

93. Lomax, P., Green, M. D. 1975. Histamine and temperature regulation. See Ref. 3, pp. 85–94

94. Brezenoff, H. E., Lomax, P. 1970. Temperature changes following microinjection of histamine into the thermoregulatory centers of the rat. *Experientia* 26:51–52

95. Shaw, G. G. 1971. Hypothermia produced in mice by histamine acting on the central nervous system. *Br. J. Pharmacol.* 42:205–14

96. Schwartz, J.-C., Lampart, C., Rose, C. 1973. Histamine formation in rat brain in vivo: effects of histidine loads. *J. Neurochem.* 19:801–10

97. Taylor, K. M., Snyder, S. H. 1972. Dynamics of the regulation of histamine levels in mouse brain. *J. Neurochem.* 18:341–54

98. Green, M. D., Simon, M. L., Lomax, P. 1975. Histidine induced hypothermia in the rat. *Life Sci.* 16:1293–99

99. Cox, B., Green, M. D., Lomax, P. 1976. Thermoregulatory effects of histamine. *Experientia* 32:498–500

100. Green, M. D., Cox, B., Lomax, P. 1975. Histamine H_1- and H_2-receptors in the central thermoregulatory pathways of the rat. *J. Neurosci. Res.* 1:353–59

101. Green, M. D., Cox, B., Lomax, P. 1976. Sites and mechanisms of action of histamine in the central thermoregulatory pathways of the rat. *Neuropharmacology* 15:321–24

102. Clark, W. G., Cumby, H. R. 1975. Biphasic effect of centrally injected histamine on body temperature in the cat. *Pharmacologist* 17:256

103. Cox, B., Green, M. D., Cheserak, W., Lomax, P. 1976. The effect of 4-methylhistamine on temperature regulation in the rat. *J. Thermal Biol.* 1:205–7

104. Green, M. D., Lomax, P. 1976. Behavioral thermoregulation and neuroamines in fish (*Chromus chromus*). *J. Thermal Biol.* 1:237–40

105. Feldberg, W. 1975. Summing up a symposium. See Ref. 3, pp. 393–95

Ann. Rev. Pharmacol. Toxicol. 1977. 17:355–67
Copyright © 1976 by Annual Reviews Inc. All rights reserved

PHARMACOLOGY
OF LAXATIVES

❖6685

Henry J. Binder
Department of Internal Medicine, Yale University, New Haven, Connecticut 06510

INTRODUCTION

Effective laxative action results in an increase in fecal water excretion, and increased fecal water excretion is usually secondary to altered intestinal fluid and electrolyte movement. Both an understanding of the process(es) by which laxatives work and a classification of laxatives therefore should be based on the mechanism(s) by which cathartics either increase fecal water excretion or alter intestinal fluid and electrolyte movement. Since most laxatives were initially introduced into clinical practice on an empirical basis, the traditional classification of laxatives found in textbooks of pharmacology and therapeutics employ arbitrary categories that do not reflect the pathophysiological principles of altered intestinal fluid and electrolyte transport (1–3).

Diarrhea, as well as laxative action, is characterized by increased fecal water excretion. Recent studies of intestinal fluid and electrolyte movement in patients with various diarrheal illnesses have revealed alteration of water and sodium movement (4–6). Dihydroxy bile acids and ricinoleic acid are classical laxatives and have also been implicated in the pathophysiology of diarrhea of ileal resection and the diarrhea of steatorrhea respectively (7, 8). Further, laxative abuse has been identified as responsible for an occasional case of previously undiagnosed watery diarrhea (9, 10). Although clinicians are now beginning to consider diarrhea in terms of increased fecal water excretion, altered intestinal electrolyte movement, and intestinal electrolyte secretion, much less attention has been given to similar considerations in regard to the pharmacology of laxatives (11). This review summarizes recent observations of the effect of laxatives on intestinal function, which indicate that most laxatives alter intestinal electrolyte transport, and provides a basis for the development of a classification of laxatives based on the effect of these drugs on intestinal electrolyte transport.

ALTERATION OF ELECTROLYTE MOVEMENT

Since an increase in fecal water excretion is common to both laxatives and diarrhea, I first review certain aspects of intestinal fluid and electrolyte movement that are derived from studies of patients with diarrhea in order to provide a basis for a discussion of the effect of laxatives on intestinal water and electrolyte transport.

When segmental perfusions of the intestine are performed in normal subjects, net absorption of fluid and electrolytes is demonstrated. In contrast, when these studies are performed in patients with diarrhea of various etiologies, either a decrease in fluid and electrolyte movement or fluid and electrolyte accumulation is observed in the involved segment of intestine (4–6, 12–15). Therefore, the phenomenological observation is either a decrease in fluid absorption or luminal fluid accumulation (which often is referred to as secretion[1]). Demonstration of either of these two phenomena (i.e. diminished absorption or fluid accumulation) does not provide any information regarding the mechanism(s) responsible for these events. For example, a decrease in net absorption may be secondary either to a decrease in the active absorptive process or to an increase in the active secretory process. Conversely, more than one mechanism may be responsible for the phenomena of net fluid accumulation; that is, active electrolyte secretion is not the only mechanism that can result in net fluid accumulation. Increased osmolarity of luminal contents can result in net fluid accumulation and probably accounts for the diarrhea and fluid accumulation that occur in patients with lactose intolerance (16). Inhibition of an active absorptive process alone should not result in net fluid accumulation unless a coexisting secretory process is also present. Whether stimulation of an active secretory process results in either a decrease in net absorption or net fluid accumulation depends on the magnitude of the secretory process.

Active Ion Secretion

Several substances stimulate active ion secretion which may result in either fluid accumulation or decreased net fluid absorption. These secretory stimulants (secretogogues) can be grouped as either (a) bacterial enterotoxins, (b) enteric and nonenteric hormones, or (c) certain luminal products. The best-known and most thoroughly studied secretogogue is cholera enterotoxin (17–20). It is currently accepted that cholera enterotoxin stimulates adenylate cyclase and the resulting increased mucosal cyclic AMP then stimulates, by processes that are totally unknown at present, an active secretory process. In addition to cholera enterotoxin, there are at least six other bacterial enterotoxins that stimulate net fluid accumulation (21, 22), but not all bacterial enterotoxins activate secretion by means of the

---

[1]I prefer to employ the term fluid and electrolyte *accumulation* rather than *secretion* to describe the addition of water to a solution perfusing a segment of intestine. I restrict the term *secretion* to describe the active transport process that is stimulated, for example, by cholera enterotoxin. Significant confusion has resulted from the use of *secretion* to describe both the phenomena of fluid accumulation and the active transport process.

cyclic AMP system (23). Of the several hormones associated with net fluid accumulation, vasoactive intestinal polypeptide (VIP) has gained significant attention in recent years and probably produces fluid accumulation in a manner similar to cholera enterotoxin (24, 25). Other hormones that stimulate fluid accumulation include gastric inhibitory polypeptide, cholecystokinin, secretin, thyrocalcitonin, prostaglandin E_1, and glucagon (26–31). Many of these hormones have been implicated as the causative agents in the watery diarrhea syndrome (pancreatic cholera) (32–34). Perfusion of the lumen of intestine with several substances such as bile acids, fatty acids, and hydroxy fatty acids will also provoke net fluid accumulation (35–41). These agents have been implicated in the pathophysiology of certain diarrheal illnesses and have also been employed as laxatives. Other luminal compounds besides bile acids and fatty acids which may induce fluid accumulation include caffeine, which inhibits cyclic nucleotide phosphodiesterase activity resulting in increased mucosal cyclic AMP levels, and several laxatives (42).

Role of Motility

The exact role of motility in the production of alterations of fluid and electrolyte movement is ill defined and requires further study. Many drugs alter intestinal motor function both in vitro and in vivo and affect intestinal transit (43–45), and changes in motility accompany various diarrheal illnesses. There is, however, no direct evidence that changes in motility, motor function, or transit alter intestinal electrolyte absorption. Although an increase in transit may diminish absorption, an increase in intestinal transit (i.e. a decrease in transit time) alone should never result in fluid and electrolyte accumulation. It is possible that increased luminal flow which occurs secondary to alteration of intestinal electrolyte movement may be responsible for the observed changes in motility. Therefore, additional studies are required to determine whether motility affects fluid absorption, especially if changes of fluid and electrolyte movement and transit are observed simultaneously. This information is extremely important to an understanding of laxative action since the general assumption has been that laxatives are effective by their action on intestinal motility.

In contrast, an opposite effect on motility (i.e. a decrease in intestinal transit) may alter absorption. Pharmacological agents (e.g. codeine), which decrease transit or increase transit time, may decrease fecal water excretion but probably do so by increasing the time that the absorbing surface is exposed to luminal contents. There is no experimental evidence to date that indicates that drugs like codeine directly affect absorptive or secretory transport processes.

Mucosal Permeability

Several different mechanisms may result in net fluid and electrolyte accumulation and therefore increase fecal water excretion. Active electrolyte secretion, a hyperosmolar load, and a decrease in the absorptive process as already mentioned may result in net fluid accumulation. Additional mechanisms have also been implicated as possible causative factors in the production of net fluid accumulation and include increased hydrostatic pressure and increased mucosal permeability. Although increased hydrostatic pressure is not responsible for cholera enterotoxin–induced fluid accumulation (46), Lifson and associates have provided convincing evidence that increased hydrostatic pressure in the in vitro canine jejunum results in net serosal to mucosal sodium movement (47, 48). Whether this phenomenon occurs in vivo is not known. Increased mucosal permeability has also been suggested to cause net fluid accumulation; however, an alteration of permeability should result in equal increases in solute and fluid movement in *both* lumen to plasma and plasma to lumen directions without any change in net movement. Although an increase in permeability is present during both bile acid and fatty acid–induced fluid accumulation, altered mucosal permeability is not required for fluid accumulation per se since in cholera enterotoxin–induced fluid accumulation, an increase in tissue resistance is found (20), and no change in mucosal permeability is noted in the fluid accumulation that is secondary to an hyperosmolar load (49). Therefore, the importance of increased mucosal permeability in the genesis of intestinal fluid accumulation is uncertain. It would be intriguing to speculate that increased hydrostatic pressure becomes a driving force for net fluid accumulation only in the presence of increased mucosal permeability—a circumstance that may explain the diminished net absorption observed following volume expansion in experimental animals (50, 51).

Mucosal Damage

The role of intestinal mucosal damage or morphological abnormalities on the production of fluid accumulation is also difficult to assess. The decrease in net absorption or net fluid accumulation that is associated with intestinal morphological changes may directly reflect a decrease in an absorptive process or stimulation of a secretory process secondary to mucosal injury. Alternatively, certain substances may be responsible for both the morphological abnormalities and stimulation of secretory process or inhibition of the absorptive process. If an increase in mucosal permeability is also present, this may only reflect the mucosal damage. The pathophysiological role of histologic changes in the intestinal mucosa in the production of altered fluid movement is therefore unclear.

When fluid accumulation or diminished absorption is present simultaneously with alteration of several different processes of intestinal function, it may be difficult to define which particular factor or factors are primarily responsible for the alteration of fluid and electrolyte movement. As is discussed subsequently, this is presently the primary problem in the determination of the mechanism(s) responsible for the fluid accumulation produced by several laxatives.

TRADITIONAL CLASSIFICATION OF LAXATIVES

The present classification of laxatives neither reflects these pathophysiologic considerations concerning alteration of intestinal fluid and electrolyte transport nor possesses any other logical basis to explain laxative action. Various textbooks on pharmacology offer a variety of differing and overlapping classifications (1–3). The Food and Drug Administration's over-the-counter drug panel on laxatives, antidiarrheal, antiemetic, and emetic products (52) adapted a classification of laxatives similar to most other classifications and suggested five categories: (*a*) stimulant or irritant, (*b*) stool softeners, (*c*) saline, (*d*) bulk, and (*e*) lubricant. It is evident that this classification does not relate to mechanisms responsible for either increasing fecal water excretion or altering intestinal fluid movement (11).

Stimulants

The largest member of laxatives belong to the stimulant or irritant category, and most recent studies of laxatives have evaluated the effect of these agents on intestinal function. The terms *stimulant* and *irritant* are not mechanisms of altered intestinal fluid and electrolyte movement, but rather are used to suggest that these agents possess laxative properties by virtue of their "stimulation" of peristalsis by "irritation" of colonic mucosa. However, recent studies of four of the most common laxatives in this category provide compelling evidence that these laxatives alter fluid and electrolyte absorption in both man and experimental animals and that net fluid accumulation is often observed. These four laxatives are ricinoleic acid which is the active ingredient of castor oil, dihydroxy bile acids, bisacodyl, and oxyphenisatin. These laxatives are surface-active compounds and appear to possess a similar pattern of action with multiple effects on intestinal function. These agents can convert net fluid and electrolyte absorption to net fluid accumulation; in addition they alter mucosal permeability, induce certain changes in intestinal motor activity, on occasion produce mucosal damage, and in the case of dihydroxy bile acids stimulate active anion secretion.

BILE ACIDS   Investigations of the effect of bile acids on intestinal electrolyte transport are more extensive than those of fatty acids and hydroxy fatty acids. Bile acids have well-known laxative properties and are often included in multiple-ingredient preparations. Further, diarrhea is a significant side effect of chenodeoxycholic acid therapy when given to dissolve cholesterol gallstones (53), and bile acid alteration of colonic electrolyte transport has been implicated as the causative factor in cholerrheic enteropathy which is the diarrhea that occurs in patients with ileal dysfunction (7).

Several different bile acids alter fluid transport although dihydroxy bile acids such as deoxycholic acid are more effective than trihydroxy bile acids, and unconjugated bile acids may be more effective than conjugated bile acids (35–37, 54–56). Perfusion of the human colon and ileum with deoxycholic acid results in net fluid and electrolyte accumulation. Similar changes have been noted in the jejunum of human volunteers. Several, although not all studies, have indicated that significant histological damage is present in colonic mucosa following perfusion with unconjugated dihydroxy bile acids (54, 57). Bile acids also produce marked alteration of colonic mucosal permeability. Evidence of these changes of mucosal permeability include (*a*) a decrease in electrical potential difference (PD), (*b*) an increase in the passage of inulin from plasma to lumen, (*c*) an increase in the movement of EDTA from serosa to mucosa, (*d*) an increase in urea and oxalate absorption, and (*e*) an increase in oxalate clearance by the colon (58–60).

Evidence has been obtained recently that dihydroxy bile acids stimulate active anion secretion (61). These studies suggest that bile acids stimulate secretion in a manner analogous to the secretion produced by cholera enterotoxin because the colon possesses a cyclic AMP–mediated secretory system and because in in vitro studies bile acids decrease net sodium absorption, produce net chloride secretion, and increase mucosal cyclic AMP levels (61, 62). Additional studies have confirmed that dihydroxy bile acids stimulate adenylate cyclase activity in the colon (63), and bile acids also increase mucosal cyclic AMP in the small intestine (64). In contrast to the studies with cholera enterotoxin, which increases tissue resistance, bile acids increase mucosal permeability in addition to stimulating active anion secretion.

Therefore, bile acids produce fluid and electrolyte accumulation, and stimulation of active anion secretion may be the primary driving force responsible for the net fluid accumulation. The importance of increased mucosal permeability, mucosal damage, and changes in motor activity in the genesis of fluid accumulation must be considered (65). As already suggested, motility changes cannot result in net fluid accumulation. Increased permeability should result in an increase in both lumen to plasma and plasma to lumen movement without a resulting change in net movement unless there is also an increase in hydrostatic pressure. Morphological damage is not a constant observation. Therefore, although these changes in permeability, morphology, and motility may contribute to the production of net fluid accumulation, active anion secretion, which is probably mediated by cyclic AMP, is likely to be the primary determinant of these changes in fluid and electrolyte movement.

HYDROXY FATTY ACIDS Recent detailed studies have clearly indicated that ricinoleic acid influences intestinal fluid and electrolyte movement, alters colonic slow wave activity, increases mucosal permeability, and produces morphological changes that are observed on scanning electron microscopy (38–41, 67–73). Which of these changes are responsible for the increased fecal water excretion that occurs following castor oil ingestion is uncertain but several tentative conclusions can be made.

Study of the effect of ricinoleic acid and other hydroxy and nonhydroxy fatty acids on fluid and electrolyte movement has indicated that several fatty acids alter fluid absorption (38–41). In both the human and rodent colon, perfusion with ricinoleic acid diminishes net fluid absorption or produces net fluid and sodium accumulation. Further, hydroxy fatty acids are more effective than nonhydroxy fatty acids. Although hydroxy fatty acids are not absorbed as effectively as nonhydroxy fatty acids, and therefore their intraluminal concentrations may be higher than those of the nonhydroxy fatty acids, there is little correlation between absorption of fatty acids and their alterations of fluid movement. Perfusion of the dog ileum also results in similar effects on fluid absorption, and perfusion of the jejunum in human volunteers reveals that ricinoleic acid produces net fluid accumulation. In contrast, octanoic acid, a medium chain fatty acid which when employed therapeutically in medium-chain triglycerides often decreases diarrhea, does not alter fluid and electrolyte movement (40, 58). These experiments provide conclusive evidence that ricinoleic acid can reverse net fluid absorption to net fluid accumulation and suggest that this production of fluid accumulation is related to the laxative properties of ricinoleic acid. However, these studies do not provide information concerning the mechanism by which ricinoleic acid induces fluid accumulation. In contrast to bile acids there is no conclusive evidence that ricinoleic acid stimulates an active secretory process. We have attempted to study the effect of ricinoleic acid on isolated intestinal epithelia utilizing the methods employed in previous studies with both bile acids and cholera enterotoxin, but the mucosal requirement for calcium has prevented the addition of ricinoleic acid to the mucosal solution (H. J. Binder, unpublished observations). Direct demonstration of the effect of ricinoleic acid on ion transport in vitro is still required although preliminary reports indicate that ricinoleic acid increases mucosal cyclic AMP in the colon (66; H. J. Binder, unpublished observations).

In other studies ricinoleic acid decreases both motility in vivo and muscular contractility in vitro (67–69). In addition, ricinoleic acid may uncouple the basal electrical rhythm (BER) of circular muscle of the isolated cat colon (70). The recent observation that similar changes of BER were present in the colon of cats with spontaneous diarrhea suggests that this change in slow wave activity may be a nonspecific effect secondary to increased fecal water excretion (71). Ricinoleic acid also increases colonic mucosal permeability as demonstrated by an increase in inulin clearance and a decrease in the electrical PD (38). Finally, Gaginella & Phillips have shown that focal abnormalities of surface epithelial cells are apparent in both ileal and colonic mucosa in the rabbit when examined by scanning electron microscopy following exposure of the mucosa to ricinoleic acid (72, 73). These histological changes may represent a toxic effect of ricinoleic acid on the surface epithelia, and the changes in mucosal permeability may then be secondary to these anatomical observations. Again it must be emphasized that the relationship of these changes in permeability, morphology, and motility to the production of net fluid accumulation is unknown. A unifying though unproven hypothesis is that fatty acids and hydroxy fatty acids, like bile acids, stimulate a cyclic AMP–mediated active secretory process which is the driving force for net fluid accumulation and increased fecal water excretion.

OTHER AGENTS   Other compounds that are usually included in the irritant or stimulant category alter fluid and electrolyte movement and also affect more than one aspect of intestinal function. Bisacodyl has recently been studied in considerable detail (74–79). Perfusion of both the dog and the human colon with bisacodyl results in net fluid and electrolyte accumulation (74, 75). Further, perfusion of the small intestine of human volunteers and the rat also results in altered fluid and electrolyte movement (76). Focal changes in intestinal epithelial cells recently have been observed following exposure of colonic mucosa to bisacodyl (77). In addition, bisacodyl inhibits glucose absorption and intestinal Na-K-ATPase activity; changes in motor activity are also evident (78–80). It is not known as yet whether bisacodyl alters mucosal permeability. Studies of the effect of bisacodyl on in vitro ion transport, adenylate cyclase, and mucosal cyclic AMP are awaited.

Phenolphthalein is a classical American laxative. There is but one report available that has evaluated the effect of phenolphthalein on fluid and electrolyte movement. In the isolated rabbit ileum, 1 mM phenolphthalein converted net sodium absorption to net sodium secretion and at a rate similar to that produced by 10 mM ricinoleic acid (81). Although the laxative action of phenolphthalein has usually been ascribed to an effect on peristalsis, it is important to recognize that phenolphthalein and bisacodyl have very similar chemical structures. Since phenolphthalein inhibits Na-K-ATPase activity (79), this effect on fluid movement may be mediated in part by inhibition of sodium absorption. Oxyphenisatin was a popular laxative until its recent removal from distribution by the FDA because of its association with chronic active hepatitis. Oxyphenisatin also has a chemical structure similar to both phenolphthalein and bisacodyl and significantly alters intestinal fluid and electrolyte movement. In experimental animals oxyphenisatin has produced net fluid accumulation and in parallel studies, oxyphenisatin markedly increased mucosal permeability and inhibited glucose absorption (79, 82, 83). Once more it is tempting to ascribe the fluid accumulation produced by oxyphenisatin to active ion secretion, but further studies are required to substantiate this possibility.

Stool Softeners

Another major category of laxatives is the stool softeners. The principal drug in this group is dioctyl sodium sulfosuccinate (DSS). Of note is that DSS as well as bile acids and fatty acids are detergents. Although unequivocal evidence of the efficacy of DSS as a laxative in man is still lacking, we have recently reported that DSS produces net fluid and electrolyte accumulation in the rat cecum in addition to increasing mucosal permeability (84). In these studies DSS increased mucosal cyclic AMP and altered ion transport in a manner similar to bile acids. Cyclic AMP–mediated active anion secretion may then be the driving force for the observed net fluid accumulation produced by DSS. In other studies DSS also altered both fluid and electrolyte movement in the human and murine small intestine and the histological appearance of the surface cells of the colon (85). Therefore, DSS clearly alters fluid movement which may then be related to and responsible for its laxative effects. Clearly, the term *stool softener* could apply to all laxatives for if effective, all laxatives should result in "stool softening." I suspect that DSS was categorized as a stool softener since it is less potent in altering fluid and electrolyte movement than other laxatives.

Saline

Magnesium salts are described as saline or osmotic laxatives, and their laxative effect has been attributed to their poor absorbability with resulting hyperosmolarity. This proposed mechanism of laxative action is unproven. Isosmolarity is present at the ligament of Trietz following ingestion of hyperosmolar or hyposmolar meals, and magnesium salts are effective laxatives at relatively low concentrations. It has been proposed as an intriguing, though totally unproven, speculation that the laxative action of magnesium may be mediated by cholecystokinin (CCK) (86). CCK is a secretagogue that alters fluid movement and stimulates intestinal motor activity and is released from duodenal mucosa by both magnesium and amino acids (27). Recent studies suggest that magnesium decreases both circular smooth muscle contractility of the ileum and decreases transit time (67, 87). Additional studies are required to assess the effects of magnesium on fluid absorption.

Bulk

Several different products are classified as bulk laxatives. The recent interest in dietary fiber has brought increased attention to these agents. There are no direct data to indicate that these products directly affect mucosal electrolyte transport. The general assumption has been that bulk laxatives work by virtue of their ability to adsorb fluid resulting in less fluid available for absorption. The recent demonstration that bran changes the composition of fecal bile acids suggests that other possible explanations may account for the laxative action of various bulk products (88).

CONCLUSION

Laxative action must be considered in terms of increases in fecal water excretion. Despite twenty-five years of emphasis on motility abnormalities it is uncertain (a) how various laxatives affect motility, (b) how changes in motor activity alter fluid and electrolyte movement, and (c) how changes in motor function result in fecal water excretion. Most of the laxatives studied to date alter intestinal fluid and electrolyte movement, and net fluid and electrolyte accumulation is often observed. Alteration of fluid and electrolyte movement, which often results in fluid accumulation, is central to effective laxative action. We propose that active ion secretion stimulated by laxative agents may be the driving force for the fluid accumulation produced by many of these drugs. Studies in the future should focus on the effect of various laxatives on ion transport with emphasis on their ability to stimulate active secretory processes or to inhibit active absorptive processes or both. Studies are also required to determine the possible contribution of other laxative-induced changes in intestinal function to alterations of electrolyte movement. Therefore, future classifications should be based on the pathophysiological mechanisms by which laxatives alter fluid and electrolyte movement.

ACKNOWLEDGMENTS

Studies that were performed in the author's laboratory were supported in part by USPHS grant AM 14669 from the National Institute of Arthritis, Metabolism, and Digestive Disease and grants from the John A. Hartford Foundation and the Connecticut Digestive Disease Society. Ms. Diane Whiting provided expert bibliographic assistance.

1. Fingl, E. 1970. In *The Pharmacological Basis of Therapeutics,* ed. L. S. Goodman, A. Gilman, 1020–24. New York: Macmillan. 1794 pp.
2. Bonnycastle, D. D. 1971. In *Drill's Pharmacology in Medicine,* ed. J. R. DiPalma, 975–91. New York: McGraw-Hill. 1920 pp.
3. Goth, A. 1972. *Medical Pharmacology Principles and Concepts,* 429–34. St. Louis: Mosby. 704 pp.
4. Hendrix, T. R., Bayless, T. M. 1970. Digestions: Intestinal secretion. *Ann. Rev. Physiol.* 32:139–64
5. Phillips, S. F. 1972. Diarrhea: A current view of the pathophysiology. *Gastroenterology* 63:495–518
6. Binder, H. J. 1975. In *Functions of the Stomach and Intestine,* ed. M. H. F. Friedman, 247–58. Baltimore: Univ. Park Press. 469 pp.
7. Hofmann, A. F., Poley, J. R. 1969. Cholestyramine treatment of diarrhea associated with ileal resection. *N. Engl. J. Med.* 281:397–402
8. Binder, H. J. 1973. Fecal fatty acids—mediators of diarrhea? *Gastroenterology* 65:847–50
9. Heizer, W. D., Warshaw, A. L., Waldmann, T. A., Laster, L. 1968. Protein-losing gastroenteropathy and malabsorption associated with factitious diarrhea. *Ann. Int. Med.* 68:839–52
10. LaRusso, N. F., McGill, D. B. 1975. Surreptitious laxative ingestion. Delayed recognition of a serious condition: A case report. *Mayo Clin. Proc.* 50:706–8
11. Binder, H. J., Donowitz, M. 1975. A new look at laxative action. *Gastroenterology* 69:1001–5
12. Fordtran, J. S., Rector, F. C., Locklear, T. W., Ewton, M. F. 1967. Water and solute movement in the small intestine of patients with sprue. *J. Clin. Invest.* 46:287–98
13. Pierce, N. F., Banwell, J. G., Rupak, D. M., Mitra, R. C., Caranasos, G. J., Keimowitz, R. I., Mondal, A., Manji, P. M. 1968. Effect of intragastric glucose-electrolyte infusion upon water and electrolyte balance in Asiatic cholera. *Gastroenterology* 55:333–43
14. Harris, J., Shields, R. 1970. Absorption and secretion of water and electrolytes by the intact human colon in diffuse untreated protocolitis. *Gut* 11:27–33
15. Turnberg, L. A. 1971. Abnormalities in intestinal electrolyte transport in congenital chloridorrhea. *Gut* 12:544–51
16. Christopher, N. L., Bayless, T. M. 1971. Role of the small bowel and colon in lactose-induced diarrhea. *Gastroenterology* 60:845–52
17. Hendrix, T. R., Banwell, J. G. 1969. Pathogenesis of cholera. *Gastroenterology* 57:751–55
18. Carpenter, C. C. J. 1971. Cholera enterotoxin—recent investigations yield insights into transport processes. *Am. J. Med.* 50:1–7
19. Field, M., Fromm, D., Al-Awqati, Q., Greenough, W. B. 1972. Effect of cholera exterotoxin on ion transport across isolated ileal mucosa. *J. Clin. Invest.* 51:796–804
20. Kimberg, D. V., Field, M., Johnson, J., Henderson, A., Gershon, E. 1971. Stimulation of intestinal mucosal adenyl cyclase by cholera enterotoxin and prostaglandins. *J. Clin. Invest.* 50:1218–30
21. Banwell, J. G., Sheer, H. 1973. Effect of bacterial enterotoxins on the gastrointestinal tract. *Gastroenterology* 65:467–97
22. Klipstein, F. A., Horowitz, I. R., Engert, R. F., Schenk, E. A. 1975. Effect of Klebsiella pneumoniae enterotoxin on intestinal transport in the rat. *J. Clin. Invest.* 56:799–807
23. Donowitz, M., Keusch, G. T., Binder, H. J. 1975. Effect of shigella enterotoxin on electrolyte transport in rabbit ileum. *Gastroenterology* 69:1230–37
24. Said, S. I. 1974. Vasoactive intestinal polypeptide. *Gastroenterology* 67:735–37
25. Schwartz, C. J., Kimberg, D. V., Sheerin, H. E., Field, M., Said, S. I. 1974. Vasoactive intestinal peptide stimulation of adenylate cyclase and active electrolyte secretion in intestinal mucosa. *J. Clin. Invest.* 54:536–44
26. Barbezat, G. O., Grossman, M. I. 1971. Intestinal secretion: Stimulation by peptides. *Science* 174:422–24
27. Matuchansky, C., Huet, P. M., Mary, J. Y., Rambaud, J. C., Bernier, J. J. 1972. Effects of cholecystokinin and metoclopramide on jejunal movements of water and electrolytes and on transit time of luminal fluid in man. *Eur. J. Clin. Invest.* 2:169–75
28. Moritz, M., Finkelstein, G., Meshkinpour, H., Fingerut, J., Lorber, S. H. 1973. Effect of secretin and cholecys-

tokinin on the transport of electrolyte and water in human jejunum. *Gastroenterology* 64:76–80

29. Gray, T. K., Biederdorf, F. A., Fordtran, J. S. 1973. Thyrocalcitonin and the jejunal absorption of calcium, water and electrolytes in normal subjects. *J. Clin. Invest.* 52:3084–88

30. Matuchansky, C., Bernier, J. J. 1973. Effect of prostaglandin E_1 on glucose, water and electrolyte absorption in the human jejunum. *Gastroenterology* 64:1111–18

31. Hicks, T., Turnberg, L. A. 1974. Influence of glucagon on the human jejunum. *Gastroenterology* 67:1114–18

32. Said, S. I., Faloona, G. R. 1975. Elevated plasma and tissue levels of vasoactive intestinal polypeptide in the watery diarrhea syndrome due to pancreatic, bronchogenic and other tumors. *N. Engl. J. Med.* 293:155–60

33. Schmitt, M. G., Soergel, K. H., Hensley, G. T., Chey, W. Y. 1975. Watery diarrhea associated with pancreatic islet cell carcinoma. *Gastroenterology* 69:206–16

34. Rambaud, J. C., Modigliani, R., Matuchansky, C., Bloom, S., Said, S., Pessayre, D., Bernier, J. J. 1975. Pancreatic cholera. Studies on tumoral secretions and pathophysiology of diarrhea. *Gastroenterology* 69:110–22

35. Mekhjian, H. S., Phillips, S. F., Hofmann, A. F. 1971. Colonic secretion of water and electrolytes induced by bile acids: Perfusion studies in man. *J. Clin. Invest.* 50:1569–77

36. Krag, E., Phillips, S. F. 1974. Active and passive bile acid absorption in man. Perfusion studies of the ileum and jejunum. *J. Clin. Invest.* 53:1686–94

37. Wingate, D. L., Phillips, S. F., Hofmann, A. F. 1973. Effect of glycine-conjugated bile acids with and without lecithin on water and glucose absorption in perfused human jejunum. *J. Clin. Invest.* 52:1230–36

38. Bright-Asare, P., Binder, H. J. 1973. Stimulation of colonic secretion of water and electrolytes by hydroxy fatty acids. *Gastroenterology* 64:81–88

39. Ammon, H. V., Phillips, S. F. 1973. Inhibition of colonic water and electrolyte absorption by fatty acids in man. *Gastroenterology* 65:744–49

40. Ammon, H. V., Phillips, S. F. 1974. Inhibition of ileal water absorption by intraluminal fatty acids. Influence of chain length, hydroxylation, and conjugation of fatty acids. *J. Clin. Invest.* 53:205–10

41. Ammon, H. V., Thomas, P. H., Phillips, S. F. 1974. Effects of oleic and ricinoleic acid on net jejunal water and electrolyte movement. *J. Clin. Invest.* 53:374–79

42. Wald, A., Bayless, T. M. 1975. The effect of caffeine on the small intestine. *Gastroenterology* 68:1008 (Abstr.)

43. Hendrix, T. R., Atkinson, M., Clifton, J. A., Ingelfinger, F. J. 1957. The effect of 5-hydroxytryptamine on intestinal motor function in man. *Am. J. Med.* 23:886–93

44. Misiewicz, J. J., Waller, S. L., Eisner, M. 1966. Motor responses of human gastrointestinal tract to 5-hydroxytryptamine in vivo and in vitro. *Gut* 7:208–16

45. Fishlock, D. J. 1966. Effect of bradykinin on the human isolated small and large intestine. *Nature* 212:1533–35

46. Carpenter, C. C. J., Greenough, W. B. III, Sack, R. B. 1969. The relationship of superior mesenteric artery blood flow to gut electrolyte loss in experimental cholera. *J. Infect. Dis.* 119:182–93

47. Hakim, A. A., Lifson, N. 1969. Effects of pressure on water and solute transport by dog intestinal mucosa in vitro. *Am. J. Physiol.* 216:276–84

48. Yablonski, M. E., Lifson, N. 1976. Mechanism of production of intestinal secretion by elevated venous pressure. *J. Clin. Invest.* 57:904–15

49. Kinsey, M. D., Formal, S. B., Giannella, R. A. 1975. Role of altered permeability in the pathogenesis of Salmonella diarrhea. *Gastroenterology* 68:926 (Abstr.)

50. Humphreys, M. H., Earley, L. E. 1971. The mechanism of decreased intestinal sodium and water absorption after acute volume expansion in the rat. *J. Clin. Invest.* 50:2355–67

51. Higgins, J. T., Blair, N. P. 1971. Intestinal transport of water and electrolytes during extracellular volume expansion in dogs. *J. Clin. Invest.* 50:2569–79

52. Food Drug Adm. Over-the-Counter Drugs. 1975. Proposal to establish monographs for OTC laxative, antidiarrheal, emetic and antiemetic products. *Fed. Regist.* 40:12902–44

53. Iser, J. H., Dowling, R. H., Mok, H. Y. I., Bell, G. D. 1975. Chenodeoxycholic acid treatment of gallstones. A followup report and analysis of factors influencing response to therapy. *N. Engl. J. Med.* 293:378–83

54. Teem, M. V., Phillips, S. F. 1972. Perfusion of the hamster jejunum with conjugated and unconjugated bile acids: Inhibition of water absorption and effects on morphology. *Gastroenterology* 62:261–67

55. Mekhjian, H. S., Phillips, S. F. 1970. Perfusion of the canine colon with unconjugated bile acids: Effect on water and electrolyte transport, morphology and bile acid absorption. *Gastroenterology* 59:120–29

56. Sladen, G. E., Harries, J. T. 1972. Studies on the effects of unconjugated dihydroxy bile salts on rat small intestinal function in vivo. *Biochim. Biophys. Acta* 288:443–50

57. Saunders, D. R., Hedges, J. R., Sillery, J., Esther, L., Matsumura, K., Rubin, C. E. 1975. Morphological and functional effects of bile salts on rat colon. *Gastroenterology* 68:1236–45

58. Dobbins, J. W., Binder, H. J. 1976. Effect of bile salts and fatty acids on the colonic absorption of oxalate. *Gastroenterology* 70:1096–1100

59. Nell, G., Forth, W., Rummel, W., Wanitschke, R. 1972. In *Bile Acids in Human Diseases*, ed. P. Back, W. Gerok, 263–67. Stuttgart: Schattauer. 271 pp.

60. Rummel, W., Nell, G., Wanitschke, R. 1975. In *Intestinal Absorption and Malabsorption*, ed. T. Z Csáky, 209–27. New York: Raven. 308 pp.

61. Binder, H. J., Rawlings, C. L. 1973. Effect of conjugated dihyroxy bile salts on electrolyte transport in rat colon. *J. Clin. Invest.* 52:1460–66

62. Binder, H. J., Filburn, C., Volpe, B. T. 1975. Bile salt alteration of colonic electrolyte transport: Role of cyclic adenosine monophosphate. *Gastroenterology* 68:503–8

63. Conley, D. R., Coyne, M. J., Bonorris, G. G., Chung, A., Schoenfield, L. 1976. Bile acid stimulation of colonic adenylate cyclase and secretion in the rabbit. *Am. J. Dig. Dis.* 21:453–58

64. Mertens, R. B., Mayer, S. E., Wheeler, H. O. 1976. Effect of cholera toxin on mucosal adenylate cyclase activity and in vivo fluid transport in rabbit gallbladder. *Gastroenterology* 70:919 (Abstr.)

65. Kirwan, W. O., Smith, A. N., Mitchell, W. D., Falconer, J. D., Eastwood, M. A. 1975. Bile acids and colonic motility in the rabbit and the human. *Gut* 16:894–902

66. Binder, H. J. 1974. Cyclic adenosine monophosphate controls bile salt and hydroxy fatty acid-induced colonic electrolyte secretion. *J. Clin. Invest.* 53:7–8a (Abstr.)

67. Stewart, J. J., Gaginella, T. S., Olsen, W. A., Bass, P. 1975. Inhibitory actions of laxatives on motility and water and electrolyte transport in the gastrointestinal tract. *J. Pharmacol. Exp. Ther.* 192:458–467

68. Gaginella, T. S., Stewart, J. J., Gullikson, G. W., Olsen, W. A., Bass, P. 1976. Inhibition of small intestinal mucosal and smooth muscle cell function by ricinoleic acid and other surfactants. *Life Sci.* 16:1595–1606

69. Stewart, J. J., Gaginella, T. S., Bass, P. 1975. Actions of ricinoleic acid and structurally related fatty acids on the gastrointestinal tract. I. Effects on the smooth muscle contractility in vitro. *J. Pharmacol. Exp. Ther.* 195:347–54

70. Christensen, J., Freeman, B. W. 1972. Circular muscle electromyogram in the cat colon: Local effect of sodium ricinoleate. *Gastroenterology* 63:1011–15

71. Christensen, J., Weisbrodt, N. W., Hauser, R. L. 1972. The electrical slow wave of the proximal colon of the cat in diarrhea. *Gastroenterology* 62:1159–66

72. Gaginella, T. S., Phillips, S. F. 1976. Ricinoleic acid (castor oil) alters intestinal surface structure. A scanning electronmicroscopic study. *Mayo Clin. Proc.* 51:6–12

73. Gaginella, T. S., Lewis, J. C., Phillips, S. F. 1976. Ricinoleic acid produces mucosal damage in the rabbit colon: Scanning electron microscopic (SEM) appearances. *Gastroenterology* 70:886 (Abstr.)

74. Ewe, K., Holker, B. 1974. Einflu eines diphenolischen laxans (Bisacodyl) aug den Wasser-und Elektrolyt-transport im menschlichen colon. *Klin. Woschenschr.* 52:827–33

75. Ewe, K. 1972. Effect of laxatives on intestinal water and electrolyte transport. *Eur. J. Clin. Invest.* 2:283

76. Rachmilewitz, D., Saunders, D. R., Rubin, C. E., Tytgat, G. N. 1976. Pharmacology of laxatives: Effects of Bisacodyl (Bis) on structure and function of intestinal mucosa. *Gastroenterology* 70:928 (Abstr.)

77. Meisel, J. L., Bergman, D., Saunders, D. R., Graney, D. 1976. Human rectal mucosa: Proctoscopic and morphologic changes caused by laxatives. *Gastroenterology* 70:918 (Abstr.)

78. Hart, S. L., McColl, I. 1967. The effect of purgative drugs on the intestinal ab-

sorption of drugs. *J. Pharm. Pharmacol.* 19:70–71

79. Chignell, C. F. 1968. The effect of phenolphthalein and other purgative drugs on rat intestinal (Na+-N+)-adenosine triphosphatase. *Biochem. Pharmacol.* 17:1207–12

80. Hardcastle, J. D., Mann, C. V. 1968. Study of large bowel peristalsis. *Gut* 9:512–20

81. Phillips, R. A., Love, A. H. G., Mitchell, T. G., Neptune, E. M. 1965. Cathartics and the sodium pump. *Nature* 206:1367–68

82. Nell, G., Overhoff, H., Forth, W., Kulenkampff, H., Specht, W., Rummel, W. 1973. Influx and efflux of sodium in jejunal and colonic segments of rats under the influence of oxyphenisatin. *Naunyn-Schmiedebergs Arch. Pharmacol.* 277:53–60

83. Nell, G. Forth, W., Rummel, W., Wanitschke, R. 1976. Pathway of sodium moving from blood to intestinal lumen under the influence of oxy-

phenisatin and deoxycholate. *Naunyn-Schmiedebergs Arch. Pharmacol.* 293:31–37

84. Donowitz, M., Binder, H. J. 1975. Effect of dioctyl sodium sulfosuccinate on colonic fluid and electrolyte movement. *Gastroenterology* 69:941–50

85. Saunders, D. R., Sillery, J., Rachmilewitz, D. 1975. Effect of dioctyl sodium sulfosuccinate on structure and function of rodent and human intestine. *Gastroenterology* 69:380–86

86. Harvey, R. F., Read, A. E. 1973. Saline purgatives act by releasing cholecystokinin. *Lancet* 2:185–87

87. Wanitschke, R., Ammon, H. V. 1976. Effects of magnesium sulfate on transit time and water transport in the human jejunum. *Gastroenterology* 70:949 (Abstr.)

88. Pomare, E. W., Heaton, K. W., Lowbeer, T. S., White, C. 1974. Effect of wheat bran on bile salt metabolism and bile composition. *Gut* 15:824–25 (Abstr.)

Ann. Rev. Pharmacol. Toxicol. 1977. 17:369–86
Copyright © 1977 by Annual Reviews Inc. All rights reserved

PHARMACOLOGICAL IMPLICATIONS OF BRAIN ACETYLCHOLINE TURNOVER MEASUREMENTS IN RAT BRAIN NUCLEI

❖6686

D. L. Cheney and E. Costa

Laboratory of Preclinical Pharmacology, National Institute of Mental Health,
Saint Elizabeths Hospital, Washington DC 20032

INTRODUCTION

The action of drugs on cholinergic mechanisms can be evaluated electrophysiologically (1–3) or biochemically (4–7). In brain, there are a few cholinergic pathways amenable to an electrophysiological investigation. Among them are the septal-hippocampal (8) and the habenulo-interpeduncular pathways (9). However, most of the important cholinergic mechanisms of brain elude this method of study. For instance, it is not possible to study electrophysiologically the intrinsic cholinergic systems of striatum and *N. accumbens*. Striatum and *N. accumbens* are the subject of greater interest in psychopharmacology because it is currently believed that by understanding the way drugs act on these intrinsic cholinergic systems we may learn how to minimize the extrapyramidal side effects of antipsychotics (10). Thus, with the present technical development it appears possible that progress in this area will stem from biochemical studies rather than from electrophysiological research.

The action of drugs on cholinergic systems in the brain can be inferred by measuring the acetylcholine (ACh) turnover rate in vivo (4, 5), or the V_{max} of choline (Ch) uptake (11) or the rate of ACh release using a push-pull cannula (6). The use of ACh turnover rate measurements to estimate the cholinergic neuronal activity stems from the belief that the turnover rate of ACh increases or decreases when the activity of cholinergic neurons is enhanced or depressed, respectively. Historically, this belief developed as a result of the demonstration that in cat

369

superior cervical ganglion the turnover rate of ACh at rest never exceeded 20% of the maximum rate that could be attained during electrical stimulation of preganglionic nerves (12). Since the ACh stored in cat sympathetic ganglia is located in terminal axons, the ganglion was a good model to correlate the neuronal activity with the ACh turnover rate. Unfortunately the whole brain cannot be used as a model for this correlation because of the intricate network of cholinergic neurons.

It is highly unlikely that drugs would simultaneously change the activity of every cholinergic neuron in brain in the same direction unless they act directly on Ch acetyltransferase (CAT) or acetylcholinesterase. Hence, the nonuniformity and intricacy of the brain cholinergic network make measurements of ACh turnover in whole brain devoid of any significance in the study of the action of analgesics, neuroleptics, hypnotics, etc. In contrast, measurements of ACh turnover rates in specific brain nuclei containing small, intrinsic cholinergic neurons or important cholinergic projections are of value in understanding how drugs change the cholinergic function at the level of specific synapses. Furthermore, when such studies are carried out in several nuclei of the brain simultaneously one might be able to elucidate whether a drug given chronically or acutely acts primarily on cholinergic mechanisms or whether the involvement of cholinergic neurons is secondary to a drug-induced modification of the synaptic input mediated by other transmitters, i.e. serotonin, dopamine, γ-aminobutyric acid (GABA), substance P, etc. These results allow drug actions to be described in terms of their effects on the integration of different synaptic mechanisms. Thus a given drug effect may be expressed in terms of the changes in the biochemical correlate of various transmitter systems in selected brain nuclei. Only recently have suitable methods become available to measure ACh content (13) and its turnover rate in brain parts or nuclei (14, 15) in which the ACh and Ch content have been stabilized by killing the rats with microwave radiation focused on the skull (16). This procedure kills the animals instantaneously and rapidly inactivates the enzymes responsible for the synthesis and degradation of ACh and its precursor, Ch (16). Moreover, the use of microwave radiation has imposed a reevaluation of older reports on drug effects on ACh and Ch content of brain nuclei. This review attempts to bring into focus the new concepts that are emerging from currently ongoing experiments to study the molecular dynamics of cholinergic transmission.

METHODS TO MEASURE ACh TURNOVER RATE

Over the past several years the methods proposed to study the regulation of cholinergic transmission in vivo have required the labeling of the ACh and Ch stored in neurons by injecting labeled precursors of ACh and by measuring simultaneously the changes with time in the specific activities of Ch and ACh (4, 5, 14, 15, 17–22). In addition to these isotopic methods, various nonisotopic approaches have been suggested to estimate the fractional rate constant of ACh efflux (6, 23–29). Some of the nonisotopic methods used drugs to instantaneously inhibit synthesis, metabolism, or transport of ACh, its precursor, or metabolites (30). A flaw common to all the methods involving the use of inhibitors derives from the widely spread assumption that drugs are so specific that even in high doses they selectively inhibit a given metabolic step. Obviously such specificity is exceptional; more often drugs that inhibit ACh metabolism exert collateral actions on other processes which directly or indirectly regulate a number of other metabolic steps. The isotopic methods which use tracer doses of a precursor of ACh are devoid of such an assumption but may be plagued by other conceptual flaws. Therefore, they are not devoid of problems; in fact they include a number of other tacit assumptions concerning the dynamics and compartmentation of ACh and its precursors which are open to critique. The assumption implicit in all of these techniques, whether isotopic or nonisotopic, is that at steady state the newly taken up pool of Ch is in rapid equilibrium with the pool of Ch that is the precursor of ACh. Moreover, it is assumed that the rates of synthesis and degradation of ACh are in equilibrium, and therefore principles of steady state kinetics can be used to calculate ACh turnover rate.

Nonisotopic Methods

RELEASE RATES OF ACh   MacIntosh (12) reported that in the absence of changes in tissue concentrations of ACh and after inhibition of ACh metabolism, the efflux of ACh from a perfused superior cervical ganglion of cats would describe the rate of ACh renovation in the ganglion. He further suggested that this same approach might be valid in brain (see 31). A rate constant for ACh release from brain slices was determined by measuring the release of ACh elicited by electrical stimulation in the presence or absence of eserine and/or atropine (23). However, in view of the rapid postmortem increase in tissue Ch concentrations (16, 32) and considering that an increase in Ch content (33, 34) increases ACh synthesis because CAT is not saturated, the heuristic value and physiological significance of methods which measure in vitro the ACh turnover rate by measuring release rates of ACh are open to question. A more reliable estimation of the dynamic state of ACh stores can be obtained by in vivo perfusion of limited areas of exposed cerebral cortex (24–26), cerebellum (27), striatum (28), and hippocampus (29) of rabbits, cats, and rats using specifically constructed cups perfused with Ringer's solution. However, with this perfusion method the size of the tissue being perfused is unknown. Hence, it is impossible to calculate turnover rate because the number of neurons contributing to the ACh efflux may change during the experiment and because it is impossible to prove that steady state is maintained during perfusion when drugs are administered. The use of the push-pull cannulae (6), which limit perfusion to small areas, has been preferred, but even in this case it is practically impossible to estimate the turnover rate of the ACh stores being studied. However, with the push-pull cannula, neurotransmitter efflux from various brain regions of the awake, gallamine-immobilized, or unrestrained cat can be measured [see references in (6)]. The effluxes can be compared in the presence or absence of various drugs, which, if needed, can even be added to the perfusion fluid. However, intervening edema or other dynamic problems may change the size of the brain tissue from which the efflux is being collected.

Since the amount of tissue perfused cannot be quantitated with any degree of accuracy, the ACh dynamics can be expressed neither in terms of fractional rate constant nor as a turnover rate. Moreover, it is almost impossible to assess whether during a push-pull cannula operation the ACh store in the tissue perfused is maintained at steady state.

As an example of the problems involved in the push-pull cannula experiments, we recall that atropine increases the rates of ACh efflux from the cerebral cortex when given either systemically (12, 26, 35–39) or topically (35, 37–41). It has, therefore, been concluded that atropine increases ACh turnover rate. However a number of laboratories have reported that atropine also lowers ACh content in brain structures (42–45). Thus the increased rate of ACh release following atropine reflects the decreased steady state content while synthesis is unchanged. Although push-pull cannula experiments give useful indications, one must be prepared to deal with the problem that drugs may increase efflux rates as they are compensating for decrease in steady state; thereby the synthesis rate of ACh is constant (45).

INHIBITION OF ACh SYNTHESIS   In brain the fractional rate constant of a transmitter efflux can be measured from the slope of the decline of the transmitter content elicited by complete and instantaneous blockade of its synthesis (30). By definition, this rate constant multiplied by the ACh content at steady state yields the turnover rate. Hemicholinium C-3 (HC-3), which is believed to block ACh synthesis (46), has been injected intraventricularly to measure the turnover rate of brain ACh (47). However, it appears that the main action of HC-3 is not a blockade of synthesis but a competitive inhibition of Ch uptake (46, 49). In addition, HC-3 may inhibit ACh synthesis by competing with Ch for acetylation (49), by blocking Ch kinase (50), or by diverting Ch to phospholipid formation (51). Since HC-3 inhibits Ch uptake and does not inhibit CAT completely and instantaneously, the essential requirements of the postulate for the use of HC-3 in the measurement of ACh turnover are not fulfilled. In line with this conclusion is the observation that the decline of ACh after HC-3 injection is not exponential but reaches a plateau after partial depletion at 30 min postinjection.

Calculations of ACh turnover rate from the ACh decline elicited by HC-3 thus far have been made from a single time point taken at a fixed interval after HC-3 injection (47) without assessing whether or not the ACh declines at maximal rates and follows first order kinetics. Thus what has been published on the ACh turnover using HC-3 is not adequate and the method does not have great future potential.

POSTMORTEM CHANGES IN ACh CONTENT   Some investigators have proposed that in rats killed by decapitation drugs may change brain ACh content when they have changed the ACh turnover rate before death (52, 53). Thus, an increase in striatal ACh content in rats which were decapitated at a certain time after the injection of dopamine receptor agonists (1, 54–58) has been interpreted to indicate a decrease in the turnover rate of striatal ACh. On the other hand, it has been reported that a decrease of striatal ACh content following the injection of dopamine receptor antagonists (1, 54, 56, 58) or after cerebral hemisection (1) indicates an increase in ACh turnover rate. When the rats are killed by microwave irradiation which stabilizes Ch content, the injection of dopamine receptor agonists or antagonists fails to change striatal ACh content (10, 59).

When the enzymes involved in ACh metabolism are not inactivated instantaneously and irreversibly, the ACh content of brain structures may change considerably because of the rapid postmortem metabolism of ACh and the increase of brain Ch content (16). Focused microwave irradiation (16) prevents the postmortem accumulation of free Ch in brain and blocks ACh destruction. Since the stability of ACh levels depends on the method used to kill the rats, predictions made concerning the turnover rate of ACh based on ACh content may or may not be correct. A decrease of striatal ACh content occurs after injection of ACh receptor blockers although they do not decrease ACh turnover rate (10, 59).

CHANGES IN V_{MAX} OF SODIUM-DEPENDENT HIGH AFFINITY Ch UPTAKE
Various lines of evidence suggest that sodium-dependent high affinity Ch uptake may be a rate-limiting step in the synthesis of ACh (60–62). This uptake (60, 61, 63, 64) appears to play an important role in the functioning of cholinergic terminals where it is located (65, 66), shows a specificity for a free hydroxyl group and a quaternary nitrogen (67), and does not transport ACh (68–70). Since it is functionally coupled to CAT (62) and to a releasable pool of ACh (71) the Ch uptake is an integral part of the regulation of ACh turnover (72). Hence, changes in the V_{max} of the high affinity Ch uptake measured in vitro after drug treatment may indicate changes in the ACh synthesis which have occurred in vivo following drug treatment (73, 74).

Unfortunately this method does not give a quantitative measure of synthesis rate. It only indicates the direction of the change. At least theoretically it appears possible to decrease or increase the availability of Ch without changing the V_{max} of Ch uptake by changing the affinity of the uptake for Ch. This method is rapid and simple and gives some important information on neuronal activity. Since in these studies fresh tissue must be used, the rapid postmortem increase in tissue Ch content might introduce artifacts and cause problems in interpretation. It must be emphasized that data available on drug effects on Ch uptake (74) parallel the data on the action of drugs on ACh synthesis obtained by other methods (25, 26, 31, 45, 75–80).

Isotopic Methods

GENERAL CONSIDERATIONS   The rate of ACh efflux from endogenous stores, including the efflux from neuronal stores, can be measured by labeling the ACh at steady state (17). The rate-limiting step of ACh synthesis is the uptake of Ch (60–62). This Ch in part is transported from plasma and in part is generated from the hydrolysis of ACh. Since this recycling of Ch could cause a reutilization of the label which would interfere with the estimation of ACh turnover based on principles of steady state kinetics, one must minimize the interference created by the recycling of labeled Ch (4, 5).

Calculations of the efflux rates of ACh are made by applying principles of steady state kinetics. Since the labeling procedures do not alter the steady state of the precursor, we are monitoring the rate of synthesis and degradation of ACh by measuring the change with time of the abundance of label in Ch and ACh. It is imperative in this method that the total amounts of Ch and ACh do not change while the relative abundance of a given isotope in the chemical composition of Ch and ACh changes. Furthermore, this approach requires that the enzymes responsible for the synthesis and degradation of ACh and Ch are instantaneously inactivated at the time of sacrifice, preferably with microwave irradiation. Even the 20 seconds that are required to freeze the brain following the immersion of rats in liquid nitrogen could cause a variability in the measurement of Ch concentrations which would not be tolerable for the measurement of ACh turnover with isotopic methods.

Although these methods eliminate some of the drawbacks associated with the nonisotopic methods, the isotopic methods are based on the following assumptions which are not yet entirely documented by experimental evidence (4, 5, 19, 22):

1. Plasma Ch is assumed to be preferentially transferred to a pool of free brain Ch which in turn equilibrates with the various metabolic pools of brain Ch at a rate proportional to their intrinsic metabolic rates. The pool size of Ch that functions as a precursor for ACh is very small. Since the rate of ACh synthesis is fast, the specific activity of free brain Ch would mirror with a certain accuracy the specific activity of Ch serving as ACh precursor.
2. A simple kinetic model based on a single open metabolic compartment of ACh store is assumed. Some equations are derived from this assumption and used to calculate turnover.
3. With the constant rate of label infusion and the time limits proposed in this model, the feedback due to recycling of labeled Ch formed from the hydrolysis of ACh is insignificant and fails to exceed the noise of the methods available to measure isotopic abundance.
4. The rate of conversion of free brain Ch into brain ACh is assumed to be much more rapid than the turnover rates which describe the other Ch metabolic pathways.

PULSE INJECTION OF ISOTOPIC LABEL   This approach utilizes the measurement of the specific radioactivity of ACh and its precursor Ch or the percentage of incorporation of deuterated ACh and Ch at various times after the pulse injection of labeled Ch or a labeled precursor of Ch (17–22). Both radioactive and stable isotopes of Ch have been used to pulse label brain ACh and measure the turnover rate of ACh in whole mouse brain (21, 75), whole rat brain (17), or in large brain regions (78).

The injections of radiolabeled Ch necessary to label the ACh content of small brain areas may change the steady state of Ch; hence phosphorylcholine has been used to bypass this difficulty (4, 5, 14, 19, 22, 76, 81). In fact in plasma and brain there is a large pool of phosphorylcholine (83, 83). Perhaps in brain tissue phosphorylcholine may be even a natural precursor of brain Ch (84). Radioactive phosphorylcholine efficiently labels brain Ch (19).

With pulse injections of labeled phosphorylcholine one can measure the ACh turnover rate in samples of brain tissue weighing about 100–300 mg (22). However, it is impossible to label ACh in brain nuclei with pulse injections of isotopically labeled phosphorylcholine because the amount of ^{14}C or deuterium that can be incorporated into ACh at steady state is too small to be detectable.

CONSTANT RATE INFUSION OF DEUTERIUM OR ^{14}C LABELED PHOSPHORYL-CHOLINE   Intravenous infusion of radiolabeled Ch or phosphorylcholine at constant rate for several minutes allows for a sufficient labeling of endogenous stores of Ch and ACh, and ACh turnover rate can be measured in various regions of rat brain (4, 5, 20). Although this approach is valid to measure ACh turnover rates in 100–200 mg brain samples, it cannot be used to measure the turnover rate of ACh in brain samples of 0.5–10 mg tissue (34; G. Racagni and D. L. Cheney, unpublished observations). To measure ACh turnover rate in such small tissue samples mass fragmentography and deuterium labeling must be used. A constant rate infusion with deuterated phosphorylcholine can label the Ch and ACh content in tissues weighing about 1 mg without changing the steady state content of either ACh or Ch (14, 15). Considering that a brain nucleus usually contains a few picomoles of ACh, the detection of a labeling of 10% of the molecules of Ch and ACh implies a measurement of the variant atomic species of molecules in the range of 200–300 femtomoles. This range is the lower limit of mass fragmentographic detection of ACh (85).

ACTIONS OF DRUGS ON ACh TURNOVER

Parasympathomimetics

Muscarinic agonists appear to increase ACh content in brain of rats or mice whether killed by microwave irradiation or by decapitation (10, 45, 76, 78, 86, 87). Pilocarpine (86), arecoline (86), and oxotremorine (18, 76) reduce the conversion of labeled precursor into ACh in mouse brain. Since this reduced conversion does not compensate for the increased brain ACh content, the turnover rate of ACh is decreased. It should be noted that the V_{max} of low K_m Ch uptake (74) and the release of ACh are also reduced by oxotremorine (87). The biosynthesis of ACh in cerebellum, medulla oblongata, midbrain, hippocampus, and cerebral cortex (88) is decreased by oxotremorine. Analgesics, dopamine receptor agonists, and GABA receptor agonists reduce the ACh turnover in certain structures, but not in others (see specific references later). In contrast, oxotremorine reduces ACh turnover in every structure tested and by the same extent (78). This finding suggests that Ch uptake is regulated by ACh hydrolysis occurring in the synaptic cleft, which in turn regulates the ACh turnover rate. It can be inferred that when ACh receptors are occupied by the agonist, little or no ACh is released and hydrolized. As a result of some unknown regulatory mechanism when the ACh synthesis is not utilized, the ACh content of the tissue increases and the ACh synthesis is reduced. By analogy with dopamine neurons this finding suggests that there are presynaptic cholinergic receptors which regulate ACh synthesis. Since this regulatory mechanism is diffuse to every cholinergic synapse, one might infer that these regulatory receptors may be closely associated with Ch uptake located presynaptically.

Acetylcholinesterase inhibitors increase the brain concentration of ACh (10, 45, 76, 89–91) even when the animals are killed by microwave irradiation (10, 75). Physostigmine reduced the Ch uptake in whole mouse brain and in rat hippocampus (74) and decreases the ACh turnover rate in mouse brain (76). Perhaps these acetylcholinesterase inhibitors reduce Ch uptake thereby causing a decrease in ACh synthesis.

The ganglionic stimulant, nicotine (92), increases the ACh release from cerebral cortex while the ganglionic blocker, hexamethonium (93), reduces the release of ACh from neocortex.

Parasympatholytics

Muscarinic receptor blockers increase the ACh release from the cerebral cortex (36, 38, 94–97), caudate (96), and hippocampus (96). These drugs also increase the V_{max} of the high affinity Ch uptake (11), lower the ACh content of striatum (45, 98), and increase the rate of conversion of labeled Ch into labeled ACh (45, 98) in mouse brain. Since this increase in the rate of conversion of labeled Ch to ACh is counterbalanced by the reduction in the size of the ACh pool, no change in the turnover rate of ACh ensues. Other anticholinergics, benztropine, trihexyphenidyl, and clozapine, in high doses decrease ACh striatal concentrations and increase the fractional rate constant for ACh efflux without changing the turnover rate of ACh in rat striatum (10). Some reports have suggested that clozapine in high oral doses reduces ACh turnover rate in cerebral cortex (99).

Inhibitors of Acetylcholine Synthesis

Only a few drugs have been found that will acutely inhibit Ch acetyltransfease in vivo (100). The most specific of these is 4-(1-napthylvinyl) pyridine (100, 101). This drug decreases the ACh content of mice killed by quick freezing in liquid nitrogen (45) but fails to change the brain content of ACh in mice killed by microwave irradiation (102). However, in animals killed with microwave, napthylvinylpyridine depresses the conversion of intravenous labeled Ch into ACh (45, 102). That the brain ACh content is not lowered by an extensive inhibition of CAT suggests that this enzyme is not rate limiting (60, 62, 103) and must be inhibited almost totally before the ACh content is decreased.

Hemicholinium competitively blocks the Ch transport in cholinergic axon terminals, thereby limiting the synthesis of ACh available for release (93, 104). Intraventricular injections of HC-3 deplete brain ACh by 80% (77). This depletion can be prevented by prior administration of Ch (77). While CAT inhibition does not reduce brain ACh, HC-3 injection reduces the ACh content to 20% of the level of non-treated rats and the ACh turnover rate by 70% (24, 31). This finding suggests that Ch plays an important role in the regulation of cholinergic fraction; when the Ch uptake is reduced (16, 61) the release of ACh from neocortex is also diminished.

Barbiturates and Anesthetics

Pentobarbital inhibits the release of ACh from the cerebral cortex of rabbit (39) and sheep (36) and increases the ACh content of cortex (105), striatum (105), and whole brain of rats (43, 89). In anesthetic doses barbiturates reduce the Ch uptake (74, 105) and decrease ACh turnover rate in mouse brain (18, 105–107). In rats pentobarbital inhibits the rate of brain ACh decline following intraventricular HC-3 (47), reduces the Ch uptake in cerebral cortex (11, 74, 105), hippocampus (11, 94), and hypothalamus (11), but not in striatum (74, 105) or in brain stem (105), and reduces the rate of conversion of labeled Ch into ACh in cerebral cortex and in striatum (105). Thus, pentobarbital does not alter striatal ACh turnover rate while it depresses the cortical and, perhaps, hippocampal turnover rate of ACh. This is a clear indication that barbiturates change ACh turnover by an indirect, perhaps transsynaptic mechanism. Similar inferences can also be made for other general anesthetics, thus raising the possible theoretical suggestion that a mimicry of some endogenous inhibitory transmitters is a possible mechanism of action of some anesthetics.

Ketamine decreases the turnover rate of ACh in caudate and hippocampus without changing that of the cerebral cortex or the thalamic-hypothalamic region (108). Chloralose (31) decreases the release of ACh from neocortex. The local anesthetic, cocaine (94), also decreases the release of ACh from cerebral cortex. The gaseous anesthetics, ether (36), cyclopropane (36), and halothane-N_2O (35) have been reported to inhibit the release of ACh from cerebral cortex in sheep and cat. Halothane also decreases the turnover rate of ACh measured by infusion of isotopic ACh precursors in cerebral cortex, caudate, hippocampus, and thalamic-hypothalamic region (108). In contrast, enflurane decreases the ACh turnover rate only in cerebral cortex (108).

In fact, other nongaseous anesthetics also depress ACh turnover rate in various regions of rat brain. Chlorohydrate and γ-butyrolactone cause a 50–80% reduction in Ch uptake in hippocampus (11), and chlorohydrate reduces the turnover rate of ACh also in the whole brain (109).

Narcotic Analgetics

Narcotic analgetics inhibit the release of ACh from cerebral cortex of cats (24, 31) and mice (110) and from striatum of cats (28). Morphine also inhibits the HC-3–induced decline of rat brain ACh content and the uptake of Ch in rat occipital cortex but fails to change the uptake of Ch in rat striatum (74). Furthermore, an ED_{50} for analgesia of morphine, meperidine, viminol R_2, and azidomorphine decreases the turnover rate of ACh measured by infusion of isotopic precursors in cerebral cortex and hippocampus of rats but not in rat striatum (111) or whole mouse brain (112). In more detailed studies performed in tissue punches from brains of morphine-treated rats, an ED_{80} dose of morphine for analgesia decreased the ACh turnover rate in *N. accumbens,* cerebral cortex, and hippocampus but failed to change that of striatum, septum, dorsal raphe, or locus coeruleus (15). The observation that morphine reduces the ACh turnover rate in the hippocampus but not in the septum raises an interesting point. The septum contains the cell bodies of the cholinergic neurons that innervate the hippocampus (1). The transsynaptic mechanisms triggered by opiate receptor activation may control the synthesis and degradation of the ACh in terminals located in hippocampus but not that of ACh in cell bodies. If this were the case the metabolism of ACh in terminals would change in parallel with changes in neuronal activity, whereas no changes of ACh turnover would occur with activity changes in cell bodies. A similar conclusion was reached by measuring uptake of Ch: uptake changes with turnover rate of ACh in terminals (70) but not in cell bodies (69).

Psychotomimetics

Tetrahydrocannabinol decreases the release of ACh from cerebral cortex, reduces the Ch uptake in hippocampus but not in cerebral cortex (74), diminishes the HC-3–elicited depletion of ACh in whole brain (113), and reduces the conversion of labeled Ch into ACh in slices of rat striatum, hypothalamus, and cerebral cortex (114). Further studies are needed to assess the reliability of predictions concerning the activity of cholinergic neurons made from measurements of conversion rates of Ch into ACh in slices of brain. Judging from studies on tetrahydrocannabinol, conversion of Ch into ACh in brain slices and uptake studies of Ch yield discrepant results. Since uptake studies have a reasonable level of predictability (see Table 1) one must suspect that as a result of the changes in the sizes of the Ch pool the conversion in vitro fails to yield reliable information concerning drug actions on ACh from turnover.

Ethyl alcohol (115) decreases the release of ACh from neocortex.

Dopamine Receptor Agonists

As we mentioned in our discussion of the effects of anesthetics on ACh turnover, many drugs may alter the ACh turnover rate through an action on synaptic mechanisms which control the activity of the cholinergic neurons. In striatum, there is evidence for an interaction between DA and cholinergic neurons (116, 117). Thus, (+)-amphetamine (25, 118), a DA releaser, and L-DOPA (119), which is a potent dopamine receptor agonist, decrease the turnover rate of ACh in striatum but not in cortex. Similar results have been obtained with push-pull cannulae except by measuring the ACh release from cerebral cortex of guinea pig and cat it has been found that (+)-amphetamine and L-DOPA release ACh (118, 119). Stimulation of dopaminergic receptors directly with apomorphine fails to alter the turnover rate

Table 1 Comparison of drug effects on sodium-dependent high affinity Ch uptake (51) and ACh turnover rate (phosphorylcholine infusion) (4, 64, 89)

	Ch uptake			ACh turnover rate		
	Cortex	Caudate	Hippocampus	Cortex	Caudate	Hippocampus
Haloperidol		↑		→	↑	↓
Morphine	↓	→	↓	↓	→	↓
Pentobarbital	↓	→	↓	↓	→	

of ACh in rat cerebral cortex but reduces the ACh turnover rate in striatum (80). Also amantadine (118), which releases catecholamines from their intraneural storage site and possibly inhibits their reuptake, decreases the release of ACh from neocortex. Although the results obtained with Ch uptake, push-pull cannula, and isotopic measurement of ACh turnover show a good correlation, apomorphine fails to decrease the Ch uptake in striatum (74) whereas it decreases the ACh turnover rate in striatum (80).

Dopamine Receptor Blockers

When dopaminergic receptors are blocked by either chlorpromazine or haloperidol the turnover rate (79) and release (52) of ACh increases in striatum but not in cortex. Using mice and high doses of chlorpromazine, Jenden (120) demonstrated a decrease in the ACh turnover of whole brain. In more detailed studies using pharmacological doses of chlorpromazine it was found that this drug and haloperidol increase the ACh turnover rate of *N. caudatus* and *N. accumbens* but fail to change that of *N. interpeduncularis*, amygdala, raphe dorsalis, locus coeruleus, and septum (10). Clozapine, another potent dopaminergic receptor blocker endowed with antipsychotic activity, fails to change ACh turnover rate in caudate and *N. accumbens*; this apparent discrepancy was explained by the muscarinic receptor blockade elicited by clozapine (10). In fact the increase of ACh turnover elicited by haloperidol in striatum can be reduced by administration of either muscarinic receptor blockers or clozapine.

Haloperidol, clozapine, and chlorpromazine fail to change ACh turnover in substantia nigra but decrease the turnover rate of ACh in globus pallidus (121). Since drugs which share a defined pharmacological property on dopamine receptors affect differently the ACh turnover in specific brain nuclei, it is possible to retain some of the pharmacological effects associated with dopamine receptor blockade and to eliminate other effects by increasing certain pharmacological characteristics of the molecules. This appears to be the case in the association of the ACh and dopamine receptor–blocking activity of clozapine. Clozapine possesses anticholinergic and antidopaminergic actions and retains the antipsychotic activity that derives from the dopamine receptor–blocking action but loses the cataleptogenic action of pure dopamine receptor blockers. It is important to note that dopaminergic receptor blockers can increase the turnover of striatal ACh when they fail to block muscarinic receptors. In contrast, all the antipsychotics with dopamine receptor–blocking activity reduce the turnover rate of ACh in globus pallidus whether or not they block cholinergic receptors. These results suggest that the increase of ACh turnover in striatum is an index of the extrapyramidal liability of antipsychotics and that the decrease of ACh turnover in globus pallidus is a characteristic property related to the antipsychotic action.

It may be mentioned here that all antipsychotics increase GABA turnover in globus pallidus (122), suggesting that the GABA output from striatum to pallidus is facilitated by antipsychotics and that perhaps these GABA neurons may impinge on cholinergic neurons causing their inhibition (122). By measuring turnover rate of various transmitters in different nuclei and by obtaining the profiles of drug action on various synaptic mechanisms, it is possible to foster our understanding and make predictions from animal studies on the therapeutic action and the intensity of possible side effects of various antipsychotics.

GABAergic Receptor Stimulants

Diazepam and muscimol reduce the ACh turnover rate measured by infusion of an isotopic precursor of ACh in cortex and midbrain but fail to change that of ACh in striatum or hippocampus (123). Since muscimol and diazepam (124, 125) activate GABA receptors, these results invite speculation on the possibility that GABA regulates ACh transsynaptically in cortex and midbrain but not in striatum and hippocampus.

Central Nervous System Stimulants

Strychnine, picrotoxin, and pentylenetetrazol are thought to exert their primary action through noncholinergic transmitter systems. Nevertheless, they all have similar actions on cholinergic mechanisms. Strychnine (25), which may act by blocking glycine receptors (126), increases ACh release from the cerebral cortex (25). Pentylenetetrazol (96, 123, 128) and hexamethylenetetrazol (25, 29, 36) increase ACh release from cerebral cortex, caudate, and hippocampus and increase the low K_m Ch uptake of brain homogenates (11, 74).

CONCLUSION

Various techniques have been employed to study how drugs affect the dynamic regulation of cholinergic function. The various studies carried out with these techniques have contributed new ways to study the action of drugs on the CNS. By measuring ACh turnover rate in various brain nuclei the profiles of the synaptic actions of drugs can be traced. Thus side effects and therapeutic activity of drugs can be categorized in terms of their action at various synapses in different nuclei of rat brain. Of the techniques discussed in this review the measurement of the V_{max} of the low K_m uptake of Ch and the measurement of deuterium incorporation into Ch and ACh of various nuclei of rat brain, following the infusion at constant rate with deuterated phosphorylcholine, appear to be the methods of choice for these studies. Table 1 illustrates the analogies between the results obtained with the Ch uptake and deuterium incorporation measurements. Although there are some discrepancies, the number of analogies is encouraging. A drawback of the uptake method is the limited sensitivity (10 mg tissue or more) and the impossibility of relating quantitatively this response to the amount of drug injected. Although more complicated, the mass fragmentographic method gives reliable dose-response relationships and allows measurements in 0.5 mg tissue samples. By understanding the profile of drug actions on various synaptic mechanisms of brain nuclei it might be possible to design new screening procedures whereby unwanted side effects of therapeutically useful drugs can be predicted and therefore eliminated in careful structure-activity studies. With the present understanding of neuropharmacology this appears to be an important practical contribution of the in vitro turnover rate measurements of ACh.

Literature Cited

1. Rommelspacher, H., Kuhar, M. 1975. Effects of dopaminergic drugs and acute medial forebrain bundle lesions on striatal acetylcholine levels. *Life Sci.* 16: 65–70
2. Gage, F. H., Olton, D. S. 1975. Hippocampal influence on hyperreactivity induced by septal lesions. *Brain Res.* 98:311–25
3. Kuhar, M. J., DeHaven, R. N., Yamamura, H. I., Rommelspacher, H., Simon, J. R. 1975. Further evidence for cholinergic habenulo-interpeduncular neurons: Pharmacologic and functional characteristics. *Brain Res.* 97:265–75
4. Racagni, G., Cheney, D. L., Trabucchi, M., Wang, C., Costa, E. 1974. Measurement of acetylcholine turnover rate in discrete areas of the rat brain. *Life Sci.* 15:1961–75
5. Cheney, D. L., Trabucchi, M., Racagni, G., Costa, E. 1974. Effects of acute and chronic morphine on regional rat brain acetylcholine turnover rate. *Life Sci.* 15:1977–90
6. Bartholini, G., Stadler, H., Gadea-Ciria, M., Lloyd, K. G. 1976. The use of the push-pull cannula to estimate the dynamics of acetylcholine and catecholamines within various brain areas. *Neuropharmacology* 15:515–19
7. Dross, K., Kewitz, H. 1972. Concentration and origin of choline in the rat brain. *Naunyn Schmiedebergs Arch. Pharmacol.* 274:91–106
8. Lewis, P. R., Shute, C. C. D. 1967. The cholinergic limbic system: Projections to hippocampal formation, medial cortex, nuclei or the ascending cholinergic reticular system, and the subfornical organ and supra-optic crest. *Brain Res.* 90:521–42
9. Kataoka, K., Nakamura, Y., Hassler, R. 1973. Habenulointerpeduncular tract: A possible cholinergic neuron in rat brain. *Brain Res.* 62:264–67
10. Racagni, G., Cheney, D. L., Trabucchi, M., Costa, E. 1975. *In vivo* actions of clozapine and haloperidol on the turnover rate of acetylcholine in rat striatum. *J. Pharmacol. Exp. Ther.* 196: 323–32
11. Simon, J. R., Atweh, S., Kuhar, M. J. 1976. Sodium-dependent high affinity choline uptake: A regulatory step in the synthesis of acetylcholine. *J. Neurochem.* 26:909–22
12. MacIntosh, F. C. 1963. Synthesis and storage of acetylcholine in nervous tissue. *Can. J. Biochem. Physiol.* 41: 2555–71
13. Cheney, D. L., LeFevre, H. F., Racagni, G. 1975. Choline acetyltransferase activity and mass fragmentography measurement of acetylcholine in specific nuclei and tracts of rat brain. *Neuropharmacology* 14:801–9
14. Costa, E., Cheney, D. L., Racagni, G., Zsilla, G. 1975. An analysis at synaptic level of the morphine action in striatum and n. accumbens: Dopamine and acetylcholine interactions. *Life Sci.* 17:1–8
15. Zsilla, G., Racagni, G., Cheney, D. L., Costa, E. 1977. Constant rate infusion of deuterated phosphorylcholine to measure the effects of morphine on acetylcholine turnover rate in specific nuclei of rat brain. *Neuropharmacology.* In press
16. Guidotti, A., Cheney, D. L., Trabucchi, M., Doteuchi, M., Wang, C., Hawkins, R. A. 1974. Focussed microwave radiation: A technique to minimize post mortem changes in cyclic nucleotides, DOPA and choline and to preserve brain morphology. *Neuropharmacology* 13:1115–22
17. Dross, K., Kewitz, H. 1966. Der einbau von i.v. zugefuhrtem cholin in das acetylcholin des gehirns. *Naunyn-Schmiedebergs Arch. Pharmakol. Exp. Pathol.* 255:10–11
18. Schuberth, J., Sparf, B., Sundwall, A. 1969. A technique for the study of acetylcholine turnover in mouse brain *in vivo. J. Neurochem.* 16:695–700
19. Hanin, I., Cheney, D. L., Trabucchi, M., Massarelli, R., Wang, C. T., Costa, E. 1973. Applications of principles of steady state kinetics to measure acetylcholine turnover rate in rat salivary glands: Effects of diafferentation and duct ligation. *J. Pharmacol. Exp. Ther.* 187:68–77
20. Saelens, J. K., Simke, J. P., Allen, M. P., Conroy, C. A. 1973. Some of the dynamics of choline and acetylcholine metabolism in rat brain. *Arch. Int. Pharmacodyn.* 203:305–12
21. Jenden, D. J., Choi, L., Silverman, R. W., Steinborn, J. A., Roch, M., Booth, R. A. 1974. Acetylcholine turnover estimation in brain by gas chromatography-mass spectrometry. *Life Sci.* 14: 55–63
22. Cheney, D. L., Costa, E., Hanin, I., Trabucchi, M., Wang, C. T. 1975. Application of principles of steady state ki-

netics to the *in vivo* estimation of acetyl-choline turnover rate in mouse brain. *J. Pharmacol. Exp. Ther.* 192:288–96

23. Szerb, J. C. 1975. The release of acetyl-choline from central cortical slices in the presence or absence of an anti-cholinesterase. In *Cholinergic Mechanisms*, ed. P. G. Waser, 213–16. New York:Raven

24. Pepeu, G., Garau, L., Mulas, M. L., Marconcini-Pepeu, I. 1975. Stimulation by morphine of acetylcholine output from the cerebral cortex of septal rats. *Brain Res.* 100:677–80

25. Hemsworth, B. A., Neal, M. J. 1968. The effect of central stimulant drugs on acetylcholine release from rat cerebral cortex. *Br. J. Pharmacol.* 34:543–50

26. Celesia, G. G., Jasper, H. H. 1966. Acetylcholine released from cerebral cortex in relation to state of activation. *Neurology* 16:1053–63

27. Mitchell, J. F. 1960. Release of acetylcholine from the cerebral cortex and the cerebellum. *Proc. Physiol. Soc.* 155:22P

28. Yaksh, T. L., Yamamura, H. I. 1975. Blockade by morphine of acetylcholine release from the caudate nucleus in the mid-pontine pretrigeminal cat. *Brain Res.* 83:520–24

29. Smith, C. M. 1972. The relase of acetylcholine from the rabbit hippocampus. *Br. J. Pharmacol.* 45:172P

30. Costa, E., Neff, N. H. 1966. Isotopic and nonisotopic measurement of the rate of catecholamine biosynthesis. In *Biochemistry and Pharmacology of the Basal Ganglion*, ed. E. Costa, L. Cote, M. D. Yaks, 141–56. New York:Raven

31. Beleslin, D., Polak, R. L. 1965. Depression by morphine and chloralose of acetylcholine release from the cats brain. *J. Physiol. London* 177:411–19

32. Butcher, S. G., Butcher, L. L. 1974. Acetylcholine and choline levels in rat corpus striatum after microwave irradiation. *Proc. West. Pharmacol. Soc.* 17:37–39

33. Cohen, E. L., Wurtman, R. J. 1976. Brain acetylcholine: Control by dietary choline. *Science* 191:561–62

34. Racagni, G., Trabucchi, M., Cheney, D. L. 1975. Steady-state concentrations of choline and acetylcholine in rat brain parts during a constant rate infusion of deuterated choline. *Naunyn-Schmiedebergs Arch. Pharmacol.* 290:99–105

35. Dudar, J. D., Szerb, J. C. 1969. The effect of topically applied atropine on resting and evoked cortical acetylcholine release. *J. Physiol.* 203:741–62

36. Mitchell, J. F. 1963. The spontaneous and evoked release of acetylcholine from the cerebral cortex. *J. Physiol.* 165:98–118

37. Phillis, J. W., Chong, G. C. 1965. Acetylcholine release from the cerebral and cerebellar cortices: Its role in cortical arousal. *Nature* 207:1253–55

38. Szerb, J. C. 1964. The effect of tertiary and quaternary atropine on cortical acetylcholine output and on the electroencephalogram in cats. *Can. J. Physiol. Pharmacol.* 42:303–14

39. Beani, L., Bianchi, C., Santinoceto, L., Marchetti, P. 1968. The cerebral acetylcholine release in conscious rabbits with semi-permanently implanted epidural cups. *Int. J. Neuropharmacol.* 7:469–81

40. Collier, B., Mitchell, J. F. 1966. The central release of acetylcholine during stimulation of the visual pathway. *J. Physiol. London* 184:239–54

41. Phillis, J. W. 1968. Acetylcholine release from the cerebral cortex: Its role in cortical arousal. *Brain Res.* 7:378–89

42. Holmstedt, B., Lundgren, G., Sundwall, A. 1963. Tremorine and atropine effects on brain acetylcholine. *Life Sci.* 10:731–39

43. Consolo, S., Ladinsky, H., Peri, G., Garattini, S. 1972. Effect of central stimulants and depressants on mouse brain acetylcholine and choline levels. *Eur. J. Pharmacol.* 18:251–55

44. Giarman, N. J., Pepeu, G. 1964. The influence of centrally acting cholinolytic drugs on brain acetylcholine levels. *Br. J. Pharmacol.* 23:123–26

45. Saelens, J. K., Simke, J. P. Schuman, J., Allen, M. P. 1974. Studies with agents which influence acetylcholine metabolism in mouse brain. *Arch. Int. Pharmacodyn. Ther.* 209:250–58

46. Gardiner, J. E. 1961. The inhibition of acetylcholine synthesis in brain by a hemicholinium. *Biochem. J.* 81:297–303

47. Domino, E. F., Wilson, A. E. 1972. Psychotropic drug influences on brain acetylcholine utilization. *Psychopharmacologia* 25:291–98

48. Buterbaugh, G. G., Spratt, J. L. 1968. Effect of hemicholinium on choline uptake in the isolated perfused rabbit heart. *J. Pharmacol. Exp. Ther.* 159:255–60

49. Rodriquez deLores Arnaiz, G., Zieher, L. M., DeRobertis, E. 1970. Neurochemical and structural studies on the

mechanism of action of hemicholinium-3 in central cholinergic synapses. *J. Neurochem.* 17:221–29

50. Ansell, G. B., Spanner, S. 1975. The origin and metabolism of brain choline. See Ref. 23, pp. 117–29

51. Gomez, M., Domino, E. F., Sellinger, O. Z. 1970. Effect of hemicholinium on choline distribution *in vivo* in the canine caudate nucleus. *Biochem. Pharmacol.* 19:1753–60

52. Stadler, H., Lloyd, K. G., Gadea-Ciria, M. 1973. Enhanced striatal acetylcholine release by chlorpromazine and its reversal by apomorphine. *Brain Res.* 55:476–80

53. Guyenet, P. G., Agid, Y., Javoy, F., Beaujouan, J. C., Bossier, J., Glowinski, J. 1975. Effects of dopaminergic receptor agonists and antagonists on the activity of the neostriatal cholinergic system. *Brain Res.* 84:227–44

54. Sethy, V. H., VanWoert, M. H. 1974. Modification of striatal acetylcholine concentration by dopamine receptor agonist and antagonists. *Res. Commun. Chem. Pathol. Pharmacol.* 8:13–28

55. Ladinsky, H., Consolo, S., Garattini, S. 1974. Increase in striatal acetylcholine levels in vivo by Piribedil, a new dopamine receptor stimulant. *Life Sci.* 14:1251–60

56. McGeer, P. L., Grewaal, D. S., McGeer, E. G. 1974. Influence of non-cholinergic drugs on rat striatal acetylcholine levels. *Brain Res.* 80:211–17

57. Consolo, S., Ladinsky, H., Garattini, S. 1974. Effect of several dopaminergic drugs and trihexyphenidyl on cholinergic parameters in rat striatum. *J. Pharm. Pharmacol.* 26:275–77

58. Guyenet, P., Agid, Y., Javoy, F., Beaujouan, J. C., Glowinski, J. 1974. Action selective des neuroleptiques sur les neurones cholinergiques du neostriatum chez le rat: Antagonisme vis-à-vis de l'apomorphine. *C. R. Acad. Sci. Paris* 278:2679–82

59. Cheney, D. L., Racagni, G., Zsilla, G., Costa, E. 1976. Differences in the action of various drugs on striatal acetylcholine and choline content in rats killed by decapitation or microwave radiation. *J. Pharm. Pharmacol.* 28:75–77

60. Yamamura, H. I., Snyder, S. H. 1973. High affinity transport of choline into synaptosomes of rat brain. *J. Neurochem.* 21:1355–74

61. Guyenet, P., Lefresne, P., Rossier, J., Beaujouan, J. C., Glowinski, J. 1973. Inhibition by hemicholinium-3 of C^{14}

acetylcholine synthesis and H^3 choline high affinity uptake in rat striatal synaptosomes. *J. Mol. Pharmacol.* 9:630–39

62. Barker, L. A., Mittag, T. W. 1975. Comparative studies of substrates and inhibitors of choline transport and choline acetyltransferase. *J. Pharmacol. Exp. Ther.* 192:86–94

63. Haga, T., Noda, H. 1973. Choline uptake systems of rat brain synaptosomes. *Biochem. Biophys. Acta* 291:564–75

64. Carroll, P. T., Buterbaugh, G. G. 1975. Regional differences in high affinity choline transport velocity in guinea-pig brain. *J. Neurochem.* 24:229–32

65. Kuhar, M. J., Sethy, V. H., Roth, R. H., Aghajanian, G. K. 1973. Choline: Selective accumulation by central cholinergic neurons. *J. Neurochem.* 20:581–93

66. Pert, C. B., Snyder, S. H. 1974. High affinity transport of choline into the myenteric plexus of guinea pig intestine. *J. Pharmacol. Exp. Ther.* 191:102–8

67. Simon, J. R., Mittag, T. W., Kuhar, M. J. 1975. Inhibition of synaptosomal uptake of choline by various choline analogs. *Biochem. Pharmacol.* 24:1139–42

68. Kuhar, M. J., Simon, J. R. 1974. Acetylcholine uptake: Lack of association with cholinergic neurons. *J. Neurochem.* 22:1135–37

69. Suszkiw, J. B., Beach, R. L., Pilar, G. R. 1976. Choline uptake by cholinergic neuron cell somas. *J. Neurochem.* 26:1123–31

70. Suszkiw, J. B., Pilar, G. 1976. Selective localization of a high affinity choline uptake system and its role in ACh formation in cholinergic nerve terminal. *J. Neurochem.* 26:1133–38

71. Mulder, A. H., Yamamura, H. I., Kuhar, M. J., Snyder, S. H. 1974. Release of acetylcholine from hippocampal slices by potassium depolarization: Dependence on high. affinity choline uptake. *Brain Res.* 70:372–76

72. Guyenet, P. G., Lefresne, P., Beaujouan, J. C., Glowinski, J. 1975. The role of newly taken up choline in the synthesis of acetylcholine in rat striatal synaptosomes. See Ref. 23, pp. 137–44

73. Simon, J., Kuhar, M. J. 1975. Impulse-flow regulation of high affinity choline uptake in brain cholinergic nerve terminals. *Nature* 255:162–63

74. Atweh, S., Simon, J. R., Kuhar, M. J. 1975. Utilization of sodium-dependent high affinity choline uptake *in vitro* as a measure of the activity of cholinergic neurons *in vivo*. *Life Sci.* 17:1535–44

75. Sparf, B. 1973. On the turnover of acetylcholine in the brain. *Acta Physiol. Scand. Suppl.* 397:1–47
76. Trabucchi, M., Cheney, D. L., Hanin, I., Costa, E. 1975. Application of principles of steady-state kinetics to the estimation of brain acetylcholine turnover rate: Effects of oxotremorine and physostigmine. *J. Pharmacol. Exp. Ther.* 194:57–64
77. Freeman, J. J., Choi, R. L., Jenden, D. J. 1975. The effects of homicholinium on behavior and on brain acetylcholine and choline in the rat. *Psychopharmol. Commun.* 1:15–27
78. Choi, R. L., Roch, M., Jenden, D. J. 1973. A regional study of acetylcholine turnover in rat brain and the effect of oxotremorine. *Proc. West. Pharmacol. Soc.* 16:188–90
79. Trabucchi, M., Cheney, D. L., Racagni, G., Costa, E. 1974. Involvement of brain cholinergic mechanisms in the action of chlorpromazine. *Nature* 249:664–66
80. Trabucchi, M., Cheney, D. L., Racagni, G., Costa, E. 1975. In vivo inhibition of striatal acetylcholine turnover by L-Dopa, apomorphine and amphetamine. *Brain Res.* 86:130–34
81. Cheney, D. L., Trabucchi, M., Hanin, I., Costa, E. 1975. Morphine dependence and *in vivo* turnover rate in whole mouse brain. *J. Pharmacol. Exp. Ther.* 195:288–95
82. Dawson, R. M. C. 1955. Phosphorylcholine in rat tissues. *Biochem. J.* 60:325–28
83. Ansell, G. B., Spanner, S. 1975. The origin and metabolism of brain choline. See Ref. 23, pp. 117–29
84. Ansell, G. B., Spanner, S. 1971. Studies on the origin of choline in the brain of the rat. *Biochem. J.* 122:741–50
85. Koslow, S., Racagni, G., Costa, E. 1974. Mass fragmentographic measurement of norepinephrine, dopamine, serotonin and acetylcholine in seven discrete nuclei of the rat tel-diencephalon. *Neuropharmacology* 13:1123–30
86. Haubrich, D. R., Reid, W. D., Gillette, J. R. 1972. Acetylcholine formation in mouse brain and effect of cholinergic drugs. *Nature New Biol.* 238:88–89
87. Szerb, J. C., Somogyi, G. T. 1973. Depression of acetylcholine release from cerebral cortical slices by cholinesterase inhibition and by oxotremorine. *Nature New Biol.* 241:121–22
88. Nordberg, A., Sundwall, A. 1976. Effects of oxotremorine on endogenous

89. Giarman, N. J., Pepeu, G. 1962. Drug-induced changes in brain acetylcholine. *Br. J. Pharmacol.* 19:226–34
90. Pazzagli, A., Pepeu, G. 1964. Amnesic properties of scopolamine and brain acetylcholine in the rat. *Int. J. Neuropharmacol.* 4:291–99
91. Milosevic, M. P. 1969. Acetylcholine content in the brain of rats treated with paraoxon and pyridinium-2-aldoxime methylchloride. *J. Pharm. Pharmacol.* 21:469–70
92. Armitage, A. K., Hall, G. H., Sellers, C. M. 1969. Effects of nicotine on electrical activity and acetylcholine release from the cat cerebral cortex. *Br. J. Pharmacol. Chemother.* 35:152–60
93. Rao, K. S., Bhatt, H. V., Gopalakrishna, G., Haranth, P. S. R. K. 1970. Influences of intracarotid infusions of hexamethonium on acetylcholine release from perfused cerebral ventricles in anesthetized dogs. *Indian J. Med. Res.* 58:1279–84
94. Bartolini, A., Pepeu, G. 1967. Investigating into acetylcholine output from the cerebral cortex of the cat in the presence of hyoscine. *Br. J. Pharmacol. Chemother.* 31:66–73
95. Polak, R. L. 1965. Effect of hyoscine on the output of acetylcholine into perfused cerebral ventricles of cats. *J. Physiol. London* 181:317–23
96. Yaksh, T. L., Yamamura, H. I. 1975. The release in vivo of [³H] acetylcholine from cat caudate nucleus and cerebral cortex by atropine pentylenetetrazol, K⁺- depolarization and electrical stimulation. *J. Neurochem.* 25:123–30
97. Domino, E. F., Bartolini, A. 1972. Effects of psychotromimetic agents on the EEG and acetylcholine release from the cerebral cortex of brainstem transected cats. *Neuropharmacology* 11:703–13
98. Lundholm, B., Sparf, B. 1975. The effect of atropine on the turnover of acetylcholine in the mouse brain. *Eur. J. Pharmacol.* 32:287–92
99. Haubrich, D. R., Wang, P. F. L., Herman, R. L., Clody, D. E. 1975. Acetylcholine synthesis in rat brain: Dissimilar effects of clozapine and chlorpromazine. *Life Sci.* 17:739–48
100. Smith, J. C., Cavallito, C. J., Foldes, F. F. 1967. Choline acetyltransferase inhibitors: A group of styrylpyridine ana-

logs. *Biochem. Pharmacol.* 16:2438–41
101. Salama, A. I., Goldberg, M. E. 1975. Elevation of amphetamine levels in rat brain after administration of the choline acetyltransferase inhibitor 4-(1-naphthylvinyl) pyridine (NVP). *Arch. Int. Pharmacodyn. Ther.* 215:197–201
102. Haubrich, D. R., Wang, P. F. L. 1976. Inhibition of acetylcholine synthesis by juglone and 4-(1-napthylvinyl) pyridine. *Biochem. Pharmacol.* 25:669–72
103. Hebb, C. 1972. Biosynthesis of acetylcholine in nerve tissue. *Physiol. Rev.* 52:918–57
104. Birks, R., MacIntosh, F. C. 1961. Acetylcholine metabolism of a sympathetic ganglion. *Can. J. Biochem.* 39:787–827
105. Trabucchi, M., Cheney, D. L., Racagni, G., Costa, E. 1975. Pentobarbital *in vivo* turnover rate of acetylcholine in mouse brain and in regions of rat brain. *Pharmacol. Res. Commun.* 7:81–94
106. Trabucchi, M., Cheney, D. L., Hanin, I., Costa, E. 1973. Effect of various sedative drugs on levels of choline and acetylcholine and on turnover rate of acetylcholine in mouse brain. *Proc. APHA Acad. Pharm. Sci.,* San Diego, Abstr.
107. Nordberg, A., Sundwall, A. 1975. Effect of pentobarbital on endogenous acetylcholine and biotransformation or radioactive choline in different brain regions. See Ref. 23, p. 229
108. Ngai, S. H., Cheney, D. L., Finck, A. D. 1976. Effects of halothane, enflurane, and ketamine on acetylcholine concentrations and turnover in rat brain structures. *Proc. Ann. Meet. Am. Soc. Anesthesiol.,* Abstr., p. 427
109. Atweh, S., Kuhar, M. J. 1975. Effects of impulse flow alterations of the *in vivo* synthesis of ^{3}H-acetylcholine in the rat hippocampus. *Pharmacologist* 17:255
110. Jhamandas, K., Dickinson, G. 1973. Modification of precipitated morphine and methadone abstinence in mice by acetylcholine antagonists. *Nature New Biol.* 245:219–21
111. Zsilla, G., Cheney, D. L., Racagni, G., Costa, E. 1976. Correlation between analgesia and the decrease of acetylcholine turnover rate in cortex and hippocampus elicited by morphine, meperidine, viminol R_2 and azidomorphine. *J. Pharmacol. Exp. Ther.* 199:662–68
112. Cheney, D. L., Costa, E., Hanin, I., Racagni, G., Trabucchi, M. 1975. See Ref. 23, pp. 217–28
113. Domino, E. F. 1971. Neuropsychopharmacologic studies of marihuana and natural THC derivatives in animals and man. *Ann. NY Acad. Sci.* 191:166–91
114. Friedman, E., Hanin, I., Gershon, S. 1976. Effect of tetrahydrocannabinols on ^{3}H-acetylcholine biosynthesis in various rat brain slices. *J. Pharmacol. Exp. Ther.* 196:339–45
115. Graham, D. T., Erickson, C. K. 1971. The effect of ethanol on the output of cerebral acetylcholine *in vivo. Fed. Proc.* 30:622 (Abstr.)
116. Anden, N. E., Bedard, P. 1971. Influences of cholinergic mechanisms on the function and turnover rate of brain dopamine. *J. Pharm. Pharmacol.* 23:460–62
117. Stadler, H., Lloyd, K. G., Gadea-Ciria, M., Bartholini, G. 1973. Enhanced striatal acetylcholine release by chlorpromazine and its reversal by apomorphine. *Brain Res.* 55:476–80
118. Beani, L., Bianchi, C. 1973. Effect of amantadine on cerebral acetylcholine release and content in the guinea pig. *Neuropharmacology* 12:283–89
119. Pepeu, G., Bartholini, A. 1968. Effect of psychoactive drugs on the output of acetylcholine from the cerebral cortex of the cat. *Eur. J. Pharmacol.* 4:254–63
120. Jenden, D. J. 1974. Effects of chlorpromazine on acetylcholine turnover in vivo. In *The Phenothiazines and Structurally Related Drugs,* ed. I. S. Forrest, C. J. Carr, E. Usdin. New York:Raven
121. Cheney, D. L., Zsilla, G., Costa, E. 1977. Dopamine and acetylcholine interactions in *N. accumbens, N. caudatus, Globus pallidus* and *Substantia nigra:* Pharmacological implications. In *Non-striatal Dopamine,* ed. E. Costa, G. L. Gessa, 179–86. New York:Raven
122. Mao, C. C., Marco, G., Revuelta, A., Bertilsson, L., Costa, E. 1977. The turnover rate of γ-aminobutyric acid in the nuclei of telencephalon: Implications in the pharmacology of antipsychotics and of a minor tranquilizer. *Biol. Psychiatry.* In press
123. Zsilla, G., Cheney, D. L., Costa, E. 1976. Regional changes in the rate of turnover of acetylcholine in rat brain receiving diazepam or muscimol. *Naunyn Schmiedebergs Arch. Pharmacol.* 294:251–55
124. Johnston, G. A. R., Curtis, D. R., DeGroat, W. C., Duggan, A. W. 1968. Central actions of ibotenic acid and

muscimol. *Biochem. Pharmacol.* 17: 2488–89

125. Costa, E., Guidotti, A., Mao, C. C., Suria, A. 1975. New concepts on the mechanism of action of benzodiazepines. *Life Sci.* 17:167–86

126. Curtis, D. R., Hosli, L., Johnston, G. A. R., Johnston, I. H. 1968. The hyperpolarization of spinal motoneurons by glycine and related amino acids. *Exp. Brain Res.* 5:238–62

127. Obata, K., Takeda, K., Shinozaki, H. 1970. Further study on pharmacological properties of the cerebellar-induced inhibition of Deiter's neurons. *Exp. Brain Res.* 11:327–42

128. Nicoll, R. A., Padjen, A. 1976. Pentylenetetrazol: An antagonist of GABA at primary afferents of the isolated frog spinal cord. *Neuropharmacology* 15: 69–72

Ann. Rev. Pharmacol. Toxicol. 1977. 17:387–409
Copyright © 1977 by Annual Reviews Inc. All rights reserved

THE PHARMACOLOGY OF EXPERIMENTAL MYOPATHIES

♦6687

Michael B. Laskowski[1, 2] *and Wolf-D. Dettbarn*
Department of Pharmacology, Vanderbilt University, School of Medicine,
Nashville, Tennessee 37232

A large group of disorders affect striated muscle in man. The direct approach to the study of these diseases presents major difficulties. Biopsies can be useful in diagnosing a muscle disease and in confirming its progress. However, at a time when muscle weakness and other neurologic abnormalities become obvious, the myopathy is usually well advanced. It is also impossible to provide adequate controls to follow the development of the myopathy in man and its reversibility with experimental techniques. Consequently, a wide variety of animal models of human muscle diseases have been developed. These models include myopathies occurring spontaneously in highly inbred strains of mice, hamsters, goats, and other mammals. However, a new and rapidly expanding area of inquiry involves the pharmacologically induced myopathies developed with a wide variety of drugs. This review is concerned with this second area of research, that of pharmacologically induced experimental myopathies.

A survey of the literature of the past ten years reveals many attempts to reproduce pharmacologically human myopathies in animals. Three areas have been particularly active. These include experimental myotonia, experimental Duchenne's muscular dystrophy, and general neuromuscular disorders.

PHARMACOLOGICALLY INDUCED MYOTONIA

Of all the pharmacologic myopathies that have been attempted, experimental myotonia bears the closest resemblance to its human counterpart. When rats are injected with 2,4-dichlorophenoxyacetic acid or fed a diet containing 20,25-diazocholesterol, muscle fibers develop abnormal membrane parameters closely resembling those in patients with myotonia. A similar abnormality is observed in the myotonic goat.

---

[1]Dr. Laskowski's present address is Department of Physiology, St. Louis University School of Medicine, St. Louis, Missouri 63104.
[2]The survey of literature for this review was completed June 1, 1976.

Similarities Between Human and Drug-Induced Forms of Myotonia

In man, myotonia is characterized by sustained contraction of muscle produced either by a voluntary contraction, percussion with an instrument, or electrical stimulation of the muscle (1, 2). The irritability of the muscle is markedly increased after insertion of a needle electrode. Electromyography reveals the typical "dive-bomber" bursting of muscle action potentials, but the myotonic effect is reduced by repeated contractions ("warm up period"). Myotonia is particularly evident in myotonia congenita which is an autosomal inherited disease (2).

Myotonic effects are produced experimentally by a wide variety of compounds including the monocarboxylic acids (3), cholesterol derivatives (4), veratrum alkaloids (5), acridine (6), several amines (7), and indoleacetic acid (8). Closer examination at the membrane level reveals that only a few of these agents, monocarboxylic acids and cholesterol derivatives, produce effects approximating those seen in myotonia congenita (3).

The effects of two drugs in particular have been examined in detail. These are 2,4-dichlorophenoxyacetic acid (2,4-D) and 20,25-diazocholesterol (20,25-D).

The Myotonic Effects of 2,4-Dichlorophenoxyacetic Acid

2,4-D is a monocarboxylic aromatic acid which was also a widely used weed killer (9). Accidental ingestion of this drug by animals and man has led to symptoms of myotonia (10). When given to rats (200 mg/kg i.p.), 2,4-D produces a myotonic electromyogram (EMG) pattern within 30 min (11). Similar effects are observed when normal diaphragm muscles are perfused in vitro with 2.5 mM 2,4-D (4, 12). These studies have revealed several major changes in muscle contraction produced by 2,4-D: (a) Within the first few minutes of exposure to the drug, the peak amplitude of a single contraction is increased severalfold. Shortly thereafter there is a ten to twenty fold increase in the duration of contraction. (b) These effects are augmented when a tetanic burst of stimuli, instead of a single pulse, is given to the muscle. (c) A conditioning or "warm up" stimulus reduces the myotonic effect of a subsequent stimulus. (d) The prolonged contraction is associated with a prolonged series of spontaneous repetitive muscle action potentials (12). These major observations produced in vitro by 2,4-D closely parallel the abnormal muscle contractions observed in human myotonia (2) and in the goat (13).

The Myotonic Effects of 20,25-Diazocholesterol

The second drug that induces a myotonic-like condition in rats is 20,25-diazocholesterol (20,25-D). This drug inhibits the enzyme desmosterol reductase (14), resulting in decreased plasma cholesterol and increased plasma desmosterol, a precursor of cholesterol (15). The myotonia-inducing side effects of this drug were first observed in patients being treated for hypercholesterolemia (16, 17). Muscle cramping and spasm, together with EMG patterns similar to myotonia, were reported. In the experimental animal model, the drug is given in the diet or through an esophageal tube for 5 to 8 weeks (4, 18). Several other cholesterol analogues including 25-azocholesterol can be injected s.c. for a similar period to produce the same effect (19–21). Like 2,4-dichlorophenoxyacetic acid, the 20,25-D animal model closely parallels human myotonia with respect to abnormal contractile properties, as well as changes in electromyography.

Membrane Abnormalities in Experimental Myotonia

The underlying membrane abnormalities in both inherited and experimental myotonia are similar. Myotonic fibers of both man and the goat have an increased membrane resistance (3). In addition, the mean resting chloride conductance is significantly less than in normal fibers, while the potassium conductance is increased. However, muscle resting membrane potential was unaffected (3, 22). The myotonia produced experimentally in the rat with 2,4-D or 20,25-D displays similar changes in membrane cable properties (4, 23). There is an increase in specific membrane resistance and a fall in chloride conductance. Like inherited myotonia, muscle fiber resting membrane potential is normal or somewhat higher than normal (3, 4, 23–26). However, unlike human and goat myotonia, the myotonia produced by 20,25-D does not display increased potassium conductance (23). We have found no report on the effect of 2,4-D on potassium conductance. The effect on potassium conductance may depend on the type of myotonia-inducing drug employed since several monocarboxylic aromatic acids other than 2,4-D increase potassium conductance (3).

An abnormally low resting chloride conductance by itself could account for both increased membrane resistance and the spontaneous firing of action potentials (27, 28). When untreated rat diaphragm muscles were exposed to low chloride solutions, the muscles fibers became myotonic within 5 min (23). Membrane resistance increased with no change in potassium conductance. Spontaneous firing and the warm-up phenomenon (reduced myotonia with exercise) occurred during the first half hour. A short burst of stimulating pulses produced an augmentation and a prolongation of tension. Unlike the resting membrane potential in nerves, a major component of membrane conductance in skeletal muscle is chloride conductance. In frog muscles that do not display myotonia (3), chloride provides approximately 70% of the resting membrane conductance (29). Chloride is an even greater factor in mammalian muscle where it accounts for up to 85% of resting membrane conductance (30, 31).

Sites of Action of Myotonia-Inducing Drugs

The foregoing evidence indicates that the primary defect in inherited myotonia is an abnormally low membrane conductance to chloride ions, and that many of the properties of myotonic fibers can be reproduced in vitro with low chloride solutions or with various drugs. It appears that a wide variety of chemical agents with little structural similarity are all capable of producing a very specific effect, namely the reduction of chloride conductance. What is needed is a careful examination of the altered cable properties produced by each drug and a comparison of these effects with abnormal membrane characteristics in inherited myotonia. As previously mentioned, the monocarboxylic acids in general and 2,4-D in particular are capable of reproducing the myotonia-like condition in animals (3). On the basis of potency in blocking chloride conductance, Bryant & Morales-Aguilera (3) have determined the chemical requirements for agents that block the chloride channel and have suggested a steric block of the channel. Much less is known about the binding potency of cholesterol derivatives other than that 20,25-diazocholesterol also produces a reduced chloride conductance and increased membrane resistance (23). Most studies of membrane biophysics during experimental myotonia have been devoted to only 2,4-D and other monocarboxylic aromatic acids. On the other hand, biochemical studies have considered almost exclusively the inhibition of cholesterol biosynthesis, primarily 20,25-D. Consequently, it is difficult to make meaningful comparisons of their respective sites of action on muscle membranes. While the simplicity of a common mechanism of action for both groups of drugs is appealing, it appears that 2,4-D and 20,25-D may act at different membrane sites.

In sarcolemmal membranes isolated from 20,25-diazocholesterol–treated skeletal and cardiac muscle, the amount of cholesterol is reduced and desmosterol is increased (32). The myotonic effect is highly dependent on membrane cholesterol, since including cholesterol in the diets of 20,25-D–treated rats reverses the myotonia (19). Membrane cholesterol levels have not been reported after 2,4-D or other monocarboxylic acids.

Most reports show that Na^+-, K^+–stimulated ATPase activity is increased in 20,25-D–treated rats (15, 18, 32, 33), with one exception which demonstrates a decrease in activity (33). Sarcolemmal Ca-stimulated ATPase activity was also increased after 20,25-D treatment (18, 32). In contrast to the action of 20,25-D, 2,4-dichlorophenoxyacetic acid had no effect on Na^+, K^+-stimulated ATPase but increased the activity of basic p-nitrophenylphosphatase (p-NPPase) activity (34). There is evidence that this sarcolemmal enzyme may regulate the gate for passive flux of K ions (34). Increased activity of p-NPPase increases K^+ efflux from leukocytes (35). This may explain the increased K conductance observed after some monocarboxylic acids (3). The activity of p-NPPase in human or myotonic goat muscle has not been described, nor has the effect of 20,25-diazocholesterol been evaluated with respect to p-NPPase activity. Until this area is further explored, no unifying hypothesis can be put forward. Clarification of this point will be essential in determining the importance of altered potassium conductance.

A logical step in analyzing the mechanism of myotonia is to look for morphological abnormalities. Unlike human myotonic dystrophy, myotonia congenita is not associated with any generalized structural abnormalities. In the goat one minor change was an increased density of T-tubules (37). Similarly, rats fed 20,25-diazocholesterol did not show abnormal morphological correlates of altered function (38). However, a nonspecific toxic side effect of 20,25-D was observed, possibly due to the drug's effect on muscle sterols.

The Relationship of the Nerve to Drug-Induced Myotonia

The myotonic response does not involve the neuromuscular junction (39). Myotonia can still be induced pharmacologically in the presence of curare (11, 40). Rats treated with 25-azocholesterol demonstrate a tendency toward neuromuscular failure which may contribute to muscle weakness, but this is separate from the typical myotonic effect seen clinically and in vitro (21). However, an intact nerve supply may be required for the development of experimental myotonia (41–43).

Once established, the myotonia produced by 2,4-D was not affected by subsequent nerve section. However, section of the sciatic nerve 7 days prior to administration of 2,4-D prevented the typical repetitive discharges and the waxing and waning of activity (41). Caccia et al (43) have observed a similar dependence on innervation for the myotonia produced by 20,25-D. However, when treatment with 20,25-D was extended for several weeks after denervation, EMG and muscle contractile behavior closely approximated myotonia (44). A difference is that typical myotonic potentials were rare.

The alteration in membrane cable properties following denervation is highly complex. Muscle membrane depolarization begins within a few hours after nerve section, followed after 3 to 4 days by increases in membrane resistance, capacitance, and time constant (45, 46). The increase in membrane resistance has been attributed to a reduction in potassium conductance (47–49). It is during this period of increased membrane resistance that 2,4-D no longer produces myotonia in diaphragm muscles (42). An explanation for this may lie in the observation that untreated muscles in chloride-free media display typical myotonia activity (27, 23). This spontaneous activity is abolished in high K^+ solutions where K conductance would be lower (28). Thus the relative insensitivity of denervated muscles to 2,4-D may be due to decreased K^+ conductance. However, much more work is required with both 2,4-D and 20,25-D treated animals before the subtleties of neural regulation of myotonia can be defined.

The pharmacologic model of myotonia congenita closely parallels its human inheritable form. While a wide variety of unrelated drugs produce myotonia symptoms in rats, those few drugs that have been closely studied show a common action on muscle membrane involving altered chloride conductance and possibly potassium as well. A more thorough examination of membrane transport proteins may also reveal a common biochemical change in the sarcolemma.

Myotonic changes in man precede the histologic changes in dystrophia myotonica (2). The slight histopathologic changes which have been reported in myotonia congenita are very similar to early changes observed in dystrophia myotonica (36). Recent studies show that chronic treatment with a myotonic drug, 2,4-D, began to reproduce some of the histopathologic abnormalities of dystrophia myotonica (50). The significance of the myotonia model may lie in the long-term effects of these drugs and the possibility of providing an animal model for the more severe disease, dystrophia myotonica.

PHARMACOLOGIC MODELS OF DUCHENNE'S MUSCULAR DYSTROPHY

The development of experimental models for progressive muscular dystrophies, of which the most debilitating is Duchenne's, has been much more difficult to achieve than the model for myotonia congenita. Myotonia is primarily a membrane-related dysfunction with minimal histopathologic abnormalities. Duchenne's muscular dystrophy is far more complex in both its etiology and its pathology. At the present time no animal model, either genetic or pharmacologic, accurately reproduces all aspects of Duchenne's muscular dystrophy. However, a first approximation to the disease has been achieved with several drug-induced myopathies.

For an animal model to reproduce accurately the pathology of Duchenne's dystrophy, several minimal criteria must be met: (*a*) Initial histopathologic changes in biopsies of Duchenne's patients include grouped fiber necrosis surrounded by normal muscle fibers (51). (*b*) As the disease progresses there is a wide variation in fiber diameter and an infiltration of endomysial connective tissue and fat (51, 53). (*c*) There is a fluctuating increase in serum levels of many enzymes including creatine phosphokinase (CPK), glutamic-oxaloacetic transaminase (GOT), glutamic-pyruvic transaminase (GPT), and lactic dehydrogenase (LDH) (52). (*d*) The proximal muscles of the pelvis and lower extremities are the first affected (53).

Some of these criteria are met by the genetically developed dystrophies in a wide variety of animals, of which the mouse and chicken have been studied most extensively (54). An alternative approach to simulating Duchenne's dystrophy in a genetic model has been the recent development of the pharmacologically induced experimental myopathies. Two general approaches have been followed. The first was based upon the initial studies of Hathaway et al (55), which involved circulatory obstruction with or without treatment with various monoamines. A second approach has been strictly pharmacologic. Either pharmacologic model meets several of the above listed criteria for Duchenne's dystrophy. In addition, they offer greater control in analyzing the basic mechanisms that produce the myopathy.

The Vascular Model of Duchenne's Dystrophy

A unique and diagnostic characteristic of a muscle biopsy from a patient in an early stage of Duchenne's dystrophy is the characteristic grouped fiber necrosis (51). This has led to the suggestion that the circumscribed area of necrotic fibers surrounded by normal muscle may represent the field of perfusion by a dysfunctioning terminal blood vessel (55). This vascular hypothesis is supported by histopathologic abnormalities in blood vessels of some patients in the early stage of the disease (55, 56), but others have not been able to confirm this (57).

Complete ligation of the femoral artery and vein yields no histologic abnormalities in the muscles of the lower extremity of rabbits (55). However, the relative ischemia produced by injection of 20μ–80μ dextran particles has led to a nearly complete reproduction of the histopathology of Duchenne's muscular dystrophy (55). Two weeks after an injection of the particles, early changes such as grouped fiber necrosis and phagocytosis occurred, and areas of regeneration were surrounded by fibers of normal appearance. The muscles of animals sacrificed 3 months after the initial treatment showed characteristic middle- and end-stage lesions such as proliferation of endomysial connective tissue, fatty infiltration, and a wide range of muscle fiber diameters. Occasional thickened walls of arterioles and some occluded vessels were also noted. These observations suggested that the histopathologic picture of Duchenne's muscular dystrophy could be reproduced experimentally by producing a relative ischemic condition in muscle.

A similar development of necrosis and phagocytosis at the light microscopic level was reproduced by aortic ligation by itself in rats (58). However, a thorough examination of the myopathy at electron microscopic level revealed significant differences from the ultrastructural changes seen in human Duchenne's dystrophy. The authors also noted that aortic ligation was selectively destructive to soleus muscle when compared to gastrocnemius muscle. This selectivity was presumably due to the higher oxidative metabolic demand of soleus muscles, since increasing the work load by contralateral denervation or tenotomy exacerbated the myopathy. The experimental methods of producing the partial ischemia differ greatly between the two studies. Consequently, until the ultrastructure of muscles treated with the microsphere approach is examined, the "relative ischemia" hypothesis cannot be fully accepted.

Ligation Plus Serotonin Model

Because very few abnormalities are seen in arteriolar walls of Duchenne's muscle biopsies, a new approach was developed combining aortic ligation plus the vasoactive agent serotonin (5-HT) (59). The rationale to using this combined approach has been given added significance in view of the observation that in Duchenne's patients, the platelet uptake of serotonin is greatly diminished (60). Serotonin itself has been suggested as a causative agent in carcinoid myopathy (61). Contrary to earlier observations (59), rats given 5-HT alone display some histopathologic abnormalities (62). In the rat, normal circulating levels of serotonin are too low to contract vascular smooth muscle (63). However, when the isolated rat hind limb was perfused with 2 to 50 mg/liter serotonin (5-HT creatinine sulfate) a decrease in blood flow in the femoral artery occurred (59). The combination of aortic ligation plus 20–75 mg/kg 5-HT, was given to rats for 5 days to 3 months either acutely or chronically. Either method alone produced no muscle necrosis, but in combination, a histopatholic picture reminiscent of Duchenne's dystrophy was produced (59). No structural abnormality was observed in blood vessel walls, leading the authors to suggest that a functional inadequacy rather than a structural lesion is responsible for the relative ischemia. Aortic ligation in the rat previously has been reported to render skeletal muscle more susceptible to vasoactive agents (64). The same characteristic pattern of muscle lesions has been reproduced with aortic ligation and another vasoactive agent, 3 mg/kg norepinephrine (59, 65).

Additional evidence for the "functional ischemic" model of Duchenne's dystrophy was obtained by examining plasma enzyme levels in rats given serotonin after aortic ligation (65). Aortic ligation itself produced some increase in plasma enzymes which returned to control levels within 72 hr. Administration of serotonin produced a marked increase in creatine phosphokinase (CPK), glutamic-oxaloacetic transaminase (GOT), glutamic-pyruvic transaminase (GPT), and lactic dehydrogenase (LDH). Enzyme levels returned to normal within 48–72 hr, but repeated injections produced a return to elevated enzyme levels (65). These data suggested that a second requirement for the animal model for Duchenne's dystrophy was achieved, that of increased levels of muscle enzymes. Damaged liver as a source for these enzymes was ruled out because there was no increase in alkaline phosphatase. Ligation plus norepinephrine was also effective in increasing enzyme levels (66). Pretreatment with phenoxybenzamine and chlorpromazine, both α-adrenergic blockers, prevented the elevated enzyme levels. Pretreatment with imipramine which blocks the preterminal amine uptake pump (67) had a paradoxical effect. Low doses (1–2 mg/kg) maintained low plasma enzyme levels whether noradrenaline or serotonin was studied. However, high doses of imipramine (20 mg/kg) actually increased the plasma enzyme levels elevated by norepinephrine (66). This interaction between imipramine and norepinephrine must be explored adequately before firm conclusions can be made with respect to overstimulation of α-receptors. In apparent conflict with these results, Melmed & Karpati (68) observed that phenoxybenzamine plus aortic ligation significantly increased the ischemic myopathy. It is quite clear that further studies are required to explain the fundamental difference between the myopathic effects of aortic ligation between the two groups. It is likely a difference in ligating techniques, but the question must be resolved before detailed pharmacology is explored. In addition, it will also be necessary to provide a more complete pharmacologic analysis in the prevention or exacerbation of histopathologic changes. Depletion of amines with reserpine, blockage of synthesis with p-chlorophenylalanine, and destruction of aminergic nerve terminals with 6-hydroxydopamine all must be thoroughly tested.

It has been emphasized recently that increased serum enzyme levels actually precede significant muscle necrosis in Duchenne's dystrophy (69). Significant abnormalities have been observed in dystrophic muscle and erythrocyte membrane composition and transport. It is conceivable that an expressed genetic error in membranes may be the earliest stage in the pathogenesis of Duchenne's dystrophy (69, 82). It should be noted that peak increases in enzyme levels occurred 12 hr after 5-HT, that is, well before the first lesions were apparent (66). Much work needs to be done to clarify early abnormalities in membrane transport and composition during the initial hours after drug treatment and before the development of lesions.

Vasoactive Amines and the Development of Myopathies

Two more specific pharmacologic approaches have been attempted. The first combined imipramine and serotonin. The second studied the myopathic effects of the monoamine oxidase (MAO) inhibitor, pargyline. Imipramine is a tricyclic antidepressant which blocks the uptake of primarily serotonin but also other amines into nerve terminals (67). Parker & Mendell (70) have succeeded in reproducing the characteristic histopathology of Duchenne's dystrophy by pretreating rats for three days with imipramine (10 mg/kg). On the fourth day serotonin was given (100 mg/kg). This 4-day procedure was repeated each week for eleven weeks. The combination of drugs closely reproduced the early and midstage lesions of Duchenne's dystrophy with the addition that proximal muscles were selectively affected. This procedure also raises plasma enzyme levels of CPK (71). When untreated muscle was perfused in vitro with imipramine and 5-HT, ^{14}C-labeled serotonin was taken up 3 times faster than control. However, oxygen uptake and the amino acid analogue γ-aminoisobutyric acid were both significantly reduced (71).

When rats were injected with the MAO inhibitor pargyline, soleus muscles contained a flurorescent material generally characterized by the Falck-Hillarp technique as catecholamines (72). Duchenne's dystrophy is the only human myopathy known to contain catecholamine-fluorescent fibers (73). It is not known, however, whether the ligation-plus-5-HT or imipramine-plus-5-HT myopathies contain fluorescence. The pargyline myopathy displayed grouped fiber necrosis and, with seven-day treatment, significant connective tissue formation in the endomysium (72). It is very much unlike Duchenne's dystrophy in that only the soleus is affected with no lesions produced in the gastrocnemius (72), or diaphragm, or quadriceps muscles (M. B. Laskowski and W. D. Dettbarn, unpublished observations). Denervation reduced the myopathy, which was assumed to be "neurogenic." This approach is questionable since both motor, sensory, and sympathetic innervation are nonselectively removed and, of course, muscle activity and metabolic requirements are significantly reduced. In none of the above-mentioned experimental myopathies has any significant ultrastructural examination of the muscle, blood vessels, or nerve been reported. It is clear that before the 5-HT model can be accepted as a replica of Duchenne's dystrophy a thorough point-by-point comparison must be made with biopsied dystrophic muscle at the fine structural level.

Recent reports have suggested that an abnormal axoplasmic flow in motor nerves may be responsible for several of the myopathies produced by vasoactive amines (74, 75). Two MAO inhibitors, pargyline and phenelzine, were reported to increase the rate of fast axoplasmic transport (75). The increased flow rate was partially prevented by pretreatment with α-methylparatyrosine. Aortic ligation with or without 5-HT produced a similar increase in axoplasmic transport (74). However, Komiya & Austin (76) found that ligation of the iliac artery plus 5-HT did not alter flow rate although the myopathy was fully developed in the gastrocnemius muscle. It should be noted that in the reports of increased fast transport mentioned above, confirmatory histologic examination of muscle lesions was not described. Resolution of the controversy will add valuable information as to whether or not a trophic material from the motor nerve might be augmenting or reducing the myopathy.

Recently a "neurovascular hypothesis" has been proposed to explain the mechanism of the myopathies produced by vasoactive amines (77). A single genetic deficit was proposed, that of reduced effectiveness of sympathetic vasoconstriction. According to this hypothesis, the normal reflex vasoconstriction during exercise is impaired, resulting in an overperfusion of unused muscles (78). Reduced blood flow to exercising muscle in Duchenne's patients has been observed (79, 80). Such patients also display reduced oxygen tension in exercising muscles (81). While the hypothesis is simple and attractive, much more work is required at the pharmacologic and ultrastructural levels before it can be accepted. Sympathetic innervation of biopsies of Duchenne's patients must be examined at the electron microscopic level. In addition, more thorough pharmacologic analyses must be made of the "functional ischemia" experimental myopathies. What is required at this point is very basic and thorough work to help clarify the origin of ischemic lesions and the way these are enhanced with vasoactive amines. Such studies will provide pharmacologic models that will be an even closer approximation to Duchenne's dystrophy. This approach will certainly provide a potentially productive area for drug development and testing.

GENERAL NEUROMUSCULAR DISEASES

Investigation of the involvement of the neuromuscular junction in muscle disease had been active before the development of electron microscopic techniques. Based upon preliminary work at the light microscopic level, ultrastructural investigations have revealed a frequent involvement of the motor end-plate in a wide variety of muscle diseases (82). Zacks (83) has written a thorough review of this topic. In a majority of muscle diseases, motor end-plate degeneration is secondary either to a primary myopathy or to motor nerve degeneration. Myasthenia gravis is a prominent exception (83). Less frequently occurring diseases that specifically affect the neuromuscular junction are carcinomatous neuromyopathy (84–86), amyotonia congenita syndrome (87), Isaacs' syndrome (88), Coxsackie B virus (89), and a variety of neurotoxins (83).

Experimental myasthenia gravis is being pursued in several laboratories. Such studies involve the myasthenic dog (90, 91) and rats made chronically autoimmune to ACh receptors (92). In recent years we have been actively pursuing studies of end-plate–mediated myopathies using a variety of cholinesterase inhibitors and cholinomimetic drugs (93–97). Rather than developing a model for a specific disease entity, this approach permits an examination of the delicate nerve-muscle relationship and explains how altering this relationship can initiate muscle lesions.

Neural Control of Muscle Properties

The now classic work of Buller, Eccles & Eccles (98, 99) revealed the significant influence that motor nerves have over the structural, functional, and biochemical properties of muscles they innervate. The trophic function of nerves was originally defined as a function that is not mediated by nerve impulses (100). However, only a few of these trophic actions are independent of nerve impulse transmission and muscle contraction (101, 102). The level of muscular activity influences contractile properties, content of specific enzymes, its sensitivity to ACh, and its ability to accept further innervation. The structural and functional integrity of skeletal muscle depends on the presence and normal function of neuromuscular transmission. Problems may arise from pharmacologic manipulation of neuromuscular transmission and may lead to changes in the development, maintenance, and integrity of the end-plate and muscle fiber. The physiology of neuromuscular transmission can be affected in several ways. The amount of the transmitter acetylcholine which is released may be increased or reduced by a wide variety of drugs (103–108). Postsynaptic sensitivity may be changed by altering the number of ACh receptors. Pharmacologic manipulation of the input resistance of the muscle fiber membrane will alter the threshold for generation of muscle action potentials. Variation in one of these factors or in combination with one another can be contributing causes to neuromuscular degeneration and can be altered experimentally (109–113).

Some of the changes that are seen after denervation may be due to disuse rather than loss of the trophic function of nerve. Other experimental procedures will interrupt various aspects of nerve-muscle interaction, while leaving the neuromuscular junction and its nerve structurally intact. Some of these approaches such as the use of vinblastine and colchicine block axoplasmic transport without interfering with the synthesis and release of ACh or the propagation and transmission of impulses (114). The effects of these compounds are almost similar to those of denervation. Total disuse of the neuromuscular junction can be induced by chemical application of local anesthetics (102) inducing block of conduction and transmission without changing structure and function of the neuromuscular junction. Such treatment also induces phenomena seen after denervation.

Cholinesterase Inhibition and Transmitter Release

Altered acetylcholine release or a reduction of its hydrolysis by loss in cholinesterase activity is observed as early pathophysiologic changes in murine dystrophy (115, 116), chicken dystrophy (117), atrophy (118), some experimental myopathies (93), and some forms of human muscle disease (119, 120). There has been considerable debate as to whether the nerve terminal or the postsynaptic region of muscle is the primary site of action of anti-ChE drugs (121), and whether either or both of these sites are affected by neuromuscular disease processes, such as muscular dystrophy and myasthenia gravis (112).

Few reports have been published on the effects of anticholinesterases, especially organophosphorus agents, on miniature end-plate potential (MEPP) frequency and end-plate potential (EPP) quantum content. Neostigmine increased MEPP frequency over a narrow concentration range but at higher doses decreased frequency (122, 123). Edrophonium was found to have similar effects on MEPP frequency (123, 124). These drugs, however, contain a quaternary ammonium ion which by itself is capable of increasing MEPP frequency (125). Indirect estimates of quantum content during neostigmine, edrophonium, and ambenonium, drugs that facilitate neuromuscular transmission, indicate that quantum content is elevated (123). Recent work has shown, however, that the method of paralyzing the muscle for intracellular recording affects the estimate of quantum content in edrophonium (124, 126).

Paraoxon, an irreversible organophosphorus inhibitor of ChE activity when injected into rats, causes (a) an augmentation of spontaneous transmitter release, (b) a reduction in quantum content, and (c) spontaneous and evoked antidromic nerve action potentials (94). Similar effects were observed when paraoxon was applied in vitro (94, 127).

A critical question is whether paraoxon produces these effects directly or acts indirectly through its inhibition of cholinesterase. The strongest evidence indicating that paraoxon acts through ChE inhibition comes from the experiments with pyridine-2-aldoxime methiodide (2-PAM). Reactivation of inhibited ChE with 2-PAM reduces the paraoxon-augmented MEPP frequency and eliminates antidromic nerve activity. Another organophosphorus compound diisopropylfluorophosphate (DFP) was without effect on MEPP frequency (128). However, these experiments were conducted while basal MEPP frequency was artifically accelerated with 10 mM K ion. Paraoxon depolarized muscle membranes by approximately 15 mV (127). This depolarizing effect was partly reversed with 10^{-6} M tetrodotoxin (TTX) and totally abolished in combination with α-bungarotoxin. The depolarizing effects of paraoxon are due to the combined depolarization of ACh receptors and extrajunctional receptors controlling Na-conductance channels. Paraoxon has no effect on the K-conductance channels (127).

Tetrodotoxin reduced the paraoxon-accelerated MEPP frequency but did not alter spontaneous release in control preparations. It has been reported previously that TTX blocks nerve and muscle action potentials while leaving the depolarization-release mechanism intact (129). Consequently, an intact action potential generating system must be present for paraoxon to yield its full effect. Whether the faster MEPP frequency is produced by reinvasion of nerve terminals with spontaneous nerve impulses or some other mechanism remains to be determined.

Acute Cholinesterase Inhibition and Muscle Fiber Degeneration

Irreversible inhibitors of the ChE activity such as paraoxon, DFP, tabun, sarin, soman, and parathion, as well as reversible inhibitors such as physostigmine and neostigmine, inhibit AChE activity at the neuromuscular junction. This loss of enzyme activity blocks the hydrolysis of ACh and leads to increased activity and stimulation of the skeletal muscle fiber. Reports from several laboratories have shown that all of the above-mentioned ChE inhibitors are myopathic (130–135).

The earliest evidence relating ChE inhibitors to necrotic lesions of skeletal muscle was in a report by Carey (130). Since then this observation has been repeated by several investigators; however, not all of them were aware of previous investigations (93, 131–134). Injection of paraoxon produces a progressive myopathy in the rat diaphragm, soleus, gastrocnemius, and quadriceps muscles. The diaphragm is the most severely affected of these muscles (133, 135), followed by the soleus and the gastrocnemius muscles. The earliest lesions noted were focal areas of abnormality close to the surface of the muscle fiber (93, 133). On H-E stain this area appeared to be more basophilic. The trichrome stain demonstrated an area of red-staining, and the normal basic pattern of mitochrondria, usually identified with LDH and NADH reactions, was disrupted by clumping of highly reactive material. These focal changes progressed to a generalized breakdown of fiber architecture, characterized by a loss of staining quality followed finally by phagocytosis. Longitudinal sections indicated that the early changes in a focal necrosis affected only a small segment of fiber lengths. The later stages affected progressively greater lengths of muscle fibers (95).

Following i.p. application of soman (methylpinacolyloxyphosphoryl fluoride), local necrotic lesions are seen scattered throughout the diaphragm muscle. Some fibers displayed severe lesions characterized by loss of cytoarchitecture and phagocytosis (131).

Within 2 hr of an injection of DFP or tabun the earliest light miscroscopic changes are seen characterized by localized eosinophilia, swelling of the sarcoplasm, and loss of striations in several muscle fibers. Approximately 12 hr after the i.v. injection a complete but localized necrosis has developed in the affected fibers (133). A delayed neuropathy beginning at the nerve terminals develops within three weeks after exposure to DFP (136, 137). At this time muscle contractile strength is returning toward normal.

Ultrastructural Changes Produced by Cholinesterase Inhibitors

Motor nerve terminals showed varying degrees of changes within 30 min to 2 hr after injection of soman and paraoxon (131, 138). Some nerve terminals appear relatively normal with the exception of slightly swollen mitochondria. These nerve terminal abnormalities are more severe after soman than after paraoxon. More obvious changes are seen in the subsynaptic area and the surrounding muscle fiber. More severely affected nerve terminals display myelin figures, membrane enclosures, and an increase in the number of large coated vesicles. Soman, paraoxon, and neostigmine initiate the formation of vesicular structure in the primary and secondary subsynaptic cleft (95, 131, 139). Occasionally some of these are seen in the sarcoplasm. Many of the cleft vesicles are similar in density and size to synaptic vesicles but with considerable variations in diameter. The severity of lesions in the subsynaptic folds varies even within the same muscle. Normal subsynaptic clefts with few cleft vesicles are seen side by side with subsynaptic clefts with many cleft vesicles and a widening of the cleft itself (95, 131).

The ChE inhibitors, in addition to the changes seen in the region of the end-plate, cause changes in the muscle fiber itself. Muscle surrounding the motor end-plate shows a disruption of cytoarchitectural organization. Initially the first changes are in the mitochondria which show swelling leading to lysis of the central cristae. Myelin figures beneath the end-plate are frequently observed while the region more distal to the end-plate is less affected. The nucleoli of the muscle cell nucleus are enlarged and move to the periphery of the nucleus. There is an increase in the sarcoplasmic ribosomes, the sarcoplasmic reticulum becomes dilated followed by a loss of striation of the myofibrils, and later total destruction of the myofilaments and fragmentation of Z bands occurs (95, 131).

Muscle Lesions Developing During Chronic Cholinesterase Inhibition

Treatment of rats with paraoxon over a period of seven consecutive days produces a progressive myopathy (93, 95, 135). In the diaphragm a maximal effect is seen after 3 days of treatment. All stages of the myopathic process were maximal at this point and 6.5% of all fibers were found to be affected. By day 7 the muscle appeared to be relatively normal. In soleus muscle the maximum number of lesions was seen at day 3, but only 0.7% of the total fiber population was affected. The gastrocnemius muscle, unlike the diaphragm and the soleus, exhibited maximal lesions on days 5 to 7. The total number of fibers involved at this time was 0.8%. In all muscles studied, maximal loss of ChE activity occurred during the first 30 min after the initial paraoxon treatment. Within 24 hr of each injection of paraoxon, the enzyme activity in diaphragm and soleus muscle had recovered to about 50% of control activity, while in gastrocnemius muscle the ChE activity had returned to 67% of control.

There is a marked difference in the susceptibility of muscle type to the paraoxon action. The muscles tested are distinct from each other as to predominant fiber type, rate of firing, speed of contraction, and inherent metabolism. The myopathy is much more severe in the diaphragm, which is predominantly a slow contracting, tonic or red muscle, than it is in soleus, which consists of a majority of intermediate fibers, or in the gastrocnemius, which is a fast contracting phasic or white muscle (97, 135).

Modification of the Myopathy

In animals undergoing right sciatic or left phrenic nerve transection 4–7 days prior to the application of the irreversible inhibitor, the innervated muscles showed a slight increase in the number of lesions, while the denervated muscles were protected against the myopathic process and instead underwent typical denervation atrophy (93, 97, 133). Animals that were given hemicholinium, an inhibitor of cholineacetyl-transferase, did not demonstrate any histologic abnormalities in the muscles to paraoxon. The maximum number of lesions was significantly reduced as compared with animals receiving a similar dose of paraoxon without the hemicholinium (93). Internal skeletal fixation by pinning the right ankle and knee three days before treatment with paraoxon protected the soleus from the paraoxon-induced myopathy and potentiated the myopathy in the soleus of the unfixed limb, which had assumed a greater weight-bearing function.

A normal, untreated diaphragm is capable of sustaining a 10-sec tetanic contraction at indirect stimulation frequencies of 25, 50, 100, and 200 per second. A diaphragm removed from a DFP-treated rat 2 to 4 hr after the injection has lost the ability to sustain a contraction at 200 stimuli per second, and performs subnormally at 100 stimuli per second. Unilateral stimulation of the sciatic nerve with 5 stimuli per second during 6 hr in anesthetized DFP-treated rats produced extensive necrosis on the stimulated side only (133). Curare prevented the necrosis when given every 2 hr during the 6 hr indirect stimulation period. Necrosis developed, however, when the curare concentration was reduced. The muscles were still insensitive to indirect stimulation, but apparently sensitive to the necrotic effects of ACh (133).

Reactivation of Phosphorylated ChE

When given at a concentration of 0.23 mg/kg s.c. to rats, paraoxon produced an 85% inhibition of neuromuscular ChE of the diaphragm, and the enzyme remained at this level of inhibition for the next 2 hr. Administration of 2-PAM (20–60 mg/kg i.p.), a reactivator of phosphorylated ChE, at various time intervals after the paraoxon injection (10–120 min) increased ChE activity to 75% of control. When administered between 10–30 min after paraoxon, 2-PAM totally prevented the development of the paraoxon myopathy. At longer intervals between paraoxon and PAM there was a time related increase in muscle necrosis. If ChE inhibition proceeded uninterrupted for 2 hr prior to PAM administration, the muscle necrosis occurred in 4.2% of the fibers. The myopathic process depends upon the degree and duration of ChE inhibition (134, 135).

Rats treated with 2-PAM within 2 hr after DFP or soman poisoning showed no necrosis; if the PAM injection was postponed, the necrosis developed as usual (133, 134).

Reversible Cholinesterase Inhibition and Myopathies

Long-term treatment of rats with prostigmine sulfate for 42 to 150 days showed degeneration of postsynaptic folds, mainly in red muscle fiber and less so in white muscle (139, 140). The postsynaptic membrane profile concentration was decreased by 29% in red muscle fibers and by 10% in white muscle fibers. The mean miniature end-plate potential amplitude was decreased by 29%. Frequency, quantum content, and muscle resting membrane potential were not affected by neostigmine (139).

In acute experiments, prostigmine as well as physostigmine in concentrations between 0.2 to 0.6 mg/kg cause muscle fiber necrosis, not unlike that seen with the irreversible inhibitor of ChE. The number of necrotic fibers rises with increasing inhibitor concentration. The total number of necrotic fibers, however, is less than that caused by paraoxon (M. B. Laskowski and W-D. Dettbarn, unpublished observations). Signs of cholinergic intoxication, such as salivation, diarrhea, as well as body tremor and pronounced muscle fasiculation, are seen only for about 30 min after reversible inhibition of ChE. The same symptoms can be observed for over 2 hr after irreversible inhibition of the enzyme. Repeated application of the reversible inhibitor, i.e. 3 times during a given 1.5 hr period, leads to an increasing number of lesions.

Mechanisms for the Development of Myopathies

The observations reported above indicate the reversible or irreversible inhibition of ChE at the neuromuscular junction produces a progressive myopathy, primarily associated with the motor end-plate region. Possible mechanisms for this myopathy include the following. (a) The myopathy is the result of the abnormal functioning of the myoneural junction when ChE activity is reduced as a consequence of the presence of increased amounts of ACh. (b) Increased circulating catecholamines may cause local ischemia. (c) The inhibitors may act directly on the postsynaptic membrane or other components of the muscle cell. (d) The inhibitors may exert nonspecific toxicity. Besides diffusion, the enzyme AChE is responsible for the rapid removal of ACh from end-plate receptors. Thus, inhibition of this enzyme allows ACh to accumulate, to react longer, and interact with a larger area of the motor end-plate. The end result is an increase in amplitude and duration of the MEPPs. Formation of these leads to action potentials and spontaneous twitching of muscle fibers. Similar effects on end-plate potentials may be observed. In addition, as is the case with paraoxon, the frequency of MEPPS is drastically increased (94). The effect of the ChE inhibitors leads to increased excitability of the nerve terminal and therefore increased antidromic activity (141–147). The back response to a single nerve stimulus and the repetitive muscle action potentials are prolonged and intensified. The myopathy-inducing action of guanidine (96), which does not inhibit ChE but causes an increased release of ACh per impulse and produces spontaneous muscle twitching by inducing spontaneous multiquantal end-plate potentials, again supports the role of ACh in the genesis of this myopathy. By inhibiting antidromic activity, curare prevents the increased MEPP frequency, blocks neuromuscular transmission and spontaneous muscle twitching, and thus prevents the ChE inhibitor–induced myopathy. Additional support for the role of ACh as the myopathy-inducing agent comes from the experiments with 2-PAM, a reactivator of phosphorylated ChE. 2-PAM when given within 10–30 min after the organophosphorus ChE inhibitor not only reactivates the enzyme, but also greatly reduces antidromic firing and the MEPP frequency. It also completely prevents the myopathy, unless given after a critical time, usually between 60–90 min (133–135). Hemicholinium has been shown to reduce the amount of ACh in the quantum released and reduces significantly the severity of the myopathy (93).

By inhibiting ChE in vitro, cholinergic as well as adrenergic stimulation is achieved. All preganglionic nerve fibers, as well as motor nerves, are cholinergic and the preganglionic transmitter is ACh. Under conditions when ChE is inhibited, simultaneous stimulation of postganglionic cholinergic and adrenergic and motor nerves will occur. This results in an increased release of ACh or norepinephrine from postganglionic fibers. Under these conditions not enough blood may be supplied to the most active muscle fibers and thus relative ischemia might result. This could lead to ischemic changes, leakage of muscle enzymes, and eventual necrosis. The effects of prolonged cholinergic vasodilation in combination with reduced adrenergic vasoconstrictor tone during the periods of increased ChE inhibitor-induced muscle activity could lead to functional ischemia in certain hyperactive muscle fibers and not in others. Less active muscle may have normal oxygen requirements, but may receive the same blood supply. The functional ischemia could appear during the period of the ACh-induced muscle fiber activity. This could also explain the prevention of necrosis by denervation due to immobilization of the denervated muscle.

It is generally accepted that two groups on the enzyme are essential for hydrolysis, the esteratic and anionic site. The anionic site interacts by ionic binding with the cationic head of the ACh molecule. There is good evidence that part of the chemical forces binding ACh to the enzyme are more or less similar to those between ACh and its receptor. It is therefore not surprising that drugs that inhibit ChE may, to some extent, also react with the ACh receptor. DFP, for instance, in higher concentrations than needed to inhibit enzyme activity has a curare-like action which may block neuromuscular transmission (128). In contrast to ChE inhibition, this latter effect is reversible on washing. Furthermore, it has not been shown as yet whether this higher concentration is due to direct action on the receptor or on the ionophore which controls the permeability once the receptor has been activated, an effect not unlike that of local anesthetic. The myopathic effects of the ChE inhibitors can be explained entirely on the basis of their inhibition of the enzyme and the increased action of ACh on pre- and postganglionic receptor sites. Other effects that have been described occur at a much higher concentration of the inhibitor.

Besides their inhibition of ChE, or interaction with the ACh receptor and or the ionic conductance modulator, organophosphates may have direct effects on the muscle. We have observed that paraoxon directly depolarizes muscle membranes (127), and subsarcolemmal abnormalities of muscle fine structure are occasionally seen not associated with an end-plate (95). This unspecific action as a cause of the myopathy could not explain the selectivity of the myopathy, since only 6–8% of the fibers are affected.

The importance of studying the myopathies produced by cholinesterase inhibitors derives not from the accurate reproduction of a specific human disease but rather from the insight they provide into the myopathic effects of altering the delicate nerve-muscle relationship. With this approach it is possible to follow a highly controllable disease process from its origin at the end-plate within 30 min after the drug, to its completion with necrosis and phagocytosis after 24 hr. The crucial questions may lie with the mechanisms which spare most fibers, rather than the disease process itself.

CONCLUSIONS

Within the last ten years there have been major developments in the field of experimental models of human muscle disease. Recently models of Duchenne's muscular dystrophy have been pursued most actively because of the particularly sinister nature of the disease. It is essential now to define carefully the mechanisms underlying the generation of these myopathies and to clarify major areas of controversy. This will require a multidisciplinary approach combining physiology, ultrastructure, and biochemistry, using the same drug under the same experimental conditions. Duchenne's dystrophy is a multisystem disease. The significance of pursuing the pharmacologic models rests with the development of drugs important to combating muscle degeneration.

The models for myotonia present a different problem. The pharmacology of these experimental myopathies has been examined in considerable detail. A review of the literature demonstrates that membrane physiology has been examined thoroughly in one model and biochemistry in another. Again, what is required is a multidisciplinary investigation of each model toward the end of defining whether a single common defective mechanism is responsible for the myotonic state.

Finally the myopathies induced by experimental alteration of nerve-muscle relationships have been developed to analyze the basic pathophysiology of muscle degeneration. The most actively studied of these have been the experimental myopathies induced by cholinesterase inhibitors. Muscles respond to insult with a limited arsenal of physiological and histological alterations. In-depth multidisciplinary analyses of the very earliest of these myopathic processes can provide insight into some of the basic mechanisms underlying muscle fiber degeneration.

Literature Cited

1. Thomsen, J. 1875. Tonische Krampfe in willkurlichen beweglichen Muskeln in Folge von erebterpsychischer Disposition (Ataxia muscularis?). *Arch. Psychiatr. Nervenkr.* 6:706–18
2. Merritt, H. H. 1973. *A Textbook of Neurology,* 531–36. Philadelphia: Lea & Febiger
3. Bryant, S. H., Morales-Aguilera, A. 1971. Chloride conductance in normal and myotonic muscle fibers and the action of monocarboxylic aromatic acids. *J. Physiol.* 219:367–83
4. Rudel, R., Senges, J. 1972. Experimental myotonia in mammalian skeletal

muscle: Changes in membrane properties. *Pfluegers Arch.* 331:324–34
5. Ulbricht, W. 1969. The effect of veratridine on excitable membranes of nerve and muscle. *Ergeb. Physiol. Biol. Chem. Exp. Pharmacol.* 61:18–71
6. Udenfriend, S. 1962. *Fluorescence Assay in Biology and Medicine.* New York: Academic
7. Seiler, D., Kuhn, E. 1969. Experimentelle Myotonie durch Amine Veranderungen am Fettsaurenmuster der Phosphatide im Rattenmuskel. *Klin. Wochenschr.* 47:1114–15
8. Fuller, R. W., Lacefield, W. B., Kattau, R. W., Nickander, R. C., Snoddy, H. D.

1971. Myotonia produced by indole-acetic acid. Studies with related compounds and correlation with drug levels in tissues. *Arch. Int. Pharmacodyn.* 193:48–60

9. Hildebrand, E. M. 1946. War on weeds. *Science* 103:465–68

10. Berwick, P. 1970. 2,4-dichlorophenoxyacetic acid poisoning in man: Some interesting clinical and laboratory findings. *J. Am. Med. Assoc.* 214:1114–17

11. Eyzaguirre, C., Folk, B. P., Zierler, K. L., Lilienthal, J. L. Jr. 1948. Experimental myotonia and repetitive phenomena: the veratrinic effects of 2,4-dichlorophenoxyacetic acid (2,4-D) in the rat. *Am. J. Physiol.* 155:69–77

12. Senges, J., Rudel, R. 1972. Experimental myotonia in mammalian skeletal muscle: Changes in contractile properties. *Pfluegers Arch.* 331:315–23

13. Brown, G. L., Harvey, A. M. 1939. Congenital myotonia in the goat. *Brain* 62:341–63

14. Steinberg, D., Avigan, J. 1960. Studies of cholesterol biosynthesis. *J. Biol. Chem.* 235:3127–29

15. Peter, J. B., Andiman, R. M., Bowman, R. L., Nagatomo, T. 1973. Myotonia induced by diazocholesterol: Increased (Na^+, K^+)-ATPase activity of erythrocyte ghosts and development of cataracts. *Exp. Neurol.* 41:738–44

16. Somers, J. E., Winer, N. 1966. Reversible myopathy and myotonia following administration of a hypocholesterolemic agent. *Neurology* 16:761–65

17. Winer, N., Martt, J. M., Somers, J. E., Wolcott, L., Dale, H. E., Burns, T. W. 1964. Induced myotonia in man and goat. *J. Lab. Clin. Med.* 64:1019–20

18. Fiehn, W., Seiler, D., Kuhn, E., Bartles, D. 1975. Transport ATPases of cardiac sarcolemma in 20,25-diazocholesterol induced myopathy. *Eur. J. Clin. Invest.* 5:327–30

19. Winer, N., Klachko, D. M., Baer, R. D., Langley, P. L., Burns, T. W. 1966. Myotonic response induced by inhibitors of cholesterol biosynthesis. *Science* 153:312–13

20. Goodgold, J., Eberstein, A. 1968. An electromyographic study of induced myotonia in rats: after contraction and prolonged relaxation time. *Exp. Neurol.* 21:159–66

21. Mrozek, K., Kwiecinski, H. 1975. Neuromuscular failure in myotonic rats. *Eur. Neurol.* 13:47–53

22. McComas, A. J., Mrozek, K. 1968. The electrical properties of muscle fiber membranes in dystrophia myotonica and myotonia congenita. *J. Neurol. Neurosurg. Psychiatry* 31:441–47

23. Rudel, R., Senges, J. 1972. Mammalian skeletal muscle: Reduced chloride conductance in drug-induced myotonia and introduction of myotonia by low-chloride solution. *Naunyn Schmiedebergs Arch. Pharmacol.* 274:337–47

24. Riecker, G., Dobbelstein, H., Rohl, D., Botte, H. D. 1964. Messungen des Membranpotentials einzelner quergestreifter Muskelzellen bei Myotonia congenita (Thomsen). *Klin. Wochenschr.* 42:519–22

25. Lipicky, R. J., Bryant, S. H., Salmon, J. H. 1971. Cable parameters, sodium, potassium, chloride, and water content, and potassium efflux in isolated external intercostal muscle of normal volunteers and patients with myotonia congenita. *J. Clin Invest.* 50:2091–2103

26. Bryant, S. H. 1969. Cable properties of external intercostal muscle fibers from normal and myotonic goats. *J. Physiol.* 204:530–50

27. Falk, G., Landa, J. F. 1960. Prolonged response of skeletal muscle in the absence of penetrating anions. *Am. J. Physiol.* 198:289–99

28. Falk, G., Landa, J. F. 1960. Effects of potassium on frog skeletal muscle in a chloride deficient medium. *Am. J. Physiol.* 198:1225–31

29. Hodgkin, A. L., Horowicz, P. 1959. The influence of potassium and chloride ions on the membrane potentials of single fibers. *J. Physiol.* 148:127–60

30. Hutter, O. F., Noble, D. 1960. The chloride conductance of frog skeletal muscle. *J. Physiol.* 151:89–102

31. Eisenberg, R. S., Gage, P. W. 1969. Ionic conductances of the surface and transverse tubular membranes of frog sartorius fibers. *J. Gen. Physiol.* 53:279–97

32. Peter, J. B., Fiehn, W. 1973. Diazocholesterol myotonia: Accumulation of desmosterol and increased adenosine triphosphatase activity of sarcolemma. *Science* 179:910–12

33. Seiler, D. 1971. The ATPases of the sarcolemma from skeletal muscle in experimental myotonia. *Experientia* 27:1170–71

34. Brody, I. A. 1973. Myotonia induced by monocarboxylic aromatic acids: A possible mechanism. *Arch. Neurol.* 28:243–46

35. Woodin, A. M., Wieneke, A. A. 1968. Role of leucocidin and triphosphoinositide in the control of potassium permeability. *Nature* 221:283–86
36. Wohlfart, G. 1951. Dystrophia myotonica and myotonia congenita. Histopathologic studies with special reference to changes in the muscles. *J. Neuropathol. Exp. Neurol.* 10:109–24
37. Olson, W. H., LeQuire, V., Freeman, J. A., Fenichel, J. A. 1977. A t-system abnormality in the myotonic goat. *Neurology.* In press
38. Schroder, J. M., Kuhn, E. 1968. Zur Ultrastruktur der Muskelfaser bei der experimentellen Myotonie mit 20,25-diazocholesterin. *Virchows Arch. A* 344:181–95
39. Hofmann, W. W., Alston, W., Rowe, G. 1966. A study of individual neuro-muscular junctions in myotonia. *Electroencephalogr. Clin. Neurophysiol.* 21:521–37
40. Tang, A. H., Schroeder, L. A., Keasling, H. H. 1968. U-23, 223 (3-chloro-2,5,6-trimethylbenzoic acid), a veratrinic agent selective for the skeletal muscles. *Arch Int. Pharmacodyn. Ther.* 175:319–29
41. Iyer, V., Whiting, M., Fenichel, G. 1976. Neural influence in experimental myotonia. *Neurology* 26:384
42. Ranish, N. A., Dettbarn, W-D., Iyer, V. 1977. The influence of nerve stump length on 2,4-dichlorophenoxyacetic acid induced myotonia. In press
43. Caccia, M. R., Boiardi, A., Andreussi, L., Cornelio, F. 1975. Nerve supply and experimental myotonia in rats. *J. Neurol. Sci.* 24:145–50
44. Eberstein, A., Goodgold, J., Johnston, R. 1976. Myotonia induced in denervated muscles. *Exp. Neurol.* 51:266–70
45. Albuquerque, E. X., McIsaac, R. J. 1970. Fast and slow mammalian muscles after denervation. *Exp. Neurol.* 26:183–202
46. Albuquerque, E. X., Schuh, F. T., Kauffman, F. C. 1971. Early membrane depolarization of the fast mammalian muscle after denervation. *Pfluegers Arch.* 328:36–50
47. Lullman, H. 1960. Uber die Ursache spontaner Fibrillationen Denervierter Skeletmusculatur. *Klin. Wochenschr.* 38:1169–71
48. Thesleff, S. 1963. Spontaneous electrical activity in denervated rat skeletal muscle. In *The Effect of Use and Disuse on Neuromuscular Function,* ed. E. Gut-mann, P. Hnik, 41–51. Prague: Publ. House Czech. Acad. Sci.
49. Ware, F. Jr., Bennett, A. L., McIntyre, A. R. 1954. Membrane resting potential of denervated mammalian skeletal muscle measured *in vivo. Am. J. Physiol.* 177:115–18
50. Danon, J. M., Karpati, G., Carpenter, S., Wolfe, L. S. 1976. Experimental myotonic myopathy. *Neurology* 26:384
51. Engel, W. K. 1967. Muscle biopsies in neuromuscular diseases. *Pediatr. Clin. North Am.* 14:963–95
52. Pearce, J. M. S., Pennington, R. J., Walton, J. N. 1964. Serum enzyme studies in muscle disease. II. Serum creatine kinase activity in muscular dystrophy and in other myopathic and neuropathic disorders. *J. Neurol. Neurosurg. Psychiatry* 27:96–99
53. Chason, J. L. 1971. Nervous system and skeletal muscle. In *Pathology,* ed. W. A. D. Anderson, p. 1781. St. Louis: Mosby
54. Telford, I. R. 1971. *Experimental Muscular Dystrophies in Animals: A Comparative Study.* Springfield, Ill.: Thomas. 250 pp.
55. Hathaway, P. W., Engel, W. K., Zellweger, H. 1970. Experimental myopathy after microarterial embolization: Comparison with childhood X-linked pseudohypertrophic muscular dystrophy. *Arch. Neurol.* 22:365–78
56. Erb, W. H. 1891. Dystrophia muscularis progressiva. Klinische und pathologisch-anatomische Studien. *Dtsch. Z. Nervenheilkd.* 1:13–94
57. Koehler, J. P. 1974. Blood vessel structure in Duchenne muscular dystrophy. *Neurology* 24:354
58. Karpati, G., Carpenter, S., Melmed, C., Eisen, A. A. 1974. Experimental ischemic myopathy. *J. Neurol. Sci.* 23:129–61
59. Mendell, J. R., Engel, W. K., Derrer, E. C. 1971. Duchenne muscular dystrophy: Functional ischemia reproduces its characteristic lesions. *Science* 172:1143–45
60. Murphy, D. L., Mendell, J. R., Engel, W. K. 1973. Serotonin and platelet function in Duchenne muscular dystrophy. *Arch Neurol.* 28:239–42
61. Swash, M., Fox, K. P., Davidson, A. R. 1975. Carcinoid myopathy: Serotonin induced muscle weakness in man? *Arch. Neurol.* 32:572–74
62. Munsat, T. L., Hudgson, P., Johnson, M. 1976. Serotonin myopathy. *Neurology* 26:384

63. Altura, B. M. 1967. Evaluation of neurohumoral substances in local regulation of blood flow. *Am. J. Physiol.* 212:1447–54

64. Selye, H. 1965. A muscular dystrophy induced by cold following restriction of the arterial blood supply. *Experientia* 21:610–11

65. Mendell, J. R., Engel, W. K., Derrer, E. C. 1972. Increased plasma enzyme concentrations in rats with functional ischaemia of muscle provide a possible model of Duchenne muscular dystrophy. *Nature* 239:522–24

66. Engel, W. K., Derrer, E. C. 1975. Drugs blocking the muscle-damaging effects of 5-HT and noradrenaline in aorta-ligatured rats. *Nature* 254:151–52

67. Pletscher, A. 1973. The impact of monoamine research on drug development. In *Frontiers in Catecholamine Research,* ed. E. Usdin, S. H. Snyder, pp. 27–37. New York: Pergamon

68. Melmed, C., Karpati, G. 1973. Unpublished data, referred to in Ref. 58

69. Rowland, L. P. 1976. Pathogenesis of muscular dystrophies. *Arch. Neurol.* 33:315–21

70. Parker, J. M., Mendell, J. R. 1974. Proximal myopathy induced by 5-HT-imipramine simulates Duchenne dystrophy. *Nature* 247:103–4

71. Silverman, L. M., Gruemer, H-D., Mendell, J. R. 1975. Experimental model for Duchenne dystrophy. *Clin. Chem.* 21:1026

72. Yu, M. K., Wright, T. L., Dettbarn, W-D., Olson, W. H. 1974. Pargyline-induced myopathy with histochemical characteristics of Duchenne muscular dystrophy. *Neurology* 24:237–44

73. Wright, T. L., O'Neill, J. A., Olson, W. H. 1973. Abnormal intrafibrillar monoamines in sex-linked muscular dystrophy. *Neurology* 23:510–17

74. Wood, P. L., Boegman, R. J. 1975. Increased axoplasmic flow in experimental ischemic myopathy. *Exp. Neurol.* 48:136–41

75. Boegman, R. J., Wood, P. L., Pinaud, L. 1975. Increased axoplasmic flow associated with pargyline under conditions which induce a myopathy. *Nature* 253:51–52

76. Komiya, Y., Austin, L. 1975. Axoplasmic flow of protein in the sciatic nerve of mice with experimentally induced myopathy. *Exp. Neurol.* 47:307–15

77. Appenzeller, O., Ogin, G. 1975. Pathogenesis of muscular dystrophies: Sympathetic neurovascular components. *Arch. Neurol.* 32:2–4

78. Roddie, I. C., Shepherd, J. T. 1963. Nervous control of the circulation in skeletal muscle. *Br. Med. Bull.* 19: 115–19

79. Demos, J. 1961. Mesures des temps de circulation chez 79 myopathes. Étude statistique des resultats. Role du degre de l'atteinte musculaire clinique, du mode evolutif de la maladie, du sexe du malade, des saisons. *Rev. Fr. Etud. Clin. Biol.* 6:876–87

80. Demos, J., Treumann, F., Schroeder, W. 1968. Anomalies de regulation de la micro-circulation musculaire chez les enfants atteints de dystrophie musculaire progressive par rapport a des enfants normaux du meme age. *Rev. Fr. Etud. Clin. Biol.* 13:467–83

81. Kunze, K. 1970. Hypoxia: A possible cause in the development of muscle disease. In *Muscle Disease, Proc. Int. Congr.,* ed. J. Walton, pp. 327–31. Amsterdam: Excerpta Med.

82. Bickerstaff, E. R., Evans, J. V., Woolf, A. L. 1959. Ultrastructure of the myoneural junction in myasthenia gravis. *Nature* 184:1500

83. Zacks, S. I. 1973. *The Motor End-Plate,* 318–83. Huntington, NY: Krieger

84. Eaton, L. M., Lambert, E. H. 1957. Electromyography and electric stimulation of nerves in diseases of motor unit: Observations on the myasthenic syndrome associated with malignant tumors. *J. Am. Med. Assoc.* 163:1117–24

85. Santa, T., Engel, A. G., Lambert, E. H. 1972. Histometric study of neuromuscular junction ultrastructure. II. Myasthenic syndrome. *Neurology* 22:370–76

86. Elmqvist, D., Lambert, E. H. 1968. Detailed analysis of neuromuscular transmission in a patient with the myasthenic syndrome sometimes associated with bronchogenic carcinoma. *Mayo Clin. Proc.* 43:689–713

87. Coers, C., Pelc, S. 1954. Un cas d'amyotonie congenitale caracterise par une anomalie histologique et histochimique de la jonction neuromusculaire. *Acta Neurol. Belg.* 54:166–73

88. Isaacs, H. 1961. A syndrome of continuous muscle-fibre activity. *J. Neurol. Neurosurg. Psychiatry* 24:319–25

89. Sanz-Ibanez, J. 1951. Estudios sobre el comportamiento de las cepas A y B del virus Coxsakie. *Trab. Inst. Cajal Invest. Biol.* 43:165–88

90. Zacks, S. I., Shields, D. R., Steinberg, S. A. 1966. A myasthenic syndrome in the

dog: A case report with electron microscopic observations on motor endplates and comparisons with the fine structure of endplates in myasthenia gravis. *Ann. NY Acad. Sci.* 135:79–97

91. Omrod, A. N. 1961. Myasthenia gravis in a cocker spaniel. *Vet. Rec.* 73:489–90

92. Engel, A. G., Lindstrom, J. M., Lambert, E. H., Lennon, V. A. 1976. Ultrastructural localization of the acetylcholine receptor in myasthenia gravis and in its experimental autoimmune model. *Neurology* 26:371

93. Fenichel, G. M., Kibler, W. B., Olson, W. H., Dettbarn, W-D. 1972. Chronic inhibition of cholinesterase as a cause of myopathy. *Neurology* 22:1026–33

94. Laskowski, M. B., Dettbarn, W-D. 1975. Presynaptic effects of neuromuscular cholinesterase inhibition. *J. Pharmacol. Exp. Ther.* 194:351–61

95. Laskowski, M. B., Olson, W. H., Dettbarn, W-D. 1975. Ultrastructural changes at the motor end-plate produced by an irreversible cholinesterase inhibitor. *Exp. Neurol.* 47:290–306

96. Fenichel, G. M., Dettbarn, W-D., Newman, T. M. 1974. An experimental myopathy secondary to excessive acetylcholine release. *Neurology* 24:41–45

97. Fenichel, G. M., Kibler, W. B., Dettbarn, W-D. 1974. The effect of immobilization and exercise on acetylcholine-mediated myopathies. *Neurology* 24:1086–90

98. Buller, A. J., Eccles, J. C., Eccles, R. M. 1960. Differentiation of fast and slow muscles in the cat hind limb. *J. Physiol.* 150:399–416

99. Buller, A. J., Eccles, J. C., Eccles, R. M. 1960. Interactions between motorneurons and muscles in respect of the characteristic speeds of their responses. *J. Physiol.* 150:417–39

100. Gutmann, E., Hnik, P. 1963. *The Effect of Use and Disuse on Neuromuscular Functions.* Amsterdam: Elsevier. 576 pp.

101. Drachman, D. B., Witzke, F. 1972. Trophic regulation of acetylcholine sensitivity of muscle: Effect of electrical stimulation. *Science* 176:514–16

102. Lomo, T., Rosenthal, J. 1972. Control of ACh sensitivity by muscle activity in the rat. *J. Physiol.* 221:493–513

103. Birks, R., MacIntosh, F. C. 1961. Acetylcholine metabolism of a sympathetic ganglion. *Can. J. Biochem. Physiol.* 39:787–827

104. Drachman, D. B. 1972. Neurotrophic regulation of muscle cholinesterase.

Effects of botulinum toxin and denervation. *J. Physiol.* 226:619–27

105. Edstrom, A., Mattsson, H. 1972. Rapid axonal transport *in vitro* in the sciatic system of the frog of fucose- glucoseamine and sulfate-containing material. *J. Neurochem.* 19:1717–29

106. Otsuka, M., Endo, M. 1960. The effect of guanidine on neuromuscular transmission. *J. Pharmacol. Exp. Ther.* 128:273–82

107. Otsuka, M., Nonomura, Y. 1963. The action of phenolic substances on motor nerve endings. *J. Pharmacol. Exp. Ther.* 140:41–45

108. Feng, T. P. 1937. Studies on the neuromuscular junction. VII. The eserine-like effects of barium on motor nerve endings. *Chin. J. Physiol. Rep. Ser.* 12:177–96

109. Roberts, D. V., Thesleff, S. 1969. Acetylcholine release from motor nerve endings in rats treated with neostigmine. *Eur. J. Pharmacol.* 6:281–85

110. Chang, C. C., Chen, T. F., Chuang, S. T. 1973. Influence of chronic neostigmine treatment on the number of acetylcholine receptors and the release of acetylcholine from the rat diaphragm. *J. Physiol.* 230:613–18

111. Fleming, W. W., McPhillips, J. J., Westfall, D. P. 1973. Postjunctional supersensitivity and subsensitivity of excitable tissues to drugs. *Ergeb. Physiol. Biol. Chem. Exp.* 68:55–119

112. Fambrough, D. M., Drachman, D. B., Satyamurti, S. 1973. Neuromuscular junction in myasthenia gravis: decreased acetylcholine receptors. *Science* 182:293–95

113. Wecker, L., Dettbarn, W-D. 1975. Effects of atropine and neostigmine on receptor interactions at the neuromuscular junction. *Arch. Int. Pharmacodyn. Ther.* 217:236–45

114. Albuquerque, E. X., Warnick, J. E., Tasse, J. R., Sansone, F. M. 1972. Effects of vinblastine and colchicine on neural regulation of the fast and slow skeletal muscles of the rat. *Exp. Neurol.* 37:607–34

115. Conrad, J. T., Glaser, G. H. 1962. Neuromuscular fatigue in dystrophic muscle. *Nature* 196:4858

116. Glaser, G. H., Seashore, M. R. 1967. End-plate cholinesterase in dystrophic muscle. *Nature* 214:1351

117. Jedrzejczyk, J., Wieckowski, J., Rymaszewska, T., Barnard, E. A. 1972. Dystrophic chicken muscle: altered synap-

tic acetylcholinesterase. *Science* 180: 406–8

118. Crone, H. D., Freeman, S. E. 1972. The acetylcholinesterase activity of the denervated rat diaphragm. *J. Neurochem.* 19:1207–8

119. McComas, A. J., Sica, R. E. P., Currie, S. 1971. An electrophysiological study of Duchenne dystrophy. *J. Neurol. Neurosurg. Psychiatry* 34:461–68

120. Sica, R. E. P., McComas, A. J. 1971. An electrophysiological investigation of limb girdle and facioscapulohumeral dystrophy. *J. Neurol. Neurosurg. Psychiatry* 34:469–74

121. Riker, W. F., Okamoto, M. 1969. Pharmacology of motor nerve terminals. *Ann. Rev. Pharmacol.* 9:173–208

122. Boyd, I. A., Martin, A. R. 1956. Spontaneous subthreshold activity at mammalian neuromuscular junctions. *J. Physiol.* 132:61–73

123. Blaber, L. C., Christ, D. D. 1967. The action of facilitatory drugs on the isolated tennuissimus muscle of the cat. *Int. J. Neuropharmacol.* 6:473–84

124. Blaber, L. C. 1972. The mechanism of the facilitatory action of edrophonium in cat skeletal muscle. *Br. J. Pharmacol.* 46:498–507

125. Furukawa, T., Furukawa, A., Takagi, T. 1957. Fibrillation of muscle fibers produced by ammonium ions and its relation to the spontaneous activity at the neuromuscular junction. *Jpn. J. Physiol.* 7:252–63

126. Hubbard, J. I., Schmidt, R. F., Yokota, T. 1965. The effect of acetylcholine upon mammalian motor nerve terminals. *J. Physiol.* 181:810–29

127. Laskowski, M. B., Adler, M., Albuquerque, E. X., Dettbarn, W-D. 1977. An electrophysiological analysis of the effects of paraoxon on mammalian skeletal muscle. *J. Pharm. Exp. Ther.* In press

128. Kuba, K., Albuquerque, E. X., Daly, J., Barnard, E. A. 1974. A study of the irreversible cholinesterase inhibitor diisopropylfluorophosphate on time course of end-plate currents in frog sartorius muscle. *J. Pharmacol. Exp. Ther.* 189:499–512

129. Katz, B., Miledi, R. 1969. Tetrodotoxin-resistant electric activity in presynaptic terminals. *J. Physiol.* 203:459–87

130. Carey, E. J. 1944. Studies on ameboid motion and secretion of motor end-plates. III. Experimental histopathology of motor end-plates produced by quinine, curare, prostigmine, acetylcholine, strychnine, tetraethyl lead and heat. *Am. J. Pathol.* 20:341–93

131. Preusser, H. J. 1967. Die Ultrastruktur der motorischen Endplatte im Zwerchfell der Ratte und Veranderungen nach Inhibierung der Acetylcholinesterase. *Z. Zellforsch. Mikrosk. Anat.* 80: 436–57

132. Fischer, G. 1968. Inhibierung und Restitution der Azetylcholinesterase an der motorischen Endplatte im Zwerchfell der Ratte nach Intoxikation mit Soman. *Histochemie* 16:144–49

133. Ariens, A. T., Meeter, E., Wolthuis, O. L., van Benthem, R. M. J. 1969. Reversible necrosis at the end-plate region in striated muscles of the rat poisoned with cholinesterase inhibitors. *Experientia* 25:57–59

134. Fischer, G. 1970. Die Azetylcholinesterase an der motorischen Endplatte des Rattenzwerchfells nach Intoxikation mit Paraoxon und Soman bei Applikation von Oximen. *Experientia* 26: 402–3

135. Wecker, L., Dettbarn, W-D. 1976. Paraoxon induced myopathy: muscle specificity and acetylcholine involvement. *Exp. Neurol.* 51:281–91

136. Lowndes, H. E., Baker, T., Riker, W. F., Jr. 1974. Motor nerve dysfunction in delayed DFP neuropathy. *Eur. J. Pharmacol.* 29:66–73

137. Lowndes, H. E., Baker, T., Riker, W. F., Jr. 1975. Motor nerve terminal response to edrophonium in delayed DFP neuropathy. *Eur. J. Pharmacol.* 30: 69–72

138. Laskowski, M. B., Olson, W. H., Dettbarn, W-D. 1976. Motor end-plate degeneration coincident with cholinesterase inhibition and increased frequency of miniature end-plate potentials. *Fed. Proc.* 35:800

139. Engel, A. G., Lambert, E. H., Santa, T. 1973. Study of long-term anticholinesterase therapy. Effects on neuromuscular transmission and motor end-plate fine-structure. *Neurology* 23: 1273–81

140. Lytle, R. B. 1970. Increased synaptic area of neuromuscular junction in neostigmine-treated rats. *Anat. Rec.* 166: 339

141. Masland, R. L., Wigton, R. S. 1940. Nerve activity accompanying fasciculation produced by prostigmine. *J. Neurophysiol.* 3:249–75

142. Barstad, J. A. B. 1962. Presynaptic effects of the neuromuscular transmitter. *Experientia* 18:579–81

143. Randic, M., Straughn, D. W. 1964. Antidromic activity in the rat phrenic nerve-diaphragm preparation. *J. Physiol.* 173:130–48

144. Feng, T. P., Li, T. H. 1941. Studies on the neuromuscular junction XXIII. A new aspect of the phenomena of eserine potentiation and post-tetanic facilitation in mammalian muscles. *Chin. J. Physiol.* 16:37–56

145. Van Deer Meer, C., Meeter, E. 1956. The mechanism of action of anticholinesterases. II. The effect of di-ido-propylfluorophosphate (DFP) in the isolated rat phrenic nerve diaphragm preparation. *Acta Physiol. Pharmacol. Neerl.* 4:454–71

146. Riker, W. F. Jr., Roberts, J., Standaert, F. G., Fujimori, H. 1957. The motor nerve terminal as the primary focus for drug-induced facilitation of neuromuscular transmission. *J. Pharmacol. Exp. Ther.* 121:286–312

147. Blaber, L. C., Bowman, W. C. 1963. Studies on the repetitive discharges evoked in motor nerve and skeletal muscle after injection of anticholinesterase drugs. *Br. J. Pharmacol.* 20:326–44

Ann. Rev. Pharmacol. Toxicol. 1977. 17:411–24
Copyright © 1977 by Annual Reviews Inc. All rights reserved

THE EFFECTS OF PSYCHOPHARMACOLOGICAL AGENTS ON CENTRAL NERVOUS SYSTEM AMINE METABOLISM IN MAN

♦6688

James W. Maas
Department of Psychiatry, Yale University School of Medicine,
New Haven, Connecticut 06510

INTRODUCTION AND CAVEATS

In assessing the effects of psychopharmacological agents on the disposition and turnover of biogenic amines in the central nervous system (CNS) of man, investigators are ethically limited to the use of indirect experimental approaches. Most investigators have focused on changes in concentrations of amine metabolites in cerebrospinal fluid (CSF) that are associated with drug administration, and the greatest attention has been paid to 3-methoxy-4-hydroxyphenethyleneglycol (MHPG), homovanillic acid (HVA), and 5-hydroxyindoleacetic acid (5-HIAA) as these are the principal metabolites of norepinephrine (NE), dopamine (DA), and serotonin (5-HT), respectively, in the CNS. To a lesser extent, changes in the concentration of urinary MHPG in relationship to drug administration have also been studied in an attempt to understand the effects of psychotropic agents upon CNS NE metabolism. Each of these approaches has certain advantages and inherent limitations, which are briefly reviewed below. It is thought that such comments will help to place in better perspective the data obtained by using these techniques with human subjects.

There is a gradient between ventricular CSF HVA and lumbar CSF HVA of approximately 10:1 (1). Obstructions to flow between the cistern and lumbar spaces are associated with a marked reduction in the concentration of CSF HVA (2–4). DA is found in the spinal cord in very low concentrations (5, 6) and there is a barrier to the movement of HVA from blood into CSF (7, 8). As a group, these studies suggest that HVA in lumber CSF originates principally in structures within brain. The degree to which various structures in brain contribute to lumber CSF HVA is

411

unknown but it is likely that a significant proportion of the HVA originates in structure that are close to the ventricles, e.g. the caudate nucleii (4, 9). Following the administration of probenecid (which blocks the efflux of HVA from brain), there is a lag time of approximately four hours before lumbar CSF HVA levels begin to increase (10). While this supports the conclusion that most of the lumbar CSF HVA originates in brain it also suggests that relatively transient changes in the functional activity of DA neurons in brain may not be readily detected by examination of concentrations of HVA in lumbar CSF.

There is a barrier to the movement of 5-HIAA from blood to CSF (11, 12) and there is a ventriculolumbar gradient for 5-HIAA of approximately 5:1 (1). Although it has been found that there is a lag between probenecid administration and the increase in CSF 5-HIAA (10), there is a controversy as to the brain versus spinal cord origins of lumbar CSF 5-HIAA. Some investigators have found that with a complete block of the subarachnoid space at the thoracic level lumbar CSF 5-HIAA levels were normal (3, 4), whereas in another study it was found that the concentration of 5-HIAA was significantly reduced below complete blocks (2). A variety of other experimental techniques have been utilized to resolve the question of the brain versus cord origins of 5-HIAA, but because of apparent differences in methodology and perhaps species differences the issue remains unsettled. On balance it would appear that lumbar CSF 5-HIAA is partially derived from brain and partially from cord, but the relative contributions of each is uncertain. [For a review of the data dealing with this problem, see (13).]

There is no ventriculolumbar gradient for MHPG (14). Spinal cord transection in humans is associated with the lowering of lumbar CSF MHPG whereas a block of CSF flow between higher and lower centers is associated with no decrement in lumbar CSF MHPG (3). It has also been noted that CSF MHPG is continually lost through capillaries within the spinal cord and that the degree of this loss differs as a function of the depth of the region within the spinal cord; that is, the deeper the site of production of the metabolite the smaller the proportion that would be expected to reach CSF. For these reasons it seems unlikely that lumbar CSF MHPG will provide an index of NE metabolism in brain. The degree to which lumbar CSF MHPG will reflect NE metabolism in cord has also been questioned (15).

Depending upon the particular technique used as well as the species of animal, estimates of the quantity of urinary MHPG which is derived from the CNS varies. In the rat it has been estimated that between 10 and 30% of urinary MHPG comes from CNS NE (16–18), whereas in the dog and monkey the estimates are in the range of 25–65% (19, 20). In man exact figures are not available but it has been suggested that the amount of urinary MHPG originating in CNS NE metabolism may be quite large (21, 22). All of the methods used are indirect and require certian assumptions and inference. Until more definitive data are available, a reasonably exact idea of the fraction of urinary MHPG originating in brain versus periphery must remain an open question.

Probenecid has been found to block the efflux of weak organic acids from brain and as such it has been reasoned that increases in concentrations of HVA or 5-HIAA which are associated with probenecid may give some measure of the turnover of the amine under investigation. [Changes in human CSF MHPG following probenecid are either absent or modest and the probenecid technique has not been used extensively in studies of this metabolite (23, 24).] In evaluating data obtained with the probenecid technique the following points should be noted. The administration of probenecid is frequently a stressful experience for the patient in that it is often associated with nausea and vomiting. In at least one case, it has been demonstrated that a psychopharmacological agent alters CSF levels of probenecid (25) and hence the interaction between the effectiveness of the probenecid block and the preceding drug treatment is a question which is of importance but not often studied. The kinetics of the changes in CSF HVA and 5-HIAA produced by probenecid are complicated and the relationship of baseline to postprobenecid concentrations of metabolites may be of importance. However, because of the practical and clinical problems raised by repeating the lumbar puncture, in practice, CSF samples are often obtained only after probenecid administration. In summary, while probenecid is of use in studying the actions of drugs on DA and 5-HT metabolism the data obtained may be semiquantitative.

Despite the problems associated with each of the above approaches, important data have been obtained with these techniques. It should be noted that these data as to the effects of psychopharmacological agents on amine metabolism in patients are of special value in that in contrast to many animal studies they have frequently been obtained from subjects receiving therapeutic doses of drugs for the period of time usually required to obtain therapeutic effects. In addition, these drugs, by definition, have been given to patients having specific psychiatric illnesses rather than normal experimental animals.

This review is limited to effects associated with the use of antipsychotic drugs and agents used in the treatment of affective disorders (mania and/or depression) or other psychotic states, e. g. schizophrenia. Finally, wherever possible the implications of the data for an increase in our understanding of the biological bases of psychopathology is noted.

ANTIPSYCHOTIC DRUGS AND HUMAN CNS AMINE METABOLISM

In 1963 Carlsson & Lindqvist concluded from a series of animal studies that while the antipsychotic drugs chlorpromazine or haloperidol did not alter endogenous brain stores of NE or DA they did produce increases in the metabolites of these amines. Furthermore, these changes were not produced by a phenothiazine, promethazine, which does not possess antipsychotic properties. Although there is still debate as to the mechanisms by which this increase in turnover is produced, results from a number of animal studies are consistent with the original observations by Carlsson & Lindqvist (26). Given these observations that emerged from acute experiments with animals, interest was aroused as to the effects of a number of different antipsychotic drugs upon DA and 5-HT metabolism in patients suffering from a variety of psychotic disorders. In these studies, which are summarized below, the focus has been primarily upon the metabolites of DA and 5-HT in CSF.

In 1968 Persson & Roos (27) reported that two schizophrenic patients who previously had been treated with neuroleptics without effect and who were unmedicated at the time of the study were accidentally given 20 and 40 mg of haloperidol respectively. It was noted that the patient who had received the 40 mg of haloperidol had a twofold increase in CSF HVA, whereas in the other patient CSF HVA did not change. In a subsequent and more systematic study they examined the effects on CSF HVA and 5-HIAA of antipsychotic drugs of the phenothiazine type in 40 chronic schizophrenic patients (28). The patients were divided into groups according to whether they had received high, medium, or low doses of the drugs. All patients were then taken off medication for four days and samples of CSF were obtained. It was found that those patients who had been receiving high or medium doses of drugs had significantly greater levels of CSF HVA than did those patients who had received the low doses of the drugs. There were no differences noted in CSF 5-HIAA.

Bowers et al (29) examined the effects of phenothiazine treatment (equivalent to 600 mg per day of chlorpromazine) on CSF 5-HIAA and HVA levels. They found no significant differences between the predrug and treatment values. It should be noted, however, that all of the schizophrenic patients in this study had received some phenothiazines prior to admission and that the drug treatment CSF specimens were obtained one to four months after the patients had been started on a phenothiazine drug. This last issue is important because of the development of "biochemical" tolerance, as is discussed later in this review. The authors further note that the values for CSF HVA both before and during drug treatment were high and make the comment that this is consistent with data from animal studies that indicate that these drugs produce an increased turnover of brain DA. It is thus possible that the lack of a difference in the quantities of CSF in HVA between the pretreatment and treatment periods was due to the treatment of the schizophrenic patients with antipsychotic drugs prior to entry into the study and/or the development of tolerance. No differences in CSF 5-HIAA were noted between the pretreatment and treatment periods.

Fyrö et al (30) examined the effects of chlorpromazine on CSF HVA levels of schizophrenic patients using a more sensitive and specific method, i. e. mass fragmentography. Further, the patients in this study had an extended washout period of two months and were given a single drug, chlorpromazine, in the range of 200 to 600 mg per day for 12 days. They found that women had significantly higher HVA levels than did men, but that for both sexes treatment with chlorpromazine produced a twofold or greater increase in CSF HVA. Interestingly enough, they also found a negative correlation between the dose of chlorpromazine and the increase in CSF HVA; that is, the lower the dose of chlorpromazine the greater the increase in HVA during treatment.

Chase et al (31) examined the effects of antipsychotic drugs on CSF HVA and 5-HIAA in a chronic schizophrenic patient group with particular emphasis upon the relationship of amine metabolites to drug-induced extrapyramidal disorders. Three patients groups were chosen. Group one was composed of chronic schizophrenic patients who had received no drug treatment for at least two weeks. Groups two and three were patients who had been on a variety of phenothiazine drugs for periods of greater than one year with patients in Group two being those who had no extrapyramidal signs and those in Group three being patients with extrapyramidal disorders. It was found that there were differences between Groups one and two in terms of CSF HVA and 5-HIAA; that is, these metabolites were increased in the group of patients receiving drugs. In contrast, many of those patients who had extrapyramidal side effects had metabolite levels similar to those in Group one. The authors speculated that compensatory increases in amine metabolism may be impaired in subjects having extrapyramidal disorders. If one excludes the issue of motoric dysfunctions as induced by the drugs, the data from this study are generally supportive of the concept that phenothiazine drugs in man produce an increased turnover of DA and perhaps 5-HT.

Beginning in 1972 a series of studies appeared in which the problem of DA and 5-HT metabolism as influenced by the antipsychotic drugs was again evaluted but with the use of probenecid. Sjöstrom & Roos (32) examined the effects of probenecid versus probenecid plus methylperidol (a neuroleptic). They found that the probenecid plus the methylperidol produced a further increase in 5-HIAA which was significant, whereas there was only a trend toward a further increment in HVA. In another study they determined CSF HVA and 5-HIAA during a baseline period, following probenecid, and finally following probenecid plus methylperidol. The results of this second study were similar to those obtained in the first one. In addition, Sjöstrom & Roos used as their control subjects patients who had a variety of neurological diseases; they noted that many of these comparison subjects had been taking neuroleptics of the phenothiazine or butyrophenone type for some time and that there was no differences in CSF HVA or 5-HIAA between those subjects who did, and those who did not, take neuroleptics.

Using the probenecid technique, Bowers (33) examined the effect on CSF 5-HIAA and HVA in patients treated with phenothiazines, haloperidol, and in some cases benztropine. Twenty-five acutely psychotic patients made up the study group and patients were maintained off drugs for at least two weeks prior to obtaining the baseline CSF specimens. Following the institution of antipsychotic drug treatment, CSF specimens were again obtained after a two to six month period. It was found that HVA but not 5-HIAA was significantly increased by drug treatment. There was, however, no correlation between the increase in HVA and the dosage of medication used, nor did the use of the anticholinergic agent, benztropine, appear to have a relationship to changes in HVA. Parenthetically, it should be noted that Guldberg et al found that ventricular quantities of CSF HVA or 5-HIAA were not changed by some commonly used anticholinergic drugs (34).

Bowers noted that in several of the studies that examined the relationship between antipsychotic drugs and changes in CSF metabolites, there was a significant incidence of extrapyramidal side effects that occurred in conjunction with the use of these drugs, and as such, the question arose as to whether or not the noted changes of HVA in CSF occurred as a function of the extrapyramidal side effects or as a function of the antipsychotic properties of the drugs. He approached this problem via the use of thioridazine which has a low incidence of extrapyramidal disorders associated with its usage. In this study, fourteen patients diagnosed as being within the schizophrenic spectrum were maintained drug free for two weeks and a CSF specimen following probenecid was obtained. Thioridazine treatment was then started, and another CSF specimen following probenecid was obtained 18 to 44 days after the beginning of treatment. It was noted that significant extrapyramidal side effects were found in only one patient but that there was a significant increase in CSF HVA induced by thioridazine. Bowers also found that treatment with thioridazine resulted in a significant reduction of 5-HIAA in CSF; however, he also found that the drug produced a decrease in CSF probenecid levels and concluded that the effects of 5-HIAA were probably artifactual (25). The finding that this particular drug can influence CSF levels of probenecid should serve as a note of warning to future investigators that it cannot be assumed that antipsychotic drugs have no effect upon probenecid levels in the CSF.

Gerlach et al (35) examined the relationship between extrapyramidal reactions and amine metabolites in CSF during haloperidol and clozapine treatment of schizophrenic patients. This study was particularly well designed in that it was done in a double-blind fashion with drug crossovers, and CSF specimens were obtained at 0, 4, and 21 days for both drugs. Furthermore, there was a washout period of three weeks prior to the beginning of the first and second drugs. It was found that with haloperidol treatment the HVA levels were increased over baseline at four days and there was a tendency to return toward baseline by 21 days. Clozapine induced a fall in HVA of 34%, which was statistically significant, but after 21 days of treatment the CSF HVA levels were not significantly different from baseline. The concentration of 5-HIAA was not affected by treatment with haloperidol but was significantly decreased after four days of treatment with clozapine, although after 21 days of treatment the levels of 5-HIAA were not significantly different from baseline. CSF probenecid levels were not assayed in this study.

Post & Goodwin (36) focused specifically upon the temporal effects of antipsychotic drug administration in relationship to changes in CSF HVA levels. Their patients were not followed longitudally and the number of patients treated for the short period of time was relatively small; however, their data are generally consistent with that of other investigations; that is, after 15–19 days of treatment with phenothiazines there was an increase in CSF HVA, but there was no significant difference after treatment for 25 to 77 days. These investigators also examined five patients who were treated with pimozide and found that in three of these patients the initial elevation in HVA that occurred between days five and twelve of treatment were not seen after 16 to 26 days of treatment.

Rüther et al (38) studied the temporal relationships between changes in CSF HVA and 5-HIAA and shifts in psychopathological states (paranoid-hallucinatory syndrome) associated with treatment with haloperidol. They found significant differences in CSF HVA (but not 5-HIAA) five days after drug treatment although the change in psychotic symptoms was slight. After 15 days of treatment significant antipsychotic effects were observed, but there was only a trend toward a significant difference in CSF HVA. In another study from the same group, Schilkrut et al (37) examined the relationships between changes in psychopathological symptoms, extrapyramidal side effects, and CSF HVA and 5-HIAA during treatment with haloperidol. They found at 15 days that there were significant antipsychotic effects, that parkinsonism scores had increased slightly, and that CSF HVA, but not 5-HIAA, was significantly increased.

In summary, the following statements may be made regarding the effects of the antipsychotic drugs on central nervous system amine metabolism in man.

1. Although there are exceptions, most investigators have found increases in human lumbar CSF HVA following the administration of structurally dissimilar drugs which have in common, however, antipsychotic properties. This increase in CSF HVA is probably due to an increased turnover of DA. This finding is consistent with data that have been obtained by more direct approaches in experimental animals.

2. The study by Gerlach et al (35) is particularly important in that these investigators have found that clozapine, an antipsychotic drug, produced a decrement rather than an increment in CSF HVA and 5-HIAA when given acutely. Since clozapine possesses antipsychotic properties the decrement (rather than an increment) in CSF HVA poses problems for a DA theory of schizophrenia.

3. The situation with 5-HIAA is less clear than with HVA. Several investigators have not found changes in CSF 5-HIAA, with or without probenecid, following the administration of antipsychotic drugs but there are some important exceptions. In general, where changes in 5-HIAA have been found, they appear to be less dramatic than those that occur with HVA.

4. Increases in CSF HVA following the administration of antipsychotic drugs occur even though extrapyramidal symptoms are not present.

5. Inspection of the data presented in several reports indicates that with chronic adminstration of the antipsychotic drugs there is a tendency for amine metabolite concentrations to return toward predrug levels. This development of "tolerance" is also compatible with data obtained from experiments with animals.

6. A relationship between drug-induced changes in CSF amine metabolites and alterations in clinical state has not been established. This issue of CSF amine metabolite concentration and therapeutic change has not, however, been intensively studied.

ANTIDEPRESSANT DRUGS AND HUMAN CNS AMINE METABOLISM

In an initial report, Bowers et al (29) noted that patients who were being treated with amitriptyline had significant reductions in CSF 5-HIAA relative to a baseline period. In contrast, no significant differences in homovanillic acid concentration during the two periods were seen. In a subsequent study Bowers (39) used the probenecid technique to further examine the effects of amitriptyline upon the accumulation of 5-HIAA and HVA in lumbar CSF. In this study the patient group consisted of 11 subjects who were diagnosed as having unipolar depressions with the dose range of amitriptyline being 150–300 mg per day. Baseline and repeat CSF specimens (after probenecid) were taken after six to eight weeks of drug treatment.

It was found that during the period of drug treatment there was a significant decrease in CSF 5-HIAA and a trend toward a decrease in HVA. In another study Bowers further found that levels of L-tryptophan in the CSF before and during treatment with amitriptyline were the same, suggesting that the differences in CSF 5-HIAA during drug treatment were not secondary to precursor availability (40).

Papeschi & McClure (41) also noted similar significant decreases in CSF 5-HIAA but not homovanillic acid following two weeks of imipramine treatment. Post & Goodwin (42) noted that the treatment of patients with amitriptyline or imipramine was associated with a decreased accumulation of 5-HIAA in CSF, but they found no differences for HVA. Sjöstrom & Roos (32) compared the effects of antidepressant tricyclic drugs (not further specified) versus some other "adequate medication" for depressed subjects but found no differences for the two groups between CSF 5-HIAA and HVA. Mendels et al (43) noted that there was a small increase in CSF 5-HIAA after treatment of manic-depressive, depressed patients and a slight drop in 5-HIAA after treatment of the manic patients. In constrast, it was noted that in a small number of subjects there was an increase in CSF HVA after the treatment. Although it can be assumed that some specific form of antimanic or antidepressant treatment was given, the type of drugs used was not indicated and hence the data are difficult to evaluate.

Jori et al (44) examined the effects of ECT and imipramine treatment on the concentrations of CSF 5-HIAA and HVA of depressed patients. Lumbar punctures were performed both before and after probenecid administration prior to and after antidepressant treatment. The pretreatment lumbar punctures were performed five to seven days apart and the third and fourth lumbar punctures were performed seven days after the ECT or the last dose of imipramine and the fourth and final lumbar punctures (with probenecid) five to seven days later. It was found that ECT treatment was associated with an increase in the absolute (preprobenecid) values of CSF HVA and 5-HIAA whereas imipramine treatment was not. When the accumulation of the two acids as a function of probenecid administration was examined it was found that there were no significant differences between the pretreatment and treatment periods for either ECT or imipramine. It should be noted, however, that the fourth lumbar puncture in this study was performed two weeks following the cessation of drug treatment and this artifactual washout period may account for the discrepancy between the results found by this group of investigators and those of others.

Asberg et al (45) examined the effects of nortriptyline administration on CSF 5-HIAA and IAA. In this study the metabolites were assayed using the method of mass fragmentography and all patients had been on medication for three weeks prior to the performance of the second lumbar puncture. It was found that during treatment the concentrations of 5-HIAA and IAA decreased significantly, but the decrements were not correlated with plasma levels of nortriptyline. Bertilsson et al (46) determined CSF MHPG and 5-HIAA levels in CSF both before and during the treatment of depressed patients with chlorimipramine or nortriptyline. The second CSF specimen (during treatment with one of the noted antidepressant drugs) was obtained three weeks after the beginning of treatment. It was found that MHPG levels in CSF decreased significantly with treatment with either chlorimipramine or nortriptyline. Nortriptyline treatment was also associated with a decrement in CSF MHPG, but in contrast to the earlier study of Asberg et al (45) there was no change in CSF 5-HIAA during the treatment with nortriptyline.

Three separate groups of investigators (47–49) have demonstrated that treatment of patients with imipramine results in marked decrements in the urinary excretion of vanilylmandelic acid (VMA) and an increment in urinary normetanephrine (NM) (which did not, however, equal the decrement in VMA). The experimental approaches in these investigations did not allow for a definitive interpretation as to the mechanisms that might be involved, although it appeared that a decrement in overall synthesis of catecholamines was being produced by imipramine. If therapeutic outcome is ignored (see later), imipramine treatment is not associated with a significant change in urinary MHPG.

In addition to the above-noted general pharmacological effects on amine metabolism of a variety of tricyclic antidepressant drugs, there are preliminary data that suggest that the changes in amine metabolism and/or dispostion that occur with treatment with the tricyclic drugs may vary with the repsonse of the patient to a particular drug and conversely that pretreatment amine metabolite levels may be associated with response, or a failure of response, to a particular drug.

As an example, Maas et al (49) reported that patients who responded well to imipramine or desmethylimipramine had low pretreatment 24-hr urinary MHPG values and that when MHPG was assayed during the fourth week of treatment with these drugs, the level of MHPG in the urine for the responder group showed modest increments or no change. In marked contrast were those patients who had normal or high pretreatment MHPG concentrations; that is, these patients tended not to respond to imipramine or desmethylimipramine, and during the fourth week of treatment there was a marked decrement in urinary MHPG. While pretreatment urinary NM was not associated with a response to imipramine or desmethylimipramine those patients who responded particularly well to imipramine or desmethylimipramine had marked increases in NM during the fourth week of treatment relative to baseline periods. There was a significant decrement in urinary VMA whether or not the patients responded to treatment. Schildkraut et al (50) found in a preliminary study that high or normal baseline urinary MHPG was associated with a favorable response to amitriptyline. Beckmann & Goodwin (51) also found that low pretreatment urinary MHPG concentrations were associated with a good response to imipramine and a failure to respond to amitriptyline. They also noted that normal or greater than normal amounts of MHPG in urine were associated with a favorable response to amitriptyline and failure of response to imipramine. However, in contrast to the findings of Maas et al (49), imipramine treatment was associated with a decrease in urinary MHPG in the responder group.

Asberg et al (45) made the observation that while as a group nortriptyline produced a decrement in 5-HIAA and IAA in CSF, if one looked at the patients in terms of those having low versus high CSF 5-HIAA levels, a different pattern emerged. In seven of the patients who had pretreatment 5-HIAA levels below 15 ng/ml of CSF, the 5-HIAA concentration increased in five patients and decreased in two. In contrast, in the 13 patients with an initial 5-HIAA concentration higher than 15 ng/ml the 5-HIAA levels decreased in all.

Van Praag & Korf (52) have published preliminary data indicating that the therapeutic response of patients to 5-hydroxytryptophan may be associated with the pretreatment rate at which patients accumulate 5-HIAA in CSF following probenecid; that is, those depressed patients having the smallest increments in 5-HIAA accumulation after probenecid do best when given 5-hydroxytryptophan. Goodwin & Post (53) observed that tricyclic drug treatment was associated with a slight increase in CSF MHPG among those patients who were classified as responders but that there was a significant decrease in MHPG among the nonresponders. They note that the responder/nonresponder difference in the tricyclic effect on MHPG was highly significant ($P<0.001$). They also note that patients who subsequently responded to treatment with the tricyclic drugs had higher pretreatment accumulations of 5-HIAA and HVA following probenecid as compared with those who did not respond (the types of tricyclic drugs used in these studies were not specified).

The above studies are of interest because they indicate that some types of biochemical responses that one obtains with treatment with a particular drug may vary as a function of the therapeutic outcome. In addition, these reports support the concept that depression is a biochemically heterogeneous illness and have led to the suggestion that there are biochemical and pharmacological criteria by which two types of depression may be separated (54).

In summary the following CNS amine metabolite changes have been found with antidepressant drug treatment.

1. Most investigators have found that amitriptyline or imipramine administration to depressed patients for three weeks or longer is not associated with changes in CSF HVA accumulation following probenecid. This finding is in agreement with animal studies which indicate that at doses similar to those that are used therapeutically the tricyclic antidepressants have little effect upon brain DA systems.

2. Although there are discrepant findings, it would appear that treatment of depressed patients with amitriptyline or imipramine for three weeks or longer is associated with a decrement in the accumulation of CSF 5-HIAA after probenecid administration. This finding is consistent with data from animal studies that indicate that these two drugs produce a decrease in brain 5-HT turnover.

3. Changes in MHPG associated with tricyclic antidepressant drug treatment have been less well studied than those of 5-HIAA and HVA. There is some suggestive evidence, however, which indicates that this metabolite may change as a function of the therapeutic response of the patient, i.e. patients who respond well to treatment may have modest increments in MHPG whereas nonresponders have marked decrements. Further, there is agreement among different groups of investigators that pretreatment levels of urinary MHPG are predictive of a response, or failure of response, to amitriptyline versus imipramine. It thus appears that there may be interactions between pretreatment amine metabolism, the type of tricyclic drug used, therapeutic response, and the type of biochemical change associated with the drug being used.

LITHIUM TREATMENT AND CNS AMINE METABOLISM

In 1971 Mendels reported that two manic patients who had been treated with lithium for 85 and 57 days had a marked increment in CSF 5-HIAA during the treatment period as compared to the prelithium period (55). Wilk et al noted that there was a sharp increase in CSF 5-HIAA with a moderate increase in HVA in two manic patients who were treated with lithium carbonate. The time of treatment in this study was not specified (56). In contrast to these preliminary findings neither Bowers (29) nor Sjöstrom & Roos (32) found any effects on 5-HIAA or HVA in CSF as a consequence of lithium treatment. It should be noted, however, that in the Bowers et al study the time on lithium was not specified. In addition, in the Sjöstrom & Roos study 57 manic patients were studied but one third of these had been on lithium before inclusion in the research and some of the manic patients received antipsychotic drugs during the time of treatment. Some of these design and pharmacological problems may have confounded the results.

Fyro et al (57) studied a group of 13 acutely manic or hypomanic patients. None of the patients had received any drugs for at least one month prior to study. CSF specimens were obtained both prior to beginning lithium and 12 days after the start of lithium treatment. Plasma levels were maintained within the therapeutic range of 0.7 and 1.4 meq/liter. It was found that the quantities of CSF 5-HIAA as well as HVA increased significantly during the treatment period.

Goodwin & Post (58) in contrast to the other studies examined the effects on CSF metabolites of lithium carbonate in depressed rather than manic patients. They found that during the treatment period depressed patients had probenecid-induced accumulations of 5-HIAA which were low in comparison to the prelithium period. HVA was not significantly altered between the treatment and nontreatment periods. It is of interest that the changes in 5-HIAA induced by or accompanying lithium treatment in depressed patients were in the opposite direction of those found with manic subjects.

Wilk et al (56) found that treatment with lithium carbonate of two manic patients produced a marked decrease in CSF MHPG. Both patients had good clinical responses to lithium. Schildkraut (59) noted that there was a sharp increase in urinary MHPG which occurred coincident with the beginning of lithium treatment and lasted for approximately seven to ten days. Even though the patient was continued on lithium, however, the urinary MHPGs then returned toward baseline levels and remained there for the next 35 days. Beckmann et al (60) treated ten depressed patients (eight bipolar and two unipolar) with lithium carbonate and looked at both the therapeutic responses of the patients and the changes in urinary MHPG that occurred during the lithium treatment. In their group they found that there were four patients who were unequivocal responders and six patients who were nonresponders to lithium treatment. They noted that during the first week there was no consistent change in urinary MHPG but looking at the third to fourth week of treatment all of the responders had increases in urinary MHPG values and all nonresponders had a decrement in urinary MHPG or no change in this NE metabolite.

In summary there are relatively few studies of the effects of lithium upon CNS amine metabolism in man but taking into account a variety of methodological issues it appears that lithium treatment of manic patients is associated with an increase in CSF 5-HIAA and HVA. This finding is consistent with the report that lithium induces an increased turnover of brain amines in animals. However, the finding by Goodwin et al (58) that depressed patients in contrast to manic patients have a *decrement* in CSF 5-HIAA accumulation during treatment with lithium indicates that the pharmacological response of patients may vary as a function of the type or phase of the illness. The report (60) which indicates that depressed patients who respond to lithium have changes in MHPG that differ from those of nonresponders again raises this issue.

Literature Cited

1. Moir, A. T. B., Ashcroft, G. W., Crawford, T. B. B., Eccleston, D., Guldberg, H. C. 1970. Cerebral metabolites in cerebrospinal fluid as a biochemical approach to the brain. *Brain* 93:357–68
2. Curzon, G., Gumpert, E. J. W., Sharpe, D. M. 1971. Amine metabolites in the lumbar cerebrospinal fluid of humans with restricted flow of cerebrospinal fluid. *Nature New Biol.* 231:189–91
3. Post, R. M., Goodwin, F. K., Gordon, E., Watkin, D. M. 1973. Amine metabolites in human cerebrospinal fluid: Effects of cord transsection and spinal fluid block. *Science* 179:897–99
4. Garelis, E., Sourkes, T. L. 1973. Sites of origin in the central nervous system of monoamine metabolites measured in human cerebrospinal fluid. *J. Neurol. Neurosurg. Psychiatry* 4:625–29
5. Atack, C. V. 1973. The determination of dopamine by a modification of the dihydroxyindole fluorimetric assay. *Br. J. Pharmacol.* 48:699–714
6. Stanton, E. S., Smolen, P. M., Nashold, B. S. Jr., Dreyer, D. A., Davis, J. N. 1975. Segmental analysis of spinal cord monoamines after thoracic transection in the dog. *Brain Res.* 89:93–98
7. Bartholini, G., Pletscher, A., Tissot, R. 1966. On the origin of homovanillic acid in the cerebrospinal fluid. *Experientia* 22:609–10
8. Guldberg, H. C., Yates, C. M. 1968. Some studies of the effects of chlorpromazine, reserpine, and dihydroxyphenylalamine on the concentrations of homovanillic acid, 3,4-dihydroxyphenylacetic acid and 5-hydroxyindol-3-acetic acid in ventricular cerebrospinal fluid in the dog using the technique of serial sampling of the cerebrospinal fluid. *Br. J. Pharmacol.* 33:457–71

9. Sourkes, T. L. 1973. On the origin of homovanillic acid (HVA) in the cerebrospinal fluid. *J. Neural Transm.* 34:153–57
10. Tamarkin, N. R., Goodwin, F. K., Axelrod, J. 1970. Rapid elevation of biogenic amine metabolites in human CSF following probenecid. *Life Sci.* 9:1397–1408
11. Bulat, M., Zivkovic, B. 1973. Penetration of 5-hydroxyindoleacetic acid across the blood cerebrospinal fluid barrier. *J. Pharm. Pharmacol.* 29:178–79
12. Ashcroft, G. W., Dow, R. C., Moir, A. T. B. 1968. The active transport of 5-hydroxyindol-3-acetic acid and 3-methoxy-4-hydroxyphenylacetic acid from a recirculatory perfusion system of the cerebral ventricles of the unanesthesized dog. *J. Physiol. London* 199:397–425
13. Garelis, E., Young, S. N., Lal, S., Sourkes, T. L. 1974. Monoamine metabolites in lumbar CSF: the question of their origin in relation to clinical studies. *Brain Res.* 79:1–8
14. Chase, T. N., Gordon, E. K., Ng, L. K. Y. 1973. Norepinephrine metabolism in the central nervous system of man: Studies using 3-methoxy-4-hydroxyphenethyleneglycol in cerebrospinal fluid. *J. Neurochem.* 21:581–87
15. Kessler, J. A., Fenstermacher, J. D., Patlak, C. S. 1976. 3-Methoxy-4-hydroxyphenylene glycol (MHPG) transport from the spinal cord during spinal subarachnoid perfusion. *Brain Res.* 102:131–41
16. Bareggi, S. R., Marc, V., Morselli, P. L. 1974. Urinary excretion of 3-methoxy-4-hydroxphenylglycol sulfate in rats after intraventricular injection of 6-OHDA. *Brain Res.* 75:177–80

17. Karoum, F., Wyatt, R., Costa, E. 1974. Estimation of the contribution of peripheral and central noradrenergic neurons to urinary 3-methoxy-4-hydroxyphenylglycol in the rat. *Neuropharmacology* 13:165–76

18. Breese, G. R., Prange, A. J., Howard, J. L., Lipton, M. A. 1972. Noradrenaline metabolite excretion after central sympathectomy with 6-hydroxydopamine. *Nature New Biol.* 240:286–87

19. Maas, J. W., Landis, D. H. 1968. In vivo studies of the metabolism of norepinephrine in the central nervous system. *J. Pharmacol. Exp. Ther.* 163:147–62

20. Maas, J. W., Dekirmenjian, H., Garver, D., Redmond, D. E. Jr., Landis, D. H. 1973. Excretion of catecholamine metabolites following intraventricular injection of 6-hydroxydopamine in the *Macaca* speciosa. *Eur. J. Pharmacol.* 23:121–30

21. Maas, J. W., Landis, D. H. 1971. The metabolism of circulating norepinephrine by human subjects. *J. Pharmacol. Exp. Ther.* 177:600–12

22. Ebert, M. H., Kopin, I. J. 1975. Differential labelling of origins of urinary catecholamine metabolites by dopamine-[14]C. *Trans. Assoc. Am. Physicians* 88:256–64

23. Korf, J., Van Praag, H. M., Sebens, J. B. 1971. Effect of intravenously administered probenecid in humans on the levels of 5-hydroxyindoleacetic acid, homovanillic acid and 3-methoxy-4-hydroxyphenylglycol in cerebrospinal fluid. *Biochem. Pharmacol.* 20:659–68

24. Gordon, E. K., Oliver, J., Goodwin, F. K., Chase, T. N., Post, R. M. 1973. Effect of probenecid on free 3-methoxy-4-hydroxyphenethyleneglycol (MHPG) and its sulfate in human cerebrospinal fluid. *Neuropharmacology* 12:391–96

25. Bowers, M. B. Jr. 1975. Thioridazine: Central dopamine turnover and clinical effects of antipsychotic drugs. *Clin. Pharmacol. Ther.* 17:73–78

26. Carlsson, A., Lindqvist, M. 1963. Effect of chlorpromazine or haloperidol on formation of 3-methoxytyramine and noremetanephrine in mouse brain. *Acta Pharmacol. Toxicol.* 20:140–44

27. Persson, T., Roos, B-E. 1968. Clinical and pharmacological effects of monoamine precursors or haloperidol in chronic schizophrenia. *Nature* 217:854

28. Persson, T., Roos, B-E. 1969. Acid metabolites from monoamines in cerebrospinal fluid of chronic schizophrenics. *Br. J. Psychiatry* 115:95–98

29. Bowers, M. B. Jr., Heninger, G. R., Gerbode, F. 1969. Cerebrospinal fluid 5-hydroxyindoleacetic acid and homovanillic acid in psychiatric patients. *Int. J. Neuropharmacol.* 8:255–62

30. Fyrö, B., Wode-Helgodt, B., Borg, F., Sedvall, G. 1974. The effect of chlorpromazine on homovanillic acid levels and cerebrospinal fluid of schizophrenic patients. *Psychopharmacologia* 35:287–94

31. Chase, T. N., Schnur, J. A., Gordon, E. K. 1970. Cerebrospinal fluid monoamine metabolites in drug induced extrapyramidal disorders. *Neuropharmacology.* 9:265–68

32. Sjöstrom, R., Roos, B-E. 1972. 5-Hydroxyindoleacetic acid and homovanillic acid in cerebrospinal fluid in manic depressive psychosis. *Eur. J. Clin. Pharmacol.* 4:170–76

33. Bowers, M. B. Jr. 1973. 5-Hydroxyindoleacetic acid (5-HIAA) and homovanillic acid (HVA) following probenecid in acute psychotic patients treated with phenothiazines. *Psychopharmacologia* 28:309–18

34. Guldberg, H. C., Turner, J. W., Hanieh, A., Ashcroft, G. W., Crawford, T. B. B., Perry, W. L. M., Gillingham, F. J. 1967. On the occurrence of homovanillic acid and 5-hydroxyindoleacetic acid in the ventricular spinal fluid of patients suffering from Parkinsonism. *Confin. Neurol.* 29:73–77

35. Gerlach, J., Thorsen, K., Fog, R. 1975. Extrapyramidal reactions and amine metabolites in cerebrospinal fluid during haloperidol and clozapine treatment of schizophrenic patients. *Psychopharmacologia* 40:341–50

36. Post, R. M., Goodwin, F. K. 1975. Time dependent effects of phenothiazines on dopamine turnover in psychiatric patients. *Science* 190:488–89

37. Schilkrut, R., Rüther, E., Ackenheil, M., Even, E., Hippius, H. 1976. Clinical and biochemical parameters during neuroleptic treatment. *Pharmakopsychiatr. Neuro Psychopharmakol.* 9:37–42

38. Rüther, E., Schilkrut, R., Ackenheil, M., Even, E., Hippius, H. 1976. Clinical and biochemical parameters during neuroleptic treatment. *Pharmakopsychiatr. Neuro Psychopharmakol.* 9:33–36

39. Bowers, M. B. Jr. 1972. Cerebrospinal fluid 5-hydroxyindoleacetic acid (5-

HIAA) and homovanillic acid (HVA) following probenecid in unipolar depressives treated with amitriptyline. *Psychopharmacologia* 23:26–33

40. Bowers, M. B. Jr. 1974. Amitriptyline in man: Decreased formation of central 5-hydroxyindoleacetic acid. *Clin. Pharmacol. Ther.* 15:167–70

41. Papeschi, R., McClure, D. J. 1971. Homovanillic and 5-hydroxyindoleacetic acid in cerebrospinal fluid of depressed patients. *Arch Gen. Psychiatry* 25:354–58

42. Post, R. M., Goodwin, F. K. 1974. Effects of amitriptyline and imipramine on amine metabolites in the cerebrospinal fluid of depressed patients. *Arch. Gen. Psychiatry* 30:234–39

43. Mendels, J., Frazer, A., Fitzgerald, R. J., Ramsey, T. A. Stokes, J. W. 1972. Biogenic amine metabolites in cerebrospinal fluid of depressed and manic patients. *Science* 175:1380–82

44. Jori, A., Dolfini, E., Casati, C., Argenta, G. 1975. Effect of ECT and imipramine treatment on the concentration of 5-hydroxyindoleacetic acid (5-HIAA) and homovanillic acid (HVA) in the cerebrospinal fluid of depressed patients. *Psychopharmacologia* 44:87–90

45. Asberg, M., Bertilsson, L., Tuck, D., Cronholm, B., Sjöqvist, F. 1973. Indolamine metabolites in the cerebrospinal fluid of depressed patients before and during treatment with nortriptyline. *Clin. Pharmacol. Ther.* 14:277–86

46. Bertilsson, L., Asberg, M., Thoren, P. 1974. Differential effect of chlorimipramine and nortriptyline on metabolites of serotonin and noradrenalin in the cerebrospinal fluid of depressed patients. *Eur. J. Clin. Pharmacol.* 7: 365–68

47. Schildkraut, J. J., Gordon, E. K., Durell, J. 1965. Catecholamine metabolism in affective disorders. I. Noremetanephrine and VMA excretion in depressed patients treated with imipramine. *J. Psychiatr. Res.* 3:213–28

48. Prange, A. J. Jr., Wilson, I. C., Knox, A. E., McClane, T. K., Breese, G. R., Martin, B. R., Alltop, L. P., Lipton, M. A. 1971. Thyroid-imipramine interaction: clinical results and basic mechanism. In *Brain Chemistry and Mental*

Disease, ed. B. T. Ho, W. M. McIsaac, p. 208. New York: Plenum

49. Maas, J. W., Fawcett, J. A., Dekirmenjian, H. 1972. Catecholamine metabolism, depressive illness and drug response. *Arch. Gen. Psychiatry* 26: 252–62

50. Schildkraut, J. J. 1973. Norepinephrine metabolites as biochemical criteria for classifying depressive disorders and predicting responses to treatment: Preliminary findings. *Am. J. Psychiatry* 130:695–99

51. Beckmann, H., Goodwin, F. K. 1975. Antidepressant response to tricyclics and urinary MHPG in unipolar patients. *Arch. Gen. Psychiatry* 32:17–21

52. Van Praag, H. M., Korf, J. 1974. 5-Hydroxytryptophan as an antidepressant. *J. Nerv. Ment. Dis.* 158:331–37

53. Goodwin, F. K., Post, R. M. 1975. Studies of amine metabolites in affective illness and in schizophrenia: A comparative analysis. In *Biology of the Major Psychoses: A Comparative Analysis,* ed. D. X. Freedman. New York: Raven

54. Maas, J. W. 1975. Biogenic amines and depression. *Arch. Gen. Psychiatry* 32:1357–61

55. Mendels, J. 1971. Relationship between depression and mania. *Lancet* 1:342

56. Wilk, S., Shopsin, B., Gershon, S., Suhl, M. 1972. Cerebrospinal fluid levels of MHPG in affective disorders. *Nature* 235:41–44

57. Fyro, B., Petterson, U., Sedvall, G. 1975. The effect of lithium treatment on manic symptoms and levels of monoamine metabolites in cerebrospinal fluid of manic depressive patients. *Psychopharmacologia* 44:99–103

58. Goodwin, F. K., Post, R. M., Sack, R. L. 1975. Clinical evidence for neurochemical adaptation to psychotropic drugs. In *Neurobiological Mechanisms of Adaptation and Behavior,* ed. A. J. Mandell. New York: Raven

59. Schildkraut, J. J. 1974. The effects of lithium on norepinephrine turnover and metabolism: Basic and clinical studies. *J. Nerv. Ment. Dis.* 158:348:60

60. Beckmann, H., St.-Laurent, J., Goodwin, F. K. 1975. The effect of lithium on urinary MHPG in unipolar and bipolar depressed patients. *Psychopharmacologia* 42:277–82

PUTATIVE PEPTIDE NEUROTRANSMITTERS

♦6689

Masanori Otsuka and Tomoyuki Takahashi

Department of Pharmacology, Faculty of Medicine, Tokyo Medical and Dental University, Yushima, Bunkyo-ku, Tokyo, Japan

The purpose of this review is to examine the present status of peptides as putative neurotransmitters. Special emphasis is placed on the evaluation of evidence for or against the transmitter role of peptides, particularly in mammalian CNS, according to the well-established criteria for transmitter identification (1, 2). The field of peptide transmitters is a new and rapidly developing one, and therefore, we can derive from the available results only tentative views as to whether or not certain peptides are likely to be transmitters. Although a number of peptides are known to influence various neural activities such as behavior and sleep (3–5), this review deals only with the peptides of known structures for which there is certain or definite neurochemical as well as electrophysiological evidence implicating their transmitter functions.

The notion that certain nerve cells secrete peptides from their axon terminals has been well known in the field of endocrinology since the early 1950s (6). Bargmann et al (7) proposed the term *peptidergic neuron* for hypothalamic neurosecretory cells, and suggested that these neurons not only release peptide hormones into the blood stream but also form peptidergic synapses on endocrine epithelial cells. Recent discovery of the powerful effects of physalaemin (8) and vasopressin on central neuronal activities (9) in 1971 sparked interest in the possibility that certain peptides may serve as neurotransmitters in mammalian CNS (10). This was timely because the recent progress in peptide chemistry was ready to promote the subsequent development of the field of peptide neuropharmacology. A considerable amount of data has accumulated that suggests the transmitter role of certain peptides. Particularly good evidence has been obtained for two peptides, substance P and proctolin, which are described below in detail.

SUBSTANCE P

In 1931, Euler & Gaddum (11) detected a smooth muscle–stimulating and vasodilating agent in extracts of equine brain and intestine. This agent was called substance P (12, 13) and was shown to be of peptide nature (14). Studies of substance P distribution in the early 1950s (15–19) revealed that mammalian spinal dorsal root contains a larger amount of substance P than the ventral root. Based on these results, Lembeck proposed a hypothesis that substance P may be an excitatory transmitter of primary sensory neurons (16). The studies of substance P, however, had long been hampered by the ambiguity of its chemical nature. In fact, no pure substance P preparation was available, and for many years Lembeck's hypothesis could not be properly tested. In the early study of Galindo et al (20) with the crude preparation, no direct action of substance P on cat central neurons could be detected.

A breakthrough in this field was made by the recent studies of Leeman and her colleagues, who succeeded in purifying substance P from bovine hypothalamus, determining its structure as an undecapeptide (Arg-Pro-Lys-Pro-Gln-Gln-Phe-Phe-Gly-Leu-Met-NH$_2$), and synthesizing the peptide (21–23). Before the discovery of the structure of the undecapeptide substance P, the definition of substance P was based on its pharmacological activities (24). Thus so-called substance P was postulated to comprise multiple peptides (25–27). However, it is now generally agreed that substance P denotes the peptide characterized by Chang et al (22).

Evidence for a Transmitter of Primary Sensory Neurons

PRESENCE OF SUBSTANCE P IN PRIMARY SENSORY NEURONS   Preferential distribution of substance P in spinal dorsal root as opposed to ventral root (15–19) was confirmed by recent studies using radioimmunoassay as well as bioassay combined with column chromatography (28–30). Thus it was revealed that the concentration of substance P in bovine and feline dorsal root is 9–27 times higher than that in the ventral root. Furthermore, the chemical, pharmacological, and immunological properties of substance P extracted from bovine dorsal root were shown (28, 29) to be identical with those of substance P extracted from hypothalamus and characterized by Chang et al (22). In order to examine further the relation between substance P and primary sensory neurons, Takahashi & Otsuka (30, 31), using bioassay, examined the distribution of substance P in cat spinal cord. It was thus shown that substance P is particularly concentrated in dorsal horn where a large part of the primary afferent fibers terminates and forms synapses (32). The highest level of substance P was found in the dorsal part of dorsal horn. After sectioning the incoming dorsal roots, the level of the peptide in the dorsal horn was markedly reduced. Furthermore, when the dorsal root was ligated, a large amount of substance P accumulated on the ganglion side of the ligature, which suggests that substance P is synthesized in spinal ganglia and transported through the dorsal root to their nerve terminals in the cord (30, 31). All these findings by bioassay were recently confirmed by immunohistochemical studies of Hökfelt and his colleagues, who showed that substance P-like immunoreactivity is selectively localized in nerve fibers of laminae I–III of spinal cord of the rat and cat (33, 34). The latter finding agrees with the results of subcellular fractionation studies using bioassay (35–37) as well as radioimmunoassay (38, 39), which indicate that substance P is most concentrated in synaptosomal fraction.

ACTION OF SUBSTANCE P ON SPINAL NEURONS   Application of synthetic substance P in quite low concentration induced a depolarization of motoneurons in isolated frog spinal cord (28, 40, 41). The depolarizing potency of substance P was, on a molar basis, about 200 times higher than that of L-glutamate, another excitatory transmitter candidate (42). Substance P-induced depolarization of frog spinal motoneurons was accompanied by the increase of membrane conductance (41). In order to examine the possibility that substance P may depolarize the motoneurons by a transsynaptic mechanism, substance P was applied after the synaptic transmission in the spinal cord was blocked by reducing Ca concentration in the medium or by adding tetrodotoxin (40, 41). Substance P still induced similar depolarizing responses indicating that the peptide acts directly on the motoneurons.

Recently the effect of substance P on mammalian spinal cord was studied. For this purpose, an isolated spinal cord preparation of the newborn rat was developed (43). Substance P was applied into the perfusion bath in known concentrations and the effects were recorded either extracellularly from the ventral root or intracellularly from the motoneurons. Substance P again induced a depolarization accompanied by high frequency spike discharges of the motoneurons (44–46). The depolarizing potency of substance P was 1000–9000 times higher than that of L-glutamate. When the preparation was soaked in a low Ca (0.2 mM) and high Mg (5 mM) medium, the spinal reflexes were completely blocked. Repetitive stimulation of the dorsal root did not produce any detectable synaptic potentials when recorded from the ventral root. Under such conditions, substance P still produced a similar depolarizing response although the dose-response curve was slightly displaced to the right. These results suggest that substance P causes the depolarization of rat motoneurons by both direct effect on the motoneurons and indirect effect activating the excitatory interneurons synapsing with the motoneurons (44–46; S. Konishi and M. Otsuka, unpublished). There is also evidence that substance P activates the inhibitory interneurons in the spinal cord (44). Electrophoretic application of substance P also produced an excitant effect on dorsal horn neurons and cuneate neurons of the cat (47, 48).

ANTAGONISTS OF SUBSTANCE P Several substances, e.g. AMP, cystine-di-β-naphthylamide, and trimethaphan camphorsulfonate (Arfonad®), were reported to antagonize the action of substance P on guinea pig ileum (49). It may be interesting to see whether or not these compounds antagonize the excitant action of substance P on central neurons. It was recently reported that baclofen [β-(4-chlorophenyl)-γ-aminobutyric acid, Lioresal®] antagonizes the depolarizing action of substance P on rat spinal motoneurons (45, 46). The depolarizing action of L-glutamate was also reduced, but to a smaller extent (45, 46; cf 50). Since baclofen readily blocked the monosynaptic and polysnaptic reflexes as well as the dorsal root potential (45, 46, 50–52), it was proposed that baclofen blocks the primary afferent transmission by antagonizing the transmitter action of substance P (45, 46). The antagonism between baclofen and substance P was also observed by electrophoretic application on neurons of cat spinal cord and brain, although the excitant effects of L-glutamate and acetylcholine were also depressed by baclofen in some but not all cells (53–55). Further studies are needed to clarify the mechanism of action of baclofen.

STRUCTURE-ACTIVITY RELATIONSHIP   From the studies on frog and rat spinal motoneurons, it has become evident that the C-terminal amino acid sequence is essential for the motoneuron-depolarizing activity of substance P (40, 46, 56, 57). Omission of one to five amino acids at the N-terminus did not cause any serious loss of the motoneuron-depolarizing activity. Two C-terminal analogues of substance P, i.e. hepta- and hexapeptides, were considerably more active than the undecapeptide substance P. By contrast, when the C-terminal methionine was omitted, the depolarizing activity was completely lost (46,57). Hypotensive and gut-contracting activities of the substance P analogues were roughly parallel with their motoneuron-depolarizing activities (58).

RELEASE OF SUBSTANCE P   Early studies of Angelucci (59) and Ramwell et al (60) showed the presence of substance P-like activity in the perfusate of frog spinal cord. Recently, the isolated spinal cord of newborn rat was perfused, and the perfusates were analyzed by radioimmunoassay for substance P (61). Repetitive stimulation of dorsal roots caused a marked increase of substance P–like immunoreactivity in the perfusate. By contrast, when the preparation was perfused with a low Ca and high Mg medium where the synaptic transmission was completely blocked, the same stimulation of dorsal roots produced no change of the immunoreactivity. Perfusion of the spinal cord with high K (55 mM) solution caused a large increase in release of substance P–like immunoreactivity. Potassium-evoked release of substance P–like immunoreactivy was also observed from rat hypothalamic slices, and this release was completely abolished in the low Ca and high Mg medium (62).

INACTIVATION OF SUBSTANCE P   There are two kinds of mechanisms known to inactivate transmitter substances, i.e. enzymatic breakdown and reuptake. When slices of rat spinal cord, substantia nigra, and hypothalamus were incubated with ^{125}I-labeled substance P, no accumulation of the peptide into the tissues could be detected (33, 62, 63). On the other hand, the presence of substance P-inactivating enzyme system in various regions of CNS, e.g. basal ganglia, hypothalamus, and spinal cord, was reported by many workers (64–70). The inactivating enzyme was extracted and partially purified from mammalian brain (69, 70). Studies of detailed distribution of this enzyme in nervous system will help to elucidate its physiological role. Furthermore, it will be interesting to find specific inhibitors of the substance P–inactivating enzyme and to examine their effect on primary afferent transmission in the spinal cord. In this connection, Krivoy reported that lysergic acid diethylamide (LSD-25) inhibits the enzymatic inactivation of substance P by neural tissue extracts, and also enhances the fourth wave of the dorsal root potential in the cat (67, 71).

STATUS OF SUBSTANCE P AS A SENSORY TRANSMITTER   Among the criteria for transmitter identification, the presence in presynaptic neurons and the release in response to presynaptic stimulation have been fairly well established for substance P as a transmitter of primary afferent fibers. Further studies are needed to clarify the details of substance P action, e.g. the reversal potential and ionic mechanism, its inactivation process at synaptic site, and its synthesis. However, judging from the data available at the present time, substance P seems likely to be an excitatory transmitter of spinal dorsal root fibers.

The question arises whether substance P is a transmitter of all dorsal root fibers or of only a part of them. Immunohistochemical studies of Hökfelt et al (34, 72) showed that only 10–20% of neurons in the rat spinal ganglia were substance P–positive. However, the possibility cannot be excluded that many more spinal ganglion cells contain substance P, because in the cat spinal ganglia the substance P–positive fluorescence could be demonstrated in the cell bodies only after preventing the axonal transport of the peptide (33). Henry (54, 73) showed that electrophoretically applied substance P caused excitation of cat spinal neurons which were activated by noxious stimuli applied to the skin and suggested that substance P is specifically related to nociception.

An important question is whether or not substance P is an excitatory transmitter of Group Ia fibers that monosynaptically excites spinal motoneurons. Some observations are consistent with the transmitter role of the peptide in this place. Namely, substance P exerts a direct depolarizing action on spinal motoneurons (40, 41, 44, 46); spinal monosynaptic reflex is blocked by baclofen which antagonizes the depolarizing action of substance P (45, 46); and the level of substance P in the ventral horn is slightly reduced after the section of dorsal roots (30). To settle this question it may be crucial to find the drugs that correspond to curare or eserine in cholinergic synapse, and then to examine the effect of these drugs on monosynaptic excitatory postsynaptic potential (EPSP) recorded in the motoneurons.

When substance P was applied to the isolated rat spinal cord, the time course of the depolarization of motoneurons was slightly slower than that of glutamate-induced depolarization (44-46). This may be at least partly due to the diffusion of the peptide through the cord tissue. Krnjević and his colleagues (47, 48), on the other hand, reported that the excitant effect of electrophoretically applied substance P on cuneate and spinal neurons appeared with a delay of 10–30 sec and persisted for 1–2 min after the end of application. In the experiment of Walker et al (74) in brain stem neurons, however, the effect of electrophoretically applied substance P appeared within 4 sec and subsided with a similarly fast time course. It would be desirable to examine the effect of substance P by iontophoretic application on synaptic sites of central neurons under visual control (75), possibly by using thin tissue slices or neurons in cell culture.

Henry et al (48) showed that substance P potentiated the excitant effect of glutamate on cat spinal neurons, and proposed that the function of substance P is a form of sensitization or modulation. However, the simultaneous application of substance P and L-glutamate on the motoneurons in isolated rat or frog spinal cord produced a simply additive effect (41, 46).

Other Possible Transmitter Functions of Substance P

Substance P is widely and selectively distributed in mammalian CNS (17–19, 76–78). Particularly high levels of substance P were found in trigeminal nerve nucleus, hypothalamus, substantia nigra, etc. Immunohistochemical studies of Nilsson et al (79) suggested that substance P is concentrated in nerve endings in hypothalamus and other regions of rat CNS. Electrophoretic application of substance P on cerebral cortical as well as substantia nigral neurons caused excitatory responses (55, 74, 80). Duffy & Powell (81) reported that substance P stimulates the brain adenylate cyclase activity.

An interesting possibility is that substance P may be released from the peripheral nerve terminals of primary sensory neurons and may serve as a transmitter of axon reflex vasodilatation. Dale in 1935 already suggested that the transmitter of axon reflex vasodilatation is closely related to the transmitter released by sensory neurons at the central synapse (82). In this connection, Hökfelt et al (33) found substance P–positive fibers around blood vessels in the cat skin.

Substance P exerts a powerful stimulant action on various smooth muscles (11, 23, 29, 83). Immunohistochemical studies of Nilsson et al (84) showed the occurrence of substance P–positive fibers in mammalian gastrointestinal tract. Substance P extracted from equine intestine was shown by Studer et al (85) to be identical with substance P isolated from hypothalamus and characterized by Chang et al (22).

The above results suggest that substance P may serve as a transmitter in many places in mammalian central and peripheral nervous system.

PROCTOLIN

Brown (86) found in the extract of cockroach gut a substance that causes a contraction of longitudinal muscle of the gut. This factor was first called *gut factor*. The concentration of the gut factor in the nerves innervating intestinal muscle was up to 150 times greater than that in the thoracic peripheral nerves which innervate somatic muscle. This gut factor is present in considerable amount in the rectum, and it is depleted from the rectum after surgical section of the innervating nerves, which suggests that the gut factor is of neural origin. In the homogenate of rectum, the gut factor is associated with subcellular particles which may correspond to synaptic vesicles. Based on these findings, Brown proposed that the gut factor functions as an excitatory transmitter in insect intestinal muscle.

Recently the gut factor was purified and its structure determined as a pentapeptide (Arg-Tyr-Leu-Pro-Thr), which was named proctolin (87, 88). Synthetic proctolin in quite a low concentration (10^{-9} M) produced a contraction of the rectum, and the peptide was fully active on tetrodotoxin-treated or surgically denervated muscle, indicating that proctolin acts directly on muscle membrane. Tyramine (10^{-6} M) suppressed the responses evoked both by proctolin and by nerve stimulation. Furthermore, when a nerve-rectum preparation was perfused, an active substance with similar pharmacological activity as proctolin was released during repetitive nerve stimulation. Although further experiments are needed for elucidating, for example, the reversal potential of proctolin action and the identification of the active substance released from the nerve-rectum preparation, the above results provide impressive evidence for proctolin as a transmitter in cockroach gut. Starratt & Brown (88) found that a substance chemically indistinguishable from proctolin is present in eight other species of insects and proposed that proctolin is a universal constituent of the Insecta.

CARNOSINE

The cell bodies of primary olfactory neurons lie in the nasal olfactory epithelium, and send their axons to the olfactory bulb where these axons form synapses with mitral and periglomerular cells. Margolis (89, 90) and Neidle & Kandera (91) found that carnosine (β-alanyl-L-histidine) is highly concentrated in the olfactory bulb of mouse, rat, and guinea pig. The concentration of carnosine in the olfactory bulb of the mouse was about 20 times higher than that in cerebral hemisphere (91). Carnosine occurs also in olfactory epithelium in uniquely high concentration (89, 90). Degeneration studies showed that both carnosine and carnosine synthetase are highly localized in the primary olfactory pathway (89, 90, 92). Based on these findings, Margolis proposed a hypothesis that carnosine is a neurotransmitter of the primary olfactory pathway (89, 90, 92). A crucial test of this hypothesis would be to see the effect of carnosine on mitral and periglomerular cells, but this has not yet been performed.

OTHER PEPTIDES

Several peptides occur in mammalian CNS and exert either excitant or depressant action on central neurons when applied by microiontophoresis. Although these peptides were proposed as central neurotransmitters, evidence is still far from convincing. It would be desirable to examine the possible transmitter role of each of these peptides at anatomically defined synapses according to the criteria of transmitter identification.

Enkephalin

The presence of the opiate receptor, which specifically binds to morphine agonists and its antagonist, was recently shown in mammalian brain and intestine (93–95). These findings prompted several workers to search for an endogenous substance which acts on this receptor and has pharmacological properties similar to morphine (96–98). Consequently, a peptide factor, termed *enkephalin* (98), was found from brain extract. Enkephalin inhibits competitively the binding of dihydromorphine and naloxone, a morphine antagonist, to opiate receptor (96, 99, 100). Like morphine, enkephalin inhibits neurally evoked contractions of vas deferens, and this effect is antagonized by naloxone (97, 98). Enkephalin is unevenly distributed in mammalian CNS and its distribution parallels that of the opiate receptor (97, 99, 101). Recently enkephalin was shown to be localized in the synaptosomal fraction (99, 102).

Hughes et al (103) identified enkephalin as comprising two pentapeptides, methionine enkephalin (Tyr-Gly-Gly-Phe-Met) and leucine enkephalin (Tyr-Gly-Gly-Phe-Leu). Although the hypothesis was proposed that enkephalin might serve as a neurotransmitter (100, 104), the hypothesis depends largely on the assumption that morphine acts at certain synapses as an agonist of the transmitter, and this remains to be seen. Effects of enkephalin on neural activities were studied. Intracerebroventricular administration of enkephalin to mice resulted in an analgesic effect (105). Iontophoretic application of methionine enkephalin produced a depressant effect on brain stem neurons of the rat and cat, and this effect was blocked by naloxone in the rat (106) but not in the cat (107).

Hypothalamic Releasing Factors

So far three hypothalamic releasing factors were structurally identified, i.e. thyrotropin- releasing hormone (TRH) (108, 109), luteinizing hormone–releasing hormone (LHRH) (110, 111), and somatostatin (growth hormone release inhibiting factor) (112). TRH and somatostatin are widely distributed in mammalian hypothalamic and extrahypothalamic brain tissues (113–116) as well as in the spinal cord (72, 117, 118). With immunofluorescence and immunoperoxidase techniques, evidence was obtained that these releasing factors are localized in certain nerve terminals (72, 117–120). Hökfelt et al (72, 117) observed that somatostatin-like immunoreactivity is present in certain neuronal cell bodies in spinal ganglia and in fibers in the dorsal horn of the spinal cord, and suggested that somatostatin may play a role as a transmitter of primary sensory neurons. When administered by microiontophoresis, TRH, LHRH, and somatostatin produced a depressant or excitant effect on neurons of different regions of CNS (121–124).

Neurohypophysial Peptides

Vasopressin is synthesized primarily in supraoptic neurosecretory cells and released into the circulation from their axon terminals which are located in the neurohypophysis. Nicoll & Barker (5, 9) found that vasopressin administered by microiontophoresis decreased the firing rate of supraoptic neurosecretory cells. Based on this and other findings they proposed a hypothesis that this posterior pituitary hormone might also be released from recurrent collaterals of the supraoptic neurons and serve as the transmitter of recurrent inhibition. This hypothesis was supported by the observation of Vincent & Arnauld (125) that recurrent inhibition of supraoptic neurosecretory cells in the monkey disappeared after 5 days of water deprivation when a total depletion of vasopressin is expected to occur. However, a doubt as to the hypothesis has recently been raised by Dreifuss et al (126) who observed the recurrent inhibition of supraoptic neurosecretory cells in the Brattleboro strain of rats, which do not synthesize vasopressin.

Moss et al (127) observed that iontophoretically applied oxytocin excited selectively the paraventricular neurosecretory cells that produce oxytocin. The physiological meaning of this observation is unknown.

Angiotensin II

Mammalian brain contains angiotensin I and II (128, 129) as well as angiotensin-converting enzyme (130). Electrophoretic application of angiotensin II on supraoptic neurosecretory cells as well as on neurons of subfornical organ produced an excitant effect (131–134). The question remains whether this effect of angiotensin reflects the transmitter action on these neurons or the response to the circulating angiotensin.

CONCLUSIONS

It now seems likely that a new class of substances, peptides, must be added to the list of neurotransmitters. Considerable evidence is available that substance P and proctolin are excitatory transmitters in mammalian primary sensory neurons and in insect peripheral nerves respectively. In view of the relatively small molecular weights of the established neurotransmitters, it may appear rather unexpected that a peptide of more than 1000 daltons serves a transmitter function. However, if we consider the many common characteristics shared by neurotransmission and neurosecretion (135), together with the fact that neurosecretory cells secrete various peptides, then the idea of peptide neurotransmitters may not be novel. In fact, it has been suggested by many authors that certain neurosecretory cells release peptides as hormones or releasing factors from some nerve endings into the circulation and the same peptides as neurotransmitters from other nerve endings at synapses (9, 121, 123, 125). This may be parallel with the case of primary sensory neurons which probably release substance P as excitatory transmitter from their intraspinal nerve endings and the same peptide as transmitter of axon reflex vasodilatation from the peripheral nerve endings contacting the blood vessels.

A particular advantage for the study of peptide neurotransmitters is the availability of immunological techniques. With a highly specific radioimmunoassay, it is possible to determine as little as 10^{-15} moles of substance P (38, 58, 136). Furthermore, immunohistochemical techniques enable one to locate specific peptide immunoreactivities at the light microscopic as well as electron microscopic level (33, 72, 117–120). Such techniques will provide a useful means for mapping specific neurons in CNS, and may also be useful in chemical pathology for revealing abnormalities in diseases.

Another promising field which may possibly be introduced by peptide transmitters is its pharmacology. Little is known about the possible pharmacological manipulation of peptidergic neurotransmission. With modern techniques of peptide chemistry it is probably not difficult to synthesize various peptides which act as agonists or antagonists of peptide transmitters. If we can synthesize peptides that penetrate into the CNS, a group of new drugs acting on the CNS may be introduced.

The question remains why the nervous system needs relatively large and possibly expensive molecules such as undecapeptide to transmit either an excitatory or inhibitory effect if precise neuronal connections are assured by anatomical contacts at synapses. For example, do primary afferent fibers need diverse peptides for mediating different modalities of sensation? Future studies will clarify whether or not the functions of peptide transmitters are explicable in terms of traditional concepts of chemical transmission.

Literature Cited

1. Eccles, J. C. 1964. *The Physiology of Synapses.* Berlin: Springer. 316 pp.
2. Werman, R. 1966. Criteria for identification of a central nervous system transmitter. *Comp. Biochem. Physiol.* 18:745–66
3. de Wied, D., Witter, A., Greven, H. M. 1975. Behaviorally active ACTH analogues. *Biochem. Pharmacol.* 24:1463–68
4. Pappenheimer, J. R., Koski, G., Fencl, V., Karnovsky, M. L., Krueger, J. 1975. Extraction of sleep-promoting factor S from cerebrospinal fluid and from brains of sleep-deprived animals. *J. Neurophysiol.* 38:1299–1311
5. Barker, J. L. 1976. Peptides: Roles in neuronal excitability. *Physiol. Rev.* 56:435–52
6. Scharrer, E., Scharrer, B. 1954. Hormones produced by neurosecretory cells. *Recent Prog. Horm. Res.* 10:183–240
7. Bargmann, W., Lindner, E., Andres, K. H. 1967. Über Synapsen an endokrinen Epithelzellen und die Definition sekretorischer Neurone. *Z. Zellforsch. Mikrosk. Anat.* 77:282–98
8. Konishi, S., Otsuka, M. 1971. Actions of certain polypeptides on frog spinal neurons. *Jpn. J. Pharmacol.* 21:685–87
9. Nicoll, R. A., Barker, J. L. 1971. The pharmacology of recurrent inhibition in the supraoptic neurosecretory system. *Brain Res.* 35:501–11
10. Bloom, F. E. 1972. Amino acids and polypeptides in neuronal function. *Neurosci. Res. Program Bull.* 10:127–251
11. Euler, U.S.v., Gaddum, J. H. 1931. An unidentified depressor substance in certain tissue extracts. *J. Physiol. London* 72:74–87
12. Chang, H. C., Gaddum, J. H. 1933. Choline esters in tissue extracts. *J. Physiol. London* 79:255–85
13. Gaddum, J. H., Schild, H. 1934. Depressor substances in extracts of intestine. *J. Physiol. London* 83:1–14
14. Euler, U.S.v. 1936. Untersuchungen über Substanz P, die atropinfeste, darmerregende und gefäßerweiternde Substanz aus Darm und Hirn. *Naunyn-Schmiedebergs Arch. Exp. Pathol. Pharmakol.* 181:181–97
15. Hellauer, H. 1953. Zur Charakterisierung der Erregungssubstanz sensibler Nerven. *Naunyn-Schmiedebergs Arch. Exp. Pathol. Pharmakol.* 219:234–41

16. Lembeck, F. 1953. Zur Frage der zentralen Übertragung afferenter Impulse. III. Mitteilung. Das Vorkommen und die Bedeutung der Substanz P in den dorsalen Wurzeln des Rückenmarks. *Naunyn-Schmiedebergs Arch. Exp. Pathol. Pharmakol.* 219:197–213
17. Pernow, B. 1953. Studies on substance P—purficiation, occurrence, and biological actions. *Acta Physiol. Scand.* 29:Suppl. 105, pp. 1–90
18. Kopera, H., Lazarini, W. 1953. Zur Frage der zentralen Übertragung afferenter Impulse. *Naunyn-Schmiedebergs Arch. Exp. Pathol. Pharmakol.* 219:214–22
19. Amin, A. H., Crawford, T. B. B., Gaddum, J. H. 1954. The distribution of substance P and 5-hydroxytryptamine in the central nervous system of the dog. *J. Physiol. London* 126:596–618
20. Galindo, A., Krnjević, K., Schwartz, S. 1967. Micro-iontophoretic studies on neurones in the cuneate nucleus. *J. Physiol. London* 192:359–77
21. Chang, M. M., Leeman, S. E. 1970. Isolation of a sialogogic peptide from bovine hypothalamic tissue and its characterization as substance P. *J. Biol. Chem.* 245:4784–90
22. Chang, M. M., Leeman, S. E., Niall, H. D. 1971. Amino-acid sequence of substance P. *Nature New Biol.* 232:86–87
23. Tregear, G. W., Niall, H. D., Potts, J. T. Jr., Leeman, S. E., Chang, M. M. 1971. Synthesis of substance P. *Nature New Biol.* 232:87–89
24. Lembeck, F., Zetler, G. 1971. Substance P. In *International Encyclopedia of Pharmacology and Therapeutics,* ed. J. M. Walker, Sect. 72. 1:29–71. Oxford:Pergamon. 305 pp.
25. Zetler, G. 1961. Zwei neue pharmakologisch aktive Polypeptide in einem Substanz P-haltigen Hirnextrakt. *Naunyn-Schmiedebergs Arch. Exp. Pathol. Pharmakol.* 242:330–52
26. Meinardi, H., Craig, L. C. 1966. Studies of substance P. In *Hypotensive Peptides,* ed. E. G. Erdös, N. Back, F. Sicuteri, A. F. Wilde, 594–607. Berlin: Springer. 660 pp.
27. Iven, H., Zetler, G. 1973. Comparison of crude bovine subcortical substance P with synthetic substance P. *Naunyn-Schmiedebergs Arch. Exp. Pathol. Pharmakol.* 276:123–31

28. Otsuka, M., Konishi, S., Takahashi, T. 1972. A further study of the montoneuron-depolarizing peptide extracted from dorsal roots of bovine spinal nerves. *Proc. Jpn. Acad.* 48:747–52

29. Takahashi, T., Konishi, S., Powell, D., Leeman, S. E., Otsuka, M. 1974. Identification of the motoneuron-depolarizing peptide in bovine dorsal root as hypothalamic substance P. *Brain Res.* 73:59–69

30. Takahashi, T., Otsuka, M. 1975. Regional distribution of substance P in the spinal cord and nerve roots of the cat and the effect of dorsal root section. *Brain Res.* 87:1–11

31. Takahashi, T., Otsuka, M. 1974. Distribution of substance P in cat spinal cord and the alteration following unilateral dorsal root section. *Jpn. J. Pharmacol.* 24: Suppl., p. 105

32. Sprague, J. M., Ha, H. 1964. The terminal fields of dorsal root fibers in the lumbosacral spinal cord of the cat, and the dendritic organization of the motor nuclei. In *Organization of the Spinal Cord, Progr. Brain Res.*, ed. J. C. Eccles, J. P. Schadé, 11:120–54. Amsterdam: Elsevier. 285 pp.

33. Hökfelt, T., Kellerth, J. O., Nilsson, G., Pernow, B. 1975. Experimental immunohistochemical studies on the localization and distribution of substance P in cat primary sensory neurons. *Brain Res.* 100:235–52

34. Hökfelt, T., Kellerth, J. O., Nilsson, G., Pernow, B. 1975. Substance P: Localization in the central nervous system and in some primary sensory neurons. *Science* 190:889–90

35. Inouye, A., Kataoka, K. 1962. Subcellular distribution of the substance P in the nervous tissues. *Nature* 193:585

36. Cleugh, J., Gaddum, J. H., Mitchell, A. A., Smith, M. W., Whittaker, V. P. 1964. Substance P in brain extracts. *J. Physiol. London* 170:69–85

37. Ryall, R. W. 1962. Sub-cellular distribution of pharmacologically active substances in guinea pig brain. *Nature* 196:680–81

38. Powell, D., Leeman, S. E., Tregear, G. W., Niall, H. D., Potts, J. T. Jr. 1973. Radioimmunoassay for substance P. *Nature New Biol.* 241:252–54

39. Duffy, M. J., Mulhall, D., Powell, D. 1975. Subcellular distribution of substance P in bovine hypothalamus and substantia nigra. *J. Neurochem.* 25:305–7

40. Konishi, S., Otsuka, M. 1974. The effects of substance P and other peptides on spinal neurons of the frog. *Brain Res.* 65:397–410

41. Nicoll, R. A. 1976. Promising peptides. *Neurosci. Symp.* 1:99–122

42. Graham, L. T. Jr., Shank, R. P., Werman, R., Aprison, M. H. 1967. Distribution of some synaptic transmitter suspects in cat spinal cord: glutamic acid, aspartic acid, γ-aminobutyric acid, glycine, and glutamine. *J. Neurochem.* 14:465–72

43. Otsuka, M., Konishi, S. 1974. Electrophysiology of mammalian spinal cord in vitro. *Nature* 252:733–34

44. Konishi, S., Otsuka, M. 1974. Excitatory action of hypothalamic substance P on spinal motoneurones of newborn rats. *Nature* 252:734–35

45. Saito, K., Konishi, S., Otsuka, M. 1975. Antagonism between Lioresal and substance P in rat spinal cord. *Brain Res.* 97:177–80

46. Otsuka, M., Konishi, S. 1976. Substance P and excitatory transmitter of primary sensory neurons. *Cold Spring Harbor Symp. Quant. Biol.* 40:135–43

47. Krnjević, K., Morris, M. E. 1974. An excitatory action of substance P on cuneate neurones. *Can. J. Physiol. Pharmacol.* 52:736–44

48. Henry, J. L., Krnjević, K., Morris, M. E. 1975. Substance P and spinal neurones. *Can. J. Physiol. Pharmacol.* 53:423–32

49. Stern, P., Huković, S. 1961. Specific antagonists of substance P. In *Symposium on Substance P,* ed. P. Stern, 83–88. Sarajevo: Sci. Soc. Bosnia Herzegovina. 143 pp.

50. Davidoff, R. A., Sears, E. S, 1974. The effects of Lioresal on synaptic activity in the isolated spinal cord. *Neurology* 24:957–63

51. Pedersen, E., Arlien-Søborg, P., Grynderup, V., Henriksen, O. 1970. GABA derivative in spasticity (β-(4-chlorophenyl)-γ-aminobutyric acid, Ciba, 34.647-Ba). *Acta Neurol. Scand.* 46:257–66

52. Pierau, F. K., Zimmermann, P. 1973. Action of a GABA-derivative on postsynaptic potentials and membrane properties of cats' spinal motoneurones. *Brain Res.* 54:376–80

53. Phillis, J. W. 1976. Is β-(4-chlorophenyl)-GABA a specific antagonist of substance P on cerebral cortical neurons? *Experientia* 32:593–94

54. Ben-Ari, Y., Henry, J. L. 1976. Effects of the para-chlorophenyl derivative of GABA on spinal neurones in the cat. *J. Physiol. London* 259:46–47P
55. Davies, J., Dray, A. 1976. Substance P in the substantia nigra. *Brain Res.* 107:623–27
56. Otsuka, M., Konishi, S., Takahashi, T. 1972. The presence of a motoneuron-depolarizing peptide in bovine dorsal roots of spinal nerves. *Proc. Jpn. Acad.* 48:342–46
57. Otsuka, M., Konishi, S. 1977. Electrophysiological and neurochemical evidence for substance P as a transmitter of primary sensory neurons. In *Substance P*, ed. U.S.v. Euler, B. Pernow. New York: Raven. In press
58. Yanaihara, N., Yanaihara, C., Hirohashi, M., Sato, H., Hashimoto, T., Sakagami, M., Iizuka, Y. 1976. Substance P analogues: Synthesis and biological and immunological properties. See Ref. 57
59. Angelucci, L. 1956. Experiments with perfused frog's spinal cord. *Br. J. Pharmacol.* 11:161–70
60. Ramwell, P. W., Shaw, J. E., Jessup, R. 1966. Spontaneous and evoked release of prostaglandins from frog spinal cord. *Am. J. Physiol.* 211:998–1004
61. Otsuka, M., Konishi, S. 1976. Release of substance P-like immunoreactivity from isolated spinal cord of newborn rat. *Nature* 264:83–84
62. Iversen, L. L., Jessell, T., Kanazawa, I. 1976. Release and metabolism of substance P in rat hypothalamus. *Nature* 264:81–83
63. Segawa, T., Nakata, Y. 1976. Substance P in rabbit brain and spinal cord: Regional and subcellular distribution and evidence for lack of high-affinity uptake system. *Jpn. J. Pharmacol.* 26: Suppl., 100 P.
64. Gullbring, B. 1943. Inactivation of substance P by tissue extracts. *Acta Physiol. Scand.* 6:246–55
65. Umrath, K. 1953. Über die fermentative Verwandlung von Substanz P aus sensiblen Neuronen in die Erregungssubstanz der sensiblen Nerven. *Pflügers Arch.* 258:230–42
66. Eber, O., Lembeck, F. 1956. Über den enzymatischen Abbau der Substanz P. *Naunyn-Schmiedebergs Arch. Exp. Pathol. Pharmakol.* 229:139–47
67. Krivoy, W. A. 1957. The preservation of substance P by lysergic acid diethylamide. *Br. J. Pharmacol.* 12:361–64

68. Hooper, K. C. 1962. The catabolism of some physiologically active polypeptides by homogenate of dog hypothalamus. *Biochem. J.* 83:511–17
69. Claybrook, D. L., Pfiffner, J. J. 1968. Purification and properties of a substance P-inactivating enzyme from bovine brain. *Biochem. Pharmacol.* 17:281–93
70. Benuck, M., Marks, N. 1975. Enzymatic inactivation of substance P by a partially purified enzyme from rat brain. *Biochem. Biophys. Res. Commun.* 65:153–60
71. Krivoy, W. A. 1961. Potentiation of substance P by lysergic acid diethylamide in vivo. *Br. J. Pharmacol.* 16:253–56
72. Hökfelt, T., Elde, R., Johansson, O., Luft, R., Nilsson, G., Arimura, A. 1976. Immunohistochemical evidence for separate populations of somatostatin-containing and substance P-containing primary afferent neurons in the rat. *Neuroscience* 1:131–36
73. Henry, J. L. 1976. Excitation of spinal nociceptive neurons by substance P. *Nobel Symp. 37, Substance P, Stockholm*, pp. 29–31 (Abstr.)
74. Walker, R. J., Kemp, J. A., Yajima, H., Kitagawa, K., Woodruff, G. N. 1976. The action of substance P on mesencephalic reticular and substantia nigral neurones of the rat. *Experientia* 32:214–15
75. Dennis, M. J., Harris, A. J., Kuffler, S. W. 1971. Synaptic transmission and its duplication by focally applied acetylcholine in parasympathetic neurons in the heart of the frog. *Proc. R. Soc. London Ser. B.* 177:509–39
76. Zetler, G., Schlosser, L. 1955. Über die Verteilung von Substanz P und Cholinacetylase im Gehirn. *Naunyn-Schmiedebergs Arch. Exp. Pathol. Pharmakol.* 224:159–75
77. Paasonen, M. K., Vogt, M. 1956. The effect of drugs on the amounts of substance P and 5-hydroxytryptamine in mammalian brain. *J. Physiol. London* 131:617–26
78. Kanazawa, I., Jessell, T. 1976. Postmortem changes and regional distribution of substance P in the rat and mouse nervous system. *Brain Res.* 117:362–67
79. Nilsson, G., Hökfelt, T., Pernow, B. 1974. Distribution of substance P-like immunoreactivity in the rat central nervous system as revealed by immunohistochemistry. *Med. Biol.* 52:424–27

80. Phillis, J. W., Limacher, J. J. 1974. Substance P excitation of cerebral cortical Betz cells. *Brain Res.* 69:158–63

81. Duffy, M. J., Powell, D. 1975. Stimulation of brain adenylate cyclase activity by the undecapeptide substance P and its modulation by the calcium ion. *Biochim. Biophys. Acta* 385:275–80

82. Dale, H. 1935. Pharmacology and nerve-endings. *Proc. R. Soc. Med.* 28:319–32

83. Euler, U.S.v., Hedqvist, P. 1974. Effects of substance P on the response of guinea pig vas deferens to transmural nerve stimulation. *Acta Physiol. Scand.* 90: 651–53

84. Nilsson, G., Larsson, L.-I., Håkanson, R., Brodin, E., Pernow, B., Sundler, F. 1975. Localization of substance P-like immunoreactivity in mouse gut. *Histochemistry* 43:97–99

85. Studer, R. O., Trzeciak, A., Lergier, W. 1973. Isolierung und Aminosäuresequenz von Substanz P aus Pferdedarm. *Helv. Chim. Acta* 56:860–66

86. Brown, B. E. 1967. Neuromuscular transmitter substance in insect visceral muscle. *Science* 155:595–97

87. Brown, B. E. 1975. Proctolin: A peptide transmitter candidate in insects. *Life Sci.* 17:1241–52

88. Starratt, A. N., Brown, B. E. 1975. Structure of the pentapeptide proctolin, a proposed neurotransmitter in insects. *Life Sci.* 17:1253–56

89. Margolis, F. L. 1974. Carnosine in the primary olfactory pathway. *Science* 184:909–11

90. Margolis, F. L., Roberts, N., Ferriero, D., Feldman, J. 1974. Denervation in the primary olfactory pathway of mice: Biochemical and morphological effects. *Brain Res.* 81:469–83

91. Neidle, A., Kandera, J. 1974. Carnosine —an olfactory bulb peptide. *Brain Res.* 80:359–64

92. Margolis, F. L., Ferriero, D., Herding, J. 1975. Carnosine (β-alanyl-L-histidine) in the olfactory nerve: A putative transmitter candidate. *Proc. Int. Congr. Pharmacol., 6th, Helsinki* 2:61–69

93. Terenius, L. 1973. Characteristics of the "receptor" for narcotic analgesics in synaptic plasma membrane fraction from rat brain. *Acta Pharmacol. Toxicol.* 33:377–84

94. Pert, C. B., Snyder, S. H. 1973. Opiate receptor: Demonstration in nervous tissue. *Science* 179:1011–14

95. Simon, E. J., Hiller, J. M., Edelman, I. 1973. Stereospecific binding of the potent narcotic analgesic [³H]etorphine to rat-brain homogenate. *Proc. Natl. Acad. Sci. USA* 70:1947–49

96. Terenius, L., Wahlström, A. 1975. Search for an endogenous ligand for the opiate receptor. *Acta Physiol. Scand.* 94:74–81

97. Hughes, J. 1975. Isolation of an endogenous compound from the brain with pharmacological properties similar to morphine. *Brain Res.* 88:295–308

98. Hughes, J., Smith, T., Morgan, B., Fothergill, L. 1975. Purification and properties of enkephalin—the possible endogenous ligand for the morphine receptor. *Life Sci.* 16:1753–58

99. Pasternak, G. W., Goodman, R., Snyder, S. H. 1975. An endogenous morphine-like factor in mammalian brain. *Life Sci.* 16:1765–69

100. Simantov, R., Snyder, S. H. 1976. Isolation and structure identification of a morphine-like peptide "enkephalin" in bovine brain. *Life Sci.* 18:781–88

101. Simantov, R., Kuhar, M. J., Pasternak, G. W., Snyder, S. H. 1976. The regional distribution of a morphine-like factor enkephalin in monkey brain. *Brain Res.* 106:189–97

102. Simantov, R., Snowman, A. M., Snyder, S. H. 1976. A morphine-like factor "enkephalin" in rat brain: Subcellular localization. *Brain Res.* 107:650–57

103. Hughes, J., Smith, T., Kosterlitz, H. W., Fothergill, L. A., Morgan, B. A., Morris, H. R. 1975. Identification of two related pentapeptides from the brain with potent opiate agonist activity. *Nature* 258:577–79

104. Kosterlitz, H. W., Hughes, J. 1975. Some thoughts on the significance of enkephalin, the endogenous ligand. *Life Sci.* 17:91–96

105. Büscher, H. H., Hill, R. C., Römer, D., Cardinaux, F., Closse, A., Hauser, D., Pless, J. 1976. Evidence for analgesic activity of enkephalin in the mouse. *Nature* 261:423–25

106. Bradley, P. B., Briggs, I., Gayton, R. J., Lambert, L. A. 1976. Effects of microiontophoretically applied methionine-enkephalin on single neurones in rat brainstem. *Nature* 261:425–26

107. Gent, J. P., Wolstencroft, J. H. 1976. Effects of methionine-enkephalin and leucine-enkephalin compared with those of morphine on brainstem neurones in cat. *Nature* 261:426–27

108. Burgus, R., Dunn, T. F., Desiderio, D., Ward, D. N., Vale, W., Guillemin, R. 1970. Characterization of ovine hypo-

thalamic hypophysiotropic TSH-releasing factor. *Nature* 226:321–25

109. Nair, R. M. G., Barrett, J. F., Bowers, C. Y., Schally, A. V. 1970. Structure of porcine thyrotropin releasing hormone. *Biochemistry* 9:1103–6

110. Schally, A. V., Arimura, A., Baba, Y., Nair, R. M. G., Matsuo, H., Redding, T. W., Debeljuk, L., White, W. F. 1971. Isolation and properties of the FSH and LH-releasing hormone. *Biochem. Biophys. Res. Commun.* 43:393–99

111. Amoss, M., Burgus, R., Blackwell, R., Vale, W., Fellows, R., Guillemin, R. 1971. Purification, amino acid composition and N-terminus of the hypothalamic luteinizing hormone releasing factor (LRF) of ovine origin. *Biochem. Biophys. Res. Commun.* 44:205–10

112. Brazeau, P., Vale, W., Burgus, R., Ling, N., Butcher, M., Rivier, J., Guillemin, R. 1973. Hypothalamic polypeptide that inhibits the secretion of immunoreactive pituitary growth hormone. *Science* 179:77–79

113. Jackson, I. M. D., Reichlin, S. 1974. Thyrotropin-releasing hormone (TRH): Distribution in hypothalamic and extrahypothalamic brain tissues of mammalian and submammalian chordates. *Endocrinology* 95:854–62

114. Oliver, C., Eskay, R. L., Ben-Jonathan, N., Porter, J. C. 1974. Distribution and concentration of TRH in the rat brain. *Endocrinology* 96:540–46

115. Winokur, A., Utiger, R. D. 1974. Thyrotropin-releasing hormone: Regional distribution in rat brain. *Science* 185:265–67

116. Brownstein, M., Arimura, A., Sato, H., Schally, A. V., Kizer, J. S. 1975. The regional distribution of somatostatin in the rat brain. *Endocrinology* 96:1456–61

117. Hökfelt, T., Elde, R., Johansson, O., Luft, R., Arimura, A. 1975. Immunohistochemical evidence for the presence of somatostatin, a powerful inhibitory peptide, in some primary sensory neurons. *Neurosci. Lett.* 1:231–35

118. Hökfelt, T., Fuxe, K., Johansson, O., Jeffcoate, S., White, N. 1975. Thyrotropin releasing hormone (TRH)-containing nerve terminals in certain brain stem nuclei and in the spinal cord. *Neurosci. Lett.* 1:133–39

119. Hökfelt, T., Fuxe, K., Johansson, O., Jeffcoate, S., White, N. 1975. Distribution of thyrotropin-releasing hormone (TRH) in the central nervous system as

revealed with immunohistochemistry. *Eur. J. Pharmacol.* 34:389–92

120. Pelletier, G., Labrie, F., Puviani, R., Arimura, A., Schally, A. V. 1974. Immunohistochemical localization of luteinizing hormone-releasing hormone in the rat median eminence. *Endocrinology* 95:314–17

121. Dyer, R. G., Dyball, R. E. J. 1974. Evidence for a direct effect of LRF and TRF on single unit activity in the rostral hypothalamus. *Nature* 252:486–88

122. Renaud, L. P., Martin, J. B. 1975. Thyrotropin releasing hormone (TRH): Depressant action on central neuronal activity. *Brain Res.* 86:150–54

123. Renaud, L. P., Martin, J. B., Brazeau, P. 1975. Depressant action of TRH, LH-RH and somatostatin on activity of central neurones. *Nature* 255:233–35

124. Kawakami, M., Sakuma, Y. 1974. Responses of hypothalamic neurons to the microiontophoresis of LH-RH, LH and FSH under various levels of circulating ovarian hormones. *Neuroendocrinology* 15:290–307

125. Vincent, J. D., Arnauld, E. 1975. Vasopressin as a neurotransmitter in the central nervous system: Some evidence from the supraoptic neurosecretory system. *Prog. Brain Res.* 42:57–66

126. Dreifuss, J. J., Nordmann, J. J., Vincent, J. D. 1974. Recurrent inhibition of supraoptic neurosecretory cells in homozygous Brattleboro rats. *J. Physiol. London* 237:25 P

127. Moss, R. L., Dyball, R. E. J., Cross, B. A. 1972. Excitation of antidromically identified neurosecretory cells of the paraventricular nucleus by oxytocin applied iontophoretically. *Exp. Neurol.* 34:95–102

128. Ganten, D., Marquez-Julio, A., Granger, P., Hayduk, K., Karsunky, K. P., Boucher, R., Genest, J. 1971. Renin in dog brain. *Am. J. Physiol.* 221:1733–37

129. Fischer-Ferraro, C., Nahmod, V. E., Goldstein, D. J., Finkielman, S. 1971. Angiotensin and renin in rat and dog brain. *J. Exp. Med.* 133:353–61

130. Yang, H-Y. T., Neff, N. H. 1972. Distribution and properties of angiotensin converting enzyme of rat brain. *J. Neurochem.* 19:2443–50

131. Nicoll, R. A., Barker, J. L. 1971. Excitation of supraoptic neurosecretory cells by angiotensin II. *Nature New Biol.* 233:172–74

132. Sakai, K. K., Marks, B. H., George, J., Koestner, A. 1974. Specific angiotensin II receptors in organ-cultured canine supra-optic nucleus cells. *Life Sci.* 14:1337–44

133. Felix, D., Akert, K. 1974. The effect of angiotensin II on neurones of the cat subfornical organ. *Brain Res.* 76: 350–53

134. Felix, D. 1975. Peptide and acetylcholine action on neurones of the cat sub-fornical organ. *Naunyn-Schmiedebergs Arch. Exp. Pathol. Pharmakol.* 292:15–20

135. Bern, H. A., Knowles. F. G. W. 1966. Neurosecretion. In *Neuroendocrinology,* ed. L. Martini, W. F. Ganong, 1:139–86. New York: Academic. 774 pp.

136. Nilsson, G., Pernow, B., Fischer, G. H., Folkers, K. 1976. Radioimmunoassay of substance P. *Nobel Symp. 37, Substance P, Stockholm,* p. 8 (Abstr.)

Ann. Rev. Pharmacol. Toxicol. 1977. 17:441–77
Copyright © 1977 by Annual Reviews Inc. All rights reserved

SELECTIVE CYCLIC   ❖6690
NUCLEOTIDE PHOSPHODIESTERASE
INHIBITORS AS POTENTIAL
THERAPEUTIC AGENTS

Benjamin Weiss and William N. Hait
Department of Pharmacology, Medical College of Pennsylvania,
Philadelphia, Pennsylvania 19129

INTRODUCTION

Not thirty years have passed since Earl Sutherland, Ted Rall, and their co-workers first suggested that a heat-stable cyclic nucleotide mediates the actions of certain hormones and neurotransmitters. This original handful of cyclic nucleotide enthusiasts has now swelled to hundreds and encompasses biologists of every discipline. As one might expect, the early studies concentrated largely on the biochemical and physiological actions of cyclic nucleotides and on the enzymes responsible for their biosynthesis (nucleotide cyclases) and hydrolysis (cyclic nucleotide phosphodiesterases); relatively little was done to manipulate the intracellular concentrations of cyclic nucleotides by pharmacological means. Now, however, in the face of mounting evidence that cyclic nucleotides may be involved in the etiology or pathogenesis of certain diseases, increasing numbers of investigators have turned their attention to finding pharmacologic agents that will selectively alter the intracellular concentration or the action of cyclic nucleotides. These agents fall into three general categories: compounds that alter the activity of the nucleotide cyclases, the cyclic nucleotide phosphodiesterases, or the cyclic nucleotide–dependent protein kinases.

The evidence that the cyclic nucleotide phosphodiesterases exist in several molecular forms and that these isozymes are unequally distributed in tissue makes the phosphodiesterases particularly suitable targets for pharmacologic manipulation, for it suggests that by finding selective inhibitors of the different phosphodiesterase isozymes, one may be able to raise the concentration of cyclic nucleotides in discrete cell types. Through the selective inhibition of the major phosphodiesterase isozyme of a diseased tissue, it may then be possible to alter the course of diseases characterized by an abnormal metabolism of cyclic nucleotides.

The present paper reviews the findings that suggest that cyclic nucleotides may be involved in certain diseases and summarizes the experimental results that support the notion that certain inhibitors of cyclic nucleotide phosphodiesterase might serve as effective and specific therapeutic agents.

ROLE OF CYCLIC NUCLEOTIDES IN BIOLOGY

The cyclic nucleotides, adenosine cyclic 3',5'-monophosphate (cyclic AMP), and guanosine cyclic 3',5'-monophosphate (cyclic GMP) have been shown to regulate innumerable biological processes [for reviews see (1–15)]. Cyclic AMP not only mediates the actions of most biogenic amines and polypeptide hormones (16, 17), but also appears to influence such fundamental processes as cell division (18), fertilization (19), embryonic growth and differentiation (20), blood production (21–23), smooth muscle tone (24, 25), cardiac contractility and metabolism (26–28), the function of the central nervous system (29) and autonomic nervous system (30), vision (31), immunological responses (32, 33), gonadal function (34), and the release of stored intracellular materials such as insulin (35–37), histamine (38, 39), and lysosomal enzymes (40).

Several of the actions of cyclic GMP appear to be opposite to those of cyclic AMP. These observations have prompted the so-called yin-yang hypothesis (41).

Since the cyclic nucleotides influence the most basic processes in biology, any abnormality in the intracellular concentration of these compounds might disrupt normal physiological function and lead to disease. The following sections explore this possibility and suggest certain approaches by which one may use drugs to restore the proper balance in the cyclic nucleotide system.

ROLE OF CYCLIC NUCLEOTIDES IN DISEASE

As mentioned earlier, there are three major sites at which the cyclic nucleotide system may be altered in diseases and, accordingly, three general sites at which drugs may interact to modulate disease processes. One site is on the cyclic nucleotide cyclases which catalyze the synthesis of cyclic nucleotides from the high energy phosphate compounds, adenosine triphosphate and guanosine triphosphate; another is at the level of the cyclic nucleotide phosphodiesterases, a group of hydrolytic enzymes, which exist in several molecular forms and catalyze the degradation of cyclic nucleotides; and a third site is on the cyclic nucleotide–dependent protein kinases which, when activated by the cyclic nucleotides, cause the phosphorylation of other intracellular proteins leading ultimately to a biological response.

Diseases Associated with Defects in the Cyclic Nucleotide System

Table 1 outlines the diseases which are associated with abnormalities in each of the different steps of cyclic nucleotide physiology. An example of a disease which is associated with an abnormality in adenylate cyclase is nephrogenic diabetes insipidus. In this disorder, which is characterized by an inability to concentrate urine in response to antidiuretic hormone (ADH), the adenylate cyclase receptor in the

Table 1 Diseases associated with abnormalities in the concentration or metabolism of cyclic nucleotides

| Disease | Tissue | Cyclic nucleotide concentration | | | Enzyme activity | | | | | | References |
		cyclic AMP basal	stim.[a]	cyclic GMP	Phosphodiesterase cyclic AMP	cyclic GMP	Adenylate cyclase basal	stim.[b]	Guanylate cyclase	Protein kinase	
ASTHMA	leucocytes								decrease		265
	leucocytes		decrease								213
	leucocytes							decrease			266
	leucocytes		decrease								267
	urine		decrease								268
CANCER	adrenal cortex				decrease						269
	adrenal cortex	decrease				decrease					47
	glioblastoma			increase			increase				280
	hepatoma	increase									270
	hepatoma						decrease	decrease			271
	hepatoma	decrease		increase	decrease						65
	hepatoma	increase					increase				272
	hepatoma	increase									273
	hepatoma									decrease	66
	hepatoma				c						274
	hepatoma						decrease				275
	hepatoma				c						276
	hepatoma	decrease									183
	hepatoma								d		277
	thymus						increase	decrease			50,278
	thymus	decrease			increase						50
	lymphocytes	decrease									184

Table 1 *(Continued)*

| Disease | Tissue | Cyclic nucleotide concentration | | | Enzyme activity | | | | | | References |
		cyclic AMP basal	stim.[a]	cyclic GMP	Phosphodiesterase cyclic AMP	cyclic GMP	Adenylate cyclase basal	stim.[b]	Guanylate cyclase	Protein kinase	
	lymphocytes	decrease									264
	leukocytes							decrease			49
	lymphocytes				increase	increase					60,61
	spleen				decrease						279
	mammary	decrease									281
	mammary				increase	increase					156
	mammary	increase			increase						282
	mammary						increase				283
	mammary	increase									284
	plant				increase						285
	skin	increase	decrease								286
	skin melanoma						decrease				287
	skin	decrease									288
	skin	increase			increase	increase					289
	thyroid							decrease			48
	transformed cells						decrease				45
	transformed cells						decrease				290
	transformed cells						decrease				291
	transformed cells						decrease				44

Table 1 *(Continued)*

Tissue / Condition								Ref.
transformed cells	decrease							292
transformed cells			decrease					293
transformed cells		decrease		decrease				51
transformed cells			decrease	decrease	decrease			275
transformed cells			increase		increase			181
transformed cells			increase		increase			294
transformed cells			decrease		decrease			294
CARDIOVAS-CULAR								
Atherosclerosis cardiac	increase							295
Congestive failure cardiac	increase					decrease		242–245, 296
cardiac					decrease	decrease		243
Hypertension amniotic fluid	increase				increase			297
aorta	decrease	decrease			decrease			298
aorta	decrease	increase			decrease			299
aorta	decrease							52
cardiac	increase	decrease			decrease			300
plasma	increase							86
urine	increase							301
Myocardial infarction plasma	increase							85

Table 1 *(Continued)*

| Disease | Tissue | Cyclic nucleotide concentration | | | Enzyme activity | | | | | | References |
		cyclic AMP basal	stim.[a]	cyclic GMP	Phosphodiesterase cyclic AMP	cyclic GMP	Adenylate cyclase basal	stim.[b]	Guanylate cyclase	Protein kinase	
DOWN'S SYNDROME	saliva	increase									88
ENDOCRIN-OPATHIES											
Diabetes insipidus	kidney						decrease				43
	urine	decrease					decrease				42
	urine	decrease									77
Diabetes mellitus	adipocytes				decrease						54
	heart				decrease						56
	liver	increase									56
	pancreas				decrease						54
	plasma				decrease						55
	saliva	decrease									87
Hyperpara-thyroidism	urine	increase									73–75, 302,303
Hypopara-thyroidism	urine	decrease									73–75, 302,303
Hyperthyroid-ism	urine	increase									71,304
	urine		increase								72

Table 1 *(Continued)*

	Tissue					Ref.
Hypothyroidism	adipocytes	decrease				305
Pseudohypoparathyroidism	urine	decrease				75
EYE DISEASE	retina		increase			57,58
	retina	decrease		decrease		306
NEUROPSYCHIATRIC DISEASES						
CNS damage	CSF				increase	307
Depression	CSF				decrease	80
	urine				decrease	79–81
Epilepsy	cerebrum	decrease				309
	CSF				increase	307
	forebrain				increase	308
Mania	CSF				increase	80
	urine				increase	79–81
OBESITY	adipose tissue	decrease	increase			53
	adipose tissue			decrease		232
PSORIASIS	epidermis	decrease				204
	epidermis	decrease	increase			205
	epidermis		increase	decrease	decrease	207
	epidermis		increase			208

^a Hormonally stimulated increase in cyclic AMP concentration.
^b Hormonally stimulated increase in adenylate cyclase activity.
^c Increase in low K_m phosphodiesterase and decrease in high K_m phosphodiesterase.
^d Increase in particulate guanylate cyclase and decrease in soluble guanylate cyclase.

renal tubule is insensitive to ADH (42, 43). Similarly, several forms of cancer, which have abnormally low intracellular concentrations of cyclic AMP, have a reduction in adenylate cyclase activity or a reduction in its hormonal responsiveness (44–50). Other forms of cancer reportedly have a reduced activity of guanylate cyclase as well (51).

There is also evidence that tissues of animals with certain diseases have an abnormal activity of cyclic AMP phosphodiesterase. These include aortas of spontaneously hypertensive rats (52), adipocytes of congenitally obese mice (53), pancreas and adipose tissue of spontaneously diabetic mice (54), plasma (55) and hearts (56) of diabetic rats, and retina of mice with an inherited retinal degenerative disease (57, 58). Our studies have shown that the activities of both cyclic AMP phosphodiesterase and cyclic GMP phosphodiesterase are increased tenfold in leukemic lymphocytes compared with that of normal lymphocytes (59–61).

Certain diseases may also have a defect in the major site at which cyclic nucleotides act, i.e. at the protein kinases. For example, in a variant of pseudohypoparathyroidism (Type II), although cyclic AMP is produced in response to parathyroid hormone, the cyclic nucleotide fails to induce the normal physiological response (62). A similar effect is seen in certain murine lymphomas. Whereas in most lymphomas cyclic AMP is cytotoxic, in a mutant cell line lacking a specific cyclic AMP–dependent protein kinase, cyclic AMP fails to exert a carcinostatic effect (63, 64). Abnormalities in the intracellular binding of cyclic nucleotides have also been seen in other forms of cancer (65–67) and in diabetes (68).

Measurement of Cyclic Nucleotides in Tissue and Extracellular Fluid As a Diagnostic Aid

The findings that certain diseases are associated with an abnormal metabolism of cyclic nucleotides suggests that one might find a different concentration of cyclic nucleotides in the diseased tissue or in one of the extracellular fluid compartments (e.g. plasma, urine, or cerebrospinal fluid) of diseased individuals. This proved to be the case (for review see ref. 69). For example, in studies of the urinary excretion of cyclic nucleotides it was reported that the concentration of cyclic AMP in urine is increased in patients with diabetes (70), hyperthyroidism (71, 72), and hyperparathyroidism (73, 74). Moreover, injection of parathyroid hormone causes a large increase in urinary cyclic AMP in patients with hypoparathyroidism but not in patients with pseudohypoparathyroidism (75, 76). Urinary cyclic AMP does not increase in response to ADH in patients with nephrogenic diabetes insipidus (42) but does increase in response to ADH in patients who are ADH deficient (77). The reports of urinary excretion of cyclic AMP in manic patients are conflicting. Some showed an increase in cyclic AMP excretion in mania (79–81), whereas more recent studies failed to find such differences (82, 83). Finally, it has been found that the concentration of cyclic GMP in urine of rats bearing hepatomas is increased in proportion to the rate of tumor growth (84).

In studies of the concentration of cyclic nucleotides in plasma of diseased individuals, it was found that cyclic AMP increased following massive myocardial infarction (85) and increased in patients with hypertension (86). In cerebrospinal fluid, cyclic AMP was reported to be elevated during the manic phase and decreased during the depressive phase of manic depressive disease (80). In gingival fluid, cyclic AMP was decreased in diabetic patients (87). In saliva, cyclic AMP was increased in children with Down's syndrome (88).

With the exception of the case of hypoparathyroidism, none of the above studies has as yet resulted in the development of specific diagnostic tests. Nevertheless, the potential of finding an early diagnostic test based on a correlation between the concentration of cyclic nucleotide in extracellular fluids with a particular disease state still exists, and this area of study should continue to be explored.

These studies point to the possibility that cyclic nucleotides are important factors in the etiology or pathogenesis of many diseases and suggest that by restoring the imbalance in the intracellular concentration of cyclic nucleotides, one may eliminate the cause or alleviate the symptoms of the disease. The enormous problem presented to the pharmacologist is not only how to alter the intracellular concentration of cyclic nucleotides, but more importantly, how to alter the concentration of each of the cyclic nucleotides selectively in discrete cell types.

DEVELOPMENT OF THERAPEUTIC AGENTS THAT ALTER CYCLIC NUCLEOTIDE METABOLISM

General Considerations

A major problem in using drugs affecting cyclic nucleotide metabolism to alter physiological responses is the ubiquitous nature of the cyclic nucleotides and the wide variety of responses they produce. (For other reviews of this topic see ref. 89–93.) It is difficult to conceive how one can alter the function of a specific cell type by manipulating cyclic nucleotide metabolism without also changing the concentration of cyclic nucleotides in other cells and, consequently, altering their function as well. Fortunately, this problem may be overcome because the metabolism of the cyclic nucleotides is controlled by an extremely complex system of enzymes consisting of many isozymes and receptor subunits. Moreover, the characteristics of these enzyme systems differ between tissues and even between cell types (94). The development of pharmacological agents which could take advantage of these characteristic differences in the enzymes might result in the selective alteration of cyclic nucleotide metabolism only in the diseased tissue. To do this, one must first gain a firm understanding of the fundamental properties of these enzymes.

Adenylate Cyclase

Adenylate cyclase, the enzyme that catalyzes the conversion of ATP to cyclic AMP, consists of a catalytic subunit facing the interior of the cell and one or more receptors in contact with the intracellular fluid (97). (For reviews of this topic see ref. 6, 93, 95, 96.) The catalytic portion of adenylate cyclase of all mammalian cells is activated by sodium fluoride. Hormones and neurotransmitters, on the other hand, are thought to interact with specific receptor sites, present only on certain cell membranes. Thus, a given hormone activates only the adenylate cyclase contained in the tissue in which the hormone exerts a physiological action, thereby explaining the specificity of hormonal actions (reviewed in 93).

Since variations in the properties of the receptor, rather than of the catalytic moiety of adenylate cyclase, apparently are responsible for the specificity with which different hormones can activate the various adenylate cyclases, one might be able to develop specific drugs that inhibit adenylate cyclase activity by preventing the hormone's interaction with the receptor. Unfortunately, little progress has been made in this promising area of research [see (93) for a more detailed discussion of agents that activate or inhibit adenylate cyclase].

Recently, a heat-stable, calcium-dependent protein, originally shown to increase phosphodiesterase activity (98), has been demonstrated to activate adenylate cyclase as well (99, 100). Whether this observation can be exploited to develop other types of selective agents for inhibiting specific adenylate cyclases must await further investigation. This endogenous activator of phosphodiesterase is discussed further in a subsequent section.

Guanylate Cyclase

Guanylate cyclase catalyzes the formation of cyclic GMP from GTP. (See ref. 93, 101, 102 for reviews.) This enzyme apparently exists in more than one form since guanylate cyclase activity isolated from soluble and particulate fractions migrate differently on gel filtration columns and respond differently to detergents and ions (103, 104).

The general, albeit greatly simplified, consensus relating the nucleotide cyclases to the function of the autonomic nervous system is that adenylate cyclase mediates β-adrenergic responses whereas guanylate cyclase is involved in cholinergic transmission. This is based largely on the results showing that sympathomimetic agents, as a rule, elevate cyclic AMP in adrenergically innervated structures (97, 105), whereas cholinergic agents cause an increase in the concentration of cyclic GMP (106, 107, 110).

Although it is well established that adenylate cyclase is activated by a wide variety of substances, only recently has it been demonstrated that guanylate cyclase can be stimulated in vitro (108, 109). However, there is substantial evidence that several hormones and neurotransmitters can increase the concentration of cyclic GMP (106, 107, 110, 111).

The development of agents that can selectively inhibit the activity of guanylate cyclase is still in its infancy but will surely progress as one gains a clearer understanding of the factors controlling the normal function of this enzyme. One important obstacle which must be overcome is the lack of hormonal responsiveness of guanylate cyclase in broken cell preparations.

Cyclic Nucleotide Phosphodiesterase

DISTRIBUTION   Cyclic nucleotide phosphodiesterase activity is found in virtually all living cells, its relative activity varying greatly among different tissues (114, 115). (For reviews see ref. 93, 112, 113.) The regional and subcellular distribution of cyclic

GMP phosphodiesterase generally parallels that of cyclic AMP phosphodiesterase. Both enzyme activities are found in all subcellular fractions with most of the activity being in the 100,000 xg supernatant fluid (61, 114, 116–120).

Although phosphodiesterase is largely a soluble enzyme, some investigators have suggested that the particulate enzyme may be of greater physiological importance since the particulate fraction contains a high affinity form of the enzyme (112, 113, 121). However, the soluble fraction also contains a high affinity form of phosphodiesterase (94, 122–124). Moreover, it is not uncommon to achieve cyclic AMP concentrations of 10^{-4} M and more in whole tissue and cells in response to hormones (125–127). Thus, even if there were no intracellular compartmentalization of cyclic nucleotides, which in fact there is (128), it would not be difficult to achieve concentrations of cyclic nucleotides in at least the 0.1 millimolar range at the active site of phosphodiesterase. In our view, it is more likely that both the low and high K_m forms of phosphodiesterase play a role in regulating the intracellular concentration of cyclic nucleotides, the low K_m form of the enzyme being responsible for the basal levels and the high K_m form controlling the cyclic nucleotide concentrations following hormonal stimulation of the nucleotide cyclases (124).

SUBSTRATE SPECIFICITY   The cyclic nucleotide phosphodiesterases are not completely substrate specific since some of the purified phosphodiesterase isozymes can hydrolyze cyclic AMP and cyclic GMP as well as a number of other cyclic nucleotides. However, the different isozymes of phosphodiesterase do have different relative affinities for the various cyclic nucleotides (129–137).

KINETIC PROPERTIES   Phosphodiesterase exhibits anomalous kinetic behavior, suggesting either the existence of a single enzyme form with the property of negative cooperativity (138) or the existence of at least two forms of phosphodiesterase, one having a low affinity (high K_m) for cyclic AMP and the other having a high affinity (low K_m) (94, 124, 130, 139–143). The evidence suggests that both possibilities are true. On the one hand, it has been shown that there are different molecular forms of phosphodiesterase (see below) and, on the other hand, it has been shown that even highly purified isozymes of phosphodiesterase exhibit negative or positive cooperativity, suggesting that there are allosteric sites on the enzyme that influence the catalytic site (132, 138, 144, 145).

MULTIPLE MOLECULAR FORMS   The existence of multiple molecular forms of phosphodiesterase has been demonstrated in many tissues by numerous investigators using a variety of techniques (94, 119, 125, 143, 146–156). The pattern and ratio of these phosphodiesterase isozymes vary with the specific tissue (94, 130, 148, 149, 156) and cell type (94, 157), and their activity can be altered both chronically and acutely. Chronically, it has been shown that a specific form of phosphodiesterase can be induced by treating astrocytoma cells with norepinephrine (157). Other studies have demonstrated that one of the phosphodiesterase isozymes increases with the age of the animals (143). Acutely, it has been demonstrated that the different phosphodiesterase isozymes can be selectively inhibited and activated by drugs (94,

120, 158–160). This phenomenon is discussed in detail in a later section and forms the basis of our hypothesis that drugs can be developed that selectively alter cyclic nucleotide metabolism in a diseased tissue.

ENDOGENOUS ACTIVATOR   While purifying phosphodiesterase from heart, Cheung (98, 161) noticed that the phosphodiesterase activity decreased as the enzyme became more pure, suggesting that a factor that activates phosphodiesterase was being removed during the purification process (reviewed in 162). This activator has now been isolated and has been the subject of numerous investigations (137, 163–168). The activator is a heat-stable, calcium-dependent protein (149, 166, 169–171) with a molecular weight of between 11,000 and 40,000 (161, 172). The mechanism by which the activator increases phosphodiesterase activity is quite complex and is still controversial (171, 173–175). At low concentrations, the activator increases the maximum velocity of hydrolysis (V_{max}) of cyclic AMP phosphodiesterase (158, 173) and cyclic GMP phosphodiesterase (137), whereas at high concentrations the activator appears to decrease the apparent Michaelis constant (K_m) for cyclic AMP (137, 173, 174) and cyclic GMP (137).

This endogenous activator is of particular interest to us because it is extremely potent and highly selective. Less than 1 μg of activator is capable of increasing the activity of one of the molecular forms of phosphodiesterase more than tenfold, while the activity of other isozymes of phosphodiesterase isolated from the same tissue remains essentially unaltered (158). Moreover, this activable form of phosphodiesterase is not present in all tissues (60, 61, 120), and where it is found, it is present in different amounts relative to the other phosphodiesterase isozymes (149, 176). Therefore, by interfering with the activation process, one may be able to inhibit selectively phosphodiesterase activity in one tissue and not in another. Recent studies from our laboratory indicate that certain phenothiazine antipsychotics, in fact, do act by preventing the activation of phosphodiesterase (158, 159, 168).

The proposal that the interaction of the activator with the activable form of phosphodiesterase is controlled by a protein kinase–mediated release of activator from the membrane (177) suggests yet another site at which drugs might act to alter the metabolism of cyclic nucleotides.

To summarize, the properties of the cyclic nucleotide phosphodiesterase system pertinent to our discussion are the following: (a) the enzymes exist in several different molecular forms; (b) these isozymes are unequally distributed among the various tissues; (c) they have different kinetic properties and different substrate affinities; (d) they can be selectively activated by an endogenous protein; (e) they can be selectively inhibited by drugs; and (f) they possess allosteric sites that can influence their activity.

These properties of the cyclic nucleotide phosphodiesterases suggest to us that drugs could be developed which would interfere with phosphodiesterase activity through a variety of different mechanisms, namely: Drugs could act (a) by interfering with the binding of substrate to the active site of the enzyme by competing with the substrate for the active site, (b) by altering allosteric sites on the enzyme, or

(c) by interfering with the release or binding of activators. Drugs acting by these mechanisms may prove to be highly selective in modifying the phosphodiesterase activity and, consequently, the intracellular concentration of cyclic nucleotides in discrete cell types, and may, therefore, constitute a new class of pharmacologic agents useful in the treatment of diseases.

USE OF PHOSPHODIESTERASE INHIBITORS IN THE TREATMENT OF DISEASE

Drugs that inhibit phosphodiesterase activity have been used for decades in treating diseases [for recent reviews see (89, 120, 178)]. Although it is obvious that not all of the beneficial effects of these drugs can be explained by their inhibition of phosphodiesterase, nevertheless some drugs clearly act by inhibiting phosphodiesterase activity. The findings that several diseases are associated with an abnormal metabolism of cyclic nucleotides suggest that it might be possible to alter the course of diseases with specific phosphodiesterase inhibitors. We concentrate our discussion on the use of phosphodiesterase inhibitors only in those diseases in which there is good evidence of abnormalities in cyclic nucleotide metabolism.

Cancer Chemotherapeutic Agents

Of the many diseases associated with an abnormality in cyclic nucleotide physiology, neoplasia has received the most attention and offers one of the best examples of how, by controlling the metabolism of cyclic nucleotides, one might eventually alter the course of a disease (reviewed in 154, 179, 180). Generally, it has been found that malignant or transformed cells have a lower concentration of cyclic AMP when compared with normal or nontransformed cells (50, 181–184). Moreover, cyclic AMP or agents that increase the concentration of cyclic AMP, such as activators of adenylate cyclase or inhibitors or phosphodiesterase, reduce the growth rate of malignant cells (185–191), and, in some cases, revert the morphological and biochemical characteristics of these cells toward those of normal cells (192–195). Pertinent to our discussion are studies showing a correlation between phosphodiesterase inhibition and carcinostasis. For example, Hsie et al (196) have shown that dibutyryl cyclic AMP, which reduces the growth rate of transformed Chinese hamster ovary cells, also inhibits a low K_m phosphodiesterase in these cells. Tisdale & Phillips (197, 198) have demonstrated that the carcinostatic effect of alkylating agents, such as chlorambucil and melphalan, may be due, at least in part, to their inhibition of phosphodiesterase. They demonstrated that chlorambucil increased the concentration of cyclic AMP only in those cell lines in which it inhibited cell growth; it had no effect on the concentration of cyclic AMP in chlorambucil-resistant cell lines. These results could be explained by the ability of alkylating agents to inhibit a low K_m form of phosphodiesterase; this form of the enzyme apparently is deficient in the drug-resistant cell lines.

Determination of the mechanism by which cyclic AMP reverts malignant cells toward the normal phenotype may provide the key to the pathogenesis of certain forms of cancer. One clue into the mechanism by which cyclic AMP exerts its carcinostatic effects was derived from studies on mutant cells. Cyclic AMP failed to produce a carcinostatic effect in mutant lymphoma cells that lack a specific cyclic AMP-dependent protein kinase, suggesting that activation of protein kinase was essential for the growth-inhibitory effects of cyclic AMP (63, 64). Activation of protein kinase could, in turn, lead to the phosphorylation of histones (199) which could account for the increased DNA-mediated RNA synthesis (200), increased protein synthesis (201), and changes in the properties of the cell membrane (202, 203) seen in malignant cells treated with agents that increase the intracellular concentration of cyclic AMP.

Drugs Used in the Treatment of Psoriasis

Psoriasis is a disease of the skin characterized by an increased proliferation and a decreased differentiation of epidermal epithelium and by an increased accumulation of glycogen in these cells. Stimulated by the observations that cyclic AMP inhibits cellular proliferation (185), induces cellular differentiation (192–195), and stimulates the breakdown of glycogen (16), Voorhees and his co-workers (204, 205) have studied the concentration and metabolism of cyclic nucleotides in the skin of psoriatic patients. They demonstrated that the concentration of cyclic AMP was significantly decreased in psoriatic lesions (204), whereas the levels of cyclic GMP was increased (205). They also showed that β-adrenergic agonists such as isoproterenol inhibited epidermal cell division and that this effect was associated with a concomitant increase in cyclic AMP (206).

Studies of the adenylate cyclase system of psoriatic skin have not yielded conclusive results (207, 208). However, studies of the phosphodiesterase system showed a threefold increase in cyclic AMP phosphodiesterase activity in psoriatic lesions (208). The increased phosphodiesterase activity could explain the decreased concentrations of cyclic AMP and suggests that phosphodiesterase inhibitors may be effective clinical agents in treating psoriasis. This concept gains support from the recent clinical study showing that topically applied papaverine, a potent inhibitor of phosphodiesterase, was effective in the treatment of psoriasis (209).

Antiasthmatics

One suggestion concerning the etiology of asthma is that there is an intrinsic defect in the β-adrenergic receptor–adenylate cyclase complex. In the bronchioles this defect results in a decreased response to the smooth muscle relaxant effects of catecholamines (210). Support for this notion is derived from experiments showing that asthmatics have a diminished hyperglycemic (211) and lipolytic (212) response to epinephrine, and that leucocytes from these patients show a decreased accumulation of cyclic AMP in response to catecholamines (213). This hypothesis is supported further by studies showing that several agents that are effective in treating asthma, both acutely and prophylactically, increase the intracellular concentration of cyclic AMP. For example, the most effective agents for treating the acute asthmatic attack are epinephrine and isoproterenol, potent stimulators of adenylate cyclase. The phosphodiesterase inhibitor, theophylline, theophylline-containing compounds, such as aminophylline, and several other phosphodiesterase inhibitors (214–216) are also effective in treating experimentally induced asthmatic reactions. Since theophylline often potentiates the effects of agents that stimulate adenylate cyclase activity in vitro (217), it would not be surprising to find that the concomitant administration of a catecholamine and theophylline is more effective than using either drug alone.

In individuals with allergic or intrinsic asthma, the asthmatic attack is precipitated by the binding of an allergen to a specific immunoglobulin on sensitized mast cells which results in the release of pharmacologically active substances such as histamine, bradykinin, and slow-reacting substances of anaphylaxis. The release of these agents appears to be controlled by the cyclic nucleotides since drugs that increase the intracellular concentration of cyclic AMP inhibit the antigen-induced release of histamine from sensitized tissues (218–220). In contrast, compound 48/80, which promotes the release of histamine, decreases the intracellular concentration of cyclic AMP (221), presumably by increasing phosphodiesterase activity (222).

A logical approach to the prophylactic treatment of asthma, therefore, would be through the use of drugs that would raise the intracellular levels of cyclic AMP in mast cells, thereby preventing the release of anaphylactoid mediators from these cells. The recently developed drug, sodium dichromoglycate, may act through this mechanism since it has been shown to be an inhibitor, albeit a weak one, of phosphodiesterase activity (223). Moreover, lymphocytes of patients receiving disodium chromoglycate do, in fact, have lower activities of phosphodiesterase than do those of untreated or theophylline-treated patients (224).

Certain steroids used prophylactically in treating asthma may also act by altering the metabolism or action of cyclic nucleotides. This would be predictable since glucocorticoids augment many physiological responses mediated by cyclic AMP, such as lipolysis and glycogenolysis (225). In this regard, hydrocortisone (226) and dexamethasone (227) have been reported to inhibit phosphodiesterase activity. However, since these agents are relatively weak phosphodiesterase inhibitors, they may be acting by increasing adenylate cyclase activity or by increasing the synthesis of a cyclic AMP–dependent-protein kinase.

Anti-Inflammatory Agents

The role of cyclic nucleotides in the inflammatory process has been reviewed recently by Ignarro et al (40). They and other investigators (228, 229) have demonstrated that cyclic AMP stabilizes lysosomal membranes, and cyclic GMP labilizes these membranes. Moreover, they have shown that the release of endogenous substances that mediate the inflammatory response is inhibited by agents which increase the intracellular concentration of cyclic AMP. Based on these results, one would predict that certain cyclic AMP phosphodiesterase inhibitors might have antiinflammatory properties. In fact, it has been shown that the antiinflammatory compounds, indomethacin and several of its analogues (230), arylaceticade, mefenemic acid, flufenic acid, quinolone compounds, and pyrazolones (230, 231) inhibit phosphodiesterase of chicken cartilage.

Drugs Used in the Treatment of Obesity

Cyclic AMP mediates the effect of catecholamines and other lypolytic agents (217). Evidence that some forms of obesity may be due to a defect in the metabolism of cyclic nucleotides comes from the study of Kupiecki & Adams (232) who showed that the adenylate cyclase system of adipocytes of genetically obese mice was poorly responsive to the stimulatory effects of catecholamines, and from that of Lovell-Smith & Sneyd (53) who showed an increased activity of phosphodiesterase in these mice as well as a decreased responsiveness of adenylate cyclase to catecholamines. This suggests that drugs which inhibit the specific phosphodiesterase isozyme in adipocytes may be of benefit in certain forms of obesity.

Drugs Used in the Treatment of Cardiovascular Disease

SMOOTH MUSCLE RELAXANTS   Evidence for a role of cyclic AMP in the relaxation of smooth muscle has been reviewed by Somlyo et al (24). This evidence is based, in part, on the observations that several drugs that relax smooth muscle inhibit phosphodiesterase activity. These agents include papaverine (233, 234), isobutylmethylxanthine (235), diazoxide (236, 237), and chromonar (238). Wells et al (155, 160) have isolated two phosphodiesterase isozymes from porcine coronary arteries and have demonstrated that only one of the isozymes was activated by the endogenous protein activator. They also found that papaverine was a potent inhibitor of this activable isozyme whereas isobutylmethylxanthine was a more potent inhibitor of the nonactivable isozyme. Thus, as in the brain (see section on drugs used in the treatment of neuropsychiatric diseases), the isozymes of phosphodiesterase in coronary arteries can be selectively activated and inhibited by drugs. It would be important to learn whether the increased activity of phosphodiesterase seen in arteries of hypertensive animals (52) is due to a selective increase in one of these isozymes. If this were so, and one could find a drug that selectively inhibits this phosphodiesterase isozyme, a more potent and specific class of therapeutic agents for relaxing smooth muscle would evolve.

DIURETICS   The hypothesis that cAMP is involved in diuresis is derived largely from experiments showing that cAMP increases the water permeability of toad bladder (239). The pharmacological evidence supporting this notion is based on the observations that clinically effective diuretics such as the benzothiadiazine derivatives inhibit phosphodiesterase activity (236, 237). Other classes of diuretics such as the mercurials (240), furosemide and bendroflumethiazide (89), ethacrynic acid, chlorthalidone, and acetazolamide (241) inhibit phosphodiesterase activity. However, since antidiuretic hormone, as well as diuretic agents, elevates cAMP, it is not readily apparent how inhibition of phosphodiesterase activity could explain the mechanism of action of diuretics. Perhaps this apparent contradiction could be clarified by determining the effects of all these agents on the specific phosphodiesterase isozymes in the cells on which these drugs are thought to act to produce their diuretic effects.

CARDIAC GLYCOSIDES   There is abundant evidence that cyclic AMP plays a role in the inotropic effects of the heart (26, 242). The observation that cardiac tissue from experimental animals and humans with congestive heart failure exhibits a reduced accumulation of cyclic AMP in response to glucagon (242–244) and norepinephrine (245) suggests that specific phosphodiesterase inhibitors might be of benefit in this disease. Support for this proposal was provided by Lippmann (246) who demonstrated that certain analogues of cardiac glycosides were more potent inhibitors of phosphodiesterase than was theophylline. In contrast, several naturally occurring and pharmacologically inactive glycosides were less potent inhibitors of this enzyme.

ANTIATHEROSCLEROTIC AGENTS   The possible role of cyclic AMP in the pathogenesis of atherosclerosis has been reviewed by Shimamato (247). He suggested that a decreased concentration of cyclic AMP in arterial endothelial cells may be responsible for the accumulation of lipids in these cells. This accumulation of lipid and the development of atherosclerosis in rabbits was inhibited by dibutyryl cyclic AMP, and phthalazinol and its derivatives, agents that inhibit phosphodiesterase activity (247). The hypolipidemic agent, eritadenine [2(R)-dihydroxy-Y-(9-adenyl)-butyric acid], has also been shown to inhibit phosphodiesterase activity (248).

Oral Hypoglycemic Agents

Cyclic AMP induces the release of insulin from pancreatic islets (37). The therapeutic consequences, therefore, of inhibiting pancreatic phosphodiesterase would predictably be an increase in the release of insulin and a hypoglycemic effect. Accordingly, it was not surprising to find that several oral hypoglycemic agents such as the sulfonylureas inhibit phosphodiesterase activity (249–251). Agents that inhibit the dominant isozyme of phosphodiesterase present in pancreas might be still more effective and specific for treating adult onset diabetes.

Antiviral Agents

The antiviral agent, N-methyl-isatin-β semicarbazone, inhibited phosphodiesterase in peripheral blood lymphocytes but not in lymphoma cells (252). However, the role of cyclic nucleotides in viral infections is unclear.

Drugs Used in the Treatment of Neuropsychiatric Diseases

ANTIPSYCHOTIC AGENTS   The effects of cyclic nucleotides in the central nervous system and their role in neuropsychiatric disorders have been reviewed recently (29). The pharmacologic evidence supporting a role for these cyclic nucleotides in the central nervous system is based largely on the actions of psychotropic drugs, such as the phenothiazine antipsychotics and butyrophenones, on the cyclic nucleotide system of brain. Apparently, these drugs have two distinct effects on the enzymes catalyzing the biosynthesis and hydrolysis of cyclic nucleotides. On the one hand, they inhibit specific norepinephrine- (253) and dopamine- (254) sensitive adenylate cyclases, effects that would prevent the rise of cyclic AMP induced by these agents. On the other hand, they inhibit a specific activator-sensitive phosphodiesterase in brain (158, 159, 168), an effect that would tend to increase the intracellular concentration of cyclic nucleotides. Therefore, the net effect of these agents on the concentration of cyclic nucleotides in each area of the brain would depend on the relative quantity of the catecholamine-sensitive adenylate cyclases and the activator-sensitive phosphodiesterase in each of these brain areas. This theory predicts that antipsychotics might increase the level of cyclic AMP in one region of the brain and reduce it in another, an effect which, in fact, has recently been demonstrated (255).

The unusual specificity of antipsychotics for inhibiting a single phosphodiesterase isozyme in brain is discussed in more detail in a subsequent section.

ANTIANXIETY AGENTS   Antianxiety agents such as the benzodiazepines have also been shown to inhibit phosphodiesterase of brain (168, 256). The effects of these drugs on the phosphodiesterase of several areas of cat brain varied with the specific brain area studied (257).

TRICYCLIC ANTIDEPRESSANTS   Several dibenzazepines also inhibit phosphodiesterase activity. These agents were found to be competitive with cyclic AMP (256, 258, 259) and were more potent than theophylline (260), a finding which should not be viewed as remarkable since, despite its widespread use, theophylline is a relatively weak inhibitor of phosphodiesterase.

A FEASIBLE APPROACH TO THE SELECTIVE ALTERATION OF CYCLIC NUCLEOTIDE METABOLISM

Drugs that exert their effect by indiscriminately altering cyclic nucleotide metabolism would have little clinical utility since they would alter the function of many different types of cells. Ideally, the drug should be able to alter the concentration of specific cyclic nucleotides in a diseased tissue without substantially affecting the concentration of these cyclic nucleotides in normal tissue.

We feel that there is a good possibility of realizing this ideal. We base our optimism on the following observations: there are different patterns and ratios of the phosphodiesterase isozymes in different tissues; these isozymes can be selectively altered by drugs; certain diseases are associated with an abnormal metabolism of cyclic nucleotides; and drugs that alter the intracellular concentrations of cyclic nucleotides already have been shown to be fairly selective and effective therapeutic agents.

Some of the evidence in support of these statements has already been reviewed briefly. A more detailed discussion of the distribution and selective inhibition of the phosphodiesterase isozymes is presented below.

Several studies have shown that drugs could differentially inhibit the phosphodiesterase activity of different tissues (89, 90, 253, 259, 261, 262). For example, Uzunov & Weiss (253) showed that trifluoperazine was more effective in inhibiting the phosphodiesterase of cerebrum than that of cerebellum, and Pichard et al (259) demonstrated that dipyridamole, an inhibitor of platelet aggregation, is a more potent inhibitor of the phosphodiesterase of platelets than that of the brain, while the tricyclic antidepressants, opipramol, nortryptyline, and imipramine were more potent inhibitors of the phosphodiesterase of brain than that of platelets. These and other studies suggested that the selectivity of the phosphodiesterase inhibitors was due to a difference in the distribution or in the sensitivity of the phosphodiesterase isozymes to inhibitors.

Distribution of Phosphodiesterase Isozymes

It is now clear that there are marked differences in the distribution of the various cyclic nucleotide phosphodiesterase isozymes among different tissues and cell types (see section on multiple molecular forms). For example, the rat cerebellum was found to have six forms of phosphodiesterase (149), cerebrum four forms (94), and caudate nucleus two forms (119). The lung (120) also had two forms of phosphodiesterase activity but the types and ratio of these isozymes were different from those of the caudate nucleus. A cloned astrocytoma cell line (C21) had two forms of phosphodiesterase as well, but the type and ratio of these isozymes was unlike that found in the caudate nucleus or in lung (94). Finally, cloned neuroblastoma cells were shown to have a single isozyme of phosphodiesterase, and this isozyme was different from either of the two forms found in the C21 astrocytoma cell lines (94).

Selective Activation and Inhibition of the Phosphodiesterase Isozymes

The other important property of these isozymes that must be satisfied before phosphodiesterase inhibitors can be clinically useful is that they must be selectively activated or inhibited by drugs. Studies from our laboratory demonstrated that some of the phosphodiesterase isozymes can, in fact, be selectively inhibited and activated by endogenous and exogenous agents (94, 119, 120, 144, 149, 158, 159), a finding that has recently been confirmed by other laboratories (160, 175). For example, of the four isozymes of phosphodiesterase isolated from the rat cerebrum (94) (isozymes were designated as Peaks I to IV according to the order of their emergence from a preparative polyacrylamide gel column), Peak I, which hydrolyzes cyclic AMP and not cyclic GMP, is relatively resistant to the commonly used inhibitors of phosphodiesterase (120, 158, 159). Peak II, which is the major form of phosphodiesterase in cerebrum (94, 158, 159), is of great pharmacological and biological interest, since it is the only major isozyme which is activated by the endogenous activator of phosphodiesterase (94, 158). This isozyme, which is sensitive to the inhibitory effects of cyclic GMP and is particularly sensitive to the effects of trifluoperazine and other antipsychotic agents when it is in the activated form, has been examined in some detail (94, 137, 158, 168; see below). Peak III phosphodiesterase was not significantly activated by the protein activator and was relatively sensitive to theophylline and papaverine (158). Peak IV phosphodiesterase was more sensitive to papaverine than to trifluoperazine or theophylline (158). A summary of these studies is presented in Table 2.

Table 2 Selective inhibition of the multiple forms of cyclic AMP phosphodiesterase of rat cerebrum[a]

Peak	Ki values (μM)			
	Theophylline	Trifluoperazine	Papaverine	Cyclic GMP
I	2000	1000	180	730
II (not activated)	350	250	100	20
II (activated)	350	10	100	10
III	180	250	60	25
IV	600	75	25	—

[a] The phosphodiesterase isozymes were prepared from the soluble 100,000 × g supernatant fraction of rat cerebrum. Each peak of phosphodiesterase was identified by its electrophoretic mobility on a polyacrylamide gel column (149). Phosphodiesterase activity was determined by the luciferin-luciferase technique (140). The Peak II isozyme was assayed in the absence and presence of optimum amounts of the calcium-dependent activator. The activator produced approximately a tenfold increase in phosphodiesterase activity. (Taken in part from 158.)

Mechanism for the Selective Inhibition of the Phosphodiesterase Isozymes

One obvious explanation for the selective inhibition of the phosphodiesterase isozymes is that the phosphodiesterase inhibitors are acting by different mechanisms. Therefore, considerable effort was spent in studying the mechanism of action of these agents. Thus far, evidence has been obtained for four distinct mechanisms of action. The drugs may act (a) by competing with the cyclic nucleotide substrate; (b) by acting at the substrate site noncompetitively; (c) by acting at an allosteric site to increase or decrease the affinity of the enzyme for its substrate; and (d) by acting on one of the endogenous activators or cofactors for the enzyme.

Methylxanthines, like theophylline, which have a structural similarity to the cyclic nucleotides, competitively inhibit phosphodiesterase. This was shown initially in cardiac tissue (115) and more recently in isolated phosphodiesterase isozymes of brain (94, 158). Low concentrations of papaverine also competitively inhibit the phosphodiesterase isozymes (158), whereas high concentrations appear to act noncompetitively (158). Other phosphodiesterase inhibitors such as SQ 20,009 also have been reported to act both competitively and noncompetitively (262).

A compound that apparently acts at an allosteric site to alter the activity of cyclic AMP phosphodiesterase is the cyclic nucleotide, cyclic GMP (132, 144, 145). This latter observation suggests that the concentration of one cyclic nucleotide may influence the metabolism of another cyclic nucleotide.

The final mechanism by which compounds may act is by interfering with the endogenous activator of phosphodiesterase. This mechanism may prove to be one of the most specific since the activity of only one major form of phosphodiesterase is increased by this endogenous activator (149, 158–160, 175). Since trifluoperazine was a particularly effective inhibitor of the Peak II isozyme of phosphodiesterase, and since this is the only major phosphodiesterase isozyme which is activated by the endogenous activator of phosphodiesterase, we examined the influence of tri-fluoperazine on Peak II in the presence and absence of the phosphodiesterase activator. The phenothiazine was found to be 25 times more potent an inhibitor of activated Peak II than of the unactivated form (Table 2). Moreover, this inhibition of phosphodiesterase by trifluoperazine (158) or chlorpromazine (168) could be overcome by adding excess activator; kinetic analysis of these data revealed that these phenothiazines were competitive inhibitors of the activation of Peak II phos-phodiesterase. Other centrally acting drugs were also shown to be highly specific inhibitors of the activated form of phosphodiesterase (169).

The specific mechanisms by which phenothiazine antipsychotics block the activa-tion of phosphodiesterase has recently been studied in our laboratory where it was shown that the phenothiazines act by binding to the endogenous activator (R. Levin and B. Weiss, unpublished). Since the same protein that increases phosphodiesterase activity apparently is responsible for the activation of adenylate cyclase, our results may explain why phenothiazine antipsychotics inhibit the activity of both adenylate cyclase (253, 254, 263) and phosphodiesterase.

These results suggest again that drugs, by selectively inhibiting the phosphodiester-ase isozymes, may be able to raise the intracellular concentration of cyclic AMP in discrete tissues. For example, phenothiazine antipsychotics should raise the con-centration of cyclic AMP in cerebral cortex, which has a high proportion of Peak II phosphodiesterase (94, 158), but should have little effect on peripheral tissues that have little or none of this isozyme (60, 61, 144). Papaverine, on the other hand, may exert a greater effect on tissues with a high proportion of Peak III or Peak IV phosphodiesterase. Studies of this type might also yield compounds that exert a selective inhibitory action on either the cyclic GMP phosphodiesterase or cyclic AMP phosphodiesterase (160), a result which would render even greater specificity of action to these compounds.

Possible Clinical Application of the Selective Inhibition of Phosphodiesterase Isozymes

Although the extrapolation of these basic studies to therapeutic applications is a long way off, the goal is clear, that is, to find drugs that will selectively inhibit or activate the major isozyme of phosphodiesterase in each tissue. If a disease is caused by a defect in the metabolism of cyclic nucleotides, these drugs may be able to restore the concentration of cyclic nucleotides in that tissue without adversely affecting other tissue.

Recently, we have begun to test this approach in an attempt to alter selectively the cyclic nucleotide metabolism of malignant cells. The investigations to be de-scribed were based on the assumptions that (a) an abnormality in cyclic nucleotide physiology was a characteristic and perhaps a causative factor in neoplastic disease; (b) the major isozyme of malignant tissue may be different from that of normal tissues; (c) this abnormal metabolism might be corrected by the selective manipula-tion of phosphodiesterase isozymes; (d) this isozyme could be selectively manipu-lated by drugs; and (e) the correction of cyclic nucleotide metabolism would result in the restoration of normal growth and differentiation of neoplastic tissue and would, therefore, provide a new therapeutic approach to malignant disease.

For these studies we chose the murine leukemias, L5178Y and L1210, because there was substantial evidence to suggest that these and other leukemic lymphocytes had an abnormal cyclic nucleotide system (see Table 1). For example, Monahan and co-workers (264) demonstrated that unlike normal cells, which accumulate cyclic AMP at high cell density and exhibit contact inhibition of growth, L5178Y cells do not. The addition of exogenous cyclic AMP to these cells, however, does inhibit their growth (187). Our studies showing that both L5178Y and L1210 leukemic lymphocytes had approximately a tenfold increase in activity in both cyclic AMP phosphodiesterase and cyclic GMP phosphodiesterase compared with that of normal lymphocytes (59, 60, 61) provided one explanation for the inability of cyclic AMP to accumulate in these leukemic lymphocytes.

To determine whether this increased phosphodiesterase activity of leukemic lymphocytes was due to a specific elevation of one of the phosphodiesterase isozymes, we separated the phosphodiesterases of these lymphocytes by gel electrophoresis according to the procedure of Uzunov & Weiss (149). Three major forms of phosphodiesterase were found. One peak, which constituted about 5% of the total activity, was found in fractions 30–35; a second peak, also having about 5% of the activity, was in fractions 40–50; the third peak (fractions 80–100) accounted for about 90% of the activity recovered from the gel electrophoresis column. This pattern of phosphodiesterase activity was clearly different from that of all other tissues we have studied thus far. For example, leukemic lymphocytes do not contain the major form of phosphodiesterase found in most brain areas, i.e. the activator-sensitive Peak II, nor do they have substantial quantities of the isozyme which is the predominant form found in salivary gland. Thus, the mouse salivary gland had only two major forms of phosphodiesterase activity. The first peak (fractions 40–50) accounted for about 60% of the activity and the second peak (fractions 60–70) for about 40% of the recovered activity. The different isozymic pattern of phosphodiesterase activity of leukemic lymphocytes suggested that the phosphodiesterase in this tissue might be selectively inhibited by drugs.

To test this hypothesis we compared the effects of a phenothiazine (chlorpromazine), a methylxanthine (isobutylmethylxanthine), a benzylisoquinolone (papaverine), and a pyrazole derivative (SQ 20,009) on the phosphodiesterase activity of cerebrum, salivary gland, and leukemic lymphocytes. As predicted from earlier experiments, the phosphodiesterase of cerebrum, which is rich in the Peak II isozyme, was very sensitive to the inhibitory effects of chlorpromazine ($I_{50} = 30 \mu M$) whereas the phosphodiesterase of leukemic lymphocytes, which is essentially devoid of Peak II phosphodiesterase, was totally resistant to the phenothiazine (61). Papaverine, which is a potent inhibitor of Peak III phosphodiesterase of cerebrum (159), produced a marked inhibition of the major phosphodiesterase isozyme of leukemic lymphocytes. SQ 20,009, a drug which also has been shown to be a selective inhibitor of isolated phosphodiesterase isozymes (120), was 10 times more potent an inhibitor of the major form of phosphodiesterase of salivary gland than that of leukemic lymphocytes (Figure 1). In contrast, isobutylmethylxanthine was a more specific inhibitor of the major phosphodiesterase isozyme of leukemic lymphocytes than that of the major isozyme of salivary gland (Figure 2). These studies,

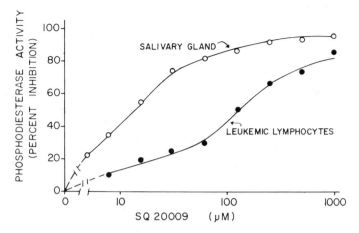

Figure 1   Effect of SQ 20,009 on purified isozymes of phosphodiesterase from mouse salivary gland and leukemic lymphocytes. Tissue was homogenized in 50 mM glycylglycine buffer, pH 8.0, and centrifuged at 100,000 xg for 60 min. The phosphodiesterase isozymes in the supernatant fraction were separated by preparative polyacrylamide gel electrophoresis (149). The activity of phosphodiesterase was assayed by the firefly luciferin-luciferase technique (140) with 100 μM cyclic AMP as substrate. The figure shows the effects of varying concentrations of SQ 20,009 [1-ethyl-4-(isopropylidenehydrazino)-1H-pyrazolo-(3,4-b)-pyridine-5-carboxylic acid, ethyl ester] on the major phosphodiesterase isozyme isolated from salivary gland (fractions 40–50) and leukemic lymphocytes (fractions 80–100).

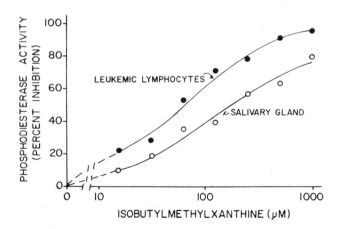

Figure 2   Effect of isobutylmethylxanthine on purified isozymes of phosphodiesterase from mouse salivary gland and leukemic lymphocytes. The tissue and isozymes were prepared as described in the legend to Figure 1. The major phosphodiesterase isozymes of salivary glands and leukemic lymphocytes were assayed in the absence and presence of varying concentrations of isobutylmethylxanthine.

combined with the evidence that cyclic AMP is cytotoxic to leukemic lymphocytes (63, 64), suggest that the development of selective inhibitors of the major phosphodiesterase isozyme of leukemic lymphocytes, may yield new agents for treating certain forms of leukemia.

Moreover, these studies support the hypothesis that by identifying and characterizing the major form of phosphodiesterase in each tissue, it may be possible to predict which drug would selectively inhibit the phosphodiesterase of that tissue. Further studies on the mechanisms by which these agents act and on the structure-activity relationship of these drugs will surely lead to more potent and more selective inhibitors of the individual phosphodiesterase isozymes.

SUMMARY

The cyclic nucleotides, cyclic AMP and cyclic GMP, influence a wide variety of biological functions, and many diseases apparently are associated with or may even be caused by an abnormal intracellular concentration of these cyclic nucleotides. This abnormal concentration of cyclic AMP or cyclic GMP in diseased tissue has been shown to be due to an alteration in the enzymes that catalyze their synthesis (nucleotide cyclases) or hydrolysis (cyclic nucleotide phosphodiesterases). Accordingly, by correcting the defect in cyclic nucleotide metabolism, the course of a disease may be favorably altered.

The cyclic nucleotide phosphodiesterases, which hydrolyze cyclic AMP and cyclic GMP, are instrumental in controlling the concentration of these cyclic nucleotides. Since these enzymes exist as a complex system of isozymes having characteristic differences among tissues, they represent excellent targets for selective pharmacological manipulation. Recent studies showed that the individual isozymes can be selectively activated and inhibited and that this selective alteration of enzyme activity is due to differences in the mechanisms by which these agents act. For example, methylxanthines inhibit phosphodiesterase activity by competing with the cyclic nucleotide substrates, SQ 20,009 inhibits phosphodiesterase activity both competitively and noncompetitively, cyclic GMP activates cyclic AMP phosphodiesterase by binding to an allosteric site, and the phenothiazine antipsychotics inhibit a specific isozyme of phosphodiesterase by interfering with an endogenous protein activator of this phosphodiesterase isozyme.

Since each tissue has its own peculiar pattern and ratio of the phosphodiesterase isozymes, drugs may be developed that will inhibit the major isozyme in each tissue, resulting in the selective alteration of the concentration of cyclic nucleotides in this tissue. As an example, our studies showed that leukemic lymphocytes have a markedly increased activity of phosphodiesterase compared with that of normal lymphocytes. This increase was due to an elevation of one of the phosphodiesterase isozymes. Since this isozyme can be inhibited by drugs which have relatively little action on the major phosphodiesterase isozymes of other tissue, one would predict that the concentration of cyclic nucleotides would be elevated in the leukemic cells but not in normal tissue. And since malignant cell growth can be repressed by increasing the intracellular concentration of cyclic AMP, specific phosphodiesterase inhibitors may inhibit the growth and induce the differentiation in these leukemic lymphocytes without adversely affecting the function of other tissue.

Thus, the evidence reviewed in this paper favors the conclusion that the determination of the biochemical properties of the phosphodiesterase isozymes in normal and diseased tissue and the continued search for new and more selective inhibitors of each phosphodiesterase isozyme may lead to the development of a new class of selective therapeutic agents, ones that act by altering the metabolism of cyclic nucleotides.

ACKNOWLEDGMENT

This investigation was supported in part by Grant Number CA15883, awarded by the National Cancer Institute, DHEW. We thank Ms. J. S. Siew for her help in typing the manuscript.

Literature Cited

1. Weiss, B. 1970. In *Biogenic Amines as Physiological Regulators,* ed. J. J. Blum, 35–73. New Jersey: Prentice-Hall
2. Greengard, P., Costa, E., eds. 1970. *Adv. Biochem. Psychopharmacol.* 3:11–381
3. Weiss, B., Crayton, J. W. 1970. *Adv. Biochem. Psychopharmacol.* 3:217–39
4. Robison, G. A., Butcher, R. W., Sutherland, E. W. 1971. *Cyclic AMP.* New York: Academic
5. Hardman, J. G., Robison, G. A., Sutherland, E. W. 1971. Cyclic nucleotides. *Ann. Rev. Physiol.* 33:311–36
6. Weiss, B. 1971. Cyclic AMP and cell function. *Ann. NY Acad. Sci.* 185:507–19
7. Hittelman, K. J., Butcher, R. W. 1972. In *Effects of Drugs on Cellular Control Mechanisms,* ed. B. R. Rabin, R. B. Freedman, 153–74. Baltimore: Univ. Park Press
8. Greengard, P., Paoletti, R., Robison, G. A., eds. 1972. *Adv. Cyclic Nucleotide Res.,* Vol. 1. 590 pp.
9. Rall, T. 1972. Role of adenosine 3',5'-monophosphate (cyclic AMP) in actions of catecholamines. *Pharmacol. Rev.* 24:399–409
10. Bitensky, M. W., Gorman, R. E. 1973. Cellular responses to cyclic AMP. *Prog. Biophys. Mol. Biol.* 26:411–61
11. Kahn, R. H., Lands, W. E. M., eds. 1973. *Prostaglandins and Cyclic AMP: Biological Actions and Clinical Applications.* New York: Academic. 304 pp.
12. Greengard, P., Robison, G. A., eds. 1973. *Adv. Cyclic Nucleotide Res.,* Vol. 3. 383 pp.
13. Greengard, P., Robison, G. A. eds. 1974. *Adv. Cyclic Nucleotide Res.,* Vol. 4. 461 pp.
14. Braun, W., Lichtenstein, L. M., Parker, C. W., eds. 1974. *Cyclic AMP, Cell Growth and the Immune Response.* New York: Springer. 411 pp.
15. Drummond, G. I., Greengard, P., Robison, G. A., eds. 1975. *Adv. Cyclic Nucleotide Res.,* Vol. 5. 841 pp.
16. Robison, G. A., Butcher, R. W., Sutherland, E. W. 1968. Cyclic AMP. *Ann. Rev. Biochem.* 37:149–74
17. Weiss, B., Kidman, A. D. 1969. *Adv. Biochem. Psychopharmacol.* 1:131–64
18. Ryan, W. L., Heidrick, M. L. 1968. Inhibition of cell growth in vitro by adenosine 3',5'-monophosphate. *Science* 162:1484–85
19. Castañeda, M., Tyler, A. 1968. Adenyl cyclase in plasma membrane preparations of sea urchin eggs and its increase in activity after fertilization. *Biochem. Biophys. Res. Commun.* 33:782–87
20. Zalin, R. J., Montague, W. 1975. Changes in cyclic AMP, adenylate cyclase and protein kinase levels during the development of embryonic chick skeletal muscle. *Exp. Cell Res.* 93:55–62
21. Bottomley, S. S., Whitcomb, W. H., Smithee, G. A., Moore, M. Z. 1971. Effect of cyclic adenosine 3',5'-monophosphate on bone marrow Δ-aminolevulinic acid synthetase and erythrocyte iron uptake. *J. Lab. Clin. Med.* 77:793–801
22. Rodgers, G. M., Fisher, J. W., George, W. J. 1975. Renal cyclic AMP accumulation and adenylate cyclase stimulation

by erythropoietic agents. *Am. J. Physiol.* 229:1387–92

23. Norris, A., Gorshein, D., Besa, E. C., Leonard, R. A., Gardner, F. H. 1974. Stimulation and suppression of erythropoiesis in the plethoric mouse by cyclic nucleotides. *Proc. Soc. Exp. Biol. Med.* 145:975–78

24. Somylo, A. P., Somlyo, A. V., Smiesko, V. 1972. *Adv. Cyclic Nucleotide Res.* 1:175–94

25. Bar, H. P. 1974. *Adv. Cyclic Nucleotide Res.* 4:195–237

26. Kukovetz, W., Poch, G. 1972. *Adv. Cyclic Nucleotide Res.* 1:261–90

27. Entman, M. L., Levey, G. S., Epstein, S. E. 1969. Mechanism of action of epinephrine and glucagon on the canine heart: Evidence for increase in sarcotubular calcium stores mediated by cyclic 3',5'-AMP. *Circ. Res.* 25:429–38

28. Mayer, S. E., Dobson, J. G., Gross, S. R., Khoo, J. C., Steinberg, D. 1975. In *Cyclic Nucleotides in Disease*, ed. B. Weiss, 105–16. Baltimore: Univ. Park Press

29. Weiss, B., Greenberg, L. H. 1975. See Ref. 28, pp. 269–320

30. Greengard, P., McAfee, D. A., Kebabian, J. W. 1972. *Adv. Cyclic Nucleotide Res.* 1:337–56

31. Bitensky, M. W., Miller, W. H., Gorman, R. E., Neufeld, A. H., Robinson, R. 1972. *Adv. Cyclic Nucleotide Res.* 1:317–36

32. Singh, J. N., Dhalla, N. S. 1975. *Adv. Cyclic Nucleotide Res.* 5:759–70

33. Parker, C. W., Sullivan, T. J., Wedner, H. J. 1974. *Adv. Cyclic Nucleotide Res.* 4:1–79

34. Marsh, J. M., Butcher, R. W., Savard, K., Sutherland, E. W. 1966. The stimulatory effect of luteinizing hormone on adenosine 3',5'-monophosphate accumulation in corpus luteum slices. *J. Biol. Chem.* 241:5436–40

35. Malaisse, W. J., Pipeleers, D. G., Levy, J. 1974. The stimulus-secretion coupling of glucose-induced insulin release. XVI. A glucose-like and calcium-independent effect of cyclic AMP. *Biochim. Biophys. Acta* 362:121–28

36. Turtle, J. R., Littleton, G. K., Kipnis, D. M. 1967. Stimulation of insulin secretion by theophylline. *Nature* 213:727–28

37. Kuo, J. F., Kuo, W-N. 1975. See Ref. 28, pp. 211–26

38. Sullivan, T. J., Parker, K. L., Stenson, W., Parker, C. W. 1975. Modulation of cyclic AMP in purified rat mast cells. I.

Responses to pharmacologic, metabolic, and physical stimuli. *J. Immunol.* 114:1473–79

39. Sullivan, T. J., Parker, K. L., Eisen, S. A., Parker, C. W. 1975. Modulation of cyclic AMP in purified rat mast cells. II. Studies on the relationship between intracellular cyclic AMP concentrations and histamine release. *J. Immunol.* 114:1480–85

40. Ignarro, L. J. 1975. See Ref. 28, pp. 184–210

41. Goldberg, N. D., Haddox, M. K., Nicol, S. E., Glass, D. B., Sanford, C. H., Kuehl, F. A. Jr., Estensen, R. 1975. *Adv. Cyclic Nucleotide Res.* 5:307–30

42. Fichman, M. P., Brooker, G. 1972. Deficient renal cyclic AMP production in nephrogenic diabetes insipidus. *J. Clin. Endocrinol. Metab.* 35:35–47

43. Dousa, T. P., Rowland, R. G., Carone, F. A. 1973. Renal medullary adenylate cyclase in drug-induced nephrogenic diabetes insipidus. *Proc. Soc. Exp. Biol. Med.* 142:720–22

44. Burk, R. R., 1968. Reduced adenyl cyclase activity in a polyoma virus transformed cell line. *Nature* 219:1272–75

45. Weiss, B., Shein, H. M., Snyder, R. 1971. Adenylate cyclase and phosphodiesterase activity of normal and SV_{40} virus-transformed hamster astrocytes in cell culture. *Life Sci.* 10:1253–60

46. Allen, D. O., Munshower, J., Morris, H. P., Weber, G. 1971. Regulation of adenyl cyclase in hepatomas of different growth rates. *Cancer Res.* 31:557–60

47. Ney, R. L., Hochella, N. J., Grahame-Smith, D. G., Dexter, R. N., Butcher, R. W. 1969. Abnormal regulation of adenosine 3',5'-monophosphate and corticosterone formation in an adrenocortical carcinoma. *J. Clin. Invest.* 48:1733–39

48. Macchia, V., Meldolesi, M. F., Chiariello, M. 1972. Adenyl-cyclase in a transplantable thyroid tumor: Loss of ability to respond to TSH. *Endocrinology* 90:1483–91

49. Polgar, P., Vera, J. C., Kelley, P. R., Rutenburg, A. M. 1973. Adenylate cyclase activity in normal and leukemic human leukocytes as determined by a radioimmunoassay for cyclic AMP. *Biochim. Biophys. Acta* 297:378–83

50. Kemp, R. G., Hsu, P-Y., Duquesnoy, R. J. 1975. Changes in lymphoid cyclic adenosine 3':5'-monophosphate metabolism during murine leukemogenesis. *Cancer Res.* 35:2440–45

51. Nesbitt, J. A. III, Anderson, W. B., Miller, Z., Pastan, I., Russell, T. R., Gospodarowicz, D. 1976. Guanylate cyclase and cyclic guanosine 3':5'-monophosphate phosphodiesterase activities and cyclic guanosine 3':5'-monophosphate levels in normal and transformed fibroblasts in culture. J. Biol. Chem. 251:2344–52

52. Amer, M. S. 1973. Cyclic adenosine monophosphate and hypertension. Science 179:807–9

53. Lovell-Smith, C. J., Sneyd, J. G. T. 1974. Lipolysis and adenosine 3',5'cyclic monophosphate in adipose tissue of the New Zealand obese mouse; the activities of adipose tissue adenyl cyclase and phosphodiesterase. Diabetologia 10:655–59

54. Kupiecki, F. P. 1969. Reduced adenosine 3',5'-monophosphate phosphodiesterase activity in the pancreas and adipose tissue of spontaneously diabetic mice. Life Sci. 8:645–49

55. Hemington, J. G., Chenoweth, M., Dunn, A. 1973. Cyclic nucleotide phosphodiesterase activity in the plasma and erythrocytes of normal and diabetic rats. Biochim. Biophys. Acta 304:552–59

56. Das, I. 1973. Effect of diabetes and insulin on the rat heart adenyl cyclase, cyclic AMP phosphodiesterase and cyclic AMP. Hormone Metab. Res. 5:330–33

57. Schmidt, S. Y., Lolley, R. N. 1973. Cyclic-nucleotide phosphodiesterase: An early defect in inherited retinal degeneration of C3H mice. J. Cell Biol. 57:117–23

58. Farber, D. B., Lolley, R. N. 1973. Proteins in the degenerative retina of C3H mice: Deficiency of a cyclic-nucleotide phosphodiesterase and opsin. J. Neurochem. 21:817–28

59. Hait, W. N., Weiss, B. 1975. Increased activity of cyclic AMP and cyclic GMP phosphodiesterase in lymphocytic leukemia. Clin. Res. 23:595A

60. Hait, W. N., Weiss, B. 1976. Increased cyclic nucleotide phosphodiesterase activity in leukemic lymphocytes. Nature 259:321–23

61. Hait, W. N., Weiss, B. 1977. Characterization of the cyclic nucleotide phosphodiesterases of normal and leukemic lymphocytes. Biochim. Biophys. Acta. In press

62. Drezner, M., Neelon, F. A., Lebovitz, H. E. 1973. Pseudohypoparathyroidism Type II: A possible defect in the reception of the cyclic AMP signal. N. Engl. J. Med. 289:1056–60

63. Daniel, V., Litwack, G., Tomkins, G. M. 1973. Induction of cytolysis of cultured lymphoma cells by adenosine 3',5'-cyclic monophosphate and the isolation of resistant variants. Proc. Natl. Acad. Sci. USA 70:76–79

64. Coffino, P., Bourne, H. R., Tomkins, G. M. 1975. Mechanism of lymphoma cell death induced by cyclic AMP. Am. J. Pathol. 81:199–204

65. Goldberg, M. L., Burke, G. C., Morris, H. P. 1975. Cyclic AMP and cyclic GMP content and binding in malignancy. Biochem. Biophys. Res. Commun. 62:320–27

66. Criss, W. E., Morris, H. P. 1973. Protein kinase activity in Morris hepatomas. Biochem. Biophys. Res. Commun. 54:380–86

67. Prasad, K. M., Fogleman, D., Gaschler, M., Sinha, P. K., Brown, J. L. 1976. Cyclic nucleotide-dependent protein kinase activity in malignant and cyclic AMP-induced "differentiated" neuroblastoma cells in culture. Biochem. Biophys. Res. Commun. 68:1248–55

68. Zapf, J., Waldvogel, M., Froesch, E. R. 1973. Protein kinase and cyclic AMP-binding activities in liver and adipose tissue of normal, streptozotocin-diabetic and adrenalectomized rats. FEBS Lett. 36:253–56

69. Murad, F. 1973. Adv. Cyclic Nucleotide Res. 3:355–87

70. Tucci, J. R., Lin, T., Kopp, L. E. 1973. Urinary cyclic 3',5'-adenosine monophosphate levels in diabetes mellitus before and after treatment. J. Clin. Endocrinol. Metab. 37:832–35

71. Lin, T., Kopp, L. E., Tucci, J. R. 1973. Urinary excretion of cyclic 3',5'-adenosine monophosphate in hyperthyroidism. J. Clin. Endocrinol. Metab. 36:1033–36

72. Guttler, R. B., Shaw, J. W., Otis, C. L., Nicoloff, J. T. 1975. Epinephrine-induced alterations in urinary cyclic AMP in hyper- and hypothyroidism. J. Clin. Endocrinol. Metab. 41:707–11

73. Murad, F., Pak, C. 1972. Urinary excretion of adenosine 3',5'-monophosphate and guanosine 3',5'-monophosphate. N. Engl. J. Med. 286:1832–37

74. Schmidt-Gayk, H., Roher, H. D. 1973. Urinary excretion of cyclic adenosine monophosphate in the detection and diagnosis of primary hyperparathyroidism. Surg. Gynecol. Obstet. 137:439–44

75. Chase, L. R., Melson, G. L., Aurbach, G. D. 1969. Pseudohypoparathyroidism: Defective excretion of 3',5'-AMP in response to parathyroid hormone. *J. Clin. Invest.* 48:1832–44
76. Chase, L. R., Aurbach, G. D. 1967. Parathyroid function and the renal excretion of 3',5'-adenylic acid. *Proc. Natl. Acad. Sci. USA* 58:518–25
77. Bell, N. H., Clark, C. M., Avery, S., Sinha, T., Trygstad, C. W., Allen, D. O. 1974. Demonstration of a defect in the formation of adenosine 3',5'-monophosphate in vasopressin-resistant diabetes insipidus. *Pediatr. Res.* 8:223–30
78. Fireman, P. 1973. Metabolic abnormalities in asthma-decreased urinary cyclic AMP. *Int. Arch. Allergy Appl. Immunol.* 45:123–27
79. Paul, M. I., Ditzion, B. P., Pauk, G. L., Janowsky, D. S. 1970. Urinary adenosine 3',5'-monophosphate excretion in affective disorders. *Am. J. Psychiatry* 126:1493–97
80. Abdulla, Y. H., Hamadah, K. 1970. 3',5'-Cyclic adenosine monophosphate in depression and mania. *Lancet* 1:378–81
81. Paul, M. I., Cramer, H., Bunney, W. E. Jr. 1971. Urinary adenosine 3',5'-monophosphate in the switch process from depression to mania. *Science* 171:300–3
82. Jenner, F. A., Sampson, G. A., Thompson, E. A., Sommerville, A. R., Beard, N. A., Smith, A. A. 1972. Manic depressive psychosis and urinary excretion of cyclic AMP. *Br. J. Psychiatry* 121:236–37
83. Brown, B. C., Salway, J. G., Albano, J. P., Hullin, R. P., Ekins, R. P. 1972. Urinary excretion of cyclic AMP and manic-depressive psychosis. *Br. J. Psychiatry* 120:405–8
84. Murad, F., Kimura, H., Hopkins, H. A., Looney, W. B., Kovacs, C. J. 1975. Increased urinary excretion of cyclic guanosine monophosphate in rats bearing Morris hepatoma 3924A. *Science* 190:59–60
85. Rabinowitz, B., Kligerman, M., Parmley, W. W. 1974. Plasma cyclic adenosine 3',5'-monophosphate (AMP) levels in acute myocardial infarction. *Am. J. Cardiol.* 34:7–11
86. Hamet, P., Kuchel, O., Fraysse, J., Genest, J. 1974. Plasma adenosine 3',5'-cyclic monophosphate in human hypertension. *Can. Med. Assoc. J.* 111:323–28
87. Grower, M. F., Ficara, A. J., Chandler, D. W., Kramer, G. D. 1975. Differences in cAMP levels in the gingival fluid of

diabetics and nondiabetics. *J. Periodontol.* 46:669–72
88. Sproles, A. C. 1973. Cyclic AMP concentration in saliva of normal children and children with Down's syndrome. *J. Dent. Res.* 52:915–17
89. Weinryb, I., Chasin, M., Free, C. A., Harris, D. N., Goldenberg, H., Michel, I. M., Paik, V. S., Phillips, M., Samaniego, S., Hess, S. M. 1972. Effects of therapeutic agents on cyclic AMP metabolism in vitro. *J. Pharm. Sci.* 61:1556–67
90. Amer, M. S., McKinney, G. R. 1973. Possibilities for drug development based on the cyclic AMP system. *Life Sci.* 13:753–67
91. Breckenridge, B. M. 1970. Cyclic AMP and drug action. *Ann. Rev. Pharmacol.* 10:19–34
92. Weiss, B., ed. 1975. *Cyclic Nucleotides in Disease.* Baltimore: Univ. Park Press
93. Weiss, B., Fertel, R. 1977. *Adv. Pharmacol. Chemother.* 14:189–283
94. Uzunov, P., Shein, H. M., Weiss, B. 1974. Multiple forms of cyclic 3',5'-AMP phosphodiesterase of rat cerebrum and cloned astrocytoma and neuroblastoma cells. *Neuropharmacology* 13:377–91
95. Rall, T. W. 1969. In *The Role of Adenyl Cyclase and Cyclic 3',5'-AMP in Biological Systems, Fogerty Int. Proc., 4th, Natl. Inst. Health, Bethesda, Md.,* ed. T. W. Rall, M. Rodbell, P. Condliffe, pp. 7–15
96. Perkins, J. P. 1973. *Adv. Cyclic Nucleotide Res.* 3:1–64
97. Robison, G. A., Butcher, R. W., Sutherland, E. W. 1967. Adenyl cyclase as an adrenergic receptor. *Ann. NY Acad. Sci.* 139:703–23
98. Cheung, W. Y. 1970. Cyclic 3',5'-nucleotide phosphodiesterase. Demonstration of an activator. *Biochem. Biophys. Res. Commun.* 38:533–38
99. Brostrom, C. O., Huang, Y-C., Breckenridge, B. M., Wolff, D. J. 1975. Identification of a calcium-binding protein as a calcium-dependent regulator of brain adenylate cyclase. *Proc. Natl. Acad. Sci. USA* 72:64–68
100. Cheung, W. Y., Bradham, L. S., Lynch, T. J., Lin, Y. M., Tallant, E. A. 1975. Protein activator of cyclic 3':5'-nucleotide phosphodiesterase of bovine or rat brain also activates its adenylate cyclase. *Biochem. Biophys. Res. Commun.* 66:1055–62
101. Goldberg, N. D., O'Dea, R. F., Had-

dox, M. K. 1973. *Adv. Cyclic Nucleotide Res.* 3:155–224

102. Strada, S. J., Kirkegaard, L., Thompson, W. J. 1975. Studies of rat pineal gland guanylate cyclase. *Neuropharmacology* 15:261–66

103. Kimura, H., Murad, F. 1974. Evidence for 2 different forms of guanylate cyclase in rat heart. *J. Biol. Chem.* 249:6910–16

104. Chrisman, T. D., Garbers, D. L., Parks, M. A., Hardman, J. G. 1975. Characterization of particulate and soluble guanylate cyclases from rat lung. *J. Biol. Chem.* 250:374–81

105. Weiss, B., Costa, E. 1968. Selective stimulation of adenyl cyclase of rat pineal gland by pharmacologically-active catecholamines. *J. Pharmacol. Exp. Ther.* 161:310–19

106. George, W. J., Polson, J. B., O'Toole, A. G., Goldberg, N. D. 1970. Elevation of guanosine 3',5'-cyclic phosphate in rat heart after perfusion with acetylcholine. *Proc. Natl. Acad. Sci. USA* 66:398–403

107. Ferrendelli, J. A., Steiner, A. L., McDougal, D. B. Jr., Kipnis, D. M. 1970. The effect of oxotremorine and atropine on cGMP and cAMP levels in mouse cerebral cortex and cerebellum. *Biochem. Biophys. Res. Commun.* 41:1061–67

108. Thompson, W. J., Williams, R. H., Little, S. A. 1973. Activation of guanyl cyclase and adenyl cyclase by secretin. *Biochim. Biophys. Acta* 302:329–37

109. Rudland, P. S., Gospodarowicz, D., Seifert, W. 1974. Activation of guanyl cyclase and intracellular cyclic GMP by fibroblast growth factor. *Nature* 250:741–43

110. Stoner, J., Manganiello, V. C., Vaughan, M. 1974. Guanosine cyclic 3',5'-monophosphate and guanylate cyclase activity in guinea pig lung: Effects of acetylcholine and cholinesterase inhibitors. *Mol. Pharmacol.* 10:155–61

111. Ignarro, L. J., George, W. J. 1974. Mediation of immunologic discharge of lysosomal enzymes from human neutrophils by guanosine 3',5'-monophosphate. *J. Exp. Med.* 140:225–38

112. Appleman, M. M., Thompson, W. J., Russell, T. R. 1973. *Adv. Cyclic Nucleotide Res.* 3:65–98

113. Amer, M. S., Kreighbaum, W. E. 1975. Cyclic nucleotide phosphodiesterases: Properties, activators, inhibitors, structure-activity relationships, and possible role in drug development. *J. Pharm. Sci.* 64:1–37

114. Weiss, B., Costa, E. 1968. Regional and subcellular distribution of adenyl cyclase and 3',5'-cyclic nucleotide phosphodiesterase in brain and pineal gland. *Biochem. Pharmacol.* 17:2107–16

115. Butcher, R. W., Sutherland, E. W. 1962. Adenosine 3',5'-phosphate in biological materials. I. Purification and properties of cyclic 3',5'-nucleotide phosphodiesterase and use of this enzyme to characterize adenosine 3',5'-phosphate in human urine. *J. Biol. Chem.* 237:1244–50

116. Nair, K. G. 1966. Purification and properties of 3',5'-cyclic nucleotide phosphodiesterase from dog heart. *Biochemistry* 5:150–57

117. Campbell, M. T., Oliver, I. T. 1972. 3',5'-cyclic nucleotide phosphodiesterase in rat tissues. *Eur. J. Biochem.* 28:30–37

118. Beavo, J. A., Hardman, J. G., Sutherland, E. W. 1970. Hydrolysis of cyclic guanosine and adenosine 3',5'-monophosphates by rat and bovine tissues. *J. Biol. Chem.* 245:5649–55

119. Fertel, R., Weiss, B. 1974. A microassay for guanosine 3',5'-monophosphate phosphodiesterase activity. *Anal. Biochem.* 59:386–98

120. Fertel, R., Weiss, B. 1976. Properties and drug responsiveness of cyclic nucleotide phosphodiesterases of rat lung. *Mol. Pharmacol.* 12:678–87

121. Clark, J. F., Morris, H. P., Weber, G. 1973. Cyclic adenosine 3',5'-monophosphate phosphodiesterase activity in normal, differentiating, regenerating and neoplastic liver. *Cancer Res.* 33:356–61

122. Brooker, G., Thomas, L. J. Jr., Appleman, M. M. 1968. The assay of adenosine 3',5'-cyclic monophosphate and guanosine 3',5'-cyclic monophosphate in biological materials by enzymatic radioisotopic displacement. *Biochemistry* 7:4177–81

123. Lagarde, A., Colobert, L. 1972. Cyclic 3',5'-AMP phosphodiesterase of human blood lymphocytes. *Biochem. Biophys. Acta* 276:444–53

124. Weiss, B., Strada, S. J. 1972. *Adv. Cyclic Nucleotide Res.* 1:357–74

125. Clark, R. B., Perkins, J. P. 1971. Regulation of adenosine 3',5'-cyclic monophosphate concentration in cultured human astrocytoma cells by catecholamines and histamine. *Proc. Natl. Acad. Sci. USA* 68:2757–60

126. Gilman, A. G., Nirenberg, M. 1971. Effect of catecholamines on the adenosine 3',5'-cyclic monophosphate concentration in clonal satellite cells of neurons. *Proc. Natl. Acad. Sci. USA* 68:2165–68

127. Strada, S. J., Klein, D. C., Weller, J., Weiss, B. 1972. Effect of norepinephrine on the concentration of adenosine 3',5'-monophosphate of rat pineal gland in organ culture. *Endocrinology* 90:1470–75

128. Pan, P., Bonner, J. T., Wedner, H. J., Parker, C. W. 1974. Immunofluorescence evidence for the distribution of cyclic AMP in cells and cell masses of the cellular slime molds. *Proc. Natl. Acad. Sci. USA* 71:1623–25

129. Rosen, O. M. 1970. Interaction of cyclic GMP and cyclic AMP with a cyclic nucleotide phosphodiesterase of the frog erythrocyte. *Arch. Biochem. Biophys.* 139:447–49

130. Thompson, W. J., Appleman, M. M. 1971. Characterization of cyclic nucleotide phosphodiesterases of rat tissue. *J. Biol. Chem.* 246:3145–50

131. Song, S-Y., Cheung, W. Y. 1971. Cyclic 3',5'-nucleotide phosphodiesterase: properties of the enzyme of human blood platelets. *Biochim. Biophys. Acta* 242:593–605

132. Beavo, J. A., Hardman, J. G., Sutherland, E. W. 1971. Stimulation of adenosine 3',5'-monophosphate hydrolysis by guanosine 3',5'-monophosphate. *J. Biol. Chem.* 246:3841–46

133. Sung, C. P., Wiebelhaus, V. D., Jenkins, B. C., Adlercreutz, P., Hirschowitz, B. I., Sachs, G. 1972. Heterogeneity of 3',5'-phosphodiesterase of gastric mucosa. *Am. J. Physiol.* 223:648–50

134. Miller, J. P., Boswell, K. H., Muneyama, K., Simon, L. N., Robins, R. K., Shuman, D. A. 1973. Synthesis and biochemical studies of various 8-substituted derivatives of guanosine 3',5'-cyclic phosphate, inosine 3',5'-cyclic phosphate and xanthosine 3',5'-cyclic phosphate. *Biochemistry* 12:5310–19

135. Amer, M. S., Mayol, R. F. 1973. Studies with phosphodiesterase III. Two forms of the enzyme from human blood platelets. *Biochim. Biophys. Acta* 309:149–56

136. Russell, T. R., Terasaki, W. L., Appleman, M. M. 1973. Separate phosphodiesterases for the hydrolysis of cyclic adenosine 3',5'-monophosphate and cyclic guanosine 3',5'-monophosphate in rat liver. *J. Biol. Chem.* 248:1334–40

137. Brostrom, C. O., Wolff, D. J. 1976. Calcium-dependent cyclic nucleotide phosphodiesterase from brain: Comparison of adenosine 3',5'-monophosphate and guanosine 3',5'-monophosphate as substrates. *Arch. Biochem. Biophys.* 172:301–11

138. Russell, T. R., Thompson, W. J., Schneider, F. W., Appleman, M. M. 1972. 3',5'-cyclic adenosine monophosphate phosphodiesterase: Negative cooperativity. *Proc. Natl. Acad. Sci. USA* 69:1791–95

139. Loten, E. G., Sneyd, J. G. T. 1970. An effect of insulin on adipose tissue adenosine 3',5'-cyclic monophosphate phosphodiesterase. *Biochem. J.* 120:187–93

140. Weiss, B., Lehne, R., Strada, S. 1972. Rapid microassay of adenosine 3',5'-monophosphate phosphodiesterase activity. *Anal. Biochem.* 45:222–35

141. Schonhofer, P. S., Skidmore, I. F., Bourne, H. R., Krishna, G. 1972. Cyclic 3',5'-AMP phosphodiesterase in isolated fat cells. *Pharmacology* 7:65–77

142. Weiss, B., Strada, S. J. 1973. In *Fetal Pharmacology*, ed. L. Boreus, 205–32. New York: Raven

143. Strada, S. J., Uzunov, P., Weiss, B. 1974. Ontogenetic development of a phosphodiesterase activator and the multiple forms of cyclic AMP phosphodiesterase of rat brain. *J. Neurochem.* 23:1097–1103

144. Hait, W. N., Weiss, B. 1977. Isolation, characterization and selective inhibition of the multiple forms of phosphodiesterase of normal and leukemic lymphocytes. In preparation

145. Franks, D. J., MacManus, J. P. 1971. Cyclic GMP stimulation and inhibition of cyclic AMP phosphodiesterase from thymic lymphocytes. *Biochem. Biophys. Res. Commun.* 42:844–49

146. Thompson, W. J., Appleman, M. M. 1971. Multiple cyclic nucleotide phosphodiesterase activities from rat brain. *Biochemistry* 10:311–16

147. Goren, E. N., Hirsch, A. H., Rosen, O. M. 1971. Activity stain for the detection of cyclic nucleotide phosphodiesterase separated by polyacrylamide gel electrophoresis and its application to the cyclic nucleotide phosphodiesterase of beef heart. *Anal. Biochem.* 43:156–61

148. Monn, E., Christiansen, R. O. 1971. Adenosine 3',5'-monophosphate phosphodiesterase: Multiple molecular forms. *Science* 173:540–42

149. Uzunov, P., Weiss, B. 1972. Separation of multiple forms of cyclic adenosine

3',5'-monophosphate phosphodiesterase in rat cerebellum by polyacrylamide gel electrophoresis. *Biochim. Biophys. Acta* 284:220–26

150. Klotz, U., Berndt, S., Stock, K. 1972. Characterization of multiple cyclic nucleotide phosphodiesterase activities of rat adipose tissue. *Life Sci.* 11:7–17

151. Schroder, J., Rickenberg, H. V. 1973. Partial purification and properties of the cyclic AMP and the cyclic GMP phosphodiesterase of bovine liver. *Biochim. Biophys. Acta* 302:50–63

152. Pichard, A. L., Hanoune, J., Kaplan, J. C. 1973. Multiple forms of cyclic adenosine 3',5'-monophosphate phosphodiesterase from human blood platelets. *Biochem. Biophys. Acta* 315:370–77

153. Pledger, W. J., Stancel, G. M., Thompson, W. J., Strada, S. J. 1974. Separation of multiple forms of cyclic nucleotide phosphodiesterases from rat brain by isoelectrofocusing. *Biochim. Biophys. Acta* 370:242–48

154. Strada, S. J., Pledger, W. J. 1975. See Ref. 28, pp. 3–34

155. Wells, J. N., Baird, C. E., Wu, Y. J., Hardman, J. G. 1975. Cyclic nucleotide phosphodiesterase activities of pig coronary arteries. *Biochim. Biophys. Acta* 384:430–42

156. Singer, A. L., Sherwin, R. P., Dunn, A. S., Appleman, M. M. 1976. Cyclic nucleotide phosphodiesterases in neoplastic and nonneoplastic human mammary tissues. *Cancer Res.* 36:60–66

157. Uzunov, P., Shein, H. M., Weiss, B. 1973. Cyclic AMP phosphodiesterase in cloned astrocytoma cells: Norepinephrine induces a specific enzyme form. *Science* 180:304–6

158. Weiss, B., Fertel, R., Figlin, R., Uzunov, P. 1974. Selective alteration of the activity of the multiple forms of cyclic 3',5'-AMP phosphodiesterase of rat cerebrum. *Mol. Pharmacol.* 10:615–25

159. Weiss, B. 1975. *Adv. Cyclic Nucleotide Res.* 5:195–211

160. Wells, J. N., Wu, Y. J., Baird, C. E., Hardman, J. G. 1975. Phosphodiesterases from porcine coronary arteries: Inhibition of separated forms by xanthine, papaverine and cyclic nucleotides. *Mol. Pharmacol.* 11:775–83

161. Cheung, W. Y. 1971. Cyclic 3',5'-nucleotide phosphodiesterase evidence for and properties of a protein activator. *J. Biol. Chem.* 246:2859–69

162. Cheung, W. Y., Lin, Y. M., Liu, Y. P., Smoake, J. A. 1975. See Ref. 28, pp. 321–50

163. Kakiuchi, S., Yamazaki, R., Nakajima, H. 1970. Properties of a heat-stable phosphodiesterase activating factor isolated from brain extract. Studies on cyclic 3',5'-nucleotide phosphodiesterase II. *Proc. Jpn. Acad.* 46:587–92

164. Goren, E. N., Rosen, O. M. 1971. The effect of nucleotides and a non dialyzable factor on the hydrolysis of cyclic AMP by a cyclic nucleotide phosphodiesterase from beef heart. *Arch. Biochem. Biophys.* 142:720–23

165. Teo, T. S., Wang, J. H. 1973. Mechanism of activation of a cyclic adenosine 3',5'-monophosphate phosphodiesterase from bovine heart by calcium ions: Identification of the protein activator as a Ca^{2+} binding protein. *J. Biol. Chem.* 248:5950–55

166. Wolff, D. J., Brostrom, C. O. 1974. Calcium-binding phosphoprotein from pig brain: Identification as a calcium dependent regulator of rat brain nucleotide phosphodiesterase. *Arch. Biochem. Biophys.* 163:349–58

167. Wickson, R. D., Boudreau, R. J., Drummond, G. I. 1975. Activation of 3',5'-cyclic adenosine monophosphate phosphodiesterase by calcium ion and a protein activator. *Biochemistry* 14:669–75

168. Levin, R. M., Weiss, B. 1976. Mechanism by which psychotropic drugs inhibit cyclic AMP phosphodiesterase of brain. *Mol. Pharmacol.* 12:581–89

169. Kakiuchi, S., Yamazaki, R. 1970. Calcium dependent phosphodiesterase activity and its activating factor (PAF) from brain. Studies on cyclic 3',5'-nucleotide phosphodiesterase (III). *Biochem. Biophys. Res. Commun.* 41:1104–11

170. Wang, J. H., Teo, T. S., Ho, H. C., Stevens, F. C. 1975. *Adv. Cyclic Nucleotide Res.* 5:179–95

171. Lin, Y. M., Liu, Y. P., Cheung, W. Y. 1975. Cyclic 3',5'-nucleotide phosphodiesterase Ca^{2+}-dependent formation of bovine brain enzyme-activator complex. *FEBS Lett.* 49:356–60

172. Teshima, Y., Kakiuchi, S. 1974. Mechanism of stimulation of Ca^{2+} plus Mg^{2+}-dependent phosphodiesterase from rat cerebral cortex by the modulator protein and Ca^{2+}. *Biochem. Biophys. Res. Commun.* 56:489–95

173. Teo, T. S., Wang, J. H. 1973. Mechanism of activation of a cyclic adenosine 3',5'-monophosphate phosphodiesterase from bovine heart by calcium ions. *J. Biol. Chem.* 248:5950–55

174. Uzunov, P., Lehne, R., Revuelta, A. V., Gnegy, M. E., Costa, E. 1976. A kinetic analysis of the cyclic nucleotide phosphodiesterase regulation by the endogenous protein activator. A study of rat brain and frog sympathetic chain. *Biochim. Biophys. Acta* 422:326–34

175. Pledger, W. J., Thompson, W. J., Strada, S. J. 1975. Isolation of an activator of multiple forms of cyclic nucleotide phosphodiesterase of rat cerebrum by isoelectric focusing. *Biochim. Biophys. Acta* 391:334–40

176. Greenberg, L. H., Weiss, B. 1976. Activatable phosphodiesterase in various areas of rat brain. *Am. Soc. Neurochem.* 7:115

177. Uzunov, P., Revuelta, A., Costa, E. 1975. A role for the endogenous activator of 3'5';-nucleotide phosphodiesterase in rat adrenal medulla. *Mol. Pharmacol.* 11:506–10

178. Amer, M. S. 1975. Cyclic nucleotides in disease; On the biochemical etiology of hypertension. *Life Sci.* 17:1021–38

179. Ryan, W. L., Heidrick, M. L. 1974. *Adv. Cyclic Nucleotide Res.* 4:81–116

180. Johnson, G. S. 1975. See Ref. 28, pp. 35–44

181. Anderson, W. B., Russell, T. R., Carchman, R. A., Pastan, I. 1973. Interrelationship between adenylate cyclase activity, adenosine 3',5'-cyclic monophosphate phosphodiesterase activity, adenosine 3',5'-cyclic monophosphate levels, and growth of cells in culture. *Proc. Natl. Acad. Sci. USA* 70:3802–5

182. Rein, A., Carchman, R. A., Johnson, G. S., Pastan, I. 1973. Simian Virus 40 rapidly lowers cAMP levels in mouse cells. *Biochem. Biophys. Res. Commun.* 52:899–904

183. Hickie, R. A., Walker, C. M., Croll, G. A. 1974. Decreased basal cyclic adenosine 3',5'-monophosphate levels in Morris Hepatoma 5123 t.c.(h). *Biochem. Biophys. Res. Commun.* 59:167–73

184. Monahan, T. M., Marchand, N. W., Fritz, R. R., Abell, C. W. 1975. Cyclic adenosine 3',5'-monophosphate levels and activities of related enzymes in normal and leukemic lymphocytes. *Cancer Res.* 35:2540–47

185. Ryan, W. L., Heidrick, M. L. 1968. Inhibition of cell growth by adenosine 3',5'-monophosphate. *Science* 162:1484–85

186. Gericke, D., Chandra, P. 1969. Inhibition of tumor growth by nucleoside cyclic 3',5'-monophosphates. *Hoppe-Seylers Z. Physiol. Chem.* 350:1469–71

187. Yang, T. J., Vas, S. I. 1971. Growth inhibitor effects of adenosine 3',5'-monophosphate on mouse leukemia L–5178–Y–R cells in culture. *Experientia* 27:442–44

188. Webb, D., Braun, W., Plescia, O. J. 1972. Antitumor effects of polynucleotides and theophylline. *Cancer Res.* 32:1814–19

189. Van Wijk, R., Wicks, W. D., Clay, K. 1972. Effects of derivatives of cyclic 3',5'-adenosine monophosphate on the growth, morphology, and gene expression of hepatoma cells in culture. *Cancer Res.* 32:1905–11

190. Keller, R., Keist, R. 1973. Suppression of growth of P–815 mastocytoma cells in vitro by drugs increasing cellular cyclic 3',5'-adenosine monophosphate. *Life Sci.* 12:97–105

191. Cho-Chung, Y. S., Gullino, P. M. 1974. In vivo inhibition of growth of two hormone-dependent mammary tumors by dibutyryl cyclic AMP. *Science* 183:87–88

192. Hsie, A. W., Puck, T. T. 1971. Morphological transformation of Chinese hamster cells by dibutyryl adenosine cyclic 3',5'-monophosphate and testosterone. *Proc. Natl. Acad. Sci. USA* 68:358–61

193. Johnson, G. S., Friedman, R. M., Pastan, I. 1971. Restoration of several morphological characteristics of normal fibroblasts and sarcoma cells treated with adenosine-3',5'-cyclic monophosphate and its derivatives. *Proc. Natl. Acad. Sci. USA* 68:425–29

194. Prasad, K. M., Hsie, A. W. 1971. Morphologic differentiation of mouse neuroblastoma cells induced in vitro by dibutyryl adenosine 3',5' cyclic monophosphate. *Nature New Biol.* 233:141–42

195. Ortiz, J., Yamada, T., Hsie, A. 1973. Induction of the stellate configuration in cultured iris epithelial cells by adenosine and compounds related to adenosine 3',5' cyclic monophosphate. *Proc. Natl. Acad. Sci. USA* 70:2286–90

196. Hsie, A., Kawashima, K., O'Neil, J. P., Schroder, C. H. 1975. Possible role of adenosine cyclic 3',5'-monophosphate phosphodiesterase in the morphological transformation of Chinese hamster ovary cells mediated by N^6,O^2-dibutyryl adenosine cyclic 3',5'-monophosphate. *J. Biol. Chem.* 250:984–89

197. Tisdale, M. J., Phillips, B. J. 1975. Inhibition of cyclic 3',5'-nucleotide phosphodiesterase—a possible mechanism of action of bifunctional alkylating

agents. *Biochem. Pharmacol.* 24:211–17
198. Tisdale, M. J. 1975. Characterisation of cyclic adenosine 3',5'-monophosphate phosphodiesterase from Walker carcinoma sensitive and resistant to bifunctional alkylating agents. *Biochim. Biophys. Acta* 397:134–43
199. Langan, T. A. 1969. Histone phosphorylation stimulation by adenosine 3',5'-monophosphate. *Science* 162:579–80
200. Bordy, S. C., Prasad, K. N., Purdy, J. L. 1974. Neuroblastoma: Drug induced differentiation increases proportion of cytoplasmic RNA that contains polyadenylic acid. *Science* 186:359–61
201. Fuhr, J. E., Overton, M., Yang, T. J. 1976. Stimulatory effect of 3',5'-adenosine monophosphate on protein synthesis in heat shocked murine leukemia lymphoblasts. *J. Natl. Cancer Inst.* 56:189–91
202. Willingham, M., Pastan, I. 1975. Cyclic AMP modulates microvillus formation and agglutinability in transformed and normal mouse fibroblasts. *Proc. Natl. Acad. Sci. USA* 72:1263–67
203. Tchao, R., Leighton, J. 1976. Inhibitory effect of dibutyryl cyclic AMP and theophylline on the aggregation of human breast tumor cell line BT-20. *Nature* 259:220–22
204. Voorhees, J. J., Duell, E. A., Bass, L. J., Powell, J. A., Harrell, E. R. 1972. Decreased cyclic AMP in the epidermis of lesions of psoriasis. *Arch. Dermatol.* 105:695–701
205. Voorhees, J. J., Stawiski, M., Duell, E. A., Haddox, M. K., Goldberg, N. D. 1973. Increased cyclic GMP and decreased cyclic AMP levels in the hyperplastic abnormally differentiated epidermis of psoriasis. *Life Sci.* 13:639–53
206. Powell, J. A., Duell, E. A., Voorhees, J. J. 1971. Beta adrenergic stimulation of endogenous epidermal cyclic AMP formation. *Arch. Dermatol.* 104:359–65
207. Wright, R. K., Mandy, S. H., Halprin, K. M., Hsia, S. L. 1973. Defects and deficiency of adenyl cyclase in psoriatic skin. *Arch. Dermatol.* 107:47–53
208. Voorhees, J. J., Duell, E. A., Stawiski, M., Creehan, P., Harrell, E. R. 1975. See Ref. 28, pp. 79–101
209. Stawiski, M. A., Powell, J. A., Lang, F. G., Schork, M. A., Duell, E. A., Voorhees, J. J. 1975. Papaverine: Its effects on cyclic AMP in vitro and psoriasis in vivo. *J. Invest. Dermatol.* 64:124–27
210. Szentivanyi, A. 1968. The beta adrenergic theory of the atopic abnormality in bronchial asthma. *J. Allergy* 42:203–32

211. Cookson, D. U., Reed, C. E. 1963. A comparison of the effects of isoproterenol in the normal and asthmatic subject. *Am. Rev. Respir. Dis.* 88:636–43
212. Kirkpatrick, C. H., Keller, C. 1967. Impaired responsiveness to epinephrine in asthma. *Am. Rev. Respir. Dis.* 96:692–99
213. Parker, C. W., Smith, J. W. 1973. Alterations in cyclic adenosine monophosphate metabolism in human bronchial asthma. *J. Clin. Invest.* 52:48–59
214. Taylor, W. A., Francis, D. H., Sheldon, D., Roitt, I. M. 1974. Anti-allergic actions of disodium cromoglycate and other drugs known to inhibit cyclic 3',5'-nucleotide phosphodiesterase. *Int. Arch. Allergy Appl. Immunol.* 47:175–93
215. Tateson, J. E., Trist, D. G. 1976. Inhibition of adenosine 3',5'-cyclic monophosphate phosphodiesterase by potential antiallergic compounds. *Life Sci.* 18:153–62
216. Davies, G. E., Evans, D. P. 1973. Studies with two new phosphodiesterase inhibitors (ICI 58, 301 and ICI 63, 197) on anaphylaxis in guinea pigs, mice and rats. *Int. Arch. Allergy Appl. Immunol.* 45:467–78
217. Weiss, B., Davies, J. I., Brodie, B. B. 1966. Evidence for a role of adenosine 3',5'-monophosphate in adipose tissue lipolysis. *Biochem. Pharmacol.* 15:1553–61
218. Lichtenstein, L. M., Margolis, S. 1968. Histamine release in vitro: Inhibition by catecholamines and methylxanthines. *Science* 161:902–3
219. Ishizuka, M., Braun, W., Matsumoto, T. 1971. Cyclic AMP and immune responses: I. Influence of poly A:U and cAMP on antibody formation in vitro. *J. Immunol.* 107:1027–35
220. Bourne, H. R., Lichtenstein, L. M., Melmon, K. L. 1972. Pharmacologic control of allergic histamine release in vitro: Evidence for an inhibitory role of 3',5'-adenosine monophosphate in human leukocytes. *J. Immunol.* 108:695–705
221. Gillespie, E. 1973. Compound 48/80 decreases adenosine 3',5'-monophosphate formation in rat peritoneal mast cells. *Experientia* 29:447–48
222. Sullivan, T., Parker, C. W. 1973. Cyclic AMP phosphodiesterase activation by the histamine releasing agent, compound 48/80. *Biochem. Biophys. Res. Commun.* 55:1334–39

474   WEISS & HAIT

223. Roy, A. C., Warren, B. T. 1974. Inhibition of cAMP phosphodiesterase by disodium cromoglycate. *Biochem. Pharmacol.* 23:917–20
224. Lavin, N., Rachelefsky, G. S., Kaplan, S. A. 1975. An action of disodium cromoglycate: Inhibition of cyclic 3',5'-AMP phosphodiesterase. *J. Allergy Clin. Immunol.* 57:80–88
225. Brodie, B. B., Davies, J. I., Hynie, S., Krishna, G., Weiss, B. 1966. Interrelationships of catecholamines with other endocrine systems. *Pharmacol. Rev.* 18:273–89
226. Lavin, N., Rachelefsky, G., Kaplan, S. A. 1975. Inhibition of cyclic AMP phosphodiesterase in human lymphocytes by physiological concentrations of hydrocortisone. *Horm. Metab. Res.* 7:253–58
227. Manganiello, V., Vaughan, M. 1972. An effect of dexamethasone on adenosine 3',5'-monophosphate content and adenosine 3',5'-monophosphate phosphodiesterase activity of cultured hepatoma cells. *J. Clin. Invest.* 51:2763–67
228. Weissman, G., Zurier, R. B., Hoffstein, S. 1974. See Ref. 14, pp. 176–88
229. Lichtenstein, L. M., 1974. See Ref. 14, pp. 142–62
230. Stefanovich, V. 1974. Inhibition of 3',5'-cyclic AMP phosphodiesterase with anti-inflammatory agents. *Res. Commun. Chem. Pathol. Pharmacol.* 7:573–82
231. Newcombe, D. S., Thanassi, N. M., Ciosek, C. P. Jr. 1974. Cartilage cyclic nucleotide phosphodiesterase: Inhibition by anti-inflammatory agents. *Life Sci.* 14:505–19
232. Kupiecki, F. P., Adams, L. D. 1974. The lipolytic system in adipose tissue of Toronto-KK and C57BL/KₛJ diabetic mice. Adenylate cyclase, phosphodiesterase and protein kinase activities. *Diabetologia* 10:633–37
233. Kukovetz, W. R., Poch, G. 1970. Inhibition of cyclic 3',5'-nucleotide phosphodiesterase as a possible mode of action of papaverine and similarly acting drugs. *Arch. Pharmakol.* 267:189–94
234. Markwardt, F., Hoffmann, A. 1970. Effects of papaverine derivatives on cyclic AMP phosphodiesterase of human platelets. *Biochem. Pharmacol.* 19:2519–20
235. Beavo, J. A., Rogers, N. L., Crofford, O. B., Hardman, J. G., Sutherland, E. W., Newman, E. V. 1970. Effects of xanthine derivatives on lipolysis and adenosine 3',5'-monophosphate phosphodiesterase activity. *Mol. Pharmacol.* 6:597–603
236. Schultz, G., Senft, G., Losert, W., Sitt, R. 1966. Biochemische grundlagen der diazoxidhyperglykamie. *Naunyn Schmiedeberg's Arch. Exp. Pathol. Pharmacol.* 253:372–87
237. Moore, P. F. 1968. The effects of diazoxide and benzothiadiazine diuretics upon phosphodiesterase. *Ann. NY Acad. Sci.* 150:256–60
238. Nitz, R. E., Schraven, E., Trottnow, D. 1968. Hemmung der Phosphodiesterase aus Rattenherzen durch Intensain. *Experientia* 24:334–35
239. Orloff, J., Handler, J. S. 1962. The similarity of effects of vasopressin, adenosine 3',5'-phosphate (cyclic AMP) and theophylline on the toad bladder. *J. Clin. Invest.* 41:702–9
240. Gadd, R. E. A., Clayman, S., Herbert, D. 1973. Inhibition of cyclic 3',5'-nucleotide phosphodiesterase activity by diuretics and other agents. *Experientia* 29:1217–19
241. Senft, G., Schultz, G., Munske, K., Hoffmann, M. 1968. Effects of glucocorticoids and insulin on 3',5'-AMP phosphodiesterase activity in adrenalectomized rats. *Diabetologia* 4:330–35
242. Levey, G. S. 1975. See Ref. 28, pp. 157–64
243. Sobel, B. E., Henry, P. D., Robison, A., Bloor, C., Ross, J. Jr. 1969. Depressed adenyl cyclase activity in the failing guinea pig heart. *Circ. Res.* 24:507–12
244. Gold, H. K., Prindle, K. H., Levey, G. S., Epstein, S. E. 1970. Effects of experimental heart failure on the capacity of glucagon to augment myocardial contractility and activate adenyl cyclase. *J. Clin. Invest.* 49:999–1006
245. Sulakhe, P. V., Dhalla, N. S. 1972. Adenyl cyclase activity in failing hearts of genetically myopathic hamsters. *Biochem. Med.* 6:471–82
246. Lippmann, W. 1974. Inhibition of beef heart and rat brain nucleoside-3',5'-monophosphate phosphodiesterase by 3 β-14-dihydroxy-21-oxo-23-desoxo-5-β-card-20(22)-enolide 3 acetate (AY-17,605) and structurally related compounds. *Experientia* 30:237–39
247. Shimamoto, T. 1975. Hyperactive arterial endothelial cells in atherogenesis and cyclic AMP phosphodiesterase inhibitor in prevention and treatment of atherosclerotic disorders. *Jpn. Heart J.* 16:76–97
248. Iwai, H. 1974. Inhibition of protein kinase and cyclic AMP phosphodiester-

ase by eritadenine isoamyl ester. *J. Biochem.* 76:419–29

249. Goldfine, I. D., Perlman, R., Roth, J. 1971. Inhibition of cyclic 3',5'-AMP phosphodiesterase in islet cells and other tissues by tolbutamide. *Nature* 234:295–96

250. Rosen, O., Hirsch, A., Goren, E. N. 1971. Factors which influence cyclic AMP formation and degradation in an islet cell tumor of the Syrian hamster. *Arch. Biochem. Biophys.* 146:660–63

251. Ashcroft, S. J. H., Randle, P. J., Taljedal, I. B. 1972. Cyclic nucleotide phosphodiesterase in normal mouse pancreatic islets. *FEBS Lett.* 20:263–65

252. Webb, D. R., Bourne, H. R., Levinson, W. 1974. New phosphodiesterase inhibitors in human lymphocytes N-methylisatin-beta-thiosemicarbazone. *Biochem. Pharmacol.* 23:1663–67

253. Uzunov, P., Weiss, B. 1971. Effects of phenothiazine tranquilizers on the cyclic 3',5'-adenosine monophosphate system of rat brain. *Neuropharmacology* 10:697–708

254. Kebabian, J. W., Petzold, G. L., Greengard, P. 1972. Dopamine-sensitive adenylate cyclase in caudate nucleus of rat brain, and its similarity to the "dopamine receptor." *Proc. Natl. Acad. Sci. USA* 69:2145–49

255. Palmer, G. C., Jones, D. J., Medina, M. A., Stavinoha, W. B. 1975. Action of psychoactive drugs on cyclic AMP levels in mouse crebral cortex and lung following microwave irradiation. *Pharmacologist* 17:233

256. Beer, B., Chasin, M., Clody, D. E., Vogel, J. R., Horovitz, Z. P. 1972. Cyclic adenosine monophosphate phosphodiesterase in brain: Effect on anxiety. *Science* 176:428–30

257. Dalton, C., Crowley, H. J., Sheppard, H., Schallek, W. 1974. Regional cyclic nucleotide phosphodiesterase activity in cat central nervous system: Effects of benzodiazepines (37820). *Proc. Soc. Exp. Biol. Med.* 145:407–10

258. Berndt, S., Schwabe, U. 1973. Effect of psychotropic drugs on phosphodiesterase and cyclic AMP level in rat brain in vivo. *Brain Res.* 63:303–12

259. Pichard, A. L., Hanoune, J., Kaplan, J. C. 1972. Human brain and platelet cyclic adenosine 3',5'-monophosphate phosphodiesterases: Different response to drugs. *Biochim. Biophys. Acta* 279:217–20

260. Muschek, L. D., McNeill, J. H. 1971. The effect of tricyclic antidepressants

and promethazine on 3',5'-cyclic AMP phosphodiesterase from rat brain. *Fed. Proc.* 30:330

261. Vernikos-Danellis, J., Harris, C. G. III. 1968. The effect of in vitro and in vivo caffeine, theophylline and hydrocortisone on the phosphodiesterase activity of the pituitary, median eminence, heart, and cerebral cortex of the rat. *Proc. Soc. Exp. Biol. Med.* 128:1016–21

262. Chasin, M., Harris, D. N., Phillips, M. B., Hess, S. M. 1972. 1-Ethyl-4-(isopropylidenehydrazino)-1H-pyrazolo-(3,4-b)-pyridine-5-carboxylic acid, ethyl ester, hydrochloride (SQ 20,009)—A potent new inhibitor of cyclic 3',5'-nucleotide phosphodiesterases. *Biochem. Pharmacol.* 21:2443–50

263. Palmer, G. C., Robison, G. A., Sulser, F. 1971. Modification by psychotropic drugs of the cyclic adenosine monophosphate response to norepinephrine in rat brain. *Biochem. Pharmacol.* 20:236–39

264. Monahan, T. M., Fritz, R. R., Abell, C. W. 1973. Levels of cyclic AMP in murine L5178Y lymphoblasts grown in different concentrations of serum. *Biochem. Biophys. Res. Commun.* 11:642–46

265. Coffey, R. G., Logsdon, P. S., Middleton, E. 1973. Leucocyte adenyl cyclase and ATPase in asthma: Effect of corticosteroid therapy. *Chest* 63:25–35

266. Alston, W. C., Patch, K. R., Kerr, J. W. 1974. Response of leucocyte adenyl cyclase to isoprenaline and effects of alpha blocking drugs in extrinsic bronchial asthma. *Br. Med. J.* 1:90–93

267. Gillespie, E., Valentine, M. D., Lichtenstein, L. M. 1974. Cyclic AMP metabolism in asthma: Studies with leucocytes and lymphocytes. *J. Allergy Clin. Immunol.* 53:27–33

268. Fireman, P., Palm, C. R., Friday, G. A. 1970. Metabolic responses to epinephrine in asthmatic, eczematous and normal subjects. *J. Allergy* 45:117

269. Sharma, R. K. 1972. Studies on adrenocortical carcinoma of rat cyclic nucleotide phosphodiesterase activities. *Cancer Res.* 32:1734–36

270. Thomas, E. W., Murad, F., Looney, W. B., Morris, H. P. 1973. Adenosine 3',5'-monophosphate and guanosine 3',5'-monophosphate: Concentrations in Morris hepatomas of different growth rates. *Biochim. Biophys. Acta* 297:564–67

271. Boyd, H., Louis, C. J., Martin, T. J. 1974. Activity and hormone responsiveness of adenyl cyclase during induction of tumors in rat liver with 3'-methyl-4-dimethylaminoazobenzene *Cancer Res.* 34:1720–25

272. Chayoth, R., Epstein, S. M., Field, J. B. 1973. Glucagon and prostaglandin E$_1$ stimulation of cyclic adenosine 3',5'-monophosphate levels and adenylate cyclase activity in benign hyperplastic nodules and malignant hepatomas of ethionine treated rates. *Cancer Res.* 33:1970–74

273. Chayoth, R., Epstein, S. M., Field, J. B. 1972. Increased cyclic AMP levels in malignant hepatic nodules of ethionine treated rats. *Biochem. Biophys. Res. Commun.* 49:1663–70

274. Clark, J. F., Morris, H. P., Weber, G. 1973. Cyclic adenosine 3',5'-monophosphate phosphodiesterase activity in normal, differentiating, regenerating and neoplastic liver. *Cancer Res.* 33:356–61

275. Makman, M. H. 1971. Conditions leading to enhanced response to glucagon, epinephrine, or prostaglandins by adenylate cyclase of normal and malignant cultured cells. *Proc. Natl. Acad. Sci. USA* 68:2127–30

276. Hickie, R. A., Walker, C. M., Datta, A. 1975. Increased activity of low-Km cyclic adenosine 3',5'-monophosphate phosphodiesterase in plasma membranes of Morris hepatoma 5123tc. *Cancer Res.* 35:601–5

277. Kimura, H., Murad, F. 1975. Increased particulate and decreased soluble guanylate cyclase activity in regenerating liver, fetal liver and hepatoma. *Proc. Natl. Acad. Sci. USA* 72:1965–69

278. Kemp, R. G., Duquesnoy, R. J. 1974. Thymus adenylate cyclase activity during murine leukemogenesis. *Science* 18:218–19

279. Konings, A. W. T., Pierce, D. A. 1974. Hydrolysis of 2'3'-cAMP and 3',5' cAMP in subcellular fractions of normal and neoplastic mouse spleen. *Life Sci.* 15:491–99

280. Perkins, J. P., Macintyre, E. H., Riley, W. D., Clark, R. B. 1971. Adenyl cyclase, phosphodiesterase and cyclic AMP dependent protein kinase of malignant glial cells in culture. *Life Sci.* 10:1069–80

281. Cohen, L., Chan, P-C. 1974. Intracellular cAMP levels in normal rat mammary gland and adenocarcinoma in vivo vs. in vitro. *Life Sci.* 16:107–15

282. Chatterjee, S. K., Kim, U. 1976. Biochemical properties of cyclic nucleotide phosphodiesterase in metastasizing and non-metastasizing rat mammary carcinomas. *J. Natl. Cancer Inst.* 56:105–10

283. Brown, H. D., Chattopadhyay, S. K., Spjut, H. J., Spratt, J. S. Jr., Pennington, S. N. 1969. Adenyl cyclase activity in dimethylamino biphenyl-induced breast carcinoma. *Biochim. Biophys. Acta* 192:372–75

284. Minton, J. P., Wisenbaugh, T., Matthews, R. H. 1974. Elevated cyclic AMP levels in human breast cancer tissue. *J. Natl. Cancer Inst.* 53:283–84

285. Raymond, M. K., Schmitt, G., Galsky, A. G. 1975. Cyclic AMP phosphodiesterase in crown gall tumor formation. *Biochem. Biophys. Res. Commun.* 66:222–26

286. Verma, A. K., Murray, A. W. 1974. The effect of benzo(a)pyrene on the basal and isoproterenol stimulated levels of cyclic adenosine 3',5'-monophosphate in mouse epidermis. *Cancer Res.* 34:3408–13

287. Lincoln, T., Vaughan, G. L. 1975. The role of adenosine 3',5'-monophosphate in the transformation of Cloudman mouse melanoma cells. *J. Cell. Physiol.* 86:543–52

288. Belman, S., Troll, W. 1974. Phorbol-12-myristate-13-acetate effect on cyclic adenosine 3',5'-monophosphate levels in mouse skin and inhibition of phorbol myristate acetate promoted tumor genesis. *Cancer Res.* 34:3446–55

289. Verma, A. K., Froscio, M., Murray, A. 1976. Croton oil-and benzo(a) pyrene-induced changes in cyclic adenosine 3',5'-monophosphate and cyclic guanosine 3',5'-monophosphate phosphodiesterase activities in mouse epidermis. *Cancer Res.* 36:81–87

290. Anderson, W. B., Johnson, G. S., Pastan, I. 1973. Transformation of chickembryo fibroblasts by wild-type and temperature-sensitive Rous sarcoma virus alters adenylate cyclase activity. *Proc. Natl. Acad. Sci. USA* 70:1055–59

291. Otten, J., Bader, J., Johnson, G. S., Pastan, I. 1972. A mutation in a Rous sarcoma virus gene that controls adenosine 3',5'-monophosphate levels and transformation. *J. Biol. Chem.* 247:1632–33

292. Otten, J., Johnson, G. S., Pastan, I. 1972. Regulation of cell growth by cyclic adenosine 3',5'-monophosphate. Effect of cell density and agents which alter cell growth on cyclic adenosine

3',5'-monophosphate levels in fibro-blasts. *J. Biol. Chem.* 247:7082–87

293. Lynch, T. J., Tallant, E. A., Cheung, W. Y. 1975. Marked reduction of cyclic GMP phosphodiesterase activity in vi-rally transformed mouse fibroblasts. *Biochem. Biophys. Res. Commun.* 65:1115–22

294. Peery, C. V., Johnson, G. S., Pastan, I. 1971. Adenyl cyclase in normal and transformed fibroblasts in tissue cul-ture: Activation by prostaglandins. *J. Biol. Chem.* 246:5785–90

295. Augustyn, J. M., Ziegler, F. D. 1975. Endogenous cyclic adenosine mono-phosphate in tissues of rabbits fed an atherogenic diet. *Science* 187:449–50

296. Goldstein, R. E., Skelton, C. L., Levy, G. S., Glancy, D. L., Beiser, G. D., Ep-stein, S. E. 1971. Effects of chronic heart failure on the capacity of glucagon to enhance contractility and adenyl cy-clase activity of human papillary mus-cles. *Circulation* 44:638–47

297. Ling, W. Y., Marsh, J. M., Spellacy, W. N., Thresher, A. J., Lemaire, W. J. 1974. Adenosine 3',5'-monophosphate in amniotic fluid from pregnancy com-plicated by hypertension. *J. Clin. Endo-crinol. Metab.* 39:479–86

298. Klenerova, V., Albrecht, I., Hynie, S. 1975. The activity of adenylate cyclase and phosphodiesterase in hearts and aortas of spontaneous hypertensive rats. *Pharmacol. Res. Commun.* 7:453–62

299. Ramanathan, S., Shibata, S. 1974. Cy-clic AMP in blood vessels of the sponta-neously hypertensive rat. *Blood Vessels* 11:312–18

300. Ramanathan, S., Shibata, S., Tasaki, T. K., Ichord, R. N. 1976. Cyclic AMP metabolism in the cardiac tissue of the spontaneously hypertensive rat. *Bio-chem. Pharmacol.* 25:223–25

301. Hamet, P., Kuchel, O., Genest, J. 1973. Effect of upright posture and iso-proterenol infusion on cyclic adenosine

monophosphate excretion in control subjects and patients with labile hyper-tension. *J. Clin. Endocrinol. Metab.* 36:218–26

302. Kaminsky, N. I., Broadus, A. E., Hard-man, J. G., Jones, D. J., Ball, J. H., Sutherland, E. W., Liddle, G. W. 1970. Effects of parathyroid hormone on plasma and urinary adenosine 3',5'-monophosphate in man. *J. Clin. Invest.* 49:2387–95

303. Taylor, A. L., Davis, B. B., Pawlson, L. G., Josinovich, J. B., Mintz, D. H. 1970. Factors influencing the urinary excre-tion of 3',5'-adenosine monophosphate in humans. *J. Clin. Endocrinol. Metab.* 30:316–24

304. Rosen, O. M. 1972. Urinary cyclic AMP in Grave's disease. *N. Engl. J. Med.* 287:670–71

305. Grill, V., Rosenqvist, U. 1975. Accu-mulation of cyclic AMP in hypothyroi-dism. Decreased sensitivity to norepi-nephrine in rat adipocytes. *Acta Endo-crinol.* 78:39–43

306. Farber, D. B., Lolley, R. N. 1974. Cy-clic guanosine monophosphate: Eleva-tion in degenerating photoreceptor cells of the C3H mouse retina. *Science* 186:449–51

307. Myllyla, V. V., Heikkinen, E. R., Vapaatalo, H., Hokkanen, E. 1975. Cy-clic AMP concentration and enzyme activities of cerebrospinal fluid in pa-tients with epilepsy or central nervous system damage. *Eur. Neurol.* 13:123–39

308. Sattin, A. 1971. Increase in the content of adenosine 3',5'-monophosphate in mouse forebrain during seizures and prevention of the increase by methyl-xanthines. *J. Neurochem.* 18:1087–96

309. Skolnick, P., Daly, J. W. 1974. The ac-cumulation of adenosine 3',5'-mono-phosphate in cerebral cortical slices of the quaking mouse, a neurologic mu-tant. *Brain Res.* 73:513–25

Ann. Rev. Pharmacol. Toxicol. 1977. 17:479–98
Copyright © 1977 by Annual Reviews Inc. All rights reserved

THE PHARMACOLOGICAL EFFECTS OF HYMENOPTERA VENOMS

❖6691

Richard M. Cavagnol
Natural Sciences Division, Johnson County Community College, Overland Park, Kansas 66210

In all things there is a poison and there is nothing without poison. It only depends upon the dose whether a poison is a poison or not.

Paracelsus (1)

INTRODUCTION

The Hymenoptera form one of the largest and most highly developed orders of the class Insecta. As members of the Arthropoda phylum, which contains about 85% of the known animal world, these invertebrates exhibit segmented bodies, jointed appendages, and hard exoskeletons. The female of various Hymenoptera have evolved modified ovipositors, capable of delivering a venom to adversaries. This venom is a complex mixture of biochemical compounds ranging from simple amines to complicated proteins and enzymes. Because of their painful and sometimes fatal reactions in humans, Hymenoptera venoms are of interest to the clinician and researcher.

The terms *venom* and *poison* were used interchangeably in early writings. The word *venom* is thought to have originated from the Latin *veneneum,* meaning a magical charm relating to Venus (2). A *poison* was originally a harmless draught or drink, the term probably derived from the Greek *potos* (3). From *potos* evolved the Latin *potum,* to drink, and possibly potion, potable, and even pot, a vessel from which to drink. The fatal meaning of poison came about as a result of the ancient practice of giving a lethal potion, or drink, to one's enemies.

Works of ancient alchemists and physicians (4) described the clinical effects of venoms and envenomation, but it was not until the eighteenth century that anything approaching a scientific investigation of venom was attempted. Robert Mead, an English physician, injected venon into animals and observed and recorded their effects (5). Several venoms he tested on himself, placing small quantities on the tip of his tongue and recording the effects.

During the last two centuries, many advances have been made in the fields of analytical chemistry, biochemistry, and pharmacology. Even with our sophisticated techniques of isolation, purification, and identification of biochemical compounds, several venom components remain to be isolated and identified.

CLINICAL MANIFESTATIONS OF ENVENOMATION

Envenomation by Hymenoptera is characterized by symptoms that depend upon the inflicting species, the quantity of injected venom, the degree of hypersensitivity of the victim, and, to some extent, the site of the sting. The reaction of victims to the stings of bees, wasps, hornets, or ants is usually painful, local, and brief, but occasionally is systemic and potentially fatal.

The local reaction to single stings is described by many as a sharp prick when the sting pierces the skin, followed by mild pain lasting several minutes. A small red area, surrounded by a white zone and a red flare, gradually appears around the sting site. A wheal forms, accompanied a few hours later by itching, tenderness, swelling, and generalized erythema.

More severe reactions from multiple stings are documented (6). Systemic poisoning from the venom is manifested as swollen and tender joints with accompanying urticaria, petechial hemorrhages, dizziness, weakness, nausea, diarrhea, abdominal cramps, and constriction of the chest. These symptoms are often accompanied by involuntary muscle spasm and convulsions. A man suffering over 2000 bee stings within a period of minutes displayed generalized edema, hemoglobinuria, severe hypotension, incontinence, and shock (7). The symptoms subsided 72 hours later.

The greatest threat to life posed by Hymenoptera venom is the anaphylactic reaction elicited in hypersensitive individuals by antigens in the venom. Large molecular weight substances, usually proteins, produce the life-threatening immunological reaction in sensitive individuals. The reaction is characterized by a dry, hacking cough, labored breathing, constriction of the throat and chest, flushing of the skin, edema of the glottis, and hypotension (8). Postmortem findings in fatal cases disclosed severe visceral and pulmonary congestion, cerebral edema, and laryngeal edema with obstruction. Precipitin antibodies to Hymenoptera venom were demonstrated in the serum of these individuals by Ouchterlong technique (8).

It is suspected that insects are responsible for many more deaths than are actually recorded or recognized by physicians. Many deaths attributed to shock, allergy, or laryngeal edema were, in fact, preceded by stings from Hymenoptera (9). Hymenoptera are believed responsible for 50% of the fatalities resulting from envenomation (10).

BEE VENOM

The earliest recorded investigation of venom from the honeybee, *Apis mellifera*, was conducted by two German chemists, Brandt and Ratzburg in 1837, during the infancy of chemistry and pharmacology. They observed bee venom to be bitter to the taste, soluble in water but not alcohol, and to leave a gummy residue upon evaporation (11).

The first thorough chemical examination of bee venom, from the same species, *Apis mellifera*, was undertaken in 1897 by Langer. Dropping the poison sacs together with the sting and glands into alcohol, he found the watery extract of the dried precipitate to be acidic in nature and bitter to the taste. Subcutaneous injection of venom droplets into rabbits, hand squeezed from 12,000 bees and collected in water, produced minute localized necrosis surrounded by edema and hyperemia (12).

Analyzing the alcoholic precipitate isolated from bee venom by Langer, Flury (13) detected what he believed to be various unsaturated fatty acids, choline, phosphoric acid, and other nitrogenous compounds. Pharmacological activity, which included inflammation upon injection and hemolysis of red blood cells in vitro, was confined to a nitrogen-free fraction.

Intrigued by the discoveries of Langer and Flury, Essex and co-workers (14) allowed the venom from avulsed *Apis mellifera* stinging apparatus to diffuse into a Ringer-glycerine solution, which was subsequently injected into prepared dogs. They observed a rapid fall in systemic blood pressure, while in guinea pigs, i.v. injections of the venom solution produced bronchospasms, often terminating in death. The isolated virgin guinea pig uterus showed a maximal contraction when perfused with the venom solution, while the isolated rabbit heart ceased beating. Addition of the venom solution to heparized dog blood resulted in considerable hemolysis. These effects were attributed to histamine in combination with other protoplasmic poisons.

Quantitation of the bee venom potency was attempted by Lacaillade (15) using cytolysis of *Paramecium caudatum* and hemolysis of horse erythrocytes as in vitro indices. Intradermally injected guinea pigs served as in vivo models for comparison. The degree of necrosis in guinea pigs was correlated with cytolysis of *Paramecium* and hemolysis of erythrocytes. Dilutions of 1:48,000 were effective in both systems. Bees were found to contain approximately 0.3 mg of venom, composed of an inflammatory substance, histamine, proteases, and surface-active components. Other investigators suggested that histamine, acting together with protease and other "intestinally active" principles, were responsible for the clinical symptoms of bee sting (16).

In an attempt to characterize the symptomatology of bee venom poisoning, Feldberg & Kellaway (17) attributed the hypotension observed in intact dogs, after i.v. administration of venom, to histamine released from tissues by lysolecithin. Subsequent experiments involving isolated organs of dogs and guinea pigs perfused with bee venom in a physiological solution showed that the venom depleted 40–75% of their endogenous histamine stores. Bee venom was also shown to release epinephrine from the isolated adrenals of rabbits, an action attributed to the lytic action of lysolecithin produced by the venom's lecithinase (18).

When whole venom was applied to the isolated guinea pig jejunum, a complex contraction composed of a fast and a slow component was observed (17). The rapid contraction was attributed to histamine, while the prolonged, slow contraction and the altered reactivity to histamine after several venom exposures was attributed to some unknown substance.

Formic acid extracts of the venom were found to contain nitrogen, sulfur, and phosphorus, while whole venom had an isoelectric point of pH 8.7 (19). The existence of pharmacologically active peptides in bee venom was becoming evident. Further purification of the formic acid extract with ethanol allowed the isolation of two components after extensive dialysis (20). The dialyzable component, 40% by weight of the crude venom, produced severe convulsions and death in mice receiving i.v. injections. The nondialyzable portion of the venom produced death in mice by respiratory paralysis, with no evidence of convulsion.

Investigating the possibility that neuromuscular blockade produced the respiratory paralysis previously observed in mice, Hofmann (21) added diluted (1:1000) bee venom to isolated rat phrenic nerve-diaphragm preparations and observed a contraction followed by partial relaxation. The block appeared to be more of the decamethonium- than of the curare-type as it was resistant to physostigmine and was accompanied by contracture. It differed from decamethonium block by lack of reversibility. Nerve conduction appeared unaffected, even by strongly contracting doses of bee venom. After prolonged contact with venom (2 hr) the muscles became unresponsive to direct electrical stimulation.

In 1953, Fischer & Neumann (22) separated the picric acid precipitate of bee venom into two fractions by paper chromatography, and found that each fraction possessed hemolytic activity. Fraction I, devoid of any S-amino acids, hemolyzed serum-free, washed erythrocytes. This direct lytic factor differed from the component of Fraction II, which required serum or lecithin for lysis of erythrocytes. Further investigation of the indirect lytic factor showed it to be phospholipase A, the lecithinase first detected by Feldberg & Kellaway in 1937 (23).

Research on venoms intensified and with the advent of new biochemical techniques, more effective separation of these highly complex substances was realized. Neumann & Habermann (24) separated whole bee venom by paper electrophoresis into five cathodal fractions: histamine, F0, FI, FII, and K. Pharmacological analysis of these fractions showed F0 devoid of any biological activity, while FI, designated melittin, hemolyzed serum-free, washed erythrocytes, lowered surface tension at air-water interfaces, produced pain and inflammation on injection, and increased the permeability of skin capillaries for i.v.-administered Evans blue (25). Animals receiving i.v. melittin injections displayed a profound drop in arterial blood pressure, while isolated preparations of frog abdominus rectus muscle and guinea pig ileum responded to melittin with strong contractions. The isolated rat phrenic nerve-diaphragm showed a transient excitation followed by blockade subsequent to melittin, an effect identical with that observed earlier by Hofmann (21) with whole bee venom.

Melittin was later isolated and purified by gel filtration on Sephadex ® G-50 and chromatography on carboxymethyl cellulose (26, 27). The physiochemical properties of melittin (strong basicity, high surface activity, and absorbability to organic constituents) could be manifestations of the peptide's primary structure. Amino acid analysis revealed 26 amino acids, with a calculated molecular weight of 2840 (28). Enzyme degradation of the linear peptide by trypsin, chymotrypsin, and pepsin, as well as partial Edman degradation, revealed that amino acids in positions 1–20 were principally neutral and hydrophobic, while positions 21–26 contained basic, hydrophilic amino acids (29). Convenient associations between hydrophobic portions of the molecule and acyl chains of membrane phospholipids may be predicted, making melittin a "structural" poison (30). The broad spectrum of pharmacological activities manifested by melittin undoubtedly results from its general attack on cellular membranes.

Melittin was found to be highly toxic to *Drosophila melanogaster* larvae, manifested by violent muscle contractions occurring in the vicinity of the injection site (31). Chronic reactions to melittin, injected in the larvae's anterior three segments, included slowing of growth, lethargy, anorexia, and loss of weight. It was suggested that these effects were due to the peptide's interaction with the excitable membrane of the brain, ganglia, and ring gland, resulting in an alteration of the membrane's permeability to ions. More rigorous fractionation of melittin disclosed another peptide, minimine, found to be responsible for the lethargy and anorexia in larvae (32). Metamorphosis of treated larvae yielded miniature adult flies, reduced in size as much as 75%, of controls. They were, however, normal with respect to feeding, mobility, and production of progeny, who were of normal size.

Intra-arterial administration of melittin to cats produced a profound depression of recorded EEG activity (33). This EEG depression was followed shortly by an elevation of blood pressure and the cessation of respiration. Later, blood pressure dropped to shock levels.

Cytotoxicity of melittin on cultured cells has been observed. These include the reduction of DNA, RNA, and protein synthesis in ascites cells (34); inhibition of colony-forming ability of mouse bone-marrow cells (35); and antibacterial action against *Staphylococcus aureus* (36).

The gel filtration technique used by Fischer, Neumann, Habermann, and Reiz to separate and purify melittin also permitted the resolution of the F0 fraction into three distinct but unidentified proteins. In addition, a small basic peptide, named apamine, was eluted between histamine and melittin on the Sephadex column. This peptide was previously concealed in the FI fraction because of similar electrophoretic motility and low content relative to melittin. Unlike melittin, the pharmacological effects of apamine were rather specific and were confined primarily to the central nervous system. Mice injected with apamine exhibited long-lasting central nervous system excitation characterized by uncoordinated, uninterupted movements, culminating in generalized convulsion (37–39). Death ensued from lack of coordinated respirations.

Cats, transected at various spinal levels and injected with apamine, showed an increase in amplitude of recorded reflex potentials as compared to controls (40). This suggested that apamine augments polysynaptic reflexes and increases the effectiveness of excitatory polysynaptic pathways over inhibitory pathways.

Biochemical analysis of apamine showed it to contain 18 amino acids, with four half-cysteine residues and no aromatic amino acids (41). Trypsin and chymotrypsin-digested fragments were examined and the amino acid sequence determined (42). The peptide has a calculated molecular weight of 2036.

The cathodal fraction FII of Neumann & Habermann (24) was found to contain the enzymes phospholipase A (PLA) and hyaluronidase. These enzymes were shown to be, in large part, responsible for the anaphylactic reaction to bee venom (43).

Purified PLA was examined for pharmacological activity (44, 45) and found to have an i.v. LD_{50} in mice of 10–20 mg/kg. Death occurred from convulsions following respiratory paralysis. Anesthetized cats receiving i.v. PLA responded with a fall in systemic arterial pressure. The isolated guinea pig ileum contracted upon exposure to PLA, but showed marked tachyphylaxis to subsequent doses. The isolated frog heart and rectus abdominus were not affected by PLA. Washed guinea pig erythrocytes, but not those from humans, were hemolyzed when incubated with PLA.

Dramatic cardiovascular changes were observed in anesthetized dogs receiving PLA intravenously (46). The enzyme produced ventricular fibrillation, increased the central venous pressure, left atrial pressure, systemic vascular resistance, and ventricular stroke work within five minutes of administration. Death followed within ten minutes. Under similar experimental conditions, Slotta and co-workers (47) found that 1 mg/kg PLA introduced intravenously in dogs produced a sharp fall in arterial pressure accompanied by a marked rise in central venous pressure. Simultaneously, a short period of apnea and profound bradycardia ensued, accompanied by complete loss of cortical EEG activity.

The activity of PLA is attributed to its reaction products, lysophosphatide and free fatty acid, produced from PLA's hydrolysis of 2-acyl bonds of natural phosphatidyl choline, ethanolamine, and serine. The surfactant character of the formed lysophospholipids is thought to result from the combination between the hydrophobic aliphatic acyl chain and the hydrophilic phosphorylated base (30). Such a molecule is capable of solubilizing tissue and disrupting membrane structures, resulting in nonspecific permeability changes. PLA constitutes a significant percentage (approximately 12%) of dried bee venom, and it is reasonable to assume that a part of bee sting symptomatology results from pharmacologically active substances liberated through nonspecific membrane damage by lysolecithin (30, 48).

It was demonstrated earlier (17) that bee venom exerted some type of histamine-releasing activity on animal tissues. PLA and later melittin were thought to be the agents in bee venom responsible for the release of histamine and the resulting physiological consequences (48). Histamine released through lysolecithin-mediated membrane destruction required no energy, as demonstrated in vitro by the failure of dinitrophenol (DNP) or the withdrawal of glucose to influence PLAs releasing action. No degranulation of mast cells was observed after PLA treatment. While degranulation of mast cells did occur after melittin treatment, histamine liberation was not affected by DNP or glucose-free medium (48).

Since the physiological release of histamine from mast cells is thought to proceed by activation of an energy-requiring degranulation process (49), the existence of a third histamine-releasing factor in bee venom was suspected. Fredholm & Haegermark (50), working with bee venom fraction obtained by gel filtration, discovered a basic polypeptide with histamine-releasing properties similar to compound 48/80. The degranulating activity of the peptide prompted the name mast cell degranulating (MCD)-peptide. The possibility that this peptide might be melittin was ruled out by its high susceptibility to the metabolic inhibitors DNP and NEM (N-ethyl maleimide) (51, 52). The lack of central nervous system stimulation in mice receiving a dose of MCD-peptide ten times the LD_{50} reported for apamine discounted apamine as the mastocytolytic component.

Concurrently, Breithaupt & Habermann (53) purified the MCD-peptide and identified it as one of the basic F0-peptides. Acid hydrolysis of the purified peptide revealed 22 amino acids with a molecular weight of 2855. Haux (54) determined the amino acid sequence and found that the amino acids in positions 3–6 corresponded exactly to the sequence of position 1–4 in apamine. However, no central neurotoxicity was detected with MCD-peptide. It was further distinguished from melittin by its inability to release serotonin from platelets, failure to hemolyze red blood cells, and by its LD_{50}, which, in mice, exceeds 40 mg/kg.

Purified MCD-peptide has been shown to reduce carrogeenin-induced edema in the rat paw (55). The anti-inflammatory activity of MCD-peptide is not abolished by pretreatment with antagonists of histamine, serotonin, or adrenergic agents. The anti-inflammatory activity persists after regional denervation or adrenalectomy. A direct action of MCD-peptide on vascular walls to reduce their permeability is suggested as the mechanism of action.

Several biogenic amines have been isolated from bee venom (56). Gel filtration and ion-exchange chromatography of whole bee venom yielded several fractions, one of which was found to contain norepinephrine and dopamine.

Other investigators (57) have isolated a cardioactive substance identified as cardiopep (cardiac peptide). When applied to isolated perfused hearts, the heart rate increased 50% and the force of contraction increased by 150%. In hearts with intrinsic arrhythmias, cardiopep produced an immediate restoration to normal rhythm. The identity of the compound is not known, but it is not a peptide, as originally thought.

Venom produced by the honeybee *Apis mellifera* is a highly complex mixture of pharmacologically active agents. Included among the identified constituents are the enzymes phospholipase A and hyaluronidase, the biogenic amines histamine, norepinephrine, and dopamine, and the peptides melittin, apamine, MCD-peptide, and minimine. Free amino acids, sugars, lipids, free bases, a cardioactive substance, and other unidentified compounds whose contribution to the toxicity of bee venom await determination, constitute the remainder of the venom (58).

WASP VENOM

Research on wasp venom was initiated by Jaques & Schachter (59,60) after their discovery of a potent histamine liberator in alcoholic extracts of sea anemone tentacles. Wasp stings were known to be extremely painful and to manifest many of the symptoms of bee stings. The presence of pharmacologically active agents in wasp venom was therefore suspected.

Crude venom from the yellow jacket *Vespa vulgaris* produced a biphasic contraction of the isolated guinea pig ileum (60). Mepyramine partially antagonized the response, suggesting histamine as one of the venom components. Paper chromatography of the crude venom revealed distinct spots corresponding to histamine and serotonin standards in R_f values and color reactions. When eluates of the spots were tested on isolated preparations, mepyramine blocked the ileal contractions produced by the histamine spot. The serotonin eluate failed to contract the tryptamine-desensitized ileum. But neither block was complete, and small amounts of the crude venom still contracted the ileum rendered insensitive to histamine and serotonin. It was concluded that wasp venom contained a third substance responsible for the slow contraction seen as the second component of the biphasic ileal response. The slow-contracting substance remained after trichloroacetic acid (TCA) precipitation but was destroyed after treatment of the TCA-soluble venom fraction with boiling hydrochloric acid.

Because of the similarity of the slow-contracting substance to bradykinin, Schachter & Thain named it wasp kinin. Further studies with wasp venom, involving atropinized and mepyramine-treated rats and rabbits, confirmed the presence of a potent pharmacological agent whose effects on smooth muscle were direct and not mediated through the release of other compounds (61).

In a comparative study of wasp kinin, bradykinin, and kallidin, all three substances exhibited qualitatively similar pharmacological properties (62). Wasp kinin differed from the other kinins in that it was partially inactivated by trypsin, while kallidin and bradykinin were unaffected. Differences in rate of migration and R_f value between wasp kinin and bradykinin, kallidin and substance P on paper chromatograms were also noted.

Wasp kinin from *Vespa vulgaris* was resolved by ion-exchange chromatography into a single major and two minor components (63). All three components reacted with azocarmine and ninhydrin, exhibited similar pharmacological activity on guinea pig ileum and rat uterus preparations, and were completely inactivated by chymotrypsin. Incubation with trypsin greatly reduced activities of the three components. Like kallidin and bradykinin, wasp kinins appeared to be polypeptides.

Venom from other wasps was examined for kinins and other pharmacologically active substances. Extensive chemical analysis of venom from *Polistes annularis, P. fusicatus,* and *P. exclamanus* demonstrated three kinins readily separable on columns of carboxymethyl cellulose or carboxymethyl Sephadex (64). *Polistes* kinin 1 and 2 bore remarkable chemical and pharmacological similarities to bradykinin and kallidin. *Polistes* kinin 3, or simply *Polistes* kinin, the most abundant fraction, possessed the highest biological activity on guinea pig ileum, rat blood pressure, and rat duodenum. Treatment of *Polistes* kinin with trypsin changed its chromatographic properties and increased biological activity as opposed to the kinins from *Vespa vulgaris*, which were partially inactivated. The activity of trypsin-treated *Polistes* kinin was recovered as a single peak from carboxymethyl Sephadex. Amino acid analysis of the active tryptic peptide revealed glycyl-bradykinin in addition to other amino acids. The structure of *Polistes* kinin has been elucidated and confirmed by synthesis to be Pyr-Thr-Asn-Lys-Lys-Lys-Arg-Gly-(Bradykinin) (65). This suggests that *Polistes* kinin is actually a kininogen-like substance whose pharmacological activity is liberated by tryptic enzymes present in the envenomated organism.

Recent investigation of venoms from various social wasps has revealed the presence of the catecholamines norepinephrine, epinephrine, and dopamine, with dopamine the most abundant (66). Small quantities of serotonin have also been identified in the venoms.

The parasitic solitary wasps of the suborder *Terebrantes* and *Aculeato* dispense a venom that is rather unique in its ability to paralyze, but not kill, the intended prey. Beard (67), investigating the toxicological effects of *Habrabracon juglandis* venom on wax moth larvae, discovered that one part venom in 2×10^8 parts insect hemolymph was sufficient to induce spreading paralysis. Oscillographic recordings of muscle and nerve action potentials indicated that the paralysis resulted from impairment of excitatory processes of the body-wall musculature, while internal organs remained unaffected. The effects of the venom on larvae paralleled the effects of curare on mammalian neuromuscular transmission. The venom was postulated to interfere with neuromuscular transmission in insects by chelation of copper, thus inactivating a copper-containing mediator of neuromuscular transmission. To date, no such mediator has been identified.

The paralysis observed in insects after envenomation by the paralytic wasps may be either transient or permanent, depending upon the species of wasp. The effects of *Microbracon hebetor* and *Philanthus triangulum* venoms on in vivo and in vitro insect preparations include a reversible locomotor paralysis, with the central nervous system, internal organs, and muscle fibers unaffected (68). The neuromuscular junction is cited as the venom's proposed site of action.

Electrophysiological investigation of miniature excitatory postsynaptic potentials (MEPP) recorded from the flight muscles of *Philosamia cynthia* indicate that *Microbracon hebetor* venom markedly decreases the frequency but not the amplitude of the spontaneous potentials (69). The end-plate potential measured in the neuromuscular junction is thought to be composed of a large number of smaller potentials, corresponding with the quantal release of the transmitter substance (70). The miniature end-plate potentials presumably are the direct postsynaptic result of spontaneous release of one or few transmitter-substance quanta (71). The predominant effect of *M. hebetor* venom on MEPP frequency suggested that the venom had a presynaptic site of action.

Rathmayer (72) observed a progressive paralysis in *Apis mellifera* stung by *Philanthus triangulum* and concluded that the venom was carried by the prey's hemolymph to the locomotor organs where it exerted its paralytic action. Venom from *P. triangulum* was later shown to decrease the frequency of MEPP recorded from *Shistocercia gregoria* flight muscles, similar to the effect observed by Piek & Engles (69) with *M. hebetor* venom. This led Piek (73) to propose a similar site of action for *P. triangulum* venom. It was observed that nerve stimulation during venom produced a faster onset of muscle paralysis, suggesting that the venom might be interfering with the synthesis of transmitter or its storage (73).

Both *Microbracon hebetor* and *Philanthus triangulum* venoms have proven extremely difficult to analyze chemically. Visser & Spanjer (74) partially purified *P. triangulum* venom and recovered a toxin of 700 molecular weight from gel filtration. *M. hebetor* venom was reported to contain amino acids, enzymes, and peptides, none of which were identified (74).

Limited success has been achieved in chemical analysis of venom from *Sceliphron caementarium*. Histamine, serotonin, and acetylcholine, three low molecular weight agents previously demonstrated in other Hymenoptera venoms, were absent from *S. caementarium* venom (75). This is consistent with the mild reaction experienced by humans after receiving a sting. Small amounts of histidine, methionine, and pipecolic acid, all of unknown function, were identified by paper chromatography. Proteins isolated from *S. caementarium* venom by disc electrophoresis showed no antigenic cross-reactivity with venom proteins from *Polistes apachus* (wasp), *Vespula pennsylvanica* (yellow jacket), *Vespula arenario* (yellow hornet), or *Apis mellifera* (honeybee) (76). Solvent extraction of the purified venom followed by different chromatographic procedures disclosed 22 components, which accounted for 96 ± 8% of the dry venom weight (77). The paralyzing factor was not isolated and was believed to result from cooperative interaction of some or all of the venom constituents.

The pharmacological activities of *Vespula* and *Polistes* venoms may be attributed to histamine and serotonin acting synergistically with bradykinin-like polypeptides and venom enzymes (41). Venoms from the solitary wasps apparently exert their paralytic effect presynaptically at the neuromuscular junction, but the active components have yet to be isolated and identified (78).

HORNET VENOM

Investigation of hornet venom began in 1960, shortly after the discovery of potent pharmacological agents in the venom of wasps and other stinging Hymenoptera. Venom from the European hornet *Vespa crabo* was shown, by parallel assay, to contract the isolated guinea pig ileum and frog rectus absominus muscle (79, 80). The antagonism of these effects by atropine and *d*-tubocurarine, respectively, suggested that the venom contained an acetylcholine-like compound not previously demonstrated in venoms of other Hymenoptera. Paper chromatograms of acetylcholine standards and alcoholic extracts of hornet venom revealed spots with identical R_f's. When the venom spot was eluted and injected into rabbits, a profound hypotensive effect was observed. This effect was blocked by pretreatment of the animals with atropine.

Bhoola and co-workers (80) also detected histamine in the hornet venom by assay on the atropinized guinea pig ileum. A spot with an R_f value identical with histamine was eluted and applied to the ileum preparation. The contraction produced by the spot was completely abolished by mepyramine.

The whole-venom chromatograph also showed a spot with an R_f value very close to serotonin. The spot gave a blue-gray color when sprayed with dimethylaminobenzaldehyde, indicating a positive Ehrlich reaction for indoles. Eluates of the spot contracted the isolated guinea pig ileum and rat uterus, the latter reaction being partially antagonized with LSD. Preincubation of the eluate with chymotrypsin destroyed the LSD-resistant component. The effects observed were attributed to serotonin and a peptide with chromatographic mobility similar to serotonin in the solvent systems used (80).

Further chromatographic investigation with different solvent systems resulted in the isolation of the new peptide. Named hornet kinin by Bhoola because of its pharmacological activity and sensitivity to chymotrypsin, it differed from wasp kinin by its insensitivity to trypsin inactivation (61). Hornet kinin demonstrated a remarkable similarity to bradykinin when tested on the rat uterus, rat duodenum, and rat arterial pressure, but was only one tenth as active on the guinea pig ileum. Hornet venom has been shown to contain phospholipase A (30) and is suspected to contain other peptides, amino acids, and enzymes as yet unidentified.

A pharmacological evaluation of *Vespa orientalis* venom was started by Edery and co-workers in 1972 (81) and has been continued by Ishay. Venom injected into mice produced akinesia and paralysis which lasted until the death of the animals. While the paralyzing effect of Hymenoptera venom on other insects has been well documented (68, 69, 73, 82), there have been no reported instances of insect venom causing neuromuscular disturbances in mammals. Intra-arterial injections of the venom into cats blocked directly and indirectly induced single twitches of gastronemius-soleus and tibialis anterior muscles, without affecting conduction in the sciatic or semitendinosus nerve. A blockade of neuromuscular transmission was suggested as the mechanism of action.

Whole venom produced bronchiolar constriction when injected into guinea pigs and increased capillary permeability in rabbits and rats receiving intradermal injections. The presence in the venom of histamine or histamine-releasing agents as well as other potent biogenic amines was suspected, since these substances had been demonstrated in other hornets and wasps. Histamine, serotonin, and acetylcholine were identified by their actions on the guinea pig ileum and rat uterus, with antagonism by mepyramine, 2-bromolysergic acid tartrate, and atropine, respectively. The venom continued to elicit a slow, sustained contraction of smooth muscle preparations in the presence of the three antagonists. Incubation of the venom with chymotrypsin abolished the ileal contraction while trypsin did not affect the kinin's activity. It appears that kinin from *Vespa orientalis* is related to that of *Vespa crabo*, but differs from wasp kinins which are sensitive to trypsin. The presence in *V. orientalis* venom of a histamine-releasing agent was explored using rat peritoneal mast cells incubated with hornet venom or compound 48/80. No histamine remained in the mast cells after incubation, while substantial quantities of histamine could be liberated from controls.

Edery and his group found norepinephrine, epinephrine, and dopamine in small quantities after biochemical analysis of the venom and venom sacs of *V. orientalis*

(81). These agents had been previously demonstrated in the venom sacs, but not venom, of bees and wasps (83). It was suggested that they prolong the local action of the venom by constriction of cutaneous capillaries and venules.

Ishay and co-workers have continued the investigation of the venom and venom sac extract (VSE) of the Oriental hornet, *Vespa orientalis*. Intravenous administration of VSE to cats produce a drop in blood sugar. This effect was attributed to a nondialyzable protein or protein-bound substance in the VSE that is heat sensitive (84).

The hornet VSE was shown to have in vivo and in vitro anticoagulant properties (85). VSE inhibited in vitro formation of thrombin and thromboplastin when incubated with human plasma. Intravenous administration of VSE to dogs reduced the clottability of whole blood. The anticoagulant factor has not been identified, but it is inactivated at high temperature and alkaline pH.

The hornet venom produced dramatic cardiovascular effects when administered intravenously to prepared dogs (86). Effects seen 10 sec after administration of the venom included increased respiration and cardiac output, while mean aortic pressure and peripheral resistance decreased. Pretreatment of dogs with methysergide prior to the administration of the venom abolished all of the effects except vasodilation. This appears to confirm the presence of serotonin in hornet venom as previously reported by Edery (81). The vasodilation seen after blockade of the serotonin effects were attributed to a kinin-like substance, previously isolated by other investigators (61).

The local reaction to hornet sting, characterized by pain, inflammation, and edema result from the potent amines and polypeptides present in the venom. In addition, the presence of the enzymes hyaluronidase and phospholipase A, as well as a histamine liberator, probably contribute to the reaction by promoting the spread of the venom.

ANT VENOM

Ant venoms fall into two categories, proteinaceous and nonproteinaceous, and are found among species of primitive subfamilies where the sting mechanism is highly developed. The majority of ant stings are only slightly painful but those inflicted by *Myrmecia* or *Solenopsis* ants result in both localized necrosis and systemic reactions of severe intensity. Within the classification of ant venom, *Myrmecia* produces a proteinaceous venom, while *Solenopsis* secretes a venom devoid of detectable protein. As with venom from other stinging Hymenoptera, the greatest threat to human life lies in the allergic reaction exhibited by sensitive individuals. The severity of the reaction depends on the degree of sensitivity of the individual, with death occurring as a consequence of anaphylactic shock.

Initial studies on the venom of the fire ant *Solenopsis saevissina* revealed the absence of ninhydrin-positive reactants, suggesting a nonproteinaceous venom (87). The pure venom was insoluble in water, dispersing as fine, milky-white globules on the water surface. The venom was soluble in most organic solvents. While the fire ant is not susceptible to its own venom, several species of mites and weevils, as well as *Drosophila melanogaster* and *Musca domestica*, are.

Pharmacological investigation of crude *Solenopsis* venom was undertaken with the aim of isolating and identifying the necrotoxic principle(s) (88). The venom showed marked hemolytic activity on washed rabbit erythrocytes, and the active component was thought to be nonprotein in nature because no loss of activity was observed after exposure to 100°C for 1 hr. Isolation of the hemolytic component was accomplished by solvent extraction which yielded white crystals melting at 144–145°C. These crystals gave a positive test for a tertiary amine.

The pustules produced by experimental ant sting being bacteriologically sterile (89), the crystalline hemolytic component was screened for antimycotic activity utilizing 21 different human pathogens (90). Susceptible pathogens included *Candida albicans, Blastomycese dermatitis*, and *Cryptococcus neoforus*, as determined by the zone of inhibition surrounding a crystal on the agar plate.

The first chemical analysis of the hemolytic component (91) suggested the compound 2-methyl-3-hexadecyl-pyrrolidine. More recent experimental analysis, utilizing gas chromatography, mass spectroscopy, and NMR, has led investigators to propose *trans*-2-methyl-6-*n*-undecylpiperidine named *Solenopsin A*, as the active hemolytic component (92). The structure was verified after synthesis of Solenopsin A.

In contrast to *Solenopsis* venom, the clear, colorless liquid obtained from the venom reservoirs of *Myrmecia gulosa* was readily soluble in water, was insoluble in organic solvents, and gave a positive ninhydrin reaction (93). Its protein nature was further supported by absorbance at 277–282 mμ of the UV spectrum.

Separation of the crude venom into eight fractions was accomplished with paper electrophoresis. Fraction I corresponded to histamine by comparative paper chromatography. Hyaluronidase activity was detected in Fractions IV and V, as was a kinin-like substance which contracted the guinea pig ileum and rat uterus. Fraction VII contained a direct hemolytic factor found to be heat labile. No cholinesterase, 5-nucleotidase, or protease was detected in the venom.

Similar investigative efforts have been directed toward venoms from other members of the Myrmeciinae subfamily. Precise identification of the extract species sometimes proved difficult. Venom collected from *Myrmecia forficata*, later identified as *M. pyriformis*, produced a contraction of the isolated rat uterus characterized by a prolonged delay in recovery when compared with serotonin and acetylcholine (94). Incubation of the venom with trypsin abolished the activity on the uterus, but had no effect on the response of the guinea pig ileum. Mepyramine completely antagonized the latter action. The presence of histamine was confirmed by paper chromatography of whole venom. One spot produced a positive reaction to ninhydrin, had an R_f identical with the histamine standard, and was resistant to boiling in strong mineral acid. This latter treatment had no effect upon the ileum-contracting ability of the spot eluate, although mepyramine completely abolished the activity. The prolonged response seen with the other chromatogram spot on the rat uterus was suggestive of a kinin-like substance.

Myrmecia sting is characterized by a pronounced local reaction, suggesting that the venom might contain a histamine-releasing compound (95). Normal saline extracts of *Myrmecia pyriformis* venom sacs, when incubated with rat peritoneal mast cells, showed considerable histamine-liberating activity. Ten micrograms of venom, about the amount present in one good ant bite, released 56% of the mast cells' histamine, as compared to 74% released by an equal concentration of compound 48/80. Increasing the venom concentration tenfold resulted in 95% depletion of mast cell histamine. This histamine-releasing activity might be involved with the prolonged spasmogenic activity of ant venom on smooth muscle and the long-lasting erythema and localized edema seen after envenomation.

A more detailed investigation of *M. pyriformis* venom, aimed at characterizing the various components, was undertaken by Lewis & de la Lande (96). Crude venom contracted the isolated rat uterus, toad rectus abdominus muscle, and guinea pig ileum, and constricted the vessels of the isolated rabbit ear. A marked hypotensive effect was observed in anesthetized cats after administration of the venom. Histamine identified previously in other experiments was believed partially responsible for the isolated organ activity. The persistence, however, of a slow contractile response on histamine-insensitive uterus and mepyramine-treated ileum suggested another active component. The crude venom released histamine from isolated peritoneal mast cells, lysed washed red blood cells, and showed hyaluronidase activity. All four activities were destroyed by boiling the venom, while a marked loss of all activities was noted after incubation with trypsin or chymotrypsin. The involvement of polypeptides as mediators of the above responses was suspected.

Paper chromatography allowed the separation of histamine from the other active substances, but failed to separate the smooth-muscle stimulant from either the red-cell lysing fraction or the histamine-releasing component.

A possible correlation of the single substance in ant venom that stimulates smooth muscle, lyses red blood cells, and releases histamine to the bee peptide, melittin, has been suggested (97).

The ability of purified *M. pyriformis* to split lecithin was demonstrated by in vitro incubation of the venom with plant and liver lecithin (98). Thin-layer chromatography of precipitated lysolecithin from the ant venom incubation produced spots identical in R_f with lysolecithin from phospholipase A hydrolysis. The components of ant venom appear very similar in activity to the substances found in the venom of the honeybee, *Apis mellifera* (99).

Venom is but one of the exocrine secretions produced by ants. Ant venom has been shown to contain histamine, a histamine-releasing substance, a nonhistamine smooth-muscle stimulant, a direct red-cell lysing factor, hyaluronidase, phospholipase, and other complex chemical substances (97).

SUMMARY

Venoms from the hymenopteran superfamilies Apoidea, Vespoidea, Sphecoidea, and Formicoidea constitute a group of toxic substances that have been of concern to man since prehistoric times. Even now, after seventy-five years of research on hymenopteran venoms, it is difficult to make any meaningful generalizations concerning their composition except to say that they contain pharmacologically active components that fall into one of three general categories: (a) biogenic amines, (b) nonenzymatic proteins and polypeptide toxins, and (c) enzymes. Venoms from different families and species of Hymenoptera have been biochemically separated, and some components isolated and evaluated pharmacologically by a multiplicity of techniques, resulting in a rather fragmentary picture of venom composition.

A highly specialized apparatus serves to secrete, store, and eject the venom. Venom, produced in the venom glands of the female, is stored in a venom reservoir until needed, at which time it is ejected through a hollow, pointed aculeus, or stinger, into the intended victim. The entire maneuver is controlled by a series of muscles located in the abdomen of the Hymenoptera. The morphology of the sting apparatus varies slightly between different families.

The venom of the honeybee, *Apis mellifera*, has received the greatest research attention over the years, and as a result, more is known about this venom than the others. Histamine was the first pharmacological agent identified in bee venom, along with other substances that produced slow, sustained contractions of the guinea pig ileum and released epinephrine from perfused cat adrenals. The latter action was attributed to lecithinase, previously discovered in cobra venom, and later found in bee venom. Other factors present in bee venom included a hemolytic component and a convulsant factor.

Among the more sophisticated techniques of separation employed by venom researchers, paper electorphoresis proved the most fruitful. Whole bee venom was separated into five fractions: FO, FI, FII, H, and K. Analysis of these fractions revealed histamine, phospholipase A, hyaluronidase, and a polypeptide, melittin, as components of bee venom. Comprising 50% of total dry bee venom by weight, melittin was believed to be responsible for most of the pharmacological actions of whole bee venom. These included direct hemolysis of washed erythrocytes, liberation of histamine and serotonin from mast cells and platelets, contraction of smooth muscle, and ganglionic blockade. The amino acid sequence of melittin has been determined and the peptide recently synthesized. It has been suggested that pharmacological properties of melittin are directly related to its primary structure, that of an invert soap, giving melittin strong surface-active characteristics.

Continued investigation of bee venom has led to the discovery of several other peptides of pharmacological interest. The dialyzable convulsant factor, first recognized by Hahn and Ledelschke in 1937, was isolated and named apamine. This peptide had rather specific actions; it produced long-lasting central excitation in mice and increased the permeability of rat cutis for Evans blue dye. The central excitation is thought to result from apamine's augmentation of central excitatory pathways. The amino acid sequence of apamine has been described and the peptide synthesized.

A specific mast cell degranulating peptide (MCD-peptide) was isolated by Breithaupt and Habermann from their electrophoretic fraction FO, previously described as biologically inactive. At the same time, Fredholm discovered a similar active principle in his bee venom fractions. The two substances were found to be identical and to exert their histamine-releasing action in a manner similar to compound 48/80. The amino acid sequence of MCD-peptide has been elucidated. Bee venom, therefore, acts to release histamine by three mechanisms: (a) phospholipase A, acting indirectly by forming lysolecithin from extracellular lecithin; (b) melittin, disrupting mast cells directly by surface activity; and (c) MCD-peptide, producing degranulation similar to 48/80.

A fourth peptide, minimine, has been detected in bee venom. Minimine produced lethargy and anorexia when injected into *Drosophila melanogaster* larvae. Adult flies emerging from the treated larvae were one fourth the normal size, although they appeared normal with respect to feeding, motility, and progeny.

Recently, a cardioactive substance, cardiopep, has been found in bee venom. It has been shown to increase the rate and the force of contraction of the heart.

Venom from the wasp *Vespa vulgaris* was found to contain histamine, serotonin, phospholipases, and a substance that produced slow, sustained contractions of the guinea pig ileum. The slow contracting substance bore a remarkable pharmacological resemblance to bradykinin and kallidin, but differed from these peptides in that it was susceptible to trypsin inactivation. The substance was named wasp kinin and was shown to be a peptide.

A peptide with properties similar to the wasp kinin from *V. vulgaris* was isolated from the venom of *Polistes* wasps by fractionation on carboxymethyl cellulose. *Polistes* kinin differed from the Vespa kinin in that its activity was enhanced by trypsin. Amino acid analysis of the trypsin fragment showed it to be glycyl-bradykinin, suggesting that Polistes kinin is actually a kininogen-like substance whose pharmacological activity is unmasked by the host's enzyme system. The complete structure of *Polistes* kinin recently has been described and confirmed by synthesis.

Wasps of the family *Sphecoidea* elaborate a venom that is paralytic in action and devoid of the usual pain-producing substances. The paralytic component reportedly acts presynaptically at the insect neuromuscular junction and has proven resistant to isolation attempts.

Hornet venom of the species *Vespa crabo* and *Vespa orientalis* contain histamine, serotonin, phospholipase A, hyaluronidase, and substantial quantities (10% by weight of dried venom) of acetylcholine. Both venoms contain a kinin sensitive to chymotrypsin but insensitive to trypsin. Norepinephrine, epinephrine, and dopamine, previously reported as constituents of bee and wasp venom sacs, were present in small quantities in hornet venom. The amines are thought to prolong the local action of the venom by constricting cutaneous capillaries and venules.

Ant venoms may be classified as proteinaceous and nonproteinaceous. *Myrmecia gulosa* produces a proteinaceous venom that was separated electrophoretically into eight components. Histamine, hyaluronidase, and a direct lytic factor were identified among the constituents. Another species of *Myrmecia, M. pyriformis,* elaborates a venom containing a potent histamine liberator, a hemolytic component, a smooth-muscle stimulant, and hyaluronidase. Except for hyaluronidase, none of the components have been identified.

Venom devoid of detectable protein is produced by the fire ant, *Solenopsis saevissina*. It contains a powerful hemolytic agent that has been crystallized and identified as *trans*-2-methyl-6-*n*-undecylpiperidine.

Hymenoptera venoms are highly concentrated mixtures of pharmacologically active substances that may be of value in the study of agents activated or released by tissue damage. Venoms may be for the pharmacologist

> ...an instrument which associates and analyzes the most delicate phenomena of the living machine and in studying attentively the mechanism of death ... [reveals] by an indirect route the physiological mechanism of life.

Claude Bernard (100)

ACKNOWLEDGMENT

I am grateful to Carla Z. Schade and Marty Levi for assistance in preparing this manuscript.

Literature Cited

1. Guterman, N. 1958. *Paracelsus: Selected Writings,* p. 95. New York: Pantheon. 360 pp.
2. Witkop, B. 1965. Poisonous animals and their venoms. *J. Wash. Acad. Sci.* 55:53–58
3. Wain, H. 1958. *The Story Behind the Word,* p. 252. Springfield: Thomas. 342 pp.
4. Adams, F. 1847. On the preservatives from venomous animals in general. In *The Seven Books of Paulus Aegineta,* II (Book V): 157–61. London: Sydenham Soc. 511 pp.
5. Mead, R. 1745. *A Mechanical Account of Poisons,* pp. 88–89. London: Feathers. 319 pp.
6. Schaffer, J. 1961. Stinging insects—a threat to life. *J. Am. Med. Assoc.* 177:473–79
7. Murray, J. 1964. A case of multiple bee stings. *Cent. Afr. J. Med.* 10:249–51
8. McCormick, W. 1963. Fatal anaphylactic reaction to wasp sting. *Am. J. Clin. Pathol.* 39:485–91
9. Swinny, B. 1950. Severe reactions to insect stings. *Tex. Med. J.* 46:639–40
10. Parish, H. 1963. Analysis of 460 fatalities from venomous animals in the United States. *Am. J. Med. Sci.* 245:129–41
11. Benson, R., Semenov, A. 1930. Allergy and its relation to bee sting. *J. Allergy* 1:105–16
12. Langer, J. 1897. On the venom of our honeybees. *Naunyn-Schmiedeberg's Arch. Exp. Pathol. Pharmakol.* 38: 381–96
13. Flury, F. 1920. On the chemical nature of bee venom. *Naunyn-Schmiedebergs Arch. Exp. Pathol. Pharmakol.* 85: 319–26
14. Essex, H., Markowitz, J., Mann, F. 1930. The physiological action of the venom of the honeybee (*Apis mellifera*). *Am. J. Physiol.* 94:209–14
15. Lacaillade, C. 1933. The determination of potency of bee venom *in vitro. Am. J. Physiol.* 105:251–56
16. Reinert, M. 1936. Bee venom. *Festschr. Emil C. Barell* 1936:407–21
17. Feldberg, W., Kellaway, C. 1937. The liberation of histamine and its role in the symptomatology of bee venom poisoning. *Aust. J. Exp. Biol. Med. Sci.* 15:461–89
18. Feldberg, W. 1940. The action of bee venom, cobra venom, and lysolecithin on the adrenal medulla. *J. Physiol. London* 99:104–18
19. Haverman, R., Wolff, K. 1937. The protein nature of bee and crotalus poison. *Biochem. Z.* 290:354–59
20. Hahn, G., Ledilschke, B. 1937. Bee venom. III. Separation of venom into two components. *Ber. Dtsch. Chem. Ges.* 70B:681–86
21. Hofmann, H. 1952. Neuromuscular effect of bee toxin on the isolated rat diaphragm. *Naunyn-Schmiedebergs Arch. Exp. Pathol. Pharmakol.* 216: 250–57
22. Fischer, F., Neumann, W. 1953. The poison of the honeybee. *Biochem. Z.* 324:447–75
23. Neumann, W., Habermann, E., Hansen, H. 1953. Differentiation of two hemolytic factors in bee venom. *Naunyn-Schmiedebergs Arch. Exp. Pathol. Pharmakol.* 217:130–43

24. Neumann, W., Habermann, E. 1954. Active substances in bee venom. *Naunyn-Schmiedebergs Arch. Exp. Pathol. Pharmakol.* 222:367–87
25. Neumann, W., Habermann, E. 1956. Paper electrophoresis separation of pharmacologically and biochemically active components of bee venom. In *Venoms.* ed. E. Buckley, N. Porges, 171–74. Washington DC: Am. Assoc. Adv. Sci. 467 pp.
26. Habermann, E. 1956. The action of animal toxins and of lysolecithin at interfaces. *Z. Gesamte Exp. Med.* 130:19–26
27. Fischer, F., Neumann, W. 1961. The venom of the honeybee. III. Chemistry of melittin. *Biochem. Z.* 335:51–61
28. Habermann, E., Reitz, K. 1965. Biochemistry of the bee poison peptides melittin and apamine. *Biochem. Z.* 343:192–203
29. Habermann, E., Jentsch, J. 1967. Sequence analysis of melittin from tryptic and peptic fragments. *Hoppe-Seylers Z. Physiol. Chem.* 348:37–50
30. Habermann, E. 1972. Bee and wasp venoms. *Science* 177:314–22
31. Mitchell, H. Lowy, P. Sarmiento, L., Dickson, L. 1971. Melittin: Toxicity to *Drosophila* and inhibition of acetylcholinesterase. *Arch. Biochem. Biophys.* 145:344–48
32. Lowy, P., Sarmiento, L., Mitchell, H. 1971. Polypeptides minimine and melittin from bee venom: Effects on *Drosophila. Arch. Biochem. Biophys.* 145:338–44
33. Ishay, J., Ben-Shachar, D., Elazar, Z., Kaplinsky, E. 1975. Effects of melittin on the central nervous system. *Toxicon* 13:277–84
34. Jentsch, J. 1969. Biological activity of bee venom melittin. *Z. Naturforsch. Teil B* 24:33–35
35. Cole, L., Shipman, W. 1968. Cytotoxicity of bee venom and some of its chromatographic fractions for mouse bone marrow stem cells (Abstr.) *US Nav. Radiol. Def. Lab. Rep.–Tr–68–82.* In *US Gov. Res. Dev. Rep.* 68(21):63
36. Fennell, J., Shipman, W., Cole, L. 1968. Antibacterial action of melittin, a polypeptide from bee venom. *Proc. Soc. Exp. Biol. Med.* 127:707–10
37. Habermann, E., Reitz, K. 1964. Apamine, a basic, centrally stimulatory polypeptide from bee venom. *Naturwissenschaften* 51:61
38. Habermann, E., Reitz, K. 1965. A new method for the separation of the components of bee venom, especially the centrally active peptide, apamine. *Biochem. Z.* 343:192–203
39. Habermann, E., Cheng-Raude, D. 1975. Central toxicity of apamine, crotamin, phospholipase A, and α-amanitin. *Toxicon* 13:465–73
40. Wellhoner, H. 1969. Spinal actions of apamine. *Naunyn-Schmiedebergs Arch. Exp. Pathol. Pharmakol.* 262:29–41
41. Habermann, E. 1965. Recent studies on Hymenoptera venoms. In *Recent Advances in the Pharmacology of Toxins,* ed. H. Raudonat, J. Vanecek, 53–62. New York: Macmillan. 240 pp.
42. Haux, P., Sawerthal, H., Habermann, E. 1967. Sequence analysis of the bee venom neurotoxin, apamine, from its tryptic and chymotryptic fragments. *Hoppe-Seylers Z. Physiol. Chem.* 350:737–38
43. Shkenderov, S. 1974. Anaphylactogenic properties of bee venom and its fractions. *Toxicon* 12:529–34
44. Habermann, E., Neumann, W. 1956. Purification of phospholipase A from bee toxin. *Naturwissenschaften* 43:84
45. Habermann, E. 1957. Pharmacology of phospholipase. *Naunyn-Schmiedebergs Arch. Exp. Pathol. Pharmakol.* 230:538–46
46. Phillips, S. 1972. The effects of snake and bee venom on cardiovascular hemodynamics and function. In *Toxins of Animal and Plant Origin,* ed. A. de Vries, E. Kochva, II:682–701. New York: Gordon & Breach. 331 pp.
47. Slotta, K., Vick, J., Ginsberg, N. 1971. Enzymatic and toxic activity of phospholipase A. In *Toxins of Animal and Plant Origin,* ed. A. de Vries, E. Kochva, I:401–18. New York: Gordon & Breach. 489 pp.
48. Rothschild, A. 1965. Histamine release by bee venom phospholipase A and melittin in the rat. *Br. J. Pharmacol.* 25:59–66
49. Hogberg, B., Uvnas, B. 1957. The mechanism of the disruption of mast cells produced by the compound 48/80. *Acta Physiol. Scand.* 41:345–69
50. Fredholm, B., Haegermark, O. 1967. Histamine release from mast cells induced by a mast cell degranulating fraction in bee venom. *Acta Physiol. Scand.* 69:304–12
51. Fredholm, B., Haegermark, O. 1967. Histamine release from rat mast cell granules induced by bee venom fractions. *Acta Physiol. Scand.* 71:357–67
52. Fredholm, B., Haegermark, O. 1969. Studies on the histamine releasing effect

of bee venom fractions and compound 48/80 on skin and lung tissue of the rat. *Acta Physiol. Scand.* 76:288–98

53. Breithaupt, H., Habermann, E. 1968. MCD-peptide from venom: Isolation, biochemical and pharmacological properties. *Naunyn-Schmiedebergs Arch. Exp. Pathol. Pharmakol.* 261:252–70

54. Haux, P. 1969. Amino-acid sequence of MCD-peptide, a specific mast cell degranulating peptide of bee venom. *Hoppe-Seylers Z. Physiol. Chem.* 350:536–46

55. Hanson, J., Morley, J., Soria-Herrera, C. 1974. Anti-inflammatory property of 401 (MCD-peptide), a peptide from the venom of the bee, *Apis mellifera. Br. J. Pharmacol.* 50:383–92

56. Banks, B., Hanson, J. Sinclair, N. 1976. The isolation and identification of noradrenaline and dopamine in the venom of the honeybee, *Apis mellifera. Toxicon* 14:117–26

57. Vick, J., Shipman, W., Brooks, R. 1974. Beta adrenergic and antiarrhythmic effects of cardiopep, a newly isolated substance from whole bee venom. *Toxicon* 12:139–44

58. Habermann, E. 1972. Chemistry, pharmacology and toxicology of bee, wasp and hornet venom. In *Venomous Animals and Their Venoms*, ed. W. Bücherl, E. Buckley, III: 61–93. New York: Academic. 535 pp.

59. Jaques, R., Schachter, M. 1954. A sea anemone extract (thalassine) which liberates histamine and a slow contracting substance. *Br. J. Pharmacol.* 9:49–52

60. Jaques, R., Schachter, M. 1954. The presence of histamine, 5-hydroxytryptamine and a potent slow contracting substance in wasp venom. *Br. J. Pharmacol.* 9:53–58

61. Schachter, M., Thain, E. 1954. Chemical and pharmacological properties of the slow contracting substance kinin in wasp venom. *Br. J. Pharmacol.* 9:352–59

62. Holdstock, D., Mathias, A. Schachter, M. 1957. A comparative study of kinin, kallidin, and bradykinin. *Br. J. Pharmacol.* 12:149–58

63. Mathias, A., Schachter, M. 1958. The chromatographic behavior of wasp venom kinin, kallidin, and bradykinin. *Br. J. Pharmacol.* 13:326–29

64. Prado, J., Tamura, Z., Furano, E., Pisano, J., Udenfriend, S. 1966. Characterization of kinins in wasp venom. In *Hypotensive Peptides*, ed. E. Erdos, N.

Black, F. Sicuteri, 95–104. New York: Springer. 660 pp.

65. Pisano, J. 1970. Kinins of non-mammalian origin. In *Handbook of Experimental Pharmacology*, ed. E. Erdos, XXV: 589–95. New York: Springer. 786 pp.

66. Ishay, J., Zalman, A., Grunfeld, Y., Gitter, S. 1974. Catecholamines in social wasps. *Comp. Biochem. Physiol.* 48:369–73

67. Beard, R. 1957. The study of *Habrabracon* venoms: A study of natural insecticides. *Bee World* 38:193–98

68. Piek, T. 1966. Site of action of venom of *Microbracon hebetor* Say. *J. Insect. Physiol.* 12:561–68

69. Piek, T., Engles, E. 1969. Action of the venom of *Microbracon hebetor* Say on larvae and adults of *Philosamia cynthia* Hubn. *Comp. Biochem. Physiol.* 28: 603–18

70. Dudel, J., Kuffler, S. 1961. The quantal nature of transmission and spontaneous miniature potentials at the crayfish neuromuscular junction. *J. Physiol. London* 155:514–29

71. Katz, B. 1962. The transmission of impulses from nerve to muscle, the subcellular unit of synaptic action. *Proc. R. Soc. London Ser. B* 155:455–77

72. Rathmayer, W. 1962. Paralysis caused by the digger wasp *Philanthus. Nature* 196:1148–51

73. Piek, T. 1969. Action of the venom of *Philanthus triangulum* on the neuromuscular transmission in insects. *Acta Physiol. Pharmacol. Neerl.* 15:104–5

74. Visser, B., Spanjer, W. 1969. Biochemical studies of two paralyzing insect venoms. *Acta Physiol. Pharmacol. Neerl.* 15:82–83

75. O'Connor, R., Rosenbrook. W. 1963. The venom of the mud dauber wasp. I. *Sceliphron caementarium:* Preliminary separations and free amino acid content. *Can. J. Biochem. Physiol.* 41: 1943–48

76. Rosenbrook, W., O'Connor, R. 1964. The venom of the mud dauber wasp. II. *Sceliphron caementarium:* Protein content. *Can. J. Biochem.* 42:1005–10

77. Rosenbrook, W., O'Connor, R. 1964. The venom of the mud dauber wasp. III. *Sceliphron caementarium:* General character. *Can. J. Biochem.* 42:1567–75

78. Piek, T., Thomas, R. 1969. Paralyzing venoms of solitary wasps. *Comp. Biochem. Physiol.* 30:13–31

79. Bhoola, K., Calle, J., Schachter, M. 1960. The identification of acetycho-

line, 5-hydroxytryptamine and other substances in hornet venom. *J. Physiol. London* 151:35P–36P

80. Bhoola, K., Calle, J., Schachter, M. 1961. Identification of acetylcholine, 5-hydroxytryptamine and a new kinin in hornet venom (*V. crabo*). *J. Physiol. London* 159:167–82

81. Edery, H., Ishay, J., Lass, I., Gitter, S. 1972. Pharmacological activity of Oriental hornet (*Vespa orientalis*) venom. *Toxicon* 10:13–24

82. Beard, R. 1963. Insect toxins and venoms. *Ann. Rev. Entomol.* 8:1–18

83. Owen, M. 1971. Insect venoms: Identification of dopamine and noradrenaline in wasp and bee strings. *Experientia* 27:544–45

84. Ishay, J. 1975. Hyperglycemia produced by the *Vespa orientalis* venom sac extract. *Toxicon* 12:221–26

85. Joshua, H., Ishay, J. 1975. The anticoagulant properties of an extract of the Oriental hornet venom sac. *Toxicon* 13:11–20

86. Kaplinsky, E., Ishay, J., Gitter, S. 1974. Oriental hornet venom: Effects on cardiovascular dynamics. *Toxicon* 12:69–74

87. Blum, M., Walker, J., Callahan, P., Novak, A. 1958. Chemical, insecticidal, and antibiotic properties of fire ant venom. *Science* 128:306–7

88. Adrouny, G., Derbes, V., Jung, R. 1959. Isolation of a hemolytic component of fire ant venom. *Science* 130:449–50

89. Caro, M., Derbes, V., Jung, R. 1957. Skin response to sting of the imported fire ant (*Solenopsis saevissima*). *Arch. Dermatol.* 75:475–88

90. Sinski, J., Adrouny, G., Derbes, V., Jung, R. 1959. Further characterization of the hemolytic component of fire ant

venom: Mycological aspects. *Proc. Soc. Exp. Biol. Med.* 102:659–60

91. Adrouny, G. 1966. The fire ant's fire. *Tulane Univ. Med. Fac. Bull.* 25:67

92. MacConnell, J., Blum, M., Fales, H. 1970. Alkaloid from fire ant venom: Identification and synthesis. *Science* 168:840–41

93. Cavill, G., Robertson, P., Whitfield, F. 1964. Venom and venom apparatus of the bull ant *Myrmecia gulosa*. *Science* 146:79–80

94. de la Lande, I., Thomas, D., Tyler, M. 1965. Pharmacological analysis of the venom of the "bulldog" ant *Myrmecia forficata*. In *Recent Advances in the Pharmacology of Toxins*, ed. H. Raudonat, J. Vanacek, 71–75. New York: Macmillan. 240 pp.

95. Thomas, D., Lewis, J. 1965. Histamine release by the ant. *Aust. J. Exp. Biol. Med. Sci.* 43:275–76

96. Lewis, J., de la Lande, I. 1967. Pharmacological and enzymatic constituents of the venom of the Australian "bulldog" ant, *Myrmecia pyriformis*. *Toxicon* 4:225–34

97. Wanstall, J., de la Lande, I. 1974. Fractionation of "bulldog" ant venom. *Toxicon* 12:649–56

98. Lewis, J., Day, A., de la Lande, I. 1968. Phospholipase A in the venom of the Australian "bulldog" ant, *Myrmecia pyriformis*. *Toxicon* 6:109–12

99. O'Connor, R., Henderson, G., Nelson, D., Parker, R., Peck, M. 1967. The venom of the honeybee (*Apis mellifera*). I. General character. In *Animal Toxins*, ed. F. Russell, P. Sanders, 17–22. New York: Pergamon. 428 pp.

100. Bernard, C. 1864. Etudies physiologiques sur quelques poisons American: I. Le curare. *Rev. Deux Mondes* 53:164–90

Ann. Rev. Pharmacol. Toxicol. 1977. 17:499–510
Copyright © 1977 by Annual Reviews Inc. All rights reserved

THE EFFECT OF HYPOLIPIDEMIC DRUGS ON PLASMA LIPOPROTEINS

♦6692

Robert I. Levy

National Heart, Lung, and Blood Institute, National Institutes of Health,
Bethesda, Maryland 20014

In recent years advances in the study of normal and abnormal lipid metabolism have resulted in a broader understanding of the mechanisms and effects of hypolipidemic drugs (1). A clearer concept of how lipid is transported in the blood has helped clarify the etiology of the lipid disorders, which in turn has provided fresh insights into the reasons for the efficacy of lipid-lowering agents. Thus, the management of hyperlipidemia has become increasingly precise and the selection of therapy more rational.

It is now known that the major blood lipids—cholesterol, triglycerides, and phospholipids—are insoluble and do not circulate freely in aqueous solution. Rather, they are solubilized by proteins and are transported through the plasma as lipid-protein complexes or lipoproteins (2). The levels of these lipoproteins are subject to dynamic changes. The major lipoprotein families, separated according to electrophoretic mobility or density, are all interrelated within a complex metabolic system. The pathway of very low density lipoproteins (VLDL), intermediate density lipoproteins (IDL), and low density lipoproteins (LDL) is of particular interest in the study of hyperlipoproteinemia and hypolipidemic drugs. VLDL, the main carrier of triglyceride, originates in the liver and small intestine from endogenous sources (Figure 1). It is catabolized rapidly into a transient intermediate form (IDL), which is further degraded into LDL (3) (Figure 2). Thus, LDL (which is 50% cholesterol by weight) appears to be in part, if not entirely, a remnant of VLDL and is presumably cleared by the liver (4). Transport of lipoproteins through the plasma then is not a passive affair; dynamic metabolic changes are occurring throughout their passage in the bloodstream.

It is now recognized that the lipid disorders are related to problems in lipoprotein metabolism (1). Specifically, excess lipid levels can occur because of either overproduction or faulty removal of one or more lipoproteins. Numerous mechanisms may

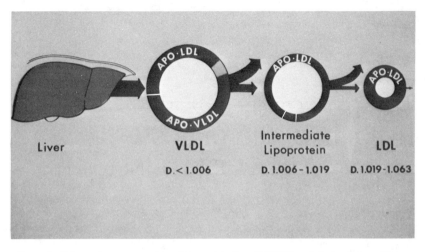

Liver   VLDL   Intermediate Lipoprotein   LDL

D.<1.006   D. 1.006-1.019   D. 1.019-1.063

Figure 1   Schematic representation of the metabolism of VLDL and chylomicrons. FFA = free fatty acids. From Levy et al (13). Reproduced by permission.

be responsible for the resulting hyperlipoproteinemia: increased influx of exogenous cholesterol or triglyceride entering from the intestine as chylomicrons; increased amounts of endogenous cholesterol or triglyceride released from the liver and small intestine as VLDL; defects in the clearing enzymes at sites of catabolism; abnormalities in plasma solubility or in the lipoproteins themselves (5). Other modifying factors include the state of carbohydrate or protein metabolism in general and the activity of hormones promoting lipogenesis or lipolysis in the muscle, liver, and adipose tissue.

The hyperlipoproteinemias are heterogeneous not only in etiology, but in clincial signs, prognosis, and responsiveness to therapy as well (1). *Hypercholesterolemia* and *hypertriglyceridemia* are nonspecific terms that do not identify either the site or the nature of the disorder. However, by translating these hyperlipidemias into hyperlipoproteinemia, it is possible to localize the area of lipid transport that is disordered. Patterns of hyperlipoproteinemia have been differentiated (6). A typing system represents a convenient code for the identification of lipoproteins that are present in excess (Table 1). None of the types is unique, however. To determine the disease mechanism in each case it is necessary first to rule out possibile secondary causes for the hyperlipoproteinemia such as alcoholism, myxedema, liver disease, diabetes mellitus, renal disease, stress, and dietary excess. In addition, each type when genetically determined may be associated with different modes of inheritance. Certain kinds of primary hyperlipoproteinemia have been linked with a greatly increased risk of premature atherosclerosis. Because of the multiplicity of possible origins for each hyperlipoproteinemia, there is no single diet or drug that is effective for all the types (7, 8). Some drugs may actually increase lipid levels in certain disorders. Looking at blood lipid abnormalities in terms of the lipoprotein or lipo-

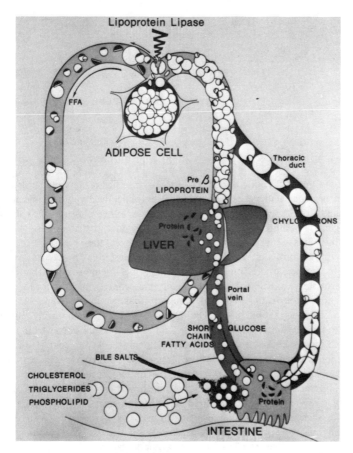

Figure 2 Schema of normal lipoprotein metabolism. From Levy & Rifkind (7). Reproduced by permission.

proteins present in excess has helped eliminate much of the guesswork involved in selecting appropriate therapy. Management of hyperlipoproteinemia should always begin with a diet specific for the lipoprotein excess. Diet is the cornerstone of therapy that will reduce, and sometimes obviate, the need for potentially toxic drugs. If a drug is introduced, the diet should be continued since the combined effects of both forms of therapy are additive.

In the past, studies of drug efficacy focused primarily on how hypolipidemic drugs affected cholesterol biosynthesis and catabolism and bile acid formation (Figure 3). Moreover, no distinction was made between the various forms of hypercholesterolemia and hypertriglyceridemia. Thus, what would work for one patient would fail to work for another. The principal drawbacks of this approach included the failure to appreciate the heterogeneity of blood fat disorders as well as a failure to

Table 1   Types of HLP

Type	Abnormality
I	↑ Chylomicrons
IIa	↑ LDL
IIb	↑ LDL and VLDL
III	↑ IDL
IV	↑ VLDL
V	↑ VLDL and chylomicrons

explain the mode of action and the reason for the effectiveness of the drugs. For instance, nicotinic acid was recognized as a highly effective hypolipidemic agent but which had no clearly demonstrable influence on either cholesterol synthesis or catabolism. The efficacy of cholestyramine was originally attributed to its capacity to bind bile acids in the gastrointestinal tract and prevent their reabsorption, thereby increasing their turnover and the breakdown of cholesterol. This concept was challenged by further studies on cholestyramine which demonstrated that de novo cholesterol biosynthesis in the liver was increasing concomitantly with the catabolism of cholesterol, so that the total cholesterol balance in the liver remained unchanged. Why then should plasma cholesterol levels fall so dramatically? In seeking a reply to this question, the focus of drug studies began to shift away from lipid and fatty acid biosynthesis toward lipoprotein metabolism. At the root of this change in direction was the simple fact that the plasma lipid levels are dependent upon the amounts of circulating lipoproteins. Thus, the amount of lipoproteins entering the plasma and the amount being cleared determine how much lipid is found at any time in the plasma. The utility of hypolipidemic drugs in each disorder should then be sought in their effect—whether primary or secondary—upon *lipoprotein*, rather than lipid, concentrations (9). On the basis of this concept, the hypolipidemic drugs currently available can be classified into two basic categories: (*a*) those that effect lipoprotein production, and (*b*) those that affect lipoprotein removal (Figure 4).

DRUGS THAT AFFECT LIPOPROTEIN PRODUCTION

Nicotinic Acid

Nicotinic acid has been a consistently effective lipid-lowering agent when given in doses exceeding its requirement as a vitamin. Its mode of action had long been a puzzle because no direct effect by the drug could be demonstrated on cholesterol biosynthesis, catabolism, or bile acid formation (10). Recent studies have shown that nicotinic acid acts primarily by depressing VLDL synthesis and subsequently that of its plasma products, IDL and LDL. Plasma triglyceride levels generally fall within 4 to 6 hr as a direct result of the decreased VLDL production. Plasma cholesterol levels are lowered because of the decreased rate of LDL snythesis. This latter effect, however, occurs only after several days, undoubtedly because of the longer half-life of LDL (11).

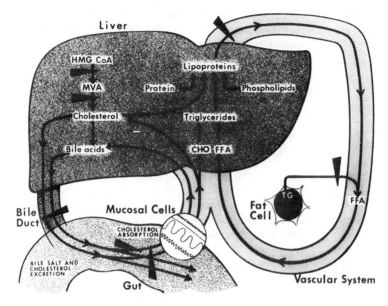

Figure 3 Schematic representation of the systems involved in endogenous lipid transport. *Arrows* indicate previously proposed sites of action of hypolipidemic drugs. From Levy & Langer (8a). Reproduced by permission.

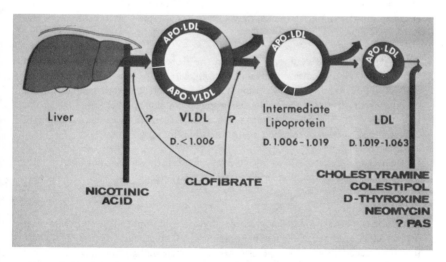

Figure 4 Possible site of action of hypolipidemic drugs. From Levy & Rifkind (7). Reproduced by permission.

Reports on the use of nicotinic acid in hypercholesterolemic subjects have demonstrated a reduction in cholesterol ranging from 15–30% (10). The effect of nicotinic acid on plasma triglyceride has been variable, but decreases of over 60% have been noted (12). In studies conducted at the National Institutes of Health Clinical Center, nicotinic acid was found to be effective in treating homozygous type II patients in combination with diet and cholestyramine therapy (13). Nicotinic acid given in divided doses of 55 and 87 mg/kg body weight per day reduced total plasma cholesterol from 19 to 49% in five out of six patients. In severe heterozygotes who had responded inadequately to a diet and cholestyramine regimen, cholesterol levels were normalized with the use of larger doses of nicotinic acid (4 to 6 g/day).

INDICATIONS   Primary indications for nicotinic acid include any hyperlipidemic states characterized by increases in VLDL or its products, IDL and LDL.

DOSE   Nicotinic acid is available in tablets of 100 and 500 mg. The 100 mg tablet is generally absorbed better. The initial dose is 100 mg orally three times a day, incremented by 300 mg/day every four to seven days until a maintenance dose of 3 to 9 g/day is attained. The drug should be taken at mealtimes to reduce gastric irritation.

SIDE EFFECTS   The most common and annoying effect of nicotinic acid therapy is intense cutaneous flushing and pruritus which generally develop within one to two hours of a dose. This symptom disappears in 85% of patients within one to two weeks. Other transitory side effects may include nausea, vomiting, and diarrhea.

More troublesome side effects that can occur are hepatotoxicity, abnormal glucose tolerance, glycosuria, and hyperuricemia. These normally regress after the drug is discontinued. Prolonged therapy may also cause hyperpigmentation, dry skin, and acanthosis nigricans.

OTHER EFFECTS   Recent evidence from the Coronary Drug Project (CDP), a secondary coronary prevention trial in subjects with a previous history of myocardial infarctions, shows that nicotinic acid did not affect overall mortality from coronary heart disease in these subjects, in spite of a significant decrease in recurrent infarctions (14). Moreover, the drug was associated with an excess incidence of arrhythmias, as well as skin and gastrointestinal findings.

DRUG INTERACTIONS   Nicotinic acid may increase the vasodilating and postural hypotensive effect of ganglioplegic antihypertensive agents.

Clofibrate

Clofibrate is a branched fatty acid ester (ethyl-parachlorophenoxyisobutyrate) that can affect a wide range of metabolic activites of lipids and lipoproteins. These include reduced cholesterol synthesis, decreased hepatic lipoprotein secretion, decreased free fatty acid and triglyceride synthesis, increased triglyceride catabolism, decreased hepatic cholesterogenesis from glucose but not pyruvate, inhibition of microsomal reduction of hydroxymethylglutamyl COA to mevalonate, increased excretion of fecal neutral and acid sterols, and increased cholesterol efflux from tissues (15–26).

The principal hypolipidemic action of clofibrate is the reduction of VLDL concentrations, both by inhibiting the synthesis and by increasing the clearance of this lipoprotein. Recent reports, however, suggest that the latter effect may be dominant. VLDL and IDL levels usually fall predictably but the effect on LDL is variable. The rise in cholesterol levels which has been reported (27) would seem to emphasize the effect of clofibrate on VLDL catabolism rather than production. In hypertriglyceridemic states, clofibrate has been shown to decrease triglyceride levels by 10–40% (13), but its ability to reduce cholesterol varies from 5–20% (28). In a recent report, clofibrate lowered triglycerides and depressed cholesterol levels below baseline in subjects with type IV hyperlipoproteinemia. It reduced VLDL but raised LDL levels (29).

Clofibrate can also produce changes in blood coagulation and fibrinolysis (30, 31), which may have clinical implications independent of its lipid-lowering abilities.

INDICATIONS   Because of its beneficial effect on VLDL and IDL levels, clofibrate has been most useful in the treatment of type III and some subjects with types IV and V hyperlipoproteinemia. Because of its unpredictable influence on cholesterol, its usefulness in type II has been limited.

DOSE   Clofibrate is prepared in tablets of 500 mg and is administered in two or four divided doses. The total daily dose is 2 g/day.

SIDE EFFECTS   Clofibrate has been associated with relatively few overt side effects. It can occasionally cause nausea, diarrhea, and weight gain but these usually disappear quickly. Rare side effects include skin rash, myositis, weakness, giddiness, and alopecia. Liver function tests may be slightly elevated.

OTHER EFFECTS   The most important effects associated with clofibrate use reported to date were found by the Coronary Drug Project group. The drug was linked with a twofold increase in cholelithiasis and a significant increase in arrhythmias, new angina, increased heart size, heart failure, and thromboembolism in patients with existing cardiovascular disease. No beneficial effect on cardiac or overall mortality was observed (14).

DRUG INTERACTIONS   Clofibrate can enhance the hypoprothrombinemic effects of warfarin sodium, necessitating an adjustment in warfarin dosage.

DRUGS THAT AFFECT LIPOPROTEIN CATABOLISM

Cholestyramine

Cholestyramine is the quaternary ammonium chloride salt of a high molecular-weight copolymer composed of a styrene 2% divinyl benzene skeleton. It is hydrophilic but insoluble in water and remains completely unchanged in the gastrointestinal tract. The drug is an anion exchange resin that binds bile acids in the small intestine, thus interfering with their enterohepatic circulation. The resulting increases in bile acid production and cholesterol catabolism, however, are compensated for by an increase in de novo cholesterol synthesis (32). Thus, the cholesterol-lowering effect of cholestyramine cannot be explained by its action on cholesterol metabolism, since the total cholesterol balance remains unchanged.

Recent studies have demonstrated that the primary effect of cholestyramine is on the low density lipoprotein. Turnover experiments using ^{125}I-labeled LDL have shown that the drug increases the fractional catabolic rate of the apoprotein moiety (33). No changes were observed in the rate of synthesis of the lipoprotein, nor in its intravascular distribution.

Cholestyramine has been consistently reported to reduce total plasma cholesterol levels by 20–25% in subjects with type II hyperlipoproteinemia (13, 34–36). In a double-blind trial conducted at NIH comparing the effects of cholestyramine versus placebo in patients with primary type II, the drug lowered plasma cholesterol by 20.6% and LDL cholesterol by 27.3% (37). A more recent report further confirms earlier findings that the total cholesterol reduction obtained with cholestyramine therapy is due to a decrease in LDL concentrations (38).

In subjects with hypercholesterolemia due to increased VLDL or IDL, cholestyramine may actually increase cholesterol levels (12, 36, 37). Its effect on triglyceride levels is variable; transient, usually insignificant, to marked triglyceride increases have been observed (34–38).

INDICATIONS   Cholestyramine is the drug of choice for treatment of primary type II hyperlipoproteinemia, particularly IIa where LDL alone is elevated. It is contraindicated in states characterized by VLDL or IDL excesses (types III, IV, V) because it may increase the production of these lipoproteins.

DOSE   The initial dose of cholestyramine is 16 g/day given in two to four divided doses. This is generally incremented by 4–8 g every 2–3 weeks until a maximum of 32 g/day is achieved.

SIDE EFFECTS   Gastrointestinal side effects are the most common, particularly constipation in older patients, and often make this agent difficult to use. Other symptoms include nausea, vomiting, cramps, and abdominal distention. Rare side effects which have been reported include steatorrhea, alkaline phosphatase elevations, and gastrointestinal obstruction.

DRUG INTERACTIONS   Cholestyramine may interfere with the absorption of fat-soluble vitamins and acidic compounds. It is recommended that drugs such as phenylbutazone, digitalis, iron, warfarin, thiazides, tetracycline, and thyroid preparations be taken at least one hour prior to cholestyramine.

D-Thyroxine

Dextrothyroxine sodium is the sodium salt of the dextrorotatory isomer of thyroxine. Thyroid active agents increase both the production and clearance of hepatic cholesterol. D-Thyroxine lowers plasma cholesterol by reducing LDL concentrations (39). Reductions of 15–25% in total cholesterol are generally reported. It is suspected that the drug acts primarily by accelerating LDL catabolism.

INDICATIONS   D-Thyroxine is indicated for disorders caused by LDL elevations (type II). Its effects on VLDL and IDL have not been fully evaluated.

DOSE   The initial dose is 2 mg daily with increases of 1 to 2 mg per month. The adult maintenance dose is generally 4 to 8 mg per day.

SIDE EFFECTS   The most serious effect of D-thyroxine is its cardiotoxicity, which limits its utility as a hypolipidemic agent. Originally selected for trial by the Coronary Drug Project, the drug was abandoned because of excessive morbidity and mortality in the D-thyroxine treatment group (40).

Other symptoms associated with the drug include neutropenia, glucose intolerance, glycosuria, and abnormal liver function.

DRUG INTERACTIONS   D-Thyroxine increases the hypoprothrombinemic effect of warfarin sodium, requiring up to 30% reduction in warfarin dosage.

OTHER HYPOLIPIDEMIC DRUGS

β-Sitosterol

β-Sitosterol is a plant sterol with a structure similar to that of cholesterol, except for the substitution of an ethyl group at the C-24 of its side chain. Like most plant sterols it is unabsorbed in man. Although the mechanism of its hypolipidemic effect is unknown, it is suspected that the drug inhibits cholesterol absorption competitively. Its special effect on lipoprotein metabolism has not been studied, but its primary efficacy is in states characterized by LDL excess. The drug probably affects LDL clearance.

It is available as a liquid with a recommended dose of 30 cc one half hour before meals and at bedtime. A mild laxative effect may occur; diarrhea and nausea have also been noted.

Colestipol

Colestipol is a bile acid sequestrant with an action similar to that of cholestyramine. It has not yet been approved by the FDA for use in lipid lowering. It is an insoluble, high molecular weight granular copolymer of tetraethylenepentamine and epichlorhydrate. Like cholestyramine, it has a high binding capacity for bile acids. Both drugs have a similar effect on plasma cholesterol levels. Colestipol has had no demonstrably significant effect on plasma triglycerides (41, 42). Its effects on lipoprotein metabolism are unclear.

The drug is prepared as water-insoluble beads. The usual dose is 4 to 5 g three or four times per day.

PAS-C

Para-aminosalicylic acid recrystallized in vitamin C (PAS-C) is a highly purified new agent that is still being investigated. PAS was first found to have a hypocholesterolemic effect in patients being treated for pulmonary tuberculosis (43). Recently, the new preparation with ascorbic acid was reported to be successful in lowering serum cholesterol and triglycerides in patients with type IIa and IIb hyperlipoproteinemia (44). Although its effect on lipoprotein metabolism has not been studied, PAS-C has been found to reduce LDL levels.

The maintenance dose generally used is 8–9 g/day for adults, 5–6 g/day for children. Some gastrointestinal effects were reported but the drug is generally well tolerated and remains effective for prolonged periods. Excessive alcohol intake can offset the hypolipidemic effect of the drug.

Neomycin

Neomycin is an antibiotic produced from *Streptomyces gradiar* which has a hypolipidemic effect only when administered orally (45). This effect is not dependent on its antibiotic action in intestinal flora, but seems to be secondary to the formation of insoluble complexes with bile acids in the intestine (46). It is suspected that the mechanism of neomycin is similar to that of cholestyramine by increasing bile acid excretion and LDL clearance. Cholesterol reduction of 15–25% has been reported with little or no change in triglyceride levels (47, 48).

Neomycin has been administered in divided doses of 0.5–2.0 g/day. Ninety-seven percent of an oral dose remains unabsorbed. Mild diarrhea may occur and there have been some reports of serious oto- and nephrotoxicity, although these are rare. Further studies into its potential long-term toxicity are needed before the drug can be recommended for general use.

Combined Chemotherapy

The combination of hypolipidemic agents has proven clinically efficacious in certain cases, particularly in controlling the more severe forms of hyperlipoproteinemia. For instance, cholestyramine combined with nicotinic acid—two drugs that act by alternate mechanisms—has been useful in treating patients with homozygous type II in whom diet and cholestyramine alone had proved inadequate (13). Other combinations that have been used successfully include cholestyramine and clofibrate, nicotinic acid and clofibrate, as well as others, but these are still under investigation.

CONCLUSION

Much has been learned about lipid-transport physiology and lipid disorders in recent years. This in turn has shed light on the effects and mechanisms of hypolipidemic agents, so that therapy of hyperlipoproteinemia has become increasingly more precise. A dietary prescription should always be tried first but if lipid lowering is inadequate, drug therapy may be added. Drugs should be used with caution, however, because all are associated with side effects. Further studies are needed to determine the molecular defects underlying the lipid disorders so that the mode of action of the drugs may be clarified further.

Literature Cited

1. Fredrickson, D. S., Levy, R. I. 1972. Familial hyperlipoproteinemia. *The Metabolic Basis of Inherited Disease,* ed. J. B. Stanbury, J. B. Wyngaarden, D. S. Fredrickson., 545–614. New York: McGraw-Hill. 3rd ed.
2. Fredrickson, D. S., Levy, R. I., Lees, R. S. 1967. Fat transport in lipoproteins—an integrated approach to mechanisms and disorders. *N. Engl. J. Med* 276:34–44, 94–103, 148–56, 215–26, 273–81
3. Levy, R. I., Bilheimer, D. W., Eisenberg, S. 1971. The structure and metabolism of chylomicrons and very low density lipoproteins (VLDL) In *Plasma Lipoproteins—Biochem. Soc. Symp. No. 33 (1971),* ed. R. M. S. Smellie, 3–17. London & New York: Academic
4. Havel, R. J. 1972. Mechanisms of hyperlipoproteinemia. *Adv. Exp. Biol. Med.* 26:57–70
5. Levy, R. I., Langer, T. 1969. Mechanisms involved in hyperlipidemia. *Mod. Treat.* 6:1313–27
6. WHO Memorandum. 1972. Classification of hyperlipidemias and hyperlipoproteinemias. *Circulation* 45:501–8
7. Levy, R. I., Rifkind, B. M. 1973. Lipid lowering drugs and hyperlipidemia. *Drugs* 6:12–45
8. Levy, R. I., Morganroth, J., Rifkind, B. M. 1974. Drug therapy—treatment of hyperlipidemia. *N. Engl. J. Med.* 290:1295–1301
8a. Levy, R. I., Langer, T. 1971. Hypolipidemic drugs and hyperlipoproteinemia. *Ann. NY Acad. Sci.* 179:475–80
9. Levy, R. I., Langer, T. 1972. Hypolipidemic drugs and lipoprotein metabolism. In *Pharmacological Control of Lipid Metabolism,* W. L. Holmes, R. Paoletti, D. Kritchevsky, 155–63. New York: Plenum.
10. Kritchevsky, D. 1971. Effect of nicotinic acid and its derivatives on cholesterol metabolism: A review. In *Metabolic Effects of Nicotinic Acid and Its Derivatives,* K. F. Gey, L. A. Carlson, H. Bern, Stuttgart & Vienna: Huber
11. Langer, T., Levy, R. I. 1970. Effect of nicotinic acid on beta lipoprotein metabolism. *Clin. Res.* 18:458 (Abstr.)
12. Parsons, W. B. 1971. Use of nicotinic compounds in treatment of hyperlipidemia. In *Treatment of Hyperlipidemic States,* ed. H. R. Casdorph, 333–45. Springfield, Ill.: Thomas
13. Levy, R. I., Fredrickson, D. S., Shulman, R., Bilheimer, D. W., Breslow, J.

L., Stone, N.J., Lux, S. E., Sloan, H. R., Krauss, R. M., Herbert, P. N. 1972. Dietary and drug treatment of primary hyperlipoproteinemia. *Ann. Int. Med.* 77:267–94
14. Coronary Drug Proj. Res. Group. 1975. Clofibrate and niacin in coronary heart disease. *J. Am. Med. Assoc.* 231:4–25
15. Cheng, C. Y., Feldman, E. B. 1971. Clofibrate, inhibitor of intestinal cholesterogenesis. *Biochem. Pharmacol.* 20:3509–19
16. Gans, J. H., Carter, M. R. 1971. Metabolic effects of clofibrate and of cholestyramine administration to dogs. *Biochem. Pharmacol.* 20:3321–29
17. White, L. W. 1971. Regulation of hepatic cholesterol biosynthesis by clofibrate administration. *J. Pharmacol. Exp. Ther.* 178:361–70
18. Gould, R. G., Swyryd, E. A., Coan, B. J., Avoy, D. R. 1966. Effects of chlorophenozyisobutyrate (CPIB) on liver composition and triglyceride synthesis in rats. *J. Atheroscler. Res.* 6:555–64
19. Rifkind, B. M. 1966. Effect of CPIB ester on plasma free fatty acid levels in man. *Metabolism* 15:673–75
20. Hunninghake, D. B., Azarnoff, D. L. 1968. Clofibrate effect on catecholamine-induced metabolic changes in humans. *Metabolism* 17:588–95
21. Barrett, A. M., Thorp, J. M. 1968. Studies on the mode of action of clofibrate: Effect on hormone-induced changes in plasma free fatty acids, cholesterol, phospholipids and total esterified fatty acids, in rats and dogs. *Br. J. Pharmacol.* 32:381–91
22. Bierman, E. L., Brunzell, J. D., Bagdade, J. D., Lerner, R. L., Hazzard, W. R., Prite, D. 1970. On the mechanism of action of atromid-S on triglyceride transport in man. *Trans. Assoc. Am. Physicians* 83:211–22
23. Adams, L. L., Webb, W. W., Fallon, H. J. 1971. Inhibition of hepatic triglyceride formation by clofibrate. *J. Clin. Invest.* 50:2339–46
24. Sodhi, H. S., Kudchodkar, B. J., Horlick, L. 1971. Effect of chlorophenoxyisobutyrate on the metabolism of endogenous glycerides in man. *Metabolism* 20:309–18
25. Grundy, S. M., Ahrens, E. H. Jr., Salen, G., Quintao, E. 1969. Mode of action of atromid-S on cholesterol metabolism in man. *J. Clin. Invest.* 48:33a (Abstr.)

26. Horlick, L. L., Kudchodkar, B. J., Sodhi, H. S. 1971. Mode of action of chlorophenoxyisobutyric acid on cholesterol metabolism in man. *Circulation* 43:299–309
27. Strisower, E. H., Adamson, G., Strisower, B. 1968. Treatment of hyperlipidemias. *Am. J. Med.* 45:488–501
28. Levy, R. I., Quarfordt, S. H., Brown, W. V., Sloan, H. R., Fredrickson, D. S. 1969. The efficacy of clofibrate (CPIB) in familial hyperlipoproteinemias. In *Drugs Affecting Lipid Metabolism,* ed. L. A. Carlson, W. L. Holmes, R. Paoletti, 377–87. New York: Plenum
29. Dujovne, C. A., Azarnoff, D. L., Huffman, D. H., Pentikainen, P., Hurwitz, A., Shoeman, D. W. 1976. One-year trials with halofenate, clofibrate and placebo. *Clin. Pharmacol. Ther.* 19:352–59
30. Gilbert, J. B., Mustard, J. F. 1963. Some effects of Atromid on platelet economy and blood coagulation in man. *J. Atheroscler. Res.* 3:623–26
31. Sweet, B., Rifkind, B. M., McNichol, G. P. 1965. The effect of Atromid-S on the fibrinolytic enzyme system. *J. Atheroscler. Res.* 5:347–50
32. Moutafis, C. D., Myant, N. B. 1969. The metabolism of cholesterol in two hypercholesterolemic patients treated with cholestyramine. *Clin. Sci.* 37:443–54
33. Langer, T., Levy, R. I., Fredrickson, D. S. 1969. Dietary and pharmacologic perturbation of beta lipoprotein (βLP) turnover. *Circulation* 40:111–14
34. Fallon, H. J., Woods, J. W. 1968. Response of hyperlipoproteinemia to cholestyramine resin. *J. Am. Med. Assoc.* 204:1161–64
35. Glueck, C. J., Steiner, P. M., Scheel, D., Ford, S. 1971. U-26, 597A and cholestyramine: comparative effects in familial type II hyperlipoproteinemia. *Circulation* 43–44: Suppl. II, p. 197
36. Casdorph, H. R. 1971. Cholestyramine. See Ref. 12, pp. 234–67
37. Levy, R. I., Fredrickson, D. S., Stone, N. J., Bilheimer, D. W., Brown, W. V., Glueck, C. J., Gotto, A. M., Herbert, P. N., Kwiterovich, P. O., Langer, T., LaRosa, J., Lux, S. E., Rider, A. K., Shulman, R. S., Sloan, H. R. 1973. Cholestyramine in type II hyperlipo-

proteinemia: A double-blind trial. *Ann. Int. Med.* 79:51–58
38. Oro, L., Olsson, A. G., Rossner, S., Carlson, L. A. 1975. Cholestyramine, clofibrate and nicotinic acid as single or combined treatment of type IIa and IIb hyperlipoproteinemia. *Postgrad. Med. J.* 51: Suppl. 8, pp. 76–79
39. Strisower, E. H. 1962. Hypolipoproteinemic effect of d-thyroxine. *Fed. Proc.* 21:96
40. The Coronary Drug Project. 1972. Findings leading to further modifications of its protocol with respect to dextrothyroxine. 220:996–1008
41. Ryan, J. R., Jain, A. 1972. The effect of colestipol or cholestyramine on serum cholesterol and triglycerides in a long-term controlled study. *J. Clin. Pharmacol.* 12:268–73
42. Rubulis, A., Lim, E. C., Faloon, W. W. 1972. Effect of a bile acid sequestrant, colestipol, on serum cholesterol, fecal bile acids and neutral sterols in human subjects. *Fed. Proc.* 31:727
43. Riska, N. 1955. The effect of PAS on the cholesterol level in the blood. *Acta Tuber. Scand.* 30:134–43
44. Kuo, P. T., Fan, W. C., Kostis, J. B., Hayase, K. 1976. Combined paraaminosalicylic acid and dietary therapy in long-term control of hypercholesterolemia and hypertriglyceridemia (types IIa and IIb hyperlipoproteinemia). *Circulation* 53:338–41
45. Samuel, P., Steiner, A. 1959. Effect of neomycin on serum cholesterol level of man. *Proc. Soc. Exp. Biol. Med.* 100:193–95
46. Faloon, W. W., Paes, I. C., Woolfolk, D., Nankin, H., Wallace, K., Haro, E. N. 1966. Effect of neomycin and kanamycin upon intestinal absorption. *Ann. NY Acad. Sci.* 132:879–83
47. Leveille, G. A., Powell, R. C., Sauberlich, H. E., Nunes, W. T. 1963. Effect of orally and parenterally administered neomycin on plasma lipids of human subjects. *Am. J. Clin. Nutr.* 12:421–25
48. Samuel, P., Holtzman, C. M., Meilman, E., Sekowski, I. 1970. Reduction of serum cholesterol and triglyceride levels by the combined administration of neomycin and clofibrate. *Circulation* 41:109–14

Ann. Rev. Pharmacol. Toxicol. 1977. 17: 511–27

CLINICAL PHARMACOLOGY ❖6693
OF SYSTEMIC CORTICOSTEROIDS

James C. Melby

Section of Endocrinology and Metabolism, Boston University School of Medicine, Boston, Massachusetts 02118

It is more than a quarter of a century since Hench showed the prompt and dramatic reversal of the inflammatory manifestations of rheumatoid arthritis after the administration of cortisone. In 1971, Christy (1) estimated that more than 5 million patients were treated with corticosteroids yearly. From this enormous experience and from a massive literature, concepts have evolved regarding the safe and effective use of these agents. An obvious generalization is that corticosteroid therapy is most often *temporary* and adjunctive. The corticosteroids allow the host to recover in self-limited conditions and to suppress some manifestations of chronic diseases that reappear when corticosteroids are withdrawn. It is predominantly in patients with chronic diseases that the deleterious effects of the corticosteroids are most prominent.

In the discussion to follow, the clinical pharmacology of systemic corticosteroid administration and concepts of systemic corticosteroid therapy are examined. The special problem of suppression of the hypothalamic-pituitary-adrenal system is emphasized.

ACTIONS OF THE CORTICOSTEROIDS

Cortisol and its synthetic analogues—prednisolone, methylprednisolone, triamcinolone, dexamethasone, betamethasone, and paramethasone—are known to exhibit many important physiological and biochemical effects. The multiplicity of activities that have been observed are so disparate that no unitary hypothesis of corticosteroid hormone action has been possible. It is often difficult to relate the cellular actions of the corticosteroids to their effects on physiology generally. Most interesting to the clinician are studies of the anti-inflammatory and antiallergic actions of the corticosteroids. Of almost equal importance, however, is the knowledge of biochemical actions of the corticosteroids, particularly in excessive concentrations that ac-

511

count for the undesirable side effects in the course of anti-inflammatory corticosteroid therapy.

Biochemical and Metabolic Effects of the Corticosteroids

Cortisol and certain of its synthetic analogues are also referred to as "glucocorticoids" because of action of the corticosteroids increasing hepatic glucose output by stimulating hepatic gluconeogenesis while depressing protein synthesis or stimulating protein catabolism in muscle. It is highly likely that one of the most primal and important events in corticosteroid biochemical action is the inhibition of amino acid incorporation into protein in peripheral tissues. After the administration of glucocorticoids, alanine is released from muscle, massively, leading to a transient rise in plasma alanine concentration. The alanine derived from muscle and other peripheral tissues released in response to acute doses of corticosteroids is derived from glucose and muscle glycogen, and the nitrogen from the catabolism of amino acids within the muscle cell. Hyperalaninemia not only provides a marked increment in substrate for hepatic gluconeogenesis, but also is implicated in the increased secretion of glucagon by the pancreatic α cells (2). Hyperglucagonemia has been shown after corticosteroid administration; the increment in plasma glucagon levels may exceed 50% of the basal level, and responsiveness to amino acid infusions (alanine) may quadruple. Whether or not hyperaminoaciduria is the proximate stimulus for glucagon elaboration by the pancreatic α cell is not known, but it is likely that the hyperglucagonemia accounts, in part, for the marked increment in hepatic glucose output after the administration of corticosteroids.

A number of hepatic enzymes concerned with gluconeogenesis exhibit marked increases in activity after the administration of glucocorticoids. Among these enzymes are glucose-6-phosphatase, fructose-6-diphosphatase, and phosphoenolpyruvate carboxykinase. The increased activities of these enzymes apparently are caused by an actual increase in the amount of enzyme protein. It has long been argued that the increase in the gluconeogenic enzymes in the liver results from induction by excessive substrate or amino acids derived from peripheral tissues. Since the corticosteroids had been shown to diminish the peripheral use of glucose and amino acid uptake, there seemed little need to posit a hepatic enzyme as a primary action of the glucocorticoid; however, corticosteroids now have been shown to increase hepatic gluconeogenesis in vitro and to increase the activities of tyrosine aminotransferase and tryptophan pyrrolase (3). The induction of these specific proteins results from the corticosteroids' promoting the transcription of messenger RNA for the two enzymes, tyrosine aminotransferase and tryptophan pyrrolase. Hepatic enzyme induction is believed to be a model for the mechanism of action of the glucocorticoids (4). The glucocorticoid enters the cell and binds to a specific cytoplasmic receptor protein. The steroid-protein receptor complex after alteration enters the nucleus of the cell, either associated with a cytoplasmic receptor or after interchange with a nuclear receptor, as described by Baxter & Tomkins in 1971 (5). A unitary hypothesis cannot explain the diverse effects of corticosteroids. Corticosteroid inhibition of amino acid incorporation into protein of peripheral tissues may be the dominant expression of glucocorticoid action.

The effects of corticosteroids on the metabolism of fat are even less clear than those for protein and carbohydrate metabolism. Glucocorticoids, independently, seem to have no effect on basal lipolysis as measured by glycerol production; but, lipolysis induced by epinephrine or any of the catecholamines is markedly potentiated by the administration of glucocorticoids. In isolated epididymal fat cells treated with dexamethasone, it was found that a small cAMP-dependent protein kinase was stimulated, as demonstrated by Lamberts et al in 1975 (6). Corticosteroids seem to have opposite effects in specific tissues. For example, the corticosteroids seem to sensitize the subcutaneous fat cells of the tissues of the arms and legs to the fat-mobilizing action of the catecholamines, and lipogenesis is inhibited, because glucose entry into fat cells is prevented by corticosteroids. On the other hand, the subcutaneous fat tissue of the abdomen and the dorsal fat pad manifest predominantly lipogenesis in response to corticosteroid administration (7).

The corticosteroids also have been shown to induce negative calcium balance, oppose the action of vitamin D on the intestine, and produce both osteoporosis and osteomalacia.

The principal biochemical actions of the glucocorticoids or the corticosteroids are the stimulation of hepatic gluconeogenesis, inhibition of peripheral tissue protein synthesis, and stimulation and induction of protein synthesis in the liver. These actions could explain many of the manifestations of Cushing's syndrome, either spontaneously or exogenously induced, with glucocorticoid or corticosteroid excess.

Anti-Inflammatory and Antiallergic Actions of the Corticosteroids

The anti-inflammatory and antiallergic activities of the corticosteroids are the most important reason for their clinical application in disease states. Suppression of the inflammatory response by corticosteroids has long been investigated without yielding a unifying concept of how the corticosteroids modify reaction. Although the precise mechanism of corticosteroid protection against cellular damage of inflammation is not understood, certain characteristics of this action can be enumerated.

1. Corticosteroid protection against cellular damage and suppression of the inflammatory response is nonspecific with regard to the kind of noxious stimulus, such as bacterial products, histamine and other by-products of the antigen-antibody union, metallic ions such as calcium, hypoglycemia, and snake venom. Pretreatment of several species of experimental animals with sufficient doses of corticosteroids will inhibit the inflammatory reaction to nearly any type of injury (8).

2. Corticosteroid action is local in that unaltered hormone must be present at the site of inflammation. It is not known whether cortisol must enter the nucleus of the cell to exert its anti-inflammatory effect. When cortisol is linked to agarose beads as cortisol hemisuccinyl sepharose, it remains outside the cell or in approximation to the cell wall. This preparation of cortisol can inhibit entry of glucose into adipose tissue; therefore, one of its biochemical actions can occur without penetration.

3. The degree of suppression of the inflammatory response and subsequent cellular injury is proportionate to the concentration of corticosteroids in a given volume of inflammatory tissue. The possibility of interference with the inflammatory re-

sponse by a remote effect of the corticosteroids cannot be excluded with certainty and could involve the lymphocytopenia and eosinopenia observed with corticosteroids (8).

Many corticosteroid effects on the inflammatory response have been described. The relative importance of each and the mechanism of action have not been explained. A few of these features of corticosteroid suppression of the inflammatory response are listed below.

MAINTENANCE OF INTEGRITY OF THE MICROCIRCULATION   Corticosteroids block the increased permeability of endothelium of capillaries induced by acute inflammation. There is a reduction both in the leakage of edematous fluid and in the transport of proteins into the areas of injury. Thus, tissue swelling is minimized, if not prevented. Exudation of inflammatory cells, including white cells and mast cells, is markedly inhibited.

MAINTENANCE OF CELL MEMBRANE OR PLASMA MEMBRANE INTEGRITY   Corticosteroids prevent the sequestration of water intracellularly and swelling and destruction of cells. In patients with Addison's disease, water intoxication may lead to death. In the local inflammatory response, intracellular transfer of water occurs with the swelling of the cytoplasmic organelles. Direct cellular injury by toxins, proteolytic enzymes, and mechanical factors may be inhibited by the presence of high concentrations of corticosteroids.

STABILIZATION OF LYSOSOMES   Lysosomes are small, bag-like organelles of the cell, usually spherical, contained in the cytoplasm. They contain a variety of enzymes that are hydrolytic for protein, carbohydrate, and fat and are known collectively as acid hydrolases. Enzymes are stored in the organelle by a single lipoprotein membrane. With cellular injury, the lysosomal membrane ruptures, and there is a release of the acid hydrolases that digest the cell contents and enlarge and perpetuate the inflammatory response by attacking extracellular protein substituents. Secondary tissue damage from the rupture of the lysosomes after cellular injury and attendant inflammatory response can be modified or eliminated in the presence of high concentrations of corticosteroids. The corticosteroids stabilize the lysosomal membrane and protect it from rupture in cellular injury. Whether the corticosteroids are attached to the lysosomal membrane or whether they exert some more remote effect is unknown. The action of the corticosteroids, then, is to interrupt the progressive cycle of inflammatory response by inhibiting the progressive digestion and disruption of the connective tissue and cells. The lysosomal participation in the inflammatory response has been likened to the "domino" theory. Corticosteroids interfere at some point with the "domino" of inflammation.

INHIBITION OF NEUTROPHILIC CHEMOTAXIS   Pharmacologic doses of the corticosteroids induce neutrophilic leukocytosis associated with eosinopenia, monocytopenia, and lymphocytopenia. This matter has been reviewed recently by Fauci et al (9). In studies on suppression of inflammation by corticosteroids, one of the most important mechanisms appears to be corticosteroid impedance of neutrophils and monocytes when arriving at the inflammatory site. Suppression of the acute inflammatory response involves inhibition of in vivo chemotaxis, including a reduction of the volume of inflammatory fluid, lysosomal and lactic dehydrogenase enzymes, as well as neutrophils (10). The mechanism by which corticosteroids inhibit in vivo chemotaxis is not understood and cannot be explained by steroid genome interaction.

Regulation of the Circulation by Corticosteroids

In acute adrenal insufficiency, glucocorticoids are most effective in restoring circulatory competence when shock has supervened. Mineralocorticoids such as aldosterone do not have this activity. Corticosteroids in high doses may restore circulatory function in shock associated with hemorrhage, endotoxin, snake venom, anaphylaxis, and trauma. The mechanism of the corticosteroid-induced improvement in the major circulation is not completely known. Corticosteroids exhibit an inotropic effect on the myocardium. In myocardial tissue, there exist receptors with high affinity for glucocorticoids. Glucocorticoid receptors have been demonstrated in the cytosol in a number of species by Ballard & Ballard in 1974 (11). Cytoplasmic receptors for mineralocorticoids (aldosterone) have not been demonstrated in the myocardium. Glucocorticoids incubated in vitro with myocardial cells improve utilization of fatty acids for energy metabolism. The administration of dexamethasone to dogs with severe low cardiac output syndrome resulted in a 50% decrement in mortality and improvement in cardiac function. Improvement in cardiac function in the low output syndrome in animals treated with dexamethasone was attributed to an increase in myocardial linolenic acid content and a decrease in prostaglandin content (12). It is possible that the corticosteroids in various shock states, such as in acute adrenal insufficiency, may restore cardiac function and increase cardiac output. It is possible that the therapeutic effect of corticosteroids in certain shock states may be related to improvement of cardiac function.

Antiallergic and Anti-Immunologic Effects of Corticosteroids

It is both surprising and intriguing that the corticosteroids exert a suppressive effect at each stage of the immune response (13). Corticosteroids seem to interfere with the phagocytosis of antigens and their subsequent intracellular digestion or processing. Corticosteroids also inhibit the migration of cells to areas of inflammation. The corticosteroids in large doses suppress cell-mediated hypersensitivity reaction.

It should be recalled that cell-mediated immunity is derived from the lymphocyte population that is thymus-processed or -dependent, and these lymphocytes are referred to as T cells. These T cells transform to lymphoblasts that incorporate antibody into their surface membrane but do not secrete humoral or free antibody. It is the thymus-dependent cell system that subserves the function of cell-mediated immunity. The thymus system is necessary for the development of specialized cells that are chiefly small lymphocytes which play the vital part in contact sensitivity, homograft rejection, and delayed hypersensitivity. The small lymphocytes and the thymocytes are most vulnerable to the action of corticosteroids and, in some species, permit modification of the immune cell-mediated immune response (14). The small lymphocytes of man are much less sensitive to the effects of corticosteroids. There is ample evidence that corticosteroids are taken up by lymphoid cells and bound to specific receptors.

There are steroid-sensitive and steroid-resistant species of lymphocytes. Some of the lymphocytic steroid receptors, when occupied by a corticosteroid, undergo cytolosis; others exhibit an inhibition of metabolism of the cell. In man, thymus-derived lymphocytes are more susceptible to the effects of corticosteroids than the bursa-derived lymphocytes that elaborate humoral antibody. Thus antibody reproduction is rarely reduced significantly, except with very large doses of corticosteroids, whereas cell-mediated immunity is modified at lower corticosteroid concentrations.

In recent years the importance of cell-mediated immunity has been amplified by organ transplantation. Corticosteroids are most effective in promoting homograft acceptance and survival. There is no evidence that the union of antigen and antibody is prevented, but the inflammatory response to this union is suppressed by corticosteroid therapy. Certainly the effects of corticosteroids in the reversal of an acute rejection episode is probably related to suppression of the inflammatory response and not so much to the cell-mediated immune mechanism.

The corticosteroids inhibit antigen processing by macrophages, cell-mediated immunity, and the inflammatory response after antigen-antibody union. Only in enormous doses do corticosteroids alter gamma globulin production by plasma cells in circulation. These properties of the corticosteroids resulted in their application to a variety of disorders in which alterations of the immune response are paramount, and it is in these disorders that corticosteroid therapy is probably most appropriate.

PHARMACOLOGY OF NATURAL AND SYNTHETIC CORTICOSTEROIDS

Structural alterations of cortisol have resulted in increased biological potency of its synthetic derivatives. It is generally agreed that prednisolone, methylprednisolone, triamcinolone, betamethasone, dexamethasone, and paramethasone share an advantage over cortisol in that sodium retention is not as marked at equipotent anti-inflammatory doses, although all of the other undesirable side effects of cortisol overdosage have been observed with the synthetic analogues.

Prednisolone, triamcinolone, methylprednisolone, betamethasone, and dexamethasone possess certain theoretical advantages over cortisol in relation to their availability to the tissues. Cortisol, the major corticosteroid product of the normal human adrenal cortex, circulates in the blood at a concentration from 5 to 25 μg per 100 ml of plasma. Eighty percent of the circulating cortisol is bound to an α-globulin, transcortin (corticosteroid-binding globulin), which represents an inactive transport complex. A smaller moiety is bound to albumin, and it is only this albumin-bound portion that may diffuse into the extravascular fluid that bathes tissue cells at any given moment. The synthetic analogues of cortisol do not compete for the binding sites of cortisol on the protein storage complex, transcortin. The synthetic analogues of cortisol are less extensively bound to plasma albumin and diffuse more completely into the tissue than does cortisol. It is possible that they exert their biological effect at the tissue receptor site earlier than does cortisol.

All of the synthetic analogues of cortisol are metabolized more slowly than cortisol by the liver because of the alterations of the steroid molecule in each instance and the rapid equilibration in blood with peripheral tissues.

The relative biological potency of the synthetic analogues of cortisol is compared with cortisol in Table 1, as are the plasma half-life and biological half-life of action for each of the corticosteroids (8). The plasma biological half-life of the corticosteroid represents the time elapsed before one half of the concentration of the given steroid disappears at any given point. It is generally accepted that the biological half-life in plasma of the corticosteroid reflects roughly the rate of degradation of the steroid by liver enzymes and hence is probably related in some way to the duration of activity and the metabolic stability of the corticosteroid at the receptor site. Thus, dexamethasone and betamethasone, with the longest biological half-lives, exhibit the longest duration of measurable biological activity in man, and cortisol, the shortest. In addition, relative anti-inflammatory potencies are also approximately correlated with the plasma half-times.

The duration of anti-inflammatory activity of cortisol and its synthetic analogues when administered orally approximates the duration of hypothalamic-pituitary-adrenal suppression. No synthetic or natural glucocorticoid has been found in which the anti-inflammatory potency and the hypothalamic-pituitary-adrenal suppressibility do not approximately parallel each other in terms of degree and duration. Apparently, the substituents of the glucocorticoid molecule necessary for attachment to the receptors in the hypothalamus are the same as those required for attachment to the receptors in the peripheral tissues. It has been possible to estimate the duration of therapeutic effects of cortisol and its analogues by examining the hypothalamic pituitary-adrenal suppressive activity that can be quantitated readily.

Table 1 Relative anti-inflammatory potencies and plasma and biological half-lives of cortisol and its synthetic analogues

	Anti-inflammatory potency	Plasma half-life (min)	Biological half-life (hr)
Cortisol	1	90	8–12
Prednisolone	3–5	200 or greater	12–36
Methylprednisolone	3–5	200 or greater	12–36
Triamcinolone	3–5	200 or greater	12–36
Paramethasone	10		
Betamethasone	20–30	300 or greater	36–54
Dexamethasone	20–30	300 or greater	36–54

In Table 1, biological half-lives of cortisol and its synthetic analogues are compared. These biological half-lives have been determined by the duration of suppression of hypothalamic-pituitary-adrenocortical secretory activity. Except for replacement therapy, cortisol is generally not used as a therapeutic agent for nonendocrine disorders because of its propensity for sodium retention in susceptible individuals. The sodium-retaining ability of cortisol, however, is but a tiny fraction of that of aldosterone (less than one one-hundredth). The most commonly administered corticosteroids are those with intermediate and prolonged biological half-lives. Prednisolone, methylprednisolone, and triamcinolone exhibit unusually variable biological half-lives. This group of steroids is used in alternate-day dosage regimens, although it is apparent that biological activity could persist well into the alternate off-day of the regimen. Nevertheless, a single dose of any of this group of steroids, administered in the early morning, generally will not induce hypothalamic-pituitary suppression on the day in which no steroid is given. Alternate-day steroid therapy is the preferred schedule in chronic conditions requiring pharmacologic doses of steroids. Betamethasone and dexamethasone exhibit prolonged anti-inflammatory and hypothalamic-pituitary-adrenal suppressibility and are ideally suited for the treatment of disorders requiring inhibition of the pituitary ACTH secretion but are not suitable for alternate-day schedules. If intermittent therapy or periodic steroid therapy is desirable, betamethasone or dexamethasone can be given once every 3 or 4 days.

MODALITIES OF CORTICOSTEROID THERAPY

The emphasis in this discussion is on the modalities of corticosteroid therapy and not specific indications. On assessing each modality of corticosteroid therapy, I attempt to suggest regimens that will provide sufficient therapeutic benefits with minimum complicating side effects.

Replacement

The treatment of primary (Addison's disease) and secondary adrenocortical insufficiency in the chronic state requires little comment. In primary adrenocortical insufficiency, one should administer enough cortisol by mouth daily to diminish hyperpigmentation and to abolish postural hypotension, the hallmark of adrenal insufficiency even in the chronic state. The mean amount of cortisol for this task is 20 mg/day, and aldosterone replacement must be in the form of 9α-fluorocortisol (Florinef ®) at 0.1 mg/day.

Secondary adrenocortical insufficiency occurs in hypopituitarism and in patients receiving corticosteroid therapy for nonendocrine diseases. There are approximately 5 million persons in the United States receiving doses of corticosteroid sufficient to produce hypothalamic-pituitary-adrenocortical insufficiency. It is unfortunate, but true, that patients with secondary adrenocortical insufficiency are not ordinarily severely symptomatic until an acute precipitating event results in the development of the adrenocortical insufficiency. The only manifestation is that of arterial hypotension and low cardiac output. Abnormalities in potassium metabolism and hyperpigmentation are not present to identify the patient as having adrenocortical insufficiency. It is often necessary to treat the patient without a confirmed diagnosis. A bolus of 100 mg of cortisol, as cortisol phosphate or succinate esters, should be given intravenously, and an infusion of cortisol phosphate or succinate at a rate of 15 mg/hr for the first 24 hr with saline as a vehicle should be used. Restoration of the blood pressure may be apparent within minutes and should be apparent by 1 hr.

We have studied many patients with Gram-negative septic shock and disseminated intravascular coagulation and a few patients who died with what seemed to be replacement of the adrenal glands by intra-adrenal hemorrhage (8, 15). These patients met the criteria of the Waterhouse-Friderichsen syndrome, yet in every instance their plasma cortisol levels were elevated, with a mean of 73 μg/100 ml, and their plasma cortisol levels were further increased to between 100 and 120 μg/100 ml with injections of ACTH. Isolated reports of actual adrenal failure with hemorrhagic replacement of the adrenals do exist, but only one or two have documentation of cortisol deficiency. Acute adrenal insufficiency is not a usual feature of the Waterhouse-Friderichsen syndrome.

Intensive Short-Term Therapy

Prompt, intensive corticosteroid therapy may reduce morbidity and mortality of potentially lethal conditions in which the inflammatory response itself has imperiled the host. Such may be true for certain allergic emergencies, infectious shock, necrotizing vasculitis, and the metabolic upheaval accompanying water intoxication, central hyperthermia, hypoglycemic coma, and acute hypercalcemia associated with vitamin D intoxication and hormone therapy for metastatic cancer of the breast.

The use of corticosteroids in septic shock is controversial. If the pathophysiology of septic shock is related to endotoxin shock in animals, then corticosteroid therapy must be pushed to its ultimate. There is little doubt that restoration of cardiac output may result after a massive infusion of corticosteroids in some patients with septic shock. Hardly anyone would dispute the value of intensive corticosteroid therapy in acute allergic emergencies, but the rejoinder should be made that β-adrenergic stimulators and bronchodilators must be used as needed with corticosteroid therapy. Intensive short-term corticosteroid therapy in severe exacerbations of bronchial asthma does not induce an earlier remission than more conventional dosage forms. McFadden et al in 1976 (16) failed to demonstrate any objective improvement in pulmonary function with massive doses of cortisol succinate when compared to the administration of isoproterenol alone during the first 6 hr of treatment. In those situations in which circulatory failure is prominent, one can usually observe the restoration of blood pressure after a single dose, which may not need to be repeated. The advantage of the longer-acting corticosteroid esters, bethamethasone and dexamethasone, is that a single dose is usually all that is required.

The complications of brief, intensive corticosteroid therapy, which should be limited to a maximum 48-hr period, include burning and itching at mucocutaneous junctions and rarely, multifocal premature ventricular contractions (17), precipitation of diabetic ketoacidosis (in a genetic diabetic), and superficial punctate ulcerations of the gastric mucosa with hemorrhage. One need *not* taper the dosage of steroid at all, and it may be withdrawn abruptly if the underlying disease is not exacerbated as a result. It is the activity of the underlying or precipitating condition that determines whether or not any tapering is required. It is best to withdraw the steroids as abruptly as they were begun.

Prolonged, High Dose, Suppressive Therapy

Because of the duration of therapy and the doses of corticosteroids used, complications with prolonged, high dose, suppressive corticosteroid therapy are more frequently encountered. This modality of corticosteroid therapy is indicated and efficacious to treat asthma, ulcerative colitis, subacute hepatic necrosis, chronic active hepatitis, severe alcoholic hepatitis, gluten-sensitive enteropathy, autoimmune hemolytic anemia, idiopathic thrombocytopenic purpura, acute lymphocytic leukemia, disseminated Hodgkin's disease, nephrotic syndrome, acute rejection after tissue homotransplantation; central nervous system involvement, nephritis, hemolytic anemia, and thrombocytopenic purpura accompanying disseminated lupus erythematosus, polymyositis, atypical dermatomyositis, and temporal arteritis (giant cell).

In these disorders erratic coricosteroid dosage is hazardous, and rapid withdrawal of corticosteroids is often associated with an exacerbation of the underlying disease. Nearly all patients on prolonged, high dose steroid therapy (more than 15 mg of prednisolone daily) require gradual tapering of dosage when therapy is to be withdrawn. It is emphasized that although these patients are vulnerable to acute secondary adrenal insufficiency, abrupt withdrawal of steroid therapy produces secondary adrenal insufficiency only indirectly, by exacerbating the underlying disease. Prednisolone dosage varies in these disorders from 15 to 120 mg/day, and this amount of corticosteroid when given for more than two weeks may result in prolonged suppression of the hypothalamic-pituitary-adrenal axis and one or more undesirable side effects of corticosteroid therapy (see below). To avoid these complications, alternate-day steroid therapy is recommended whenever possible, and if alternate-day therapy is not effective, then the total daily dose should be given in the morning.

Low Dose, Chronic, Palliative Therapy

Low dose, chronic, palliative therapy involves ingestion, each morning, of 2–10 mg of prednisolone as an adjuvant to other therapy (such as salicylates in rheumatoid arthritis and lupus erythematosus).

This form of therapy may be used in a few patients with rheumatoid arthritis, when excruciating, unrelenting pain that is unresponsive to salicylate therapy occurs, or if systemic vasculitis and fever are predominant. Salicylate therapy remains central, and corticosteroids should not be given as a first form of therapy. The same constraints apply to the treatment of lupus erythematosus in which arthritis is the principal manifestation. Regional enteritis may respond to modest doses of corticosteroid as adjunctive therapy. Corticosteroid-treated patients with rheumatoid arthritis are particularly vulnerable to the complication of peptic ulcer (18). Erratic corticosteroid dosage or withdrawal may precipitate a panmesenchymal reaction—

"steroid pseudorheumatism" (19). Withdrawal of corticosteroids is tedious, and to avoid rheumatoid exacerbation reduction in dosage should not exceed 1 mg of prednisolone each one to two months.

It is of interest that corticosteroids apparently increase the metabolic disposition of the salicylates as the steroids enhance salicylate clearance by the kidneys (20). Toxic blood levels of salicylates have occurred in patients whose corticosteroid dosage has been reduced.

Chronic Inhibition of Pituitary ACTH Secretion

Betamethasone and dexamethasone are ideally suited for the treatment of patients with disorders of cortisol biosynthesis or idiopathic hirsutism, because the suppression of hypothalamic-pituitary-adrenocortical secretion is desired. This can best be accomplished by the administration of between 0.5 and 0.75 mg of betamethasone or dexamethasone at bedtime each night. Very few side effects are observed at the lower dose, and a good control of urinary 17-ketosteroid excretion is achieved.

COMPLICATIONS OF CORTICOSTEROID THERAPY

Prolonged, high dose, suppressive, daily corticosteroid therapy may be associated with a host of complications and side effects. Some of the more important complications are listed in Table 2, and the nonendocrine complications of corticosteroid therapy are detailed elsewhere (1, 20).

Not included in the complications listed in Table 2 is the peculiar steroid-associated entity, "steroid pseudorheumatism" or steroid-induced panmesenchymal reaction, or the steroid withdrawal syndrome. This term is used to describe musculoskeletal aching, fever, malaise, emotional lability, lupus-like syndrome, hypertension, and general debility that occurs in patients, particularly with rheumatoid arthritis, in whom erratic steroid dosage has been used or for that in which high doses of steroids have been used in the treatment of rheumatoid arthritis and then are rapidly tapered, as described by Slocumb in 1953 (21). This steroid-induced disorder frequently complicated the high dose therapy that was used in the early years of corticosteroid treatment for both lupus erythematosus and rheumatoid arthritis. Hardin (22) has described a few patients in which these manifestations have occurred quite recently. It is noteworthy that patients who have so-called steroid pseudorheumatism may have positive serological tests for lupus erythematosus. This syndrome is avoided by gradual tapering of dosage and by avoiding excessive dosage of corticosteroids in the first place.

Conn & Blitzer (23) recently have challenged the long-held clinical notion that peptic ulceration of the upper gastrointestinal tract could occur following all corticosteroid therapy. The incidence of proved peptic ulceration was 1.0% in a control population of nearly 1500 patients but 1.4% in a population of 2000 steroid-treated patients. The incidence of upper gastrointestinal hemorrhage and symptoms of ulcer, however, was significant in the combined data presented. It would seem that peptic ulceration is not the hazard it was once considered.

Table 2 Complications of corticosteroid therapy

Musculoskeletal	Metabolic
Myopathy	Precipitation of clinical manifestations,
Osteoporosis–vertebral compression	including ketoacidosis, of genetic dia-
fractures	betes mellitus
Aseptic necrosis of bone	Hyperosmolar nonketotic coma
Gastrointestinal	Hyperlipidemia
Peptic ulceration (often gastric)	Induction of centripetal obesity
Gastric hemorrhage	Endocrine
Intestinal perforation	Growth failure
Pancreatitis	Secondary amenorrhea
Central Nervous System	Suppression of hypothalamic-pituitary-
Psychiatric disorders	adrenal system
Pseudocerebral tumor	Inhibition of fibroplasia
Ophthalmologic	Impaired wound healing
Glaucoma	Subcutaneous tissue atrophy
Posterior subcapsular cataracts	Suppression of the immune response
Cardiovascular and renal	Superimposition of a variety of bacter-
Hypertension	ial, fungous, viral, and parasitic infec-
Sodium and water retention–edema	tions in steroid-treated patients
hypokalemic alkalosis	

Corticosteroids given to laboratory animals early in the course of pregnancy have been found to induce a high incidence of cleft palate in the offspring. No such relationship has been noted in human pregnancy and Schatz et al (24) did not observe maternal, fetal, or neonatal mortality in 70 pregnancies and 55 asthmatic patients treated with pharmacologic doses of corticosteroid. Acute adrenal insufficiency did not supervene in the infant nor was there an increased incidence of toxemia of pregnancy in the mother. A slightly increased rate of prematurity occurred in infants born of corticosteroid-treated mothers. On the other hand, fetal mortality has been significantly reduced and previously untreated mothers were given large doses of corticosteroids if they entered premature labor (25). Neonatal experimental animals exhibit marked growth retardation, when given substantial doses of corticosteroids. Loeb (26) demonstrated that low doses of glucocorticoid induced a marked suppression of cell proliferation in growing tissues with stable cell populations, such as the liver of weanling rats. Steroid-induced suppression of somatic growth may involve the suppression of cell proliferation in stable parenchymal tissue. Infants of steroid-treated mothers do not exhibit obvious inhibition in somatic growth. Inhibition of cell proliferation by steroids appears to be a postnatal event. Pharmacologic doses of the corticosteroids inhibit pituitary discharge of certain tropic hormones—the glycoprotein hormones. Re et al (27) demonstrated that dexamethasone inhibits thyroid-stimulating hormone (TSH) secretion and responsiveness to thyrotropin-releasing hormone (TRH), whereas prolactin secretion continues to be stimulated normally by TRH during dexamethasone administration. Luteinizing hormone (LH) and follicle-stimulating hormone (FSH) levels are reduced in the postmenopausal woman given large doses of corticosteroids. It is likely that dexamethasone-induced suppression of pituitary secretion of TSH, LH, and FSH (the glycoprotein hormones) is a direct pituitary effect and not mediated through hypothalamic-releasing factors.

Suppression of the Hypothalamic-Pituitary-Adrenal System During Administration of Corticosteroids

Suppression of the hypothalamic-pituitary-adrenal system is among the most prevalent and potentially hazardous derangements induced by corticosteroids. Regulation of ACTH-dependent steroidogenesis is accomplished by long or external loop negative feedback. Corticotropin-releasing factor from the hypothalamus activates ACTH release by the anterior pituitary, and ACTH stimulates the conversion of cholesterol to cortisol in the adrenal cortex. As cortisol levels rise in blood, binding sites in the hypothalamus are occupied, and corticotropin-releasing factor is no longer elaborated, until concentrations of cortisol in the extracellular fluid decline. Levels of corticosteroids equipotent to or greater than physiological concentrations of cortisol, when maintained, activate the inhibitory feedback pathway. ACTH and cortisol secretion are negligible while supraphysiologic, constant levels of exogenous corticosteroids are continued. In 1953, Salassa, Bennett & Keating (28), in a series of postmortem examinations, showed that in a man receiving high dose steroid therapy, there is a significant reduction in adrenal weight within 5 to 10 days after the beginning of corticosteroid therapy. It is generally acknowledged that adrenal atrophy is apparent in nearly all species tested after 10 days of high dose corticosteroid therapy.

Adrenocortical atrophy appears to be completely reversible when caused by deprivation of ACTH and reduced ACTH-secretory activities, which are caused by deprivation of corticotropin-releasing factor. Hypothalamic corticoptropin-releasing factor production is variably suppressed during the first 1 to 2 weeks of steroid therapy, but, as the duration of therapy is extended, responsiveness of the hypothalamic-pituitary-adrenal system is progressively diminished and continues after steroid therapy is withdrawn. In a number of studies, inhibition of the feedback response persists up to 12 months if corticosteroid levels are maintained in the supraphysiologic range for only two weeks.

The responsiveness to stress, however, may be recovered much earlier than 12 months. We have examined many patients in this laboratory with respect to stress responsiveness and the relations between duration of therapy, dose, and length of time after cessation of therapy (29). These studies are described here and involve the use of the pyrogen test (30). Purified lipopolysaccharide (0.25 μg), derived from salmonella abortus-equi, was injected intravenously into healthy subjects, and activation of the hypothalamic-pituitary-adrenal system was apparent within 2 hr, since the plasma cortisol level increased 200%.

The results of studies in patients as compared with those of healthy controls appear in Table 3. Two of the test groups of patients were subjected to the intravenous pyrogen test, 24 hours after the last dose of corticosteroid. The duration of corticosteroid therapy in both groups varied from one month to eight years. The high dose group received 50 mg or more of cortisol or equipotent doses of its synthetic analogues daily. The low dose group received 20 mg or less of cortisol or equipotent doses of its synthetic analogues daily. High dose corticosteroid therapy abolished the hypothalamic-pituitary-adrenal response to pyrogen stress, whereas low doses of steroids produced only insignificant alterations to the response to pyrogen stress. Other studies involving testing of the negative feedback response (metyrapone test) may be abnormal even at rather modest doses of corticosteroids. Patients receiving high dose corticosteroid therapy whose corticosteroid regimen was discontinued one month before the pyrogen test was undertaken showed somewhat more variable responses, yet the 4-hr response was clearly attenuated. In patients whose corticosteroid therapy was discontinued five months before the pyrogen test was given, responsiveness to this type of stress was completely restored. Patients who had been receiving alternate-day high dose corticosteroid therapy were tested on the day they received no steroid, and no interference with pyrogen stress responsiveness was demonstrated. Apparently, prolonged negative feedback inhibition is not of clinical significance, but response to pyrogen stress more nearly relates to the problem of stress responsiveness in general.

Single, daily doses of less than 20 mg of cortisol or equipotent doses of its analogue and cessation of corticosteroid therapy for a period of 5 months are associated with normal pyrogen stress responsiveness, and acute adrenocortical insufficiency in these patients is unlikely to supervene. Similarly, patients receiving alternate-day steroid therapy have little or no attenuation of pyrogen stress response. It would seem that low dose and alternate-day steroid therapy are the most desirable modalities of therapy, since they obviate concern over diminished stress responsiveness—the most hazardous complication of corticosteroid therapy.

The question of whether or not intermittent stimulation of the adrenal cortex with corticotropin in patients treated with pharmacologic doses of corticosteroids will preserve the functional integrity of the hypothalamic-pituitary-adrenocortical axis remains unsolved. In dexamethasone-suppressed normal subjects, intermittent corticotropin administration in the form of the synthetic 1-18 corticotropin maintains a hyperresponsive secretory adrenal cortex, as indicated by the studies reported by Kolanowski et al in 1975 (31). Several studies have suggested that chronic corticotropin stimulation induces less suppression of the hypothalamic-pituitary-adrenocortical axis, but it is emphasized that in order to obtain less suppression it is necessary to stimulate repeatedly with corticotropin throughout the entire period of treatment, which is not practical. Administration of corticotropin at the end of

Table 3 Results of the pyrogen response test in steroid treated patients (34)

	Control	Low dose (< 20 mg)	High dose (> 50 mg)		Alternate day
Time since last dose of corticosteroid		24 hr	24 hr 1 month 5 months		24 hr
Plasma cortisol (µg/dl) 4 hr after pyrogen	34 ± 4.2	28±5.9	5±3.5 13.4±7.6 37±4.8		35.6±3.8
P value test vs control	–	NS	< 0.001 < 0.02 NS		NS

prolonged corticosteroid therapy is ineffective in restoring hypothalamic-pituitary-adrenocortical functional integrity.

Alternate-Day Corticosteroid Therapy

Whenever possible, in patients requiring high dose, prolonged corticosteroid therapy, the alternate-day program should be attempted. One should *not* use alternate-day palliative, low dose steroid therapy in the treatment of rheumatoid arthritis and lupus erythematosus because of the danger of precipitating the peculiar pan-mesenchymal response. It is even recommended, for patients who seem to require consecutive, daily, high dose steroid therapy, that alternate-day therapy be attempted after the underlying disease is quiescent. With alternate-day or intermittent corticosteroid therapy, the hypothalamic-pituitary-adrenal system is not disturbed, the negative calcium balance is much less intense, the negative nitrogen balance is similarly reduced, and often only the desired therapeutic effect is retained. Alternate-day corticosteroid therapy allows for the administration of much higher total dosage. An extensive literature on the virtues of alternate-day corticosteroid therapy attests to the efficacy and safety of this program.

In Table 4 are listed the disease entities that might be expected to respond to alternate-day therapy. Both bronchial asthma and ulcerative colitis have been managed on an alternate-day basis successfully, but a significant portion of patients are unable to tolerate the omission of dosage within a 24-hr period. Also listed in Table 4 are those conditions in which alternate-day therapy may, in fact, be hazardous. Hunder et al (32) found that patients with temporal or giant cell arteritis would tolerate daily solitary dosage but that one half of the patients treated on an alternate-day basis were symptomatic.

Table 4 Indications and contraindications for alternate-day corticosteroid therapy

May be effective	Ineffective
Asthma	Complications of systemic lupus erythematosus: nephritis, thrombocytopenic purpura, CNS involvement
Ulcerative colitis	
Subacute hepatic necrosis	
Chronic active hepatitis	Polymyositis
Severe alcoholic hepatitis	Polymyalgia rheumatica and temporal arteritis (giant cell)
Gluten-sensitive enteropathy	
Hemolytic anemia	Severe rheumatoid arthritis
Idiopathic thrombocytopenic purpura	
Acute lymphocytic leukemia	
Disseminated Hodgkin's disease	
Acute rejection after tissue transplantation	
Macroglobulinemia	
Sarcoidosis	
Subacute thyroiditis	
Metastatic cancer of breast, prostate	
Cerebral metastases with brain edema	

Topical and Inhalant Corticosteroids with Local Anti-Inflammatory but Little Systemic Effect

Beclomethasone dipropionate, as an aerosol, has been demonstrated to be an effective agent in the treatment of bronchial asthma (33). This steroid ester exhibits intense topical or local activity and almost no measurable systemic activity. Aerosol dosage of beclomethasone dipropionate in an inhaled dose of less than one sixth the usual oral dosage of potent corticosteroid, such as dexamethasone or betamethasone, controls the symptoms of chronic bronchial asthma as completely or more so than the oral preparations. In trials carried out in the United Kingdom with this agent, the only complication observed was a 4% incidence of oral candidiasis. Local corticosteroid-ester therapy is to be preferred if significant systemic absorption does not occur, or if local anti-inflammatory activity is apparent in the absence of systemic metabolic effects.

ACKNOWLEDGMENTS

Supported by Grants-in-Aid AM 12027-09, PO2-AM-08657-12, and HL-18318-01 (SRC) from the National Institutes of Health.

Literature Cited

1. Christy, N. P., ed. 1971. *The Human Adrenal Cortex,* p. 395. New York: Harper & Row
2. Marco, J., Calle, C., Roman, D., Diaz-Fierros, M., Villanueva, M., Valverde, I. 1973. Hyperglucagonism induced by glucocorticoid treatment in man. *N. Engl. J. Med.* 288:128–31
3. Julian, J. A., Chytil, F. 1969. A two-step mechanism for the regulation of tryptophan pyrrolase. *Biochem. Biophys. Res. Commun.* 34:734–40
4. Thompson, E. B., Lippman, M. E. 1974. Mechanism of action of the glucocorticoids. *Metabolism* 23:159–203
5. Baxter, J. D., Tomkins, G. M. 1971. Specific cytoplasmic glucocorticoid hormone receptors. *Proc. Natl. Acad. Sci. USA* 68:936–46
6. Lamberts, S. W. J., Timmermans, H. A. T., Kramer-Blankestijn, M., Birkenhäger, J. C. 1975. The mechanism of the potentiating effect of glucocorticoids on catecholamine-induced lipolysis. *Metabolism* 24:681–90
7. Krotkiewski, M., Blohme, B., Lindholm, N., Bjorntorp, P. 1976. The effects of adrenal corticosteroids on regional adipocyte size in man. *J. Clin. Endocrinol. Metab.* 42:91–98
8. Melby, J. C. 1961. Adrenocorticosteroids in medical emergencies. *Med. Clin. North Am.* 45:875–76
9. Fauci, A. S., Dale, D. C., Balow, J. E. 1976. Glucocorticosteroid therapy: Mechanism of actions and clinical considerations. *Ann. Intern. Med.* 84: 304–15
10. Wiener, S. L., Wiener, R., Urivetzky, M., Shafer, S., Isenberg, H. D., Janov, C., Meilman, E. 1975. The mechanism of action of a single dose of methylprednisolone on acute inflammation. *J. Clin. Invest.* 56:679–89
11. Ballard, P. L., Ballard, R. A. 1974. Cytoplasmic receptor—for glucocorticoids in lung of human fetus and neonate. *J. Clin. Invest.* 53:477–86
12. Bonilla, C. A., Dupont, J. 1976. Fatty acid and prostaglandin composition of left ventricular myocardium from dexamethasone-treated dogs with severe low output syndrome (LOS). *Prostaglandins* 11:935–51
13. Zurier, R., Weissman, G. 1959. Anti-immunologic effects of steroid therapy. *Med. Clin. North Am.* 43:295
14. Claman, H. N. 1972. Corticosteroids and lymphoid cells. *N. Engl. J. Med.* 287:388–97
15. Melby, J. C., Spink, W. W. 1958. Comparative studies on adrenal cortical function and cortisol metabolism in healthy adults and in patients with shock due to infection. *J. Clin. Invest.* 37:1791–98

16. McFadden, E. R. Jr., Kiser, R., de-Groot, W. J., Holmes, B., Kiker, R., Viser, G. 1976. A controlled study of the effects of single doses of hydrocortisone on the resolution of acute attacks of asthma. *Am. J. Med.* 60:52–60

17. Schmidt, G. B., Meier, M., Sadove, M. S. 1972. Sudden appearance of cardiac arrhythmias after dexamethasone. *J. Am. Med. Assoc.* 221:1402–4

18. Decker, J. L. 1964. Primer on the rheumatic diseases. *J. Am. Med. Assoc.* 190:741–51

19. Slocumb, C. H. 1952. Relative cortisone deficiency stimulating exacerbation of arthritis. *Bull. Rheum. Dis.* 3:21–22

20. David, D. S., Grieco, H., Cushman, P. Jr. 1970. Adrenal glucocorticoids after twenty years. A review of their clinically relevant consequences. *J. Chronic Dis.* 22:637–711

21. Slocumb, C. H. 1953. Rheumatic complaints during chronic hypercortisonism during withdrawal of cortisone in rheumatic patients. *Proc. Mayo Clin.* 28:655–57

22. Hardin, J. G. Jr. 1973. Steroid-induced morbidity mimicking active systemic lupus erythematosus. *Ann. Intern. Med.* 78:558–60

23. Conn, H. O., Blitzer, B. L. 1976. Nonassociation of adrenocorticosteroid therapy and peptic ulcer. *N. Engl. J. Med.* 294:473–80

24. Schatz, M., Patterson, R., Zeitz, S., O'Rourke, J., Melam, H. 1975. Corticosteroid therapy for the pregnant asthmatic patient. *J. Am. Med. Assoc.* 233:804–7

25. Editorial. 1976. Corticosteroids and the fetus. *Lancet* 1:74–75

26. Loeb, J. N. 1976. Corticosteroids in growth. *N. Engl. J. Med.* 295:547–53

27. Re, R. N., Kourides, I. A., Ridgway, E. C., Weintraub, B. D., Maloof, F. 1976. The effect of glucocorticoid administration on human pituitary secretion of thyrotropin and prolactin. *J. Clin. Endocrinol. Metab.* 43:338–46

28. Salassa, R. M., Bennett, W. A., Keating, F. R. Jr., Sprague, R. G. 1953. Postoperative adrenal cortical insufficiency; occurrence in patients previously treated with cortisone. *J. Am. Med. Assoc.* 152:1509–15

29. Melby, J. C. 1960. Assessment of adrenocorticotropic activity in man following steroid therapy. *Acta Endocrinol. Copenhagen.* 35: Suppl. 51, 347–48

30. Melby, J. C. 1959. Assessment of adrenocorticotropic activity with bacterial pyrogen in hypopituitary states. *J. Clin. Invest.* 38:1025 (Abstr.)

31. Kolanowski, J., Pizarro, M. A., Crabbe, J. 1975. Potentiation of adrenocortical response upon intermittent stimulation with corticotropin in normal subjects. *J. Clin. Endocrinol. Metab.* 41:453–65

32. Hunder, G. G., Sheps, S. G., Allen, G. L., Joyce, J. W. 1975. Daily and alternate-day corticosteroid regimens in treatment of giant cell arteritis. *Ann. Intern. Med.* 82:613–18

33. Brompton Hosp. Med. Res. Counc. Collab. Trial: Prelim. Rep. 1974. Double-blind trial comparing two dosage schedules of beclomethasone dipropionate aerosol treatment of chronic bronchial asthma. *Lancet* 2:303–8

Ann. Rev. Pharmacol. Toxicol. 1977. 17:529–43
Copyright © 1977 by Annual Reviews Inc. All rights reserved

THE CLINICAL APPLICATIONS ❖6694
OF CELL KINETICS
IN CANCER THERAPY

R. B. Livingston
Department of Medicine, University of Texas Health Science Center,
San Antonio, Texas 78284

J. S. Hart
Developmental Therapeutics, MD Anderson Hospital, Houston, Texas 77030

INTRODUCTION

The study of cell kinetics has been of interest to clinicians involved in the care of cancer patients for several reasons. An initial hypothesis which motivated this interest was that, using tools like the FLM (fraction of labeled mitoses) curve, major differences would be demonstrated between cancer cells and normal cells in terms of duration of the phases of cell cycle. Except that cancer cells in general show some prolongation in G_2, this has not been found to be the case (1). A second early hypothesis was that, in general, cancer cell populations would have a much higher proliferating fraction than normal cell populations: a major rationale for the design of S-phase active antimetabolites. In fact, human leukemic blasts usually have a *lower* level of proliferation, as measured by tritiated thymidine (^{3}HTdR) labeling, than corresponding normal bone marrow precursors (2). Most human solid tumors have a relatively low growth fraction, compared to normal host tissues like the bone marrow or gastrointestinal mucosa.

A third hypothesis, which remains viable though unresolved, is that tumor cells can be efficiently and differentially synchronized or recruited, by appropriate pretreatment with some agent, so that more of them are in a phase of the cell cycle (such as S) where they can be killed by a subsequently administered "executor" agent. A related hypothesis, now supported by several studies, is that a direct correlation exists between pretreatment proliferative state and clinical response: that patients with higher growth fraction tumors are more likely to respond than those with lower growth fraction tumors because most chemotherapeutic agents preferentially affect proliferating cells.

Recently, work from our laboratory and others has supported a hypothesis initially put forward by Sky-Peck (3): that a decrease in tumor-cell labeling index (LI) predicts for subsequent clinical response.

This brief review focuses on developments related to the viable hypotheses in cell kinetics, particularly with reference to their real or potential application in clinical cancer therapy.

ATTEMPTS AT SYNCHRONIZATION AND RECRUITMENT

Experimental Tumors

Dethlefsen et al (4) recently reviewed the use of the S-phase–specific inhibitors, cytosine arabinoside and hydroxyurea, in attempts to block cell populations in S with subsequent release of a synchronized cohort. In a variety of rodent systems, they conclude that "the published data strongly suggest that the drugs . . . which can cause good synchronization in vitro, can exert only a mild synchronizing effect in vivo and then only in tissues that have a relatively high growth fraction and short cell cycle-transit time." However, the work of Gibson & Bertalanffy (5) suggested that repeated injections of cytosine arabinoside (about 40 mg/m^2 every 2 hr for a total of 8 injections, or 16 hr: roughly twice the mean duration of S) results in marked synchronization of the B16 melanoma, a solid murine tumor with an intermediate baseline LI (19%) and growth fraction (53%).

Vinca alkaloids have been shown to arrest both tumor and normal cells in mitosis (6). Klein et al (7) demonstrated that Ehrlich ascites tumor cells in vivo could escape from the mitotic arrest produced by vincristine and travel as a synchronized cohort through at least two successive waves of mitosis. As demonstrated by labeling experiments, the second peak consisted almost entirely of cells that had been arrested by vincristine in the first peak. Thus, vincristine here produced synchronization and not recruitment of cells from a "nonproliferating pool."

It has been widely postulated that administration of a cell cycle nonspecific agent to a sensitive tumor, with resultant reduction in tumor volume, leads to an increase in growth fraction of the remaining tumor and resultant heightened sensitivity to administration of cell cycle specific therapy (8). One would expect, if this hypothesis is correct, to see an increase in LI and mitotic index (MI) at some time after administration of the first drug, presumably after it had produced tumor reduction, at least in terms of viable cell mass. There is a surprising dearth of data to support or refute this concept, from experimental systems. Schenken et al (9) recently presented preliminary data in one mouse system to support this conclusion. A number of empirical studies have reported increased therapeutic efficacy from scheduling of an alkylator followed by an antimetabolite (10–12). However, the appropriate control of simultaneous alkylator and antimetabolite was not reported, and recent work by Valeriote et al (13) suggests that, at least for phenyalanine mustard (L-PAM) and 5-FU, the reverse sequence of antimetabolite followed by alkylator may be most effective.

Work by Capizzi (14) and by Chlopkiewiez et al (15) demonstrated an apparent increase in the therapeutic index of methotrexate when it was preceded by L-asparaginase given several days before. This may be due to shutting-off of protein-dependent initiation of DNA synthesis secondary to asparaginase, with a resultant piling up of cells at the G_1-S interface which are then released when intracellular drug levels decline to a point sufficient to allow renewed DNA synthesis, resulting in progression of a temporarily synchronized cohort of tumor cells through S.

All work with drugs in synchronizing schedules, in which a second, systemically administered agent serves as the "executor," shares one problem: Synchrony of normal cell populations may occur as well, resulting in increased host toxicity. Further work is greatly needed to delineate the time sequence of synchronization and loss of synchrony in tumor versus sensitive host tissues; it may be that a sufficient differential exists to allow for therapeutic exploitation with appropriate scheduling. A different approach involves administration of a synchronizing agent, followed by *local* therapy aimed at the tumor that kills the synchronized cohort of cells most efficiently; an example is administration of radiation (most effective at killing cells in G_2 and M) after synchronization with 5-FU, as reported by Ganzer & Nitze (16). Vincristine pretreatment might be effective as well in this setting.

Human Tumors

Lampkin et al were among the first to suggest that cell synchronization techniques could increase therapeutic efficacy in acute leukemia (17). They reported that partial synchronization could be achieved with pulse doses of cytosine arabinoside in acute lymphocytic leukemia (ALL), and that "a greater therapeutic advantage can be achieved by a second cycle-dependent drug after synchronization than after the second drug alone." The time between administration of cytosine arabinoside and the peak in LI varied from 24 to 96 hr, with no synchronization observed in 4 of 20 serial studies. Lampkin et al (18) recently reported their results in 21 patients with acute myelogenous leukemia (AML) who received ara-C as an i.v. push injection of 5 mg/kg (100–180 mg/m²). Of 14 patients in whom consecutive LI and MI determinations were performed, 7 showed a significant increase in LI and 12 in MI at 18 to 24 hr after the ara-C. The patients then received 12-hr continuous infusions with ara-C 5 mg/kg every 12 hr, started at the time of maximal S-phase accumulation (usually 18–24 hr after the initial ara-C), and continued until complete remission, with escalations in ara-C dose if the patient failed to respond to lower doses. A complete remission was achieved in 12 out of 16 children and all 5 adults (81%).

Other investigators have not found evidence of synchronization after push doses of ara-C in AML (19), possibly because of lower doses, or differences in sampling time or patient population. Kremer et al (20) found an increase in LI in 11 out of 14 patients with remission or "anti-leukemic effect" who received either 1 or 3 daily push doses of ara-C, followed 48 hr after the last ara-C dose by LI determination and treatment with vincristine and methotrexate, while only 3 out of 9 patients with no response or early death demonstrated such an increase. (Five out of ten responders sampled at 24 hr and four out of eleven "nonresponders" had a similar increase.) MacKinney et al (21) used the "Lampkin AML schedule" in 23 adults with acute leukemia: They achieved complete marrow remissions in only six.

Buchner et al (22) reported a continuous infusion schedule of ara-C in patients with acute leukemia: 100 mg/m^2 per day for 48 hr. They found in 8 out of 11 patients a 1.3–4.0 fold increase in cells in the S-phase range, by DNA histogram, at the conclusion of the infusion. They employed ifosfamide as the executor drug.

More work is needed to clarify the role of ara-C as a synchronizing agent in acute leukemia, both in clinical studies and experimental models. In a homogeneous tumor cell population, the use of pulse cytophotometry to provide rapid DNA histogram analysis should allow the clinician to determine more accurately at what point synchronization is (or is not) achieved (23), and allow for more precise timing of executor agents.

Capizzi has extended his work with asparaginase and methotrexate to clinical studies in ALL (24); in several patients studied sequentially after asparaginase (dose, 40,000 units/m^2), he found evidence of initial depression in leukemic cell DNA synthesis, followed by recovery and "overshoot" at days 7–10; a similar decline in LI of normal bone marrow precursors was followed by more rapid recovery, "overshoot," and return to baseline. He has observed complete remission in 9 out of 11 adults with ALL, all of whom were "refractory" to prior methotrexate, with a median response duration of 6 months.

Marshall et al (25) reported results of LI determination after a single intravenous dose of prednisone (30–20 mg) in 10 normal and 11 acute leukemic patients: 8 out of 10 normals had a significant increase at 6 hr with a return to baseline levels at 24 and 48 hr; the leukemic marrows demonstrated peak DNA synthesis at 24 hr; with a return to baseline at > 48 hr. This provocative observation awaits confirmation and/or extension to clinical trials; that steroids produce a G_1-S block is well established (26).

In solid tumors, clinical protocols have been designed along synchronization lines using a variety of drugs and concepts. Based on the observation that continuous infusion of bleomycin for 48 hr produced an increase in LI in the nodules of patients with melanoma (27) (presumably as a result of S-G_2 arrest and subsequent release), Costanzi designed a regimen (28) in which 17 patients with disseminated carcinoma of the head and neck were treated with bleomycin as in i.v. infusion at 7.5 units/m^2/24 hr for 48 hr. Methotrexate (30 mg/m^2) and hydroxyurea (2000 mg/m^2) were administered in a single dose after a 24-hr rest period to allow the synchronized cohort to traverse G_2, M, and G_1 and reach the G_1-S interface. Tumor response was seen in 10 out of 17 (59%), not better than what one might achieve with methotrexate alone. Costanzi then adopted a 96-hr bleomycin infusion (to allow for S-G_2 trapping of more cells) and changed the rest period to 48 hr and the executor to methotrexate, 250 mg/m^2 with citrovorum factor rescue. Early results are promising, but no kinetic data are available.

Samuels (29) has compared a program in which bleomycin was given on a standard twice weekly schedule, with intermittent high dose vinblastine (VB-1), to one in which bleomycin was given as a 96-hr continuous infusion, followed by vinblastine. Patients with metastatic embryonal carcinoma of the testis appeared to fare better on VB-3, while those with teratocarcinomas responded better to VB-1. Unique toxicity (jaundice and hemolysis) was observed with bleomycin as a continuous infusion.

The observation that vincristine reliably produces stathmokinetic arrest (i.e. in G_2 and M) in human tissues 6 to 24 hr after injection, coupled with the apparent cell-kill specificity for cells in G_2 and M of bleomycin, led Livingston et al to design a two-drug combination in which the former was given 6 hr earlier (30). An encouraging response rate in this pilot study was seen in patients with lung carcinoma (4 of 15) and led to its inclusion in more complex, combination regimens designed primarily for patients with lung tumors (31, 32). Unfortunately, kinetic data were never obtained to support this hypothesis and the most recent trial involving this combination indicates that vincristine and "staggered" bleomycin adds nothing to the antitumor efficacy of a simpler, three-drug regimen (Southwest Oncology Group, unpublished data). However, encouraging results have been obtained with a similar staggered schedule in carcinoma of the cervix (33); in a study of adriamycin, vincristine, and bleomycin in testicular cancer, (34); and in Einhorn's recent study of vinblastine, bleomycin, and platinum in testicular cancer (35). It is conceivable that this combination may produce an increase in the therapeutic index of bleomycin, given (a) some degree of inherent efficacy for bleomycin against the tumor cells involved, and (b) a sufficiently large growth fraction that arrest of cells in G_2 and M by vincristine becomes meaningful, in terms of subsequent mitotic cell kill of a synchronized cohort. The lack of a suitable experimental model has prevented testing of the concept to date at a basic level.

Only one published clinical study has looked at ara-C in solid tumors as a potential synchronizing agent (36). In this study, a push dose of ara-C (200 mg/m^2) was followed by methotrexate 24 hr later, in a variety of patients who were already refractory to first-line chemotherapy. No striking evidence of synergy was seen, possibly because the empiric schedule was too imprecise or simply wrong in its timing. This study again points up the need for serial *measurements* of kinetic effects if meaningful clinical studies, seeking to demonstrate efficacy of kinetic manipulations, are to be conducted.

A number of investigators have explored "kinetically oriented" approaches in which cell-cycle nonspecific agent was followed by a cell-cycle specific one, with varying results. Burke & Owens (37) employed in acute leukemia a sequence of cyclophosphamide followed by vincristine at 24 hr and ara-C, as a 48 hr i.v. infusion begun 12 hr after vincristine. No consistent effect of cyclophosphamide was seen on LI prior to vincristine and ara-C, but it could be argued that the cyclophosphamide dose was too low and the time interval too short. Salmon recently reviewed (38) attempts to capitalize on the apparent increase in growth fraction (39), manifested as an increase in LI, after therapy with an alkylating agent in myeloma: "Despite this apparent expansion of the growth fraction, most patients do not appear to have further tumor regression induced with cycle active agents such as ara-C, azathioprine, hydroxyurea, or methotrexate, although optimal schedules and doses may not have been utilized." The other clinical study which offers laboratory support for an increase in growth fraction after alkylator therapy recently was reported by Mauer

(40). Cyclophosphamide was administered to children with disseminated neuroblastoma, at a dose of 150 mg/m²/day for seven days. The patients received adriamycin 25 mg/m² on day 8. Among 14 patients whose tumor cells could be selectively studied from bone marrow aspirates, 10 had an increase in LI after the cyclophosphamide, and all responded with a decrease in LI and complete remission after adriamycin. Furthermore, if the LI and MI decreased immediately after the 7 days of cyclophosphamide, the clinical response to the sequential regimen was poor.

Other studies with encouraging clinical results, but no kinetic measurements, have been carried out in oat-cell carcinoma of the lung (41) and non-oat-cell lung tumors (42) with the sequential combination of cyclophosphamide and methotrexate. However, equally encouraging results have been obtained in these tumor categories using simultaneous combinations of drugs without any kinetic rationale.

Klein's work with vincristine in Ehrlich ascites tumor led him to do clinical trials with two doses of vincristine, followed at various, empirically chosen intervals by cyclophosphamide (7). He treated 55 patients, of whom 39 had lymphomas, 7 had oat cell lung carcinoma, 7 had acute leukemia, and 2 had unknown primary sites. He observed a 60% complete and 90% complete plus partial response rate; although these are good results, they are not extraordinary, particularly since all but two of the complete remissions were in leukemia or lymphoma. Pouillart et al (43, 44) have also treated patients with lymphoma, lung carcinoma, and other malignancies with vincristine given twice, followed by other executor compounds, with good results but not kinetic data. As Pouillart himself has emphasized (45), some of the heightened effectiveness of the combinations may be due to pharmacodynamic interactions, rather than kinetic effects.

Early work by Rentschler et al (46) has shown encouraging results in solid tumors with sequential asparaginase and methotrexate in a regimen similar to that of Capizzi in acute leukemia. Further studies in this area, including measurement of tumor cell LI when possible, are in progress.

CORRELATION OF KINETIC PARAMETERS AND CLINICAL RESPONSE

Another use of cell kinetic data, which may prove more fruitful than the design of "kinetic" clinical protocols, lies in the possible predictive relationship of these parameters (especially LI) to response and survival.

Pretreatment LI: Response and Survival

Hart et al (47) reported that a direct relationship exists between height of the pretreatment LI and the likelihood of complete response for patients with acute leukemia, studying a population composed largely of adults with AML. Hart further found a direct relationship between LI and tumor burden, as estimated by "absolute leukemic infiltrate" (percentage of blasts X percentage of cellularity of bone marrow X 100). Thus, although patients with a high percentage of LI had a greater chance of responding to (primarily cycle-active) chemotherapy, they also tended to have *shorter* remission durations, possibly related to a greater residual "subclinical" burden of leukemia and/or inherently a more aggressive growth of residual disease. But high LI and leukemic infiltrate also correlated with longer survival, because these patients tended to be more easily reinduced and very few had early deaths. Hillen (48), Vogler (49), and Burke (37) have reported a similar correlation between pretreatment LI and response, as shown in Table 1. It is noteworthy that these regimens relied primarily on cytosine arabinoside or methotrexate, both S-phase specific agents, to induce remission.

When the "backbone" of induction therapy is ara-C plus thioguanine given simultaneously on a twice-daily schedule, the relationship of pretreatment LI to response may disappear: Vogler found no difference in LI between 45 responders and 27 nonresponders on such a regimen (50), nor did Raich (51) or Arlin (52). This suggests that thioguanine, designed as an antimetabolite but known to be incorporated into the DNA of "non-S" cells (53), may play a role in the induction of response among patients with a low LI, while ara-C is most important for those with a higher LI. However, Crowther also reported no correlation between pretreatment LI and response (54) in adult patients with AML who received a combination of daunorubicin and ara-C; moreover, in these 58 patients a *positive* correlation was reported for LI with length of remission, as well as with survival among those who achieved remission. In children with ALL, Mauer (55) has observed no relationship between pretreatment LI and response; here, of course, a major component of remission induction is the cell-cycle nonspecific agent, prednisone.

Among patients with solid tumors, data are now becoming available that suggest a relationship between pretreatment LI and response to a variety of cytotoxic drug regimens, at least for patients with breast cancer and melanoma. Sulkes et al (56) studied 56 patients with breast carcinoma and disseminated disease; among 28 with LI<8.3% prior to therapy, only 1 had > 50% tumor regression, while 12 out of 28 with LI > 8.3 responded. This difference was statistically significant, and held when the group was broken into smaller subgroups related to presence or absence of prior chemotherapy, and treatment with combinations versus single agents. Responders with a high LI also had significantly longer survival than low LI patients

Table 1 Acute leukemia: diagnosis and pretreatment kinetics versus complete remission rate

| | Labeling index % | | | | |
| | <9 | | >9 | | |
Diagnosis	#CR/TOT.[a]	(%)	#CR/TOT.	(%)	P value
AML[b]	15/71	(21)	55/75	(73)	<0.001
ALL	3/8	(38)	18/23	(78)	0.09
All patients	18/79	(23)	73/98	(74)	<0.001

[a] #CR/TOT represents number of complete remissions/total.

[b] Results represent the pooled data of Hillen, Vogler, Hart, and Burke (37, 47–49).

(as a group) or nonresponders with a high LI. The "high" and "low" LI patients were found to be comparable with respect to age, menopausal status, and dominant metastatic site. In contrast, an earlier report by Kofman et al (57) showed no correlation between the uptake of C^{14}-formate by breast tumor tissues and their subsequent response to hormone therapy. These observations support the hypotheses that, in breast carcinoma, presently available cytotoxic chemotherapy preferentially affects proliferating cells, while hormonal manipulation, if effective, affects nonproliferating cells as well as (or better than) proliferating cells.

Thirlwell et al (58) recently reported that 8 patients with melanoma who responded to regimens containing DTIC had a median LI of 8.0, compared to 3.2 for 22 patients who were nonresponders. He also found, in an analysis of 59 patients with a variety of solid tumors (excluding melanoma and breast carcinoma), that the following relationship obtained between response rate to chemotherapy and median LI respectively: > 40%, 15.8 (21 patients); 20–40%, 7.3 (15 patients); and < 20%, 3.7 (23 patients).

Further suggestion of a relationship between growth fraction and response to cytotoxic chemotherapy comes from the clinical observation that lymphomas and oat-cell carcinoma of the lung, tumors with a high degree of drug responsiveness, are also among those with the highest LI in the untreated state (59). Skipper (60) has elegantly summarized the data that support a direct relationship between the growth fraction of experimental tumors and their responsiveness, especially to agents killing cells in S phase. Against this impressive volume of clinical and experimental data stands the observation of Wolberg et al (61) that pretreatment LI failed to correlate with clinical response to 5-FU in patients, most of whom had breast or colon carcinoma. Clearly, as emphasized by Hall (62), factors other than proliferative fraction are important in whether a tumor responds to chemotherapy. Yet the importance of this factor as an independent variable seems now sufficiently well established to suggest that measurements of pretreatment LI be used as an adjunct, where possible, in deciding at least whether S-phase specific agents are indicated. The combination of LI data and information regarding the presence of estrogen receptors (63) may be very helpful in making decisions about both "adjuvant" and "advanced" regimens for patients with breast carcinoma, with regard to the role of hormones versus "cytotoxic" agents.

Changes in LI and Response

Sky-Peck (3) reported that a decrease in LI after a course of therapy correlated highly with the likelihood of subsequent clinical response to that therapy. Using a technique (64) that allowed for rapid autoradiography on representative samples of viable tumor cells, Murphy et al (65) confirmed this observation; in 63 patients with a variety of solid tumors and on numerous different chemotherapeutic regimens, clinical response was observed in 12 out of 16 patients with a significant decrease in LI after therapy, and in only 2 of 47 who failed to show such a decrease (59). Data from experimental tumors (66) also demonstrate that tumor regression after chemotherapy is accompanied by a decrease in LI; however, decreases of LI (though of lesser magnitude) have also been reported in tumors resistant to the agent employed (67, 68). Given that suppression of DNA synthesis in a tumor does not guarantee response, clinical and experimental data strongly suggest that it is a sine qua non for response to occur, at least with agents that preferentially kill proliferating cells. This appears to be true as well for radiation; in studies recently reported by Tubiana (69), among patients with head and neck tumors who underwent weekly LI determination during continuous radiation treatment, a $>$ 50% decrease in LI correlated with clinical radiosensitivity, and $<$ 50% decrease with nonresponse. Breitenecker et al (70) made a similar observation with radiation in carcinoma of the cervix.

As a clinically useful predictor of response, the study of LI pre- and post-therapy has two serious drawbacks: (a) the tumor most be accessible to repeated biopsy, and (b) the patient must be committed to a course of treatment before its effect can be evaluated. Several investigators have reported preliminary studies to test a more useful hypothesis (if correct): that drug therapy in vitro may predictably and *differentially* suppress DNA synthesis in sensitive cells. Cline (71) has summarized the conditions that should be met to test such a hypothesis: (a) the drug(s) must be in active form (or converted to it) in the in vitro system; (b) the drug(s) must be present in concentrations approximating those achieved in vivo; (c) the rate and other characteristics of DNA synthesis of the malignant cells in vivo and in vitro must be sufficiently similar so that drug effects under the two conditions are comparable; and (d) there must be sufficient time for drug action to become manifest. Zittoun et al used a test system (72) in which drugs were directly added to leukemic cells, at concentrations that produced a 50% decrease in 14-C-thymidine incorporation of control nonleukemic marrows after 2 hr; in vitro depression of labeled thymidine incorporation was more marked in those who responded to therapy than in the nonresponders. The mean decrease in 16 responders was 52% compared to 24% in 26 nonresponders (P $<$0.001). No difference was observed in depression of ^{3}H-uridine incorporation between responders and nonresponders. Lippmann et al (73) found that, when leukemic blasts from ALL patients were incubated 18 hr with dexamethasone directly added in vitro, ^{3}HTdR incorporation was significantly inhibited in glucocorticoid-sensitive, but not in glucocorticoid-resistant cells. Furthermore, the minimal concentration necessary to achieve this effect approximated that necessary to saturate steroid-binding protein receptor sites.

Problems associated with direct addition of drugs to in vitro systems include the following: (a) the drug may not be present in its active form in the in vitro system, and (b) the drug (or metabolite) concentration achievable in vivo may not be approximated under in vitro conditions, either through oversight or (commonly) lack of pharmacologic data. An attempt to circumvent these difficulties involves the use of "treated serum," defined as serum obtained from the patient shortly after drug administration, at a time when pharmacologic concentration of active metabolites may be nearly maximal. Such a technique has precedent in the use of various dilutions of host serum containing antibiotics to determine whether adequate bactericidal concentrations have been reached (74). The determination of antineoplastic activity of treated sera, for the purpose of determining duration of antitumor effect after a single dose, also has precedent in experimental systems (75).

Burns et al (76) measured ^{3}HTdR incorporation by scintillography of leukemic cells incubated with pretreatment (control) serum versus serum from the same patient obtained after 2 days of therapy with ara-C. The period of incubation with treated serum was 4 hr. All patients who had depression of thymidine uptake by 65% or more showed response, while depression by < 50% was not associated with clinical response.

It is probable that 4 hours of incubation is not, in many instances, a sufficient period of time for drug effect on DNA synthesis to become manifest. This is suggested by experimental tumor work with alkylating agents (67) which shows that maximal inhibition of DNA synthesis occurs 24-48 hr after their administration in vivo, and by the failure of systems using short-term exposure conditions to demonstrate consistent, good correlation between changes in DNA synthesis and response (77, 78). Using a 24-hr period of incubation with treated serum versus fresh and 24-hr control serum, Thirlwell et al (79) found the following: (a) the LI of tumor cells remained constant over 24 hr in 90% of controls, with no evidence of a nonspecific effect from serum itself; (b) treated sera did, in some cases, produce significant decreases in LI after 24 hr relative to controls; and (c) these decreases correlated with the subsequent observed clinical response. In 10 patients with solid tumors who had a significant decrease in vitro, who received the chemotherapy tested, 5 had partial responses and 3 improved; in 12 without a decrease, none had response, 1 improved, and 11 had progressive disease.

Other investigators have reported that depression of DNA synthesis in vitro by hormones correlates with the clinical response in patients with breast and endometrial cancer (80, 81). As with the use of cytotoxic drugs or treated serum, the results are encouraging but preliminary, and require confirmation.

FUTURE DIRECTIONS

Several areas involving measurement and manipulation of cellular proliferation have great potential for exploration. A leading possibility is to minimize cell division in the most drug-sensitive normal host tissues (usually bone marrow and gastrointestinal mucosa) in order to increase the therapeutic index of the administered drug against tumor tissue. Some ways in which this might be accomplished include: (a) intravenous hyperalimentation to reduce DNA synthesis in gastrointestinal mucosa (82, 83); (b) administration of an inhibitor of protein synthesis just prior to an S-phase specific agent (84); (c) administration of ara-C as a single injection, which reversibly and transiently suppresses bone marrow DNA synthesis, just prior to cytotoxic therapy with a short duration of action (e.g. nitrogen mustard, nitrosourea); and (d) administration of a large dose of glucocorticoid (to inhibit G_1-S transition) just prior to S-phase specific therapy. With all of these approaches, it will be critical to measure the effect on coexistent tumor cells as well; inhibition of their proliferation might negate any possible therapeutic advantage.

A second, corollary hypothesis involves maximization of bone marrow proliferation after chemotherapy, to speed recovery and allow for more intensive treatment of the tumor. This could involve (a) lithium administration (85), (b) *Corynebac-*

terium parvum (86) or other immunostimulants, (*c*) administration of stored autologous serum containing a high concentration of colony-forming units (e.g. as obtained after a previous course of myelosuppressive therapy), and (*d*) autologous marrow reinfusion (87).

Third, one may attempt hormonal or other "physiologic" stimulation of tumor growth to increase sensitivity to chemotherapy. Historically, this is illustrated by the administration of testosterone prior to radioactive phosphorus systemically, in patients with prostatic carcinoma. Experimental tumor work with organ cultures from rat mammary tumors (88) suggests that prolactin stimulates DNA synthesis in hormone-dependent but not in autonomous tissue. In addition, Kiang et al (89) have demonstrated stimulation of the DMBA-induced rat mammary tumor by low dose estrogen therapy. The provision of specific metabolites (e.g. asparagine) is another possible avenue of approach, in tumors whose dependency can be identified. Burke et al (90) studied sera containing a stimulator of leukemic and normal bone marrow cell DNA synthesis, the levels of which were maximal 9 days after administration of a massive dose (75 mg/kg) of cyclophosphamide, and suggested possible therapeutic usefulness of these growth regulators.

Young et al (91, 92) have shown that, in sensitive tumor systems, DNA synthesis is depressed in both tumor and normal tissues, but there is rapid recovery and overshoot, followed by a return to baseline values, in proliferation of the normal bone marrow and GI mucosa, with much slower recovery in DNA synthesis of the tumor. When resistance develops, this differential pattern of recovery is lost (68). This type of approach deserves application to more appropriate scheduling of chemotherapeutic agents in clinical trials, and may also indicate when relapse is imminent, in patients with serially accessible disease.

Finally, approaches toward *selective* kill of nonproliferating tumor cells can be explored and tested with appropriate measurements of kinetic parameters. They might include immunotherapy (to which S-phase cells appear most resistant) (93) or use of agents with selective toxicity toward hypoxic cells (94). In this setting one might expect to see an *increase* in the growth fraction of residual viable cells as an indicator of response.

Literature Cited

1. Mendelsohn, M. L. 1975. The cell cycle in malignant and normal tissues. In *The Cell Cycle in Malignancy and Immunity*, pp. 293–314. Springfield, Va.: Natl. Tech. Inf. Serv., US Dep. Commerce
2. Killmann, S. A. 1972. Kinetics of leukemic blast cells. *Clin. Hematol.* 1:95–113
3. Sky-Peck, H. H. 1971. Effects of chemotherapy on the incorporation of ^{3}H-thymidine into DNA of human neoplastic tissue. *Natl. Cancer Inst. Monogr.* 34:197–205
4. Dethlefsen, L. A., Ohlsen, J. D., Roti Roti, J. L. 1976. Cell synchronization in vivo: Fact or fancy? In *Growth Kinetics and Biochemical Regulation of Normal and Malignant Cells*, Houston: M. D. Anderson Hosp. Tumor Inst. In press
5. Gibson, M. H., Bertalanffy, F. D. 1972. In vivo synchrony of solid B_{16} melanoma by sytosine arabinoside, an inhibitor of DNA synthesis. *J. Natl. Cancer Inst.* 49:1007–18
6. Frei, E. III, Whang, J., Scoggins, R., Van Scott, E., Rall, D., Ben, M. 1964. The stathmokinetic effect of vincristine. *Cancer Res.* 24:1918–25

7. Klein, H. O., Lennartz, K., Gross, R., Eder, M., Fischer, R. 1972. In vivo and in vitro studies on cell kinetics and synchronization of human tumor: Their significance in tumor chemotherapy. *Dtsch. Med. Wochenschr.* 97:1273–78

8. Laster, W. R., Mayo, J. G., Simpson-Herren, L., Griswold, D. P., Lloyd, H. H., Schabel, F. M. Jr., Skipper, H. E. 1969. Success and failure in the treatment of solid tumors. II. Kinetic parameters and "cell cure" of moderately advanced carcinoma 755. *Cancer Chemother. Rep.* 53:169–88

9. Schenken, L. L., Hagemann, R. F. 1976. Recruitment oncotherapy schedules for enhanced efficacy of cycle active agents. *Proc. Am. Assoc. Cancer Res.– Am. Soc. Clin. Oncol.* 17:88

10. Griswold, D. P., Simpson-Herren, L., Schabel, F. M. Jr. 1970. Altered sensitivity of a hamster plasmacytoma to cytosine arabinoside. *Cancer Chemother. Rep.* 54:337–46

11. Maruyama, J., Lee, T. C., McMillin, R. D. 1975. Tumor age cohort variation and sensitivity to DNA synthesis directed chemotherapy. See Ref. 1, pp. 239–56

12. Schabel, F. M. Jr. 1969. The use of tumor growth kinetics in planning "curative" chemotherapy of advanced solid tumors. *Cancer Res.* 29:2384–89

13. Valeriote, F. 1976. Cell cycle dependency and scheduling of drugs. See Ref. 4

14. Capizzi, R., Summers, W., Bertino, J. 1971. L-asparaginase induced alteration of amethopterin (methotrexate) activity in mouse leukemia L5178Y. *Ann. NY Acad. Sci.* 186:302–11

15. Chlopkiewicz, B., Koziorowska, J. 1975. Role of amino acid depletion in combined treatment of neoplastic cells with methotrexate and L-asparaginase. *Cancer Res.* 35:1524–29

16. Ganzer, U., Nitze, H. 1970. Die strahlenbehandlung synchronissierter hauttumoren der maus. *Strahlentherapie* 140:711–16

17. Lampkin, B., Nagao, T., Mauer, A. 1971. Synchronization and recruitment in acute leukemia. *J. Clin. Invest.* 50:2204–14

18. Lampkin, B., McWilliams, N., Mauer, A., Flessa, H., Hake, D., Fisher, V. 1974. Manipulation of the mitotic cycle in treatment of acute myeloblastic leukemia. *Abstr. 17th Ann. Meet. Am. Soc. Hematol.*, p. 70

19. Ernst, P., Faille, A., Killmann, S-A. 1973. Perturbation of cell cycle of human leukaemic myeloblast in vivo by cytosine arabinoside. *Scand. J. Haematol.* 10:209–18

20. Kremer, W., Vogler, W., Chan, Y.-K. 1976. An attempt at synchronization of marrow cells in acute leukemia. *Cancer* 37:390–403

21. MacKinney, A., Flynn, B. 1976. Synchronization and recruitment in the treatment of adult acute leukemia. *Clin. Res.* 24:378

22. Buchner, T., Barlogie, B., Assesburg, U., Hiddemann, W., Kamanabroo, D., Gohde, W. 1974. Accumulation of S-phase cells in the bone marrow of patients with acute leukemia by cytosine arabinoside. *Blut* 28:299–300

23. Barlogie, B., Drewinko, B., Johnston, D., Buchner, T., Hauss, W., Freireich, E. 1976. Pulse cytophotometric analysis of synchronized cells in vitro. *Cancer Res.* 36:1176–81

24. Capizzi, R. 1974. Biochemical interaction between asparaginase and methotrexate in leukemia cells. See Ref. 9, 15:77

25. Marshall, G. J., Bateman, J., Gourlie, B. 1971. The effect of pulse intravenous prednisolone on marrow cell incorporation of thymidine-C-14 and deoxyuridine-C-14. *Abstr. Am. Soc. Clin. Oncol.* 8:38

26. Ernst, P., Killmann, S-A. 1970. Perturbation of generation cycle of human leukemic blast cells by cytostatic therapy in vivo: Effect of corticosteroids. *Blood* 36:689–96

27. Barranco, S., Luce, J., Romsdahl, M., Humphrey, R. 1973. Bleomycin as a possible synchronizing agent for human tumor cells in vivo. *Cancer Res.* 33:882–87

28. Costanzi, J. 1976. Bleomycin infusion as a potential synchronizing agent in carcinoma of the head and neck. See Ref. 9, 17:11

29. Samuels, M., Boyle, L., Holoye, P., Johnson, D. 1976. Intermittent vs. continuous infusion bleomycin in testicular cancer. See Ref. 9, 17:98

30. Livingston, R., Bodey, J., Gottlieb, J., Frei, E. III. 1973. Kinetic scheduling of vincristine and bleomycin in patients with lung cancer and other malignant tumors. *Cancer Chemother. Rep.* 57:219–24

31. Livingston, R., Einhorn, L., Bodey, G. Burgess, M., Freireich, E., Gottlieb, J. 1975. COMB: A four-drug combination in solid tumors. *Cancer* 36:327–32

32. Livingston, R., Fee, W., Einhorn, L., Burgess, M., Freireich, E., Gottlieb, J., Farber, M. 1976. BACON (Bleomycin, adriamycin, CCNU, Oncovin and Nitrogen Mustard) in Squamous Lung Cancer. *Cancer* 37:1237–42

33. Baker, L., Opipari, M., Izbicki, R. 1975. Mitomycin-C, vincristine and bleomycin combination therapy in treatment of disseminated cervical carcinoma. See Ref. 9, 16:35

34. Burgess, M., Einhorn, L., Gottlieb, J. 1975. Treatment of metastatic germ cell tumors with adriamycin, vincristine, and bleomycin. See Ref. 9, 16:244

35. Einhorn, L., Furnas, B., Powell, N. 1976. Combination chemotherapy of disseminated testicular carcinoma with cis-platinum, vinblastine and bleomycin. See Ref. 9, 17:240

36. Wheeler, W., Thirlwell, M. 1975. Sequential cytosine arabinoside and methotrexate in solid tumors. See Ref. 9, 16:237

37. Burke, P., Owens, A. 1971. Attempted recruitment of leukemic myeloblasts to proliferative activity by sequential drug treatment. *Cancer* 28:830–36

38. Salmon, S. 1976. Kinetics and chemotherapy of multiple myeloma. See Ref. 4

39. Salmon, S. 1975. Expansion of the growth fraction in multiple myeloma with alkylating agents. *Blood* 45:119–29

40. Hayes, A., Green, A., Mauer, A. 1976. Cell kinetic studies in children with neuroblastoma. See Ref. 9, 17:121

41. Eagan, R., Mauer, L., Forcier, R., Tulloh, M. 1973. Combination chemotherapy and radiation therapy in small cell carcinoma of the lung. *Cancer* 32:371–79

42. Straus, M. 1976. A design for combination chemotherapy in lung cancer with increased survival. See Ref. 9, 17:239

43. Pouillart, P., Mathe, G., Schwarzenberg, L. 1973. Essai de recrutement cellulaire par synchronisation partielle pour l'establishment d'une combinaison chimiotherapique. *Bull. Cancer* 60:187–90

44. Pouillart, P., Schwarzenberg, G., Amiel, J., Mathe, G., Huguenin, P., Morin, P., Baron, A., Laparre, C., Parrot, R. 1975. Combinaisons chimiotherapiques de drogues se potentialisant. *Nouv. Presse Med.* 4:10, 717–19

45. Pouillart, P., Huong, T., Brugerie, E., Lheritier, J. 1974. Sequential administration of two oncostatic drugs: Study of modalities for pharmacodynamic potentiation. *Biomedicine* 21:471–79

46. Rentschler, R., Livingston, R., Mountian, C. 1976. Methotrexate and asparaginase in drug-refractory human tumors. See Ref. 9, 17:152

47. Hart, J., George, S., Freireich, E., Bodey, G., Nickerson, R., Frei, E. III. 1976. Prognostic significance of pretreatment proliferative activity in adult acute leukemia. *Cancer.* In press

48. Hillen, H., Haanen, C., Wessels, J. 1975. Bone marrow proliferation patterns in acute myeloblastic leukemia determined by pulse cytophotometry. *Lancet* 1:609–11

49. Vogler, W., Cooper, L., Groth, D. 1971. Correlation of cytosine arabinoside induced increment in growth fraction of leukemic cells with clinical response. *Cancer* 33:603–10

50. Vogler, W., Groth, D., Garwood, F. A. 1975. Cell kinetics in acute leukemia. *Arch. Intern. Med.* 135:950–54

51. Raich, P. 1975. In vitro prediction of therapeutic response in acute leukemia. See Ref. 9, 17:182

52. Arlin, Z., Gee, T., Dowling, M., Campbell, J., Clarkson, B. 1976. Significance of pulse ^{3}H-thymidine labeling index in adult acute myeloid leukemia. See Ref. 9, 17:296

53. Nelson, J. A., Carpenter, J., Rose, L., Adamson, D. 1975. Mechanisms of action of 6-thioguanine, 6-mercaptopurine and 8-azaguanine. *Cancer Res.* 35:2872–78

54. Crowther, D., Beard, M., Bateman, C., Sewell, R. 1975. Factors influencing prognosis in adults with acute myelogenous leukaemia. *Br. J. Cancer* 32:456–63

55. Mauer, A., Murphy, S., Hayes, F. 1976. Scheduling and recruitment in leukemic populations. See Ref. 4

56. Sulkes, A., Livingston, R., Taylor, R. 1976. Pre-treatment labeling index in breast carcinoma patients as a predictor of response to combination chemotherapy. See Ref. 9, 17:59

57. Kofman, S., Sky-Peck, H., Perlia, C., Economou, S., Winzler, R., Taylor, S. 1960. A correlation between the incorporation of formate-C^{14} in tumors and the clinical course of patients with disseminated breast cancer. *Cancer* 13:425–31

58. Thirlwell, M., Mansell, P. 1976. A correlation of clinical response with in vitro pre-chemotherapy labeling index in human solid tumors. See Ref. 9, 17:307

59. Livingston, R., Sulkes, A., Thirlwell, M., Murphy, W., Hart, J. 1976. Cell kinetic parameters: correlation with clinical response. See Ref. 4
60. Skipper, H. 1971. Kinetic behavior versus response to chemotherapy. *Natl. Cancer Inst. Monogr.* 34:2–14
61. Wolberg, W., Ansfield, F. 1971. The relation of thymidine labeling index in human tumors in vitro to the effectiveness of S-fluorouracil chemotherapy. *Cancer Res.* 31:448–50
62. Hall, T. 1971. Limited role of cell kinetics in clinical cancer chemotherapy. *Natl. Cancer Inst. Monogr.* 34:15–19
63. McGuire, W. L., Pearson. W., Segaloff, A. 1975. Predicting hormone responsiveness in human breast cancer. In *Estrogen Receptors in Human Breast Cancer*, pp. 17–30. New York: Raven
64. Livingston, R., Ambus, U., George, S., Freireich, E., Hart, J. 1974. In vitro determination of thymidine-^{3}H labeling index in human solid tumors. *Cancer Res.* 34:1376–80
65. Murphy, W., Livingston, R., Ruiz, V., Gercovich, F., George, S., Hart, J., Freireich, E. 1975. Serial labeling index determination as a predictor of response in human solid tumors. *Cancer Res.* 35:1438–44
66. Wheeler, G., Alexander, J. 1964. Studies with mustards. IV. Effects of alkylating agents upon nucleic acid synthesis in bilaterally grown sensitive and resistant tumors. *Cancer Res.* 24:1338–46
67. Wheeler, G., Alexander, J. 1969. Effects of nitrogen mustard and cyclophosphamide upon the synthesis of DNA in vivo and in cell-free preparations. *Cancer Res.* 29:98–109
68. Brereton, H., Bryant, T., Young, R. 1975. Inhibition and recovery of DNA synthesis in host tissues and sensitive and resistant B_{16} melanoma after 1-(2-chloroethyl)-3-(*trans*-4-methylcychlohexyl)-1-nitrosourea, a predictor of therapeutic efficacy. *Cancer Res.* 35:2420–25
69. Tubiana, M., Guichard, M., Malaise, E. 1976. Kinetic determinants in radiotherapy. See Ref. 4
70. Breitenecker, G., Tatra, G. 1973. Histological and autoradiographical investigations during radiotherapy of carcinoma of the cervix. *Strahlentherapie* 146:664–70
71. Cline, M. 1969. In vitro test systems for anticancer drugs. *N. Engl. J. Med.* 280:955

72. Zittoun, R., Bouchard, M., Facquet-Davis, J., Percie-du-Sert, M., Bousser, J. 1975. Prediction of the response to chemotherapy in acute leukemia. *Cancer* 35:507–13
73. Lippmann, M., Halterman, R., Leventhal, G., Perry, S., Thompson, E. B. 1973. Glucocorticoid-binding proteins in human acute lymphoblastic leukemic cells. *J. Clin. Invest.* 52:1715–25
74. Dunlap, S. G. 1965. The serum dilution bactericidal test for antibiotic effectiveness. *Am. J. Med. Technol.* 31:69
75. Kline, K., Gang, M., Wodinsky, I. 1968. Duration of drug levels in mice as indicated by residual antileukemic efficacy. *Chemotherapy* 13:28–41
76. Burns, C., Armentrout, S., Stjernholm, R. 1972. Prediction of the response of patients with acute nonlymphocytic leukemia to cytosine arabinoside therapy. *Cancer Chemother. Rep.* 56:527–34
77. Volm, M., Mattern, J., Wayss, K. 1974. The effects of cytostatic drugs on transplanted tumors. An investigation of the correlation between in vivo and in vitro results. *Arch. Geschwulstforsch.* 43:137–44
78. Wayss, K., Mattern, J., Volm, M. 1975. Correlation of in vitro testing and therapeutic results after cytostatic treatment of animals with transplanted tumors. *Arzneim. Forsch.* 25:77–81
79. Thirlwell, M., Livingston, R., Murphy, W., Hart, J. 1976. A rapid in vitro labeling index method for predicting response of human solid tumours to chemotherapy. *Cancer Res.* In press
80. Nordqvist, S. R. 1974. In vitro effects of progestins on DNA synthesis in metastatic endometrial carcinoma. *Gynecol. Oncol.* 2:415–28
81. Burstein, N., Carey, R. 1974. In vitro assay for human breast cancer hormone responsiveness. *Oncology* 29:470–83
82. Hart, R. 1966. A strategy for curing cancer. *Cancer Chemother. Rep.* 50:295–96
83. Copeland, E., MacFadyen, B., Lanzotti, V., Dudrick, S. 1975. Intravenous hyperalimentation as an adjunct to cancer chemotherapy. *Am. J. Surg.* 129:167–72
84. Ben-Ishay, Z., Farber, E. 1975. Protective effects of an inhibitor of protein synthesis, cycloheximide, on bone marrow damage induced by cytosine arabinoside or nitrogen mustard. *Lab. Invest.* 32:478–90

85. Tisman, G., Herbert, V., Rosenblatt, S. 1973. Evidence that lithium induces human granulocyte proliferation. Elevated serum vitamin B_{12} binding capacity in vitro and granulocyte colony proliferative in vitro. *Br. J. Haematol.* 24: 767–71

86. Dimitrov, N., Singh, T., Cornoy, J., Suhrland, G. 1976. Combination therapy with C. parvum and adriamycin in patients with lung carcinoma. See Ref. 9, 17:292

87. Tobias, J., Tattersall, M. 1976. Perspectives in cancer research. Autologous marrow support and intensive chemotherapy in cancer patients. *Eur. J. Cancer* 12:1–8

88. Takizawa, S., Furth, J., Furth, J. 1970. DNA synthesis in autonomous and hormone-responsive mammary tumors. *Cancer Res.* 30:206–10

89. Kiang, D., Kennedy, B. 1971. Combination of cyclophosphamide and estrogen therapy in DMBA-induced rat mammary cancer. *Cancer* 28:1202–10

90. Burke, P., Karp, J., Owens, A. 1974. A timed sequential therapy based upon responsiveness of leukemic cells to normal serum growth regulators. *Abstr. 17th Ann. Meet. Am. Soc. Hematol.,* p. 152

91. Rosenoff, S., Bull, J., Young, R. 1975. The effect of chemotherapy on the kinetics and proliferative capacity of normal and tumorous tissues in vivo. *Blood* 45:107–18

92. Rosenoff, S., Bostick, F., Young, R. 1975. Recovery of normal hematopoietic tissue and tumor following chemotherapeutic injury from cyclophosphamide. *Blood* 45:465–75

93. Shipley, W. 1971. Immune cytolysis in relation to the growth cycle of Chinese hamster cells. *Cancer Res.* 31:925–29

94. Urtasun, R., Band, P., Chapman, J., Feldstein, M., Mielke, B., Fryer, C. 1976. Radiation and high-dose metronidazole in supratentorial glioblastomas. *N. Engl. J. Med.* 294:1364–67

Ann. Rev. Pharmacol. Toxicol. 1977. 17:545–59

PSYCHOPHARMACOLOGICAL   ❖6695
IMPLICATIONS OF DOPAMINE
AND DOPAMINE ANTAGONISTS:
A CRITICAL EVALUATION
OF CURRENT EVIDENCE

Oleh Hornykiewicz[1]

Department of Psychopharmacology, Clarke Institute of Psychiatry and Department of
Pharmacology, University of Toronto, Toronto, Canada M5T 1R8

Theories which combine correct and false facts are more dangerous to science than
complete errors; and hypotheses which are only "justified in a certain sense" always create
confusion because the necessary reservations cannot always be stated. Clearcut concepts
can only be formed if we ruthlessly reject everything that does not belong to them,
regardless of whether we are dealing with simple problems or with entire theories.

                                             Eugen Bleuler (1)

INTRODUCTION

The unusual attention that brain dopamine (DA) has received in the 20 years since
its identification in the mammalian brain (2) is due mainly to two factors: (*a*) the
discovery that in Parkinson's disease there is a specific deficit of nigro-striatal DA
(3) [this discovery formed the basis for the successful application of DAs precursor
L-DOPA in the treatment of Parkinson's disease (4–6)]; and (*b*) evidence implicating brain DA in psychotic disorders, especially the schizophrenic syndrome.

   Whereas the role of the nigro-striatal DA in the pathophysiology, symptomatology, and treatment of Parkinson's disease can be regarded as established (7,
8), the evidence implicating brain DA in psychotic disorders is mainly pharmacological, that is to say, indirect in nature; therefore, it has to be considered at present
as largely hypothetical.

[1]Present address: Institute of Biochemical Pharmacology, University of Vienna, A-1090
Vienna, Austria.

                                             545

Since several excellent recent reviews dealing with the role of DA in psychotic disorders, especially schizophrenia, are available (9–11), the purpose of this essay is to examine critically only the most crucial evidence and, where possible, to introduce new elements into the discussion of this complex research field. Taking into account the nature of the available evidence, the discussion concentrates on the following points: (*a*) the possible relationship between the special distribution pattern of brain DA and the anatomical substrate(s) of disturbed behavior; (*b*) the possible anatomical substrates of the schizophrenic disorders; and (*c*) the relationship between drugs mimicking or blocking DA effects respectively, their possible mechanisms of action, and their effects in patients suffering from the schizophrenic disorders.

BRAIN DA AND THE NEUROPATHOLOGY OF BEHAVIOR

There are three major DA neuron systems in the mammalian brain [for review and references cf (12)]. These are (*a*) the nigro-striatal system, which originates in the (melanin-containing) neurons of the compact zone of the substantia nigra and terminates diffusely in the caudate nucleus and putamen (the corpus striatum or striatum), and probably also in the nucleus accumbens (13); (*b*) the mesolimbic system, which originates in the ventromedial tegmentum of the mesencephalon just dorsal and lateral to the interpeduncular nucleus (area A10 of Dahlström and Fuxe, nucleus paranigralis in the human brain) and projects to the nucleus accumbens, olfactory tubercle, and the central amygdaloid nucleus [recently, a projection system probably originating in area A10 has been described as terminating in several limbic cortical regions (14–16)]; (*c*) a system consisting of short neurons, arising mainly in the anterior part of the arcuate nucleus of the hypothalamus and terminating in the external layer of the median eminence (the tubero-infundibular DA system).

There is evidence from animal experiments to show that each of these three DA systems may be involved in a variety of behavioral reactions which, by way of analogy, may be assumed to have some relevance to the behavioral disturbances seen in psychotic patients.

Over the past ten years a great deal of information has accumulated related to the role of the subcortical DA systems in the functioning of the basal ganglia (mainly corpus striatum) as well as certain structures belonging to the limbic forebrain (cf 17). The majority of these studies deals with the behavioral pharmacology of the corresponding DA systems. In this respect, it is important to stress that despite many attempts, at present the work on the role of the subcortical DA in behavior does not seem to permit a clear-cut functional distinction to be made between the striatal and the limbic DA systems. On the whole, the results of the pertinent studies suggest that the role of the subcortical structures such as the striatal complex, the nucleus accumbens, and the olfactory regions, in the elaboration of patterns of locomotor as well as stereotyped behavior is critically dependent on the intactness of their dopaminergic innervation. Similarly, various forms of conditioned avoidance behavior have been shown to depend predominantly on the activity of these dopaminergic forebrain systems. [For comprehensive review and references, cf (17).]

Recent experimental evidence also suggests that the subcortical dopaminergic systems may be critically involved in reward-seeking behavior (18) as well as mechanisms controlling memory consolidation and retention (19). The role of the recently described mesocortical (limbic) DA system has not yet been established. There is, however, preliminary evidence suggesting that this system may participate in responses of the central nervous system to stress because it seems to react to stressful procedures much more sensitively than the coritcal norepinephrine or any of the subcortical monoamine systems do (20).

The relation of the median eminence DA to behavior is suggested by the finding that, on one hand, this DA system takes part in the control of secretion of hypophyseal hormones (especially prolactin and luteinizing hormone) (cf 21); on the other hand, hypophyseal hormones recently have been postulated to exert significant actions on several behavioral parameters (22). However, details as to the behavioral consequences of disturbed functioning of the median eminence DA have not yet been worked out.

The above observations in laboratory animals on the role of brain DA in behavior furnished the basis for the notion that, by analogy, at least certain behavioral abnormalities that regularly recur in psychotic patients may in fact be related to a disturbed functioning of brain DA systems. It is obvious, however, that the question as to a possible involvement of brain DA in psychiatric disorders, particularly schizophrenia, is ultimately nothing less than the repeatedly posed question as to the neuroanatomical substrate of these disorders.

NEUROANATOMICAL SUBSTRATES OF THE SCHIZOPHRENIC DISORDER

The question whether the schizophrenic condition has an underlying cerebral neuropathology has as yet remained unanswered. At the beginning of this century, Eugen Bleuler expressed the view (1) that "complete justice to all these factors (i.e. in schizophrenia) can only be done by a concept of the disease which assumes the presence of (anatomical or chemical) disturbances of the brain." As the primary disturbance in schizophrenia Bleuler saw a disturbance of "association" and "tension." Bleuler seems to have favored a rather widespread disturbance mainly at the neocortical level since he firmly rejected all "focal" hypotheses such as those of Kleist or Wernicke as well as Berze's suggestion of a lowered or defect "energy flow" to the cortex from subcortical structures (cf 23). A detailed discussion of the various hypotheses related to a possible neuropathology of mental illness is outside the scope of this article. It is, however, relevant in this context to note that, more recently, dysfunction of two of the most important DA-rich brain parts, namely the corpus striatum and the limbic system, has been discussed in relation to a possible pathophysiology of psychotic disturbances.

Corpus Striatum and the Schizophrenic Disturbance

In 1955, Mettler (24) proposed the hypothesis that in schizophrenia there might exist a disturbed function of the striatum. He based his hypothesis on observations obtained in experimental animals showing that lesions of the striatum produced a form of physiological deficit which included, as one of its principal features, a disorder of perception. Specifically, Mettler (25–27) observed in cats with striatal lesions (which were added to a frontal cortex removal) a profoundly vacuous appearance of the animals; a visual, auditory, and labyrinthine disregard; paucity of eye movements; failure to react adaptively to situations and objects in the field of vision as well as a tendency to push forward into objects and fall down declivities. Furthermore, the animals displayed a great deal of stimulus binding (for example, they tended to follow rigidly moving objects placed directly before their eyes), cursive and essential hyperkinesias, pushing, leaping, resistance to superimposed postures, and passive movement. Also, cats with large, bilateral striatal lesions lost their ability to perform as well as to relearn tasks previously learned (28).

From these observations Mettler concluded that the striatum may be importantly involved in the organism's ability to relate itself to its environment by coordinating the shifting of attention from one source of sensory input to another. These "monitoring comparisons" of the striatum Mettler conceived of as necessary in order to maintain contact with, and make an adequate interpretation of, the source of exogenous stimuli, as well as to reinforce memory and sustain an adequate level of intellectuality. Since according to Mettler the striatum also supresses the thalamo-pallidal circuits concerned with deep afferents and vision, its overall role was to free the organism from proprioceptive dominance, thus putting it in a position to react to alternative stimulus configuration, that is, to make choices. Mettler proposed that the primary defect in schizophrenia may consist of an analogous disturbance of perception, that is, inability to shift attention from one source of sensory input to another, caused by a dysfunction of the striatal nuclei.

While Mettler's concept has to be regarded as highly speculative, recent work on the role of the caudate nucleus in complex behavior seems to furnish a certain degree of experimental basis for such a possibility. Thus, it has been convincingly demonstrated [for review and references, see (20)] that localized lesions of the caudate nucleus result in disturbances of such complex behaviors as retention of delayed responses and delayed alternation, spatial reversal, visual and auditory "go–no go" discrimination, delayed successive discrimination, object reversal, as well as bar pressing extinction, and various activity measures. Most importantly, however, the existence of a functional relation between the caudate nucleus and the prefrontal cortex has been demonstrated (cf 29); thus, lesions of the prefrontal cortex produce analogous disturbances of complex behavior like those produced by caudate lesions (see above). In the light of these experimental findings, it is conceivable that a disturbed relationship between the prefrontal cortex and the corpus striatum may produce complex behavior disturbances not dissimilar to those seen in psychotic patients.

Limbic System and the Schizophrenic Disturbance

Recently, attention has been drawn to a possible involvement of the brain's limbic system in at least some forms of schizophrenia [for review, cf (30)]. The notion that the limbic forebrain system may be relevant to psychic functions can be traced back to the concept, proposed by Papez (31) in 1937, that this forebrain system may "constitute a harmonious mechanism which may elaborate the functions of central emotion, as well as participate in emotional expression." From the anatomical point of view the limbic system, like the striatum, is unique insofar as it is mainly interconnected with the reticular formation of the fore- and midbrain, to which it sends and from which it receives all of its noncortical connections. (The connections with the thalamoneocortical apparatus are phylogenetically a more recent addition.) In particular, the strong connections between the limbic system and the hypothalamus suggest that the functional state of the latter is inseparably related to the patterns of neuronal activity in the limbic-reticular formation system as a whole (32).

In his fundamental work on the limbic system, MacLean (33, 34) has appropriately pointed out that the anatomical situation of the limbic system within the forebrain is such as to enable it to correlate and integrate every form of internal and external perception. On the experimental level, a great number of studies have convincingly demonstrated that laboratory animals with experimentally induced damage to the limbic forebrain structures exhibit a series of disturbances such as inappropriate behavior, changes in sexual drives as well as changes in emotion and affect, and impairment in the ability to screen out multiple visual stimuli [for references, see (30)]. In the light of this experimental evidence it is interesting to note that some of the early symptoms in patients with schizophrenia seem to correlate with functions of the limbic system. Specifically, disturbance of visual perception, namely, difficulty in synthesizing the incoming visual stimuli into a whole picture, has been suggested as representing a common early symptom of the disease (35). In addition, studies with implanted recording electrodes have detected electrical abnormalities specifically from limbic structures in schizophrenic patients (cf 30). Finally a relationship between the limbic system and the schizophrenic disturbance seems to be suggested by observations showing that cases with known limbic system pathology—such as temporal lobe epilepsy, as well as encephalitis and brain tumors involving limbic structures—frequently occur with schizophrenia-like symptoms (30).

In connection with the above concepts implicating the corpus striatum and the limbic system respectively, in the pathophysiology of psychotic disorders, it is important to stress that these concepts are by no means mutually exclusive. As Nauta (32) has pointed out, despite their differing anatomical structure and functional significance, the corpus striatum and the limbic forebrain system have a very important characteristic in common: they both are virtually devoid of afferent fibers from the phylogenetically more recent lemniscus systems, receiving a large part of their afferent systems directly from the reticular formation of the brain stem. Thus, Nauta visualizes the striatum and the limbic forebrain system as representing jointly the brain's "analyzer-integrator system of the second order," being interposed between the first and third order analyzer-integrator systems of the brain stem reticular formation and the thalamoneocortical apparatus respectively. The possible interrelation between the striatum and the limbic forebrain system is further underlined by the mentioned difficulty in distinguishing neurochemically and neuropharmacologically between the functional roles played by the dopaminergic systems innervating these two structures. A good example in point is afforded by the limbic area of the nucleus accumbens whose morphology as well as neurochemistry makes it in many respects nearly indistinguishable from the striatal nuclei (cf 36).

BRAIN DOPAMINE AND SCHIZOPHRENIA

The hypotheses relating the striatum and/or limbic forebrain structures with the pathophysiology of the schizophrenic disorder have provided for an obvious link between this psychotic condition and brain DA which, as discussed above, plays an important role in the functioning of these two brain regions. However, judged merely on the basis of the anatomical-functional evidence, the relation between schizophrenia and brain DA is by no means compelling. Both the striatum and the limbic structures are rich in several other important neurohumoral factors such as acetylcholine, serotonin, norepinephrine, γ-aminobutyric acid, and substance P; each of these could play an important role in normal and disturbed functioning of these brain regions. That the DA hypothesis has attracted special attention is due mainly to a number of significant pharmacological as well as pharmacological-clinical observations that favor this particular thesis. In this respect, two observations are of special importance: (a) amphetamine's action on brain DA in relation to the drug's ability to induce a psychotic state in man; and (b) the psychotherapeutic (antischizophrenic) activity of neuroleptics that have been found to possess strong DA antagonist properties.

Amphetamine Psychosis

A psychotic state, the so-called amphetamine psychosis (37), frequently develops in subjects taking amphetamine chronically. Occasionally the amphetamine psychosis may also be precipitated with a large single dose of the drug. This toxic state presents features quite similar to ("indistinguishable" from) those seen especially in paranoid schizophrenia (37–39). Amphetamine is know to release DA from its storage sites in the nerve terminals as well as to prevent its inactivation by synaptic re-uptake [for reviews, see (40)]. Thus, the idea appears attractive (41, 42) that the psychotic state produced by amphetamine abuse may be related to a dopaminergic overstimulation taking place in the DA-rich brain regions, especially the striatum and/or the limbic system regions. This possibility seems supported by clinical experience showing that both amphetamine as well as other drugs known to act on brain DA, such as L-DOPA, and several amphetamine-like compounds (e.g. methylphenidate), will produce an exacerbation of the schizophrenic symptomatology in diseased patients (43–45).

Besides its effect on brain DA, amphetamine is known to act in an analogous manner on brain norepinephrine (i.e. increased release, inhibition of re-uptake) [for reviews and references, see (40)]. Thus, the alternate possibility has to be considered that the psychotic state produced by amphetamine in man may be due to the drug's effect on brain NA mechanisms rather than brain DA or that both DA and NA are important in this respect. To resolve this dilemma, the D- and L-isomers of amphetamine have been utilized. However, the results of the corresponding studies produced confusion rather than clarification of this issue (cf 45). There seems to exist agreement regarding the observations that in inducing the psychotic state in healthy volunteers as well as exacerbating the schizophrenic symptomatology in diseased patients D- and L-amphetamine are nearly equipotent; also, both isomers seem to be nearly equipotent in inducing stereotyped behavior in laboratory animals. [This has led to the concept that the animal model of amphetamine-induced stereotypy is analogous to the amphetamine psychosis in man, representing, by inference, a model of the behavioral disturbance in schizophrenia (cf 42)].

When the amphetamine isomers were compared as to their relative potency in inhibiting the synaptosomal uptake of DA (in striatal homogenates) and NA (in homogenates of the cortex), Coyle & Snyder (46) found that both isomers were about equipotent on DA uptake; on the NA uptake D-amphetamine was ten times more potent than the L-isomer. From this the authors concluded that the psychotogenic activity of amphetamine (as well as its ability to induce stereotypies in animals) was due to an action on brain DA. In contrast to Coyle & Snyder, however, three other research groups (47–49) found that D-amphetamine was about equipotent with the L-isomer in inhibiting NA uptake (cortex) and four to five times more potent than the latter in inhibiting the striatal DA uptake. Thus, in contradistinction to Snyder's data, these data would seem to favor the opposite view, namely that rather than DA, brain NA may be involved in the amphetamine-induced psychotic disturbance. It is not even certain whether doses of amphetamine that produce all the typical behavioral effects in laboratory animals are high enough to inhibit DA or NA uptake in vivo; rather, in these (low) doses amphetamine probably has predominantly a releasing effect on the synaptically stored amines (cf 50). Likewise, it has been argued (51) that the observation that physostigmine attenuates the methylphenidate-induced psychosis but not the schizophrenic condition (52) may indicate that these two conditions are qualitatively different as to their neurochemical basis.

Although there is reason to assume that the amphetamine-induced stereotypy in laboratory animals—the animal model of amphetamine psychosis and, by inference, schizophrenia—is due to the drug's action on brain DA, it is difficult at present to decide on the precise anatomical substrate of this effect. Based on experiments with apomorphine it was suggested (53) that the DA in the limbic forebrain regions was closely related to stereotyped behavior. This was in agreement with the suggestion that several important features of amphetamine psychosis were limbic in origin (54). In contrast, recent evidence suggests that the striatal DA may be the substrate of the amphetamine stereotypy, with the limbic DA being primarily responsible in the amphetamine-induced locomotor activation (55). However, it has also been claimed that an intact striatum is not required for amphetamine to produce the typical stereotypies (56). Thus, even if the biochemical basis for the amphetamine-induced stereotyped behavior were assumed to reflect the biochemical disturbance in schizophrenia (an assumption that cannot be accepted at present without strong reservations), available experimental data would not allow a precise anatomical localization of such a hypothetical neurochemical disturbance.

In conclusion, although the animal model of amphetamine-induced stereotypy may represent a valid model of the amphetamine-induced psychosis in man, whether the latter represents a model of the schizophrenic dysfunction remains quite doubtful (57). Thus, conclusions drawn from the animal model cannot, at present, be applied directly to the problem of schizophrenia. This applies both to the biochemical as well as to the anatomical-localizational aspects of this psychotic disturbance.

Neuroleptic Drugs (DA Antagonists)

At present, the DA antagonist properties of antipsychotic drugs (i.e. the neuroleptics) probably represent the strongest argument in favor of an involvement of brain DA in schizophrenia.

With only a few exceptions, i.e. compounds with significant affinity for muscarinic receptors in the brain, such as thioridazine, clozapine, pimozide (58–60), neuroleptics of the phenothiazine and buytrophenone series in antipsychotic doses induce a parkinsonism-like syndrome in a large number of cases (cf 61). Since Parkinson's disease has been shown to be accompanied by a deficiency of DA in the nigro-striato-pallidal system (and nucleus accumbens) (3, 7, 8, 36), a relation between the parkinsonism-inducing activity of neuroleptics and a possible interference with brain DA systems suggested itself. In additon, since the relative potency of neuroleptics (with the exception of thioridazine, clozapine, pimozide; see above) for the induction of Parkinsonism correlates well with their antipsychotic activity (cf 61), involvement of brain DA in the antipsychotic effect of these drugs seemed possible.

The interference by neuroleptic drugs with brain DA mechanisms has been well established experimentally. The available evidence suggests at least three major possibilities: (*a*) blockade of the DA-sensitive adenylate cyclase, (*b*) blockade of the synaptic release of DA, and (*c*) blockade of DA receptors.

BLOCKADE OF THE DA-SENSITIVE ADENYLATE CYCLASE   The striatum as well as the dopaminergically innervated limbic forebrain structures (nucleus accumbens, olf^ctory tubercle) contain an adenylate cyclase that is specifically activated by DA (62,63). This DA-sensitive adenylate cyclase has been postulated to represent the immediate receptor molecule involved in the chain of events triggered by DA at the postsynaptic membrane, eventually resulting in a physiologic effect (62). Neuroleptics are, on the whole, strong inhibitors of the DA stimulation of the striatal and limbic adenylate cyclase. However, there seems to be a lack of a complete correlation between the inhibitory potency of the neuroleptics on the DA stimulation of this enzyme and their clinical potency in producing extrapyramidal effects (catalepsy in experimental animals, parkinsonism in man) as well as their antipsychotic activity (64). Specifically, the neuroleptically potent group of butyrophenones (e.g. haloperidol, pimozide) has proved conspicuously weak in blocking the DA effect on the enzyme (62, 62). Thus, at present, it is difficult to relate the antipsychotic activity of neuroleptics as a group with their ability to block the DA-sensitive adenylate cyclase in the DA-rich areas (striatum and/or limbic brain areas). Since neuroleptics inhibit both the striatal and limbic adenylate cyclase equally well, no conclusion can be reached as to the possible site of the drugs' antipsychotic activity.

BLOCKADE OF SYNAPTIC RELEASE OF DA   Recently, Seeman & Lee (65) provided evidence showing a striking correlation between the clinical potency of the neuroleptics (including the butyrophenones) and their ability to inhibit the stimulus-induced DA release in rat striatal slices. This action of neuroleptic compounds may be related to their well-known high efficacy in stabilizing cell membranes in general, with the brain DA neurons displaying a selective sensitivity in this respect. Thus the possibility exists that the blockade of the presynaptic coupling between nerve impulse and DA release may account for both the extrapyramidal and antipsychotic effects of all neuroleptic drugs presently available. It appears difficult, however, to reconcile this possibility with the finding obtained in vivo using the push-pull cannula technique showing that administration of neuroleptics produced an increase rather than decrease of DA release within striatal and limbic structures (66).

BLOCKADE OF DA RECEPTORS   It is reasonable to assume that in order to exert their specific (i.e. antipsychotic) actions, neuroleptics (like other drugs) have to bind in the brain to a specific site at which to exert the specific effect; this site can be called conveniently the *receptor site.* This logical proposition has prompted studies that have resulted in the demonstration that membrane fractions of brain homogenates possess "receptor binding" properties when labeled with (^{3}H)haloperidol (67, 68). Most significantly the order of affinity of a large series of neuroleptics for the (^{3}H)haloperidol binding sites (tested in preparations of calf striatal membranes) showed a highly significant correlation with the clinical (antipsychotic) potency of these drugs (69, 70). This strongly suggests that the sites in cell membranes that bind (^{3}H)haloperidol may indeed be the sites of the antipsychotic activity of the neuroleptic drugs. It is, however, important to note that the (^{3}H)haloperidol binding (as expressed in fmol/mg protein) was highest in the caudate nucleus, with the putamen and nucleus accumbens showing much lower levels; in fact, the latter two regions had values no higher than the globus pallidus (64). Thus, there seems to be little correspondence between the number of the (^{3}H)haloperidol binding sites and the density of DA terminals, the latter being (as judged from the DA levels) much higher in the putamen and nucleus accumbens (where the DA concentration is comparable to that in the caudate nucleus) than in the globus pallidus (cf 8). This poor correlation is further borne out by the observation that the order of affinity of neuroleptic drugs for (^{3}H)dopamine binding sites [tested under conditions analogous to those for (^{3}H)haloperidol binding] did not show any statistically significant correlation with the drugs' antipsychotic activity (69, 70).

The above observations would then suggest that although the clinical effect of neuroleptic drugs is produced, as would be expected, through an action on (probably) specific receptors in the brain, and these receptors may be identical with the haloperidol binding sites, the available evidence does not favor the hypothesis that the drugs' antipsychotic activity is due to brain DA receptor blockade.

ALTERNATE POSSIBILITY FOR THE MODE OF ACTION OF ANTIPSYCHOTIC DRUGS   Kornetsky (cf 57, 71, 72) has presented evidence showing that the core deficit in (at least some) schizophrenic patients involves an impairment in attention. This attentional deficit has been postulated to result from a dysfunction in those brain regions concerned with maintainence of arousal and attention, that is the brain stem reticular activating system. Thus, Kornetsky & Eliasson (72) have formulated the hypothesis that the schizophrenic patient is in a continuous state of central excitation or hyperarousal. Further, the authors proposed that the beneficial effect of neuroleptic drugs in schizophrenic patients is brought about by a suppression of the state of hyperarousal to levels consistent with optimum performance of the subject (57, 72). In this respect, the level of arousal may be related to the efficiency of performance (in experimental situations); maximum performance of which a subject is capable is usually attained with medium levels of arousal, with both under- or over-arousal eliciting poorer performance (cf "inverted U model") (73, 74).

Neuroleptic drugs have been known for a long time to inhibit effectively the behavioral as well as EEG arousal reaction produced by sensory stimulation in laboratory animals [for references see (75)]. A large body of electrophysiological evidence points to the reticular activating system of the brain stem as the site of action of this anti-arousal effect of the neuroleptic drugs. As to the mechanism(s) of the arousal-inhibiting effect of neuroleptics, the following possibilities have been considered in the literature (cf 75): (a) direct blocking effect on those mechanisms of the reticular formation that are responsible for the arousal reaction, (b) blockade of afferent impulses in the sensory collateral fibers to the brain stem reticular formation, and (c) facilitation of inhibitory "filtering" mechanisms of the reticular formation, resulting in a reduction of the sensory load reaching the cortex.

Irrespective of which of the above possibilities is given preference, the experimental neurophysiological results are consistent with Kornetsky's hypothesis that the therapeutic efficacy of neuroleptics may be due to their suppressing action on the reticular activating mechanisms. From a neurochemical point of view, it is interesting to note that the monoamine most frequently implicated as an important neurohumoral factor in the functioning of the reticular mechanisms is norepinephrine (cf 76, 77). Thus, it may be significant that, in addition to amphetamine and L-DOPA (that is, drugs that increase both dopaminergic and noradrenergic activity in the brain) tricyclic antidepressants have been observed to both activate anergic patients and exacerbate the schizophrenic symptomatology (78, 79); the latter drugs prevent the inactivation of norepinephrine (but not DA) by inhibiting its synaptic re-uptake, thereby potentiating noradrenergic effects [for reviews and references, see (40)]. Furthermore, neuroleptics, especially those of the phenothiazine series, have been known to exert antiadrenergic effects in the periphery (cf 75), and several of them have been shown to affect brain norepinephrine metabolism in a way analogous to that of brain DA (cf 80), thus suggesting a possible blockade of central norepinephrine receptors. However, the effectiveness of neuroleptics on brain norepinephrine metabolism (increase in synthesis rate) does not parallel their clinical antipsychotic potency nor do the α-adrenergic blockers (such as phenoxybenzamine or phentolamine) exert any known antischizophrenic activity. On the other hand, it is interesting to note that recently antischizophrenic activity has been claimed for propranolol (81; see also 82), a potent β-adrenergic receptor blocker. Also, the experimental data concerning the effect of neuroleptics on brain norepinephrine refer mostly to acute effects produced by single-dose administration whereas the antipsychotic effect in the schizophrenic patient typically is a function of an "irreducible minimum" of treatment time; that is to say, it is essentially chronic in nature. In this context it seems appropriate to mention the clinical observation (83) that the antipsychotic potency of neuroleptics can be increased by simultaneous administration of α-methyltyrosine, a drug known to inhibit synthesis of the catecholamines. This observation has often been quoted as supporting the DA hypothesis of antipsychotic effect of neuroleptic drugs. However, this argument rests on the assumption of a satisfactory correlation between the antipsychotic activity and the DA blocking activity of these drugs. Failing this, the above clinical observation may equally well be quoted in support of an involvement of norepinephrine; being an inhibitor of the tyrosine hydroxylase, α-methyltyrosine inhibits not only the formation of DA but also that of norepinephrine (84).

CONCLUSION

By evaluating the presently available information in a synthetic manner, the following concept seems to emerge: Accepting the premise that the schizophrenic disorder has an anatomical substrate in the brain, the corresponding neuropharmacological and behavioral studies seem to implicate three major brain systems as the most likely sites of this dysfunction: the reticular formation of the fore- and midbrain, the limbic forebrain system, and the corpus striatum. In this respect it appears significant that there exists a phylogenetically old anatomical-functional interrelationship between these three major subcortical systems (including their more recent thalamoneocortical connections); this fact underlines the crucial role of these subcortical mechanisms as important "analyzer-integrator" systems of the brain. This close anatomical-functional interrelation also makes it likely that a dysfunction of any one of these subcortical systems will find its corresponding expression in altered functioning of the other systems as well as the related thalamoneocortical mechanisms. Thus, assuming that one of these three systems may in fact be the primary "focus" of the schizophrenic disturbance, it would not be surprising to find that in the fully developed syndrome all three systems are involved. This complex relationship may explain the difficulty we face when trying to understand the pathophysiology of the schizophrenic disturbance; similarly, it makes the existence, in the fully developed syndrome, of a malfunction of a single neurohumoral factor unlikely, suggesting the possibility of a multineurohumoral disturbance as the overall biochemical feature of this disease. Specifically, the neurochemical correlate of such an anatomically extensive malfunction could be a combination of changes in the noradrenergic mechanisms in the reticular formation and dopaminergic forebrain mechanisms, especially those in the limbic-striatal systems. Moreover, disturbed functioning of the brain stem reticular formation may involve such important neurohumours as serotonin (especially in the mesencephalic-limbic subdivision) and possibly (secondarily) neuronal systems utilizing acetylcholine or γ-aminobutyric acid as their neurohumoral agents.

However, the likelihood of a multineurohumoral disturbance in schizophrenia should not be taken as a reason for evading the all-decisive question as to the primary lesion which, by definition, has to be at the root of all other biochemical alterations. Therefore, the crucial question still remains: Which of the above possibilities represents the primary anatomical and neurochemical lesion in schizophrenia? At present we do not have an answer to this question.

Although the possible existence of a multineurohumoral disturbance does not help to answer the more decisive question as to the primary neurochemical lesion, it has an important bearing on the evaluation of the current neurochemical hypotheses of mental illness in general, and schizophrenia in particular. As discussed in the preceding pages, these hypotheses are based mainly on pharmacological evidence. However, since from the pharmacological point of view beneficial or aggravating effects could be actually expected in the instance of any given drug acting on one or more of the possibly deranged neurohumoral systems, no valid hypothesis as to the underlying primary biochemical disturbance can be deduced from such clinical effects. At present, no specific drug—which would exert its antipsychotic effect by acting solely on a single specific neurochemical factor or anatomical site in the brain —seems to be available. This clearly indicates that rather than being at the endpoint of its development, the present state of the chemotherapy of psychoses is actually only in its very beginnings, thus holding some promise for further fruitful developments in this area.

Returning, at the end of this essay, to the quotation placed at the beginning, it becomes obvious that if we were to adopt, as we probably should, Eugen Bleuler's uncompromising view as to the scientific value of the current hypotheses of schizophrenia (1), the present essay would have to be replaced by nearly complete silence.

Literature Cited

1. Bleuler, E. 1911. *Dementia Praecox or the Group of Schizophrenias.* Trans. J. Zinkin, 1950, p. 465. New York: Int. Univ. 548 pp.
2. Carlsson, A., Lindqvist, M., Magnusson, T., Waldeck, B. 1958. On the presence of 3-hydroxytyramine in brain. *Science* 127:471
3. Ehringer, H., Hornykiewicz, O. 1960. Verteilung von Noradrenalin und Dopamin (3-Hydroxytyramin) im Gehirn des Menschen und ihr Verhalten bei Erkrankungen des extrapyramidalen Systems. *Klin. Wochenschr.* 38:1236–39
4. Birkmayer, W., Hornykiewicz, O. 1961. Der L-Dioxyphenylalanin (=L-DOPA) —Effekt bei der Parkinson-Akinese. *Wien. Klin. Wochenschr.* 73:787–88
5. Barbeau, A., Sourkes, T. L., Murphy, G. 1962. Les catecholamines dans la maladie de Parkinson. In *Monoamines et Systeme Neurveux Central,* ed. J. de Ajuriaguerra, 247–62. Geneva & Paris: Georg & Masson

6. Cotzias, G. C., Van Woert, M. H., Schiffer, L. M. 1967. Aromatic amino acids and modification of parkinsonism. *N. Engl. J. Med.* 276:374–79
7. Bernheimer, H., Birkmayer, W., Hornykiewicz, O., Jellinger, K., Seitelberger, F. 1973. Brain dopamine and the syndromes of Parkinson and Huntington. *J. Neurol. Sci.* 20:415–55
8. Lloyd, K. G., Davidson, L., Hornykiewicz, O. 1975. The neurochemistry of Parkinson's disease: Effect of L-dopa therapy. *J. Pharmacol. Exp. Ther.* 195:453–64
9. Snyder, S. H., Banerjee, S. P., Yamamura, H. I., Greenberg, D. 1974. Drugs, neurotransmitters, and schizophrenia. *Science* 184:1243–53
10. Snyder, S. H. 1974. Catecholamines as mediators of drug effects in schizophrenia. In *The Neurosciences, Third Study Program,* Eds-in-Chief, F. O. Schmitt, F. G. Worden, 721–32. Cambridge, Mass.: MIT Press. 1107 pp.
11. Matthysse, S. 1974. Schizophrenia: Relationships to dopamine transmission,

motor control, and feature extraction. See Ref. 10, pp. 733–37

12. Fuxe, K., Hökfelt, T., Ungerstedt, U. 1970. Morphological and functional aspects of central monoamine neurons. *Int. Rev. Neurobiol.* 13:93–126

13. Moore, R. Y., Bhatnagar, R. K., Heller, A. 1971. Anatomical and chemical studies of a nigro-neostriatal projection in the cat. *Brain. Res.* 30:119–35

14. Thierry, A. M., Blanc, G., Sobel, A., Stinus, L., Glowinski, J. 1973. Dopaminergic terminals in the rat cortex. *Science* 182:499–501

15. Hökfelt, T., Ljungdahl, A., Fuxe, K., Johansson, O. 1974. Dopamine nerve terminals in the rat limbic cortex: Aspects of the dopamine hypothesis of schizophrenia. *Science* 184:177–79

16. Lindvall, O., Björklund, A., Moore, R. Y., Stenevi, U. 1974. Mesencephalic dopamine neurons projecting to neocortex. *Brain Res.* 81:325–31

17. Laverty, R. 1974. On the role of dopamine and noradrenaline in animal behavior. *Prog. Neurobiol.* 3:31–70

18. Crow, T. J. 1972. Catecholamine-containing neurons and electrical self-stimulation: 1. A review of some data. *Psychol. Med.* 2:414–21

19. Routtenberg, A., Holzman, N. 1973. Memory disruption by electrical stimulation of substantia nigra, pars compacta. *Science* 181:83–86

20. Tassin, J. P. 1977. Qualitative and quantitative distribution of dopaminergic terminals in various areas of rat cerebral cortex. In *Symp. Non-Striatal Dopaminergic Neurons*, ed. E. Costa, G. L. Gessa. New York: Raven. In press

21. Ganong, W. F. 1972. Pharmacological aspects of neuroendocrine integration. *Prog. Brain. Res.* 38:41–57

22. DeWied, D. 1974. Pituitary-adrenal system hormones and behavior. See Ref. 10, pp. 653–66

23. Frey, T. S. 1973. A review of some important studies on schizophrenic thought disorders and their implications. *Acta Psychiatr. Scand.* 49:213–29

24. Mettler, F. A. 1955. Perceptual capacity, functions of the corpus striatum and schizophrenia. *Psychiatr. Q.* 29:89–111

25. Mettler, F. A., Mettler, C. C. 1940. Labyrinthine disregard after removal of the caudate. *Proc. Soc. Exp. Biol. Med.* 45:473–75

26. Mettler, F. A., Mettler, C. C. 1941. Role of the neostriatum. *Am. J. Physiol.* 133:594–601

27. Mettler, F. A., Mettler, C. C. 1942. The effects of striatal injury. *Brain* 65: 242–55

28. Thompson, R. L., Mettler, F. A. 1963. Permanent learning deficit associated with lesions of the caudate nuclei. *Am. J. Ment. Defic.* 67:526–35

29. Divac, I. 1972. Neostriatum and functions of prefrontal cortex. *Acta Neurobiol. Exp.* 32:461–77

30. Torrey, E. F., Peterson, M. R. 1974. Schizophrenia and the limbic system. *Lancet* II:942–46

31. Papez, J. W. 1937. A proposed mechanism of emotion. *Arch. Neurol. Psychiatry* 38:725–43

32. Nauta, J. H. 1963. Central nervous system organization and the endocrine motor system. In *Advances in Neuroendocrinology*, ed. A. V. Nalbandov, 5–21. Urbana: Univ. Illinois. 525 pp.

33. MacLean, P. D. 1949. Psychosomatic disease and the "visceral brain." *Psychosom. Med.* 11:338–53

34. MacLean, P. D. 1952. Some psychiatric implications of physiological studies on frontotemporal portion of limbic system (visceral brain). *Electroencephalogr. Clin. Neurophysiol.* 4:407–18

35. Chapman, J. 1966. The early symptoms of schizophrenia. *Br. J. Psychiatry* 112:225–51

36. Farley, I. J., Price, K. S., Hornykiewicz, O. 1977. Dopamine in the limbic regions of the human brain: normal and abnormal. See Ref. 20

37. Connell, P. H. 1958. *Amphetamine Psychosis.* London: Chapman & Hall

38. Griffith, J. D., Cavanaugh, J., Held, J., Oates, J. A. 1972. Dextro-amphetamine. *Arch. Gen. Psychiatry* 26:97–101

39. Angrist, B. M., Gershon, S. 1970. The phenomenology of experimentally induced amphetamine psychosis—preliminary observations. *Biol. Psychiatry* 2:95–107

40. Costa, E., Garattini, S., eds. 1970. *Int. Symp. Amphetamines Related Compounds.* New York: Raven. 962 pp.

41. Randrup, A., Munkvad, I. 1972. Evidence indicating an association between schizophrenia and dopaminergic hyperactivity in the brain. *Orthomolecular Psychiatry* 1:2–7

42. Snyder, S. H. 1973. Amphetamine psychosis: A model schizophrenia mediated by catecholamines. *Am. J. Psychiatry* 130:61–67

43. Janowsky, D. S., El-Yousef, M. K., Davis, J. M., Sekerke, H. J. 1973. Provocation of schizophrenic symptoms by in-

558   HORNYKIEWICZ

travenous administration of methylphenidate. *Arch. Gen. Psychiatry* 28:
185–94
44. Preston West, A. 1974. Interaction of
low-dose amphetamine use with schizophrenia in outpatients: 3 case reports.
Am. J. Psychiatry. 131:321–23
45. Matthysse, S. 1974. Dopamine and
the pharmacology of schizophrenia:
The state of the evidence. In *Symp.
Catecholamines Enzymes Neuropathol.
Schizophrenia, J. Psychiatr. Res.* 11:
107–13. Oxford: Pergamon. 364 pp.
46. Coyle, J. T., Snyder, S. H. 1969. Catecholamine uptake by synaptosomes in
homogenates of rat brain: Stereospecificity in different areas. *J. Pharmacol.
Exp. Ther.* 170:221–31
47. Ferris, R. M., Tang, F. L. M., Maxwell,
R. A. 1972. A comparison of the capaci-
ties of isomers of amphetamine, deoxy-
pipradol and methylphenidate to inhibit
the uptake of tritiated catecholamines
into rat cerebral cortex slices, synaptosomal preparations of rat cerebral
cortex, hypothalamus and striatum and
into adrenergic nerves of rabbit
aorta. *J. Pharmacol. Exp. Ther.* 181:
407–16
48. Thornburg, J. E., Moore, K. E. 1973.
Dopamine and norepinephrine uptake
by rat brain synaptosomes: Relative inhibitory potencies of l- and d- amphetamine and amantadine. *Res. Commun.
Chem. Pathol. Pharmacol.* 5:81–88
49. Harris, J., Baldessarini, R. J. 1973.
Effects of amphetamine analogs on the
uptake of (^{3}H) catecholamines by
homogenates of rat corpus striatum and
cerebral cortex. *Neuropharmacology*
12:669–79
50. Carlsson, A. 1974. Discussion. See Ref.
45, p.55
51. Hornykiewicz, O. 1974. Discussion. See
Ref. 45, p. 53
52. Davis, J. M. 1974. A two factor theory
of schizophrenia. See Ref. 45, pp. 25–29
53. McKenzie, G. M. 1972. Role of the tu-
berculum olfactorium in stereotyped
behavior induced by apomorphine in
the rat. *Psychopharmacologia* 23:
212–19
54. Ellinwood, E. H. Jr. 1968. Amphetamine psychosis. II. Theoretical implications. *Int. J. Neuropsychiatry* 4:45–54
55. Iversen, S. 1976. Behavioral implications of dopaminergic neurons in the
mesolimbic system. See Ref. 20
56. Marcus, R. J., Villablanca, J. R. 1974.
Is the striatum needed for amphetamine

induced stereotyped behavior? *Proc.
West Pharmacol. Soc.* 17:219–22
57. Kornetsky, C., Markowitz, R. 1975.
Animal models of schizophrenia. In
Model Systems in Biological Psychiatry,
ed. D. J. Ingle, H. Schein. 26–50. Cambridge, Mass.: MIT Press. 196 pp.
58. Miller, R. J., Hiley, C. R. 1974. Antimuscarinic properties of neuroleptics
and drug-induced Parkinsonism. *Nature* 248:596–97
59. Snyder, S. H., Greenberg, D., Yamamura, H. I. 1974. Antischizophrenic
drugs and brain cholinergic receptors.
Arch. Gen. Psychiatry 31:58–61
60. Yamamura, H. I., Manian, A. A., Snyder, S. H. 1976. Muscarinic cholinergic
receptor binding: Influence of pimozide
and chlorpromazine metabolites. *Life
Sci.* 18:685–92
61. Hornykiewicz, O. 1975. Parkinsonism
induced by dopaminergic antagonists.
In *Adv. Neurol., Dopaminergic Mechanisms,* ed. D. B. Calne, T. N. Chase, A.
Barbeau, 9:155–64. New York: Raven.
445 pp.
62. Kebabian, J. W., Petzold, G. L., Greengard, P. 1972. Dopamine-sensitive adenylate cyclase in caudate nucleus of rat
brain and its similarity to the "dopamine receptor." *Proc. Natl. Acad. Sci.
USA* 69:2145–49
63. Clement-Cormier, Y. C., Kebabian, J.
W., Petzold, G. L., Greengard, P. 1974.
Dopamine-sensitive adenylate cyclase
in mammalian brain: A possible site of
action of antipsychotic drugs. *Proc.
Natl. Acad. Sci. USA* 71:1113–17
64. Snyder, S. H., Creese, I., Burt, D. R.
1975. The brain dopamine receptor: Labelling with (^{3}H) dopamine. *Psychopharmacol. Commun.* 1:663–73
65. Seeman, P., Lee, T. 1975. Antipsychotic
drugs: Direct correlation between clinical potency and presynaptic action on
dopamine neurons. *Science* 188:
1217–19
66. Lloyd, K. G., Bartholini, G. 1975. The
effect of drugs on the release of endogenous catecholamines into the perfustate
of discrete brain areas of the cat brain
in vivo. Experientia 31:560–61
67. Seeman, P., Chau-Wong, M., Tedesco,
J., Wong, K. 1975. Brain receptors for
antipsychotic drugs and dopamine: Direct binding assays. *Proc. Natl. Acad.
Sci. USA* 72:4376–80
68. Burt, D. R., Enna, S. J., Creese, I., Snyder, S. H. 1975. Dopamine receptor
binding in the corpus striatum of mam-

malian brain. *Proc. Natl. Acad. Sci. USA* 72:4655–59

69. Creese, I., Burt, D. R., Snyder, S. H. 1976. Dopamine receptor binding predicts clinical and pharmacological potencies of antischizophrenic drugs. *Science* 192:481–83

70. Seeman, P., Lee, T., Chau-Wong, M., Wong, K. 1976. Antipsychotic drug doses and neuroleptic/dopamine receptors. *Nature* 261:717–18

71. Kornetsky, C., Mirsky, A. F. 1966. On certain psychopharmacological and physiological differences between schizophrenic and normal persons. *Psychopharmacologia* 8:309–18

72. Kornetsky, C., Eliasson, M. 1969. Reticular stimulation and chlorpromazine: An animal model of schizophrenic overarousal. *Science* 165:1273–74

73. Duffy, E. 1957. The psychological significance of the concept of "arousal" or "activation." *Psychol. Rev.* 64:265–75

74. Malmo, R. A. 1959. Activation: A neuropsychological dimension. *Psychol. Rev.* 66:367–86

75. Brücke, F. Th. v., Hornykiewicz, O., Sigg, E. B. 1969. *The Pharmacology of Psychotherapeutic Drugs.* New York: Springer. 157 pp.

76. Bradley, P. B., Key, B. J. 1968. The effects of drugs on arousal responses produced by electrical stimulation of the reticular formation of the brain. *Electroncephalogr. Clin. Neurophysiol.* 10:560–71

77. Boakes, J., Bradley, P. B., Candy, J. M. 1972. A neuronal basis for the alerting action of (+)-amphetamine. *Br. J. Pharmacol.* 45:391–403

78. Feldman, P. E. 1959. The treatment of anergic schizophrenics with imipramine. *J. Clin. Exp. Psychopathol.* 20: 235–42

79. Gershon, S., Angrist, B. M. 1973. Effects of alterations of cholinergic function on behavior. In *Psychopathology and Psychopharmacology,* ed. J. D. Cole, A. M. Freedman, A. J. Friedhoff, 15–36. Baltimore: John Hopkins Univ. Press. 290 pp.

80. Sedvall, G., Fyrö, B., Nybäck, H., Wiesel, F.-A. 1975. Actions of dopaminergic antagonists in the striatum. See Ref. 61, pp. 131–40

81. Jefferson, J. W. 1974. Beta-adrenergic receptor blocking drugs in psychiatry. *Arch. Gen. Psychiatry* 31:681–91

82. Yorkston, N. J., Zaki, S. A., Malik, M. K. U., Morrison, R. C., Havard, C. W. H. 1974. Propranolol in the control of schizophrenic symptoms. *Br. Med. J.* 4:633–35

83. Carlsson, A., Roos, B.-E, Walinder, J., Skott, A. 1973. Further studies on the mechanism of antipsychotic action: Potentiation by alpha-methyltyrosine of thioridazine effects in chronic schizophrenia. *J. Neural Transm.* 34:125–32

84. Udenfriend, S., Zaltzman-Nirenberg, P., Gordon, R., Spector, S. 1966. Evaluation of the biochemical effects *in vivo* by inhibitors of the three enzymes involved in norepinephrine synthesis. *Mol. Pharmacol.* 2:95–105

Ann. Rev. Pharmacol. Toxicol. 1977. 17:561–73

PEDIATRIC CLINICAL PHARMACOLOGY AND THE "THERAPEUTIC ORPHAN"

♦6696

Alan K. Done, Sanford N. Cohen, and Leon Strebel[1]
Departments of Pediatrics and Pharmacology, Wayne State University,
and Division of Clinical Pharmacology and Toxicology, Children's Hospital
of Michigan, Detroit, Michigan 48201

Despite present requirements for proof of safety and efficacy of new drugs, 78% of those marketed in the USA have not been so proved, and fully labeled for children (1). The principal reasons are the following.

1. The FDA's policy allows the marketing of drugs that have been approved in adults but not studied in children so long as labeling includes disclaimers and no instructions about pediatric use, thus creating the "therapeutic orphan" problem (2). The FDA has been urged recently to require premarketing pediatric studies of new drugs likely to be used in children (3), and guidelines have been developed for such studies (4). Also, proposed legislation would require preapproval studies in any special populations to which new drugs would have obvious application. In the meantime, the present situation forces physicians to prescribe agents that have not been proven to be safe or efficacious for children; this in itself is unreasonable, inequitable, and unethical.

2. Widespread misunderstanding of the ethical and legal implications hinders the only clinical experimental research from which reliable information can be obtained on the use of drugs in children—that which utilizes the child as the ultimate experimental subject. Enlightened investigators and institutional review boards can and have constructed pediatric clinical drug studies that can pass ethical and legal as well as scientific review. Important elements are prior informed consent from an individual qualified to act on behalf of the child, the assent of children capable of sufficient comprehension, and enrollment of a minor subject in risky or invasive studies only when the procedures or drug administration can be predicted to be for his/her own benefit (with rare exceptions).

[1]Dr. Judith Ganser assisted in the literature review.

561

3. Lack of broad categorical (as opposed to project-directed) support of pediatric clinical pharmacological research hinders the development of a core of qualified pediatric clinical pharmacology investigators and methodology for carrying out ethically acceptable pediatric drug studies. Because of the special ethical requirement that most drug studies in children be carried out in a therapeutic situation, it is crucial that there be special study procedures and units capable of focusing such techniques and appropriate pharmacologic expertise on clinical opportunities that present themselves. A number of investigators have utilized new approaches to the conduct of the type of clinical studies permissible in children, but more units with broad-based support are needed to capitalize upon the gains that have been made, and to accelerate progress toward the goal of ending the era of the therapeutic orphan.

This review examines the impact of recent pediatric clinical pharmacology studies upon the need for knowledge of pharmacokinetic parameters in pediatric patients to improve pediatric drug evaluations and usage. The aim is not only to define the current status of such clinical information, and the remaining gaps in our knowledge, but also to emphasize novel and ethically acceptable approaches that have been used. The pertinent data are scattered throughout the literature, and often indexed only according to the process or drug in question, discouraging attempts to provide comprehensive reviews. Our review is not exhaustive, but we hope adequate to serve the goals of providing a useful source of references and demonstrating the need for, and feasibility of, pediatric clinical pharmacology investigations.

PHARMACOKINETICS DURING POSTNATAL HUMAN DEVELOPMENT

Recent data concerning certain pharmacokinetic parameters in infants, children, and adults are summarized in the three tables in this chapter. These particular parameters were selected because they (a) are most often selected by pediatric clinical pharmacology investigators, (b) have the most direct and practical usefulness in determining therapeutic regimens for pediatric use, and (c) are interdependent.

Developmental Overview

Our goal is not a comprehensive discussion of these pharmacokinetic parameters, but rather to evaluate them as markers of developmental pharmacokinetic changes and as promising tools for future studies.

Plasma Concentration Half-Life

Plasma half-life and the elimination constant (K_e) have the advantages of being easily measured and of describing the overall behavior of a circulating drug in a way that permits regulation of therapeutic regimens without the need to correct for body size.

The expected prolongation of half-life for most drugs during the period of early infancy was noted (Table 1), consistent with the clinically observed need for reduced

Table 1 Comparative apparent plasma drug half-life (hours) during postnatal human development[a]

Drug	Perinatal[b] Premature	Perinatal[b] Term	Newborn[c]	Infant[d]	Child[e]	Adult[f]	Reference(s)
Anti-Infectives							
Ampicillin	3.6–6.2	2.0–4.9	1.7–2.8			[1–1.8]	5, 6
Carbenicillin	6.6	2.9–4.7	1.5–2.2			[1]	5
Cephaloridin		3.7–5.4	2.1	1.1		[1–1.5]	6
Cephalothin	2.0	2.4		0.3	0.2–0.3	[0.5–0.9]	7, 8
Chloramphenicol	(15–22)	(8–15)			4	[2.3]	6
Clindamycin					—2.4–3.4—	4.5–4.8	9
					1.5–2.2	3.2–3.5	10
Colistimethate	2.6	2.6–9.0	2.3			[4.5]	6
Doxycycline	7.6	6.9		3.7	3.2–3.7	[12–22]	11
Gentamycin	5.1–5.9	3.8–5.5	2.3–3.9	2.3–2.9		(2–3)[2]	5, 12
Kanamycin	(8.4)–18	(5.7–7.5)	(3.8)–6			2[2.2]	6, 13
Lymecycline		16.2		9.8	6.8	[(6–10)]	6
Methicillin	2.4–3.3	1.3–3.3	0.9–2.0	0.8–0.9		[0.4]	6
Neomycin	5.4		3.7				6
Oxacillin	1.6	1.5	1.2	1.1		0.7[0.4–0.7]	6
Penicillin		3.2	1.7	1.4		[0.6–0.7]	5
Streptomycin	7.0					2.7[1.9–2.7]	6
Sulfalene		135.6		53.9	51.0	63.3	6
Sulfisomidine			10.9	4.2			14
Sulfisoxazole		12.4	7.8	4.5		[6]	14
Tobramycin	8.1–8.7	4.6–6.1	3.9			2.2[2]	15
Analgesics and/or Antipyretics							
Acetaminophen					(3.1, 3.4)	(2.0–2.6)	16
		3.5–4.9[g]			4.4–4.5[g]	3.6[g]	17
Antipyrine					6.6	13.6[12–15]	18
Phenylbutazone[h]			27	17	20–40	76[71–82]	18, 19
Propoxyphene					3.4	2.7[3–7]	20
Salicylate[h]		(4.5–11.5)[g]			(2.0–3.1)	(2.0–3.5)	21
Cardiovascular drugs							
Diazoxide				(24)	(10–19)	(36, 24) [28]	22
Digoxin	90	(52, 26)	(35)–44	19–25	36–37	[31–40]	23
Sedatives/Anticonvulsants/Anesthetics							
Amobarbital		39				16[21–25]	24
Carbamazepine		(8–28)			(14, 19)	[(18–55)]	25
Clonazepam					29	[(20–60)]	26
Diazepam	75	31			18	(20–42)	27
Dipropylacetate					9.4	(15.3)	28
Ethosuximide					30–36	[56]	29, 29a
Lidocaine[h]		3				[(1.2–2.2)]	30
Mepivacaine		9				[0.12]	31
Phenobarbital	(41)–380	102–259	(67–99)	44–86	53–64	[(53)–118]	32, 42
Phenytoin[h]		17–60			5	15[21–29]	25, 33, 34
Miscellaneous							
Caffeine	(36–144)	80				3.5	35
Nortriptyline		(56)				(17) [27]	36
Theophylline	30				1.8–3.9	4.6–6.7	37–39
Tolbutamide		>30				7[6–8]	40

[a] Means, or ranges of means, are given where possible; where individual values or ranges are used, they are in parentheses.

[b] First week of life, or first 2 weeks in prematures; *premature* includes up to 37 weeks' gestation and/or low birth weight (< 2.5 kg) infants regardless of gestational age.

[c] 1 week–1 month in term infants; 2 weeks–2 months prematures.

[d] Remainder of first year.

[e] 1–16 years.

[f] Adult values in brackets are from literature cited in above references or by Pagliaro & Benet (41), and not from comparative studies in the same laboratories as the pediatric data.

[g] Determined from urinary excretion, rather than plasma levels.

[h] Dose-dependent kinetics. Values shown are for levels at or near the therapeutic, except for phenytoin, where the children had toxic levels and where different bases were used for infant $T_{1/2}$ in the studies shown.

doses and extended interdose intervals in order to achieve blood levels comparable with those in adults. Elimination of drugs from the plasma is least likely to be delayed for those mainly excreted unchanged by filtration and most likely for those that are actively secreted. For drugs that undergo extensive metabolism, elimination of drugs from the plasma varies with the efficiency of the metabolic processes involved.

Prolongations were greatest in premature infants, and for the most part declined progressively with increasing maturation such that half-life is usually within 50% of that for the adult after 1–2 months of life. Unfortunately, data are lacking for half-lives beyond early infancy for drugs with the most extreme prolongations, for example, caffeine, chloramphenicol, and cephalothin.

Somewhat unexpected was the frequency with which the half-life was shorter in children than in adults. For some, the half-life was shorter than in adults even during infancy, in which case it was also shorter in childhood.

Apparent Distribution Volume

Few data are available concerning the early development of this parameter (Table 2).

Drugs such as digoxin, anticonvulsants, sedatives, and tranquilizers have distribution volumes considerably in excess of either total body water (TBW) or extracellular water (ECW) in pediatric subjects, as in adults. The majority of drugs have a larger distribution volume during infancy and early childhood than in the adult, but the reverse was true of some drugs. Age-dependent distribution volume differences usually disappear less rapidly than those of the half-life, but here there were no

Table 2 Apparent distribution volumes (liter/kg) of drugs during postnatal human development[a]

Drug	Perinatal Premature	Perinatal Term	Newborn	Infant	Child	Adult	Study conditions[b]	References
Clindamycin					12[c]	34[c]	Therapeutic	9
Diazepam		1.8			2.6	[(0.7–2.6)]	Study	27
Digoxin	7.7	(6.0, 8.4)		15.4	16.1	[5.8]	Therapeutic	23
Dipropylacetate					0.25	(0.15)	Therapeutic	28
Ethosuximide					0.69	[0.9]	Study	29
Gentamycin	——0.52–0.56——					[0.28]	Therapeutic	12
Kanamycin	0.59–0.78	0.49–0.81	0.51–0.63			[0.19]	Therapeutic	13
Lymecycline		(1.0, 1.1)	(1.0)	(1.4–1.8)	(1.8, 2.1)		? Study	6
Phenobarbital	(0.68)	0.94		0.81	0.61	[0.7]	Therapeutic	42
Phenylbutazone[d]			0.25	0.16	0.15–0.11	[0.02–0.15]	Study	19
Phenytoin					0.78	0.78	Poisoning	34
Sulfalene		0.47		0.36	0.20	0.22	? Study	6
Sulfisomidine			0.46	0.34	0.28		Study	14
Sulfisoxazole		0.45	0.34	0.35	0.29	[0.16]	Study	14
Theophylline	0.69				0.25–0.46	0.3–0.6	Therapeutic	37–39
Total body water	0.90–0.80	0.74–0.80	0.74	0.72–0.60	0.58–0.64	0.51–0.62		43
Extracellular water	0.60–0.42	0.44–0.42	0.40	0.32–0.27	0.19–0.27	0.16–0.19		

[a] See footnotes to Table 1.

[b] Refers to the means or purpose of drug administration: Therapeutic, study (nontherapeutic) purposes, or accidental poisoning.

[c] Expressed as liters per square meter body surface area.

[d] Dose-dependent kinetics. Values shown are for levels at or near the therapeutic.

instances of reversal of the direction of age-related change from one stage of development to another.

The pattern for digoxin appears to be unique: its volume of distribution is only modestly expanded during early infancy, but is as much as threefold greater than in adults in the older infant and the child. The distribution volume for a number of drugs varies as development progresses in a manner that may be independent of the changes in body water compartments.

Additional simultaneous measurements of distribution volume and half-life would be particularly worthwhile for drugs having the most extreme or fluctuating age-related changes in either parameter and/or for which there are unusual dosage requirements for infants and children such as in the cases of dicloxacillin (44) and cloxacillin (L. Strebel, A. Dajani, A. Done, unpublished observations). Mathematical models for examining the interrelationships of changes in body water distribution, renal function, and protein binding are dealt with in detail elsewhere (43).

Drug Metabolism Processes

Even the neonate has considerable ability to carry out a number of drug metabolism processes (Table 3). While some pathways appear to be active and even capable of compensating for other reduced processes, the rates of maturation appear to vary from one type of process to another. Oxidation and hydroxylation go on relatively early, but at a reduced rate during the newborn period. N-dealkylation may be less active early and perhaps takes somewhat longer to mature. Glucuronidation of hydroxylated derivatives is perhaps the most inefficient drug metabolic pathway during early development and may take longest to mature. Other conjugations occur early in development and assume greater importance as a result of the inefficiency of other processes.

Protein Binding

Most drugs thus far studied are bound less to infant or cord blood than to normal adult serum, including salicylate (50, 54), some penicillins (54, 56), phenobarbital (56), phenytoin (36, 56), cephazolin, cephadrin, clindamycin (57), theophylline (37), sulfonamides (58, 59), lidocaine, and bupivacaine (60). For several the binding is still less with fetal than with neonatal serum (56), and binding of most drugs by infant serum is reduced still further in the presence of hyperbilirubinemia (56, 58). In contrast, diazepam (54) and digoxin (23) bind similarly to infant and adult sera. At least salicylate may be less well bound to maternal than to infant serum (55).

CLINICAL STUDY APPROACHES IN CHILDREN

References in Tables 2 and 3 to the study conditions indicate that much or most of the pharmacokinetic information needed for adequate pediatric drug use and labeling can be obtained in the therapeutic situation in ways consistent with the aforementioned caveats concerning pediatric research. We have the impression that the present constraints not only have not impeded drug research in children, but also may have improved its quality by forcing improved planning, methods development, ingenuity, and attention to detail. The hallmark of the current approach is

Table 3 Recent quantitative studies of drug metabolism during postnatal human development[a]

Drug (or substrate)	Metabolite (or process)	Units, time	Premature newborns	Term newborns	Older infants	Children	Adults	Study[b] conditions	Reference(s)
URINARY METABOLITES: as percentage of dose (d) or recovered metabolites (m)									
Acetaminophen	Unchanged	%d, 36 hr		3		4	2	Study	17
	Glucuronide			17		32–47	50		
	Sulfate			50		45–30	30		
			k=formation rate constant (hr^{-1}):						
	Unchanged	%d, 48 hr		2 k=0.005			[k=0.010]	Study	16
	Glucuronide			13 k=0.025			[k=0.171]		
	Sulfate			48 k=0.099			[k=0.076]		
	Conjugates	%d, 24 hr	14	39	52		[80]	Study	45
Salicylate	Unchanged	%m		2			[14]	Maternal	21
	Glycine conjugates	10–70 hr[c]		76			[50]		
	Glucuronide, Acyl			0			[<5–10][c]		
	Phenolic			13			[20][c]		
Salicylamide	Glucuronide	%m, 30 hr		19			[80]	Study	46
p-Aminobenzoate	Unchanged	%d, 24 hr	3	2	4	16		Study	45
	Acetate		27	22	36	16			
	Glucuronide		7	19	18	17			
	Glycine conjugates		13	27	28	47			
Benzoate Na	Glycine conjugates	%d, 6 hr	3	5	11	24		Study	45
Choramphenicol	Unchanged	%d, 24 hr		5–10			[5–15]	Therapeutic	47
	Glucuronide			ca 50			[85–95]		
Nortriptyline	Hydroxy	%m		(33–60)			(26–48)	Maternal	36
	Glucuronide	24–96 hr[c]		(40–67)			(52–74)		

Table 3 *(Continued)*

Drug (or substrate)	Metabolite (or process)	Units, time	Premature newborns	Term newborns	Older infants	Children	Adults	Study[b] conditions	Reference(s)
Diazepam	Unchanged	%d, 24 hr	0.05	0.05		0.02		Study	27
	N-Demethyl		0.06	0.17		0.05[d]			
	Glucuronide		1.0	1.4		4.4			
	Hydroxy		0	0.3		1.5	(included in glucuronide fraction)		
Phenytoin	Hydroxy, then Glucuronide	%m							
		3–124 hr[c]		91–97		>99	(99)	Maternal	25
		%m, 2–5d		88–99			[70]	Maternal	33
		%m, 6d		a b				Poison	34
Phenobarbital	Unchanged	%m a,72 hr		(70–42)			[10–25]	Therapeutic	48
	Hydroxy	b,72–192 hr		(19–26)			[Equal distribution]		
	Sulfate (of hydroxy)			(10–32)					
Caffeine	Unchanged	%m, 24 hr		(62)				Maternal	49
	Hydroxy			(32)					
	Unchanged	%m 24–48 hr[c]		(75,83)			(26)	Maternal	49
	Demethyl			(25,19)			(72)		
Lidocaine	Unchanged	%m 0–24 hr[c]		45			36	Maternal	30
	N-De-ethyl			30			10		
	De-amide, hydroxy			25			54		
Mepivacaine	Unchanged	%m 0–30 hr[c]		71			11	Maternal	31
	N-Demethyl			22			7		
	Hydroxy, then glucuronide			7			82		

Table 3 *(Continued)*

Drug (or substrate)	Metabolite (or process)	Units, time	Premature newborns	Term newborns	Older infants	Children	Adults	Study[b] conditions	Reference(s)
Tolbutamide	Oxidized	%d, 36 hr		31			53	Study	38
Diazoxide	Unchanged	%d, 24 hr			(30)	(20)	(25–35)	Therapeutic	22
Digoxin	Unchanged	%m, 5 days	—	100	—		[74–90 +]	Therapeutic	23
BLOOD OR TISSUE ENZYME ASSAYS:[e] Amount metabolized per minute									
Aspirin	Esterase	nM/ml	8	11	13	14	13	Diagnostic samples	50
Acetylcholine	Esterase (RBC)	μM/ml	4.6–5.8	5.3	7–9	9–10	10	Samples of cord blood, from indwelling catheters, etc	51
Butyrylcholine	Esterase (plasma)	μM/ml	0.3–1.1	1.2	2.0–2.3	2.1–2.5	2.0		
Phenylacetate	Arylesterase (plasma)	μM/ml	6.5	8.4	19.5	24.2	27.8		
Paraoxon	Esterase (plasma)	nM/ml	3.6	3.4		6.1	7.3		
Procaine	Esterase (plasma)	nM/ml	1–7	7	8–9	10–11	10		
Cytochrome c	Reduction (liver)	nM/mg protein		(23)	(16–21)	(14,54)		Diagnostic biopsy	52

a See footnotes to Table 1.

b Refers to drug administration or means of procuring assay specimens: therapeutic, for study (nontherapeutic) purposes, maternal drug reaching fetus, accidental poisoning, diagnostic blood or biopsy specimens.

c Hours postpartun.

d Reflects greater excretion as glucuronide; formation of this and the hydroxylated metabolites was much reduced in infants compared with children.

e Enzyme activities demonstrated to be present in the fetus, and presumably postnatal enzyme activities as well, are not included, but have recently received thorough review (53).

maximization of the potential investigative benefits afforded by therapeutic or accidental exposures of infants and children to drugs deserving of pediatric study.

Valuable sources of pharmacokinetic data, in addition to direct treatment of sick children, include studies of drugs used in labor or delivery (30, 61, 62) and of drugs received by infants transplacentally as a result of treatment either of chronic maternal disease or symptoms (21, 25, 33) or pregnancy complications (24, 48). Instances of accidental overdosage of children (32, 61, 62) or pregnant women at term (36) offer unique opportunities to study drugs or doses that could not legitimately be given to infants or children.

Nontherapeutic administration of a drug specifically for study purposes in pediatric patients, though rarely needed, seems acceptable in certain instances when the drug is being employed as a substrate for studying drug metabolism processes or broad pharmacologic problems. It is probably possible to carry out such studies when the drug(s) and dose(s) are clearly safe and often used therapeutically in the same or similar subjects, and when the study techniques do not themselves introduce risk or pain to any major extent. Appropriate peer review and consents must always be obtained. Urinary excretion of metabolites after therapeutic doses has been used under such conditions to study the status in infants and children of the detoxification processes reflected by acetaminophen (16, 17) and salicylamide (46).

A variety of techniques have been employed to capture legitimate therapeutic opportunities for investigation. The authors rely upon ongoing collaborations and prior protocol development with the clinical subspecialists who have primary responsibility for most patient care. Others have done likewise and/or have taken advantage of requests for blood-level monitoring (63); have asked parturient women about the intake of drugs of interest prior to delivery (21), or have seized such other opportunities for exceptional studies as the use of otherwise sacrificed specimens of tissue obtained at surgery (64, 65), autopsy (23, 65), or therapeutic abortion (65, 66) or cerebropinal fluid obtained for diagnostic purposes (67, 68) for studies of drug distribution, and liver biopsy materials obtained for diagnostic purposes for sensitive assays of drug metabolism enzyme activities (52).

The most generally agreed upon needs are for improving the usefulness of noninvasive procedures. Micromethods are needed so that drug measurements can be made in blood sample sizes obtainable from capillary sources, and several have been devised that require only 10 to 100 μl of serum (7, 12, 22, 24, 25, 67), and sample size can be reduced further by use of whole-blood methods (37). The use of noninvasive sampling sources (that reflect blood concentrations) such as saliva for theophylline measurements (69) also deserves further pursuit. Invasiveness can be diminished by coordinating drug-study blood samples with those obtained for diagnostic purposes and by using samples obtainable from indwelling catheters when these are employed for clinical purposes. Umbilical cord blood can sometimes be used for neonatal studies.

Levy's (21) and Roberts' (17) groups have demonstrated the ability to use urine measurements to obtain much of the needed kinetic information for at least some drugs. Cumulative urinary excretion or areas under limited-sampling serum curves often suffice for bioavailability studies in children (23). The authors agree with

Wilson (20) that where blood studies are essential, it is often satisfactory in the initial kinetic explorations to obtain limited sampling from each patient at different time intervals and to prepare scattergrams of random time intervals to approximate the profile of drug levels, in lieu of obtaining multiple samples. Pharmacokinetic predictions thus obtained can then be verified in larger therapeutic studies.

Some compromises are unavoidable, but the concern should not be with utilizing children for the initial and definitive establishment of a drug's disposition, but rather for determining whether infants or children differ significantly from adults. By the same token, efficacy should ordinarily be established in adults and pediatric studies used to verify applicability to children, a point that is often forgotten by investigators and regulatory agencies alike. The acceptability of invasive study procedures is also increased when the results can be used to regulate therapy for the individual; this necessitates a rapid turn-around time, which may be an acceptable price to pay for ability to perform the studies.

Therapeutic drug studies are undertaken usually only after adult studies have provided reasonable expectations of safety and benefit. One major safeguard stressed by a number of authors (12, 20, 67) is to leave the final decision regarding drug selection to the primary physician, when he is not the investigator, rather than with the investigator. As undesirable as concomitant medications may be, their avoidance is sometimes neither possible nor desirable in the sick patients used for pediatric studies, and it is essential that this be recognized by those who evaluate such studies particularly from a regulatory viewpoint. There is merit in obtaining kinetic studies early in the pediatric evaluation of a drug because this greatly assists further study design and provides best assurance of avoiding potentially dangerous underdosing or overdosing. It is sometimes possible in initial kinetic studies to substitute a single dose of the study drug for one of known safety and efficacy, so as not to subject the patient to undue jeopardy by prolonged exposure to an untested drug (70); the conventional "wash-out" usually sought in adult studies may not be possible.

Optimal studies in the therapeutic context require teamwork of pharmacologists, clinical specialists, and those with laboratory expertise, at least during the early stages of a drug's evaluation when it is essential to obtain sufficient kinetic data to assure the safest and most effective expansion of evaluations.

There is certainly merit in providing for more such units and in promoting individual projects. However, because of the magnitude and complexities of the pediatric drug therapy problems—involving old as well as new drugs—and the necessity for approaching most of them in the therapeutic situation, more categorical support of existing units that can provide the required types of comprehensive and sophisticated studies of large and diverse patient populations offers the greatest hope for rapid improvement in the therapeutic orphan problem.

Literature Cited

1. Wilson, J. T. 1975. Pragmatic assessment of medicines available for young children and pregnant or breast-feeding women. In *Basic and Therapeutic Aspects of Perinatal Pharmacology,* ed. P. L. Morselli, S. Garattini, F. Sereni, 411–21. New York: Raven. 440 pp.
2. Shirkey, H. 1968. Editorial comment: Therapeutic orphans. *J. Pediatr.* 72:119–20
3. Mirkin, B. L., Done, A. K., Christensen, C. N., Cohen, S. N., Howie, V. M., Lockhart, J. D. 1975. Panel on pediatric trials (in report of NAS workshop on clinical trials of drugs). *Clin. Pharmacol. Ther.* 18:657–58
4. Am. Acad. Pediatr. Comm. Drugs. 1974. *General Guidelines for the Evaluation of Drugs to be Approved for Use During Pregnancy and for Treatment of Infants and Children.* Evanston, Ill.: Am. Acad. Pediatr. 40 pp.
5. McCracken, G. H. Jr. 1974. Pharmacologic basis for antimicrobial therapy in newborn infants. *Am. J. Dis. Child.* 128:407–19
6. Sereni, F., Principi, N. 1968. Developmental pharmacology. *Ann. Rev. Pharmacol.* 8:453–66
7. Anders, M. W., Cooper, M. J., Rolewicz, T. F., Mirkin, B. L. 1975. Application of high-pressure liquid chromatography in pediatric pharmacology: Pharmacokinetics of cephalothin in man. See Ref. 1, pp. 405–9
8. Sheng, K. T., Huang, N. N., Promadhattavedi, V. 1964. Serum concentrations of cephalothin in infants and children and placental transmission of the antibiotic. *Antimicrob. Agents Chemother.* 4:200–6
9. Kauffman, R. E., Shoeman, D. W., Wan, S. H., Azarnoff, D. L. 1972. Absorption and excretion of clindamycin-2-phosphate in children after intramuscular injection. *Clin. Pharmacol. Ther.* 13:704–9
10. DeHaan, R. M., Schellenberg, D. 1972. Clindamycin palmitate flavored granules. Multidose tolerance, absorption, and urinary excretion study in healthy children. *J. Clin. Pharmacol.* 12:74–83
11. Weingartner, L., Sitka, U., Patsch, R. 1975. Zur intravenosen Verabfolgung von Doxycyclin (Vibravenos) im Kindesalter-klinische und pharmakokinetische Probleme. *Int. J. Clin. Pharmacol.* 11:245–52

12. Paisley, J. W., Smith, A. L., Smith, D. H. 1973. Gentamicin in newborn infants. *Am. J. Dis. Child.* 126:473–77
13. Howard, J. B., McCracken, G. H. Jr. 1975. Reappraisal of kanamycin usage in neonates. *J. Pediatr.* 86:949–56
14. Krauer, B. 1975. The development of diurnal variation in drug kinetics in the human infant. See Ref. 1, pp. 347–56
15. McCracken, G. H. Jr., Nelson, J. D. 1976. Commentary: An appraisal of tobramycin usage in pediatrics. *J. Pediatr.* 88:315–17
16. Levy, G., Khanna, N. N., Soda, D. M., Tsuzuki, O., Stern, L. 1975. Pharmacokinetics of acetaminophen in the human neonate: Formation of acetaminophen glucuronide and sulfate in relation to plasma bilirubin concentration and D-glucaric acid excretion. *Pediatrics* 55:818–25
17. Miller, R. P., Roberts, R. J., Fischer, L. J. 1976. Acetaminophen elimination kinetics in neonates, children and adults. *Clin. Pharmacol. Ther.* 19:284–94
18. Alvares, A. P., Kapelner, S., Sassa, S., Kappas, A. 1975. Drug metabolism in normal children, lead-poisoned children, and normal adults. *Clin. Pharmacol. Ther.* 17:179–83
19. Gladtke, E. 1968. Pharmacokinetic studies on phenylbutazone in children. *Farmaco Ed. Sci.* 23:897
20. Wilson, J. T., Atwood, G. F., Shand, D. G. 1976. Disposition of propoxyphene and propranolol in children. *Clin. Pharmacol. Ther.* 19:264–70
21. Levy, G. 1975. Salicylate pharmacokinetics in the human neonate. See Ref. 1, pp. 319–30
22. Pruitt, A. W., Dayton, P. G., Patterson, J. H. 1973. Disposition of diazoxide in children. *Clin. Pharmacol. Ther.* 14:73–82
23. Wettrell, G. 1976. Digoxin therapy in infants. A clinical pharmacokinetic study. *Acta Paediatr. Scand.* 257:7–28
24. Draffan, G. H., Dollery, C. T., Davies, D. S., Krauer, B., Williams, F. M., Clare, R. A., Trudinger, B. J., Darling, M., Sertel, H., Hawkins, D. F. 1976. Maternal and neonatal elimination of amobarbital after treatment of the mother with barbiturates during late pregnancy. *Clin. Pharmacol. Ther.* 19:271–75
25. Hoppel, C., Rane, A., Sjoqvist, F. 1975. Kinetics of phenytoin and carbamaze-

pine in the newborn. See Ref. 1, pp. 341–45

26. Dreifuss, F. E., Penry, J. K., Rose, S. W., Kupferberg, H. J., Dyken, P., Sato, S. 1975. Serum clonazepam concentrations in children with absence seizures. *Neurology* 25:255–58

27. Morselli, P. L., Mandelli, M., Tognoni, G., Principi, N., Pardi, G., Sereni, F. 1974. Drug interactions in the human fetus and in the newborn infant. In *Drug Interactions,* ed. P. L. Morselli, S. Garattini, S. Cohen, 259–70. New York: Raven

28. Schobben, F., van der Kleijn, E., Gabreels, F. J. M. 1975. Pharmacokinetics of Di-N-propylacetate in epileptic patients. *J. Clin. Pharmacol.* 8:97–105

29. Buchanan, R. A., Fernandez, L., Kinkel, A. W. 1969. Absorption and elimination of ethosuximide in children. *J. Clin. Pharmacol.* 9:393–98

29a Browne, T. R., Dreifuss, F. E., Dyken, P. R., Goode, D. J., Penry, J. K., Porter, R. J., White, B. G., White, P. T. 1975. Ethosuximide in the treatment of absence (petit mal) seizures. *Neurology* 25:515–24

30. Blankenbaker, W. L., DiFazio, C. A., Berry, F. A. Jr. 1975. Lidocaine and its metabolites in the newborn. *Anesthesiology* 42:325–30

31. Meffin, P., Long, G. J., Thomas, J. 1973. Clearance and metabolism of mepivicaine in the human neonate. *Clin. Pharmacol. Ther.* 14:218–25

32. Garrettson, L. K., Dayton, P. G. 1970. Disappearance of phenobarbital and diphenylhydantoin from serum of children. *Clin. Pharmacol. Ther.* 11:674–79

33. Reynolds, J. W., Mirkin, B. L. 1973. Urinary corticosteriod and diphenylhydantoin metabolite patterns in neonates exposed to anticonvulsant drugs *in utero. Clin. Pharmacol. Ther.* 14: 891–97

34. Garrettson, L. K., Jusko, W. J. 1975. Diphenylhydantoin elimination kinetics in overdosed children. *Clin. Pharmacol. Ther.* 17:481–91

35. Parsons, W. D., Aranda, J. V., Neims, A. H. 1976. Elimination of transplacentally acquired caffeine in full-term neonates. *Pediatr. Res.* 10:333

36. Sjöqvist, F., Bergfors, P. G., Borga, O., Lind, M., Ygge, H. 1972. Plasma disappearance of nortriptyline in a newborn infant following placental transfer from an intoxicated mother: Evidence for drug metabolism. *J. Pediatr.* 80:496–500

37. Aranda, J. V., Sitar, D. S., Parsons, W. D., Loughnan, P. M., Neims, A. H. 1976. Pharmacokinetic aspects of theophylline in premature newborns. *N. Engl. J. Med.* 295:413–16

38. Rane, A., Wilson, J. T. 1976. Clinical pharmacokinetics in infants and children. *Clin. Pharmacokinet.* 1:2–24

39. Loughnan, P. M., Sitar, D. S., Ogilvie, R. I., Eisen, A., Fox, Z., Neims, A. H. 1976. Pharmacokinetic analysis of the disposition of intravenous theophylline in young children. *J. Pediatr.* 88:874–79

40. Nitowsky, H. M., Matz, L., Berzofsky, J. A. 1966. Studies on oxidative drug metabolism in the full-term newborn infant. *J. Pediatr.* 69:1139–49

41. Pagliaro, L. A., Benet, L. Z. 1975. Critical compilation of terminal half-lives, percent excreted unchanged, and changes of half-life in renal and hepatic dysfunction for studies in humans with references. *J. Pharmacokinet. Biopharm.* 3:333–83

42. Jalling, B. 1975. Plasma concentrations of phenobarbital in the treatment of seizures in newborns. *Acta Paediatr. Scand.* 64:514–24

43. Weber, W. W., Cohen, S. N. 1975. Aging effects and drugs in man. *Hand. Exp. Pharmacol.* 28:213–33

44. Schwartz, G. J., Hegyi, T., Spitzer, A. 1976. Subtherapeutic dicloxacillin levels in a neonate: Possible mechanisms. *J. Pediatr.* 89:310–12

45. Vest, M. F., Rossier, R. 1963. Detoxification in the newborn: The ability of the newborn infant to form conjugates with glucuronic acid, glycine, acetate and glutathione. *Ann. NY Acad. Sci.* 111:183–97

46. Stern, L., Khanna, N. N., Levy, G., Yaffe, S. J. 1970. Effect of phenobarbital on hyperbilirubinemia and glucuronide formation in newborns. *Am. J. Dis. Child.* 120:26–31

47. Weiss, C. F., Glazko, A. J., Weston, J. K. 1960. Chloramphenicol in the newborn infant. A physiologic explanation of its toxicity when given in excessive doses. *N. Engl. J. Med.* 262:787–94

48. Boreus, L. O., Jalling, B., Kallberg, N. 1975. Clinical pharmacology of phenobarbital in the neonatal period. See Ref. 1, pp. 331–40

49. Horning, M. G., Butler, C. M., Nowlin, J., Hill, R. M. 1975. Drug metabolism in the human neonate. *Life Sci.* 16:651–71

50. Windorfer, A. Jr., Kuenzer, W., Urbanek, R. 1974. The influence of age on

the activity of acetylsalicylic acid–esterase and protein-salicylate binding. *Eur. J. Clin. Pharmacol.* 7:227–31

51. Ecobichon, D. J., Stephens, D. S. 1973. Perinatal development of human blood esterases. *Clin. Pharmacol. Ther.* 14: 41–47

52. Thaler, M. M., Dallman, P. R., Goodman, J. 1972. Phenobarbital-induced changes in NADPH-cytochrome c reductase and smooth endoplasmic reticulum in human liver. *J. Pediatr.* 80:302–10

53. Waddell, W. J., Marlowe, G. C. 1976. Disposition of drugs in the fetus. In *Perinatal Pharmacology and Therapeutics*, ed. B. L. Mirkin, 119–268. New York: Academic. 455 pp.

54. Krasner, J., Yaffe, S. J. 1975. Drug-protein binding in the neonate. See Ref. 1, pp. 357–66

55. Levy, G., Procknal, J. A., Garrettson, L. K. 1975. Distribution of salicylate between neonatal and maternal serum at diffusion equilibrium. *Clin. Parmacol. Ther.* 18:210–14

56. Ehrnebo, M., Agurell, S., Jalling, B., Boreus, L. O. 1971. Age differences in drug binding by plasma proteins: Studies on human foetuses, neonates and adults. *Eur. J. Clin. Pharmacol.* 3: 189–93

57. Kiosz, D., Simon, C., Malerczyk, V. 1975. Die Plasmaweissbindung von Clindamycin, Cephazolin und Cephradin bei Neugeborenen und Erwachsenen. *Klin. Paediatr.* 187:71–80

58. Chignell, C. F., Vesell, E. S., Starkweather, D. K., Berlin, C. M. 1971. The binding of sulfaphenazole to fetal, neonatal, and adult human plasma albumin. *Clin. Pharmacol. Ther.* 12:897–901

59. Ganshorn, A., Kurz, H. 1968. Unterschiede zwischen der Proteinbindung Neugeborener und Erwachsener und ihre Bedeutung fur die pharmakologische Wirkung. *Arch. Pharmakol.* 260:117–18

60. Tucker, G. T., Boyes, R. N., Bridenbaugh, P. O., Moore, D. C. 1970. Binding of anilide-type local anesthetics in

human plasma. II. Implications *in vivo,* with special reference to transplacental distribution. *Anesthesiology* 33:304–14

61. Pruitt, A. W., Zwiren, G. T., Patterson, J. H., Dayton, P. G., Cook, C. E., Wall, M. E. 1975. A complex pattern of disposition of phenytoin in severe intoxication. *Clin. Pharmacol. Ther.* 18:112–20

62. Levy, G., Yaffe, S. J. 1974. Relationship between dose and apparent volume of distribution of salicylate in children. *Pediatrics* 54:713–17

63. Rane, A., Hojer, B., Wilson, J. T. 1976. Kinetics of carbamazepine and its 10,11-epoxide metabolite in children. *Clin. Pharmacol. Ther.* 19:276–83

64. Krasula, R. W., Hastreiter, A. R., Levitsky, S., Yanagi, R., Soyka, L. F. 1974. Serum, atrial, and urinary digoxin levels during cardiopulmonary bypass in children. *Circulation* 49:1047–52

65. Gorodischer, R., Jusko, W. J., Yaffe, S. J. 1976. Tissue and erythrocyte distribution of digoxin in infants. *Clin. Pharmacol. Ther.* 19:256–63

66. Kauffman, R. E., Azarnoff, D. L., Morris, J. A. 1975. Placental transfer and fetal urinary excretion of gentamicin—comparison between an animal model and the human fetus. See Ref. 1. pp. 75–82

67. Jalling, B. 1974. Plasma and cerebrospinal fluid concentrations of phenobarbital in infants given single doses. *Dev. Med. Child. Neurol.* 16:781–93

68. Kaplan, J. M., McCracken, G. H. Jr., Horton, L. J., Thomas, M. L., Davis, N. 1974. Pharmacologic studies in neonates given large dosages of ampicillin. *J. Pediatr.* 84:571–77

69. Levy, G., Ellis, E. F., Koysooko, R. 1974. Indirect plasma-theophylline monitoring in asthmatic children by determination of theophylline concentration in saliva. *Pediatrics* 53:873–76

70. Nelson, J. D., McCracken, G. H. Jr. 1973. Clinical pharmacology of carbenicillin and gentamicin in the neonate and comparative efficacy with ampicillin and gentamicin. *Pediatrics* 52:801–13

Ann Rev. Pharmacol. Toxicol. 1977. 17:575–604
Copyright © 1977 by Annual Reviews Inc. All rights reserved

IN VITRO STUDY OF ❖6697
β-ADRENERGIC RECEPTORS

Barry B. Wolfe, T. Kendall Harden, and Perry B. Molinoff
Department of Pharmacology, University of Colorado Medical Center,
Denver, Colorado 80262

INTRODUCTION

Norepinephrine is synthesized and stored in nerve terminals in both the peripheral and central nervous systems. The release of norepinephrine from adrenergic nerves results in the modulation of a variety of cellular processes. The postsynaptic events resulting from norepinephrine release are initiated through interaction with specific membrane receptors. Interaction of norepinephrine with its specific receptor is only the first step in a complicated and incompletely understood series of events. The molecular configuration of adrenergic receptors determines the structural specificity and activity of both agonists and antagonists. Furthermore, changes in the density or properties of adrenergic receptors may be a mechanism for regulating the ultimate effects of catecholamines. Most of our knowledge of postsynaptic adrenergic mechanisms comes from studies either in whole animals or with isolated organ systems. Studies of this type can provide information only on the final events resulting from the interaction of catecholamines with adrenergic receptors. They cannot provide an understanding of the molecular interactions that occur when the receptor recognizes a specific agonist. This chapter deals with our present knowledge of the β-adrenergic receptor system. Emphasis is placed on the events that occur at or immediately distal to the receptor. In particular, the information that has accumulated during the past few years through the use of direct binding assays of β-adrenergic receptors is discussed. Several reviews of various aspects of this subject have recently appeared (1-7).

Classification of Adrenergic Receptors

The existence of multiple types of adrenergic receptors was first suggested by the results of Dale (8). He demonstrated that some of the effects of epinephrine or of sympathetic nerve stimulation were antagonised by ergot alkaloids while other responses were unaffected. In 1948, Ahlquist (9) divided adrenergic responses into two classes based on the effects elicited by a series of catecholamines. The first class of receptors, called alpha (α) were stimulated by agonists with the potency order of epinephrine $>$ norepinephrine $>$ α-methylnorepinephrine $>$ α-methyl-epinephrine $>$ isoproterenol. Stimulation of these receptors led to contraction of the nictitating membrane, to vasoconstriction, and to contraction of smooth muscle in the uterus and ureter. The second type of adrenergic receptor, called beta (β), responded with the agonist specificity of isoproterenol $>$ epinephrine $>$ α-methyl-epinephrine $>$ α-methyl-norepinephrine $>$ norepinephrine. Stimulation of these receptors resulted in positive cardiac inotropy and chronotropy, vasodilation, and relaxation of uterine smooth muscle. This classification of adrenergic receptors has been extended to include most effects mediated by catecholamines. The responses characteristic of α- and β-adrenergic receptors have been further defined through the use of specific antagonists (1, 2, 10–13). For instance, β-adrenergic responses can be divided into the subclasses β_1 and β_2 (14, 15). Epinephrine and norepinephrine are approximately equipotent activators of β_1 receptors which are preferentially inhibited by practolol (16). Epinephrine is more potent than norepinephrine in activating β_2 receptors which are inhibited by butoxamine (17, 18). A variety of antagonists including propranolol, alprenolol, and pindolol do not distinguish between β_1 and β_2 receptors (19, 20).

Relationship of Adrenergic Receptors to cAMP Formation

Sutherland and co-workers (21, 22) first introduced the concept that adenosine 3', 5'-monophosphate (cAMP) serves as a second messenger for the action of a variety of hormones. It soon became apparent to these and other workers that cAMP served as a mediator of some of the actions of catecholamines (21–23). Specifically, those actions of catecholamines mediated through β-adrenergic receptors result in increased intracellular levels of cAMP. Therefore, activation of the catalytic unit of adenylate cyclase by catecholamines can serve as a measure of β-adrenergic receptor function and permits an indirect biochemical characterization of these receptors. With the exception of the central nervous system, α-adrenergic receptor stimulation does not increase cAMP levels (22). In the brain, activation of receptors with the pharmacological characteristics of α-adrenergic receptors results in increased intracellular levels of cAMP (24–28). Therefore, norepinephrine-stimulated cAMP formation in the brain reflects the stimulation of both α- and β-adrenergic receptors.

Characterization of Direct Binding Assays for β-Adrenergic Receptors

The most direct way to characterize a receptor is to assess the interaction of a specific ligand with the receptor. On the other hand, measurement of other parameters, such as catecholamine-stimulated adenylate cyclase activity, includes several events distal to the interaction of the amine with the receptor. By directly assaying the receptor, the chemistry of the initial events involved in β-adrenergic receptor-mediated responses can be more clearly approached. Also, changes in the properties of the β-adrenergic receptor itself may play a role in regulating cell responsiveness. This possibility can be most easily examined using direct in vitro assays. And finally, by serving as a means through which β-adrenergic receptors can be followed during solubilization, isolation, and reconstitution studies, this type of assay should ultimately permit elucidation of the mechanism through which receptor occupation leads to the activation of adenylate cyclase.

Once a suitable ligand has been found, the technical aspects of establishing direct binding assays are relatively simple. There are several well-accepted methods for separating free radioactive ligand from ligand that has been specifically bound to the receptor. Equilibrium dialysis (29, 30), centrifugation (31–33), and filtration (34–37) techniques have all been used successfully in assays of β-adrenergic receptors. A greater concentration of receptors is required for equilibrium dialysis than for the other methods of quantifying bound ligand. The latter two systems offer several additional advantages since they are less time consuming than is equilibrium dialysis, and washing procedures can often be used to remove nonspecifically bound or occluded ligand from the filter or pellet. When a procedure is used that includes washing the sample, some consideration of the rate of dissociation of ligand from the receptor is required. It is theoretically possible that a wash procedure will cause dissociation of specifically bound ligand. In some cases, dissociation of specifically bound ligand has been minimized by washing with cold buffer (36, 37). In other cases, it has been advantageous to use buffer at 37° to remove ligand that is nonspecifically bound (34, 35). It is impossible to know a priori whether a given separation procedure will be appropriate. In any case, the use of a ligand with a high affinity will increase the probability that the ligand will have a slow rate of dissociation from its receptor.

Consideration of the properties of catecholamine-stimulated adenylate cyclase activity has led to the development of a set of expected criteria to characterize the in vitro binding of a reversible β-adrenergic receptor ligand to the receptor (38, 39). Thus, the binding of the radioactively labeled ligand should show saturability since only a finite number of receptors exist. If there are no spare receptors (38, 40) and a one-to-one relationship between β-adrenergic receptors and adenylate cyclase exists, the dissociation constant (K_d) of an agonist determined by inhibition of binding should be equal to the EC_{50} value determined by measuring the activation of adenylate cyclase. If spare receptors exist, the K_d should be greater than the EC_{50}. The K_d values for antagonists, determined by inhibition of binding, should be equal to the values determined from the inhibition of catecholamine-stimulated adenylate cyclase. This should be true irrespective of the existence of spare receptors. When a reversible β-adrenergic receptor ligand is used, the bound radiolabeled compound should be completely dissociable. It is important to demonstrate that a ligand that has dissociated from its binding site is chemically unchanged and will bind to membranes with properties identical with those of fresh ligand. The ratio of the kinetically derived rate constants of dissociation (k_2) and association (k_1) should be equal to the dissociation constant (K_d) determined at equilibrium ($k_2/k_1 = K_d$). Compounds that affect adenylate cyclase activity through interaction with β-adrenergic receptors should inhibit the binding of the radioligand. Conversely, compounds that are inactive at β-adrenergic receptors should not inhibit the binding of a radioligand. Finally, the binding of a ligand to the β-adrenergic receptor should be preferentially inhibited by stereoisomers having the R configuration at the β-carbon of the ethanolamine side chain. In general, this corresponds to an optical rotation in the levorotatory direction (41). Both agonist-induced activation of adenylate cyclase and inhibition of catecholamine-stimulated adenylate cyclase exhibit stereospecificity.

In any in vitro assay of a receptor, it is necessary to identify specific binding of ligand to the receptor as opposed to binding to other sites. Nonspecific bindings may include hydrophobic and hydrophilic interactions with various membrane constituents. In experiments with whole cells, the uptake of ligand must also be considered (38). To define nonspecific binding, assays are carried out in the presence of a competing β-adrenergic receptor antagonist or agonist at a concentration that will occupy essentially all of the receptor sites. In this situation, specific binding of ligand will be equal to the amount of radioactivity bound in the absence of competing ligand minus the amount of radioactivity bound in its presence. In general, when assays are carried out under conditions such that the concentrations of radioactive ligand and of receptors are both well below the K_d value for the radioactive ligand, a concentration of a competing ligand which is one hundred times its K_d value should provide a satisfactory estimate of nonspecific binding. On the other hand, when the concentration of either the radioactive ligand or of receptors approaches or exceeds the K_d value for the ligand, then a higher concentration of competing ligand will be necessary to occupy all or most of the receptor sites. The concentration can be calculated easily from the Michaelis-Menten equation (42). The need for a quantitative definition of nonspecific binding arises from the fact that too high a concentration of a competing ligand may not only block specific binding of radioligand to the β-adrenergic receptor but may also compete for nonspecific sites (38, 43).

There are other points that should be considered when establishing an in vitro assay for β-adrenergic receptors. The receptors should be found on cells that have been shown by anatomical and physiological studies to be innervated by noradrenergic neurons. With only a few exceptions (44–47), adenylate cyclase has been found to be associated with the plasma membranes of cells (4, 22). Since β-adrenergic receptors seem to be functionally connected with adenylate cyclase its distribution should parallel the distribution of plasma membrane markers, including catecholamine-stimulated adenylate cyclase.

IN VITRO ASSAYS OF β-ADRENERGIC RECEPTORS

The Use of Catecholamine Agonists

The earliest attempts to establish an in vitro binding assay for β-adrenergic receptors utilized the interaction of tritiated catecholamines with membrane preparations enriched in catecholamine-sensitive adenylate cyclase. Several tissue sources were investigated. Marinetti and co-workers (48–51) as well as Leray et al (52) studied the binding of ^{3}H-epinephrine to rat liver plasma membranes. These investigators showed that the binding was saturable and that other catecholamines were potent inhibitors of the binding. However, the binding was also inhibited by a variety of catechol-containing compounds that were not active at β-adrenergic receptors.

Also, stereospecificity was not seen, and bound radioactivity did not dissociate after the addition of strong acid. Potent β-adrenergic receptor antagonists, such as propranolol, had little effect on binding even at very high concentration (0.1 mM). Lefkowitz and co-workers investigated the interaction of ^{3}H-norepinephrine with cardiac microsomes (53–55), myocardial cells grown in tissue culture (56), and fat cell membranes (57). Inhibition of the binding of ^{3}H-norepinephrine by agonists did not show stereospecificity although binding was inhibited by a variety of catechol-containing compounds. Propranolol, at a concentration of 0.1 mM, caused only a 40% inhibition of norepinephrine binding (53, 56). Acid reversed the binding to cardiac microsomes, but the addition of a large excess of unlabeled norepinephrine did not cause the dissociation of bound ligand (55). Bilezikian & Aurbach (58, 59) as well as Schramm et al (60) studied the binding of tritiated catecholamines to turkey erythrocyte membranes, which are a rich source of β-adrenergic receptors. Binding was inhibited by several catechol-containing compounds but no evidence of stereospecificity was observed. High affinity β-adrenergic receptor antagonists did not inhibit binding. In contrast to studies with other tissues, almost total dissociation of bound ^{3}H-catecholamine from turkey erythrocytes was observed on dilution of the incubation mixture (58, 61).The concentration of binding sites determined for turkey erythrocyte ghosts ranged from 55 to 300 pmoles/mg of protein while the maximum stimulation of adenylate cyclase by isoproterenol was only 4.5 to 18 pmoles cAMP formed per milligram of protein per minute (58–60). Thus, it appeared from these studies that either the turnover number of adenylate cyclase was extremely low or there were a surprisingly high number of spare receptors.

Several reports have appeared that question the conclusion that the binding of catecholamines to membrane fragments is related to β-adrenergic receptors (61–65). The binding of ^{3}H-catecholamines to heart (61–63, 65), liver (61), adipocyte (61), skeletal muscle (65), and turkey erythrocyte membranes (61) as well as to membranes from several cell lines grown in tissue culture (62) have been studied. Binding was inhibited by a large number of catechol-containing compounds, was not affected by potent β-adrenergic receptor antagonists, and did not show stereospecificity. With a few exceptions (58, 61, 65), the binding of ^{3}H-catecholamines was almost entirely irreversible. Cuatrecasas et al (61) proposed that the binding was related to the enzyme catechol-O-methyltransferase (COMT), some of which is membrane bound (61, 66). This enzyme methylates the phenolic oxygen of a variety of catechols, and it does not show stereoselectivity. Several inhibitors of COMT inhibited the binding of catecholamines (61), and S-adenosylmethionine, a cosubstrate required for COMT activity, increased the rate of binding of ^{3}H-norepinephrine to liver and heart microsomes. An analogue of S-adenosylmethionine, S-adenosyl-homocysteine, decreased the amount of binding and also decreased the activity of COMT in liver microsomes. It is important to note that several of the COMT inhibitors studied by Cuatrecasas et al (61) were catechols. At least three groups of investigators have argued against the involvement of COMT in the binding of ^{3}H-catecholamines. Two noncatechol inhibitors of COMT had no effect on the binding of ^{3}H-epinephrine to membranes derived from rat heart (63). Although syringic acid and syringaldehyde are potent inhibitors of COMT activity, they had little effect on the binding (67). In addition, the subcellular distribution of binding activity and COMT activity were markedly different (68). It was also reported that the pH optimum for COMT differed from that of the binding reaction (68).

Maguire et al (62) showed that inhibition of oxidation by agents such as sodium metabisulfite, sodium ascorbate, EDTA, and 1,2- or 1,4-dihydroxybenzene inhibited the binding of ^{3}H-norepinephrine. Saturation of the reaction media with nitrogen caused a reduction in the rate of binding of ^{3}H-catecholamine to rat glioma cells (62). The divalent cations Mn^{2+}, Co^{2+}, and Fe^{2+} reversed the inhibitory effect of EDTA on the binding (62). Along these same lines, Wolfe et al (63) showed that the time course of oxidation of ^{3}H-epinephrine was very similar to the time course of binding to rat heart preparations. In addition, ^{3}H-epinephrine bound to bovine serum albumin with properties that were qualitatively and quantitatively similar to those of membranes derived from rat heart (63). Cuatrecasas et al (61) and Wolfe et al (63) reported that the rate of binding of ^{3}H-catecholamines was increased after tissues were boiled or stored at 4° or –22°. This increase in the rate of binding was temporally associated with an increase in the rate of tissue-catalyzed oxidation of ^{3}H-epinephrine (63). The mechanism by which storage of tissues enhances the rate of oxidation of epinephrine was not established. It may reflect the release or exposure of divalent cations associated with various tissue constituents. Finally, it was demonstrated that the addition of 30 μM pyrocatechol delayed the onset of binding of ^{3}H-epinephrine to heart membranes. Simultaneous measurements of the rate of oxidation of ^{3}H-epinephrine revealed that pyrocatechol also delayed the onset of oxidation of epinephrine (63). The two reactions occurred with an identical time course. Maguire et al (62) and Wolfe et al (63) concluded that the binding of catecholamines involves a nonspecific, probably covalent, interaction of oxidized degradation products of catechols with unspecified tissue constituents.

Lacombe & Hanoune (69) studied the binding of ^{3}H-epinephrine to liver plasma membranes in the presence of 1 mM EDTA. Similarly, Pairault & Laudat (70) studied the binding of ^{3}H-norepinephrine to membranes from rat adipocytes in the presence of 1 mM EGTA and 0.5 mM pyrocatechol. Inclusion of pyrocatechol or a chelating agent decreased the oxidation of catecholamines. In the presence of these agents the residual binding of ^{3}H-catecholamine observed was more susceptible to inhibition by propranolol than was the binding in their absence. Although the residual binding was inhibited by catecholamines, no stereospecificity was observed in these studies.

A recent report by Malchoff & Marinetti (71) described stereospecific inhibition of ^{3}H-isoproterenol binding to intact chicken erythrocytes. Specific binding was inhibited by a low concentration of propranolol (80 nM). It is likely that the high affinity of isoproterenol for β-adrenergic receptors in chicken erythrocytes permitted these workers to observe stereospecific binding. In addition, they reported that there was a dramatic increase in the amount of catecholamine bound if the reaction was performed on lysed cells. However, they were unable to demonstrate stereospecific binding in preparations of broken cells.

The studies with agonists described above suggested that in vitro assays of β-adrenergic receptors require a ligand that has a high affinity for these receptors, that can be labeled to a high specific activity, and that is resistant to oxidation. The use of a ligand with a high affinity labeled to high specific activity makes possible the assay of receptors at a low concentration of ligand. Theoretically, this should increase the proportion of total binding that is associated and with β-adrenergic receptors.

The Use of β-Adrenergic Receptor Antagonists

Many β-adrenergic receptor antagonists have affinities that are two to three orders of magnitude greater than those of catecholamine agonists. However, initial attempts to develop an in vitro β-adrenergic receptor binding assay using tritiated propranolol were unsuccessful (72, 73). These failures may have been due to the use of myocardial membranes. Levitzki et al showed that the binding of ^{3}H-propranolol (4.3 Ci/mmole) to turkey erythrocyte membranes was inhibited in a stereospecific manner by β-adrenergic receptor agonists and antagonists (29, 31). The dissociation constants of various β-adrenergic receptor ligands as determined by their ability to inhibit ^{3}H-propranolol binding were in good agreement with values obtained from measurements of adenylate cyclase activity (31, 74). Approximately 0.8 pmoles of binding sites per milligram of protein were found which was equivalent to 550 binding sites per erythrocyte (see Table 1).

More recently, Nahorski (75), using ^{3}H-propranolol with a specific activity of 21 Ci/mmol, reported stereospecifically displaceable binding to membranes from chick cerebral cortex. There were approximately 0.23 pmoles of binding sites per milligram of protein. Binding was rapid and equilibrium was reached within 2 min.

Table 1 Properties of β-adrenergic receptor binding

Tissue	Species	Ligand	K_d (nm)	pmole/mg	K_1 ($M^{-1}min^{-1}$)	K_1 (min^{-1})	Reference
Erythrocyte	Turkey	Prop	2.5	0.90	—	—	29
		IHYP	0.020–0.025	0.2–0.3	5.4×10^{10a}	0.54^a	95
	Frog	DHA	5–10	0.35	—	—	76
	Rat	IHYP	0.025	0.15	—	—	108
Heart	Dog	DHA	11	0.35	—	—	33
	Rat	IHYP	1.4	0.16	3×10^{7a}	4.75×10^{-2a}	35
Cerebral cortex	Rat	DHA	6.7	0.2	—	—	87
	Rat	IHYP	1–1.5	0.3–0.35	9.8×10^{7a}	4.5×10^{-2a}	43
	Rat	DHA	1.3	0.3	1.2×10^{8a}	0.1^b	36
	Chick	Prop	11	0.23	—	—	75
Liver	Rat	IHYP	2–3	0.039	1.2×10^{6a}	1.2×10^{-2a}	126
Adipocytes	Rat	DHA	10–20	0.24	2.4×10^{7a}	0.294	37
Lymphocytes	Human	DHA	9	0.075	—	—	88
Pineal	Rat	DHA	18	0.6	—	—	91
Cells in culture							
Glioma (C6TG1A)	Rat	IHYP	0.25	0.075	1×10^{8c}	1.7×10^{-2c}	34
Glioma (VA2)	Rat	IHYP	0.015	0.15	—	3.5×10^{-3c}	34
Astrocytoma	Human	IHYP	0.6–2	0.3–3	—	8×10^{-3a}	101
Lymphoma	Mouse	IHYP	0.033	0.028	—	6×10^{-3c}	107

^{a} = 37°.
^{b} = 23°.
^{c} = 30°.

Dissociation of bound ligand, initiated by adding excess (0.2 mM) isoproterenol, occurred with a half-time of 45 sec. One consistent problem in the studies reporting the successful use of ^{3}H-propranolol (29, 31, 74, 75) was the large amount of nonspecific binding of ligand. The low percentage of specific binding of ^{3}H-propranolol (20–45%) caused problems in quantitative studies of β-adrenergic receptors.

Lefkowitz and co-workers (32, 76, 77) reduced the unsaturated carbon-carbon double bond of (–)-alprenolol with palladium and tritium gas to obtain ^{3}H-dihydroalprenolol (DHA) with a specific activity of 17–33 Ci/mmole. The binding of DHA to frog erythrocyte membranes has been extensively characterized (32, 76, 78–86). It was inhibited stereospecifically by both β-adrenergic receptor agonists and antagonists. The binding of DHA to β-adrenergic receptors of frog erythrocyte membranes was rapid and equilibrium was reached within five min at 37° (76). Binding was reversible on addition of 10 μM propranolol or following dilution (76, 79). The half-time for dissociation at 37° was less than 30 sec. Binding was saturable with between 1000 and 2000 sites per erythrocyte. The dissociation constants of β-adrenergic receptor agonists and antagonists were determined from studies of the inhibition of DHA binding. These values were in good agreement with those obtained in studies of catecholamine-sensitive adenylate cyclase activity (76,81). Compounds not affecting catecholamine-sensitive adenylate cyclase had no effect on the binding of DHA (76).

Tritiated DHA has been used to characterize β-adrenergic receptors of several other tissues including heart (33), brain (36, 87), lymphocytes (88), pineal organ (89–91), and adipocytes (37). The properties of the binding of DHA in these systems are generally similar to those described for frog erythrocytes.

In experiments with DHA the concentration of radioligand is high relative to its K_d. Therefore, the concentration of a competing ligand that inhibits 50% of the specific binding of DHA will be greater than its true K_d value (92). In this case both the K_d of the radioligand and its concentration are needed to calculate the true K_d value for a competing ligand (81, 92, 93).

Using a slightly different approach, Aurbach et al (94) established a direct binding assay for β-adrenergic receptors in turkey erythrocytes. This group used [^{125}I]iodohydroxybenzylpindolol (IHYP), a high affinity β-adrenergic receptor antagonist, which can be purified to achieve a nearly theoretical specific activity of 2200 Ci/mmole. The binding of IHYP was inhibited in a stereoselective manner by both β-adrenergic receptor agonists and antagonists. The binding of IHYP to various tissues has been characterized. Brown et al (95, 96), using turkey erythrocyte membranes, showed that there were approximately 0.3 pmoles of binding sites per milligram of protein. This value corresponded to 400–600 sites per cell, agreeing well with the value obtained by Levitzki et al (29) using ^{3}H-propranolol as a ligand. Dissociation constants for β-adrenergic receptor agonists and antagonists were determined both by the inhibition of IHYP binding and by the measurement of catecholamine-sensitive adenylate cyclase activity. The K_d values determined by the two methods were in good agreement for antagonists. However, the K_d values for agonists, as determined by inhibition of IHYP binding were 2 to 10 times smaller than the apparent K_d values determined for the activation of adenylate cyclase (96). This discrepancy was discussed in terms of the ability of 5'-guanylimidodiphosphate (GMPPNP) to increase the apparent affinity of agonists for adenylate cyclase without affecting the binding of either agonists or antagonists to β-adrenergic receptors (96; cf section on guanyl nucleotides below).

Harden et al (35, 97) characterized β-adrenergic receptors in rat heart using IHYP. The binding of IHYP was prevented in a stereospecific manner by both agonists and antagonists and was unaffected by compounds that are not active at these receptors. There were approximately 0.2 pmoles of binding sites per milligram of protein. Approximately 40 min were required for the binding of radioligand to reach equilibrium. This slow rate was discussed in terms of the low concentrations of IHYP and of receptor used. Dissociation constants of antagonists determined by binding and by measuring adenylate cyclase activity were in good agreement. The relative order of potencies for agonists as determined by the two methods were also in good agreement. However, the absolute values of dissociation constants for agonists determined by inhibition of IHYP binding were 10–100 times less than the apparent K_d values for agonists determined from activation of adenylate cyclase. The authors suggested that homogenization resulted in a perturbation of the β-adrenergic receptor-adenylate cyclase system distal to the formation of the hormone-receptor complex (22, 35, 98–100). Additional evidence consistent with this conclusion was obtained in a study of human EH118 astrocytoma cells (101). In this study the K_d value for isoproterenol in intact cells was the same whether determined in studies of IHYP binding or in studies in which cAMP accumulation in response to isoproterenol was measured. Homogenization of the cells did not affect the K_d for isoproterenol determined by IHYP binding, but the EC_{50} determined from measurements of adenylate cyclase activity was increased approximately tenfold after homogenization.

Sporn & Molinoff (43) have characterized the binding of IHYP to membranes from rat cerebral cortex, caudate nucleus, and cerebellum. The density of sites was lower in the cerebellum than in the other two regions examined. Binding was saturable and reversible and was inhibited stereospecifically by β-adrenergic receptor ligands. These authors found that the inclusion of high concentrations of phentolamine or phenoxybenzamine (up to 0.1 mM) greatly reduced the amount of nonspecifically bound IHYP without affecting specifically bound ligand. This effect of α-adrenergic receptor antagonists was not seen in experiments with heart or liver membranes (T. K. Harden, B. B. Wolfe, and P. B. Molinoff, unpublished observations). Phentolamine (0.1 mM) inhibited specific binding in experiments with membranes from hypothalamus and brain stem and thus it could not be used with these tissues. The effect of phentolamine and phenoxybenzamine did not appear to reflect interaction with α-adrenergic receptors since (+) and (–) phenoxybenzamine were equipotent and since very high concentrations of drug were required. A similar effect of phentolamine on the small amount of nonspecific binding of IHYP to turkey erythrocyte membranes has been reported by Brown and co-workers (96).

Alexander et al (87) and Bylund & Snyder (36) have studied β-adrenergic receptors in various regions of rat brain using DHA. The properties of the binding were similar to those reported in studies of the binding of DHA to membranes from frog erythrocytes. A high density of binding sites was found in the cortex and caudate nucleus. The concentration of sites was lower in the hypothalamus and brain stem. The high density of sites in the caudate (see also 43) is surprising since there are few if any noradrenergic terminals in the caudate (102). It is not likely that the binding of DHA or IHYP in the caudate reflects the presence of a large number of dopamine receptors since dopamine was a very weak inhibitor of both DHA (36, 87) and IHYP binding (43). The presence of non-neuronal elements, which may contain these receptors (28, 103, 104), could account for the presence of binding sites in the caudate. Skolnick & Daly (105) and Markstein & Wagner (106) have recently pointed out an additional complicating factor in studying adrenergic receptors in the brain. In these studies alprenolol (105) and pindolol (106) were shown to inhibit both the α- and β-adrenergic receptor–mediated increases in brain cyclic AMP levels.

Maguire et al (34) used IHYP to study β-adrenergic receptors of several cell lines grown in tissue culture. Two types of high affinity binding sites for IHYP were found in experiments with rat glioma (C6TG1A) cells. However, binding of IHYP to only one of the sites was stereospecifically inhibited by β-adrenergic receptor ligands. This site had the properties expected of a β-adrenergic receptor. Using crude membrane preparations these workers found approximately 0.075 pmoles of binding sites per milligram of protein, corresponding to 4000 binding sites per cell. The dissociation constant determined by equilibrium binding (0.25 nM) was in good agreement with the dissociation constant (0.17 nM) determined from kinetic measurements of k_1 and k_2. Cell lines that did not respond to catecholamines with an increase in cAMP concentration did not show specific IHYP binding to β-adrenergic receptors. Conversely, stereospecifically displaceable IHYP binding was observed in cell lines that were responsive to catecholamines.

Recently Insel and co-workers (107) have suggested that the synthesis of β-adrenergic receptors and of adenylate cyclase are controlled by separate genes. With S-49 mouse lymphoma cells grown in tissue culture, it was shown that wild-type S-49 cells generated cAMP in response to catecholamines and possessed IHYP binding sites similar to those described by Maguire et al (34) for rat glioma cells. A clone of S-49 cells was isolated that did not respond to isoproterenol, PGE$_1$, or sodium fluoride by accumulating cAMP, indicating that these cells do not possess adenylate cyclase. However, these cells did contain IHYP binding sites which appeared identical with those of wild-type S-49 cells.

The idea that the synthesis of β-adrenergic receptors and catecholamine-sensitive adenylate cyclase are independently controlled has also been investigated in several studies of rat erythrocytes (108–110). In these reports both mature erythrocytes and reticulocyte-enriched preparations produced by the injection of phenylhydrazine or acetylphenylhydrazine were studied. After these treatments, approximately 90% of the cells in the blood were reticulocytes. Charness et al (108) reported that membranes obtained from reticulocyte-enriched preparations produced nine times more cAMP in response to a high concentration of isoproterenol than did membranes from mature red cells, but they possessed only 40% more IHYP binding sites. These results suggested that β-adrenergic receptors and catecholamine-stimulated adenylate cyclase activity can vary independently. On the other hand, Spiegel et al (109) reported that there was a fourfold increase in both binding sites and isoproterenol-induced cAMP accumulation in cells from acetylphenylhydrazine-pretreated animals. These authors concluded that the loss of catecholamine responsiveness as erythrocytes mature involves a concomitant loss of β-adrenergic receptors and the catalytic function of the adenylate cyclase system. However, Bilezikian & Spiegel (110) have recently reported that as reticulocytes mature, catecholamine-sensitive adenylate cyclase activity decreases more rapidly than does the concentration of β-adrenergic receptors. The authors suggested that maturation of reticulocytes is associated with an uncoupling of the β-adrenergic receptor from its biological effect.

Effects of Guanine Nucleotides

Guanine nucleotides modulate both basal and hormone-sensitive adenylate cyclase activity in a variety of systems (111–115). The naturally occurring nucleotide, GTP, increases the efficacy of catecholamines for the stimulation of adenylate cyclase activity (114). On the other hand, the synthetic analogue, 5'-guanylimidodiphosphate (GMPPNP), increases both the efficacy and the potency of catecholamines for the stimulation of adenylate cyclase activity (112, 113). It has been suggested that these nucleotides bind to a regulatory site that can affect either the interaction of agonist with the receptor or the coupling of activated receptors to the catalytic subunit of adenylate cyclase. Recently, Spiegel et al (116) and Brown et al (96) showed that incubation of turkey erythrocyte membranes with GMPPNP and various β-adrenergic receptor agonists resulted in a ten-fold decrease in the EC_{50} value for the stimulation of adenylate cyclase by catecholamines. In the presence of GMPPNP, the EC_{50} values for agonists were in good agreement with the K_d values determined by inhibition of IHYP binding. In the absence of GMPPNP, the EC_{50} values were one order of magnitude greater than the K_d values. There is substantial evidence that the effects of GMPPNP are irreversible (112, 113, 115). It is therefore difficult to interpret the effects of this agent on catecholamine-stimulated adenylate cyclase activity.

Several laboratories have reported that the presence of GMPPNP does not affect the K_d values for β-adrenergic receptor antagonists, as determined from direct-binding studies (74, 84, 96, 117). However, conflicting reports have appeared on the ability of GMPPNP to affect the K_d values of agonists. Brown et al (96) reported that GMPPNP had no effect on the ability of catecholamines to compete with IHYP for binding sites on turkey erythrocyte membranes. Maguire et al (117) have studied the effects of guanine nucleotides on the binding of IHYP to membranes of various cell lines grown in tissue culture, and more recently Lefkowitz et al (84) have studied their effects on the binding of DHA to frog erythrocyte membranes. The latter two groups of investigators reported that in the presence of GTP, GDP, or GMPPNP, the potency of agonists as determined in binding studies was decreased by approximately one order of magnitude. This subject is discussed in more detail by Maguire et al (6).

Irreversible β-Adrenergic Receptor Ligands

Irreversible blockers of muscarinic and nicotinic cholinergic receptors and α-adrenergic receptors have proved to be very useful tools in pharmacology (13, 118–121). Several irreversible β-adrenergic receptor ligands have recently been described. However, none of these compounds has been radiolabeled and tested in an in vitro assay for these receptors.

In a recent report by Takayanagi and co-workers (122), β-adrenergic receptors mediating relaxation of the guinea pig taenia coli were photoaffinity labeled with (–)-isoproterenol or 2-(2-hydroxy-3-isopropylaminopropoxy)iodobenzene. These compounds acted reversibly in the absence of photoactivation, and their interaction with the receptor was blocked by propranolol. Taenia coli were irradiated for 25 min in the presence of 6 μM (–)-isoproterenol. The tissue was then washed, and the ability of isoproterenol to cause relaxation of the taenia was determined. After irradiation the potency of isoproterenol was decreased by 20-fold although the efficacy was not altered. The authors concluded that there are a substantial number of spare receptors in this tissue. It is possible that a higher concentration of ligand or repeated irradiation would yield a decrease in the maximal response of the tissue and thus permit a quantitative estimate of the number of spare receptors. Photoaffinity inactivation together with one of the in vitro assays for β-adrenergic receptors described above could yield interesting and important data regarding the presence and number of spare receptors.

Atlas and co-workers have prepared irreversible β-adrenergic receptor blockers by bromoacetylation of free amines (123, 124). The parent compounds were reversible antagonists with dissociation constants ranging from 0.2 μM to 0.1 mM. The bromoacetyl derivatives inhibited the effect of (–)-epinephrine on adenylate cyclase activity without affecting fluoride-stimulated adenylate cyclase activity. One of the compounds, a bromoacetyl derivative of propranolol, was suggested to be an irreversible antagonist of β-adrenergic receptors of turkey erythrocyte membranes since epinephrine-sensitive enzyme activity and the capacity to bind ^{3}H-propranolol were not regained after 5 washes of the membranes (123, 124). Both (–)-epinephrine and (–)-propranolol protected receptors from the irreversible effect of the affinity label. The authors discussed the potential usefulness of irreversible ligands for the purification of β-adrenergic receptors. It should be noted, however, that bromoacetylation markedly reduced the potency of several of the antagonists studied. This may be a problem in developing an in vitro assay for β-adrenergic receptors since a low affinity irreversible ligand is likely to label nonreceptor sites in addition to β-adrenergic receptors.

Erez and his collaborators (125) have studied the ability of practolol and chloropractolol to antagonize the chronotropic response to isoproterenol seen in rat atria. The blocking actions of practolol were easily reversed, while the effects of chloropractolol were reversed only by 50% after 30 washes during a period of 30 min. The authors suggested that these results reflected an irreversible action of chloropractolol. However, IHYP, which acts reversibly (34, 35, 95), exhibits rates of dissociation in liver (126) and astrocytoma cells (101) that are similar to that reported for chloropractolol. It therefore seems likely that chloropractolol is simply a high affinity reversible antagonist with a relatively slow rate of dissociation.

A potentially exciting report has appeared describing the development of a specific antibody to β-adrenergic receptors. Wrenn & Haber (127) immunized rabbits with a deoxycholate-solubilized fraction obtained from dog heart. Serum isolated from immunized rabbits inhibited the specific binding of ^{3}H-propranolol as well as isoproterenol-stimulated adenylate cyclase activity. Preimmune serum had no effect. The inhibition appeared to be specific for the β-adrenergic receptor since serum from immunized rabbits had no effect on fluoride, GMPPNP, or glucagon-stimulated adenylate cyclase activity.

IN VITRO PROPERTIES OF β-ADRENERGIC RECEPTORS

Cooperativity of Ligand Receptor Interactions

Several laboratories have analyzed β-adrenergic receptor binding data to determine whether site-site interactions exist. Limbird et al (79) have suggested that negatively cooperative interactions occur between β-adrenergic receptors of frog erythrocyte membranes. In these studies, the time course of dissociation of DHA from its binding sites was determined. Dissociation was initiated either by a 100-fold dilution or by the addition of excess unlabeled alprenolol together with dilution. The rate of dissociation in the presence of alprenolol was greater than in its absence. Saturation data plotted by the method of Hill (128) gave a slope of 0.82, which is consistent with the existence of negative site-site interactions. A greater degree of negative cooperativity (Hill coefficient of 0.65) has been reported in a study of DHA binding to rat adipocytes (37). Maguire et al (34) in studies of cell lines maintained in culture reported Hill coefficients of about 0.8. Brown et al (95), studying the binding of IHYP to turkey erythrocyte membranes concluded from the linearity of their Scatchard plots (129) and from the agreement of K_d values determined kinetically and thermodynamically that there are no cooperative interactions among the β-adrenergic receptors of turkey erythrocyte membranes. In studies of β-adrenergic receptors of rat cerebral cortex, Hill coefficients of 1.01 (36) and 1.02 (43) were observed. Hill coefficients of 0.95 to 1.02 have been found in rat liver and heart (B. B. Wolfe, T. K. Harden, and P. B. Molinoff, unpublished observations). The difference in the results obtained in various laboratories probably reflects the differences in the tissues used.

Localization of β-Adrenergic Receptors

The anatomical and cellular complexity of a number of organs makes it difficult to interpret the results obtained when homogenates are assayed for their content of receptors. For example, in the brain β-adrenergic receptors may be associated with both neuronal (28, 130, 131) and non-neuronal elements (28, 103, 104). One way to circumvent these complexities is through the use of histological techniques. There are several possible approaches for the direct localization of β-adrenergic receptors. Melamed and his collaborators (132) have recently reported experiments carried out with a fluorescent compound, 9-amino-acridinpropranolol. This agent is a potent

($K_d = 3 \times 10^{-8}M$) inhibitor of epinephrine-stimulated adenylate cyclase activity. Following the intravenous administration of this compound, a well-defined yellow fluorescent band was seen in the cerebellar cortex in the region of the Purkinje cell layer. The highest density of fluorescence was observed on the apical dendrites of Purkinje cells. Stereospecific blockade of binding of the fluorescent ligand was demonstrated in experiments with (−) and (+)-propranolol.

Another approach to the localization of β-adrenergic receptors involves the use of the compound IHYP. This compound has a high affinity for β-adrenergic receptors and a slow rate of dissociation. Bylund et al (133) found that following the intravenous administration of IHYP to rats, radioactivity was found in the heart, brain, and lung. Binding was prevented by the prior administration of isoproterenol or propranolol. The eventual goal of these studies is to establish conditions for the autoradiographic localization of β-adrenergic receptors. A second aspect of this approach involves the labeling of cryostat tissue sections in vitro rather than injecting the ligand intravenously. This technique has been successful in preliminary experiments with adrenalectomized rat liver (J. Sporn, unpublished observations).

A third approach, which is of potential applicability to the study of β-adrenergic receptors, involves the development of fluorescein or peroxidase coupled antibodies. There has been one report of the production of an antibody to the β-adrenergic receptor (127). The immunochemical techniques needed to couple an antibody to a visual marker have been described in a variety of systems. Visualization of an antibody complex should offer no unique problems in terms of its applicability to the study of β-adrenergic receptors.

β-Adrenergic receptors are thought to be located on plasma membranes of cells since catecholamine-stimulated adenylate cyclase activity is largely restricted to these membranes (22, 134). Evidence that β-adrenergic receptors exist on the outer surface of cell membranes has been provided by experiments utilizing catecholamines immobilized on either glass beads or amino acid polymers (135, 136).

The subcellular localization of β-adrenergic receptors has been investigated in several different tissues using direct binding assays. Wolfe et al (126) found that β-adrenergic receptors copurified with fluoride-stimulated adenylate cyclase activity during subcellular fractionation of rat liver. Williams et al (37) demonstrated that DHA binding sites are associated with the plasma membrane fraction of rat adipocytes. In other studies (36, 137), DHA binding sites in rat cerebral cortex were associated with a synaptosomal fraction. The DHA binding sites in cortex copurified with the specific uptake mechanism for ^{3}H-norepinephrine. Unlike the results obtained with membranes from mammalian liver, β-adrenergic receptors in the brain did not copurify with fluoride-sensitive adenylate cyclase activity on continuous sucrose gradients (137).

Effect of Membrane-Altering Agents

The mechanism by which the interaction of catecholamines with β-adrenergic receptors leads to the activation of adenylate cyclase is not yet understood. Several approaches may lead to an understanding of these events. The effects of specific lipid perturbing agents on the sensitivity of adenylate cyclase to various hormones have been investigated (138–140). Recently, the effects of these and other agents on β-adrenergic receptors and catecholamine-sensitive adenylate cyclase of frog erythrocyte membranes have been studied (85). Several agents including phospholipases A, C, and D and amphotericin B led to a decreased ability of catecholamines to stimulate adenylate cyclase activity. A dose-dependent decrease in hormone sensitivity was paralleled by a similar decrease in the specific binding of DHA. On the other hand, the polyene antibiotic filipin decreased the ability of catecholamines to stimulate adenylate cyclase activity without significantly altering DHA binding. It was suggested that filipin acted to "uncouple" receptors from catalytic sites. A role for proteins in β-adrenergic receptor sites was suggested by a decrease in DHA binding after treatment with heat, urea, or proteolytic enzymes. Furthermore, it was suggested that both hydrophobic and hydrophilic residues were necessary for the binding of DHA to β-adrenergic receptors (7).

Solubilization of β-Adrenergic Receptors

Solubilization of the receptor is the first step in the eventual isolation and chemical characterization of the active site. Through the use of detergents, adenylate cyclase has been solubilized from a number of membrane sources (141–143). Although there has been one report of the solubilization of adenylate cyclase in a catecholamine-sensitive state (144), in most instances the soluble enzyme was no longer sensitive to hormone stimulation. From these studies, it was concluded that the loss of sensitivity to hormones after solubilization was due to a loss of protein or lipid moieties that normally exist as part of or in close association with receptors and adenylate cyclase in the plasma membrane.

A means of quantitating solubilized β-adrenergic receptors is a necessary prerequisite for their eventual purification. Recently, an in vitro assay for solubilized β-adrenergic receptors has been reported (30, 77). The plant glycoside, digitonin, was used to solubilize β-adrenergic receptors from frog erythrocyte membranes (30, 77). Equilibrium dialysis and Sephadex column chromatography were utilized to measure the binding of DHA to solubilized β-adrenergic receptors, which retain the properties of the membrane-associated receptor. Saturability, stereospecificity, and the expected effects of various pharmacological agents were observed. The solubilized β-adrenergic receptor had an apparent molecular weight of 130,000–150,000 as determined by Sepharose 6B gel chromatography. The ability to bind DHA was lost at temperatures above 4°. High concentrations of EDTA appeared to stabilize the binding sites which were denatured by guanidine hydrochloride, urea, trypsin, or phospholipase A.

REGULATION OF β-ADRENERGIC RECEPTORS

Changes in the Sensitivity of the β-Adrenergic Receptor-Adenylate Cyclase System

EFFECTS OF DENERVATION   The phenomenon of denervation supersensitivity has been described in a number of systems. If the normal afferent input is removed, the response to an appropriate transmitter is often enhanced (145). Supersensitivity has been described for the peripheral cholinergic (146–149) and adrenergic nervous systems (150–153). In the adrenergic nervous system, supersensitive responses involve two separate phenomena (150–153). There is an acute presynaptic component corresponding to the loss of the ability of the tissue to take up and inactivate catecholamines. There is also a slowly developing postsynaptic component which appears to involve changes at or beyond the site at which receptor interactions take place. Increased postjunctional responsiveness to catecholamines has been demonstrated in a number of organs after surgical, chemical, or environmental alteration of their adrenergic input. For example, an increase in catecholamine-sensitive adenylate cyclase activity was seen after the surgical denervation of dog heart (154). An increase in catecholamine-sensitive enzyme activity was also observed in homogenates of rat pineal organ after superior cervical ganglionectomy (155, 156) or after chronic exposure to light (89, 156). Chronic denervation of the rat pineal organ in vivo either by the administration of 6-hydroxydopamine or after superior cervical ganglionectomy resulted in an enhanced accumulation of cAMP in response to norepinephrine in pineal organs cultured in vitro (157).

In the mammalian brain, several investigators have reported the development of supersensitive responses to catecholamines after depletion of norepinephrine stores in nerve terminals. For example, an increase in cAMP accumulation in response to catecholamines was observed in slices of cerebral cortex following the intraventricular administration of 6-hydroxydopamine to adult rats (158–162). The subcutaneous administration of 6-hydroxydopamine to newborn rats also resulted in a marked depletion of central catecholamine stores and in an enhanced responsiveness of the adenylate cyclase system (153, 163–165). Several groups of investigators have reported that the administration of reserpine results in an enhanced accumulation of cAMP in several regions of the brain in response to a maximally effective concentration of norepinephrine (166–169). On the other hand, Palmer et al (170) observed an increase in the potency of norepinephrine after the administration of reserpine. Unilateral lesions of the medial forebrain bundle resulted in increased accumulation of cAMP in response to norepinephrine in ipsilateral rat cortical slices compared to the accumulation on the contralateral side (171).

DESENSITIZATION OF β-ADRENERGIC RECEPTOR–MEDIATED RESPONSES
Decreases in responsiveness as a consequence of exposure to catecholamines have been described in a number of systems. A decrease in the ability of isoproterenol to induce N-acetylserotonintransferase activity in cultured pineal organs was observed following the in vivo administration of isoproterenol in oil (172). In addition, injection of norepinephrine in oil prevented the development of the increased response to catecholamines seen in the pineal organ after superior cervical ganglionectomy (157). It has recently been reported that long-term treatment of rats with desipramine and other tricyclic antidepressants (173–175), or with inhibitors of monoamine oxidase (176), resulted in a 50–70% decrease in the maximal response to norepinephrine observed in slices of rat cerebral cortex. Kakiuchi & Rall (177) reported that cAMP synthesis is initially stimulated by norepinephrine but that

subsequent exposure of slices of rabbit cerebellar cortex to catecholamines does not result in a rise in cAMP levels. Daly and his collaborators have observed the same phenomenon with slices of cerebral cortex from guinea pig (178) and rat (25). It should be noted that the enhanced accumulation of cAMP in guinea pig cerebral cortex is due almost entirely to α-adrenergic receptors (24, 27, 28, 179). In a recent report by Skolnick et al (180) no refractoriness to norepinephrine was seen in experiments carried out with cortical slices from several species of rat after repeated exposure of slices to norepinephrine.

There have been a number of in vitro studies with homogeneous cell systems in which catecholamine-induced loss of cell responsiveness has been demonstrated. Incubation of lymphoid (181) or fat cells (182) with catecholamines resulted in a loss of responsiveness to a subsequent challenge with catecholamines. The same phenomenon was observed when frog erythrocytes (78, 80, 82, 83, 86), human leucocytes (183), or macrophages (184) were incubated with catecholamines. Several cultured cell lines show similar properties of agonist-induced desensitization. Cultured fibroblasts (185, 186), astrocytoma cells (187–189), and glioma cells (190) are all susceptible to catecholamine-induced refractoriness.

Changes in postsynaptic responsiveness to catecholamines could reflect alterations at any of a number of sites, including (a) changes in the affinity of catecholamines for their postsynaptic receptor sites, (b) alterations in the amount of adenylate cyclase, (c) increases or decreases in the concentration of receptors, (d) alteration in the efficiency of coupling of activated receptors to the catalytic units of adenylate cyclase, or, (e) changes in the activity of cyclic nucleotide phosphodiesterases. Alternatively, in at least one study the appearance of an endogenous inhibitor of a hormone receptor has been implicated in the regulation of cellular responsiveness (182). Within the past two years, evidence has begun to accumulate in several systems, which implicates changes in receptor density in the modulation of responsiveness to β-adrenergic receptor agonists.

β-ADRENERGIC RECEPTORS AND SUPERSENSITIVITY   The process of supersensitivity has been studied as it relates to β-adrenergic receptors in several systems. In all systems thus far examined, increased responsiveness as demonstrated by enhanced cAMP synthesis has been accompanied by an increase in the concentration of β-adrenergic receptors.

Liver   The response of rat liver adenylate cyclase to catecholamines is enhanced as a result of adrenalectomy (126, 191, 192). To determine the role of β-adrenergic receptors in this process, the properties and density of β-adrenergic receptors in rat liver were determined after adrenalectomy using IHYP as a radioligand (126). The kinetics of IHYP binding and the affinities of IHYP, propranolol, and various catecholamines were unchanged. In contrast, the concentration of β-adrenergic receptors was increased three to five fold in liver from adrenalectomized rats. The magnitude of this increase was similar to that observed when catecholamine-stimulated adenylate cyclase activity was measured in homogenates of liver from adrenalectomized rats. Both the increase in receptors and the increase in catecholamine-responsiveness were reversed by the administration of glucocorticoids in vivo. It was suggested that the increase in the density of β-adrenergic receptors following adrenalectomy may be a compensatory response of the liver to the impairment of the normal hormonal regulation of carbohydrate metabolism.

Cerebral cortex   Changes in catecholamine responsiveness in mammalian brain occur as a result of a number of physiological and pharmacological manipulations. As described above, intraventricular injection of 6-hydroxydopamine results in an enhanced response to catecholamines in the rat cerebral cortex (158–162). One week after the administration of this neurotoxin, there was an 80% greater accumulation of cAMP in treated animals in response to isoproterenol than in sham-treated controls. Using IHYP as a ligand the role of β-adrenergic receptors in this increased responsiveness has been assessed (162). Treatment with 6-hydroxydopamine resulted in a 31% increase in the density of β-adrenergic receptors in the cerebral cortex (162). During the first two days following 6-hydroxydopamine administration there was no change either in the efficacy of isoproterenol to stimulate cAMP accumulation or in the density of β-adrenergic receptors. Both parameters then began to increase reaching maximal levels by day 8 (193). An obvious disparity existed between the magnitude of the change in responsiveness and the change in receptor density. The administration of 6-hydroxydopamine also decreased phosphodiesterase activity by about 25% (160). This change may contribute to the greater change in cAMP accumulation than in the density of β-adrenergic receptors. The results suggest that 6-hydroxydopamine has multiple effects in the cerebral cortex. However, changes in receptor concentration after chemical sympathectomy appear to account for some of the observed increase in catecholamine responsiveness.

   Harden et al (194) have used the developing rat brain as a model to investigate the relationship between catecholamine responsiveness and the individual components of the β-adrenergic receptor/adenylate cyclase system. The affinities of agonists and antagonists for β-adrenergic receptors as determined by IHYP binding were the same in young and old animals. Specific binding of IHYP to β-adrenergic receptors in rat cerebral cortex was barely detectable during the first week after birth (194). Between days seven and thirteen, there was a rapid increase in the density of receptors. Adult levels were reached by the end of the second week after birth. The time course of development of catecholamine responsiveness was similar to that of β-adrenergic receptors (194, 195). Catecholamine-stimulated cAMP accumulation in slices of cerebral cortex was negligible during the first week after birth. There was a rapid increase in the ability of isoproterenol to stimulate cAMP accumulation during the second week after birth, and maximal responsiveness was attained by day fourteen (194, 195). The development of fluoride-stimulated adenylate cyclase activity in the cerebral cortex differed greatly from the development of β-adrenergic receptors and catecholamine responsiveness. Enzyme activity was 25–35% of adult levels at birth and developed gradually thereafter, reaching adult levels over the next three weeks (194, 195). The authors suggested that it is the appearance of the β-adrenergic receptor in rat cerebral cortex that allows the expression of catecholamine-sensitive adenylate cyclase activity (194). Norepinephrine stores (194, 196) and dopamine-β-hydroxylase (196) activity were 10–20% of adult levels at birth and developed with a gradual time course, reaching adult levels over the next two months. Thus, there was no correlation between the time course of development of presynaptic markers for noradrenergic nerve terminals and the postsynaptic development of β-adrenergic receptors and catecholamine responsiveness.

The administration of 6-hydroxydopamine to newborn rats prior to the development of the blood brain barrier prevents the development of noradrenergic terminals in the cerebral cortex as evidenced by a 90–95% reduction in norepinephrine levels (197). However, the time course of the ontogeny of β-adrenergic receptors was not altered by drug treatment, indicating that presynaptic input is not essential for the appearance of these receptors (197). The accumulation of cAMP in response to isoproterenol and the density of β-adrenergic receptors were both increased by 45–75% in drug-treated animals. These changes were seen in animals ranging in age from 6 to 45 days.

Pineal organ   As noted above, the rat pineal organ has been extensively utilized as a model system to investigate the influence of presynaptic sympathetic nerves on the responsiveness of a postsynaptic target organ. Axelrod and co-workers have recently evaluated the contribution of β-adrenergic receptors to changes in responsiveness of the cAMP generating system. A circadian rhythm in the sensitivity of the cAMP generating system to catecholamines has been reported (90, 158). This diurnal rhythm in responsiveness was correlated with changes in the concentration of DHA binding sites (90). Furthermore, adenylate cyclase activity in homogenates from light-adapted rats was more responsive to catecholamines than was enzyme from rats kept in the dark overnight (89, 156). The changes in catecholamine responsiveness of adenylate cyclase were paralleled by similar changes in the concentration of β-adrenergic receptors (89). The administration of cycloheximide had no effect on the alterations in catecholamine responsiveness or in receptor density, which suggested that these changes do not require the synthesis of new receptors (89, 90).

Role of β-adrenergic receptors in catecholamine-induced refractoriness   Lefkowitz and co-workers have correlated decreases in postsynaptic responsiveness with alterations in the concentration of β-adrenergic receptors. The chronic administration of catecholamines to frogs led to a decrease in adenylate cyclase activity in erythrocyte membranes in response to a subsequent in vitro challenge with isoproterenol (78, 86). The same refractoriness to catecholamines was seen if the erythrocytes were isolated and incubated in vitro with isoproterenol (80, 82). Both in vivo and in vitro desensitization was accompanied by decreased levels of β-adrenergic receptors. Furthermore, the decreases in isoproterenol-stimulated adenylate cyclase activity and in the density of β-adrenergic receptors were of similar magnitude. Cycloheximide had no effect either on the desensitization process or on the subsequent reappearance of sensitivity (86). Since the alterations in receptor concentration and catecholamine responsiveness appeared to be independent of protein synthesis, these workers suggested that desensitization of the β-adrenergic receptor/adenylate cyclase system involves "inactivation" and subsequent "reactivation" of existing receptor molecules. If this hypothesis is correct, then DHA interacts only with receptors in the functional or active configuration. The molecular basis for an alteration in existing β-adrenergic receptor molecules remains to be elucidated.

Mukherjee & Lefkowitz (83) described catecholamine-induced desensitization in a purified membrane preparation from frog erythrocytes. The desensitized receptors in this cell-free system were rapidly reactivated by exposure of the membranes to guanine nucleotides. Although the effect was most clearly seen with GTP and GMPPNP, the sensitivity of the membrane receptors was also restored by exposure to ATP. It was suggested that nucleotides induce a conformational change in adenylate cyclase which leads in turn to a conformational change in β-adrenergic receptors and to the resultant reappearance of sensitivity to catecholamines.

Perkins and co-workers (187–189, 198) have studied hormone induced refractoriness in a number of cell lines originally derived from a human astrocytoma. EH118MG astrocytoma cells showed both agonist-specific and agonist-nonspecific desensitization (198). Agonist specific refractoriness was rapid in onset. Only 20–30% of the normal response was present after incubation with 10 μM isoproterenol for 30 min (198). The role of β-adrenergic receptors in these changes has been investigated (199). Although there was a 70% decrease in isoproterenol responsiveness, the change in the density of β-adrenergic receptors was only 17%. When cells were incubated with 10 μM PGE$_1$ for 2 hr and then challenged with isoproterenol, there was a 50% decrease in the amount of cAMP that accumulated in the presence of 10 μM isoproterenol (198). Under these conditions there was no change in the density of β-adrenergic receptors. When cells which had been preincubated with PGE$_1$ for 2 hr were subsequently incubated with 10 μM isoproterenol for an additional 2 hr, a further 20% loss in responsiveness to isoproterenol occurred. This loss was accompanied by a 20% decrease in the density of β-adrenergic receptors (199). The studies with PGE$_1$ indicate that 50% of the response to isoproterenol can be lost by a mechanism not involving β-adrenergic receptors. The results with astrocytoma cells together with those with erythrocytes (78, 80, 82, 83, 86) suggest that desensitization to catecholamines may occur by one of several different mechanisms. Previous studies with cells in culture also support this premise. Although the recovery of responsiveness after desensitization to catecholamines in human diploid fibroblasts in culture was dependent on protein synthesis (186), the desensitization process in these fibroblasts was unaffected by inhibitors of protein synthesis. On the other hand, in RGC6 rat glioma cells inhibition of protein synthesis affected the development of desensitization to norepinephrine (190), but did not influence the recovery process after desensitization had taken place. With astrocytoma cells neither the onset nor the recovery of responsiveness following desensitization was affected by cycloheximide (188, 189).

Shear et al (200) studied agonist-induced desensitization in several lines of S-49 mouse lymphoma cells, including genetic variants with specific defects in the pathway of cAMP generation and function. In wild-type S-49 cells cAMP accumulation in response to isoproterenol reached a maximum within 30 min and then fell rapidly. Approximately 40–50% of the IHYP binding sites were lost following incubation with isoproterenol, which suggested that changes in β-adrenergic receptor density were involved in the desensitization process. Similar studies carried out with a clone of S-49 cells devoid of cAMP-dependent protein kinase activity yielded identical findings. Since an increase in phosphodiesterase activity was not seen following an increase in cAMP levels in kinase-deficient cells, induction of phosphodiesterase cannot account for the refractoriness. In addition, since exposure to isoproterenol led to a decrease in the density of receptors and a decrease in responsiveness to isoproterenol in kinase-deficient cells, cAMP-dependent protein kinase does not appear to be required for either of these effects. When cAMP content was increased by exposing cells to PGE_1 in the absence of isoproterenol, no decrease in either the density of IHYP binding sites or the activity of isoproterenol-stimulated adenylate cyclase was seen. Also, when an S-49 clone that lacks hormone responsive adenylate cyclase activity but still possesses a normal density of β-adrenergic receptors was incubated with isoproterenol or with isoproterenol and dibutyryl cAMP, no decrease in the density of β-adrenergic receptors was seen. Thus, receptor occupancy alone, or in combination with elevated cAMP levels is not sufficient to cause loss of responsiveness or a decrease in the density of β-adrenergic receptors. In addition, it was concluded that in this system adenylate cyclase must be present for desensitization to occur.

CONCLUSION

Progress in the study of β-adrenergic receptors has been very rapid in the last few years. From initial, largely unsuccessful, attempts to use catecholamine agonists in direct assays of β-adrenergic receptors, attention has moved to the use of high affinity antagonists labeled to high specific activity with either ^3H or ^{125}I. The use of these compounds has led to the development of valid in vitro assays for these receptors in a wide variety of mammalian and nonmammalian tissues. These assays are now being used in experiments designed to increase our understanding of the mechanisms through which cellular processes are regulated.

Attention over the next several years is likely to focus on the purification of these receptors. One report of the solubilization of β-adrenergic receptors has appeared. With affinity chromatography and other techniques, it should be possible to obtain samples of the binding component of what may turn out to be a complex, multicomponent system.

An understanding of the mechanisms by which the interaction of a catecholamine with its receptor can lead to the activation of adenylate cyclase is of primary interest to many investigators. Elucidation of this problem will be greatly facilitated by the future availability of purified receptor. It may then be possible to incorporate the binding material into membranes of either defined or complex composition. This approach should provide information as to the function of the receptor/enzyme complex at the molecular level.

ACKNOWLEDGMENTS

The authors would like to thank the following investigators for kindly supplying preprints of their work: Drs. G. D. Aurbach, J. P. Bilezikian, J. W. Daly, J. N. Davis, A. G. Gilman, P. A. Insel, R. J. Lefkowitz, A. Levitzki, G. V. Marinetti, G. C. Palmer, and S. H. Snyder. In addition, the authors are grateful to A. G. Gilman, J. P. Perkins, J. R. Sporn, and N. Weiner for carefully reviewing the manuscript and making many valuable suggestions.

The original research reported in this manuscript from the authors' laboratory was supported by grants from the USPHS (NS 13289) and the American Heart Association. TKH (NSO5126) and BBW (NSO1989) are postdoctoral fellows of the NIH. PBM is an Established Investigator of the American Heart Association.

Literature Cited

1. Furchgott, R. F. 1967. The pharmacological differentiation of adrenergic receptors. *Ann. NY Acad. Sci.* 139: 553–70
2. Furchgott, R. F. 1972. The classification of adrenoceptors (adrenergic receptors). An evaluation from the standpoint of receptor theory. In *Handbook of Experimental Pharmacology: Catecholamines,* ed. H. Blaschko, E. Muscholl, 33:283–334. Berlin: Springer
3. Molinoff, P. B., Axelrod, J. 1971. Biochemistry of catecholamines. *Ann. Rev. Biochem.* 40:465–500
4. Perkins, J. P. 1973. Adenyl cyclase. *Adv. Cyclic Nucleotide Res.* 3:1–64
5. Lefkowitz, R. J., Mukherjee, C., Limbird, L. E., Caron, M. G., Williams, L. T., Alexander, R. W., Mickey, J. V., Tate, R. 1976. Regulation of adenylate cyclase coupled β-adrenergic receptors. *Recent Prog. Horm. Res.* 32:597–629
6. Maguire, M. E., Ross, E. M., Haga, T., Biltonen, R. L., Gilman, A. G. 1977. *Adv. Cyclic Nucleotide Res.* In press
7. Lefkowitz, R. J., Limbird, L. E., Mukherjee, C., Caron, M. G. 1976. The β-adrenergic receptor and adenylate cyclase. *Biochim. Biophys. Acta* 457: 1–39
8. Dale, H. H. 1906. On some physiological actions of ergot. *J. Physiol.* 34:163–206
9. Ahlquist, R. P. 1948. A study of the adrenotropic receptors. *Am. J. Physiol.* 153:586–600
10. Powell, C. E., Slater, I. H. 1958. Blocking of inhibitory adrenergic receptors by a dichloro analog of isoproterenol. *J. Pharmacol. Exp. Ther.* 122:480–88

11. Moran, N. C., Perkins, M. E. 1958. Adrenergic blockade of the mammalian heart by a dichloro analogue of isoproterenol. *J. Pharmacol. Exp. Ther.* 124:223–37
12. Moran, N. C. 1967. The development of beta adrenergic blocking drugs: A retrospective and prospective evaluation. *Ann. NY Acad. Sci.* 139:649–60
13. Nickerson, M., Hollenberg, N. K. 1967. Blockade of α-adrenergic receptors. In *Physiological Pharmacology, Vol. 4, The Nervous System, Part D: Autonomic Nervous System Drugs,* ed. W. S. Root, F. G. Hofmann, 243–305. New York: Academic
14. Lands, A. M., Groblewski, G. E., Brown, T. G. 1966. Comparison of the action of isoproterenol and several related compounds on blood pressure, heart, and bronchioles. *Arch. Int. Pharmacodyn.* 161:68–75
15. Lands, A. M., Arnold, A., McAuliff, J. P., Luduena, F. P., Brown, T. G. 1967. Differentiation of receptor systems activated by sympathomimetic amines. *Nature* 214:597–98
16. Dunlop, D., Shanks, R. G. 1968. Selective blockade of adrenoceptive beta receptors in the heart. *Br. J. Pharmacol. Chemother.* 32:201–18
17. Burns, J. J., Salvador, R. A., Lemberger, L. 1967. Metabolic blockade by methoxamine and its analogs. *Ann. NY Acad. Sci.* 139:833–40
18. Levy, B. 1966. The adrenergic blocking activity of N-*tert*-butylmethoxamine (butoxamine). *J. Pharmacol. Exp. Ther.* 151:413–22
19. Moore, G. E., O'Donnell, S. R. 1970. A potent β-adrenoceptor blocking drug: 4-(2-hydroxy-3-isopropylaminopropox-

y) indole. *J. Pharm. Pharmacol.* 22: 180–88

20. Buckner, C. K., Patil, P. N. 1971. Steric aspects of adrenergic drugs. XVI. Beta adrenergic receptors of guinea-pig atria and trachea. *J. Pharmacol. Exp. Ther.* 176:634–49

21. Sutherland, E. W., Oye, I., Butcher, R. W. 1965. The action of epinephrine and the role of the adenyl cyclase in hormone action. *Recent Prog. Horm. Res.* 21:623–46

22. Robison, G. A., Butcher, R. W., Sutherland, E. W. 1971. *Cyclic AMP.* New York:Academic

23. Murad, F., Chi, Y-M., Rall, T. W., Sutherland, E. W. 1962. Adenyl cyclase. III. The effect of catecholamines and choline esters on the formation of adenosine 3',5'-phosphate by preparations from cardiac muscle and liver. *J. Biol. Chem.* 237:1233–38

24. Schultz, J., Daly, J. W. 1973. Adenosine 3',5'-monophosphate in guinea pig cerebral cortical slices: effects of α- and β-adrenergic agents, histamine, serotonin, and adenosine. *J. Neurochem.* 21: 573–79

25. Schultz, J., Daly, J. W. 1973. Accumulation of cyclic adenosine 3',5'-monophosphate in cerebral cortical slices from rat and mouse: Stimulatory effect of α- and β-adrenergic agents and adenosine. *J. Neurochem.* 21:1319–26

26. Perkins, J. P., Moore, M. M. 1973. Characterization of the adrenergic receptors mediating a rise in cyclic 3',5'-adenosine monophosphate in rat cerebral cortex. *J. Pharmacol. Exp. Ther.* 185:371–78

27. Sattin, A., Rall, T. W., Zanella, J. 1975. Regulation of cyclic 3',5'-monophosphate levels in guinea-pig cerebral cortex by interactions of the alpha adrenergic and adenosine receptor activity. *J. Pharmacol. Exp. Ther.* 192:22–32

28. Daly, J. 1975. Role of cyclic nucleotides in the nervous system. In *Handbook of Psychopharmacology,* ed. L. L. Iverson, S. D. Iverson, S. H. Snyder, 5:47–130. New York:Plenum

29. Levitzki, A., Atlas, D., Steer, M. L. 1974. The binding characteristics and number of β-adrenergic receptors on the turkey erythrocyte. *Proc. Natl. Acad. Sci. USA* 71:2773–76

30. Caron, M. G., Lefkowitz, R. J. 1976. β-adrenergic receptors: Solubilization of (-)[³H]-alprenolol binding sites from frog erythrocyte membranes. *Biochem. Biophys. Res. Commun.* 68:315–22

31. Atlas, D., Steer, M. L., Levitzki, A. 1974. Stereospecific binding of propranolol and catecholamines to the β-adrenergic receptor. *Proc. Natl. Acad. Sci. USA* 71:4246–48

32. Lefkowitz, R. J., Mukherjee, C., Coverstone, M., Caron, M. G. 1974. Stereospecific [³H](-)-alprenolol binding sites, β-adrenergic receptors and adenylate cyclase. *Biochem. Biophys. Res. Commun.* 60:703–9

33. Alexander, R. W., Williams, L. T., Lefkowitz, R. J. 1975. Identification of cardiac β-adrenergic receptors by (-) [³H]alprenolol binding. *Proc. Natl. Acad. Sci. USA* 72:1564–68

34. Maguire, M. E., Wiklund, R. A., Anderson, H. J., Gilman, A. G. 1976. Binding of [¹²⁵I]iodohydroxybenzylpindolol to putative β-adrenergic receptors of rat glioma cells and other cell clones. *J. Biol. Chem.* 251:1221–31

35. Harden, T. K., Wolfe, B. B., Molinoff, P. B. 1976. Binding of iodinated *beta* adrenergic antagonists to proteins derived from rat heart. *Mol. Pharmacol.* 12:1–15

36. Bylund, D. B., Snyder, S. H. 1976. β-adrenergic receptor binding in membrane preparations from mammalian brain. *Mol. Pharmacol.* 12:568–80

37. Williams, L. T., Jarett, L., Lefkowitz, R. J. 1976. Adipocyte β-adrenergic receptors. *J. Biol. Chem.* 251:3096–3104

38. Molinoff, P. B. 1973. Methods of approach for the isolation of β-adrenergic receptors. In *Frontiers in Catecholamine Research,* ed. E. Usdin, S. H. Snyder, 357–60. Elmsford, New York:Pergamon

39. Lefkowitz, R. J. 1975. Identification of adenylate cyclase-coupled beta-adrenergic receptors with radiolabeled beta-adrenergic antagonists. *Biochem. Pharmacol.* 24:1651–58

40. Goldstein, A., Aronow, L., Kalman, S. M. 1974. *Principles of Drug Action,* 101–2. New York:Wiley. 2nd ed.

41. Patil, P. N., Miller, D. D., Trendelenburg, U. 1974. Molecular geometry and adrenergic drug activity. *Pharmacol. Rev.* 26:323–423

42. Dixon, M., Webb, E. C. 1964. *Enzymes,* pp. 318–22. New York:Academic

43. Sporn, J. R., Molinoff, P. B. 1976. β-Adrenergic receptors in rat brain. *J. Cyclic Nucleotide Res.* 2:149–61

44. Rabinowitz, M., Desalles, L., Meisler, J., Lorand, L. 1965. Distribution of ade-

nyl cyclase activity in rabbit muscle fractions. *Biochim. Biophys. Acta* 97: 29–36

45. Seraydarian, K., Mommaerts, W. F. H. M. 1965. Density gradient separation of sarcotubular vesicles and other particulate constitutents of rabbit muscle. *J. Cell Biol.* 26:641–56

46. Liao, S., Lin, A. H., Tymoczko, J. L. 1971. Adenyl cyclase of cell nuclei isolated from rat ventral prostate. *Biochim. Biophys. Acta* 230:535–38

47. Soifer, D., Hechter, O. 1971. Adenyl cyclase activity in rat liver nuclei. *Biochim. Biophys. Acta* 230:539–42

48. Marinetti, G. V., Ray, T. K., Tomasi, V. 1969. Glucagon and epinephrine stimulation of adenyl cyclase in isolated rat liver plasma membranes. *Biochem. Biophys. Res. Commun.* 36:185–93

49. Tomasi, V., Koretz, S., Ray, T. K., Dunnick, J., Marinetti, G. V. 1970. Hormone action at the membrane level. II. The binding of epinephrine and glucagon to rat liver plasma membranes. *Biochim. Biophys. Acta* 211: 31–42

50. Dunnick, J. K., Marinetti, G. V. 1971. Hormone action at the membrane level. III. Epinephrine interaction with the rat liver plasma membrane. *Biochim. Biophys. Acta* 249:122–34

51. Lesko, L., Marinetti, G. V. 1975. Hormone action at the membrane level IV. Epinephrine binding to rat liver plasma membranes and rat epididymal fat cells. *Biochim. Biophys. Acta* 382:419–36

52. Leray, F., Chambaut, A.-M., Perrenoud, M.-L., Hanoune, J. 1973. Adenylate-cyclase activity of rat liver plasma membranes—Hormonal stimulations and effect of adrenalectomy. *Eur. J. Biochem.* 38:185–92

53. Lefkowitz, R. J., Haber, E. 1971. A fraction of the ventricular myocardium that has the specificity of the cardiac beta-adrenergic receptor. *Proc. Natl. Acad. Sci. USA* 68:1773–77

54. Lefkowitz, R. J., Haber, E., O'Hara, D. 1972. Identification of the cardiac beta-adrenergic receptor protein: Solubilization and purification by affinity chromatography. *Proc. Natl. Acad. Sci. USA* 69:2828–32

55. Lefkowitz, R.J., Sharp, G. W. G., Haber, E. 1973. Specific binding of β-adrenergic catecholamines to a subcellular fraction from cardiac muscle. *J. Biol. Chem.* 248:342–49

56. Lefkowitz, R. J., O'Hara, D., Warshaw, J. B. 1974. Surface interaction of [^{3}H]

norepinephrine with cultured chick embryo myocardial cells. *Biochim. Biophys. Acta* 332:317–28

57. Aprille, J. R., Lefkowitz, R. J., Warshaw, J. B. 1974. [^{3}H]Norepinephrine binding and lipolysis by isolated fat cells. *Biochim. Biophys. Acta* 373: 502–13

58. Bilezikian, J. P., Aurbach, G. D. 1973. A β-adrenergic receptor of the turkey erythrocyte. I. Binding of catecholamines and relationship to adenylate cyclase activity. *J. Biol. Chem.* 248: 5575–83

59. Bilezikian, J. P., Aurbach, G. D. 1973. A β-adrenergic receptor of the turkey erythrocyte. II. Characterization and solubilization of the receptor. *J. Biol. Chem.* 248:5584–89

60. Schramm, M., Feinstein, H., Naim, E., Lang, M., Lasser, M. 1972. Epinephrine binding to the catecholamine receptor and activation of adenylate cyclase in erythrocyte membranes. *Proc. Natl. Acad. Sci. USA* 69:523–27

61. Cuatrecasas, P., Tell, G. P. E., Sica, V., Parikh, I., Chang, K-J. 1974. Noradrenaline binding and the search for catecholamine receptors. *Nature* 247: 92–97

62. Maguire, M. E., Goldman, P. H., Gilman, A. G. 1974. The reaction of ^{3}H-norepinephrine with particulate fractions of cells responsive to catecholamines. *Mol. Pharmacol.* 10:563–81

63. Wolfe, B. B., Zirrolli, J. A., Molinoff, P. B. 1974. Binding of ^{3}H-*dl*-epinephrine to proteins of rat ventricular muscle: Nonidentity with beta-adrenergic receptors. *Mol. Pharmacol.* 10:582–96

64. Tell, G. P. E., Cuatrecasas, P. 1974. β-Adrenergic receptors: Stereospecificity and lack of affinity for catechols. *Biochem. Biophys. Res. Commun.* 57: 793–800

65. Vallieres, J., Drummond, M., Drummond, G. I. 1975. Catecholamine binding to plasma membrane enriched fractions of heart and skeletal muscle. *Can. J. Physiol. Pharmacol.* 53:458–69

66. Inscoe, J. K., Daly, J., Axelrod, J. 1965. Factors affecting the ezymatic formation of O-methylated dihydroxy derivatives. *Biochem. Pharmacol.* 14:1257–62

67. Koretz, S. H., Marinetti, G. V. 1974. Binding of *l*-norepinephrine to isolated rat fat cell plasma membranes. Evidence against covalent binding and binding to catechol-O-methyl transferase. *Biochem. Biophys. Res. Commun.* 61:22–29

68. Lefkowitz, R. J. 1974. [³H]-Norepinephrine binding: Unrelated to catechol-O-methyl transferase. *Biochem. Biophys. Res. Commun.* 58:1110–18

69. Lacombe, M.-L., Hanoune, J. 1974. Enhanced specificity of epinephrine binding by rat liver plasma membranes in the presence of EDTA. *Biochem. Biophys. Res. Commun.* 58:667–73

70. Pairault, J., Laudat, M-H. 1975. Selective identification of 'true' β-adrenergic receptors in the plasma membranes of rat adipocytes. *FEBS Lett.* 50:61–65

71. Malchoff, C. D., Marinetti, G. V. 1976. Hormone action at the membrane level. V. Binding of (±)-[³H] isoproterenol to intact chicken erythrocytes and erythrocyte ghosts. *Biochim. Biophys. Acta* 436:45–52

72. Potter, L. T. 1967. Uptake of propranolol by isolated guinea pig atria. *J. Pharmacol. Exp. Ther.* 155:91–100

73. Vatner, D., Lefkowitz, R. J. 1974. (³H) Propranolol binding sites in myocardial membranes: Nonidentity with beta adrenergic receptors. *Mol. Pharmacol.* 10:450–56

74. Levitzki, A., Sevilia, N., Atlas, D., Steer, M. L. 1975. Ligand specificity and characteristics of the β-adrenergic receptor in turkey erythrocyte plasma membranes. *J. Mol. Biol.* 97:35–53

75. Nahorski, S. R. 1976. Association of high affinity stereospecific binding of ³H-propranolol to cerebral membranes with β-adrenoceptors. *Nature* 259:488–89

76. Mukherjee, C., Caron, M. G., Coverstone, M., Lefkowitz, R. J. 1975. Identification of adenylate cyclase-coupled β-adrenergic receptors in frog erythrocytes with (−)[³H]alprenolol. *J. Biol. Chem.* 250:4869–76

77. Caron, M. G., Lefkowitz, R. J. 1976. Solubilization and characterization of the β-adrenergic receptor binding sites of frog erythrocytes. *J. Biol. Chem.* 251:2374–84

78. Mukherjee, C., Caron, M. G., Lefkowitz, R. J. 1975. Catecholamine-induced subsensitivity of adenylate cyclase associated with loss of β-adrenergic receptor binding sites. *Proc. Natl. Acad. Sci. USA* 72:1945–49

79. Limbird, L., DeMeyts, P., Lefkowitz, R. J. 1975. β-Adrenergic receptors: Evidence for negative cooperativity. *Biochem. Biophys. Res. Commun.* 64:1160–68

80. Mickey, J., Tate, R., Lefkowitz, R. J. 1975. Subsensitivity of adenylate cyclase and decreased β-adrenergic receptor binding after chronic exposure to (−) - isoproterenol *in vitro. J. Biol. Chem.* 250:5727–29

81. Mukherjee, C., Caron, M. G., Mullikin, D., Lefkowitz, R. J. 1976. Structure-activity relationships of adenylate cyclase-coupled beta adrenergic receptors: Determination by direct binding studies. *Mol. Pharmacol.* 12:16–31

82. Mickey, J. V., Tate, R., Mullikin, D., Lefkowitz, R. J. 1976. Regulation of adenylate-cyclase coupled beta adrenergic receptor binding sites by beta adrenergic catecholamines *in vitro. Mol. Pharmacol.* 12:409–19

83. Mukherjee, C., Lefkowitz, R. J. 1976. Desensitization of β-adrenergic receptors in a cell-free system: Resensitization by guanosine 5'-(β-γ-imino) triphosphate and other purine nucleotides. *Proc. Natl. Acad. Sci. USA* 73:1494–98

84. Lefkowitz, R. J., Mullikin, D., Caron, M. G. 1976. Regulation of β-adrenergic receptors by 5'-guanylimidodiphosphate and other purine nucleotides. *J. Biol. Chem.* 251:4686–92

85. Limbird, L. E., Lefkowitz, R. J. 1976. Adenylate-cyclase coupled β-adrenergic receptors: Effect of membrane lipid-perturbing agents on receptor binding and enzyme stimulation by catecholamines. *Mol. Pharmacol.* 12:559–67

86. Mukherjee, C., Caron, M. G., Lefkowitz, R. J. 1976. Regulation of adenylate cyclase coupled β-adrenergic receptors by β-adrenergic catecholamines. *Endocrinology* 99:347–57

87. Alexander, R. W., Davis, J. N., Lefkowitz, R. J. 1975. Direct identification and characterization of β-adrenergic receptors in rat brain. *Nature* 258:437–40

88. Williams, L. T., Snyderman, R., Lefkowitz, R. J. 1976. Identification of β-adrenergic receptors in human lymphocytes by (−)(³H)alprenolol binding. *J. Clin. Invest.* 57:149–55

89. Kebabian, J. W., Zatz, M., Romero, J. A., Axelrod, J. 1975. Rapid changes in rat pineal β-adrenergic receptor: Alterations in 1-(³H)alprenolol binding and adenylate cyclase. *Proc. Natl. Acad. Sci. USA* 72:3735–39

90. Romero, J. A., Zatz, M., Kebabian, J. W., Axelrod, J. 1975. Circadian cycles in binding of ³H-alprenolol to β-adrenergic receptor sites in rat pineal. *Nature* 258:435–36

91. Zatz, M., Kebabian, J. W., Romero, J. A., Lefkowitz, R. J., Axelrod, J. 1976.

Pineal beta adrenergic receptor: Correlation of binding of ^{3}H-l-alprenolol with stimulation of adenylate cyclase. *J. Pharmacol. Exp. Ther.* 196:714–22

92. Jacobs, S., Chang, K.-J., Cuatrecasas, P. 1975. Estimation of hormone receptor affinity by competitive displacement of labeled ligand: Effect of concentration of receptor and of labeled ligand. *Biochem. Biophys. Res. Commun.* 66: 687–92

93. Cheng, Y., Prusoff, W. H. 1973. Relationship between the inhibition constant (K_i) and the concentration of inhibitor which causes 50 percent inhibition (I_{50}) of an enzymatic reaction. *Biochem. Pharmacol.* 22:3099–3108

94. Aurbach, G. D., Fedak, S. A., Woodard, C. J., Palmer, J. S., Hauser, D., Troxler, F. 1974. β-Adrenergic receptor: Stereospecific interaction of iodinated β-blocking agent with a high affinity site. *Science* 186:1223–24

95. Brown, E. M., Aurbach, G. D., Hauser, D., Troxler, F. 1976. β-Adrenergic receptor interactions: Characterization of iodohydroxybenzylpindolol as a specific ligand. *J. Biol. Chem.* 251:1232–38

96. Brown, E. M., Fedak, S. M., Woodard, C. J., Aurbach, G. D., Rodbard, D. 1976. β-Adrenergic receptor interactions: Direct comparison of receptor interaction and biological activity. *J. Biol. Chem.* 251:1239–46

97. Molinoff, P. B., Wolfe, B. B., Harden, T. K. 1975. The use of radiolabeled ligands to study β-adrenergic receptors. *Proc. Sixth Int. Congr. Pharmacol.* 1:141–52

98. Hardman, J. G., Mayer, S. E., Clark, B. 1965. Cocaine potentiation of the cardiac inotropic and phosphorylase responses to catecholamines as related to the uptake of ^{3}H-catecholamines. *J. Pharmacol. Exp. Ther.* 150:341–48

99. Blinks, J. 1967. Evaluation of the cardiac effects of several beta adrenergic blocking agents. *Ann. NY Acad. Sci.* 139:673–85

100. Mayer, S. E. 1972. Effects of adrenergic agonists and antagonists on adenylate cyclase activity of dog heart and liver. *J. Pharmacol. Exp. Ther.* 181:116–25

101. Harden, T. K., Wolfe, B. B., Johnson, G. L., Perkins, J. P., Molinoff, P. B. 1976. Beta adrenergic receptors of intact and broken human astrocytoma cells. *Trans. Am. Soc. Neurochem.* 7:231

102. Swanson, L. W., Hartman, B. K. 1975. The central adrenergic system. An im-

munofluorescence study of the location of cell bodies and their efferent connections in the rat utilizing dopamine-β-hydroxylase as a marker. *J. Comp. Neurol.* 163:467–506

103. Gilman, A. G., Nirenberg, M. 1971. Effect of catecholamines on the adenosine 3',5'-cyclic monophosphate concentrations of clonal satellite cells of neurons. *Proc. Natl. Acad. Sci. USA* 68:2165–68

104. Clark, R. B., Perkins, J. P. 1971. Regulation of adenosine 3':5'-cyclic monophosphate concentration in cultured human astrocytoma cells by catecholamines and histamine. *Proc. Natl. Acad. Sci. USA* 68:2757–76

105. Skolnick, P., Daly, J. W. 1976. Antagonism of α- and β-adrenergic–mediated accumulations of cyclic AMP in rat cerebral cortical slices by the β-antagonist (–)alprenolol. *Life Sci.* 19:497–504

106. Markstein, R., Wagner, H. 1975. The effect of dihydroergotoxin, phentolamine and pindolol on catecholamine-stimulated adenyl cyclase in rat cerebral cortex. *FEBS Lett.* 55:275–77

107. Insel, P., Maguire, M. E., Gilman, A. G., Bourne, H. R., Coffino, P., Melmon, K. L. 1976. β-Adrenergic receptors and adenylate cyclase: Products of separate genes? *Mol. Pharmacol.* 12:1062–69

108. Charness, M. E., Bylund, D. B., Beckman, B. S., Hollenberg, M. D., Snyder, S. H. 1976. Independent variation of β-adrenergic receptor binding and catecholamine-stimulated adenylate cyclase activity in rat erythrocytes. *Life Sci.* 19:243–50

109. Spiegel, A. M., Bilezikian, J. P., Aurbach, G. D. 1975. Increased adrenergic receptor content in membranes of stress-induced erythrocytes. *Clin. Res.* 23:390A

110. Bilezikian, J. P., Spiegel, A. M. 1976. Identification and uncoupling of beta-adrenergic receptors during maturation of the mammalian reticulocyte. *Proc. NY Heart Assoc.* (Abstr.) In press

111. Rodbell, M., Birnbaumer, L., Pohl, S. L., Krans, H. M. J. 1971. The glucagon-sensitive adenyl cyclase system in plasma membranes of rat liver. *J. Biol. Chem.* 246:1877–82

112. Schramm, M., Rodbell, M. 1975. A persistent active state of the adenylate cyclase system produced by the combined actions of isoproterenol and guanylimidophosphate in frog erythrocyte membranes. *J. Biol. Chem.* 250: 2232–37

113. Schramm, M. 1975. The catecholamine-responsive adenylate cyclase system and its modification by 5'-guanylimidodiphosphate. *Adv. Cyclic Nucleotide Res.* 5:105–15

114. Bilezikian, J. P., Aurbach, G. D. 1974. The effects of nucleotides on the expression of β-adrenergic adenylate cyclase activity in membranes from turkey erythrocytes. *J. Biol. Chem.* 249:157–61

115. Rodbell, M., Lin, M. C., Salomon, Y., Londos, C., Harwood, J. P., Martin, B. R., Rendell, M., Berman, M. 1975. Role of adenine and guanine nucleotides in the activity and response of adenylate cyclase systems to hormones: Evidence for multisite transition states. *Adv. Cyclic Nucleotide Res.* 5:3–29

116. Spiegel, A. M., Brown, E. M., Fedak, S. A., Woodard, C. J., Aurbach, G. D. 1976. Holocatalytic state of adenylate cyclase in turkey erythrocyte membranes. Formation with guanylimidodiphosphate plus isoproterenol without effect on affinity of β-receptor. *J. Cyclic Nucleotide Res.* 2:47–56

117. Maguire, M. E., Van Arsdale, P. M., Gilman, A. G. 1976. An agonist-specific effect of guanine nucleotides on binding to the *beta* adrenergic receptor. *Mol. Pharmacol.* 12:335–39

118. Hammes, G. G., Molinoff, P. B., Bloom, F. E. 1973. Receptor biophysics and biochemistry. *Neurosci. Res. Prog. Bull.* 11:155–294

119. Hiley, C. R., Burgen, A. S. V. 1974. The distribution of muscarinic receptor sites in the nervous system of the dog. *J. Neurochem.* 22:159–62

120. Chang, C. C., Lee, C. Y. 1963. Isolation of neurotoxins from the venom of *Bungarus multicinctus* and their modes of neuromuscular blocking action. *Arch. Int. Pharmacodyn.* 144:239–57

121. Gupta, S. K., Moran, J. F., Triggle, D. J. 1976. Mechanism of action of benzilylcholine mustard at the muscarinic receptor. *Mol. Pharmacol.* 12:1019–26

122. Takayanagi, I., Yoshioka, M., Takagi, K., Tamura, Z. 1976. Photoaffinity labeling of the β-adrenergic receptors and receptor reserve for isoprenaline. *Eur. J. Pharmacol.* 35:121–25

123. Atlas, D., Levitzki, A. 1976. An irreversible blocker for the β-adrenergic receptor. *Biochem. Biophys. Res. Commun.* 69:397–403

124. Atlas, D., Steer, M. L., Levitzki, A. 1976. Affinity label for β-adrenergic receptor in turkey erythrocytes. *Proc. Natl. Acad. Sci. USA* 73:1921–25

125. Erez, M., Weinstock, M., Cohen, S., Shtacher, G. 1975. Potential probe for isolation of the β-adrenoceptor, chloropractolol. *Nature* 255:635–36

126. Wolfe, B. B., Harden, T. K., Molinoff, P. B. 1976. β-Adrenergic receptors in rat liver: Effects of adrenalectomy. *Proc. Natl. Acad. Sci. USA* 73:1343–47

127. Wrenn, S. M., Haber, E. 1976. Production and characterization of an antibody which specifically inhibits the function of the cardiac β-adrenergic receptor. *Fed. Proc.* 35:Ab1410

128. Hill, A. V. 1910. A new mathematical treatment of ionic concentration in muscle and nerve under the action of electric currents, with a theory as to their mode of excitation. *J. Physiol.* 40:190–224

129. Scatchard, G. 1949. The attractions of proteins for small molecules and ions. *Ann. NY Acad. Sci.* 51:660–72

130. Siggins, G. R., Battenberg, E. F., Hoffer, B. J., Bloom, F. E., Steiner, A. L. 1973. Noradrenergic stimulation of cyclic adenosine monophosphate in rat Purkinje neurons: An immunocytochemical study. *Science* 179:585–88

131. Kebabian, J. W., Bloom, F. E., Steiner, A. L., Greengard, P. 1975. Neurotransmitters increase cyclic nucleotides in postganglionic neurons: Immunocytochemical demonstration. *Science* 190:157–59

132. Melamed, E., Lahav, M., Atlas, D. 1976. Direct localization of β-adrenoceptor sites in rat cerebellum by a new fluorescent analogue of propranolol. *Nature* 261:420–21

133. Bylund, D. B., Charness, M. E., Snyder, S. H. 1976. Identification of β-adrenergic receptor binding in intact animals. *Trans. Am. Soc. Neurochem.* 7:229

134. Davoren, P. R., Sutherland, E. W. 1963. The cellular location of adenyl cyclase in the pigeon erythrocyte. *J. Biol. Chem.* 238:3016–23

135. Venter, J. C., Ross, J. Jr., Dixon, J. E., Mayer, S. E., Kaplan, N. O. 1973. Immobilized catecholamine and cocaine effects on contractility of cardiac muscle. *Proc. Natl. Acad. Sci. USA* 70:1214–17

136. Verlander, M. S., Venter, J. C., Goodman, M., Kaplan, N. O., Saks, B. 1976. Biological activity of catecholamines covalently linked to synthetic polymers: Proof of immobilized drug theory. *Proc. Natl. Acad. Sci. USA* 73:1009–13

137. Davis, J. N., Lefkowitz, R. J. 1976. β-Adrenergic receptor binding: Synap-

tic localization in rat brain. *Brain Res.* 113:214–18

138. Pohl, S. L., Krans. H. M., Kozyreff, V., Birnbaumer, L., Rodbell, M. 1971. The glucagon-sensitive adenyl cyclase system in plasma membranes of rat liver. III. Evidence for a role of membrane lipids. *J. Biol. Chem.* 246:4447–54

139. Rethy, A., Tomasi, V., Trevisani, A., Barnabei, O. 1972. The role of phosphatidyl serine in the hormonal control of adenylate cyclase of rat liver plasma membranes. *Biochim. Biophys. Acta* 200:58–59

140. Lefkowitz, R. J. 1975. Catecholamine stimulated myocardial adenylate cyclase: Effects of phospholipase digestion and the role of membrane lipids. *J. Mol. Cell. Cardiol.* 7:27–37

141. Sutherland, E. W., Rall, T. W., Menon, T. 1962. Adenyl cyclase. I. Distribution, preparation and properties. *J. Biol. Chem.* 237:1220–27

142. Levey, G. S. 1970. Solubilization of myocardial adenyl cyclase. *Biochem. Biophys. Res. Commun.* 38:86–92

143. Pilkis, S. J., Johnson, R. A. 1974. Detergent dispersion of adenylate cyclase from partially purified rat liver plasma membranes. *Biochim. Biophys. Acta* 341:388–95

144. Ryan, J., Storm, D. R. 1974. Solubilization of glucagon and epinephrine sensitive adenylate cyclase from rat liver plasma membranes. *Biochem. Biophys. Res. Commun.* 60:304–11

145. Cannon, B. 1939. A law of denervation. *Am. J. Med. Sci.* 198:737–50

146. Kuffler, S. W. 1943. Specific excitability of the endplate region in normal and denervated muscle. *J. Neurophys.* 6:99–110

147. Axelsson, J., Thesleff, S. 1959. A study of supersensitivity in denervated mammalian skeletal muscle. *J. Physiol.* 149:178–93

148. Miledi, R. 1960. The acetylcholine sensitivity of frog muscle fibres after complete or partial denervation. *J. Physiol.* 151:1–23

149. Brockes, J. P., Hall, Z. W. 1975. Synthesis of acetylcholine receptor by denervated rat diaphragm muscle. *Proc. Natl. Acad. Sci. USA* 72:1368–72

150. Trendelenburg, U. 1963. Supersensitivity and subsensitivity to sympathomimetic amines. *Pharmacol. Rev.* 15:225–76

151. Trendelenburg, U. 1966. Mechanisms of supersensitivity and subsensitivity to sympathomimetic amines. *Pharmacol. Rev.* 18:629–40

152. Brimijoin, S., Pluchino, S., Trendelenburg, U. 1970. On the mechanism of supersensitivity to norepinephrine in the denervated cat spleen. *J. Pharmacol. Exp. Ther.* 175:503–13

153. Perkins, J. P. 1975. Regulation of the responsiveness of cells to catecholamines: Variable expression of the components of the second messenger system. In *Cyclic Nucleotides in Disease*, ed. B. Weiss, 351–75. Baltimore: Univ. Park Press

154. Palmer, G. C., Spurgeon, H. A., Priola, D. V. 1975. Involvement of adenylate cyclase in mechanisms of denervation supersensitivity following surgical denervation of the dog heart. *J. Cyclic Nucleotide Res.* 1:89–95

155. Weiss, B., Costa, E. 1967. Adenyl cyclase activity in rat pineal gland: Effects of chronic denervation and norepinephrine. *Science* 156:1750–52

156. Weiss, B. 1969. Effects of environmental lighting and chronic denervation on the activation of adenyl cyclase of rat pineal gland by norepinephrine and sodium fluoride. *J. Pharmacol. Exp. Ther.* 168:146–52

157. Strada, S. J., Weiss, B. 1974. Increased response to catecholamines of cyclic AMP system of rat pineal gland induced by decreased sympathetic activity. *Arch. Biochem. Biophys.* 160:197–204

158. Weiss, B., Strada, S. J. 1972. Neuroendocrine control of the cyclic AMP system of brain and pineal gland. *Adv. Cyclic Nucleotide Res.* 1:357–74

159. Palmer, G. C. 1972. Increased cyclic AMP response to norepinephrine in the rat brain following 6-hydroxydopamine. *Neuropharmacology* 11:145–49

160. Kalisker, A., Rutledge, C. O., Perkins, J. P. 1973. Effect of nerve degeneration by 6-hydroxydopamine on catecholamine-stimulated adenosine 3',5'-monophosphate formation in rat cerebral cortex. *Mol. Pharmacol.* 9:619–29

161. Huang, M., Ho, A. K. S., Daly, J. W. 1973. Accumulation of adenosine cyclic 3',5'-monophosphate in rat cerebral cortical slices: Stimulatory effect of alpha and beta adrenergic agents after treatment with 6-hydroxydopamine, 2,3,5-trihydroxyphenylethylamine and dihydroxytryptamines. *Mol. Pharmacol.* 9:711–17

162. Sporn, J. R., Harden, T. K., Wolfe, B. B., Molinoff, P. B. 1976. β-adrenergic

receptor involvement in 6-hydroxy-dopamine induced supersensitivity in rat cerebral cortex. *Science* 194:624–26
163. Palmer, G. C., Scott, H. R. 1974. The cyclic AMP response to norepinephrine in young adult rat brain following post-natal injections of 6-hydroxydopamine. *Experientia* 30:520–21
164. Dismukes, R. K., Daly, J. W. 1975. Altered responsiveness of adenosine 3',5'-monophosphate-generating systems in brain slices from adult rats after neonatal treatment with 6-hydroxydopamine. *Exp. Neurol.* 49:150–60
165. Molinoff, P. B., Sporn, J. R., Harden, T. K., Wolfe, B. B., Poulos, B. K. 1976. β-Adrenergic receptors in rat cerebral cortex: Effects of 6-hydroxydopamine. *Neurosci. Abstr.* 2:712
166. Palmer, G. C., Sulser, F., Robinson, G. A. 1973. Effects of neurohumoral and adrenergic agents on cyclic AMP levels in various areas of the rat brain *in vitro*. *Neuropharmacology* 12:327–37
167. Dismukes, K., Daly, J. W. 1974. Norepinephrine-sensitive systems generating adenosine 3',5'-monophosphate increased responses in cerebral cortical slices from reserpine-treated rats. *Mol. Pharmacol.* 10:933–40
168. Williams, B. J., Pirch, J. H. 1974. Correlation between brain adenyl cyclase activity and spontaneous motor activity in rats after chronic reserpine treatment. *Brain Res.* 68:226–34
169. Palmer, G. C., Wagner, H. R., Putnam, R. W. 1976. Neuronal localization of the enhanced adenylate cyclase responsiveness to catecholamines in the rat cerebral cortex following reserpine injections. *Neuropharmacology* 15:695–702
170. Palmer, D. S., French, S. W., Narod, M. E. 1976. Noradrenergic subsensitivity and supersensitivity of the cerebral cortex after reserpine treatment. *J. Pharmacol. Exp. Ther.* 196:167–71
171. Dismukes, R. K., Ghosh, P., Creveling, C. R., Daly, J. W. 1975. Altered responsiveness of adenosine 3',5'-monophosphate generating systems in rat cortical slices after lesions of the medial forebrain bundle. *Exp. Neurol.* 49:725–35.
172. Deguchi, T., Axelrod, J. 1972. Induction and superinduction of serotonin N-acetyltransferase by adrenergic drugs and denervation in rat pineal organ. *Proc. Natl. Acad. Sci. USA* 69:2208–11
173. Vetulani, J., Sulser, F. 1975. Action of various antidepressant treatments reduces reactivity of noradrenergic cyclic

AMP-generating system in limbic fore-brain. *Nature* 257:495–96
174. Schultz, J. 1976. Psychoactive drug effects on a system which generates cyclic AMP in brain. *Nature* 261:417–18
175. Vetulani, J., Stawarz, R. J., Dingell, J. V., Sulser, F. 1976. A possible common mechanism of action of antidepressant treatments. *Naunyn-Schmiedebergs Arch. Pharmacol.* 293:109–14
176. Vetulani, J., Stawarz, R. J., Blumberg, J. B., Sulser, F. 1975. Adaptive mechanisms in the norepinephrine-sensitive cyclic AMP generating system in the slices of the rat limbic forebrain. *Fed. Proc.* 34:Ab269
177. Kakiuchi, S., Rall, T. W. 1968. The influence of chemical agents on the accumulation of adenosine 3',5'-phosphate in slices of rabbit cerebellum. *Mol. Pharmacol.* 4:367–78
178. Schultz, J., Daly, J. W. 1973. Cyclic adenosine 3',5'-monophosphate in guinea pig cerebral cortical slices. III. Formation, degradation, and reformation of cyclic adenosine 3',5'-monophosphate during sequential stimulation by biogenic amines and adenosine. *J. Biol. Chem.* 248:860–66
179. Chasin, M., Rivkin, I., Mamrak, F., Samaniego, S. G., Hess, S. M. 1971. α- and β-adrenergic receptors as mediators of accumulation of cyclic adenosine 3',5'-monophosphate in specific areas of guinea pig brain. *J. Biol. Chem.* 246:3037–51
180. Skolnick, P., Schultz, J., Daly, J. W. 1975. Repetitive stimulation of cyclic adenosine 3',5'-monophosphate formation by adrenergic agonists in incubated slices from rat cerebral cortex. *J. Neurochem.* 24:1263–65
181. Makman, M. H. 1971. Properties of adenyl cyclase of lymphoid cells. *Proc. Natl. Acad. Sci. USA* 68:885–89
182. Ho, R. J., Sutherland, E. W. 1971. Formation and release of a hormone antagonist by rat adipocytes. *J. Biol. Chem.* 246:6822–27
183. Morris, H. G., DeRoche, G. B., Caro, C. M. 1975. Response of leukocyte cyclic AMP to epinephrine stimulation *in vivo* and *in vitro*. *Adv. Cyclic Nucleotide Res.* 5:Ab812
184. Remold-O'Donnell, E. 1974. Stimulation and desensitization of macrophage adenylate cyclase by prostaglandins and catecholamines. *J. Biol. Chem.* 249:3615–21

185. Franklin, T. J., Foster, S. J. 1973. Leakage of cyclic AMP from human diploid fibroblast in tissue culture. *Nature New Biol.* 246:119–20

186. Franklin, T. J., Morris, W. P., Twose, P. A. 1975. Desensitization of beta adrenergic receptors in human fibroblasts in tissue culture. *Mol. Pharmacol.* 11:485–91

187. Clark, R. B., Su, Y-F., Ortmann, R., Cubeddu, X. L., Johnson, G. L. Perkins, J. P. 1975. Factors influencing the effect of hormones on the accumulation of cyclic AMP in cultured human astrocytoma cells. *Metabolism* 24:343–58

188. Su, Y-F., Cubeddu, X. L., Perkins, J. P. 1976. Regulation of adenosine 3':5'-monophosphate content of human astrocytoma cells: Desensitization to catecholamines and prostaglandins. *J. Cyclic Nucleotide Res.* 2:257–70

189. Su, Y-F., Johnson, G. L., Cubeddu, X. L., Leichtling, B. H., Ortmann, R., Perkins, J. P. 1976. Regulation of adenosine 3':5'-monophosphate content of human astrocytoma cells: Mechanism of agonist-specific desensitization. *J. Cyclic Nucleotide Res.* 2:271–85

190. DeVellis, J., Brooker, G. 1974. Reversal of catecholamine refractoriness by inhibitors of RNA and protein synthesis. *Science* 186:1221–23

191. Bitensky, M. W., Russell, V., Blanco, M. 1970. Independent variation of glucagon and epinephrine responsive components of hepatic adenyl cyclase as a function of age, sex and steroid hormones. *Endocrinology* 86:154–59

192. Leray, F., Chambaut, A.-M., Perrenoud, M.-L., Hanoune, J. 1973. Adenylate cyclase activity of rat liver plasma membranes—hormonal stimulations and effect of adrenalectomy. *Eur. J. Biochem.* 38:185–92

193. Sporn, J. R., Wolfe, B. B., Harden, T. K., Molinoff, P. B. 1977. Temporal relationships of the pre- and post-synaptic components of 6-hydroxydopamine-induced supersensitivity in rat cerebral cortex. Submitted for publication

194. Harden, T. K., Wolfe, B. B., Sporn, J. R., Perkins, J. P., Molinoff, P. B. 1977. Ontogeny of β-adrenergic receptors in rat cerebral cortex. *Brain Res.* In press

195. Perkins, J. P., Moore, M. M. 1973. Regulation of adenosine cyclic 3',5'-monophosphate content of rat cerebral cortex: Ontogenetic development of the responsiveness to catecholamines and adenosine. *Mol. Pharmacol.* 9:774–82

196. Coyle, J. T. 1974. Development of the central catecholaminergic neurons. In *The Neurosciences, Third Study Program,* ed. F. O. Schmitt, F. G. Worden, 877–84. Cambridge, Mass.: MIT Press

197. Harden, T. K., Wolfe, B. B., Sporn, J. R., Poulos, B. K., Molinoff, P. B. 1977. Effects of 6-hydroxydopamine on the development of the β-adrenergic receptor/adenylate cyclase system in rat cerebral cortex. *J. Pharmacol. Exp. Ther.* In press

198. Johnson, G. L., 1976. *Studies of the changes in responsiveness of hormone-sensitive adenylate cyclase in cultured cells.* PhD thesis. Univ. of Colorado Medical School, Denver

199. Wolfe, B. B., Harden, T. K., Johnson, G. L., Perkins, J. P., Molinoff, P. B. 1977. β-Adrenergic receptor density and isoproterenol-induced desensitization of adenylate cyclase. *Fed. Proc.* In press

200. Shear, M., Insel, P., Melmon, K. L., Coffino, P. 1976. Agonist-specific refractoriness induced by isoproterenol. Studies with mutant cells. *J. Biol. Chem.* 251:7572–76

Ann. Rev. Pharmacol. Toxicol. 1977. 17:605–21
Copyright © 1977 by Annual Reviews Inc. All rights reserved

PHARMACOLOGIC CONTROL   ❖6698
OF FEEDING

Bartley G. Hoebel[1]

Department of Psychology, Princeton University, Princeton, New Jersey 08540

Several forces have combined to focus research on phenethylamines. Modern research in neuroscience has concentrated on the neuroanatomy and neurochemistry of brain monoamines and their roles in psychosis, schizophrenia, anorexia nervosa, and hyperphagia. Phenethylamines such as amphetamine, fenfluramine, and phenylpropanolamine have the same basic structures as the monoamine neurotransmitters; therefore they have become useful tools in research and therapy. Phenethylamines are well known—some are infamous—for the treatment of obesity which has become prevalent in food-rich nations. Because amphetamine is now illegal in many countries, other anti-obesity drugs such as fenfluramine have been sought.

Amphetamine is primarily catecholaminergic and fenfluramine is primarily serotonergic; therefore it was our working hypothesis that somewhere in the brain, catecholamine and serotonin neurons participate in the inhibition of feeding. Depleting the appropriate neurotransmitters should release feeding from inhibition and thereby lead to obesity.

Our work has led to several findings including the following: (a) experimental obesity can follow adrenergic depletion with 6-hydroxydopamine; (b) obesity can also follow serotonergic depletion with parachlorophenylalanine; (c) adrenergic depletion causes a decrease in amphetamine anorexia, and this may be coupled with an increase in fenfluramine anorexia; (d) phenylpropanolamine may influence feeding in part by altering glucose utilization, and (e) electrical self-stimulation and stimulation-escape at certain brain sites can be used to assess the arousal and anorectic properties of anti-obesity drugs.

These findings provide new models for the study and treatment of obesity. There has developed a distinction between two kinds of hyperphagia based on monoamine

[1]The unpublished observations referred to in the text are recently completed experiments in collaboration with Robert MacKenzie, Michael Trulson, Frank Zemlan, Laurie Vollen, Rene DuCret, and Joseph Chen. This work was supported by USPHS grants MH-08493-12 and 13, NSF grant GB43407, and grants from Alleghany Pharmacal Corp., Porter-Dietsch Inc., and Thompson Medical Co.

neurochemistry, and two corresponding kinds of anorexia based on phenethylamine pharmacology. This suggests that there are different kinds of obesities that require different treatments (1, 2).

So far, these models have revealed very little about the actual brain circuitry that controls feeding. Gross depletion techniques disrupt the innervation to large areas of the brain, and it is not known whether the obesity results primarily from neural, hormonal, or metabolic alterations.

From the therapeutic point of view it might be preferable to find drugs that act to suppress appetite and hunger through a natural physiological route rather than by an action on brain neurotransmitters. The physiological route is more likely to be behaviorally specific. Therefore this review also deals with homeostatic control of feeding.

We discuss three topics: (a) amphetamine and adrenergic systems, (b) fenfluramine and serotonergic systems, and (c) phenylpropanolamine with reference to glucostatic systems.

The author previously compiled a handbook review of feeding pharmacology and neurochemistry with references by the hundred (3); therefore this review presents only selected recent work. Conference summaries of this work, including figures, are also available (1, 4, 5).

TERMINOLOGY AND ABBREVIATIONS

All researchers who have made lesions in and around the ventromedial hypothalamic nucleus agree that the medial area, not just the nucleus itself, is an effective region for inducing hypothalamic obesity; therefore we refer to these as *medial hypothalamic* (MH) lesions. The neurotoxin, 6-hydroxydopamine, is abbreviated as a dopamine (DA) analogue, 6-OH-DA, although it can kill adrenergic as well as DA neurons. *Adrenergic* refers to either or both norepinephrine (NE) or epinephrine (E) neurons; in this paper it will be important to make a distinction between the two. Unfortunately, it is often impossible to make the distinction given the state of the art at the time the research was done. The ventral bundle (VB) was originally thought to be just a NE bundle. The VB is now known to carry E, as well as NE, neurons as it travels with the medial forebrain bundle from the midbrain to the lateral hypothalamus (LH). Traversing almost the same path is part of the serotonin (5-HT) system projecting from the raphe nuclei to the hypothalamus. Our goal was to find out whether these three monoamines play a role in the normal control of food intake and in the anorexia caused by amphetamine (AMPH), fenfluramine (FEN), and phenylpropanolamine (PPA).

AMPHETAMINE AND ADRENERGIC SYSTEMS

Local Injections of Adrenergic Drugs

It was long known on the basis of brain lesion and stimulation studies that the LH is involved in initiating feeding and the MH in suppressing it (4, 6, 7). Then Grossman (8) discovered that the feeding behavior of a fully awake animal could be influenced by direct injection of drugs into the brain. Crystalline NE injected in the hypothalamus caused feeding. The effect has been confirmed with fluid doses as low as 10 nmole of the l-isomer (9). This is strictly an α-adrenergic effect, although E is more potent than NE (9, 10).

Margules (11) found that adrenergic drugs could also suppress feeding. Most of these studies used a "perifornical" injection site midway between the LH and MH. Recently Leibowitz (9) has reviewed her evidence that shows the main α-adrenergic feeding effect to be medially located, specifically, in the paraventricular nucleus; whereas the β-adrenergic synapses for satiety effects are centered in the LH.

The simplest way to incorporate this new picture with the old is to imagine that in the medial region an α-adrenergic system excites feeding by inhibiting part of the classical MH satiety system; in the lateral region a β-adrenergic system causes satiety by inhibiting part of the classical LH feeding system. The picture that will be painted in this review is more complicated than this simple outline, but compatible with it.

In accord with this view, AMPH, which has both α and β effects, elicits feeding when injected into the MH and suppresses feeding when injected in the LH (9). This may partially explain why AMPH injected systemically can increase in anorectic potency after VM lesions (12) which would block its feeding effect, and conversely, why systemic AMPH may actually induce feeding after LH lesions (13) which partially block its anorectic effect (14). However, to understand the complicated behavioral effects of AMPH more fully we need to know the anatomy of the systems it influences and the behavioral significance of these systems.

The actions of AMPH are primarily indirect via release and inhibition of uptake of endogenous catecholamines (15, 16). When Leibowitz (9) injected AMPH directly into the LH to suppress feeding, the effect was blocked by either dopaminergic or β-adrenergic blockers. Midbrain lesions also blocked the effect, presumably by killing the neurons from which AMPH would release transmitter. The same lesions did not block the anorectic effects of DA or E injected in the LH, which must have acted directly on intact postsynaptic effectors. Therefore some of the catecholamine subsystems necessary for AMPH anorexia apparently are dopaminergic or adrenergic and arise in the midbrain with terminals in the LH.

Neurochemical Depletions

When DA and NE pathways were discovered ascending from the midbrain to the hypothalamus and forebrain, Ungerstedt (17) reported a major breakthrough in the study of feeding; destruction of the DA path caused anorexia. DA depletion was like an LH lesion in many regards.

Several investigators have now proposed that the DA bundle plays a role in initiating feeding, although it is not clear which of several DA projections is responsible (18). AMPH may initiate feeding in DA depleted animals by stimulating the reticular formation or releasing the remaining stores of DA and thereby providing the behavioral arousal and sensory-motor activation necessary to eat (19, 20). The right amount of environmental or physiological stimulation may accomplish the same thing. Even in normal animals, chronic tail pinch apparently activates DA systems and can lead to obesity (21, 22). Systemic AMPH in a normal rat could release excessive amounts of DA and thereby overactivate the animal and interfere with feeding. Perhaps this is another of the reasons DA depletion reduces AMPH anorexia (23).

Recent electrophysiological evidence suggests another possibility. Excessive DA release by AMPH might overstimulate neuronal feedback that inhibits DA cells of the substantia nigra (24). The behavioral significance of this feedback system is unknown, but it is conceivable that AMPH causes diffuse DA effects at striatal DA synapses, and, at the same time by the resultant negative feedback to the substantia nigra, leads to reduced sensitivity of the DA system to its natural inputs. Thus the animal experiences a large quantity of DA stimulation which not only masks, but also actively inhibits, the natural patterns of sensory input.

Following Ungerstedt's discovery that the DA path is necessary for feeding, we reasoned that a NE pathway might be necessary for normal satiety because NE fluorescent varicosities are especially profuse in the LH where lesions block AMPH anorexia. The problem was to deplete NE but not DA. Ahlskog (25) tested the concept of an ascending NE satiety system by injecting 6-OH-DA locally into the ventral and dorsal NE bundles in the midbrain. This caused a nearly complete depletion of NE in the projection areas of the two bundles as judged by histofluorescence. Assays also showed that forebrain NE was reduced to less than 15% of normal. The animals became hyperphagic and obese. Injections that depleted only the dorsal bundle projections did not cause hyperphagia or obesity, suggesting that VB neurons were crucial (25, 26).

After 6-OH-DA injections or electrolytic lesions in the VB, an increased dose of AMPH was necessary to produce its usual anorectic effect; the dose-response curve was shifted to the right (25). We concluded that NE neurons, or recently discovered E neurons (27), in the VB are necessary for normal satiety and for a part of AMPH anorexia.

Gold (28) extended these findings to explain why MH lesions produce progressively greater hyperphagia and obesity as lesion size is increased. He suggested that lesions or knife cuts which interrupt the appropriate ascending NE system cause hyperphagia proportionate to NE damage. The same logic could apply to any other neurotransmitter necessary for satiety which is distributed in the MH region. But if the lesions or knife cuts were so big that they damage the DA system necessary for eating, then the effects would be reversed and the animal would starve, as seen after large lesions in the original studies of Anand & Brobeck (6).

We find that midbrain injections of 6-OH-DA cause a type of hyperphagia which is different from typical MH hyperphagia. First, I must warn the reader that hypothalamic hyperphagia is itself a syndrome of many faces (4, 29–31). Some MH lesions cause hyperreactivity to taste and some do not (5). Females show MH hyperphagia more readily than males, and the degree of overeating depends not only on lesion size and exact placement, but also on hormonal conditions (31, 32). Moreover, weight gain depends on preoperative weight (33). As a further complication there are chemoreceptors, such as glucoreceptors, in the hypothalamus as shown by the histotoxic effects of gold-thio-glucose in the mouse (34) and unit recording in the rat (35). The MH is also a site of pituitary control through hormone-releasing factors (36), and lesions are known to affect endocrine functions including changes in metabolism (30, 37). Some MH lesion locations are more likely to destroy these chemoreceptors and secretory cells than others.

The typical MH lesion produces overeating leading to obesity, sensory enhancement known as finickiness, larger meals, and a shift from normal circadian feeding toward feeding both day and night (4).

Our 6-OH-DA–treated VB rats depleted of NE were different than typical MH–lesioned rats. The VB rats were not finicky (38). In studies now involving hundreds of animals, they did not usually become as obese as MH rats, although some did. In a study specifically comparing the two procedures, VB rats depleted of NE by 6-OH-DA overate only at night. Unlike VB rats, the rats made obese by MH lesions were not significantly depleted of NE according to assays of the whole forebrain. Rats that were subjected to both types of neural damage, first 6-OH-DA in the VB followed later by MH lesions, showed a level of hyperphagia equal or exceeding the sum of the separate effects (39).

The pharmacology of VB obesity was also different. In MH-lesioned rats, Epstein (12) found no change or even an increase in AMPH anorexia, whereas we found a loss of AMPH anorexia in VB rats (25, 26). By all these measures MH hyperphagia and VB hyperphagia are different phenomena.

Our conclusion that hyperphagia and obesity can result from depletion of NE, or possibly E, suffers from several criticisms. The phenomenon has not yet been completely confirmed in any other laboratory although several investigators have similar findings using different techniques. Hyperphagia has been reported in rats after electrolytic lesions in the VB region (40–43). Gold (28) suggests that knife cuts that caused hyperphagia did so by transecting the VB at various levels between the mammillary bodies and hypothalamus. Ungerstedt (17) mentions hyperphagia following midbrain injections of 6-OH-DA. In geese and pigs 6-OH-DA injected intraventricularly caused hyperphagia (44) perhaps by depleting NE but not DA, whereas in rats this procedure produced NE depletion without causing hyperphagia or a reduction in AMPH anorexia (19). Panksepp (29) mentions data confirming that 6-OH-DA injections in the midbrain VB can induce hyperphagia up to a 30% increase in daily food intake.

Lorden, Oltmans & Margules (42) could not replicate 6-OH-DA obesity following VB injection, unless they used procedures designed to cause nonspecific damage (43). They suggested that the hyperphagia and obesity we obtained might not be related to NE depletion because some of their rats had NE depletion as great as we reported. Extensive NE depletion did not necessarily cause hyperphagia; however, all rats that showed hyperphagia did have some NE depletion (G. A. Oltmans, personal communication).

Perhaps different subsets of adrenergic neurons were killed in the two studies, or else nonspecific damage caused obesity in our study or blocked obesity in theirs.

It is difficult to use 6-OH-DA selectively. It readily oxidizes and must be handled with care under a nitrogen atmosphere and with ascorbic acid as an additive. In high doses, 6-OH-DA causes nonspecific damage, and even when it does not, the ascorbic acid may. Some investigators demonstrate gross damage and nonspecificity from local injections of 6-OH-DA; others demonstrate that a high degree of specificity can be obtained (43, 45, 46). This makes behavioral experiments difficult to interpret unless extensive controls are performed.

We doubt that nonspecific damage caused obesity in our study because the ascorbic acid vehicle did not cause obesity by itself; moreover desmethylimipramine, DMI, given i.p. to block 6-OH-DA uptake into adrenergic neurons prevented NE depletion and prevented the obesity. Nonspecific damage from 6-OH-DA and its vehicle should be the same with or without DMI, which leads us to the conclusion that nonspecific damage is not responsible for the phenomenon unless it occurs in conjunction with adrenergic depletion. The results strongly suggest that specific destruction of adrenergic neurons was responsible for the hyperphagia and obesity we observed.

The depleted neurotransmitter responsible for 6-OH-DA hyperphagia may be E instead of NE (9, 39, 42). Immunohistochemical studies show that a small E pathway follows the same VB path as the NE neurons (27). The experiments did not distinguish between the two because 6-OH-DA can deplete both and DMI can protect both. Leibowitz (9) also suggests that the β-adrenergic transmitter that suppresses feeding in the LH may be E. If 6-OH-DA destroys NE and E neurons in different proportions or in different subsystems depending on dose and injection site, this could explain different findings in different laboratories (46).

There is much evidence for multiple adrenergic influences on feeding. Genetically obese rats have hypothalamic NE (or E) concentration that is lower than normal in the paraventricular nucleus and higher than normal in the median eminence (47). These regional differences suggest that ascending NE pathways have subsystems that function independently. Montgomery & Singer (48) report that NE injected in the amygdala modulates the feeding effects of NE injected in the hypothalamus. Given the evidence for both adrenergic feeding and adrenergic satiety, the evidence for differential changes in adrenergic localization in genetic-obese rats, and the behavioral evidence for adrenergic modulation of adrenergic function, it seems quite possible that the relative balance of adrenergic supplies to the hypothalamus and related areas determines whether hyperphagia is or is not observed after depletion.

Experimental obesity can sometimes be blocked. Powley & Opsahl (49) blocked MH hyperphagia with vagotomy. Coscina (50) blocked it with midbrain raphe lesions. We prevented 6-OH-DA obesity by hypophysectomy (51). It is conceivable, as one more possible explanation, that 6-OH-DA lesions in the Lorden et al (42) experiments produced some such block that prevented the 6-OH-DA obesity observed by Ahlskog & Hoebel (26).

A different approach to the problem is to deplete NE by blocking dopamine-β-hydroxylase with FLA-63. The depletion produced with this drug reduced food intake and failed to affect AMPH anorexia (52). Conversely, long-lasting activation of α-adrenergic receptors with clonidine caused overeating, and reduced AMPH anorexia (53, 54). Both the FLA-63 and clonidine findings are consistent with the classical α-adrenergic feeding theory. Clonidine given intraventricularly would also inhibit adrenergic neurons that had α-adrenergic autoreceptors (55), including, perhaps, inhibition of the neurons for β-adrenergic satiety. This might contribute to the overeating.

Perfusate Collection In Vivo and In Vitro

Myers and his colleagues (56) injected perfusate from one monkey's brain into the brain of another. The state of hunger or satiety in the first monkey was reflected in the behavior of the second. They also microinjected H^3NE into the MH of a rat and then found it was preferentially released into push-pull perfusion fluid when the rat was offered food and ate a meal. A correlation between the uptake of H^3NE in vitro and the feeding pattern in rats has also been reported (57). Uptake correlated positively with feeding rate. These studies combine three valuable features: the analysis of neurotransmitter turnover, anatomical localization, and behavior. They have been difficult to interpret, however, because of their correlative nature.

Another step in analyzing E or NE systems in feeding is to study the actual membrane receptor properties in localized areas. So far this has not been done with any specific tie to feeding. It is noteworthy that pretreatment of forebrain slices with 6-OH-DA to cause neuronal damage can enhance adenylate cyclase response to NE, suggesting that at least part of NEs effect is on denervated, supersensitive, post-synaptic receptors, not just glial material (58). β-adrenergic adenylate cyclase that is more sensitive to NE than E has been isolated from homogenates of the anterior hypothalamus and other limbic forebrain structures (59). Thus it is conceivable that NE can be a β-adrenergic, as well as α-adrenergic, transmitter in the brain. There may be no necessity to say that the adrenergic suppression of feeding is mediated by endogenous E just because the effect is β-adrenergic; either NE or E could play the β role. Judging by in vitro (58) or in vivo (9) studies, some "DA blockers" can block β-adrenergic functions; therefore NE or E might also play roles sometimes attributed to DA.

Summary and Conclusion

α-Adrenergic agonists, including AMPH, induce feeding in the medial portions of the hypothalamus. AMPH probably induces feeding by releasing either NE or E; it is not clear which. Starvation has never been produced by selective, adrenergic depletion; therefore all the evidence for adrenergic feeding is based on agonist-antagonist injections and push-pull perfusion studies. This suggests that activation of the α feeding system is sufficient for feeding, but not necessary for feeding.

AMPH injected in the lateral hypothalamus suppresses feeding and the effect is β-adrenergic or dopaminergic. This agrees with the finding that systemic AMPH loses anorectic potency after dopaminergic or adrenergic depletion with 6-OH-DA.

Hyperphagia can follow adrenergic depletion. This was not the same pattern of hyperphagia or depletion seen after classical MH lesions. An overview of work from several laboratories suggests that it is possible to obtain obesity without depleting NE or vice versa, to deplete NE without obtaining obesity, or even to deplete NE to produce obesity but then block it.

We conclude from work in this laboratory that 6-OH-DA injected in the VB reduces the anorectic potency of AMPH. This procedure also depleted endogenous

NE and/or E, but not DA or 5-HT, and the procedure caused obesity. It is therefore a likely possibility that part of AMPH anorexia in the normal animal is the result of the release of endogenous NE or E at adrenergic terminals which have as one of their normal functions a suppressive effect on food intake and body weight.

FENFLURAMINE AND SEROTONERGIC SYSTEMS

Systemic Injections

FEN is structurally related to AMPH (Figure 1), but its anorectic action does not depend on catecholamines (60). For example, midbrain injections of 6-OH-DA reduced AMPH anorexia, but enhanced FEN anorexia (39), and LH lesions produced the same dissociation (14).

FEN is serotonergic. Its anorexic effect was diminished by 5-HT antagonists (61, 62), by 5-HT synthesis block with systemic parachlorophenylalanine (PCPA) (63), by depletion with an intraventricular neurotoxin, 5,6-dihydroxytryptamine (5,6-DHT) (64), or by raphe lesions (65). However, in other studies PCPA (66), 5,6-DHT (66), 5,7-DHT (63), or raphe lesions (66) failed to diminish FEN anorexia. The authors suggested that FEN can have a direct postsynaptic effect, although this has since been challenged (69), or a nonserotonergic effect, such as DA block (70), or simply that a greater degree of 5-HT depletion was needed. It is also possible that some techniques cause depletion in the wrong areas to affect FEN anorexia. It is known that systemic PCPA and various raphe lesions can have differential effects on locomotor activity, pain reactivity, and avoidance behavior (71); clearly, serotonin depletion cannot be spoken of as a unitary concept (72). Another possibility is that some of the 5-HT depletion procedures also caused catecholamine depletion which would potentiate FEN anorexia and counteract any loss of anorexia. Feeding

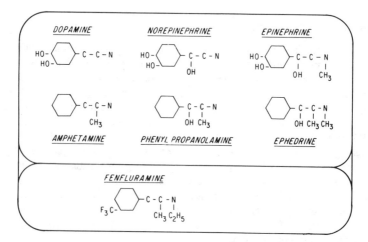

Figure 1 Structural comparison of some monoamine neurotransmitters and phenethylamine anorectics.

schedules used in anorexia tests can also influence the results (14). Another pitfall is that high doses of FEN can cause such extensive 5-HT release that FEN, itself, leads to depletion and loss of physiological function (60). In the concentrations generally used, FEN is properly considered to be a 5-HT agonist if one judges by the positive results rather than the negative. This does not necessarily mean that FEN has a straightforward action on a neural system which regulates feeding. FEN might possibly cause anorexia in part by increasing glucose utilization, enhancing lipolysis, or releasing hormones, but in any case a serotonergic basis for a major part of FEN anorexia is well established even though we do not know where it acts.

The effects of FEN on brain metabolites of monoamines suggest an action on serotonergic systems in the central nervous system (73). On the other hand a recent study of 5-HT antagonists failed to find changes in brain metabolites (74). This might have argued against a central action, except that there appears to be no neuronal feedback in brain serotonin systems to cause a compensatory change in 5-HT turnover (75). Therefore 5-HT turnover studies leave open the likelihood of central effects.

FEN injected systemically can be expected to have complicated effects in the CNS because there are many serotonin cell assemblies. Serotonin cells in the hypothalamus have recently been reported (76). Within the midbrain raphe nuclei 5-HT neurons inhibit other 5-HT-containing cell bodies (75, 77). Thus, FEN inhibits neurons in the raphe. It follows that systemic FEN may produce a 5-HT effect at 5-HT terminals in the forebrain, but at the same time inhibit the same 5-HT neurons at their source in the midbrain and render them unresponsive to normal physiological inputs. Similarly a depletor like PCPA could have a variety of effects. It becomes essential to consider factors that affect drug entry into various parts of the brain.

The usual effect of 5-HT agonists is anorexia. Hypothalamic injection of 5-HT (78), FEN to release 5-HT, a 5-HT uptake blocker to prolong synaptic action (29), or 5-HT precursor (80) all can produce anorexia, although controls for sedation are a problem.

Taken together, these facts suggest that somewhere in the chains of serotonergic neurons there may be synapses that lead to the suppression of food intake. If so, depletion of the appropriate 5-HT neurons should disinhibit food intake and cause obesity.

Neurochemical Depletions

We find that parachlorophenylalanine (PCPA) delivered into the ventricles depleted forebrain 5-HT to 25% of normal and consistently caused hyperphagia to develop (81). Brain 5-HT can be depleted with PCPA given systemically, but this failed to cause hyperphagia in many studies (81–83). The experiments may have been confounded by malaise caused by peripheral 5-HT depletion particularly in the gut, or perhaps systemic PCPA caused the wrong pattern of brain depletion.

Our PCPA-treated rats displayed hyperphagia starting three days after injection. They sometimes became overweight and continued to overeat for about two weeks. By then 5-HT levels had been partially restored. Significant changes in forebrain catecholamine levels did not occur during the period of maximum hyperphagia.

The function of 5-HT in feeding could take many forms. It is too soon to speculate whether 5-HT neurons control food intake by a direct action on a final common path for feeding, or through some circuitous neuronal or hormonal route. Another question is whether the effect is specific to feeding, or has to do with overall behavior inhibition, arousal thermoregulation, or locomotor activity (67, 84).

To begin to examine these questions, we have found that rats treated with intraventricular PCPA tend to overeat both day and night, particularly in the day when they should be sleeping (unpublished observations). The same PCPA treatment increased sexual behavior as measured by a female's tendency to assume the lordosis posture when mounted. This confirms with intraventricular PCPA an effect on mating seen earlier with systemic injections (85). Thus in female rats, only intraventricular PCPA causes hyperphagia, but either intraventricular or intraperitoneal PCPA causes hypersexuality. As confirmation that 5-HT underlies the change in sexual behavior, p-chloroamphetamine, which releases 5-HT and gradually depletes it, caused a corresponding biphasic effect on behavior. First lordosis frequency decreased, then increased (86).

Confirmation of hyperphagia following PCPA has not yet appeared; however, Saller & Stricker (87) report that serotonin depletion with the neurotoxin, 5,7-dihydroxytryptamine (5,7-DHT) given intraventricularly to young male rats caused hyperphagia and increased bone growth. PCPA and 5,7-DHT each have their own penumbra of side effects involving false transmitters, metabolites, multiple actions, and nonspecific effects. Each drug has a different set of associated problems, so it is encouraging that both produced hyperphagia. We will feel more certain of the effect if and when 5,7-DHT is shown to produce hyperphagia and obesity in females as well as males, and when the effect of PCPA and 5,7-DHT is obtained with localized injections. We have succeeded in mitigating PCPA-induced hyperphagia with systemic 5-HTP to bypass the block of 5-HT synthesis (unpublished observations). One would also expect supersensitivity to develop for serotonergic agonists after 5-HT depletion with 5,7-DHT; this has been done for simple neurological signs (88), but not for feeding behavior.

If it is true that 5-HT neurons play an important role in feeding suppression then a number of intriguing avenues are opened for exploration. Quantity and quality of food intake can cause large shifts in 5-HT levels in the brain. Theoretically, dietary additives or deficiencies or physiological imbalances that prevent tryptophan from entering the brain could deplete 5-HT and possibly cause overeating (89). The same speculation applies to sexual behavior. These behavior changes might also be caused by any environmental pollutants, genetic characteristic, or brain lesion leading to a PCPA-type action.

MH lesions can cause hyperphagia with little forebrain 5-HT depletion (39, 90) and no loss of FEN anorexia (91); nevertheless a comparison of MH hyperphagia and ventricular-PCPA hyperphagia suggests that they might have something in common. Both caused overeating that predominated in the daytime, thereby flattening the diurnal feeding cycle (5). We also have preliminary evidence that VM lesions plus intraventricular PCPA applied to the same rat produces nonadditive hyperphagia (unpublished observations). This is consistent with the possibility that a major part of the classical VM effect is similar to the action of ventricular PCPA. This is unlike the 6-OH-DA hyperphagia described earlier that occurred at night and was superimposed on the MH effect.

Summary and Speculation

FEN suppresses feeding in people as well as animals and is sold by prescription for that purpose even though it is a mild sedative. Its counterpart, cyropheptadine, a 5-HT antagonist, is marketed to promote feeding and weight gain (3).

There is no doubt that FEN anorexia depends on a different mechanism than AMPH anorexia. The FEN effect seems to be serotonergic. Some procedures designed to deplete 5-HT lead to hyperphagia but so far there is no unequivocal demonstration that any particular brain structure is necessary for FEN anorexia.

Disinhibition of feeding with midbrain 6-OH-DA and ventricular PCPA revealed different types of hyperphagia. This suggests at least two different systems that somehow suppress feeding under normal circumstances. One is adrenergic, and a normal function in the rat is to suppress feeding at night; the other is serotonergic, and it acts to suppress feeding day and night. Presumably the adrenergic one is activated by amphetamine; the serotonergic one, by fenfluramine.

Behavioral studies of AMPH and FEN also suggest a dichotomy between two feeding suppression systems. Blundell, Latham & Leshem (2) found that AMPH inhibited the initiation of meals whereas fenfluramine inhibited the continuation of meals. In other words, AMPH caused fewer meals, and FEN caused shorter meals. In another dissociation, tail pinch reversed AMPH anorexia but not FEN anorexia (92, and personal communication).

These results offer a hint that adrenergic and dopaminergic substrates control the initiation and maintenance of meals during the half of the day when most meals are taken, and that serotonergic substrates control the cessation and suppression of meals around the clock, particularly during the sleep period.

PHENYLPROPANOLAMINE AND GLUCOSTATIC SYSTEMS

PPA is intriguing for several reasons. As shown in Figure 1 it is closely related to AMPH with the addition of a hydroxyl group (β-hydroxy-AMPH). It is less potent as an anorectic by about 20-fold, but has an even greater loss of psychomotor stimulation. Because it is less stimulating it is less abused and can be sold over the counter for both weight reduction (e.g. Permathene,® Appedrine® and X-11®), and nasal decongestion (e.g. Propadrine® Allarest®, and Contac®). It was useful for studying feeding and self-stimulation in rats because some doses inhibited feeding without causing hyperactivity like AMPH or sedation like FEN (93). Therefore it was the drug of choice for our laboratory studies.

In rats with implanted electrode-cannulas, injection of crystalline PPA in the LH, but not the MH, suppressed electrically induced feeding. This suggested a possible LH site of action. However in 6-OH-DA–treated rats, PPA failed to lose anorectic potency like AMPH, or to gain potency like FEN. Therefore, if PPA acts in the brain, the mechanism is a mystery.

Ideally, an anorectic drug would act on a specific receptor system controlling feeding instead of acting on brain neurotransmitters that might be involved in many behaviors.

The glucostatic theory of feeding control suggests that anorexia could be caused by a drug with an insulin-like action or a direct excitatory action on glucoreceptors. To explore this possibility with PPA, we gave the drug to alloxan diabetic rats in a pilot study and obtained a decrease in blood sugar. Then in collaboration with Dr. Charles Hamilton, rhesus monkeys received PPA at approximately the same mg/kg dose used in humans. In normal monkeys, PPA caused anorexia with accompanying weight loss. In mildly diabetic, but not severely diabetic, monkeys PPA reduced glucosuria significantly more than could be accounted for by decreased food intake. Apparently PPA somehow increased glucose utilization. It is already known that some phenethylamines, including FEN, increase glucose utilization (94). Evidence that PPA, an over-the-counter drug, might act in this fashion is new. It is conceivable that this effect suppresses feeding.

There is currently a controversy in the United States over the issue of PPA efficacy in humans. The Post Office, Federal Trade Commission, and Food and Drug Administration want to know whether this widely sold drug produces the benefits claimed for overweight people. We found that PPA suppressed intake of a liquid lunch, and in another study that it reduced snacks and caused a statistically significant weight loss. There were no consistent reports of side effects. Average subjects lost roughly a pound in anticipation of the study, then in a one month cross-over design they lost another pound on placebo, and a third pound attributed to PPA. It is a matter of judgment whether or not this is medically significant or advisable for any given individual. It is not known whether statistical significance would be obtained in another age, economic, ethnic, educational, or racial population, or in subjects unaware of the nature of the study (3).

Given the present evidence that (a) PPA is effective as an anorectic in humans, (b) effective at the human dose in monkeys, (c) effective at relatively high doses in rats, and (d) effective in altering bronchial and nasal secretions, we conclude that there is a great need for information about this drug's effects on other behavioral and physiological systems. At the present time the millions of consumers who take PPA as a decongestant are not well informed that it may affect their appetite. We do not know what, if any, other behaviors are affected. If PPA acts primarily to facilitate energy utilization and thereby suppresses feeding, then its physiological effects on metabolism may be rather widespread and its behavioral effects rather specific. If, on the other hand, PPA turns out to be a catecholaminergic drug in the CNS at the common dose, then it can be expected to affect many behaviors that depend on brain catecholamines.

The only test of behavioral specificity for PPA so far is an indirect assessment using brain self-stimulation and stimulation-escape. This procedure for measuring "reward" and "aversion" in rats has a built-in control for overall activity changes. AMPH elevates response rates for both self-stimulation and stimulation-escape, whereas FEN lowers both. Presumably a drug that lowers self-stimulation but raises stimulation-escape is acting on behavioral reinforcement rather than on overall arousal or sedation. That is what we found with PPA; it lowered self-stimulation and raised escape rates. Tests that are independent of response rate have not yet been used to confirm this result. Instead, we repeated the experiment using two different electrodes in each rat. LH self-stimulation, which tends to vary directly with feeding, was decreased by PPA. Stimulation-escape, which tends to vary inversely with feeding, was increased by PPA. In the posterior hypothalamus, on the other hand, where self-stimulation tends to vary with sexual appetite, PPA had no effect on self-stimulation or escape (1, 93). Thus under these selected testing conditions there was evidence that PPA affected the reinforcement produced by stimulation of one part of the hypothalamus, but not another. Hernandez and I (95) obtained the same result with injections of small doses of insulin. Thus we again find PPA and insulin may have something in common.

The evidence from animal research described above suggests an application that is exciting, but untested. This over-the-counter drug could be useful in treating some mildly diabetic people. It might help them control hyperglycemia in two ways, by helping them lose weight and by increasing glucose utilization. At the present time PPA is officially contraindicated for diabetics. It might have adverse sympathomimetic effects, particularly on the cardiovascular system. Therefore it is not safe for the suggested new use until long-term tests of cardiovascular effects and controlled clinical trials are published.

SUMMARY

It has become clear that anorectic drugs vary a great deal. They act in a variety of ways and have a variety of side effects. The evidence that has been reviewed suggests that some drugs might be more appropriate than others for a given overweight individual. No one drug has emerged as best or safest for everybody. The issues raised involve central monoamine balance and peripheral metabolic state.

New neurochemical procedures for producing experimental obesity have suggested possible neurotransmitters underlying anorectic drug action. These chemical procedures are supposed to deplete only selected neurotransmitters. This has allowed research on anorectic pharmacology to be tied in conceptually with research on the neurochemistry of brain systems involved in feeding. This is a substantial advance over the state of the art when classical medial hypothalamic lesions were our best tool. However, the new techniques still have many problems and the old questions remain. For example, when we observe chemically induced hyperphagia, to what extent is it behaviorally specific (feeding versus emotion), physiologically specific (glucostasis versus lipostasis), anatomically specific (terminals versus pathways), or neurochemically specific (known transmitters versus the unknown)? In the face of these problems we have arbitrarily delved into the relation between AMPH and adrenergic systems, FEN and serotonergic systems, and PPA and glucostatic systems. Although neither the drugs nor the systems are specific to our arbitrary categories, a number of interesting relationships between the drugs, the brain, and feeding have become evident and have led to the discussion of new ideas in the pharmacologic control of feeding.

Literature Cited

1. Hoebel, B. G. 1975. Satiety: Hypothalamic stimulation, anorectic drugs, neurochemical substrates. In *Hunger: Basic Mechanisms and Clinical Implications,* ed. D. Novin, W. Wyrwicka, G. Bray, pp. 33–50. New York: Raven
2. Blundell, J. E., Latham, C. J., Leshem, M. B. 1976. Differences between the anorexic actions of amphetamine and fenfluramine—possible effects on hunger and satiety. *J. Pharm. Pharmacol.* 28:471–77
3. Hoebel, B. G. 1977. Pharmacology of feeding. In *Handbook of Psychopharmacology,* ed. L. L. Iversen, S. D. Iversen, S. H. Snyder. In press
4. Hoebel, B. G. 1975. Brain reward and aversion systems in the control of feeding and sexual behavior. In *Nebr. Symp. Motiv., 1974,* ed. J. K. Cole, T. B. Sondregger, pp. 49–112. Lincoln: Univ. Nebraska Press
5. Hoebel, B. G. 1977. Hyperphagia: A neurochemical analysis. In *Nerves and the Gut,* ed. F. P. Brooks, P. W. Evers, pp. 440–58. Thorofare, NJ: Charles Black
6. Anand, B. K., Brobeck, J. R. 1951. Hypothalamic control of food intake in rats and cats. *Yale J. Biol. Med.* 24:123–40
7. Mogenson, G. J. 1974. Changing views of the role of the hypothalamus in the control of ingestive behaviors. In *Recent Studies of Hypothalamic Function, Int. Symp. Calgary,* ed. K. Lederis, K. E. Cooper, pp. 268–93. Basel: Karger
8. Grossman, S. P. 1960. Eating or drinking elicited by direct adrenergic or cholinergic stimulation of the hypothalamus. *Science* 132:301–2
9. Leibowitz, S. F. 1976. Brain catecholamine mechanisms for controlling hunger. See Ref. 1, pp. 1–18
10. Slangen, J. L. 1974. The role of hypothalamic noradrenergic neurons in food intake regulation. *Prog. Brain Res.* 41:395–407
11. Margules, D. L. 1969. Noradrenergic synapses for the suppression of feeding behavior. *Life Sci.* 8:693–704
12. Epstein, A. N. 1959. Suppression of eating and drinking by amphetamine and other drugs in normal and hyperphagic rats. *J. Comp. Physiol. Psychol.* 52:37–45
13. Wolgin, D. L., Cytawa, J., Teitelbaum, P. 1976. The role of activation in the regulation of food intake. See Ref. 1

14. Blundell, J. E., Leshem, M. B. 1974. Central action of anorexic agents: Effects of amphetamine and fenfluramine in rats with lateral hypothalamic lesions. *Eur. J. Pharmacol.* 28:81–88
15. Baez, L. A. 1974. Role of catecholamines in the anorectic effects of amphetamine in rats. *Psychopharmacologia* 35:91–98
16. Costa, E., Garattini, S., eds. 1970. *Amphetamine and Related Compounds.* New York: Raven
17. Ungerstedt, U. 1971. Adipsia and aphagia after 6-hydroxydopamine induced degeneration of the nigro-striatal dopamine system. *Acta Physiol. Scand.,* Suppl. 367, pp. 95–121
18. Cooper, B. R., Howard, J. L., Grant, L. D., Smith, R. D., Breese, G. R. 1974. Alteration of avoidance and ingestive behavior after destruction of central catecholamine pathways with 6-hydroxydopamine. *Pharmacol. Biochem. Behav.* 2:639–49
19. Stricker, E. M., Zigmond, M. J. 1975. Brain catecholamines and the lateral hypothalamic syndrome. See Ref. 1
20. Wolgin, D. L., Cytawa, J., Teitelbaum, P. 1976. The role of activation in the regulation of food intake. See Ref. 1
21. Antelman, S. M., Szechtman, H., Chin, P., Fisher, A. E. 1975. Tail pinch-induced eating, gnawing and licking behavior in rats: Dependence on the nigrostriatal dopamine system. *Brain Res.* 99:319–37
22. Rowland, N. E., Antelman, S. M. 1976. Stress-induced hyperphagia and obesity in rats: A possible model for understanding human obesity. *Science* 191:310–21
23. Heffner, T. G., Zigmond, M. J., Stricker, E. M. 1975. Brain dopamine involvement in amphetamine-induced anorexia. *Fed. Proc.* 34:348
24. Bunney, B. S., Aghajanian, G. K. 1976. d-Amphetamine-induced inhibition of central dopaminergic neurons: Mediation by a striato-nigral feedback pathway. *Science* 192:391–93
25. Ahlskog, J. E. 1974. Food intake and amphetamine anorexia after selective forebrain norepinephrine loss. *Brain Res.* 82:211–40
26. Ahlskog, J. E., Hoebel, B. G. 1973. Overeating and obesity from damage to a noradrenergic system in the brain. *Science* 182:166–69

27. Hokfelt, T., Fuxe, K., Goldstein, M., Johansson, O. 1974. Immunohisto-chemical evidence for the existence of adrenaline neurons in the rat brain. *Brain Res.* 66:235–51

28. Gold, R. M. 1973. Hypothalamic obesity: The myth of the ventromedial nucleus. *Science* 182:488–90

29. Panksepp, J. 1975. The nature of feeding patterns—primarily in rats. See Ref. 1, pp. 369–82

30. Powley, T. L. 1977. The ventromedial hypothalamic syndrome, satiety and a cephalic phase hypothesis. *Psychol. Rev.* In press

31. Sclafani, A. 1976. Appetite and hunger in experimental obesity syndromes. See Ref. 1, pp. 281–95

32. Mook, D. G., Fisher, J. C., Durr, J. C. 1975. Some endocrine influences on hypothalamic hyperphagia. *Horm. Behav.* 6:65–79

33. Hoebel, B. G., Teitelbaum, P. 1966. Weight regulation in normal and hypothalamic hyperphagic rats. *J. Comp. Physiol. Psychol.* 61:189–93

34. Debons, A. F., Krimsky, I., From, A., Cloutier, R. J. 1969. Rapid effects of insulin on the hypothalamic satiety center. *Am. J. Physiol.* 217:1114–18

35. Oomura, Y., Takikawa, M. 1975. Input-output organization between frontal cortex and lateral hypothalamus. In *Mechanisms in Transmission of Signals for Conscious Behavior*, ed. T. Desjraju. Amsterdam: Elsevier

36. Fuller, R. W., Snoddy, H. D., Molloy, B. B. 1976. Pharmacologic evidence for a serotonin neural pathway involved in hypothalamus-pituitary-adrenal function in rats. *Life Sci.* 19:337–46

37. Panksepp, J. 1975. Central metabolic and humoral factors involved in the neural regulation of feeding. In *Central Neural Control of Eating and Obesity. Pharmacol. Biochem. Behav.* 3:Suppl. 1, 107–19

38. Ahlskog, J. E. 1976. Feeding response to regulatory challenges after 6-hydroxy-dopamine injection into the brain noradrenergic pathways. *Physiol. Behav.* 17:407–12

39. Ahlskog, J. E., Randall, P. K., Hoebel, B. G. 1975. Hypothalamic hyperphagia: Dissociation from noradrenergic depletion hyperphagia. *Science* 190:399–401

40. Mogenson, G. J. 1976. Neural mechanisms of hunger: Current status and future prospects. See Ref. 1

41. Misantone, L. J. 1976. Effects of damage to the monoamine axonal constit-

42. Lorden, J., Oltmans, G. A., Margules, D. 1976. Central noradrenergic neurons: Differential effects on body weight of electrolytic and 6-hydroxydopamine lesions in rats. *J. Comp. Physiol. Psychol.* 90:127–43

43. Oltmans, G. A., Lorden, J. F., Margules, D. L. 1976. Food intake and body weight: Effects of specific and non-specific lesions in the midbrain path of the ascending noradrenergic neurons of the rat. *Brain Res.* In press

44. Auffray, P., Marcilloux, J.-C., Bahy, C., Albe-Fessard, D. 1973. Hyperphagie in-duite chez l'oie par injections intraven-triculaires de 6-hydroxydopamine. *C. R. Acad. Sci. Ser. D* 276:347–50

45. Lidbrink, P., Jonsson, G. 1975. On the specificity of 6-hydroxydopamine-induced degeneration of central nora-drenaline neurons after intracerebral in-jection. *Neurosci. Lett.* 1:35–39

46. Willis, G. L., Singer, G., Evans, B. K. 1976. Intracranial injections of 6-OHDA. Comparison of catecholamine-depleting effects of different volumes and concentrations. *Pharmacol. Biochem. Behav.* 5:207–13

47. Cruce, J. A. F., Thoa, N. B., Jacobowitz, D. M. 1976. Catecholamines in the brains of genetically obese rats. *Brain Res.* 101:165–70

48. Montgomery, R. B., Singer, G. 1975. Functional relationship of lateral hypothalamus and amygdala in control of eating. *Pharmacol. Biochem. Behav.* 3:905–7

49. Powley, T. L., Opsahl, C. A. 1974. Ventromedial hypothalamic obesity abolished by subdiaphragmatic vagotomy. *Am. J. Physiol.* 226:25–33

50. Coscina, D. V. 1975. *Blockade of Medial Hypothalamic Hyperphagia and Weight Gain by Serotonin-Depleting Midbrain Raphe Lesions in Rats.* Presented at East. Psychol. Assoc., 46th, New York

51. Ahlskog, J. E., Breisch, S. T., Hoebel, B. G. 1974. Noradrenergic inhibition of feeding depends on pituitary function. *Fed. Proc.* 33:463

52. Franklin, K. B. J., Herberg, L. J. 1977. Amphetamine induces anorexia even after inhibition of noradrenaline synthesis. *Neuropharmacology.* In press

53. Broeckkamp, C., Van Rossum, J. M. 1972. Clonidine induced intrahypo-

620 HOEBEL

thalamic stimulation of eating in rats. *Psychopharmacologia* 25:162–68
54. Ritter, S., Wise, C. D., Stein, L. 1975. Neurochemical regulation of feeding in the rat: facilitation by α-noradrenergic, but not dopaminergic, receptor stimulants. *J. Comp. Physiol. Psychol.* 88: 778–84
55. Svensson, T. H., Bunney, B. S., Aghajanian, G. K. 1975. Inhibition of both noradrenergic and serotonergic neurons in brain by the α-adrenergic agonist clonidine. *Brain Res.* 92:291–306
56. Myers, R. D. 1975. *Handbook of Drug and Chemical Stimulation of the Brain.* New York: Van Nostrand-Reinhold
57. Van der Gugten, L., Slangen, J. L. 1975. Norepinephrine uptake by hypothalamic tissue from the rat related to feeding. *Pharmacol. Biochem. Behav.* 3:855–60
58. Blumberg, J. B., Taylor, R. E., Sulser, F. 1975. Blockage by pimozide of a noradrenaline sensitive adenylate cyclase in the limbic forebrain: Possible role of limbic noradrenergic mechanisms in the mode of action of antipsychotics. *J. Pharm. Pharmacol.* 27: 125
59. Horn, A. S., Phillipson, O. T. 1976. A noradrenaline sensitive adenylate cyclase in the rat limbic forebrain: Preparation, properties and the effects of agonists, adrenolytics and neuroleptic drugs. *Eur. J. Pharmacol.* 37:1–11
60. Barchas, J., Usdin, E., eds. 1973. *Serotonin and Behavior.* New York: Academic
61. Clineschmidt, B. V., McGuffin, J. C., Werner, A. B. 1974. Role of monoamines in the anorexigenic actions of fenfluramine, amphetamine and p-chloromethamphetamine. *Eur. J. Pharmacol.* 27:313–23
62. Jesperson, S., Scheel-Kruger, J. 1973. Evidence for a difference in mechanism of action between fenfluramine- and amphetamine-induced anorexia. *J. Pharm. Pharmacol.* 25:49–54
63. Hollister, A. S., Ervin, G. H., Cooper, B. R., Breese, G. R. 1975. The roles of monoamine neural systems in the anorexia induced by (+)-amphetamine and related compounds. *Neuropharmacology* 14:715–23
64. Clineschmidt, B. V. 1973. 5,6-Dihydroxytryptamine suppression of the anorexigenic action of fenfluramine. *Eur. J. Pharmacol.* 24:405–9
65. Samanin, R., Ghezzi, D., Valzelli, L., Garattini, S. 1972. The effects of selec-

tive lesioning of brain serotonin or catecholamine neurones on the anorectic activity of fenfluramine and amphetamine. *Eur. J. Pharmacol.* 19:318–22
66. Sugrue, M. F., Goodlet, I., McIndewar, I. 1975. Failure of depletion of rat brain 5-hydroxytryptamine to alter fenfluramine-induced anorexia. *J. Pharm. Pharmacol.* 27:950–52
67. Myers, R. D. 1975. Impairment of thermoregulation, food and water intakes in the rat after hypothalamic injections of 5,6-dihydroxytryptamine. *Brain Res.* 94:491–506
68. Hole, K., Fuxe, K., Jonsson, G. 1976. Behavioral effects of 5,7-dihydroxytryptamine lesions of ascending 5-hydroxytryptamine pathways. *Brain Res.* 107:385–99
69. Trulson, M., Jacobs, B. L. 1976. Behavioral evidence for the rapid release of CNS serotonin by PCA and fenfluramine. *Eur. J. Pharmacol.* 36:149–54
70. Fuller, R. W., Perry, K. W., Clemens, J. A. 1976. Elevation of 3,4-dihydroxyphenylacetic acid concentrations in rat brain and stimulation of prolactin secretion by fenfluramine: Evidence for antagonism and dopamine receptor sites. *J. Pharm. Pharmacol.* 28:643–44
71. Srebro, B., Lorens, S. A. 1975. Behavioral effects of selective midbrain raphe lesions in the rat. *Brain Res.* 89:303–25
72. Jacobs, B. L., Wise, W. D., Taylor, K. M. 1974. Differential behavioral and neurochemical effects following lesions of the dorsal or median raphe nuclei in rats. *Brain Res.* 79:353–61
73. Shoulson, I., Chase, T. N. 1975. Fenfluramine in man: Hypophagia associated with diminished serotonin turnover. *Clin. Pharmacol. Ther.* 17:616–21
74. Jacoby, J. H., Bryce, G. F. 1976. On the central anti-serotonergic actions of cyproheptadine and methylsergide. *Neurosci. Abstr., Soc. Neurosci.* 2:490, No. 700
75. Mosko, S. S., Jacobs, B. L. 1977. Electrophysiological evidence against negative neuronal feedback from the forebrain controlling midbrain raphe unit activity. *Brain Res.* In press
76. Beaudet, A., Descarries, L., Rossignol, S. 1976. A serotonin-containing nerve cell group in rat hypothalamus. *Neurosci. Abstr., Soc. Neurosci.* 2:479, No. 678
77. Jacobs, B. L., Mosko, S. S., Trulson, M. E. The investigation of role of serotonin in mammalian behavior. In *Neurobiology of Sleep and Memory.* ed. R. R.

PHARMACOLOGIC CONTROL OF FEEDING   621

Drucker-Colin, J. L. McGaugh. New York: Academic
78. Goldman, H. W., Lehr, D., Friedman, E. 1971. Antagonistic effects of alpha and beta-adrenergically coded hypothalamic neurones on consummatory behaviour in the rat. *Nature* 231: 453–55
79. Goudie, A. J., Thornton, E. W., Wheeler, T. J. 1976. Effects of Lilly 110140, a specific inhibitor of 5-hydroxytryptamine uptake, on food intake and on 5-hydroxytrophan-induced anorexia. Evidence for serotonergic inhibition of feeding. *J. Pharm. Pharmacol.* 28:318–20
80. Blundell, J. E., Leshem, M. B. 1975. The effect of 5-hydroxytryptophan on food intake and on the anorexic action of amphetamine and fenfluramine. *J. Pharm. Pharmacol.* 27:31–37
81. Breisch, S. T., Zemlan, F. P., Hoebel, B. G. 1976. Hyperphagia and obesity following serotonin depletion with intraventricular parachlorophenylalanine. *Science* 192:382–85
82. Panksepp, J., Nance, D. M. 1974. Effects of para-chlorophenylalanine on food intake in rats. *Physiol. Psychol.* 2:360–64
83. Borbely, A. A., Huston, J. P., Waser, P. G. 1973. Physiological and behavioral effects of parachlorophenylalanine in the rat. *Psychopharmacologia* 31:131–42
84. Messing, R. B., Phebus, L., Fisher, L. A., Lytle, L. D. 1976. Effects of p-chloroamphetamine on locomotor activity and brain 5-hydroxyindoles. *Neuropharmacology* 15:157–63
85. Zemlan, F. P., Ward, I. L., Crowley, W. R., Margules, D. L. 1973. Activation of lordotic responding in female rats by suppression of serotonergic activity. *Science* 179:1010–11
86. Zemlan, F. P., Trulson, M. E., Howell, R., Hoebel, B. G. 1977. Influence of p-

chloroamphetamine on female sexual reflexes and brain monoamine levels. *Brain Res.* In press
87. Saller, C. F., Stricker, E. M. 1976. Hyperphagia and increased growth in rats after intraventricular injection of 5,7-dihydroxytryptamine. *Science* 192: 385–87
88. Trulson, M. E., Eubanks, E. E., Jacobs, B. L. 1976. Behavioral evidence for supersensitivity following destruction of central serotonergic nerve terminals by 5,7-dihydroxytryptamine. *J. Pharmacol. Exp. Ther.* 198:23–32
89. Fernstrom, J. D., Madras. B. K., Munro, H. N., Wurtman, R. J. 1974. Nutritional control of the synthesis of 5-hydroxytryptamine in the brain. In *Aromatic Amino Acids in the Brain, Ciba Found. Symp.,* 22
90. Coscina, D. V., Godse, D. D., Stancer, H. C. 1976. Neurochemical correlates of hypothalamic obesity in rats. *Behav. Biol.* 16:365–72
91. Blundell, J. E., Leshem, M. B. 1975. Hypothalamic lesions and drug induced anorexia. *Postgrad. Med. J.* 51: Suppl. 1, pp. 45–54
92. Antelman, S. M., Caggiula, A. R., Edwards, D. J., Rowland, N. E. 1976. Tail-pinch stress reverses amphetamine anorexia. *Neurosci. Abstr., Soc. Neurosci.* 2:845, No. 1222
93. Hoebel, B. G. 1975. Brain stimulation reward and aversion in relation to behavior. In *Brain-Stimulation Reward,* ed. A. Wauquier, E. T. Rolls, pp. 335–72. Amsterdam: North-Holland
94. Turtle, J. R. 1973. Hypoglycemic action of fenfluramine in diabetes mellitus. *Diabetes* 22:858–67
95. Hernandez, L., Hoebel, B. G. 1975. Parallel effects of phenylpropanolamine and insulin on hypothalamic elicted feeding, self-stimulation, and stimulation-escape. *Neurosci. Abstr., Soci. for Neurosci.,* 1:363, No. 719

Ann. Rev. Pharmacol. Toxicol. 1977. 17:623–46

PROXIMAL TUBULAR REABSORPTION AND ITS REGULATION

❖6699

Harry R. Jacobson and Donald W. Seldin

Department of Internal Medicine, The University of Texas Health Science Center
at Dallas, Southwestern Medical School, Dallas, Texas 75235

INTRODUCTION

The early micropuncture studies of Walker et al (1) first documented that (*a*) proximal tubular reabsorption is isosmotic, and (*b*) the percentage of the filtered load reabsorbed proximally remains relatively constant, a concept referred to as proximal glomerulotubular (GT) balance. Subsequently, it was shown that proximal GT balance was not fixed but could be reset in response to factors that altered effective arterial blood volume, expansion serving to lower and contraction to enhance the fraction of filtrate reabsorbed proximally (2–5).

The present review examines the anatomic and physiologic features determining proximal reabsorption of sodium and water. Toward this end the anatomy of the proximal tubule is briefly reviewed and the concept of proximal tubule heterogeneity introduced. Next the factors determining reabsorption are divided into two major categories: (*a*) outward transport, comprised of active and passive components and (*b*) passive back-leak of reabsorbate. Net reabsorption thus represents outward transport (active plus passive) minus back-leak. Finally, some remarks are made about the regulatory factors modulating these reabsorptive processes.

PROXIMAL TUBULE HETEROGENEITY

For approximately 70 years it has been known that in most mammals, including man, two nephron populations, termed *superficial* and *deep* (or *juxtamedullary*), exist (6). The proximal tubules of both these nephron populations consist of both a convoluted and straight portion (pars recta). The superficial proximal tubules, though shorter than those of the deep nephrons, have a longer pars recta (6). It also has been shown that a gradual transition of cell types exists along the length of each proximal tubule resulting in the division of the tubule into two or three regions based

623

on cell size, height of the luminal brush border, histochemical staining, and quantity and type of intracellular organelles (7–12). Thus, it was recognized early that on a structural basis the proximal tubule exhibited two types of structural heterogeneity —intranephron and internephron heterogeneity. However, the functional significance of these structural differences was unknown.

Until recently, virtually all direct information about proximal reabsorption has been obtained from studies of the superficial proximal convolutions, owing to the inaccessibility of both the superficial pars recta and the entire deep proximal tubule to micropuncture. However, early studies of glomerular filtration rate and blood flow suggested, on the basis of highly inferential data, that superficial and deep nephrons may differ in their contribution to total kidney reabsorption (13–19). These early studies stressed that heterogeneity between nephron populations may exist with respect to glomerular filtration rate and renal plasma flow. Under various physiological circumstances, glomerular filtration and consequently the load of salt and water presented to the proximal tubule for reabsorption, may differ between superficial and deep cortical nephrons. Even though these studies served to point out possible intrarenal hemodynamic heterogeneity, they could not directly disclose whether intrinsic differences existed between tubules located in the superficial and deep cortex. *Hemodynamic heterogeneity* is not discussed further in this review. However, it is now evident that *structural heterogeneity* on a tubular level exists both within (intranephron heterogeneity) and between (internephron heterogeneity) nephron populations (20–25).

INTRANEPHRON HETEROGENEITY

In both superficial and deep nephron populations the convoluted portion has transport properties different from those of the straight portion. Kawamura et al (24) and Schafer et al (21) have studied the pars recta utilizing in vitro microperfusion of rabbit nephron segments. The former authors demonstrated, in pars recta from both superficial and deep nephrons, that net volume reabsorption in these segments is about one third to one half that of the convoluted portion. However, these studies were performed with ultrafiltrate of serum as perfusate. When the pars recta was perfused with a solution simulating in vivo conditions (perfusate without glucose and amino acids and with a bicarbonate concentration of 5 mM and a chloride concentration of 140 mM), net reabsorption was reduced to one fourth to one third of the convoluted portion. In addition to net reabsorptive differences, pars recta from both nephron populations exhibited active electrogenic[1] Na transport without

---

[1]By electrogenic sodium transport we mean the generation of a transepithelial potential difference owing to sodium movement mediated by either of two processes: 1. A rheogenic sodium-potassium exchange pump in the peritubular cell membrane may directly separate charges and generate a potential difference if the coupling is not 1:1. 2. Passive sodium transport may generate a transepithelial potential difference if the movement of sodium is coupled to substances (such as glucose or amino acids) which are actively transported; the mechanism generating the transepithelial potential difference is partial depolarization of the luminal cell membrane by the passive (though coupled) movement of sodium.

the requirement of glucose and amino acids in the perfusate, as opposed to the convoluted portions which have been shown to require these organic solutes to transport Na actively and to develop a lumen negative potential (25, 26). Finally, the superficial pars recta was shown to be more permeable to Cl than to Na as opposed to the superficial convoluted segment, which at least in its early portion is more permeable to sodium (25, 27). In these studies (24) the deep pars recta exhibited greater Na than Cl permeability similar to the subsequent demonstration of greater relative Na permeability in the deep convolution (25). The observations of Kawamura et al (24) with respect to the superficial pars recta confirmed the studies of Shafer et al (21) who had originally examined this segment and found the same reabsorptive and permeability properties.

In addition to these differences between straight and convoluted portions of the proximal tubule, functional differences exist within the superficial proximal convolution. Seely (20) first showed that the transepithelial electrical resistance varied along the length of the rat superficial proximal convolution. He postulated that this variation in resistance could reflect varying electrolyte permeabilities. Recently the superficial proximal convolution of the rabbit, studied in vitro, demonstrated varying relative Na and Cl permeabilities along its length from glomerulus to pars recta (25). In an in vivo micropuncture study, Le Grimellec (23) has demonstrated differences in electrolyte reabsorption between early and late superficial proximal convolutions. Finally, Hamburger et al (22) in another in vitro study have demonstrated differing reabsorptive rates between early and late superficial convolutions. It has thus been clearly demonstrated in both superficial and deep proximal tubules that intranephron functional heterogeneity exists. What role such intranephron heterogeneity plays in functional differences remains to be elucidated.

INTERNEPHRON HETEROGENEITY

The second major type of structural heterogeneity is internephron heterogeneity. Both the convoluted and straight portions of the superficial proximal tubule differ from their respective counterparts in the deep nephron. The superficial convolution has a varying relative Cl to Na permeability along its length, with Na being more permeant in the early portion and Cl in the later. In contrast, the deep convolution has a constant relative Na to Cl permeability along its length, with Na being more permeant (25). Similarly, the superficial pars recta has a greater Cl than Na permeability, while the deep pars recta has a greater Na than Cl permeability (24). When the later portions of the superficial convolution and pars recta are perfused in vitro with solutions simulating in vivo conditions (no glucose, no amino acids, high Cl, low HCO_3) a lumen-positive transepithelial potential is present. Similar experiments with the same segments from deep nephrons result in negative potentials (24, 25). These differences are secondary to the differing relative Na to Cl permeabilities found in these segments. In vivo micropuncture studies have confirmed the role of these permeability differences in the transepithelial potential profile of the superficial proximal tubule (28–30). To date such an in vivo study on deep nephrons has been technically impossible.

Clearly, both inter- and intranephron structural heterogeneity will influence overall proximal tubular activity. In consequence, the behavior of the renal proximal tubule cannot be reliably inferred from data obtained by a study of the convoluted portion of the superficial nephrons alone. Results from micropuncture at the end of the superficial proximal convolution cannot be automatically extrapolated to the pars recta of the same nephron. The volume and composition of fluid delivered to the thin descending limb will be changed by the transport properties of the pars recta. Moreover, even if attention is restricted to the superficial convolution, the results, whether obtained by micropuncture or microperfusion, cannot be generalized to the kidney as a whole, since the transport characteristics of similar segments differ between superficial and deep nephrons. Much of the information concerning the volume and composition of fluid delivered to the loop of Henle has been derived from micropuncture studies of superficial nephrons at the end of the accessible portion of the proximal tubule. Such studies may be seriously incomplete in the sense that (a) the reabsorptive activity of the superficial pars recta is not included; (b) if different physiologic stimuli are imposed, it cannot be assumed that the reabsorptive activity of the pars recta will change in the same manner as the convoluted portion; (c) the reabsorptive behavior of the juxtamedullary nephrons is not taken into account; (d) the response of the juxtamedullary proximal tubules to varying physiologic stimuli is uncertain.

OUTWARD TRANSPORT: ACTIVE AND PASSIVE

The proximal tubule is an example of a leaky epithelium. This conclusion is based on three distinct types of experimental evidence: (a) electrophysiological studies; (b) studies using extracellular markers; and (c) electron microscopic studies. All suggest that the proximal tubule contains a low resistance paracellular pathway that plays an important role in salt and water transport.

Windhager, Boulpaep & Giebisch (31) showed in the necturus that the transepithelial electrical resistance of the proximal tubule was at least two orders of magnitude less than the sum of the luminal and peritubular cell membranes in series. The necturus, as opposed to other species, lent itself particularly well to this type of study because its proximal tubular cells are large enough to measure directly both individual cell membrane resistances as well as transepithelial resistance. Boulpaep & Seely (32), employing micropuncture in the autoperfused dog kidney, also showed that the transepithelial resistance of the proximal tubule was quite low. Utilizing salt gradient experiments and monitoring resistance changes during bulk flow induced by osmotic gradients enabled these authors to suggest that a paracellular pathway existed for fluid and electrolyte transport. Boulpaep (33), in a series of electrophysiological and split-drop experiments on the necturus, observed the effects of saline infusion on transepithelial resistance and permeability to NaCl. During inhibition of net reabsorption caused by saline infusion, the transepithelial resistance decreased without a change in peritubular cell membrane resistance while tubular permeability to electrolytes increased. He concluded from these observations that depression of proximal sodium reabsorption during saline infusion occurred via back-leak through a low resistance paracellular shunt. In addition to these studies on the necturus and dog, Hegel et al (34) have demonstrated a low transepithelial resistance in rat proximal tubule, while Lutz et al (35), utilizing in vitro microperfusion of rabbit proximal tubules, have also demonstrated a low electrical resistance. Finally, Fromter and his collaborators (36), in a series of electrophysiological studies on the rat, have shown that (a) rat proximal tubular epithelium has the lowest electrical resistance of any known epithelium; (b) the epithelial permeabilities to K, Na, Cl, and HCO_3 are entirely different from the peritubular cell membrane permeabilities; and (c) the permeability properties of the epithelium are determined by paracellular channels.

Further support for the concept that a paracellular pathway plays an important role in proximal tubule transport is offered by several studies that have shown, under various physiological conditions, increased tubular permeability to substances normally confined to the extracellular space. Bank et al (37) showed in a micropuncture study on the rat that the inhibition of proximal reabsorption caused by renal vein constriction was associated with an increased permeability to sucrose. Lorentz et al (38) demonstrated increased proximal permeability to mannitol during elevation of ureteral pressure, partial renal venous constriction, and massive saline diuresis. In the proximal tubule of the necturus, Boulpaep (33) observed increased permeability to the extracellular marker, raffinose, during volume expansion with saline. Imai & Kokko (39) showed increased sucrose permeability in the in vitro rabbit tubule when proximal reabsorption was inhibited by hypooncotic peritubular fluid. In addition, Lorentz (40) demonstrated increased proximal permeability to mannitol in rats undergoing infusion of cyclic AMP and dibutyryl cyclic AMP. Finally, Berry & Boulpaep (41), conducting micropuncture studies in the necturus, showed that changes in proximal tubule permeability to sucrose were secondary to alteration of tight junctions and paracellular pathways and that under normal conditions a portion of lumen to peritubular volume reabsorption occurs via the paracellular space. The demonstration that three extracellular markers, mannitol, sucrose, and raffinose, which normally do not penetrate the proximal tubule to any significant degree, do penetrate the tubule under various conditions associated with decreased reabsorption constitutes strong evidence for a paracellular pathway.

The final group of studies supporting a significant role for the paracellular pathway in proximal reabsorption are morphological studies of this pathway itself. Early studies on the gall bladder, another example of a leaky epithelium, revealed widened intercellular spaces during reabsorption (42, 43). Subsequently, Whittembury & Rawlins (44), studying the doubly perfused toad kidney, demonstrated that lanthanum, an electron-dense extracellular marker, precipitated only in the paracellular space and tight junction. Bentzel (45), studying the proximal tubule of the necturus during control and volume expansion, observed a relationship between morphology and the state of net reabsorption. During volume expansion and decreased net reabsorption, the paracellular space was dilated and the zonula occludens widened. Under control conditions both the paracellular space and zonula occludens were narrowed. Bentzel correlated both the differing reabsorptive rates and morphological changes with simultaneously measured transepithelial pressure measurements. Tisher & Yarger (46) and Martinez-Palomo & Erlij (47) studied the rat and demonstrated lanthanum precipitation in the paracellular space as well as lanthanum penetration of the tight junctions in the proximal tubule. Bulger et al (48) observed widening at the tight junction in the proximal tubules of rats in which intratubular pressure had been elevated by partial renal venous constriction or elevation of ureteral pressure. More recently Rawlins et al (50) examined the width of the paracellular pathway and the movement of lanthanum through this pathway in the proximal tubule of the toad. When the tubular fluid was made hyperosmotic by the addition of urea or mannitol, the paracellular pathway and tight junction widened, allowing more lanthanum to cross the epithelium through the extracellular route. Finally, Humbert et al (51) observed widening of the tight junctions of necturus proximal tubules undergoing saline diuresis.

The exact anatomical nature of the paracellular pathway is a matter of considerable uncertainty. Tisher & Kokko (49) have recently studied the morphology of the paracellular pathway in isolated proximal tubules perfused in vitro. Alteration of the peritubular oncotic pressure, which had been shown to alter net reabsorption and permeability of the paracellular pathway to sucrose (39), was associated with changes in the morphology of the paracellular space. Specifically, widening of the paracellular pathway was observed when net reabsorption was increased by a hyperoncotic bath, while a narrowed pathway was observed when reabsorption was decreased by a hypooncotic bath. These authors, utilizing autoradiography, demonstrated significant entrance of albumin into the paracellular pathway. Because of this latter finding, they proposed that in vivo protein may exert a significant oncotic pressure effect across the lateral plasma membranes forming the boundary of the paracellular pathway, presumably affecting solute and water entry into the paracellular space from intracytoplasmic channels.

Lewy & Windhager (52), in a series of micropuncture studies that are discussed later, using the evidence for an important role of the paracellular pathway in reabsorption and combining this evidence with the model for transepithelial transport postulated by Curran & MacIntosh (53), proposed a model for proximal transport, the critical features of which are outlined in Figure 1. Adjacent proximal tubule cells are linked by a tight junction (A) which has finite permeability properties with respect to salt and water. Between cells is the lateral intercellular space (paracellular pathway) which is represented by a simple compartment (B), although in reality it exists as a complex space composed of invaginations of adjacent lateral cell membranes. Finally, at the antiluminal border of the tubule the paracellular space is separated from the blood compartment by the tubular basement membrane (C). Solutes and water are transported into the paracellular compartment by active and passive processes. This reabsorbate can meet one of two fates: first, it may be picked up by the peritubular capillaries and to this extent constitute net reabsorbate; second, it may reflux back into the luminal compartment—a process termed *back-leak*. The apportionment of reabsorbate between peritubular capillary uptake and back-leak is regulated, at least in part, by the effective hydraulic and oncotic forces acting in the peritubular environment.

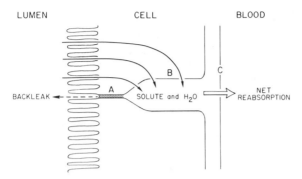

Figure 1   Simplified model to represent the role of the paracellular pathway in net reabsorption in the proximal renal tubule. *A* refers to the zonula occludens or tight junction between adjacent proximal tubular cells, *B* refers to the intercellular space, and *C* refers to the basement membrane. The *solid arrows* depict outward transport of solute and water into the paracellular space while the interrupted and *open arrows* refer to the ultimate fate of this solute and water—back-leak and net reabsorption respectively.

Movement of salt and water into the paracellular space, a process called *outward transport*, can occur by active and passive transport. Controversy still exists over the relative magnitude of each. For our purpose, transport is active if it requires energy and cannot be wholly attributed to electrochemical driving forces and bulk flow. Transport is passive if it is secondary to chemical concentration gradients, electrical driving forces, or solvent drag secondary to bulk movement of fluid.

Two major types of observation support the existence of active Na transport in the proximal tubule: (*a*) the observation of net transport in the presence of a transepithelial potential difference that is lumen negative (32, 54–59) and (*b*) the demonstration that the proximal tubule can generate and maintain a sodium concentration gradient in the presence of a nonreabsorbable solute in the lumen (27, 60, 61). The latter studies include the implicit assumption that the net electrochemical driving forces oppose passive transport. While these studies document active Na transport in a portion of the superficial proximal convoluted tubule, they clearly do not demonstrate that all the salt and water transported into the paracellular spaces of the proximal tubule is necessarily mediated by an active Na transport process. Indeed, several recent studies indicate that a significant fraction of Na transport may be passive. Moreover, the component that is active may not represent a simple direct transport of Na ions, but a complex coupling of Na and organic solute reabsorption. Finally, studies on superficial proximal convolutions cannot be extrapolated to other segments of the proximal tubule in either superficial or deep nephrons.

Micropuncture studies have shown that the majority of the filtered bicarbonate (62, 63) is reabsorbed in the early (first 25%) portion of the proximal convolution. In addition, both micropuncture (64–67) and in vitro microperfusion (68) have demonstrated that glucose reabsorption is mostly accomplished by the early proximal tubule. Finally, in vivo micropuncture studies have demonstrated that amino acids are also reabsorbed early in the proximal tubule (69–73). Knowledge of this alteration in the intraluminal fluid constituents led to studies examining the roles these substances play in the generation of the proximal tubule potential difference and volume reabsorption.

Kokko & Rector (59) first showed that the transtubular potential difference in isolated perfused segments of rabbit proximal convoluted tubules was flow dependent, the lumen negative potential approaching zero as perfusion rate was progressively decreased below 10 nl/min. They postulated transport depletion of some essential substance(s) as a possible explanation for the decline in the potential as perfusion rates were reduced. Subsequently, Kokko (26) showed that the potential in the superficial proximal convolution depended in a major way on the presence of glucose and amino acids in the lumen; indeed, the potential difference could reverse in polarity to a lumen-positive value if glucose and amino acids were removed from the luminal fluid and the majority of the bicarbonate replaced with chloride. This latter alteration of the perfusate simulates the in vivo composition of tubular fluid beyond the first quarter of the proximal convolution.

On the basis of this in vitro study the following sequence of events was proposed. Early in the proximal tubule the reabsorption of Na coupled with glucose and amino acids generates a lumen-negative potential. At the same time the bulk of the $NaHCO_3$ is reabsorbed by a process that was shown to be nonelectrogenic. This active outward transport of solute results in the osmotic flow of water into the paracellular pathway, thus reducing tubule fluid volume and maintaining isotonicity. The net result is a constant Na but elevated chloride concentration in the tubular fluid. At this point (roughly beyond 25% of the proximal convolution) the substrates for active sodium transport, the process responsible for a negative potential, have been largely depleted. The resultant high luminal Cl concentration is a force for outward diffusion of chloride down its concentration gradient, thus generating a positive potential in the remaining superficial proximal tubule. Subsequently, in vivo micropuncture studies have supported the in vitro study by showing a potential profile along the length of the superficial proximal convolution with approximately the first 25% of the tubule exhibiting a lumen-negative potential and the remainder a lumen-positive potential (28–30, 57).

The existence of this potential profile and its relationship to alteration of luminal fluid constituents have popularized one theory of proximal tubular transport originally proposed in part by Rector et al (74) and subsequently supported by Barratt (28), Maude (75), and Fromter et al (76). In essence this theory states that early in the proximal convolution, outward transport of sodium is active and coupled electrogenically to glucose, amino acids, and possibly other organic solutes and nonelectrogenically to HCO_3. These early active processes establish the conditions for two driving forces for subsequent passive outward transport: (a) electrochemical forces and (b) effective osmotic pressure forces. Luminal fluid in the later proximal tubules contains a higher Cl concentration than peritubular blood. The lumen to blood Cl concentration gradient results in Cl diffusion out of the tubule lumen. This Cl diffusion generates a lumen-positive potential which serves as a driving force for passive Na efflux.

In addition to electrochemical forces, a second type of passive driving force in the later portions of the proximal tubule is the presence of an effective osmotic gradient. The early removal of glucose, amino acids, and $NaHCO_3$ with their osmotic equivalent of water results in later luminal fluid that, from the point of freezing point depression, is in osmotic equilibrium with peritubular fluid. However, the effective osmotic pressure in the lumen may be lower. This stems from the fact that the principal solute in late proximal tubule fluid is NaCl whereas peritubular fluid has, in addition, $NaHCO_3$, glucose, and amino acids. As first pointed out by Staverman (77), the osmotic pressure that a molecule can generate across a given membrane is affected by how permeable the membrane is to the molecule. If the membrane exhibits finite permeability to the molecule, the molecule will not exert its theoretical osmotic pressure as predicted by the Van't Hoff relationship $\pi = nRTC$. Staverman (77) introduced the concept of reflection coefficient which is defined as the ratio of observed osmotic pressure to osmotic pressure predicted by the Van't Hoff relationship. The reflection coefficient for NaCl has been determined for the proximal convolution (27, 76) and is in the range of 0.7. Recently the reflection coefficients for glucose, alanine, and $NaHCO_3$ have been determined in the in vitro proximal tubule and were found to be essentially one (78). Thus, in the last two thirds to three fourths of the proximal tubule, even though luminal and peritubular fluid may have the same osmolality as determined by freezing point depression, the presence of glucose, amino acids, and bicarbonate in peritubular (presumably also in paracellular pathway) fluid generates an effective osmotic driving force for water movement. Hierholzer et al (78) have postulated that osmotic water flow generated by this process can account for at least 20% of proximal tubule NaCl reabsorption on the basis of solvent drag. Fromter, Rumrich & Ullrich (76) earlier predicted that approximately one third of proximal tubule Na transport is via solvent drag partly secondary to the effective osmotic driving force of peritubular bicarbonate.

Although the aforementioned passive driving (PD) forces (chloride concentration gradient, positive PD, and effective osmotic pressure gradients) for reabsorption in the latter two thirds of the proximal tubule could theoretically account for a large fraction of the outward transport of NaCl, actual measurements have thus far failed to demonstrate uniformly significant passive salt transport. Green & Giebisch (79), performing simultaneous perfusion of peritubular capillaries and proximal convoluted tubules in the rat, studied the ionic requirements of proximal tubular sodium transport. The authors perfused the tubules and capillaries with solutions designed to examine the role of bicarbonate, Na removal, and chloride gradients in proximal reabsorption. In addition, they examined the effect of cyanide on volume reabsorption when the chloride gradient favored passive reabsorption. They found that even in the presence of a favorable chloride gradient, cyanide inhibited the major portion of sodium and fluid reabsorption. They concluded (a) that active sodium transport accounts for the majority of proximal tubule volume reabsorption, (b) that a lumen to peritubular Cl gradient accounts for at most 20% of net transport, and (c) that normal peritubular bicarbonate concentration is essential to maintain a normal rate of volume reabsorption. Although these studies document the existence of some passive reabsorptive phenomena, they predict only a minor passive contribution. There are several difficulties with these experiments. First, no potential measurements were recorded and thus the question of a relationship between a lumen-positive potential and net reabsorption could not be examined. Second, Green & Giebisch found no effect of glucose on volume and Na flux as opposed to the findings of Burg (80) and Imai et al (81) in the isolated perfused rabbit tubule. Furthermore, Weinman and his associates (82) have demonstrated, in free-flow micropuncture studies in the rat, that glucose enhances sodium and fluid reabsorption, but the segment responsible for the glucose effect was not identified. However, in a subsequent study utilizing in vivo microperfusion of the Sprague-Dawley rat, Weinman et al (82a) demonstrated the enhancing effect of glucose on sodium and fluid reabsorption throughout the accessible portion of the proximal convolution, an effect which could be inhibited by phloridzin. Third, Green & Giebisch found that acetate, whether substituted for or added to, bicarbonate in perfusion solutions did not promote net reabsorption. This is in disagreement with the findings of Shafer and co-workers (21, 83) who found a significant component of volume reabsorption linked to acetate transport. In addition, Neumann & Rector (83a) found in the rat that acetate is capable of supporting volume reabsorption almost to the same degree as HCO_3. Although acetate was substituted for bicarbonate only in the perfusion solution, not in the peritubular fluid, it is unlikely that the amount of peritubular bicarbonate that could leak back into the tubular fluid would be sufficient to sustain normal rates of net reabsorption. Finally, Green & Giebisch did not examine directly those circumstances that pertain in vivo, specifically low HCO_3, high Cl, and no organic solutes in the tubular perfusate with normal plasma constituents in peritubular perfusate.

These latter circumstances were evaluated in a study by Cardinal et al (84). Utilizing in vitro microperfusion, these authors investigated the role of bicarbonate, organic substrates, and Cl gradients on proximal reabsorption. They observed that net volume reabsorption was two thirds normal when organic substrates were absent from tubular fluid and when a chloride concentration gradient existed from lumen to peritubular side. Under these circumstances a lumen-positive potential was observed. However, the addition of ouabain 10^{-5} M to the peritubular side inhibited net volume reabsorption without affecting the PD. This finding was interpreted to mean that despite the presence of passive driving forces, active transport, as manifested by complete inhibition of volume reabsorption by ouabain, is still responsible for all net volume reabsorption. There are three major difficulties with this group of experiments. First, whereas fluid that simulates in vivo late proximal tubule fluid was used as perfusate, no attempt was made to perfuse the late proximal tubule. With the aforementioned intranephron heterogeneity in mind, it is evident that experiments examining the effects of the composition of luminal fluid must be done in the appropriate region of the tubule. Second, in the group of experiments designed to examine the role of passive forces a significant amount of acetate was present in the perfusion fluid. This acetate may have served as a substrate for active Na transport.

Finally, these authors found no effect of HCO_3 removal from perfusate and bath on net volume reabsorption. This latter finding is in conflict with the observations of several investigators (75, 79, 85) who find a significant role for HCO_3 in proximal tubule volume reabsorption. Clearly, the type of study performed by Cardinal et al (84) should be repeated in vitro and in vivo in several species and in the appropriate nephron segments before the role of bicarbonate, chloride gradients, and chloride diffusion potentials can be defined with confidence. One study has documented significant passive reabsorption in the proximal tubule. Shafer, Patlak & Andreoli (86) perfused the superficial pars recta with fluid that simulates in vivo conditions. When active reabsorption was inhibited by ouabain, reabsorption continued at 40% the control rate. The authors attributed a major portion of this passive transport to the Cl concentration gradient, lumen-positive potential, and effective osmotic pressure of peritubular HCO_3.

In attempting to delineate the relative contributions of active and passive transport to net proximal salt and water reabsorption, proximal tubule heterogeneity must be considered. First, in vitro studies have suggested that a significant lumen-positive potential may not exist in the later portion of the deep proximal tubule because of its lower Cl permeability. This no doubt would affect the magnitude of reabsorption attributed to the passive forces of Cl concentration gradient and Cl diffusion potential. Second, net reabsorptive capacity has not been examined directly in the convoluted portion of the deep nephron. Third, various other properties of the deep convolution have not been directly quantitated. The osmotic water permeability and the reflection coefficients for NaCl, glucose, amino acid, and $NaHCO_3$ have not been determined. Knowledge of these parameters will be required to evaluate the role of passive driving forces in the deep convolution. It is clear that, coupled with as yet missing information about the deep nephron, the inter- and intranephron heterogeneity already documented (differing permeabilities to Na and Cl, differing transepithelial potentials, differing requirements for organic solutes in active Na transport) makes it premature to propose a unitary hypothesis for the mechanism of outward transport in the proximal nephron.

REGULATORY FACTORS: PASSIVE BACK-LEAK

The foregoing discussion advanced evidence that outward transport of reabsorbate had two components: (a) active outward transport accompanying the transport of HCO_3, glucose, amino acids, and possibly other organic solutes and (b) passive outward transport driven by the high luminal Cl concentration and effective osmotic gradients in the peritubular environment. Although there is admittedly great uncertainty concerning the quantitative contribution of each of these processes to outward reabsorption it is highly likely that both are operative. However, outward transport is not equivalent to net reabsorption. Indeed, several studies have demonstrated that under normal circumstances net Na reabsorption is only a fraction of outward Na transport (21, 27, 33, 87). Roughly 20% of the Na transported out of the tubular lumen is actually taken up by the peritubular capillary. The return of approximately 80% of the outward transported Na to the tubular lumen is termed *back-leak.*

Several studies have shown that a site of regulation of proximal reabsorption is in the control of this back-leak process. However, prior to the recent emphasis on the role of back-leak, a multitude of studies directed at elucidating regulatory factors proposed that such factors as tubular geometry, tubular fluid flow rate, and natriuretic hormones regulated proximal tubule reabsorption.

Gertz and his collaborators (88, 89), utilizing the shrinking-drop micropuncture technique, first proposed that tubular reabsorption varied with the cross-sectional area of the proximal tubular lumen. Rector et al (90) and Brunner et al (91), in a series of micropuncture studies on the rat examining the effects of aortic constriction and elevated ureteropelvic pressure, supported Gertz's initial hypothesis that tubular volume was critically related to net reabsorption. However, Brenner et at (92), also utilizing micropuncture in the rat, found no correlation between proximal tubule volume and reabsorption. These authors pointed out and avoided certain technical pitfalls in the earlier studies. Subsequently, Rodicio et al (93) confirmed the findings of Brenner's group and postulated that perhaps hydrostatic and oncotic pressure in peritubular capillaries were responsible for proximal glomerulotubular balance. Finally, Burg & Orloff (94) in an in vitro study failed to find a relationship between luminal volume and reabsorption.

Early in vitro studies showed that the proximal tubule potential difference was flow dependent (59). Subsequently Bartoli, Conger & Earley (95) demonstrated via in vivo microperfusion that perfusion of the rat proximal tubule with ultrafiltrate at low perfusion rates was associated with a decrease in absolute reabsorption. However, Burg & Orloff (94) in an in vitro study and Morgan & Berliner (96) and Morel & Murayama (97) in in vivo studies failed to find a correlation between reabsorption and flow rate. In spite of these differing observations, the results of these studies are not necessarily conflicting. In studies failing to find an effect of perfusion rate (94, 96, 97), rates in excess of 6 to 10 nl/min were used. In studies demonstrating an effect of perfusion rate, the effect was most pronounced at perfusion rates below 8 nl/min. A recent study by Imai, Seldin & Kokko (98), utilizing in vitro microperfusion, demonstrated that net water and unidirectional fluxes of sodium and chloride were flow dependent at perfusion rates less than 11 nl/min. Flow dependence was abolished when glucose and amino acids were removed from the perfusate. These recent observations suggest that slow flow rates, by causing substrate depletion of glucose and amino acids, may play a role in regulating proximal reabsorption, and indeed may contribute to proximal GT balance at low glomerular filtration rates (GFRs). However, glucose and amino acids are normally mostly reabsorbed in the early convolution. One would, therefore, postulate that slow flow rates would affect reabsorption only in the early proximal tubule. Presently, it is safe to say that a component of proximal reabsorption may be flow dependent but the quantitative importance and physiological significance remain to be defined.

One further postulated mechanism for controlling proximal reabsorption was the influence of a natriuretic hormone. deWardener et al (99), studying cross-circulated dogs in which the donor dog was volume expanded while receiving large doses of mineralocorticoid, suggested the presence of a humoral substance causing natriuresis. Since this early observation, several studies have both confirmed and refuted the existence of such a substance. A recent review by Levinsky (100) summarizes the evidence against a pivotal role for a natriuretic factor acting in the proximal tubule. In addition, a recent micropuncture study (101) failed to find an effect of plasma dialyzate from volume-expanded animals on sodium and water reabsorption in the proximal tubule of rats. Indeed, recent studies on the existence and physiological significance of a natriuretic hormone have focused attention on a distal site of action (102).

In the aggregate, then, these studies suggested that luminal volume, luminal fluid flow rate, and natriuretic factor do not play a major role in the regulation of proximal reabsorption. Therefore, as mentioned previously, because only a fraction of outwardly transported salt and water actually reaches the peritubular capillary, attention has recently been focused on the role of peritubular capillary uptake as a major regulator of proximal reabsorption.

Evidence for the peritubular control of proximal reabsorption was first advanced by Earley and his associates (103). Infusion of vasodilator drugs into the renal artery of the dog produced natriuresis that was greatly augmented with the superimposition of systemic blood pressure elevation by infusion of vasopressors (104). These authors initially proposed that renal vasodilation and systemic hypertension combine to increase peritubular capillary hydraulic pressure, thus reducing net reabsorption by inhibiting peritubular capillary removal of the outwardly transported salt and water (104). In further clearance studies, Earley and associates (105–107) showed that elevation of plasma oncotic pressure by albumin infusion served to cancel the natriuretic effect of vasodilatation and hypertension. Subsequently, in a group of micropuncture studies, Lewy & Windhager (52) developed the hypothesis further by proposing that net interstitial pressure was the critical factor relating peritubular capillary uptake to net reabsorption. These authors demonstrated a linear relationship between proximal reabsorption and filtration fraction. In addition, during partial renal venous occlusion, proximal fractional reabsorption was shown to remain constant at various levels of glomerular filtration. While these studies served to point out that peritubular factors may regulate proximal reabsorption, they could not determine whether the mechanism was by increased back-leak or decreased outward transport.

Such studies assigned a key role to filtration fraction (FF) in the regulation of proximal reabsorption. Filtration fraction equals glomerular filtration rate/renal plasma flow (GFR/RPF). FF is of critical importance because it influences both Starling forces acting across the postglomerular capillary. For any given afferent arteriolar protein concentration, FF determines the postglomerular oncotic pressure. In addition, since FF reflects the relationship between GFR and postglomerular blood flow, it (FF) varies inversely with postglomerular hydrostatic pressure. Thus, when FF is high postglomerular hydrostatic pressure is low and when FF is low postglomerular pressure is high.

Brenner and his associates are principally responsible for the direct demonstration by micropuncture that peritubular oncotic pressure plays a major role in the regulation of proximal reabsorption. Intra-aortic injection of colloid-free, isoncotic, and hyperoncotic solution in the rat showed that fractional and absolute reabsorption varied directly with peritubular capillary colloid osmotic pressure (108). Brenner, Troy & Daugharty (109) in an in vivo microperfusion study subsequently showed that selective elevation of peritubular oncotic pressure in volume-expanded rats almost totally reversed the inhibition of proximal reabsorption associated with volume expansion. In addition, Falchuk et al (110), measuring nephron filtration rate, absolute reabsorption, and peritubular hydrostatic pressure, examined renal vein occlusion, aortic constriction, carotid occlusion with vagotomy, and isoncotic as well as hyperoncotic albumin infusion. In all of these maneuvers, proximal reabsorption correlated with changes in peritubular oncotic and hydrostatic pressure, strongly suggesting a regulatory role for these forces. In another micropuncture study Brenner et al (111), utilizing partial aortic constriction in plasma-expanded rats, showed that glomerulotubular balance was blunted when changes in peritubular protein concentration changes were prevented. Similar findings were reported by Spitzer & Windhager (112) who, in an in vivo microperfusion study, showed under both free flow and "split-drop" conditions, that proximal reabsorption correlated with peritubular oncotic pressure as controlled by varying the concentration of dextran in peritubular capillary perfusate. Weinman et al (113), by altering the concentration in postglomerular blood, showed in the split-drop technique, a linear relationship between sodium reabsorption and peritubular capillary protein concentration. Green et al (114), in a series of in vivo microperfusion studies, confirmed the importance of peritubular protein. Although a number of investigators have failed to demonstrate an important role of peritubular oncotic pressure on regulation of proximal reabsorption, these are in the minority (61, 85, 115–120). In addition, Windhager & Giebisch (121) in a recent review, pointed out that several of these studies (61, 116–118) were beset with technical artifacts such as incomplete capillary perfusion.

Several studies have shown that in addition to effective peritubular oncotic pressure, hydraulic pressure may play a role in the regulation of proximal reabsorption. Early studies by Bank et al (122) and Aperia et al (123) on the effects of renal perfusion pressure on proximal reabsorption suggested that elevated peritubular capillary hydrostatic pressure inhibited Na reabsorption. Subsequently, Bank et al (124), in examining the role of peritubular capillary perfusion rate on proximal reabsorption in the rat, postulated that the inhibition of reabsorption observed at high peritubular capillary perfusion rates was secondary to elevated capillary hydrostatic pressure. Less inferential evidence for a direct role of peritubular hydraulic pressure in proximal reabsorption has been obtained in the necturus. Utilizing the necturus, Hayslett (125), measuring the half-time of reabsorption in the split-drop preparation as well as transepithelial potentials, demonstrated that elevated peritubular hydrostatic pressure inhibited proximal reabsorption. In addition, Grandchamp & Boulpaep (126) further strengthened the role of pressure control by demonstrating decreased proximal reabsorption in necturus during volume expansion, quantitating the contributions of changes in peritubular oncotic and hydrostatic pressures.

Finally, several investigators have postulated a role for peritubular capillary flow rate in the regulation of net reabsorption. Lewy & Windhager (52) noted a correlation between absolute proximal reabsorption and renal plasma flow during partial renal venous occlusion in the rat. Daugharty et al (127), studying the dog in which diuretic blockade of distal reabsorption was utilized, found that changes in proximal reabsorption correlated best with changes in plasma flow. Schrier & Humphreys (128), in saline-loaded and water-loaded dogs, found a close correlation between renal plasma flow and proximal reabsorption. Presumably, demonstration of plasma flow dependence in these studies is related to the fact that under a given net hydraulic and oncotic force favoring net reabsorption the slower the peritubular plasma flow rate the greater will be the dilution of peritubular protein by the reabsorbate and the sooner will be the dissipation of the oncotic driving force (129). However, the physiological importance of plasma flow dependence of proximal reabsorption remains to be defined. As pointed out by Deen et al (129), those studies demonstrating a significant role for plasma flow were associated with "reabsorptive pressure equilibrium." In other words, oncotic pressure in the peritubular capillary favoring reabsorption was approached by hydrostatic pressure in the capillary, which inhibited reabsorption. Renal plasma flow will be regulatory in proximal reabsorption when, because of sufficient slowing of flow, the peritubular oncotic pressure is diluted by the reabsorbate to the point that oncotic pressure favoring reabsorption no longer exceeds hydrostatic pressure retarding reabsorption.

A recent study by Myers et al has pointed out the potential importance of peritubular plasma flow rate (130). In this study Wistar rats, a species whose surface glomeruli offer the opportunity to study both glomerular and postglomerular hemodynamics, were studied. Infusion of pressor doses of norepinephrine and angiotensin II produced large increases in filtration fraction and thus postglomerular oncotic pressure. However, the expected increase in absolute proximal reabsorption from the large increase in peritubular oncotic pressure was not seen, because of the opposing effect of a large decrease in efferent arteriolar and thus peritubular capillary flow rate. Therefore, under the conditions of high FF and slow peritubular capillary flow rate as produced by the efferent arteriolar constriction secondary to norepinephrin and angiotensin II, proximal tubular reabsorption was maintained by the slow peritubular plasma flow rate despite Starling forces acting across the peritubular capillary bed that favored greatly increased reabsorption.

The mechanism by which alteration in peritubular physical forces effect proximal reabsorption has been studied extensively. In order to postulate a regulatory role for physical factors, the boundaries through which these forces act require certain properties. Specifically, for oncotic and hydraulic pressure to play a role, the boundary through which they exert their control should ideally be freely permeable to all substances smaller than plasma proteins and have a very high hydraulic permeability. Welling & Grantham (131) in studying the physical properties of isolated perfused tubular basement membranes documented such properties. Peritubular physical forces are thought to regulate proximal reabsorption by determining the fraction of outward transport picked up by the peritubular capillary the remainder returning via a back-leak through the paracellular pathway into the tubule lumen.

The role of peritubular oncotic pressure and the paracellular pathway in the regulation of proximal reabsorption is illustrated in Figure 2. Protein, depicted by black dots, is shown to be present in the peritubular capillary, interstitial space, and

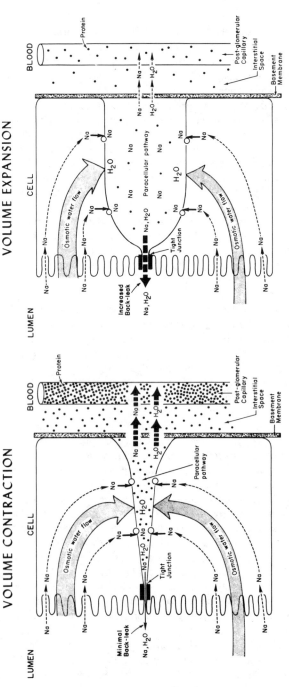

Figure 2 Depicted here is a schematic representation of how protein translates its effect on proximal tubular reabsorption through controlling backleak. On the left is the circumstance of volume contraction and its attendant increase in peritubular protein concentration due to both elevation of systemic arterial protein concentration and increased filtration fraction. The relatively high concentration of protein (*black dots*) via its oncotic pressure effect enhances movement of this salt and water from the paracellular pathway and interstitial space into the peritubular capillary. In consequence the paracellular pathway is narrowed, hydrostatic pressure within it is low, and therefore the driving force for back-leak is reduced. As depicted, the protein that enters the interstitial space and paracellular pathway may also exert an oncotic force across the lateral cell membranes (see text). On the right is the circumstance of volume expansion associated with diluted systemic arterial protein concentration and decreased filtration fraction. The less dense arrangement of black dots representing decreased protein concentration depicts the reduced driving force of peritubular (interstitial and paracellular) protein for removal of reabsorbate from the paracellular pathway, thereby causing widening of the paracellular space and increased back-leak.

paracellular pathway. This is in accord with the demonstration of the permeability of the isolated perfused basement membrane to albumin (131) together with the finding of albumin in the paracellular pathway by autoradiography (49). During volume contraction the protein concentration is elevated in the peritubular environment, being highest in the peritubular capillary. This furnishes an oncotic gradient for removal of fluid from paracellular space to peritubular capillary and diminishes the magnitude of the back-leak into tubular lumen. Because fluid is readily taken up by the peritubular capillary, the paracellular space is narrowed. By contrast, during volume expansion the protein concentration in the peritubular environment is reduced, thereby diminishing peritubular capillary uptake of reabsorbate. Therefore, fluid accumulates in the paracellular space, widening it, and thus producing a hydrostatic pressure gradient for back-leak. Hydrostatic pressure in the peritubular environment during volume contraction and expansion changes in a manner parallel to that of oncotic pressure. In volume contraction, a low peritubular capillary hydrostatic pressure promotes fluid removal from the paracellular space, while in volume expansion elevated peritubular hydrostatic pressure serves to retard fluid removal from the paracellular space.

A different set of morphologic findings was illustrated by Tisher & Kokko (49) in electron micrographs of isolated rabbit tubules exposed to a bath containing either high protein (volume contraction) or low protein (volume expansion). Their findings were the opposite of those depicted in Figure 2: widening of the paracellular pathway was observed when bath protein was high; narrowing of the paracellular pathway occurred when bath protein was low. A direct correlation among bath protein concentration, the width of the paracellular pathway, and net reabsorption was demonstrated. They therefore concluded that protein exerts its oncotic effect, not only between paracellular space and peritubular capillary, but also along the lateral walls of the paracellular pathway. Presumably, since the paracellular space is expanded when back-leak is low (volume contraction), it must be assumed that back-leak does not occur principally through the tight junction. It should be noted that the in vitro model involves only variations of oncotic pressure, and therefore differs from the actual in vivo circumstance where oncotic and hydrostatic forces act in concert. What effect the superimposition of changes in hydrostatic pressure would produce on morphologic findings is unknown. Although the width of the paracellular pathway during changes in net reabsorption observed by Tisher & Kokko are the opposite of those depicted in Figure 2, the principle of the peritubular control of back-leak by protein concentration is the same. However, the location of the area of back-leak as well as the channels through which protein exerts its effect differ. In Figure 2, protein exerts its main effect by regulating the movement of fluid between paracellular space and peritubular capillary; back-leak occurs through the tight intercellular junction when the paracellular space is widened and its hydrostatic pressure presumably increased. In the Tisher-Kokko model, protein exerts a major effect, not only on fluid movement between paracellular space and peritubular capillary, but also on fluid movement into the paracellular space across its lateral cell membranes; back-leak occurs when the paracellular space is narrowed; the principal channel of back-leak in this model is therefore not the tight junction.

Finally, a further possible modulator of the role of physical factors and the paracellular pathway on proximal reabsorption has recently been proposed. Gill & Casper (133) demonstrated inhibition of proximal reabsorption during the infusion of cyclic AMP and dibutyryl cyclic AMP into the renal arteries of dogs. Lorentz, Lassiter & Gottschalk (38) demonstrated increased proximal back-leak of extracellular markers when intrarenal pressure was elevated via elevation of ureteral pressure, partial renal venous constriction, and massive saline diuresis. Lorentz (134) subsequently showed that cyclic AMP and dibutyryl cyclic AMP also increased the permeability of the proximal tubule to extracellular markers. Finally, Lorentz (135) has reported in an abstract that parathormone increases proximal tubular permeability. These studies, in conjunction with the demonstration of increased renal cyclic AMP during volume expansion (136) and parathormone administration (137–141), constitute impressive evidence for a role of cyclic nucleotide in altering the permeability characteristics of the tight junction. These findings suggest that the control of proximal reabsorption via a back-leak may be determined by both the physical forces as well as permeability characteristics of the tight junction. It is evident that inter- and intranephron structural heterogeneity must also be considered in evaluating the role of peritubular physical forces in the regulation of proximal reabsorption. Differences in filtration fraction in different nephrons as well as possible differences in tight junction permeability characteristics would result in different degrees of back-leak and thus different net reabsorptive rates. Hamburger et al (22) have already demonstrated a differential effect of cyclic AMP on proximal reabsorption with inhibition found only in the convoluted portion.

Basically, outward transport of salt and water via active and passive processes provides substrate for net reabsorption. This substrate, which is transported to the paracellular pathway, can either be reabsorbed into the peritubular capillary and thus constitute net reabsorption or leak back through the tight junction (or through intracytoplasmic channels) into the tubular lumen. The apportionment of outwardly transported salt and water between these two fates is determined by the net Starling forces operating in the paracellular pathway—the net oncotic pressure and net hydraulic pressure—and perhaps by the permeability characteristics of the tight junction as influenced by cyclic nucleotides. Intranephron and internephron structural heterogeneity can greatly modify the influence of these factors because of intrinsic differences in active and passive permeability properties.

ACKNOWLEDGMENTS

This work was supported in part by USPHS Program Project Grant 5 PO1 HL11662.

Literature Cited

1. Walker, A. M., Bott, P. A., Oliver, J., MacDowell, M. C. 1941. The collection and analysis of fluid from single nephrons of the mammalian kidney. *Am. J. Physiol.* 134:580–95
2. Dirks, J. H., Cirksena, W. J., Berliner, R. W. 1965. The effect of saline infusion on sodium reabsorption by the proximal tubule of the dog. *J. Clin. Invest.* 44:1160–70
3. Brenner, B. M., Bennett, C. M., Berliner, R. W. 1968. The relationship between glomerular filtration rate and sodium reabsorption by the proximal tubule of the rat nephron. *J. Clin. Invest.* 47:1358–74
4. Landwehr, D. M., Schnermann, J., Klose, R. M., Giebisch, G. 1968. Effect of reduction in filtration rate on renal tubular sodium and water reabsorption. *Am. J. Physiol.* 215:687–95
5. Rodicio, J., Herrera-Acosta, J., Sellman, J. C., Rector, F. C., Seldin, D. W. 1969. Studies on glomerulotubular balance during aortic constriction, ureteral obstruction and venous occlusion in hydropenic and saline-loaded rats. *Nephron* 6:437–56
6. Huber, G. C. 1909–1910. The morphology and structure of the mammalian renal tubule. *Harvey Lect.* 5:100–49
7. Maunsbach, A. B. 1964. Ultrastructure of different segments within the rat renal proximal tubule. *Anat. Rec.* 148:387
8. Maunsbach, A. B. 1966. Observations on the segmentation of the proximal tubule in the rat kidney. Comparison of results from phase contrast, fluorescence and electron microscopy. *J. Ultrastruct. Res.* 16:239–58
9. Rhodin, J. 1962. Electron microscopy of the kidney. In *Renal Disease,* ed. D. A. K. Black. Oxford:Blackwell
10. Tisher, C. C., Rosen, S., Osborne, G. B. 1969. Ultrastructure of the proximal tubule of the rhesus monkey kidney. *Am. J. Pathol.* 56:469–93
11. Ericsson, J. L. E., Bergstrand, A., Andres, G., Bucht, H., Cinotti, G. 1965. Morphology of the renal tubular epithelium in young healthy humans. *Acta Pathol. Microbiol. Scand.* 63:361–84
12. Tisher, C. C., Bulger, R. E., Trump, B. F. 1966. Human renal ultrastructure. I. Proximal tubule of healthy individuals. *Lab. Invest.* 15:1357–94
13. Baines, A. D., Baines, C. J., deRouffignac, C. 1969. Functional heterogeneity

of nephrons I. *Pfluegers Arch.* 308:244–59
14. Baines, A. D., deRouffignac, C. 1969. Functional heterogeneity of nephrons II. *Pfluegers Arch.* 308:260–76
15. Carriere, S., Boulet, P., Mathieu, A., Brunette, M. G. 1972. Isotonic saline loading and intrarenal distribution of glomerular filtration in dogs. *Kidney Int.* 2:191–96
16. Horster, M., Thurau, K. 1968. Micropuncture studies on the filtration rate of single superficial and juxtamedullary glomeruli in the rat kidney. *Pfluegers Arch.* 301:162–81
17. Stumpe, K. O., Lowitz, H. D., Ochwadt, B. 1969. Function of juxtamedullary nephrons in normotensive and chronically hypertensive rats. *Pfleugers Arch.* 313:43–52
18. Jamison, R. L. 1970. Micropuncture study of superficial and juxtamedullary nephrons in the rat. *Am. J. Physiol.* 218:46–55
19. Jamison, R. L., Lacy, F. B. 1971. Effect of saline infusion on superficial and juxtamedullary nephrons in the rat. *Am. J. Physiol.* 221:690–97
20. Seely, J. F. 1973. Variation in electrical resistance along length of rat proximal convoluted tubule. *Am. J. Physiol.* 225:48–57
21. Schafer, J. A., Troutman, S. L., Andreoli, T. E. 1974. Volume reabsorption, transepithelial potential differences, and ionic permeability properties in mammalian superficial proximal straight tubules. *J. Gen. Physiol.* 64:582–607
22. Hamburger, R. J., Lawson, N. L., Dennis, V. W. 1974. Effects of cyclic adenosine nucleotides on fluid absorption by different segments of proximal tubule. *Am. J. Physiol.* 227:396–401
23. LeGrimellec, C. 1975. Micropunture study along the proximal convoluted tubule; electrolyte reabsorption in first convolutions. *Pfluegers Arch.* 354:133–50
24. Kawamura, S., Imai, M., Seldin, D. W., Kokko, J. P. 1975. Characteristics of salt and water transport in superficial and juxtamedullary straight segments of proximal tubules. *J. Clin. Invest.* 55:1269–77
25. Jacobson, H. R., Kokko, J. P. 1976. Intrinsic differences in various segments of the proximal convoluted tubule. *J. Clin. Invest.* 57:818–25

26. Kokko, J. P. 1973. Proximal tubule potential difference: Dependence on glucose, bicarbonate and amino acids. *J. Clin. Invest.* 52:1362–67
27. Kokko, J. P., Burg, M. B., Orloff, J. 1971. Characteristics of NaCl and water transport in the renal proximal tubule. *J. Clin. Invest.* 50:69–76
28. Barratt, L. J., Rector, F. C., Kokko, J. P., Seldin, D. W. 1974. Factors governing the transepithelial potential difference across the proximal tubule of the rat kidney. *J. Clin. Invest.* 53:454–64
29. Fromter, E., Gessner, K. 1974. Active transport potentials, membrane diffusion potentials and streaming potentials across rat kidney proximal tubules. *Pfluegers Arch.* 351:85–98
30. Seely, J. F., Chirito, E. 1975. Studies of the electrical potential difference in the rat proximal tubule. *Am. J. Physiol.* 229:72–80
31. Windhager, E. E., Boulpaep, E. L., Giebisch, G. 1967. Electrophysiological studies on single nephrons. *Proc. 3rd. Int. Congr. Nephrol.*, Washington, D.C., 1966, pp. 35–47. Basel & New York: Karger
32. Boulpaep, E. L., Seely, J. F. 1971. Electrophysiology of proximal and distal tubule in the autoperfused dog kidney. *Am. J. Physiol.* 221:1084–96
33. Boulpaep, E. L. 1972. Permeability changes of the proximal tubule of Necturus during saline loading. *Am. J. Physiol.* 222:517–31
34. Hegel, U., Fromter, E., Wick, T. 1967. Der elektrische Wandwiderstand des proximalen Konvolutes der Rattenniere. *Pfluegers Arch.* 294:274–90
35. Lutz, M. D., Cardinal, J., Burg, M. B. 1973. Electrical resistance of renal proximal tubule perfused in vitro. *Am. J. Physiol.* 225:729–34
36. Fromter, E., Muller, C. W., Wick, T. 1971. Permeability properties of the proximal tubular epithelium of the rat kidney studied with electrophysiological methods. In *Electrophysiology of Epithelial Cells*, ed. G. Giebisch, F. K. Schattauer, 119–46. Stuttgart:Verlag
37. Bank, N., Yarger, W. E., Aynedjian, H. S. 1971. A microperfusion study of sucrose movement across the rat proximal tubules during renal vein constriction. *J. Clin. Invest.* 50:294–302
38. Lorentz, W. B., Lassiter, W. E., Gottschalk, C. W. 1972. Renal tubular permeability during increased intrarenal pressure. *J. Clin. Invest.* 53:1250–57
39. Imai, M., Kokko, J. P. 1972. Effect of peritubular protein concentration on reabsorption of sodium and water in isolated perfused proximal tubules. *J. Clin. Invest.* 51:314–25
40. Lorentz, W. B. 1974. The effect of cyclic AMP and dibutyryl cyclic AMP on the permeability characteristics of the renal tubule. *J. Clin. Invest.* 53:1250–57
41. Berry, C. A., Boulpaep, E. L. 1975. Nonelectrolyte permeability of the paracellular pathway in Necturus proximal tubule. *Am. J. Physiol.* 228:581–95
42. Whitlock, R. T., Wheeler, H. O., Kaye, G. I., Lane, N. 1965. Structural-functional aspects of water transport across gall bladder epithelium. *Fed. Proc.* 24:589
43. Diamond, J. M., Tormey, J. M. 1966. Studies on the structural basis of water transport across epithelial membranes. *Fed. Proc.* 25:1458–63
44. Whittembury, G., Rawlins, F. A. 1971. Evidence of a paracellular pathway for ion flow in the kidney proximal tubule: Electron microscopic demonstration of lanthanum precipitate in the tight junction. *Pfluegers Arch.* 330:302–9
45. Bentzel, C. J. 1972. Proximal tubule structure function relationships during volume expansion in Necturus. *Kidney Int.* 2:324–35
46. Tisher, C. C., Yarger, W. E. 1973. Lanthanum permeability of the tight junction (zonula occludens) in the renal tubule of the rat. *Kidney Int.* 3:238–50
47. Martinez-Palomo, A., Erlij, D. 1973. The distribution of lanthanum in tight junctions of the kidney tubule. *Pfluegers Arch.* 343:267–72
48. Bulger, R. E., Lorentz, W. B., Colindres, R. E., Gottschalk, C. W. 1974. Morphologic changes in rat renal proximal tubules and their tight junctions with increased intraluminal pressure. *Lab. Invest.* 30:136–44
49. Tisher, C. C., Kokko, J. P. 1974. Relationship between peritubular oncotic pressure gradients and morphology in isolated proximal tubules. *Kidney Int.* 6:146–56
50. Rawlins, F. A., Gonzalez, E., Perez-Gonzalez, M., Whittembury, G. 1975. Effect of transtubular osmotic gradients on the paracellular pathway in toad kidney proximal tubule. *Pfluegers Arch.* 353:287–302
51. Humbert, F., Grandchamp, A., Pricam, C., Perrelet, A., Orci, L. 1976. Morphological changes in tight junctions of Necturus Maculosus proximal tubules

undergoing saline diuresis. *J. Cell Biol.* 69:90–96

52. Lewy, J. E., Windhager, E. E. 1968. Peritubular control of proximal tubular fluid readsorption in the rat kidney. *Am. J. Physiol.* 214:943–54

53. Curran, P. F., MacIntosh, J. R. 1962. A model system for biological water transport. *Nature* 193:347–48

54. Welbundt, W. 1938. Electrical potential difference across the wall of kidney tubules of Necturus. *J. Cell. Comp. Physiol.* 11:425–31

55. Giebisch, G. 1958. Electrical potential measurements on single nephrons of Necturus. *J. Cell. Comp. Physiol.* 51:221–39

56. Burg, M. B., Orloff, J. 1970. Electrical potential difference across proximal convoluted tubules. *Am. J. Physiol.* 219:1714–16

57. Fromter, E., Gessner, K. 1974. Free flow potential profile along rat kidney proximal tubule. *Pfluegers Arch.* 351:69–83

58. Barratt, L. J., Rector, F. C., Kokko, J. P., Seldin, D. W. 1974. Factors governing the transepithelial potential difference across the proximal tubule of the rat kidney. *J. Clin. Invest.* 53:454–64

59. Kokko, J. P., Rector, F. C. 1971. Flow dependence of transtubular potential difference in isolated perfused segments of rabbit proximal convoluted tubule. *J. Clin. Invest.* 50:2745–50

60. Kashgarian, M., Stockle, H., Gottschalk, C. W., Ullrich, K. J. 1963. Transtubular electrochemical potentials of sodium and chloride in proximal and distal renal tubules of rats during antidiuresis and water diuresis (diabetes insipidus). *Pfluegers Arch.* 277:89–106

61. Baldamus, C. A., Hierholzer, K., Rumrich, G., Stolte, H., Uhlich, E., Ullrich, K. J., Wiederholt, M. 1969. Natrium transport in den proximalen Tubuli und den Sammelrohren bei Variation der Natrium bonzentiation im umgebenden Interstitium. *Pfluegers Arch.* 310:354–64

62. Gottschalk, C. W., Lassiter, W. E., Mylle, M. 1960. Localization of urine acidification in the mammalian kidney. *Am. J. Physiol.* 198:581–85

63. Rector, F. C., Carter, N. W., Seldin, D. W. 1965. The mechanism of bicarbonate reabsorption in the proximal and distal tubules of the kidney. *J. Clin. Invest.* 44:278–90

64. Rohde, R., Deetjen, P. 1968. Die glucoseresorption in der rattenniere: Micro punktionsanalysen der Tubularan glucosekonzentration fierein fluss. *Pfluegers Arch.* 302:219–32

65. Stolte, H., Hare, D., Boylan, J. W. 1972. D-Glucose and fluid reabsorption in proximal surface tubule of the rat kidney. *Pfluegers Arch.* 334:193–206

66. Hare, D., Stolte, H. 1972. Rat proximal tubule D-glucose transport as a function of concentration, flow and radius. *Pfluegers Arch.* 334:207–21

67. Frohnert, P., Hohmann, B., Zwiebel, R., Baumann, K. 1970. Free flow micropuncture studies of glucose transport in the rat nephron. *Pfluegers Arch.* 315:66–85

68. Tune, B. M., Burg, M. B. 1971. Glucose transport by proximal renal tubules. *Am. J. Physiol.* 221:580–85

69. Bergeron, M., Morel, F. 1965. Amino acid transport in rat tubule. *Am. J. Physiol.* 216:1139–49

70. Silbernagl, S., Deetjen, P. 1972. L-Arginine transport in rat proximal tubules: Microperfusion studies on reabsorption kinetics. *Pfluegers Arch.* 336:79–86

71. Lingard, J., Rumrich, G., Young, J. A. 1973. Kinetics of L-histidine transport in the proximal convolution of the rat nephron studies using the stationary microperfusion technique. *Pfluegers Arch.* 342:13–28

72. Lingard, J., Rumrich, G., Young, J. A. 1973. Readsorption of L-glutamine and L-histidine from various regions of the rat proximal convolution studies by stationary microperfusion: Evidence that the proximal convolution is not homogeneous. *Pfluegers Arch.* 342:1–12

73. Lingard, J. M., Gyory, A. Z., Young, J. A. 1974. Analysis of the reabsorptive characteristics of neutral amino acids in the proximal convolution of the rat kidney. *Proc. Aust. Pharmacol. Soc.* 5:223–25

74. Rector, F. C., Martinez-Maldonado, M., Brunner, F. P., Seldin, D. W. 1966. Evidence for passive reabsorption of NaCl in proximal tubule of rat kidney. *J. Clin. Invest.* 45:1060

75. Maude, D. L. 1974. The role of bicarbonate in proximal tubular sodium chloride transport. *Kidney Int.* 5:253–60

76. Fromter, E., Rumrich, G., Ullrich, K. J. 1973. Phenomenologic description of Na^+, Cl^- and HCO_3^- absorption from proximal tubules of the rat kidney. *Pfluegers Arch.* 343:189–220

77. Staverman, A. J. 1951. The theory of

measurement of osmotic pressure. *Rec. Trav. Chim. Pays Bas.* 70:344–52

78. Hierholzer, K., Kawamura, S., Seldin, D. W., Kokko, J. P. 1977. Contribution of solvent drag to the reabsorption of sodium in isolated perfused proximal convoluted tubules of the rabbit kidney. Submitted for publication

79. Green, R., Giebisch, G. 1975. Ionic requirements of proximal tubular sodium transport. I. Bicarbonate and chloride. *Am. J. Physiol.* 229:1205–15

80. Burg, M. B. 1975. Mechanism of fluid absorption by proximal convoluted tubules. In *Proc. VI Int. Congr. Nephrol.,* Florence, Italy 1975. Basel: Karger

81. Imai, M., Seldin, D. W., Kokko, J. P. 1977. Effect of perfusion rate on the fluxes of water, sodium, chloride and urea across the proximal convoluted tubule. *Kidney Int.* In press

82. Weinman, E. J., Suki, W. N., Eknoyan, G. 1975. Effect of D-glucose on the reabsorption of water in the proximal tubule of the rat. *Abstr. Am. Soc. Nephrol.* 8:97

82a. Weinman, E. J., Suki, W. N., Eknoyan, G. 1976. D-Glucose enhancement of water reabsorption in the proximal tubule of the rat kidney. *Am. J. Physiol.* 231:777–80

83. Shafer, J. A., Andreoli, T. E. 1975. Anion absorption by isolated perfused proximal straight tubules. *Abstr. Am. Soc. Nephrol.* 8:94

83a. Neumann, K. H., Rector, F. C. Jr. 1976. Mechanism of NaCl and water reabsorption in the proximal convoluted tubule of the rat kidney. Role of chloride concentration gradients. *J. Clin. Invest.* 58:1110–18

84. Cardinal, J., Lutz, M. D., Burg, M. B., Orloff, J. 1975. Lack of relationship of potential difference to fluid absorption in the proximal renal tubule. *Kidney Int.* 7:94–102

85. Rumrich, G., Ullrich, K. J. 1968. The minimum requirement for the maintenance of sodium chloride reabsorption in the proximal convolution of the mammalian kidney. *J. Physiol.* 197:69–70P

86. Shafer, J. A., Patlak, C. S., Andreoli, T. E. 1975. A component of fluid absorption linked to passive ion flows in the superficial pars recta. *J. Gen. Physiol.* 66:445–71

87. Oken, D. E., Wittembury, G., Windhager, E. E., Solomon, A. K. 1963. Single proximal tubules of Necturus kidney. V. Unidirectional sodium movement. *Am. J. Physiol.* 204:372–76

88. Gertz, K. H. 1963. Transtubulare natriumchloridflusse und permeabilitat fur nichtelektrolyte im proximalen und distalen knovolut der rattenniere. *Pfluegers Arch.* 276:336–56

89. Gertz, K. H., Mangos, J. A., Braun, G., Pagel, H. D. 1965. On the glomerular tubular balance in the rat kidney. *Pfluegers Arch.* 285:360–72

90. Rector, F. C., Brunner, F. P., Seldin, D. W. 1966. Mechanism of glomerulotubular balance. I. Effect of aortic constriction and elevated ureteropelvic pressure on glomerular filtration rate, fractional reabsorption, transit time, and tubular size in the proximal tubule of the rat. *J. Clin. Invest.* 45:590–602

91. Brunner, F. P., Rector, F. C., Seldin, D. W. 1966. Mechanism of glomerulotubular balance. II. Regulation of proximal tubular reabsorption by tubular volume, as studied by stopped flow microperfusion. *J. Clin. Invest.* 45:603–11

92. Brenner, B. M., Bennett, C. M., Berliner, R. W. 1968. The relationship between glomerular filtration rate and sodium reabsorption by the proximal tubule of the rat nephron. *J. Clin. Invest.* 47:1358–74

93. Rodicio, J., Herrera-Acosta, J., Sellman, J. C., Rector, F. C., Seldin, D. W. 1969. Studies on glomerulotubular balance during aortic constriction, ureteral obstruction and venous occlusion in hydropenic and saline-loaded rats. *Nephron* 6:437–56

94. Burg, M. B., Orloff, J. 1968. Control of fluid absorption in the renal proximal tubule. *J. Clin. Invest.* 47:2016–24

95. Bartoli, E., Conger, J. D., Earley, L. E. 1973. Effect of intraluminal flow on proximal tubular reabsorption. *J. Clin. Invest.* 52:843–49

96. Morgan, T., Berliner, R. W. 1969. In vivo perfusion of proximal tubules of the rat: Glomerulotubular balance. *Am. J. Physiol.* 217:992–97

97. Morel, F., Murayama, Y. 1970. Simultaneous measurement of unidirectional and net sodium fluxes in microperfused rat proximal tubules. *Pfluegers Arch.* 320:1–23

98. Imai, M., Seldin, D. W., Kokko, J. P. 1977. Effect of perfusion rate on the fluxes of water, sodium, chloride and urea across the proximal convoluted tubule. *Kidney Int.* 11:In press

99. deWardener, H. E., Mills, I. H., Clapham, W. F., Hayter, C. J. 1961. Studies

on the efferent mechanism of the sodium diuresis which follows the administration of intravenous saline in the dog. *Clin. Sci.* 21:249–58

100. Levinsky, N. G. 1974. Natriuretic hormones. *Adv. Metab. Disor.* 7:37–71

101. Wright, F. S., Brenner, B. M., Bennett, C. M., Kermowitz, R. I., Berliner, R. W., Schrier, R. W., Verhoust, P. J., de Qardener, H. E., Holzgreve, H. 1969. Failure to demonstrate a hormonal inhibitor of proximal sodium reabsorption. *J. Clin. Invest.* 48:1107–13

102. Fine, L. G., Bourgoignie, J. J., Bricker, N. S. 1975. The influence of the natriuretic factor from uremic patients on bioelectric properties and sodium transport of the isolated mammalian collecting tubule. *Clin. Res.* 23:430A

103. Earley, L. E., Friedler, R. M. 1965. Studies on the mechanism of natriuresis accompanying increased renal blood flow and its role in the renal response to extracellular volume expansion. *J. Clin. Invest.* 44:1857–65

104. Earley, L. E., Friedler, R. M. 1966. Effects of combined renal vasodilatation and pressor agents on renal hemodynamics and the tubular reabsorption of sodium. *J. Clin. Invest.* 45:542–51

105. Earley, L. E., Martino, J. A., Friedler, R. M. 1966. Factors affecting sodium reabsorption by the proximal tubules as determined during blockade of distal sodium reabsorption. *J. Clin. Invest.* 45:1168–84

106. Martino, J. A., Earley, L. E. 1967. Demonstration of the role of physical factors as determinants of the natriuretic response to volume expansion. *J. Clin. Invest.* 46:1963–78

107. Daugharty, T. M., Belleau, L. J., Martino, J. A., Earley, L. E. 1968. Interrelationship of physical factors affecting sodium reabsorption in the dog. *Am. J. Physiol.* 215:1442–47

108. Brenner, B. M., Falchuk, K. H., Keimowitz, R. I., Berliner, R. W. 1969. The relationship between peritubular capillary protein concentration and fluid reabsorption by the renal proximal tubule. *J. Clin. Invest.* 48:1519–31

109. Brenner, B. M., Troy, J. L., Daugharty, T. M. 1971. On the mechanism of inhibition of fluid reabsorption by the renal proximal tubule of the volume-expanded rate. *J. Clin. Invest.* 50:1596–1602

110. Falchuk, K. H., Brenner, B. M., Tadokoro, M., Berliner, R. W. 1971. Oncotic hydrostatic pressure in peritubular capillaries and fluid reabsorption by proximal tubule. *Am. J. Physiol.* 220:1427–33

111. Brenner, B. M., Troy, J. L., Daugharty, T. M., MacInnes, R. M. 1973. Quantitative importance of changes in postglomerular colloid osmotic pressure in mediating glomerulotubular balance in the rat. *J. Clin. Invest.* 52:190–97

112. Spitzer, A., Windhager, E. E. 1970. Effect of peritubular oncotic pressure changes on proximal tubular fluid reabsorption. *Am. J. Physiol.* 218:1188–93

113. Weinman, E. J., Kashgarian, M., Hayslett, J. P. 1971. Role of peritubular protein concentration in sodium reabsorption. *Am. J. Physiol.* 221:1521–28

114. Green, R., Windhager, E. E., Giebisch, G. 1974. Protein oncotic pressure effects on proximal tubular fluid movement in the rat. *Am J. Physiol.* 226:265–76

115. Kuschinsky, W., Wahl, M., Wunderlich, P., Thurau, K. 1970. Different correlations between plasma protein concentration and proximal fractional reabsorption in the rat during acute and chronic saline infusion. *Pfluegers Arch.* 321:102–20

116. Lowitz, H. D., Stumpe, K. O., Ochwadt, B. 1969. Micropuncture study of the action of angtiotensin II on tubular sodium and water reabsorption in the rat. *Nephron* 6:172–87

117. Conger, J. D., Bartoli, E., Earley, L. E. 1973. No effect of peritubular plasma protein on proximal tubular volume absorption during capillary perfusion *in vivo.* In *Abstr. Proc. Ann. Meet. Am. Soc. Nephrol.,* Washington DC, p. 25

118. Holzgreve, H., Schrier, R. W. 1975. Variation of proximal tubular reabsorptive capacity by volume expansion and aortic constriction during constancy of peritubular capillary protein concentration in rat kidney. *Pfluegers Arch.* 356:73–86

119. Gyory, A. Z., Kinne, R. 1971. Energy source for transepithelial sodium transport in rat renal proximal tubules. *Pfluegers Arch.* 327:234–60

120. Knox, F. G., Willis, L. R., Strandhoy, J. W., Schneider, E. G., Navar, L. G., Ott, C. E. 1972. Role of peritubular Starling forces in proximal reabsorption following albumin infusion. *Am. J. Physiol.* 223:741–49

121. Windhager, E. E., Giebisch, G. 1976. Proximal sodium and fluid transport. *Kidney Int.* 9:121–33

122. Bank, N., Koch, K. M., Aynedjian, H. S., Aras, M. 1969. Effect of changes in renal perfusion pressure in the suppression of proximal tubular sodium reabsorption due to saline loading. *J. Clin. Invest.* 48:271–83

123. Aperia, A. C., Broberger, C. G. O., Soderlund, S. 1971. Relationship between renal artery perfusion pressure and tubular sodium reabsorption. *Am. J. Physiol.* 220:1205–12

124. Bank, N., Aynedjian, H. S., Wada, T. 1972. Effect of peritubular capillary perfusion rate on proximal sodium reabsorption. *Kidney Int.* 1:397–405

125. Hayslett, J. P. 1973. Effect of changes in hydrostatic pressure in peritubular capillaries in the permeability of the proximal tubule. *J. Clin. Invest.* 52:1314–19

126. Grandchamp, A., Boulpaep, E. L. 1974. Pressure control of sodium reabsorption and intercellular backflux across proximal kidney tubule. *J. Clin. Invest.* 54:69–82

127. Daugharty, T. M., Zweig, S. M., Earley, L. E. 1971. Assessment of renal hemohynamic factors in whole kidney glomerulotubular balance. *Am. J. Physiol.* 220:2021–27

128. Schrier, R. W., Humphreys, M. H. 1972. Role of distal reabsorption and peritubular environment in glomerulotubular balance. *Am. J. Physiol.* 222:379–87

129. Deen, W. M., Robertson, C. R., Brenner, B. M. 1973. A model of peritubular capillary control of isotonic fluid reabsorption by the renal proximal tubule. *Biophys. J.* 13:340–58

130. Myers, B. D., Deen, W. M., Brenner, B. M. 1975. Effects of norepinephine and angiotensin II on the determinants of glomerular ultrafiltration and proximal tubule fluid reabsorption in the rat. *Circ. Res.* 37:101–10

131. Welling, L. W., Grantham, J. J. 1972. Physical properties of isolated perfused renal tubules and tubular basement membranes. *J. Clin. Invest.* 51:1063–75

132. Earley, L. E., Humphreys, M. H., Bartoli, E. 1972. Capillary circulation as a regulation of sodium reabsorption and excretion. *Circ. Res.* 30 and 31:Suppl. 2, 1–18

133. Gill, J. R., Casper, A. G. T. 1971. Renal effects of adenosine 3',5'-cyclic monophosphate and dibutyryl adenosine 3',5'-cyclic monophosphate—evidence for a role for adenosine 3',5'-cyclic monophosphate in the regulation of proximal tubular sodium reabsorption. *J. Clin. Invest.* 50:1231–40

134. Lorentz, W. B. 1974. The effect of cyclic AMP and dibutyryl cyclic AMP on the permeability characteristics of the renal tubule. *J. Clin. Invest.* 53:1250–57

135. Lorentz, W. B. 1976. The effect of PTH on renal tubular permeability. *Abstr. Soc. Pediatr. Res.,* p. 838

136. Friedler, R. M., Descoeudres, C., Kurokawa, K., Kreusser, W. J., Massry, S. G. 1976. Role of cyclic AMP in the natriuresis of volume expansion. *Clin. Res.* 23:467A

137. Streeto, J. M. 1969. Renal cortical adenyl cyclase: Effect of parathyroid hormone and calcium. *Metab. Clin. Exp.* 18:968–73

138. Agus, Z. S., Puschett, J. B., Senesky, D., Goldberg, M. 1971. Mode of action of parathyroid hormone and cyclic adenosine 3',5'monophosphate on renal tubular phosphate reabsorption in the dog. *J. Clin. Invest.* 50:617–26

139. Liddle, G. W., Hardman, J. G. 1971. Cyclic adenosine monophosphate as a mediator of hormone action. *N. Engl. J. Med.* 285:560–66

140. Linarelli, L. B. 1972. Newborn urinary cyclic AMP and developmental renal responsiveness to parathyroid hormone. *Pediatrics* 50:14–23

141. Butler, D., Jard, S. 1972. Renal handling of 3',5'-cyclic AMP in the rat. *Pfluegers Arch.* 331:172–90

Ann. Rev. Pharmacol. Toxicol. 1977. 17:647-75
Copyright © 1977 by Annual Reviews Inc. All rights reserved

ETHNOPHARMACOLOGY OF ♦6700
SACRED PSYCHOACTIVE PLANTS
USED BY THE INDIANS OF MEXICO

José Luis Díaz

Centro de Investigación Interdisciplinaria y Departmento de Neurobiología, Instituto de
Investigaciones Biomédicas, Universidad Nacional Autónoma de México, México 20, D.F.

INTRODUCTION

Plants regarded as sacred or magical, which function as intermediaries between a
person and his deity, have proved to contain psychoactive agents and therefore have
been a source of extensive pharmacological scrutiny. The study of these plants has
covered, as well, other areas of research from ethnology to botany, chemistry,
neurochemistry, and psychiatry. An interdisciplinary research field, properly named
ethnopharmacology, has recently developed in an attempt to integrate the methods
of these disciplines in order to put our understanding of biodynamic plants used by
native peoples in a broader perspective.

Some Indian groups of Mexico have searched extensively for psychoactive plants
in their natural habitat. We know of about forty plants belonging to some fifteen
botanical families that are used ritually or regarded as sacred by these groups. Some
of the plants have been studied intensively but many others still present novel and
interesting topics for further research.

The body of this paper covers the general historical, botanical, and ethnological
aspects of the Mexican magic plants. A classification of the drugs based on their
reported uses and subjective effects is proposed in a section on psychopharmacology.
The specific etymological, botanical, ethnological, pharmacological, and chemical
information is summarized in a table.

HISTORY

There is extensive evidence of the use of psychotropic plants by several Indian
cultures dating from before the Spanish conquest of Mexico (1521–1525). Probably
the earliest sacred plant used was the neurotoxic *Sophora secundiflora* used by
Paleo-Indians of the desert of northern Mexico and southern Texas about 10,000

years ago (1). Polychrome ceramic pots from Casas Grandes decorated with a spiral very similar to the Huichol symbol of peyote suggests that this plant was used around the tenth century A.D. north of the Tarahumara zone (2). Codices such as the *Codex Magliabechi* (3) and *Codex Vindobonensis* (4) carry representations of mushrooms in ritual scenes associated with Indian priests and deities. The suggestion that these represent sacred mushrooms (3) is strengthened by historical evidence from Spanish colonial sources (5–7) and the modern Indian use of *Psilocybe* mushrooms (3, 8). Stones carved in the form of mushrooms with a human figure at the base or stem have been found in Mayan areas (9), but there are no data on modern usage among the Maya.

There exist two major sources referring to magic plants which date from the years following the conquest. In 1557, the Franciscan friar Bernardino de Sahagún began gathering data on Aztec culture through questionnaires and by interviews of selected informants. All the research was conducted in Náhuatl, the tongue of these learned Mesoamericans. The results of years of analysis of the material were assembled in what is known as the *Florentine Codex* (5) written in Náhuatl from which a Spanish version called *Historia General de las Cosas de la Nueva España* was made (10). In a remarkable and classic section, "Concerning Certain Herbs that Inebriate" [(5), Book 11, pp. 129–31 (see also 11)], he describes *ololiuhqui, peyote, tlápatl, tzinzintlápatl, mixitl,* and *nanácatl,* all of which have been identified (see Table 1).

Toward the end of the sixteenth century, the Spanish physician Francisco Hernández was commissioned by Philip II to collect information on medicinal plants in New Spain. His monumental report [(12) first published in 1649], the product of seven years of travel and observation, contains descriptions of a root called *peyotl de zacatecas* which "shows neither stem nor leaf over the earth and is covered by some sort of wool ... those who ingest it may divine any matter ..." [(12) Book 3, p. 92]. There is little doubt that this plant was *Lophophora williamsii.*

There are valuable descriptions appearing in the archives of the Inquisition [1536–1787 (see 13)], which date from colonial times, of magical plants used in indigenous ceremonies. The archives describe numerous trials and occasional tortures of Indians that used *peyotl, ololiuhqui,* and *pipiltzintzintli* for divinatory purposes. These writers, as well as the chroniclers Ruiz de Alarcón (14) and de la Serna (6), were eager to substitute these practices, then considered demonic, by the Catholic religion. In some cases the zeal of the friars resulted in extensive accounts of the ceremonies and "superstitions" concerning sacred plants (15); these have been very useful for purposes of comparison with modern Indian rituals. A surprising similarity of the liturgy practiced in different cultures and centuries has been found (16), indicating the strength of an oral tradition that survived through centuries of repression.

It is not until the nineteenth century that the attention of scientists was directed again to the sacred plants. In 1888 an institution was created for the study of medical resources of Mexico. A multidisciplinary group of encyclopedic botanists, chemists, physiologists, physicians, and geographers gathered information on approximately one thousand plants in 20 volumes (see 17). The works of the *Instituto Medico Nacional* (1888–1917) include botanical, chemical, and pharmacological data on *ololiuhqui* (18), *sinicuiche* (19), *peyote* (18, 20, 21), the noncactaceous *peyotes* (20), and the *Leguminosae* (22).

Numerous investigators of this century have contributed to the study of the botanical identity, chemistry, and use of magic plants: Lumholtz (23) described the use of peyote by the Tarahumara; Heffter (24) isolated mescaline from peyote buttons in 1896 and in 1919 Späth (25) elucidated its chemical structure; Reko (26) conducted important field research on many of the plants in the state of Oaxaca, a major center of divinatory plant use; Schultes (27–31) corroborated, systematized, and disseminated much valuable ethnobotanical information; Wasson (3, 8, 16, 32) discovered and carefully described the modern use of sacred mushrooms and other psychoactive flora, and Hofmann found psilocybin in the magic mushrooms (33) and ergot alkaloids in *ololiuhqui* (34).

BOTANICAL DISTRIBUTION AND IDENTIFICATION

There is extensive documentation of the existence, worldwide, of numerous ritualistic techniques and preparations employed for their mind-altering effects (30, 31). In methods of evoking changes in consciousness, ecstatic states, and mystical experiences, the New World makes more extensive use of plant materials than the Old World. The majority of known plants ceremonially used as psychotropic agents are utilized in the American continents and more than half in Mexico (30, 31). In certain regions such as the Mazatec Sierra, at least four families of psychodysleptics are currently employed (32). The disparity between Old and New World use of psychotropics is probably due to cultural factors, since many psychoactive plants grow in the Old World (31). Furst (35) has suggested that the strength of the Old World religions, primarily Christianity and Islam, may have been a decisive factor in the disappearance of shamanistic traditions in those regions. La Barre (36) has hypothesized that the New World use of plants is a survival from an ancient Paleolithic and Mesolithic shamanistic cult which he traces to the Siberian ancestors of American Indians. Other causes for the differential geographical distribution of use may include regional variations in chemical content. For example, levels of Δ^9-tetrahydrocannabinol (THC), an active factor in *Cannabis sativa*, have been found to vary widely in different locations (37). Further study of the ecology of psychoactive plants is potentially of great interest since it may shed light on some of their unresolved geographical, chemotaxonomic, and ethnologic aspects.

The function of psychoactive compounds elaborated by plants is not understood. In general, naturally occurring alkaloids have an active turnover and complex synthesis, suggesting that they are not merely inert "end products" of metabolism (38). The hypothesis that these biodynamic alkaloids could protect the plant against animal predation, even if logical, has little evidence in its favor. In fact, there appear to be many instances of deliberate association between animals and psychotropic plants (39). For example, the incidence of insect predation in *Datura stramonium* is higher than in any plant of the same econiche. The role of the tropane alkaloids in the physiology and behavior of these insects is presently under study (J. L. Díaz, unpublished data). These observations may have cultural interest, since they could be one of the mechanisms used by native man as a guide for experimenting with plants. Indeed one of the recurrent transcultural themes in the native experience of psychoactive plants is the role animals play in disclosing the psychoactive properties of plants to man (40).

The precise botanical identification of magic plants has been a necessary step to further chemotaxonomic, psychopharmacological, and neurochemical studies. The information covering the vulgar and scientific names of magic plants, their uses by Indian groups, major effects,and chemistry is summarized in Table 1. Even though identifications are often a source of academic and scholarly debate, the majority of the sacred plants referred to in the early Náhuatl sources have been identified. Thus, *péyotl* corresponds to *Lophophora williamsii* (18, 20, 21, 27); *ololiuhqui* refers to the seeds of two morning glories, *Rivea corymbosa* (18, 26, 29) and *Ipomea violacea* (32); *teonanácatl* are mushrooms mainly of the genus *Psilocybe* (3, 8); *toloatzin* corresponds to *Datura* species (41, 42) and *picietl* is the wild tobacco *Nicotiana rustica* (32). These Náhuatl names denote a reverence reserved for sacred beings or objects (see etymology in Table 1).

Three sacred plants mentioned during the time of the early colonization have not been identified to the satisfaction of all experts: *pipiltzintzintli, tlápatl,* and *poyomatli*. There are several seventeenth century references to *pipiltzintzintli*, "the venerable child." The archives of the Inquisition describe it as a cultivated shrub with male and female varieties that was dried and used for diagnosis and treatment of disease (13). A century later, in 1772, the learned priest Antonio Alzate (43) identified *pipiltzintzintli* as Indian hemp, *Cannabis indica*. This is a surprising reference since it is generally agreed that *Cannabis* was introduced in the nineteenth century and that it was cultivated neither as a source of fiber nor of drug in Mexico before that time (44). More recently it has been found that some Leguminosae are called *pipiltzintli* (45), and Wasson (32) suggested that this magic plant could correspond to *Salvia divinorum*. The identification most compatible with the data of the Inquisition archives is that of Alzate. It should be acknowledged, however, that the same name might have been given to other plants having similar effects. It is interesting that both *Cannabis sativa* and *Salvia divinorum* belong to the imagery-inducing family of psychodysleptics, as is discussed later.

Tlápatl or *tláppatl* is a word that implies "light of fire" or "red color." Sahagún (5, 10, 11) described the effects of *tlápatl* as a plant that inebriates and he adds: "if he eats it, he will go mad forever, will lose his heart, it will bewitch him" [(5) Vol. 11, p. 129]. He also mentions, *tzinzintlápatl,* a similar plant with a nonspiny fruit. Hernández (12) has included very explicit drawings and references to a group of plants to which *tlápatl, nacazul,* and *toloatzin* belong. His descriptions and drawings clearly match the genus *Datura*. About *nacazul* he states that it is "a species of *tlápatl* (which) in excess produces madness, visions and delirium . . . sometimes it is called *toloatzin*" [(12) Book 3, p. 66]. In this case we have several names referring to related plants within the same genus which give similar effects. The implication is that each name was given to a single species of *Datura*.

Much about *poyomatli* has not been elucidated beginning with its etymology. Hernández (12) writes about two *poyomatlis,* one being a root "with which, through a strange madness, Indians believe that hidden and future things are revealed"

(Book 2, p. 105). The flower of *poyomatli, poyomaxochitl,* is identified by Sahagún
(5, 10) as "the jar shape of the cacao flower. It is said that it makes the heart of
people whirl, it makes the heart of people turn, makes the heart of people jump"
(Book 11, p. 212). At that time the word "heart" referred to what is contemporarily
known as psyche (11). The "jar shape" may refer to the flower in a latter stage, or
to an early phase of the fruiting pod. Describing the cacao plant, *cacaoquavitl,* he
says: "When much is consumed, especially if it is green . . . it makes people drunk,
takes possession of people, maddens people, makes the heart of people evil" [(5),
Book 11, p. 119].

Many poems written in the Náhuatl language refer to the flower of cacao, to
poyoma and *poyomatli,* as inebriating substances. In a piece written for performance
in pantomime about the fall of Tula, a poet sings about his longing for transcendence
through his chanting, which he compares to the scent of flowers (46). Towards the
end he intones:

But the fragrant cacao flower is bursting
and smelling, Alas! Perfumed *poyomatli* falls as mist (p. 5).

The association between *poyomatli* and cacao may not be merely fortuitous since
in the same work Tlacahuipan, a brother of Moctezuma, offers cacao in flower in
the following manner: "I spread the precious blossom of *poyomatli,* the flower of
cacao" [(46) p. 25]. Reverentially, he refers to *poyomatli* as *quetzalpoyomaxochitl,*
the prefix *quetzal* denoting something exquisite or precious. With this evidence it
can be safely assumed that at least one *poyomatli* corresponds to *Theobroma cacao*
and *poyomaxochitl* to its flower. In order to determine a possible chemical basis for
emphasis on the flower and the early fruiting pod we have undertaken the study of
the content of xanthines or other possible psychoactive compounds in different parts
of the plant during different stages of development. One puzzling aspect of this plant
is that it was used as a psychoactive compound in the Valley of Mexico, far from
its tropical growing sites. This is also the case of the desert cactus, *Lophophora
williamsii.* The statement of Hernández that *poyomatli* corresponds to more than
one plant is strengthened by a testament from Xochimilco, a site in the Valley of
Mexico, in which is mentioned a *poyomacatl,* a house where *poyomatli* grows.
Perhaps this corresponds to the root encountered by Hernández (12) and to the
odorous root referred to as *puyomate* in the archives of the Inquisition (13).

In the aforementioned pantomime poems (46) there are also frequent references
to aquatic plants that inebriate. The term *quetzalaxochiacatl,* "the precious water
flower," may correspond to *Nymphea ampla* (47). This water lily is extensively
represented in Mayan art. The suggestion that it was used as a sacred psychotropic
during the classic Mayan civilization (48) is supported by analysis of the Bonampak
frescos, reports of recreational use of *N. ampla* in the Mayan highlands, and the
presence of aporphine alkaloids in the genus (47).

An interesting case of nonspecificity in Indian nomenclature is *piule,* which has
been found to refer to psychoactive seeds of *Leguminosae* and *Convulvulaceae* and
also to *Psilocybe* mushrooms (17, 32, 45). The etymology of *piule* is obscure but it
seems certain that it is not a Náhuatl word. Reko (26) thinks that it is related to

peyote, derived from *pi-yahutli,* a term denoting any psychotropic plant. Wasson agrees that *piule* might be a Zapotec derivation of *péyotl* (32).

That some of these names seem to designate several species of plants suggests two possibilities: either these Náhuatl names could have been given before the conquest to plants sharing similar properties or this nonspecificity might have resulted from the repression and subsequent dispersion of their use after 1520. There is convincing evidence in favor of the first possibility; for example, *zoapatl* is reported as a generic name of five or six plants that produce uteroconstriction. Nevertheless, some names are more specific than others, especially when they designate morphological characteristics of the plant. The common element of the Náhuatl names for psychoactive plants conveys respect or veneration. Sometimes this is evident, as in *teonanácatl* "mushroom or flesh of the gods" (3, 28) while in other cases it is implied only through association, as with *ololiuhqui,* also called *coatl xoxouhqui,* "green snake," signifying something powerful (13). Deference is also expressed through the use of the prefix *quetzal* and the suffix *tzintli.*

The concepts of darkness, the color black, or light frequently occur or are implied in the names of magic plants. For the Náhuatl the term *light* carries the same meaning as the color black. We find in the archives of the Inquisition an "*ololiuhqui* of the dark man." Its counterpart, *tlitlitzen (Ipomea violacea),* means "divine black one" (13). *Yahutli (Tagetes lucida)* also means "dark one" (47). These denominations seem to imply a dark person or a character that animates the plant which may appear after the ingestion as an image or a culturally determined stereotypic vision (40). Many names refer to the existence of such residing characters or deities of the plant who in some instances would appear or talk during its effects. This is the case with *toloatzin, pipiltzinzintli,* and "*ololiuhqui* of the dark man." When Sahagún (5, 10) says that *cacaoquavitl* takes possession of people there may be an implication of an animistic subject in the plant. Influenced by the conquest and colonization, and as a paradoxical result of repression, these indwelling characters have become transformed from pre-Columbian deities into Christian saints. As early as the seventeenth century the archives of the Inquisition identify *peyote* with the child Jesus (*Niño Jesús*) and with the Virgin Mary (13). Today, *Salvia divinorum* and *Turnera diffusa* are called *la Pastora* "the shepherdess," a possible reference to the Virgin Mary. *Tagetes lucida* is called *Flor de Santa María,* "flower of holy Mary," and the most frequent name for the morning glory seeds is *semillas de la Virgen,* "seeds of the Virgin." Other names use Christian figures such as St. Peter in *peyote de San Pedro (Mamillaria heyderii)* and St. Isidore in *San Isidro (Psilocybe cubensis)* (17).

USES AND CULTURAL ROLES

Despite colonial persecution and acculturation the magic plants are still in use among numerous Indian groups of Mexico. The intricate relationship between the effects of psychotropic plants, medicine, religion, and belief systems is just starting to be delineated.

Among modern Indian communities, shamans, *curanderos,* (healers), *brujos* (witch doctors), and *yerberos* (herbalists) know about the effects of sacred plants.

It is difficult to define the differences between these people since they are likely to share functions. The pure *yerbero* is an expert in medicinal plants; in Indian communities he will collect them himself or prescribe them to a patient. In urban Mestizo groups he will be found selling herbs in markets. On the other hand the pure *brujo* deals with magic; he uses herbs for their magical properties and his performance will be ritualistic and psychotherapeutic. The *curandero* is a Mestizo or peasant medicine man who combines the knowledge of a *yerbero* and the arts of the *brujo*. Finally, the shaman is the priest of Indian groups, an expert in states of consciousness who has direct access to the Sacred.

The role of social class in the use of psychotropic plants is important. The shaman, for example, occupies a high level in the stratification of Indian groups. The *brujo* is also respected and has special privileges, while the *curandero* and *yerbero* will be found among lower classes. In classic Indian cultures there are indications that the use of magic plants was passed from lower to higher strata of the population, where the knowledge was then concealed in highly elaborate esoteric arts and rituals (40).

One of the most frequent uses of these plants has been and is the location through divination of a lost person, domestic animal, or object (6, 13, 32, 35). In some aboriginal cultures it is common that the shaman, *brujo*, or *curandero* ingest psychodysleptics in order to diagnose illness. While under the influence of the plant the curer may receive visions of the missing item, knowledge of the cause of disease, or direct information from the residing deity of the plant. After the diagnosis the medicine man proceeds to exorcise the supernatural cause of the disease by magical means such as cleansing and suction or to treat the condition by prescribing medicinal herbs (16, 32, 35, 47, 49).

In some instances the magic plants are used to produce disease instead of healing. It is frequent that rival shamans try to damage one another by ingesting hallucinogens and performing special rites.

It has been found that psychotropic plants are used in the rituals of religious feasts. The most well-known of these is the yearly pilgrimage of the Huichols to collect and consume *peyote* (35, 50). In Mazatec country some families perform a religious ceremony with *Psilocybe* mushrooms once a year with no other apparent purpose than to experience and share the effects (47).

Independent of the specific intention, the consumption of psychedelic plants is intimately connected to religion, the central purpose being to come in contact with the Sacred (e.g. 16). In Yaqui (51) and Mazatec (47) cultures there is a protracted procedure for obtaining shamanic powers which involves the repeated ingestion of sacred plants in order to develop comprehensive empirical knowledge of their effects. Such knowledge is essential for initiation as a shaman or a *brujo*.

The magical plants are feared and respected since, as we have seen, they are believed to contain a residing deity or animate principle. The plants are handled with care, often chanted to and smoked in copal incense (32, 47, 52).

There are a series of regulations to be followed before and after the ingestion of psychodysleptic plants, usually involving fasting and sexual abstinence. The ingestion takes place most frequently in darkness and either in silence or during the long monotonous chanting of the shaman (16, 32, 35, 47). These carefully selected variables maximize the perception of effects by means of sensorial isolation, increased intestinal absorption, directed attention, and psychological expectation. Belief systems, setting, and cultural, biological, and psychological factors affect the nature of the experience (40).

The practice of the rites and ceremonies is usually concealed from the general community involving only the patient and his family, a selected group of pilgrims or the shaman himself. The presence of a guide experienced with the effects of the plants who selects the time, place, dose, and other circumstances of the ceremony is common. The guide may choose to administer the plant to the patient, consultant, apprentice, and/or to himself. During the ceremony he is likely to dance, chant, play musical instruments, or repeat the voice of the plant deity. The invocations frequently include the use of Christian names, even in remote monolingual tribes: St. Peter, St. Paul, and the Virgin Mary are the most commonly invoked (16, 47).

The continuity of the tradition surrounding and knowledge of sacred plants has been insured by the careful selection of apprentices and a rigorous training which involves experience with psychotropic plants, physical and psychological exercises, and exposure to difficult tasks (51). Thus, the shaman becomes an expert in the various states of consciousness including that of religious ecstasy (53). The shamanic flight, descent into hell, and communication with the godhead are brought about and directed by his use of magic plants.

PSYCHOPHARMACOLOGY

The effects of Mexican magic plants have been frequently classified under single labels like "narcotic," "hallucinogenic," or "psychedelic." This terminology is misleading, because our knowledge of both their cultural roles and pharmacological effects has disclosed a wide variety of actions indicating the need for reclassification. Brawley & Duffield (54) proposed in 1972 a division of what are known as hallucinogens into toxicants, deliriants, and psychomimetics. The available information points, however, to the existence of both more subtle and larger differences, even between plants within the same botanical family.

Plants may be considered as psychodysleptics, psychoanaleptics, or even psycholeptics, according to the well-accepted classification of psychotropic drugs proposed by Delay (55). In many instances it is difficult to assign a single psychopharmacological label to a plant since many either have actions that would include them in another group, produce qualitatively different biphasic effects, or have differential dose-related properties. Indeed, the same is true of some well-characterized psychotropics, for instance amphetamine, which could be considered either psychoanaleptic or psychodysleptic depending on dosage. It is of interest why plants with such a variety of actions should be regarded as sacred by Indian groups. Regardless of their differences these plants apparently have important common effects. The capacity to produce a distinct change in the quality of mentation, including light-headedness, a state of wonder, fascination with internal and external perceptions, and intensification of experience is the elementary psychopharmacological property of all the plants considered sacred or magic by the Indians who use them. These effects, which may take place accompanied by sedation, excitation, or drowsiness, are not in themselves sufficient to classify the plants as psychodysleptics. The opiates, cocaine, and ethanol can produce some of these effects and have been revered by traditional and modern cultures (56). In order to classify a plant as a psychodysleptic it must produce varying degrees of affective, perceptual, imaginative, and thought modifications. As with psycholeptics or psychoanaleptics (55), there are important differences between families of psychodysleptics. A family of psychodysleptics is defined basically by similarities in subjective effects, cross-tolerance, and structure-activity relationships. A classification of Mexican sacred plants is now proposed based on these considerations.

Psychodysleptics

VISIONARY PSYCHODYSLEPTICS The visionary plants are highly revered by Indian groups who use them as a sacrament. The compounds produce important changes in all mental areas: distortion in perception (most notably in the visual sphere); emotional changes which can encompass widely varying states such as elation, serenity, panic, or apathy; and distinct changes in thinking and memory. High doses can produce effects such as depersonalization, profound wonder, dissociative reactions, ecstasy, experience of death, or visions (57, 58). This group is the only one that could properly be called hallucinogenic. There are two groups of chemicals found in these plants which induce similar experiences with only minor differences.

Phenethylamines Several dozen different phenethylamine molecules (Figure 1, *IV*) have been isolated from cacti, especially from *Lophophora williamsii* (59, 60). This group, of which mescaline (24, 25) (Figure 1, *IV;* 3,4,5=CH$_3$O; R$_1$, R$_2$=H) is the most active compound, produces, aside from visionary effects, intense sympathomimetic responses, euphoria, decreased fatigue, and sleeplessness (21, 57). The neuropsychopharmacology of the rest of the phenethylamines and tetrahydroisoquinolines (Figure 1, *V*) discovered in the cacti family (60, 61) is virtually unknown.

Indoles The indole structure is the nucleus of several hallucinogens including phosphorylated tryptamines such as psilocin (Figure 1, *I;* 4=OH; R$_1$, R$_2$=CH$_3$) and psilocybin (Figure 1, *I;* 4=OPO$_3$H; R$_1$, R$_2$=CH$_3$) which have been isolated from the magic *Psilocybe* mushrooms (3, 33). These chemicals appear to be responsible for the psychological effects of the mushrooms (58).

Despite structural disparities the powerful semisynthetic ergot-derivative *d*-lysergic acid diethylamide (LSD) [Figure 1, *III;* R=(CH$_2$–CH$_3$)$_2$] produces mental effects remarkably similar to mescaline and psilocybin (62). A methylated tryptamine, N,N-dimethyltryptamine (Figure 1, *I;* R$_1$, R$_2$=CH$_3$), produces as intense effects as those described for high doses of the visionary psychodysleptics which begin within five minutes and end one hour after administration (63).

IMAGERY-INDUCING PSYCHODYSLEPTICS This family of compounds produces, aside from the elementary properties of the magic plants, an increase in visual imagery, sensations of weightlessness or heaviness, recent-memory disturbances, distortion in the sense of time, rapid flow of ideas, and thought disorders such as fragmentations, interruptions of the stream of thought, and occasional delusions. Three groups of chemical compounds comprise this family.

Cannabinoids   *Cannabis sativa* is the prototype of this group (64), an important economic plant (source of fiber, oil, and drug) used ritually by peoples in Asia, Africa, and America and recreationally by Westerners (56, 65) from which several dozen dibenzopyran derivatives (Figure 1, *XIII*) have been isolated (66). Δ^9-THC (Figure 1, *XIII;* 1=OH; 3=$C_5 H_{11}$; 9=CH_3) seems to be an active compound of this group (67). In the botanical family of Moraceae, *Cecropia obtusifolia* and species of *Ficus* have the reputation in Mexico of marihuana-like effects.

Coumarins   Several Compositae, especially *Calea zacatechichi* (47, 68), produce effects similar to the dibenzopyrans although they are generally milder and briefer. *C. zacatechichi* reportedly enhances dreaming, an effect used for divination by a Chontal Indian in the State of Oaxaca (47). It is suggested that coumarins could undergo chemical modifications either during smoking (the usual route of ingestion) or in vivo to produce benzopyran compounds. Interestingly, other Compositae like *Artemisia absinthium* have strikingly similar psychological actions to *Cannabis sativa* and common characteristics between the active terpenoids of both plants have been noted (69). Another coumarin-containing composite, *Tagetes lucida,* is mixed with wild tobacco (*Nicotiana rustica*) and smoked by the Huichols for alleged psychotropic effects (47, 70).

Labiatae Compounds   The prototype of the psychotropic mints, *Salvia divinorum,* produces brief colorful visual images, mild euphoria, and a sense of weightlessness (47). *Leonorus sibiricus* has been used to produce "marihuana-like effects" (47), and other members of this family are used for their psychoactive effects (47, 71). Two compounds have been detected in *S. divinorum* (47) and their structure is presently under study. Some synthetic mescaline analogues such as 3-methoxy-4,5-methylenedioxyphenylisopropylamine (Figure 1, *IV;* 3=CH_3O; 4-5=$-O-CH_2-O-$; α=CH_3; R_1, R_2=H) clearly belong to this family of psychodysleptics (72).

TRANCE-INDUCING PSYCHODYSLEPTICS   This group of compounds shares the elementary properties of the magic plants, but is uniquely characterized by producing states of physical lethargy, quietude, apathy, serenity, and abstraction of mind.

Ergot   Lysergic acid amide (Figure 1, *III;* R=H_2), its isomer iso-lysergic acid amide, and other ergot alkaloids found in members of Convolvulaceae called *ololiuhqui* (34) produce effects for several hours after the ingestion of the seeds, eventually resulting in a state of mental clarity (73, 74).

Glucosides   Various glucosides such as turbicoryn (Figure 1, *XIV;* R_1=H; R_2= O–(CH–OH)$_3$–CH_2–OH) and corymbosine (Figure 1, *XIV;* R_1=CH_2–O–(CH–OH)$_3$–CH_2–OH; R_2=H) found in the seeds of *ololiuhqui* (*Rivea corymbosa*) (75) have been reported to produce mental apathy and physical sluggishness (76).

Heimia alkaloids   A fermented potion of *Heimia salicifolia* induces a state of sedation and apathy during which the quality of perceived sound changes (19, 77).

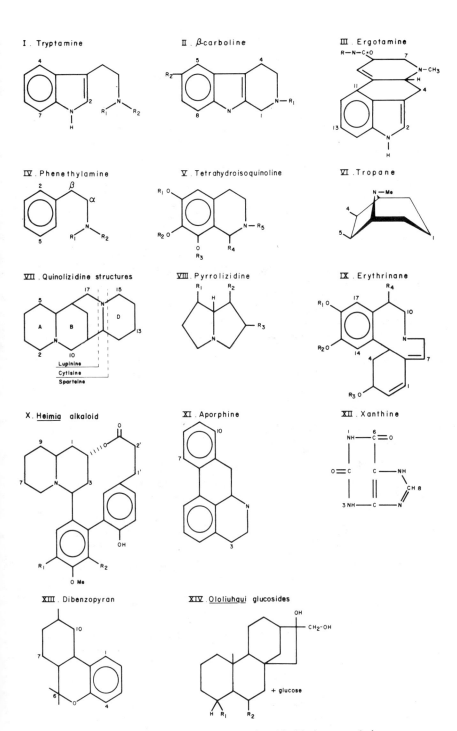

Figure 1 Basic structures of compounds found in Mexican sacred plants.

None of the alkaloids (Figure 1, *X*) found in the plant (78) have been found to be psychoactive, probably because the fermented material has not been studied and the fresh plant is inactive (47).

DELIRIANT PSYCHODYSLEPTICS   These are substances inducing confusion, thought and speech disorders, anxiety, clouding of consciousness, and hallucinations.

Tropane   The anticholinergic central nervous syndrome induced by species of tropane-containing Solanaceae is typical of the effects of this family (41, 51). Scopolamine (Figure 1, *VI;* 1=O–CO–CH (CH$_2$OH) Ø; 4–5=–O–) is an active compound responsible, at least in part, for the effects (79, 80).

NEUROTOXIC PSYCHODYSLEPTICS   This group of substances produces important effects upon motor, vegetative, and peripheral neural functions in addition to their psychological effects.

Quinolizidine   These ubiquitous chemicals (Figure 1, *VII*) found in the family Leguminosae (81) produce a state of stupor, clouding of consciousness, hallucinations, vomiting, and occasional convulsions (22, 26, 30, 45).

Erythrinane   The alkaloids of *Erythrina* (Figure 1, *IX*) have curare-like activity and share the effects of the rest of the other neurotropic Leguminosae (22, 45, 82).

Pyrrolizidine   The alkaloids of the genus *Senecio* (Figure 1, *VIII;* see 83), poorly understood as psychopharmacological agents, are reputed to be neurotoxic and in some instances to produce delusions (47, 84).

Psychoanaleptics

This class of psychopharmaca has three categories: antidepressant, excitatory, and euphoriant represented by tricyclic compounds, amphetamine, and cocaine respectively. The following Mexican herbs, considered magic, belong to the family of excitatory agents and induce some of the elementary psychopharmacological effects common to the magic plants.

EXCITATORY PSYCHOANALEPTICS   These compounds produce increased mental and physical activity, a stimulation of thought processes, and a sense of well-being.

Ephedrine   Some ephedrine-containing Malvaceae such as *Sida acuta* and *S. rhombifolia* (85) are smoked for their excitatory properties (47). The effects are similar to *kat* of the Arabs (*Katha edulis*) and the ancient Chinese *Ma Huang* (*Ephedra* spp.) (56) which contain ephedrine (Figure 1, *IV;* R$_1$=CH$_3$; R$_2$=H; α= CH$_3$; β=OH) and related compounds (85).

Xanthines   There is historical evidence that the sacred *poyomatli* used by the Náhuatl as an inebriating agent corresponds to *Theobroma cacao* which contains xanthines (Figure 1, *XII*), especially theobromine (Figure 1, *XII*; 3,7=CH₃). *Turnera diffusa,* which is used and respected by Yaqui medicine-men and traditionally regarded as an aphrodisiac (86), has been reported to contain caffeine (85). Further chemotaxonomical research is required in this group of plants to ascertain which xanthines or principles are responsible for their reputed actions.

CONCLUSION

The divine, sacred, or magic plants which function as intermediaries between some Mexican Indians and their deities contain compounds that share some elementary psychoactive properties. Six families of sacred plants can be distinguished according to their effects: visionary, imagery-inducing, trance-inducing, deliriant, neurotoxic, and excitatory agents.

After centuries of Western contact with Indian cultures and their magic plants, many of the botanical sources have been identified, chemicals considered responsible for their actions isolated, psychological effects described, and some specific neurochemical effects ascertained. While further specialized research may contribute historical, mythological, ecological, botanical, ethnological, phytochemical, psychopharmacological, and neurochemical information about each plant, it is clear that major advances can be made only by interdisciplinary groups. The capacity to design coordinated and sequential research strategies utilizing the methods of many fields should be the distinguishing characteristic of such groups. The growing field of ethnopharmacology emphasizes the need to understand the uses and effects of biodynamic plants in their cultural contexts as well as their chemical and pharmacological aspects. Social factors are considered to have an instrumental role in the modulation of biological effects of drugs.

Many areas in ethnopharmacology are suitable for interdisciplinary study. Further historical documentation of plants not clearly identified is necessary as well as a reevaluation of the cultural meaning of the ancient use of psychoactive plants. Ethnological work is needed to deepen our understanding of the modern uses of plants within specific cultural contexts, especially the nonvisionary psychodysleptics. Further botanical and chemotaxonomical research is required to isolate bioactive chemicals especially from psychoactive Compositae, Labiatae, Leguminosae, and Solanaceae. The ecology of psychotropic plants especially in relation to animal behavior is a new field. The effects of the majority of the plants and their chemical constituents upon the mind is in an embryonic state of understanding and the study of their actions upon animal behavior, brain chemistry, and physiology promises to be a productive research area in the years to come. Besides the gain in knowledge, some of the practical implications of this type of research are to be noted, especially its relevance to the mind-body problem, source of tools for neuroscience, and possible applications in psychiatry.

I hope that this review will stimulate studies that by coordinating different methods and strategies will yield a broader knowledge of the plants chosen by man to modify his mental functions, thereby expanding our understanding of such functions.

Table 1 Sacred plants used by Indian groups of Mexico

Name and etymology	Indian groups	Botanical sources	Cultural uses and effects	Phytochemistry
		Agaricaceae (Mushrooms)		
Teonanácatl (N)[a] (5) "flesh or mushroom of the Gods" (8)	Evidence of pre-Columbian use by Toltecs (3) and Náhuatl (4, 5). Mushroom stones from Mayan areas (9). Colonial references (6, 7, 14).	Initially identified as species of *Panaeolus* (26, 28) and *Stropharia* (87), these mushrooms corresponded mainly to the genus *Psilocybe* in extensive transcultural field research (3, 8).	"Makes the heart whirl. . . saddens, makes people run away, scares them, sees many horrible things or perhaps funny. He runs away, hangs himself, screams. . ." (5, 11). "They eat the mushrooms as communion. . . attribute divinity to them, drink them in *pulque*" (6).	Psilocin (I[b]; 4=OH; R_1, R_2=CH$_3$) and Psilocybin (I; 4=OPO$_3$H;R$_1$, R$_2$=CH$_3$). (33)
Teyhuinti (N) (12) "inebriant" (8)				
Quautlannanacatl (N) (6) "mushroom of the woods" (8)	Used by Náhuatl speaking people from Tenango in 1656 (6).	"Small red mushroom from the mountains" (6). Probably *Psilocybe wassonii* (3) =[c] *P. muliercula* (87).	Uses: For divination of cause and fate of disease or to resolve important problems by a shaman and suppliant. Regarded as holy in Indian communities that use them as sacraments (3, 8, 16, 32). Effects: Visionary psychodysleptics. Perception modifications.	Idem (3)
Badao-zoo, Beya-zoo (Z) "drunk mushroom" (26)	Zapotecs[d] (26)	*Panaeolus sphinctrinus* = *P. campanulatus* (26)		Idem (88)
Di-chi-to nizé, Di-nizé (Mz) "bird mushroom" (3, 90)	Mazatecs (3, 90)	*Psilocybe mexicana* (3.90)		Idem (3)
Nti-si-tho (Mz) "that which springs forth" (3, 90)	Mazatecs (3, 90)	*P. mexicana* (3, 90)	Increased visual imagery. Illusions. Hallucinations. Affective and intellectual alterations. Sympathomimetic effects (3, 89).	Idem (3)
Piule de churis (S-Z) "small narcotic" (3, 90)	Zapotecs (3, 90)	*P. mexicana* (3, 90)		Idem (3)
Cui-ya-jo-to-ki, Cui-ya-jo-o-tnu (C) "holy mushroom" (3, 90)	Chatino (3, 90)	*P. mexicana* (3, 90)		Idem (3)

Table 1 *(Continued)*

Teotlaquilnanácatl (N) (3, 90)	Nahua (3, 90)	*P. mexicana* (3, 90)	Similar effects found with psilocybin (58).	Idem (3)
Piule de barda (S) (3, 90)	Zapotecs (3, 90)	*P. mexicana* (3, 90)	Idem (3, 8, 16, 32, 58, 89)	Idem (3)
A-mo-kia (Ch) "for divination" (3, 90)	Chinantecs (3, 90)	*P. mexicana* (3) *Panaeolus sphinctrinus* (26)	Idem (3, 8, 16, 32, 58, 89)	Idem (3)
Di-chi-tó ki-shó (Mz) *Derrumbe* (S) "land slide" (3, 90)	Mazatecs (3, 90)	*Psilocybe caerulescens* var. *mazatecorum* (3)	Idem (3, 8, 16, 32, 58, 89)	Idem (3)
Razón mbei (S-Z) "mushroom of reason" (3, 90)	Zapotecs (3, 90)	*P. caerulescens* var. *mazatecorum* (3)	Idem (3, 8, 16, 32, 58, 89)	Idem (3)
Cui-ya-jo-o-su (C) "powerful sacred mushrooms" (3, 90)	Chatino (3, 90)	*P. caerulescens* var. *nigripes* (3)	Idem (3, 8, 16, 32, 58, 89)	Idem (3)
Derrumbito negro (S) "black little landslide" (3, 90)	Mazatecs (3, 90)	*P. caerulescens* var. *nigripes* (3)	Idem (3, 8, 16, 32, 58, 89)	Idem (3)
Apipiltzin (N) (3, 90)	Nahua (3, 90)	*P. aztecorum* (3)	Idem (3, 8, 16, 32, 58, 89)	Idem (3)
Siwatsitsíntli (N) "little women" (3, 90)	Nahua (3, 90)	*P. wassonii* (3) = *P. muliercula* (87)	Idem (3, 8, 16, 32, 58, 89)	Idem (3)
Santitos (S) *Netochutáta* (Mt) "sacred little ancestors" (91)	Matlazingas (91)	*P. wassonii* (3) = *P. muliercula* (87)	Idem (3, 8, 16, 32, 58, 89)	Idem (3)
Di-shi-tjo-le-rra-ja (Mz) "divine manure mushrooms" (3, 90)	Mazatecs (3, 90)	*P. cubensis* (87) = *Stropharia cubensis* (3)	Idem (3, 8, '16, 32, 58, 89)	Idem (3)
Di-nizé ta-a-ya (Mz) "mountain bird" (3, 90)	Mazatecs (87)	*P. yungensis* (87) *P. isauri* (87) *P. caerulipes* (87)	Idem (3, 8, 16, 32, 58, 89)	Psilocybin not found in *P. yungensis* (3)

Table 1 *(Continued)*

Name and etymology	Indian groups	Botanical sources	Cultural uses and effects	Phytochemistry
		Cactaceae (Cactus family)		
Peyote (S) (5) from *péyotl* (N) "covered by silk," "to prick, stimulate" (13), "bud," "shining one"	Evidence of pre-Columbian use by Chichimecas and Toltecs (5, 12) as well as north of Tarahumara area (2). Extensive evidence of use during colonial times (6, 13, 14, 21).	*Lophophora williamsii* = *Anhalonium lewinii* (20, 27)	Visionary psychodysleptic. Perception modifications. Increased visual imagery. Illusions. Hallucinations. Affective and intellectual alterations. Sympathomimetic effects. Euphoria. Decreased fatigue. Sleeplessness (21, 57).	Mescaline (*IV*; 3, 4, 5=CH_3O;R_1, R_2=H) (24, 25); biosynthesized from dopamine by activity of an O-methyltransferase (38, 59). Several dozen β-phenethylamines and isoquinolines such as anhalonidine (*V*; R_1, R_2, R_4=CH_3;R_3,R_5=H) (60).
Híkuli, Híkuli wanamé, Hikuli walula saeliami (T) (23, 52)	Tarahumara (23, 52, 92)	*Lophophora williamsii* (23)	Idem (21, 57). Used by Tarahumara long-distance runners (23, 52). Used sacramentally.	Idem (59, 60)
Hícuri (H) (35, 50, 93)	Huichol (35, 50, 93) Cora (50)	*Lophophora williamsii* (35, 50)	Idem (21, 57). Collected in yearly pilgrimage by the Huichol. Used sacramentally (35, 50).	Idem (59, 60)
Peyote cimarrón (S) *Híkuli sunami* (23) *Sunami* (T) (17)	Tarahumara (23, 52)	*Ariocarpus fissuratus* (23)	Used by runners for endurance (23).	Hordenine (*IV*; 4=OH; R_1, R_2=CH_3). N-Methyltyramine (*IV*; R_1=CH_3; R_2=H) (95).

Table 1 *(Continued)*

Falso peyote (S) (94) *Chaute* (H) (17)	Huichol (94)	*A. retusus* (94)	"Toxic." Poorly understood (94).	Idem (95)
Hikuli rosapari (T) *Hikuli mulato* (T-S) (23, 92)	Tarahumara (23, 92)	*Epithelantha micromeris* (23, 92)	Used by runners for endurance. "Increases vision" (23, 92).	—[e]
Peyote San Pedro (S) (17) *Witculiki, Wichuriki* (T) from *wichuwa-ka* (T) "madness" (52)	Tarahumara (52)	*Mammillaria heyderii* (52, 61)	Used by runners for endurance. "Clarifies vision" (52, 61).	N-methyl-3,4-dimethoxyphenethylamine (*IV*; 3,4=CH_3O; R_1=CH_3; R_2=H) (61)
Chilito, Biznaga de chilillos (S) (61)	Tarahumara (61)	*Mammillopsis senilis* (61)	Considered sacred by Tarahumara (61)	—
Bakana, Bakánawa (T) (52)	Tarahumara (52)	*Corypantha compacta* (52)	"A form of *híkuli*"; effects not defined (52).	N-methyl-3,4-dimethoxy-β-methoxyphenethylamine (*IV*; 3,4=CH_3O; R_1=CH_3; R_2=H; β=CH_3O) (96)
Híkuli (T) (52) *Pitallita* (S) (17)	Tarahumara (52)	*Echinocereus triglochidiatus* (52)	"Important mental changes" (23, 52)	Alkaloids isolated but not identified (see 52)
Chawé, Wichowaka (T) (92), *Cardón* (S) (17)	Tarahumara (52, 92)	*Pachycereus pecten-aboriginum* (52)	"Dizziness and visions" (92)	3-Hydroxy,4-methoxyphenethylamine (see 52)
Peyotillo (S) (61)	Used in San Luis Potosí (61, 97)	*Pelecyphora aselliformis* (61)	Used for fever and as a *peyote* substitute (61)	Several β-phenethylamines (61, 97), including trace amounts of mescaline (97)

Table 1 *(Continued)*

Name and etymology	Indian groups	Botanical sources	Cultural uses and effects	Phytochemistry
		Compositae (Composite family)		
Thle-pela-kano (Co) "god's leaf" (68) *Hoja madre* (S) "mother leaf" (47) *Zacatechichi*[f] (N) "bitter grass" (17)	Chontal (47, 68)	*Calea zacatechichi* (47, 68)	Imagery-inducing psychodysleptic. Brief and mild marihuana-like effects. Traditionally used to increase appetite. Used by Chontal to induce divinatory dreams (47).	Coumarins, lactones, terpenes (see 47)
Yauhtli, Yyahitl, Yyahutli (N) "dark one" (47) *Pericón*[f] (S) (17, 47)	Classic Náhuatl (5, 12)	*Tagetes lucida* (26)	Used for numbing senses of sacrificial victims (5)	Coumarins, lactones, terpenes (see 47)
Tumutsali (H) (70)	Huichol (47, 70)	*Tagetes lucida* (47, 70)	Huichol psychotropic smoking mixture with *Nicotiana rustica* (47, 70)	Coumarins, lactones, terpenes (see 47)
Peyote de Tepic (S) (18, 20)	—	*Senecio hartwegii* (18, 20)	These noncactaceous *peyotes* may have been used as psychotropic agents. Neurotoxic. Poorly defined CNS actions (47).	The genus *Senecio* is rich in pyrrolizidine alkaloids [(*VIII*), see 83].
Peyote del Valle de Mexico (S) (18, 20)	—	*Senecio* spp. (18, 20)	Idem (47)	Idem (see 83)
Peyote de Xochimilco (S) (18, 20)	—	*Senecio cardiophylus* (18, 20)	Idem (47)	Idem (see 83)
Peyote (S) (18, 20)	—	*Senecio grayanus* = *Senecio cervarifolius* (18, 20)	Idem (47)	Idem (see 83)

Table 1 *(Continued)*

Quantlapatzinzintli (N) Rabanillo (S) (84)	—	*Senecio tolucanus* (84)	Used to madden enemies (84)	Idem (see 83)
Palo loco (S) (98) "crazy stick"	—	*Senecio praecox* (98)	"Produces delusions" (98)	Idem (see 83) "Toxisenecine" (84)

Convolvulaceae (Morning Glory Family)

Ololiuhqui (N) (5, 12) "round thing" *Coaxíhuitl, Coatl xoxouhqui* (N) (5) "green snake" (13)	Used in pre-Columbian times by Náhuatl (5, 12). Documentation of use during colonial times (6, 13, 14, 99).	*Rivea corymbosa* = *Turbina corymbosa* = *Ipomoea sidaefolia* (18, 26, 29, 32)	Although the effects in the early chronicles were compared to *peyote*, these seeds are trance-inducing psychodysleptics. Biphasic effects: apathy, listlessness, sedation, fatigue, ultimately resulting in mental clarity. These effects are produced by seeds (73), ergot alkaloids, (74) and turbicoryn (75).	Ergot alkaloids, such as *d*-lysergic acid amide (*III*; $R=H_2$) and its isomer (34). Glucosides: turbicoryn (*XIV*; R_1=H; R_2=O–(CH–OH)$_3$–CH$_2$OH) and corymbosine (*XIV*; R_1=CH$_2$–O—(CH–OH)$_3$–CH$_2$–OH; R_2=H) (75).
Piule (Z) (26, 32) Semillas de la Virgen [f] (S) "seeds of the Virgin" (17, 32)	Zapotecs (26, 32)	*R.corymbosa* (26, 32)		Idem (34, 75)
A-mu-kia, Huan-mei (Ch) (29)	Chinantecs (29)	*R. corymbosa* (29)		Idem (34, 75)
No-so-le-na (Mz) (29) *Badoo, Bevan-la-si* (Z) "mystical being" (26)	Mazatecs (29) Zapotecs (26)	*R. corymbosa* (29) *R. corymbosa* (26)	Idem (73–75) Idem (73–75)	Idem (34, 75)
Tlitlitzen (N) "divine black one" (13)	Used during colonial times (13).	*Ipomoea violacea* = *I. tricolor* (32)	Idem (32)	Ergot alkaloids (34)
La'aja schnaash (Z) (32) *Badoh negro* (Mz-S) (26) *Jicama del monte* (S) "root of the mountain" (26)	Zapotecs (32) Mazatecs (26) Zapotecs (26)	*I. violacea* (32) *I. violacea* (32) *Exogonium bracteatum* (26)	Idem (32) Idem (32) Roots consumed for "narcotic effects" (26)	Idem (34) Idem (34) —

Table 1 *(Continued)*

Name and etymology	Indian groups	Botanical sources	Cultural uses and effects	Phytochemistry
		Cyperaceae (Sedge family)		
Bakánoa, Bakanawa, Bakana (T) (52)	Tarahumara (52)	*Scirpus* spp. (52)	Revered by the Tarahumara. "Profound sleep during which long distances are traveled" (52).	Harmala alkaloids [*II* (see 85)]
		Erythroxylaceae (Coca family)		
—	Yaqui (45)	*Erythroxylon* spp. *E. coca* *E. tabascence* (45)	Doubtful report of a Yaqui religious dance in which endurance was enhanced by eating bread made with coca leaves (45)	Cocaine (*VI*; 1=COO-∅; 2=COO–CH₃) (see 85)
		Labiatae (Mint family)		
Ska Pastora (Mz-S) "shepherdess leaf" (47, 71)	Mazatecs Chinantecs (26, 47, 71)	*Salvia divinorum* (100)	Used for divination and in shamanic training. Imagery-inducing, short-acting psychodysleptic. Sense of weightlessness. Affective alterations (47).	Two unidentified active compounds. Terpenes (47)
Marihuanilla (S) (47) "little marihuana" *Macho* (S) "male" (71)	Grows in Zoque territory (47) Mazatecs (71)	*Leonorus sibiricus* (47) *Coleus pumila* (71)	May be smoked as a marihuana substitute (47) Report of use similar to *Salvia divinorum* (71)	Leonurine, leonuridine (see 47) —
Nene (S) "baby" *Ahijado* (S) (71)	Mazatecs (71)	*C. blumei* (71)	Idem (71)	—

Table 1 *(Continued)*

		Lauraceae (Laurel family)		
Canela (S) "cinnamon"	Grows in the state of Chiapas	Cinnamomum zeylanicum (22)	Reports of marihuana-like effects in mixture with tobacco (45)	—
		Leguminosae (Pea family)		
Tzompanquahuitl (N) (17, 22) Colorín^f (S) Chilicote (S) Patol	May have been used in Mexico in colonial times (22, 26)	Erythrina coraloides (22)	Curare-like effects. Neurotoxic. Stupor. Convulsions. Paralysis. Hallucinations (22, 82).	Erythrinane alkaloids [IX (see 82)]
Kaposí, Aposhí (T) Chilicote^f (S) (17,52,92) coral bean	Tarahumara (52, 92)	E. flabelliformis (52)	Causes "erotic dreams." Used in medicine. Known nerve toxin (26, 52).	Idem (see 82)
—	Yaqui (101)	Cystius canariensis = Genista canariensis (101)	Used by medicine-men to induce visions (101)	Quinolizidine alkaloids, especially cytisine [VII (see 81)]
Piule (Z) (17) Negrito (S) (45)	Possible pre-Columbian representations (30). Zapotecs (26).	Rhynchosia longeracemosa = R. pyramidalis (26)	Used to produce "visions" (26)	Quinolizidine alkaloids [VII (see 81)]
Frijolillo, Chilicote (S) (1) Mescal bean, red bean	Pre-peyote cult in northeastern Mexico and southern Texas (1). Referred to by Cabeza de Vaca during the conquest (see 31).	Sophora secundiflora Sophora speciosa (V. H. Jones and W. L. Merrill, submitted for publication; see 30, 31)	Dizziness, numbness, hypothermia, stupor, visions (V. H. Jones and W. L. Merrill, submitted for publication; see 30, 31)	Quinolizidine alkaloids: cytisine, N-methylcytisine, sparteine [VII (see 102)]
Frijol del mar (S) (47) "bean of the sea"	Seeds found in graves in Oaxaca, Yucatan and Peru (300 BC – 900 AD) (103)	Canavalia maritima (47)	Smoked as a marihuana substitute on the Gulf Coast of Mexico (47)	l-Betonicine (see 47, 85)

Table 1 *(Continued)*

Name and etymology	Indian groups	Botanical sources	Cultural uses and effects	Phytochemistry
		Lythraceae (Loosestrife family)		
Sinicuiche (S) (19) from *xonocuilli* (N) "crooked foot" *Jarilla* (S) (47) *Yerba de las ánimas* (S) (17) "soul shrub"	Used by modern Nahua (19, 77) and in southern Veracruz (T. Knabb, personal communication)	*Heimia salicifolia* = *Nosoea salicifolia* (19)	As a fermented potion, produces sedation, auditory distortions. Uterotonic agent (19, 77; T. Knabb, personal communication).	*Heimia* alkaloids: Cryogenine (*X*; 1'-2;=CH=CH; R_1=OCH$_3$; R_2=H) (78). Psychoactive principles unknown (47).
		Malvaceae (Mallow family)		
Chichibe (S) *Malva de platanillo* (S) *Malva colorada* (S) (17, 98)	Used on the Gulf Coast near the Popoloca region (47)	*Sida acuta* (47)	Smoked as an energizer and marihuana substitute (47)	Ephedrine (*IV*; 3,4=OH; R_1, R_2=H; α=OOH; β=OH) (see 85)
Escobilla (S) *Huinar* (S) (17)	Idem (47)	*Sida rhombifolia* (47)	Idem (47)	Idem (see 85)
		Moraceae (Mulberry family)		
*Pipiltzintzintli*⁸ (N) (43) "venerable child" *Marihuana* (S)	Used as a psychotropic by Indians in 1772 (43). Ritually used by Tepehua and other groups (T. Knabb, unpublished observations).	*Cannabis sativa* (104)	Imagery-inducing psychodysleptic. Affective and thought alterations (64).	Dibenzopyran derivatives (*VIII*): Δ^9-tetrahydrocannabinol (*XIII*; 1=OH; 3=C$_5$ H$_{11}$; 9=CH$_3$) (67) and several dozen other cannabinoids (66)

Table.1 *(Continued)*

		Nymphaeaceae (Water lily family) / Solanaceae (Nightshade family)		
Quetzalaxochiatl[g] (N) "precious water flower" (see 47) Lila acuática (S) (17) "water lily"	Possible Mayan hallucinogen (48). Represented in ritual scenes in Mayan art (47, 48). Inebriating water plants mentioned in Náhuatl poetry (46, 47).	*Nymphea ampla* (47, 48)	Modern recreational use in Mayan areas. Reports of prolonged and powerful hallucinatory effects (47).	Aporphine alkaloids in the genus *Nymphea* [*XI* (see 47)]. One alkaloid isolated in *N. ampla* from Mayan region (47).
Tlápatl (N) "fire light," "red color," *Nacazul, Mixitl, Tolohuaxihuitl* (N) (5, 12) *Toloache*[f] (S) from *toloatzin* (N) "bowing venerable lord" and other names such as *toloachi, toloche, tolovachi, chamico* (17, 41)	Extensively used by Indian, mestizo, and urban groups from pre-Hispanic (5, 12) to colonial (99) and modern times (41, 45, 51).	*Datura* spp., section *Dutra:* *D. innoxia = D. metel;* section *Stramonium:* *D. stramonium* (30, 31, 41, 42).	Deliriant psychodysleptic. Anticholinergic CNS toxin. Delirium. Hallucinations. Anxiety. Disorientation (41). Used in shamanic training (51).	Tropane alkaloids, especially *l*-scopolamine (VI; $1{=}O{-}CO{-}CH(CH_2OH){-}\emptyset$; $4{-}5{=}{-}O{-}$) (see 79)
Dekuba, Tibuwari, Wichuri (T) (52)	Tarahumara (52)	*D. innoxia* (92)	Idem (41). Mixed with *tesguino*, a fermented maize drink. Used in shamanic rites (92).	Idem (79)
Kieli-sa (H) (35, 93)	Huichol (35, 93)	*D. stramonium* (35, 93)	Idem (41). Myths exist of a "datura person" (93).	Idem (79)

Table 1 *(Continued)*

Name and etymology	Indian groups	Botanical sources	Cultural uses and effects	Phytochemistry
Tecomaxochitl (N) *Floripondio*[f] (S) (17)	These trees are found associated with Indian houses in many areas (30, 31) (e.g. Mazatecs, Mixtecs)	*Datura* spp., section *Brugmansia*: e.g. *D. arborea, D. sanguinea, D. suaveolens* (30, 31, 42).	Intense initial agitation followed by a long disturbed sleep with vivid images (30, 31)	Idem (79)
Nexchuac (N) *Torna-loco* (S) (98) "maddening"	—	*Datura* spp., section *Ceratocaulis: D. ceratocaula* (98)	Deliriant psychodysleptic	Idem (79)
Huipatli, Tecomaxochitl (N) (98)	Ancient Náhuatl and modern use in Guerrero (98).	*Solandra guerrerensis* (98)	Deliriant psychodysleptic (98)	Idem (85)
Kieli (H) "god-plant" (105)	Huichol (105)	*Solandra brevicalix* (105)	Deliriant psychodysleptic. Worshiped as a deity. Said to produce fearful visions (105).	Idem (85)
Yetl (N) (5, 12, 13) *Quauyetl* (N) (13) tobacco	Indian religious use in pre-Columbian (5, 12) and colonial times (13, 14, 99). Widely used by modern Indian groups (32, 47).	*Nicotiana tabacum* (13)	Smoked and applied to ward off evil spirits in many Indian groups (32, 47). Suggested hallucinogenic action (106).	Nicotine, harmala alkaloids [*VI* (see 106)]
Picietl (N) (5, 12, 13) wild tobacco	Idem (5, 12, 13, 14, 32, 47, 70, 99)	*Nicotiana rustica* (13, 32)	Idem (32, 47, 106). Hallucinogenic mixture with *Tagetes lucida* used by the Huichol (47, 70).	Idem (see 106)

Table 1 *(Continued)*

Camotillo (S) from camotli (N) potato (45)	Mayan groups (45)	*Solanum tuberosum* (45)	Leaves are neurotoxic. Possible impairment of consciousness when ingested (45).	Saponine, solanine (see 45, 85)
Sterculiaceae (Chocolate family)				
Poyomatli (N) Poyomaxochitl (N) Cacaoquauitl (N) (5)	Náhuatl (5)	*Theobroma cacao* (see text)	Flower or early fruiting pod of cacao revered and used by ancient Náhuatl (5), especially Náhuatl poets [(46) see text]	Xanthine derivatives, especially theobromine (*XII*; $3,7=CH_3$) (see 85)
Turneraceae (Turnera family)				
Damiana[f] (S) (86) Hierba de la pastora (S) (17) "shepherdess herb"	Yaqui (86)	*Turnera diffusa* (86)	"Aphrodisiac." Used by northern Indians as an invigorator (86, 98)	Caffeine (*XII*; 1, 3, $7=CH_3$) (see 85)

[a] Capital letters after the name indicate language: C, Chatino; Ch, Chinantec; Co, Chontal; H, Huichol; Mt, Matlatzinga; Mz, Mazatec; N, Náhuatl; S, Spanish; T, Tarahumara; Z, Zapotec.

[b] Roman numerals correspond to chemical formulas pictured in Figure 1.

[c] Synonymous botanical denominations are denoted by an equals sign.

[d] Unless otherwise indicated, the plants are used in modern times by these groups.

[e] No information was found in regard to this category.

[f] Vulgar names used all over Mexico to designate the particular species.

[g] The identification of the vulgar name with the species is tentative.

ACKNOWLEDGMENTS

I thank the following persons for academic advice and criticism: R. Gordon Wasson, Richard E. Schultes, Efrén del Pozo, and Alfredo López Austin. Original studies in the author's laboratories were supported by a grant from Centro Mexicano de Estudios en Farmacodependencia (BC 1–73, BC 6–74, BC 9–75), the Scottish Rite Schizophrenia Research Program, and Instituto Mexicano para el Estudio de las Plantas Medicinales. I thank John Bailin for his corrections and Marcella Vogt for her careful assistance, helpful suggestions, and criticism during the preparation of this review.

Literature Cited

1. Adovasio, J. M., Fry, G. S. 1972. *Prehistoric Psychotropic Drug Use in Northeastern Mexico and Trans-Pecos Texas.* Presented at Ann. Meet. Am. Anthropol. Assoc., 71st, Toronto, Canada
2. Dipeso, C. C. 1974. *Casas Grandes, a Fallen Trading Center of the Gran Chichimeca.* Dragoon, Ariz.: Amerind Found.
3. Heim, R., Wasson, R. G. 1958. *Les Champignons Hallucinogènes du Mexique.* Paris: Arch. Mus. Natl. Hist. Nat. 324 pp.
4. Caso, A. 1963. Representaciones de hongos en los códices. *Estud. Cult. Náhuatl* 4:27–36
5. de Sahagún, B. 1950–1969. *Florentine Codex,* ed. A. J. O. Anderson, C. E. Dibble. Santa Fe, NM: Sch. Am. Res. and Univ. Utah
6. de la Serna, J. 1656. *Manual de Ministros de Indios.* Reproduced in 1892. *An. Mus. Nac. Méx.* 6:269–450
7. Motolinia, T. ca. 1541. *Historia de los Indios de Nueva España.* Reproduced in 1858–1866. *Colección de Documentos para la Historia de México,* ed. J. C. Icazbalceta. México: Andrade
8. Wasson, V. P., Wasson, R. G. 1958. *The Hallucinogenic Mushrooms.* New York: NY Bot. Gard.
9. Lowy, B. 1971. New records of mushroom stones from Guatemala. *Mycologia* 63:983–93
10. de Sahagún, B. 1956. *Historia General de las Cosas de la Nueva España.* México: Porrúa. 4 vols.
11. López-Austin, A. 1965. Descripción de estupefacientes en el Códice Florentino. *Rev. Univ. Mex.* 19:17–18
12. Hernández, F. 1942, 1943, 1946. *Historia de las Plantas de Nueva España.* México: Inst. Biol., Univ. Nac. Autón. Méx. 3 vols.
13. Aguirre Beltrán, G. 1963. *Medicina y Magia. El Proceso de Aculturación en la Estructura Colonial.* México: Inst. Nac. Indig. 443 pp.
14. Ruiz de Alarcón, H. 1629. *Tratado de las Supersticiones y Costumbres Gentilicias que oy viuen entre los Indios Naturales desta Nueua España.* Reproduced in 1892. Mexico: Imprenta Mus. Nac. Méx., pp. 125–260
15. López-Austin, A. 1967. Términos del Nahuallatolli. *Historia Mexicana.* 17:1–36, Mexico: Col. Méx.
16. Wasson, R. G., Cowan, G., Cowan, F., Rhodes, W. 1974. *María Sabina and her Mazatec Mushroom Velada.* New York & London: Harcourt Brace & Jovanovich. 279 pp.
17. Díaz, J. L. 1976. *Indice y Sinonimia de las Plantas Medicinales de México.* México: Inst. Méx. Estud. Plant. Med. 358 pp.
18. Urbina, M. 1903. El peyote y el ololiuhqui. *An. Mus. Nac. Méx.* 7:25–48
19. Calderón, J. B. 1896. Estudio sobre el arbusto llamado Sinicuiche. *Anal. Inst. Med. Nac. Mex.* 2:36–42
20. Peyotes, datos para su estudio. 1899. *Anal. Inst. Med. Nac. Mex.* 4:203–14
21. El peyote (Historia, botánica, composición química, acción fisiológica, efectos terapéuticos). 1914. *Anal. Inst. Med. Nac. Mex.* 12:183–243
22. Altamirano, F. 1876. Leguminosas indígenas medicinales. *La Naturaleza* 3:382–425
23. Lumholtz, C. 1902. *Unknown Mexico.* New York: Scribner's
24. Heffter, A. 1896. Ueber Cacteenalkaloide. *Ber. Dtsch. Chem. Ges.* Band I. 29:216–33
25. Späth, E. 1919. Ueber die Anhalonium Alkaloide. I. Anholin und Mezcalin. *Monatscshr. Chem.* 40:129–52

26. Reko, B. P. 1945. *Mitobotánica Zapoteca.* Tacubaya, Mexico, private ed.
27. Schultes, R. E. 1937. Peyote _(Lophophora williamsii)_ and plants confused with it. *Bot. Mus. Leafl. Harv. Univ.* 5:61–88
28. Schultes, R. E. 1939. Plantae Mexicanae. II. The identification of teonanácatl, a narcotic Basidiomycete of the Aztecs. *Bot. Mus. Leafl. Harv. Univ.* 7:37–54
29. Schultes, R. E. 1941. *A Contribution to Our Knowledge of Rivea corymbosa: The Ancient Narcotic Oloiuqui of the Aztecs.* Cambridge, Mass.: Bot. Mus. Harv. Univ. 45 pp.
30. Schultes, R. E. 1969. The plant kingdom and hallucinogens. *Bull. Narcotics* 21:1–56
31. Schultes, R. E., Hofmann, A. 1973. *The Botany and Chemistry of Hallucinogens.* Springfield, Ill.: Thomas
32. Wasson, R. G. 1963. Notes on the present status of ololiuhqui and other hallucinogens of Mexico. *Bot. Mus. Leafl. Harv. Univ.* 20:161–93
33. Hofmann, A., Heim, R., Brack, A., Kobel, H. 1958. Psilocybin, ein psychotroper Wirkstoff aus mexikanischen Rauschpilz *Psilocybe mexicana* Heim. *Experientia* 14:107–12
34. Hofmann, A. 1963. The active principles of the seeds of *Rivea corymbosa* and *Ipomoea violacea. Bot. Mus. Leafl. Harv. Univ.* 20:194–212
35. Furst, P. T. 1976. *Hallucinogens and Culture.* San Francisco: Chandler & Sharp. 194 pp.
36. La Barre, W .1970. Old and New World narcotics: A statistical question and an ethnological reply. *Econ. Bot.* 24:368–73
37. Small, E., Beckstead, H. D. 1973. Cannabinoid phenotypes in *Cannabis sativa. Nature* 245:147–48
38. Paul, A. G. 1973. Biosynthesis of the peyote alkaloids. *Lloydia* 36:36–45
39. Siegel, R. K. 1973. An ethologic search for self-administration of hallucinogens. *Int. J. Addict.* 8:373–93
40. Dobkin de Ríos, M. 1975. Una teoría transcultural del uso de los alucinógenos de origen vegetal. In *Etnofarmacología de Plantas Alucinógenas Latinoamericanas,* ed. J. L. Díaz, 17–34. México: Cent. Mex. Estud. Farmacodependencia
41. Safford, W. E. 1916. Narcotic plants and stimulants of the ancient Americans. *Smithsonian Report,* 387–424. Washington, D.C.: GPO
42. Matuda, E. 1952. El género Datura en Mexico. *Bol. Soc. Bot. Mex.* 14:1–13
43. Alzate y Ramirez, A. 1772. El cáñamo, algunas costumbres de los indios. *Gaz. Lit.* 4:95–102
44. *Instrucciones Para Sembrar, Cultivar y Beneficiar el Lino y el Cáñamo en Nueva España.* 1796. Manuscript in the private library of M. R. Gomez
45. Guerra, F. 1954. *Las Plantas Fantásticas de México.* México: Imprenta Diario Esp.
46. Garibay, K. A. M. 1968. *Poesía Náhuatl. Cantares Mexicanos. Manuscrito de la Biblioteca Nacional de Mexico.* Mexico: Inst. Invest. Hist., Univ. Nac. Autón. Méx. 3rd vol. 74 pp.
47. Díaz, J. L. 1975. Etnofarmacología de algunos psicotrópicos vegetales de Mexico. See Ref. 40, pp. 135–202
48. Dobkin de Ríos, M. 1973. The nonwestern use of hallucinogenic agents. In *Drug Use in America: Problem in Perspective, 2nd Rep. Natl. Comm. Marihuana Drug Abuse, Washington D.C.* Appendix, 1:1170–1235
49. Naranjo, P. 1975. Drogas psiquedélicas en Medicina Mágica. See Ref. 40, pp. 73–92
50. Nahmad, S., Klineberg, O., Furst, P. T., Meyerhoff, B. G. 1972. *El Peyote y los Huicholes.* Mexico: SEP Setentas. Secr. Educac. Pública
51. Castaneda, C. 1968. *The Teachings of Don Juan: a Yaqui Way of Knowledge.* New York: Ballantine
52. Bye, R. 1975. Plantas Psicotrópicas de los tarahumaras. See Ref. 40, pp. 49–72
53. Eliade, M. 1964. *Shamanism. Archaic Techniques of Ecstasy.* Bolingen Ser. LXXVI. Princeton: Princeton Univ. Press
54. Brawley, P., Duffield, J. C. 1972. The pharmacology of hallucinogens. *Pharmacol. Rev.* 24:31–66
55. Delay, J., Deniker, P. 1961. *Méthodes Chimiothérapeutiques en Psychiatrie. Les Neuveaux Medicaments Psychotropes.* Paris: Masson. 496 pp.
56. Von Bibra, E. F. 1855. *Die Narkotischen Genussmittel und der Mensch.* Nürnberg: Verlag von Wilhelm Schmid
57. Beringer, K. 1927. *Der Meskalinrausch; seine Geschichte und Erscheinungsweise. Monogr. Gesamtgeb. Neurol. Psychiatr.* 49:35–89, 119–315
58. Delay, J., Pichot, P., Lempérière, T., Nicolas-Charles, P. 1958. Effets psychophysiologiques de la psilocybine. *C. R. Acad. Sci.,* 247:1235–38

59. Kapadia, G. J., Fayez, M. B. E. 1970. Peyote constituents: chemistry, biogenesis and biological effects. *J. Pharm. Sci.* 59:1699–1727

60. Kapadia, G. J., Fayez, M. B. E. 1973. The chemistry of peyote alkaloids. *Lloydia* 36:9–35

61. Bruhn, J. G., Bruhn, C. 1973. Alkaloids and ethnobotany of Mexican peyote cacti and related species. *Econ. Bot.* 27:241–51

62. Hofmann, A. 1970. The discovery of LSD and subsequent investigations on naturally occurring hallucinogens. In *Discoveries in Biological Psychiatry,* ed. F. J. Ayd, B. Blackwell, 91–106. Philadelphia & Toronto: Lippincott. 254 pp.

63. Szara, S. 1956. Dimethyltryptamine: Its metabolism in man: The relation of its psychotic effect to serotonin metabolism. *Experientia* 12:441–42

64. Moreau, J. J. 1845. *Du Hachisch et de l'Aliénation Mentale. Etudes Psychologiques.* Paris: Masson. 431 pp.

65. Schultes, R. E. 1973. Man and marijuana. *Nat. Hist.* 82:59–63

66. Mechoulam, R. 1970. Marihuana chemistry. *Science* 168:1159–66

67. Mechoulam, R., Gaoni, Y. 1965. A total synthesis of dl-Δ^1-tetrahydrocannabinol, the active constituent of hashish. *J. Am. Chem. Soc.* 87:3273–75

68. MacDougall, T. A. 1968. A Compositae with psychic properties? *Gard. J.* 18:105

69. Del Castillo, J., Anderson, M., Rubottom, G. M. 1975. Marijuana, absinthe and the central nervous system. *Nature* 253:365–66

70. Siegel, R. K., Collins, P. R., Díaz, J. L. On the use of *Tagetes lucida* and *Nicotiana rustica* as Huichol smoking mixture. The Aztec "yahutli" with suggestive hallucinogenic effects. *Econ. Bot.* In press

71. Wasson, R. G. 1962. A new psychoactive drug from the mint family. *Bot. Mus. Leafl. Harv. Univ.* 20:77–84

72. Shulgin, A. T., Sargent, T., Naranjo, C. 1973. Animal pharmacology and human psychopharmacology of 3-methoxy-4, 5-methylenedioxyphenylisopropylamine (MMDD:). *Pharmacology.* 10:12–18

73. Osmond, H. 1955. *Ololiuhqui:* The ancient Aztec narcotic. *J. Ment. Sci.* 101:526–36

74. Isbell, H., Gorodetzky, C. W. 1966. Effect of alkaloids of *ololiuqui* m man. *Psychopharmacologia* 8:331–39

75. Perezamador, M. C., García Jimenez, F., Herrán, J., Flores, S. E. 1964. Structure of turbicoryn, a new glucoside from *Turbina corymbosa. Tetrahedron* 20:2999–3009

76. Hoffer, A., Osmond, H. 1967. *The Hallucinogens.* New York: Academic

77. Reko, V. A. 1936. *Magische Gifte. Rausche-und Betäubungsmittel der Neuen Welt.* Stuttgart: Ferdinand Enke Verlag

78. Dobberstein, R. H., Edwards, J. M., Schwarting, A. E. 1975. The sequential appearance and metabolism of alkaloids in *Heimia salicifolia. Phytochemistry* 14:1769–75

79. Fodor, G. 1967. The tropane alkaloids. In *The Alkaloids.* ed. R. H. F. Manske, IX:269–304. New York: Academic

80. Wangeman, C. P., Hawk, M. H. 1942. The effects of morphine, atropine and scopolamine on human subjects. *Anesthesiology* 3:24–36

81. Bohlmann, F., Schumann, D. 1967. Lupine alkaloids. See Ref. 79, pp. 175–222.

82. Hill, R. K. 1967. The Erythrina alkaloids. See Ref. 79, IX: 483–515

83. Warren, F. L. 1970. Senecio alkaloids. See Ref. 79, XII: 246–332

84. Vélez, T. 1897. Rabanillo-*Senecio tolucanus.* In *Nueva Recopilación de Monografías Mexicanas y Tesis Inaugurales de Materia Médica,* pp. 159–65. México: Folletines Estud. An. Inst. Méd. Nac.

85. Raffauf, R. F. 1970. *A Handbook of Alkaloids and Alkaloid-Containing Plants.* New York:Interscience.

86. Ramirez, J. 1903. La Damiana.-*Turnera diffusa* afrodisiaca. *An. Inst. Med. Nac. Mex.* 5:238–43

87. Singer, R. 1958. Mycological investigations on *teonanácatl,* the Mexican hallucinogenic mushroom. *Mycologia* 50:239–303

88. Ola'h, G. M. 1970. Le genre Panaeolus: Essai taxinomique et physiologique. *Rev. Mycol.* Mem. hors-serie No. 10.

89. Nieto, D. 1959. Psicosis experimentales. Efectos psíquicos del hongo *Stropharia cubensis* de Oaxaca. *Neurol. Neurochir. Psiquiatr. Mex.* 1:6–16

90. Guzmán, H. G. 1959. Sinopsis de los conocimientos sobre los hongos alucinógenos mexicanos. *Bol. Soc. Bot. Mex.* 24:14–34

91. Escalante, R., López, A. 1971. *Hongos Sagrados de los Matlatzingas.* Ser. mimiográfica No. 4. México:Mus. Nac. Antropol. 15 pp.

92. Pennington, C. W. 1963. *The Tarahumara of Mexico.* Salt Lake City:Univ. Utah Press

93. Zingg, R. M. 1938. *The Huicholes: Primitive Artists.* New York:Streckert

94. Furst, P. T. 1971. *Ariocarpus retusus* the "False Peyote" of the Huichol tradition. *Econ. Bot.* 25:182–87

95. McLaughlin, J. L. 1969. Cactus alkaloids. VI. Identification of hordenine and N-methyl-tyramine in *Ariocarpus fissuratus* varieties *fissuratus* and *lloydii. Lloydia* 32:392–94

96. Bruhn, J. G., Agurell, S., Lindgren, J.-E. 1975. Cactaceae alkaloids. XXI. Phenethylamine alkaloids of *Coryphantha* species. *Acta Pharm. Suec.* 12:199–204

97. Neal, J. M., Sato, P. T., Howald, W. N., McLaughlin, J. L. 1972. Peyote alkaloids: Identification in the Mexican cactus *Pelecyphora asselliformis* Ehrenberg. *Science* 176:1131–33

98. Martínez, M. 1945. *Las Plantas Medicinales de Mexico.* Mexico:Ediciones Botas

99. Acosta, J. 1590. *Historia Natural y Moral de las Indias.* Published in 1940. México:Fondo Cult. Econ.

100. Epling, C., Játiva, M. C. D. 1962. A new species of *Salvia* from Mexico. *Bot. Mus. Leafl. Harv. Univ.* 20:75–76

101. Fadiman, J. 1965. *Genista canarensis*— A minor psychedelic. *Econ. Bot.* 19: 383–84

102. Keller, W. J. 1975. Alkaloids from *Sophora secundiflora. Phytochemistry* 14:2305–6

103. Sauer, J., Kaplan, L. 1969. Canavalia beans in American prehistory. *Am. Antiq.* 34:417–24

104. Schultes, R. E., Klein, W. M., Plowman, T., Lockwood, T. E. 1974. *Cannabis:* an example of taxonomic neglect. *Bot. Mus. Leafl. Harv. Univ.* 23:337–67

105. Knab, T. 1976. Notes concerning use of *Solandra* among the Huichol. *Econ. Bot.* In press

106. Janiger, O., Dobkin de Ríos, M. 1973. Suggestive hallucinogenic properties of tobacco. *Med. Anthropol. Newsl.* 4:6–11

Ann. Rev. Pharmacol. Toxicol. 1977. 17:677–82
Copyright © 1977 by Annual Reviews Inc. All rights reserved

REVIEW OF REVIEWS[1]   ✦6701

Chauncey D. Leake
University of California, San Francisco, California 94143

An interesting development is occurring in the reviewing of pharmacological progress: more and more reviews of a particular field of pharmacological concern are appearing as symposia in book form. This has many advantages. It brings together current data and current opinion in that area. Yet, it cannot offer the broad coverage of pharmacological and toxicological advance as is done so well by *Annual Review of Pharmacology and Toxicology.*

It is significant that the former *Annual Review of Pharmacology* now includes *Toxicology.* This aids in keeping the discipline from fragmenting into competitive in-groups. Toxicology differs from pharmacology chiefly in a quantitative manner. Both deal with the interactions of chemical compounds, at a molecular level, with molecules of living material. These interactions proceed through the levels of organization of living material from subcellular units, cells, organ and tissues, individuals, societies to ecologies. Toxic effects can occur anywhere along the way.

Another review periodical in pharmacology, *Clinical Pharmacokinetics,* is appearing under the editorship of G. S. Avery of Auckland, New Zealand. Many significant review articles are already scheduled. The international scope of this bimonthly is indicated by its publication by Adis Press International of Hong Kong.

GENERAL

With 113 references, Hartshorn reviews interactions of psychotherapeutic agents. McMahon edits an important series of monographs on principles and methods of human research and therapeutics. These range from general principles through drug-induced toxicity, pharmacokinetics, and experimental design to special types of drugs such as cardiovascular, endocrine, and psychotherapeutic agents. Rossoff compiles a compendium of 1800 drugs used in veterinary medicine.

Pointing out that there are accessory reproductive organs in mammals, Spaziani reviews the control of cell and tissue transport by sex hormones. The six volumes of *Proceedings of the Sixth International Congress of Pharmacology* held in Helsinki

[1]This review was completed July 1, 1976, for material available at that time. References are cited by author, without numbering. Names are arranged alphabetically for convenience.

in 1975 are edited by Tuomisto & Paasonen. These go from receptors and neuro-transmission through behavioral and clinical pharmacology to mechanisms of tox-icity and metabolism. A cumulative edition of *USP Dictionary of Drug Names* appears, with listing of more than 4000 brand names and 1700 code designations of investigational drugs.

ABSORPTION, METABOLISM, AND EXCRETION OF DRUGS

Csaky edits 20 reports on intestinal absorption and malabsorption of various drugs. Dews introduces four discussions on schedule-induced olydipsia with oral intake of drugs, mostly on ethanol. With significance for drug design, Lien reviews the absorption and distribution of drugs in relation to their chemical structure.

Guldberg & Marsden review, with 442 references, the pharmacological aspects and physiological role of catechol-o-methyl transferase, with respect to its properties and wide distribution. Lindquist reviews the design of enzyme inhibitors from the standpoint of transition state analogues.

With 44 references, Mirkin reviews the placental transfer of drugs, with regard to fetal localization and neonatal disposition. Morselli, Garattini & Sereni edit an important symposium on basic and therapeutic aspects of perinatal pharmacology. This includes discussions of placental transfer, effects of narcotics, toxicity consider-ations, and developmental interactions. Rane & Wilson review clinical pharmacoki-netics in infants and children. They survey developmental body water compart-ments, kidney changes, bronchodilators, cardiac glycosides, antihypertensives, an-timicrobials, anticonvulsants, and analgesics.

The effects of oral contraceptives on vitamin metabolism are reviewed by Ander-son, Bodansky & Kappas. The metabolism of drugs administered by aerosols is surveyed by Davies.

DIAGNOSTIC DRUGS

Counsell & Ice review the design of organ-imaging radiopharmaceuticals. The design of X-ray contrast media is analyzed by Herms & Vitaenzer. Drug analysis in clinical laboratories is nicely reviewed by Wallace, Hamilton & Schwertner. With 35 references, they emphasize the increasing accuracy of rapid methods.

CHEMOTHERAPY AND ANTIBIOTICS

Some 46 surveys on the mechanism of action of antimicrobial and antitumor agents are edited by Corcoran & Hahn. Some 20 reviews of clinical cancer chemotherapy are edited by Greenspan. Rational combinations of antimetabolites for cancer che-motherapy are considered by Grindey, Moran & Werkheiser.

Walker & Weiss review the chemotherapy of treatment of malignant brain tu-mors. Warren edits six surveys of current chemotherapy from antibiotics through antifungal agents and antineoplastic agents to antiparasitic and antiviral com-pounds.

ALLERGY AND IMMUNITY

Assem makes important survey of drugs with prophylactic anti-allergy effects. Bach reviews in a welcome monograph the mode of action of immunosuppressive agents, dealing with corticosteroids, thiopurine, alkylating agents, and antilymphatic sera. He offers helpful clinical guidelines for their effective use.

DRUGS ACTING ON NERVES AND NERVOUS SYSTEMS

Eichler edits comprehensive reviews on coffee and caffeine, covering history, chemistry, biological activity, metabolism, effect of cAMP-phosphodiesterase, toxicity, and potential mutagenicity. Fielding & Lal edit 14 essays on antidepressants from chemistry and mode of action to treatment of depressive illnesses. Gordon edits five reviews on central nervous system agents, from antianxiety and narcotic antagonists to sedatives, anticonvulsants, and general anesthetics. Logan reviews neurological aspects of hallucinogenic drugs. Nicholson & Lader edit a symposium on the evaluation of psychotropic drugs, mostly on screening models and on clinical appraisal.

Nachmansohn, in discussing the chemical and molecular basis of nerve activity, considers the properties and functions of the proteins of the acetylcholine cycle in excitable membranes. He points toward a molecular model of bioelectricity. Paton edits 17 reviews on membrane transport processes utilized by noradrenaline and related amines. Singhal, Rastogi & Hrdina give a minireview on brain biogenic amines and altered thyroid function. Smithies offers an all-protein model for the molecular structure of both acetylcholine and adrenergic receptors. Usdin & Kvetnansky edit comprehensive reviews on the actions of catecholamines in stress.

ANALGESICS, NARCOTICS, AND DEPENDENCY

Burns and associates report on phenozelidine, an analgesic related to ketamine, now a street drug smoked over parsley, which causes myoclonus, vomiting, and coma. Cotten edits a symposium of 26 discussions on drug dependence, with control of drug taking by schedules of reinforcement. Dews introduces four discussions on schedule-induced polydipsia with oral intake of drugs, mostly on ethanol.

Among the 54 essays in the International Narcotic Research Club conference on opiate narcotics is an important one by Goldstein and colleagues on a peptide-like substance from the pituitary which has morphine-like effects. Iversen reviews behavioral pharmacology, using animal models in developing clinically useful drugs. Krasnegor introduces five reviews on behavioral factors in human drug abuse.

Lemberger & Rubin offer a minireview on the physiological disposition of marijuana (hemp) in humans. Lieber summarizes studies on metabolism of ethanol and of the effects of overdosage on liver cells and enzyme systems. Majchrowicz edits 18 in-depth reviews on the biochemical pharmacology of ethanol from microsomal oxidation to genetic determinants of alcohol addiction.

CARDIOVASCULAR-RENAL

Using 305 references, Dauchot & Gravenstein caution about the use of atropine in treating bradycardia after myocardial ischemia. Davies & Reid edit 26 comprehensive reviews on the central effects of drugs on blood pressure regulation, from adrenergic mechanisms to clonidine, and to the relation of reserpine to breast cancer.

Iseri, Freed & Bures review the relation of magnesium deficiency to cardiac disorders. Kritchevsky edits 10 in-depth reviews on hypolipidemic agents, ranging from cholesterol metabolism through vascular enzymes and specific drugs to the rationale for hypolipidemic therapy.

Francis offers a short review of new cardiovascular agents, while Schultz, Smith & Woltersdorf do likewise for diuretics. Needleman edits nine helpful surveys of organic nitrates, with much on metabolism. Wilson chairs a symposium on the sulphamoyl diuretic, bumetamide, with 21 reports.

TOXICOLOGY

With 79 references, Bender reviews salicylate intoxication, noting that aspirin is the most frequent drug involved in accidental poisoning. Coulston & Korte edit 30 essays on environmental quality and safety from air pollution to pesticides and herbicides. Goodman, Bischel, Wagers & Barbour describe common features of barbiturate intoxication, with pneumonia as the chief factor in morbidity and mortality. A recent report from the International Agency for Research on Cancer evaluates the carcinogenic risk of exposure to various chemicals, dealing mostly with aziridines, mustards, and selenium.

CLINICAL

Aicardi surveys drugs used in the treatment of petit mal. Cluff, Caranasos & Stewart broadly discuss various clinical problems occurring with drugs. Greenblatt edits 11 reviews on drugs used in combination with other therapies. It deals mostly with psychotropic therapy in schizophrenia, depression, and alcoholism. Hirsh, Gent & Genton review platelet suppressive drugs used in the treatment of thrombosis. A short practical review of barbiturate therapy was given by Hoskins for American Hospital Formulary Service.

With 67 references, Lunan reviews topical treatment of burn patients, mostly with silver salts and antibiotics. Simpson edits 13 reviews on drug treatment of mental disorders, from phenothiazines to lithium. Weiss edits 18 reviews on cyclic nucleotides in disease, ranging from cancer and cardiovascular disease, to endocrine and central nervous disorders.

MISCELLANEOUS

Gaetano reviews pharmacology of platelet aggregation. Goldberg & Ramwell well cover the role of prostaglandins in reproduction. With 65 references, Hemminki reviews factors influencing drug prescription, not surprisingly concluding that advertising and detailing by drug firms are most important. Houck edits 22 reviews and bibliography on chalones and their control of cell growth. Chalones may become major adjuncts to chemotherapy and immunosuppression.

Mead describes free radical mechanisms of lipid damage and resulting consequences for cell membrane injury. Mendlewicz edits selected papers dealing with genetics and psychopharmacology, such as involved in plasma dopamine β-hydroxylase. Parsons edits 21 reviews of peptide hormones from amino acid sequences to regulation of protein synthesis. With 89 references, Yosselson reviews the effects of drugs on nutritional factors from amino acids to vitamins.

IN PROSPECT

As reviews in pharmacology become more technical, and symposia volumes more diverse, an annual survey of them may aid in maintaining perspective and balance for the discipline as a whole.

Literature Cited

Aicardi, J. 1975. *Therapie* 30:161–74
Anderson, K. E., Bodansky, O., Kappas, A. 1976. *Adv. Clin. Chem.* 18:248–88
Assem, E. S. K. 1975. In *Allergy '74,* 93–107. New York: Grune & Stratton
Bach, J-F. 1975. *Mode of Action of Immunosuppressive Agents.* Amsterdam: Excerpta Med. 398 pp.
Bender, K. J. 1975. *Drug Intell. Clin. Pharm.* 9:350–60
Burns, R. S. et al 1975. *West J. Med.* 123:345–49
Cluff, L. E., Caranasos, G. J., Stewart, R. B. 1975. *Clinical Problems with Drugs.* Philadelphia: Saunders. 308 pp.
Corcoran, J. W., Hahn, F. E. 1975. *Mechanism of Action of Antimicrobial and Antitumor Agents.* New York: Springer. 750 pp.
Cotten, M. deV. 1975. *Pharmacol. Rev.* 27:291–446
Coulston, F., Korte, F. 1975. *Global Aspects of Chemistry, Toxicology and Technology as Applied to Environment.* Stuttgart: Thieme. 276 pp.
Counsell, R. E., Ice, R. D. 1975. *Drug Design* 6:172–262
Csaky, T. Z. 1975. *Intestinal Absorption and Malabsorption.* New York: Raven. 308 pp.
Dauchot, P., Gravenstein, J. S. 1976. *Anesthesiology* 44:501–18
Davies, D. S. 1975. *Lung Metabolism,* 201–18. New York: Academic
Davies, D. S., Reid, J. L. 1976. *Central Effects of Drugs on Blood Pressure Reg-*

ulation. Baltimore: Univ. Park Press. 320 pp.
Dews, P. B. 1975. *Pharmacol. Rev.* 27:447–98
Eichler, O. 1975. *Kaffee und Coffein.* Berlin: Springer. 580 pp.
Fielding, S., Lal, H., eds. 1975. *Antidepressants.* Mt. Kisco, NY: Futura. 370 pp.
Francis, J. E. 1975. *Ann. Rep. Med. Chem.* 10:61–70
Gaetano, G. 1975. *Pharmacol. Res. Commun.* 7:301–10
Goldberg, V. J., Ramwell, P. W. 1975. *Physiol. Rev.* 55:305–51
Goldstein, A. et al 1975. *The Opiate Narcotics,* 19–31. New York: Pergamon
Goodman, J. M., Bischel, M. D., Wagers, P. W., Barbour, B. H. 1976. *West. J. Med.* 124:179–86
Gordon, M. 1975. *Ann. Rep. Med. Chem.* 10:1–50
Greenblatt, M., ed. 1975. *Drugs in Combination with Other Therapies.* New York: Grune & Stratton. 202 pp.
Greenspan, E. M., ed. 1975. *Clinical Cancer Chemotherapy.* New York: Raven. 414 pp.
Grindey, G. B., Moran, R. G., Werkheiser, W. C. 1975. *Drug Design* 5:170–251
Guldberg, H. C., Marsden, C. A. 1975. *Pharmacol. Rev.* 27:135–206
Hartshorn, E. A. 1975. *Drug Intell. Clin. Pharm.* 9:536–50
Hemminki, E. 1976. *Drug Intell. Clin. Pharm.* 10:321–29
Herms, H. G., Vitaenzer, V. 1975. *Drug Design* 6:263–97

Hirsh, J., Gent, M., Genton, E. 1975. *Thrombosis* 33:406–16

Hoskins, N. M. 1976. *Am. J. Hosp. Pharm.* 33:333–39

Houck, J. C. 1976. *Chalones.* Amsterdam: North-Holland. 540 pp.

International Agency for Research on Cancer, Lyons. 1975. *Evaluation of Carcinogenic Risk of Chemicals.* 208 pp.

Iseri, L. T., Freed, J., Bures, A. R. 1975. *Am. J. Med.* 58:837–46

Iversen, S. D., Iversen, L. L. 1975. *Behavioral Pharmacology.* New York: Oxford Univ. Press. 320 pp.

Krasnegor, N. A. 1975. *Pharmacol. Rev.* 27:499–548

Kritchevsky, D. 1975. *Hypolipidemic Agents.* New York: Springer. 488 pp.

Lemberger, L., Rubin, A. 1975. *Life Sci.* 17:1637–42

Lieber, C. S. 1976. *Sci. Am.* 234:25–33

Lien, E. J. 1975. *Drug Design* 5:81–132

Lindquist, R. N. 1975. *Drug Design* 5:24–80

Logan, W. J. 1975. *Adv. Neurol.* 13:47–78

Lunan, H. N. 1975. *Am. J. Hosp. Pharm.* 32:599–605

McMahon, F. G., ed. 1974–1975. *Principles and Techniques of Human Research and Therapeutics.* Mt. Kisco, NY: Futura. 9 vols.

Majchrowicz, E. 1975. *Biochemical Pharmcology of Ethanol.* New York: Plenum. 368 pp.

Mead, J. F. 1976. *Free Radicals in Biology,* 51–68. New York: Academic

Mendlewicz, J., ed. 1975. *Genetics and Psychopharmacology.* Basel: Karger. 140 pp.

Mirkin, B. L., ed. 1976. *Perinatal Pharmacology and Therapeutics.* New York: Academic. 464 pp.

Morselli, P. L., Garattini, S., Sereni, F., eds. 1975. *Basic and Therapeutic Aspects of Perinatal Pharmacology.* New York: Raven. 440 pp.

Nachmansohn, D. 1975. *Chemical and Molecular Basis of Nerve Activity.* New York: Academic. 403 pp.

Needleman, P., ed. 1975. *Organic Nitrates.* New York: Springer. 196 pp.

Nicholson, P. A., Lader, M. H., eds. 1976. *Br. J. Clin. Pharmacol.* 3:(Suppl. 1) 109 pp.

Parsons, J. A., ed. 1976. *Peptide Hormones.* Baltimore: Univ. Park Press. 382 pp.

Paton, D. M., ed. 1975. *The Mechanism of Neuronal and Extraneuronal Transport of Catecholamines.* New York: Raven. 405 pp.

Rane, A., Wilson, J. T. 1976. *Clin. Pharmacokinetics* 1:2–24

Rossoff, I. S. 1974. *Handbook of Veterinary Drugs.* New York: Springer. 730 pp.

Schultz, E. M., Smith, R. I., Woltersdorf, O. W. 1975. *Ann. Rep. Med. Chem.* 10:71–79

Singhal, R. L., Rastogi, R. B., Hrdina, P. D. 1975. *Life Sci.* 17:1617–26

Simpson, L. L., ed. 1975. *Drug Treatment of Mental Disorders.* New York: Raven. 425 pp.

Smithies, A. R. 1975. *Int. Rev. Neurobiol.* 17:132–88

Spaziani, E. 1975. *Pharmacol. Rev.* 27:207–86

Tuomisto, J., Paasonen, M., eds. 1975. *Proc. 6th Int. Congr. Pharmacol., 6th.* Elmsford, NY: Pergamon. 6 vols. 1547 pp.

USP Convention. 1975. *USAN and USP Dictionary of Drug Names.* Rockville, Md.: USP Convention. 352 pp.

Usdin, E., Kvetnansky, R., Kopin, I. J., eds. 1976. *Catecholamines and Stress.* Elmsford, NY: Pergamon. 644 pp.

Walker, M. D., Weiss, H. D. 1975. *Adv. Neurol.* 13:149–92

Wallace, J. E., Hamilton, H. E., Schwertner, H. A. 1976. *Tex. J. Sci.* 27:7–25

Warren, G. H. 1975. *Ann. Rep. Med. Chem.* 10:109–71

Weiss, B., ed. 1975. *Cyclic Nucleotides in Disease.* Baltimore: Univ. Park Press. 410 pp.

Wilson, G. M. 1975. *Postgrad. Med. J.* 51:(Suppl. 6) 100 pp.

Yosselson, S. 1976. *Drug Intell. Clin. Pharm.* 10:8–14

AUTHOR INDEX

A

Abbott, B. J., 117-19
Abboud, F. M., 262
Abdel-Sayed, W. A., 262
Abdou, N. I., 183
Abdulla, M., 201, 204
Abdulla, Y. H., 447-49
Abell, C. W., 107, 443, 444, 453, 462
Aberg, H., 317
Abood, L. G., 35
Aboulker, P., 15
Abraham, D. J., 121
Abrams, W. B., 296, 300
Abt, A. F., 134
Abuchowski, A., 110
Aceves, J., 224, 230
Achor, R. W. P., 139
Ackenheil, M., 416
Acosta, J., 665, 670
Adam, H. M., 325, 328
Adams, D. A., 202
Adams, F., 480
Adams, H. Y., 234, 235
Adams, L. D., 447, 456
Adams, L. L., 505
Adams, T. H., 136
Adams, W. C., 215
Adamson, D., 535
Adamson, G., 505
Adir, J., 90, 91
Adler, J., 243
Adler, M., 397, 398, 402
Adler, S., 71, 189
Adlercreutz, P., 451
Admirand, W. H., 16
Adovasio, J. M., 648, 667
ADRIANI, J., 223-42; 224-40
Adrouny, G., 491
Aeling, J. L., 138
Aftergood, L., 139
Aggeler, P. M., 295, 296
Aghajanian, G. K., 346, 373, 608, 610
Agid, Y., 372
Aguirre Beltrán, G., 648, 650-53, 662, 665, 670
Agurell, S., 565, 663
Agus, Z. S., 14, 74, 640
Ahern, D. G., 268
Ahl, C. A., 183
Ahlquist, R. P., 575
Ahlskog, J. E., 608-10, 612, 614
Ahmed, A., 286
Ahrens, E. H. Jr., 505
Åhström, L., 186
Ahumada, J. J., 71
Aicardi, J., 680

Aisenberg, A. C., 186
Aitken, R. C. B., 215
Akamatsu, T. J., 239
Akert, K., 432
Al-Awquati, Q., 356
Albano, J. P., 448
Albe-Fessard, D., 609
Albers, R. W., 329, 332
Albert, A., 119
Albrecht, A. M., 107
Albrecht, I., 445
Albuquerque, E. X., 391, 397, 398, 402
Alcock, N., 78
Aldred, J. P., 74
Alessio, L., 203
Alexander, F. W., 199
Alexander, H. C., 171, 172, 174
Alexander, J., 536-38
Alexander, P., 179, 181
Alexander, R. W., 575, 577, 581-84
Alfin-Slater, R. B., 139
Alford, W. C., 84, 85
Alfredson, K. S., 68
Alfrey, A. C., 15, 16
Allen, D. O., 446, 448
Allen, D. W., 206
Allen, G. L., 525
Allen, H. J., 252
Allen, J. C., 156
Allen, J. L., 172
Allen, M. P., 370, 372-76
Allison, D., 169
Allison, J. P., 111
Alltop, L. P., 419
Allum, W., 299
Alpert, J. J., 215
Alston, W., 390
Alston, W. C., 443
Altamirano, F., 649, 658, 667
Altland, H. W., 119, 121
Altman, Y., 288
Altura, B. M., 393
Alvares, A. P., 206, 563
Alzate y Ramirez, A., 650, 668, 669
Ambache, N., 263
Ambre, J. J., 294
Ambus, U., 536
Amer, M. S., 445, 448-51, 453, 456, 458
Amiel, J. L., 189, 534
Amin, A. H., 426, 429
Aminu, J., 299
Ammann, A. J., 288
Ammon, H. V., 357, 360, 361, 363
Amoss, M., 432

Anand, B. K., 606, 608
Ananth, J. V., 139
Anast, C. S., 75, 77
Andén, N-E., 347, 378
Anders, M. W., 92, 563, 569
Anderson, E. G., 329, 331, 332
Anderson, G. H., 313
Anderson, H. J., 577, 581, 584, 586, 587
Anderson, K. E., 206, 678
Anderson, M., 656
Anderson, R. B., 170
Anderson, T. W., 138
Anderson, W. B., 444, 445, 448, 453
Andiman, R. M., 388, 390
Andreasen, F., 61
Andreoli, T. E., 624, 625, 632, 633
Andreozzi, R. J., 138
Andres, G., 624
Andres, K. H., 425
Andres, R., 53, 57
Andreussi, L., 390, 391
Angelucci, L., 428
Angervall, G., 315
Angkur, V., 183
Angrist, B. M., 550, 554
Ankermann, H., 58
Ansell, G. B., 372, 374
Ansfield, F., 536
Antelman, S. M., 608, 615
Antkiewicz, L., 347
Antoni, H., 156, 157
Aoki, M., 206
Aota, K., 130
Apajalahti, A., 295
Aperia, A. C., 636
Appenzeller, O., 395
Appleman, M. M., 444, 450, 451
Aprille, J. R., 579
Aprison, M. H., 427
Aranda, J. V., 563-65, 569
Aras, M., 636
Archer, J. A., 243
Ardaillou, R., 74
Ardoino, V., 205
Arens, A., 109
Arens, J., 235-37
Argenta, G., 418
Arias, L., 299
Ariens, A. T., 398, 400, 402
Arimura, A., 429, 432, 433
Arita, M., 300
Arlien-Soborg, P., 427
Arlin, Z., 535
Armentrout, S., 538
Armerding, G., 287
Armitage, A. K., 376

Armstrong, B., 316
Arnaud, C., 136
Arnaud, C. D., 15, 20
Arnauld, E., 432, 433
Arnold, A., 576
Arnold, D. W., 205
Arnold, L., 18
Arnsdorf, M. F., 293, 301
Aronow, L., 577
Aronson, A. L., 201
Arora, S. K., 123
Arqueros, L., 32, 34
Arthur, H. R., 121
Ary, M., 348
Asberg, M., 418, 419
Asbill, M., 249
Ash, J. F., 38
Ashcroft, G. W., 411, 412, 415
Ashcroft, S. J. H., 457
Ashkenazi, A., 288
Ashley, J. J., 55, 58, 59
Ashwell, G., 109
Asp, S., 201, 202, 204
Assem, E. S. K., 679
Assesburg, U., 532
Astley, R., 202
Åström, A., 262
Atack, C., 328
Atack, C. V., 411
Atkinson, A. J., 238, 239
Atkinson, M., 357
Atlas, D., 577, 581, 582, 585-87
Atsmon, A., 300
Atweh, S., 369, 373, 375-80
Atwood, G. F., 563, 570
Au, W. Y. W., 78
Audigier, Y., 331, 332
Auffray, P., 609
August, T., 73
Augustyn, J. M., 445
Ault, C., 252
Aungst, C. W., 189
Aurbach, G. D., 446-48, 579, 581-87
Austin, L., 395
Avant, G. R., 55, 59, 60
Averill, C. M., 68, 69
Avery, D. D., 343, 344
Avery, G. S., 108
Avery, O. T., 97
Avery, S., 446, 448
Aviado, D., 83
Avigan, J., 388
Avioli, L. V., 75, 76, 136
Avoy, D. R., 505
Axelrod, J., 265, 326, 329, 332, 333, 412, 575, 581, 582, 590, 593
Axelsson, J., 590
Axford, R. F. E., 75
Aymard, P., 75

Aynedjian, H. S., 627, 636
Azar, A., 86, 91, 199, 205
Azarnoff, D. L., 294, 505, 563, 564, 569
Azoubel, R., 134

B

Baba, Y., 432
BACH, J.-F., 281-91; 181, 281, 282, 284-88, 679
Bach, M. A., 284, 286, 287
Bach, S. J., 106
Bache, C. A., 170, 171
Bachman, B., 315
Bachta, M., 268
BACK, K.C.,83-95; 84-91
Bader, J., 444
Baehner, R. L, 201
Baer, L., 312, 317
Baer, P. G., 14
Baer, R. D., 388, 390
Baerg, R. D., 135
Baez, L. A., 607
Bagai, R. C., 188
Bagdade, J. D., 505
Bagheri, S. A., 134
Bahy, C., 609
Bailey, K. R., 294
Baines, A. D., 624
Baines, C. J., 624
Baird, C. E., 451, 452, 456, 459-61
Bajusz, E., 154
Baker, B. L., 34
Baker, F. D., 92
Baker, L., 533
Baker, P. F., 30, 31, 265
Baker, T., 398
Balant, L., 53
Baldamus, C. A., 629, 636
Baldessarini, R. J., 325, 551
Baldwin, R. W., 179, 181
Ball, G. G., 333
Ball, G. V., 207
Ball, J. H., 446
Ball, R. C., 170, 171, 174
Ballard, P. L., 515
Ballard, R. A., 515
Balow, J. E., 514
Balsan, S., 136
Baltzer, B. V., 75
Ban, T. A., 139
Band, P., 539
Banerjee, S. P., 546
Bank, N., 627, 636
Banks, B., 485
Banks, P., 28, 30, 32, 35
Banwell, J. G., 356
Bar, H. P., 442
Bar, R. S., 243
Barar, F. S. K., 299

Barbeau, A., 545
Barber, S. B., 244
Barbezat, G. O., 357
Barbin, G., 325-30
Barbour, B. H., 680
Barcelo, P., 15
Barcenas, C., 17
Barchas, J., 612, 613
Bareggi, S. R., 412
Bargmann, W., 425
Barker, E. S., 71
Barker, J. L., 425, 432, 433
Barker, L. A., 373, 376
Barker, N. W., 139
Barlogie, B., 532
Barlow, C. H., 92
Barltrop, D., 199
Barnabei, O., 588
Barnard, E. A., 397, 402
Barnes, B. A., 72
Barnes, J., 141
Barnes, J. R., 205
Barnes, M. H., 121
Barnett, A., 347
Barnett, E. V., 186
Barofsky, I., 346
Baron, A., 534
Barranco, S., 532
Barratt, L. J., 625, 629, 630
Barrett, A. M., 505
Barrett, J. F., 432
Barrett, M. B., 207
Barry, P. S. I., 200, 201
Barry, P. Z., 215, 216
Barstad, J. A. B., 401
Bartholini, A., 376, 378
Bartholini, G., 369-71, 378, 411, 553
Bartles, D., 388, 390
Bartlett, E., 300
Bartoli, E., 634, 636
Bartolini, A., 376, 377
Bartsch, P., 346
Bartter, F. C., 13, 14, 17, 20
Barzel, U. S., 19
Basch, R. S., 286
Bass, L. J., 447, 454
Bass, P., 360, 361, 363
Bassett, A. L., 293, 301
Bassett, C. A. L., 136
Bast, R. C. Jr., 188
Basticen, J. W., 74
Bateman, C., 535
Bateman, J., 532
Bates, R. B., 123
Battenberg, E. F., 587
Battistini, A., 205
Baudry, M., 326-31
Bauer, B., 156
Bauer, H., 326
Bauer, K., 104, 109
Bauer, P., 150, 155, 158

Bauernfield, J. C., 133, 134
Baum, T., 263
Baumann, I. R., 342
Baumann, K., 629
Baxter, J. D., 512
Baxter, L. A., 20
Baxter, M. G., 141
Bayard, M. A., 197
Bayless, T. M., 355-57
Baylink, D., 14
Baylink, D. J., 17
Bazzano, G., 294
Bazzano, G. S., 294
Beach, R. L., 373, 378
Beani, L., 372, 377-79
Beard, E. S., 71
Beard, M., 535
Beard, N. A., 448
Beard, R., 487, 489
Beaton, G. H., 141
Beattie, A. D., 205
Beaudet, A., 613
Beaujouan, J. C., 372, 373, 376
Beavo, J. A., 451, 456, 460
Beck, H., 49
Beck, P. S., 85, 86
Becker, D., 205
Beckett, A. H., 298
Beckman, A. L., 343, 344
Beckman, B. S., 581, 584
Beckmann, H., 419, 421, 422
Beckstead, H. D., 649
Bedard, P., 378
Beeler, G. W., 150, 157
Beer, B., 458
Beidler, L. M., 243, 247
Beiser, G. D., 445
Belcher, D. R., 90, 91
Beleslin, D., 357, 371, 373, 376, 377
Belkin, M., 117
Bell, C. L., 121
Bell, G. D., 359
Bell, N. H., 446, 448
Bellantoni, J., 92
Belleau, L. J., 635
Belman, S., 271, 444
Beltran, S. M., 200
Ben, M., 530
Ben-Ari, Y., 427, 429
Bencze, B., 139
Bend, J. R., 92
BENDER, A.D.,49-65; 49, 50, 60
Bender, F., 158, 159
Bender, K. J., 680
Bending, M. R., 318
Benedeczky, I., 34
Benedikter, L. T., 299
Benet, L. Z., 295, 298, 563
Ben-Ishay, Z., 538
Benjamin, D. M., 294

Ben-Jonathan, N., 432
Bennett, A., 270, 271
Bennett, A. L., 391
Bennett, C. M., 68, 316, 319, 623, 634, 635
Bennett, C. T., 333
Bennett, J. P., 243
Bennett, L., 36, 37
Bennett, L. L., 29
Bennett, V., 243
Bennett, W. A., 523
Bennun, M., 134
Ben-Shachar, D., 483
Benson, J., 185
Benson, R., 481
Bentzel, C. J., 627
Benuck, M., 428
Berge, K. G., 139
Berger, S. S., 133
Bergeron, M., 630
Bergert, J. H., 18
Berges, P. U., 239
Bergfors, P. G., 563, 565, 566, 569
Berglund, F., 68
Bergman, A. B., 319
Bergman, D., 361
Bergman, H., 169, 170
Bergstrand, A., 624
Bergström, S., 263
Beringer, K., 655, 662
Berk, P. D., 206
Berl, S., 38
Berlin, C. M., 565
Berlin, N. I., 206
Berliner, R. W., 68, 623, 634-36
Berman, M., 585
Bern, H. A., 433
Bernard, C., 495
Bernasconi, S., 612
Berndt, S., 451, 458
Berneis, K. H., 28
Berneske, G. M., 138
Bernhardt, I. B., 134
Bernheimer, H., 545, 552
Bernier, J. J., 357, 363
Bernlohr, R. W., 109
Bernstein, D. S., 20
Bernstein, J., 36, 37
Bernstein, R., 141
Berry, C. A., 627
Berry, F. A. Jr., 563, 567, 569
Bertalanffy, F. D., 530
Bertilsson, L., 379, 418, 419
Bertino, J. R., 107, 185
Berwick, P., 388
Berzofsky, J. A., 563
Besa, E. C., 442
Besch, H. R. Jr., 156
Bessis, M. C., 206

Bethune, J. E., 72
Better, O. S., 71
Betts, P. R., 202
Bevelle, C., 121
Beveridge, T., 294
BEYER, K.J.J.R.,1-10
Bhagat, B., 265
Bhargava, K. P., 332, 333
Bhatnagar, R. K., 546
Bhatt, H. V., 376
Bhattacharyya, M. H., 135
Bhoola, K., 488, 489
Bianchi, C., 372, 377-79
Bianchi, R. E., 30
Bianchine, J. R., 50
Bickerstaff, E. R., 394, 396
Biederdorf, F. A., 357
Biely, J., 139
Bieri, J. G., 133, 134, 138, 139
Bierling, R., 104
Bierman, E. L., 505
Bigger, J. T., 240
Bigliere, E. G., 73
Bilezikian, J. P., 579, 584, 585
Bilheimer, D. W., 499, 500, 504-6, 508
Bills, D. D., 169
Biltonen, R. L., 575, 585
BINDER, H. J., 355-67; 355-57, 359-62
Bindler, E., 28
Bingham, E., 198
Biozzi, G., 287
Birge, S. J., 136
Birkenhager, J. C., 513
Birkmayer, W., 545, 552
Birks, R., 376, 396
Birnbaumer, L., 585, 588
Bisaz, S., 20
Bischel, M. D., 680
Bischoff, S., 325-30, 333
Bitensky, M. W., 442, 591
Bjerkelund, C. J., 294
Björklund, A., 546
Bjorntorp, P., 513
Blaber, L. C., 397, 401
Black, A., 90, 91
Black, J. W., 331
Black, M. M., 183
Blackstone, M. O., 294
Blackwell, B., 319
Blackwell, R., 432
Blaese, R. M., 181
Blair, D., 294
Blair, J. A., 141
Blair, N. P., 358
Blake, D. A., 90-92
Blakeley, A. G. H., 262
Blanc, G., 546
Blanco, I., 328
Blanco, M., 591
Bland, J. H., 71

Blankenbaker, W. L., 563, 567, 569
Blanquet, R. S., 251-53
Blaschko, H., 31, 35, 38
Blaskovics, M. E., 296
Blau, G. E., 171, 172, 174
Blaufuss, A., 316, 319
Blaustein, N. P., 225, 228, 230, 232
Blaylock, W. K., 183
Blecher, M., 243
Bleifeld, W., 153
Bleifer, K., 152
Bleuler, E., 545, 547, 556
Bligh, J., 342, 345, 346
Blinks, J., 583
Blitzer, B. L., 521
Blohme, B., 513
Blondel, B., 38
Bloom, F. E., 27, 331, 332, 425, 586, 587
Bloom, S., 357
Bloomfield, T. H., 299
Bloor, C., 445, 457
Bluestone, R., 18, 19
Blum, I., 300
Blum, M., 490, 491
Blumberg, J. B., 590, 611
Blumenschein, G., 189
Blumenthal, G., 104
Bluming, A. Z., 179, 188
Blundell, J. E., 606, 607, 612-15
Boag, D. A., 250
Boakes, A. J., 299
Boakes, J., 554
Bochner, F., 60
Bockbrader, H. N., 294
Bodansky, O., 678
Bode, J., 243
Bodey, G. P., 182, 188, 533-35
Bodey, G. P. Sr., 183, 189
Boegman, R. J., 395
Bogdonoff, M. D., 86
Bohidar, N. R., 317
Bohlmann, F., 658, 667
Bohlmann, H. G., 201
Bohr, D. F., 158
Boiardi, A., 390, 391
Boissier, J. R., 325
Bolanowska, W., 200
Boldizsar, E., 107
Bolton, P. M., 183
Bondoc, C. C., 140
Bone, H., 13, 14
Bonica, J. J., 239
Bonilla, C. A., 515
Bonjour, J-P., 20
Bonner, J. T., 451
Bonnycastle, D. D., 355, 358
Bonorris, G. G., 360
Bonsignore, D., 205

Booker, J., 31
Boone, C. W., 182
Booth, R. A., 370, 374
Booth, R. S., 172, 173
Borbely, A. A., 613
Bordier, P., 20
Bordy, S. C., 454
Borella, L., 187
Boreus, L. O., 565, 567, 569
Borg, F., 414
Borga, O., 563, 565, 566, 569
Borgeat, P., 36, 37
Bornet, E. P., 156
Borsos, T., 100, 181, 182, 188
Bosanac, P., 14
Boss, S., 72
Bosshard, H. E., 243
Bossier, J., 372
Bostick, F., 539
Boswell, K. H., 451
Bott, P. A., 623
Botte, H. D., 389
Botting, J. H., 271
Bottomley, S. S., 442
Bouchard, M., 537
Boucher, R., 36, 432
Boudreau, R. J., 452
Boulet, P., 624
Boullin, D. J., 299
Boulpaep, E. L., 626, 627, 629, 633, 636
Boulu, P., 332
Boulu, R., 327, 333
Boura, A. L. A., 300
Bourgoignie, J. J., 317, 635
Bourne, H. R., 448, 451, 454, 455, 457, 464, 581, 584
Bousser, J., 537
Bovaird, J., 248, 249
Bowers, C. Y., 432
Bowers, M. B. Jr., 413-18, 421
Bowman, R. L., 388, 390
Bowman, W. C., 401
Boyce, W. H., 17, 19
Boyd, H., 443
Boyd, I. A., 397
Boyer, J. L., 134, 139
Boyes, R. N., 234, 235, 565
Boylan, J. W., 629
Boyle, I. T., 135
Boyle, L., 532
Boyse, E. A., 103, 284, 285
Brack, A., 649, 655, 660
Bradford, L. G., 134
Bradham, L. S., 450
Bradley, M. O., 38
Bradley, P. B., 432, 554
Brady, R. O., 98, 103
Brambilla, G., 99
Branch, R. A., 295
Branfman, A. R., 124, 125
Branson, D. R., 171, 172, 174

Brasted, M., 262, 265
BRATER, D.C.,293-309
Braun, G., 634
Braun, W., 442, 453, 455
Bravo, E. L., 312, 316
Brawley, P., 654
Brazeau, P., 432, 433
Breckenridge, A., 318
Breckenridge, A. M., 314, 318
Breckenridge, B. M., 449, 450
Breese, G. R., 345, 412, 419, 607, 612
Breisch, S. T., 610, 613
Breitenecker, G., 537
Breithaupt, H., 485
Brenda, P., 329
Brenner, B. M., 623, 634-37
Brereton, H., 537, 539
Breslow, J. L., 500, 504-6, 508
Breslow, N., 189
Brest, A. N., 316
Brezenoff, H. E., 332, 348
Briant, R. H., 53, 57, 299
Bricker, N. S., 635
Brickman, A. S., 71, 72, 75, 76, 78
Bridenbaugh, L. D., 228, 233
Bridenbaugh, P. O., 565
Briggs, I., 432
Briggs, M., 134
Briggs, M. H., 138
Bright-Asare, P., 357, 360, 361
Brimble, M. J., 332
Brimblecombe, R. W., 332, 344, 346
Brimijoin, S., 590
Brin, M., 133, 134
Brisson, G. R., 31
Brittain, R. T., 345-47
Brittinger, W. D., 159
Britton, R. W., 128, 129
Broadus, A. E., 446
Brobeck, J. R., 606, 608
Broberger, C. G. O., 636
Broberger, O., 137
Brochart, M., 75, 77
Brockes, J. P., 590
Brocksen, R. W., 169, 170
Brodie, B. B., 294, 296, 299, 344, 455, 456
Brodin, E., 430
Brody, I. A., 390
Brody, M. J., 262-64, 270, 327
Broeckkamp, C., 610
Brogden, R. N., 108
Bromer, L., 315, 316
Bronner, F., 136
Brooker, G., 446, 448, 451, 591, 594
Brooks, J. C., 38
Brooks, R., 485
Broome, J. D., 101, 104

Brosman, S., 179, 181, 188
Brostrom, C. O., 450-52, 459
Brown, B., 326, 327
Brown, B. C., 448
Brown, B. E., 430
Brown, D. D., 329
Brown, D. G., 328
Brown, E. M., 581-83, 585-87
Brown, G. L., 262, 267, 388
Brown, H. D., 444
Brown, J. L., 68, 448
Brown, R. S., 181
Brown, S. S., 215
Brown, T. G., 576
Brown, W. V., 505, 506
Browne, T. R., 563, 564
Brownstein, M., 432
Brownstein, M. J., 326, 333
Bruckmann, G., 62
Brugerie, E., 534
Brugmans, J., 190
Bruhn, C., 655, 663
Bruhn, J. G., 663
Bruhn, J. G., 655, 663
Bruin, W. J., 17
Bruinvels, J., 344, 345, 347
Brundin, J., 261, 265
Brunette, M., 67, 68, 70, 71
Brunette, M. G., 624
Brunner, F. P., 630, 634
Brunner, H., 317
Brunner, H. R., 312, 317
Brunzell, J. D., 505
Bruschke, G., 50
Bryan, R. F., 124, 129
Bryant, S. H., 388-90
Bryant, T., 537, 539
Bryce, G. F., 613
Buchanan, R. A., 297, 563, 564
Bucher, U. M., 331
Buchet, J. P., 203-6
Buchner, T., 532
Buchs, M., 29
Bucht, H., 624
Buck, A. T., 141
Buckalew, V. M. Jr., 19
Buckle, R. H., 77
Buckley, J. P., 269
Buckley, J. T., 36
Buckner, C. K., 576
Buhler, F. R., 312, 317
Bulat, M., 412
Bulfield, G., 327
Bulger, R. E., 624, 628
Bull, J., 539
Buller, A. J., 396
Bulpitt, C. J., 312, 317, 318
Bunney, B. S., 608, 610
Bunney, W. E. Jr., 447, 448
Burch, J. F., 19
Burchenal, J., 103
Burdick, G. E., 170

Burdick, J. F., 183
Bures, A. R., 680
Burford, G. D., 34
Burg, M. B., 625, 627, 629, 631-34
Burgen, A. S. V., 586
Burgess, M. A., 189, 533
Burgus, R., 432
Burk, D., 247
Burk, R. R., 444, 448
Burkard, W. P., 329
Burke, G. C., 443, 448
Burke, J. F., 140
Burke, P. J., 186, 533, 535, 539
Burks, T. F., 345, 347
Burn, J. H., 300
Burnet, F. M., 181
Burns, C., 538
Burns, J. J., 297, 576
Burns, R. S., 679
Burns, T. W., 75, 77, 388, 390
Burridge, K., 38
Burris, B. C., 239
Burstein, N., 538
Burt, D. R., 552, 553
Burton, A. F., 106
Burwen, S., 27
Busch, E., 159
Büscher, H. H., 432
Butcher, L. L., 371
Butcher, M., 432
Butcher, R. W., 442, 443, 448-50, 454, 460, 576, 578, 583, 588
Butcher, S. G., 371
Buterbaugh, G. G., 373, 378
Butler, C. M., 567
Butler, D., 640
Butler, V. P., 294
Butler, W. T., 188
Butson, A. R. C., 138
Butt, E. M., 200
Bye, R., 653, 662, 663, 666, 667, 669
Bygdeman, M., 261
Bylund, D. B., 577, 581-84, 587, 588
Byon, Y. K., 150, 152, 154-56, 158-60
Bystedt, U., 315

C

Cabanac, M., 341
Caccia, M. R., 390, 391
Caggiula, A. R., 615
Caillens, H., 327, 329
Calabresi, P., 183, 185
Calandra, J. C., 205
Calcutt, C. R., 325, 332
Calderón, J. B., 649, 656, 668
Caldwell, J. H., 294

Caldwell, J. L., 294
Calimlim, L. R., 50
Call, D. W., 85
Callahan, P., 490
Calle, C., 512
Calle, J., 488, 489
Calne, D. B., 347
Cambiaghi, G., 203, 205
Camerino, M., 181
Cammermeyer, J., 327
Campbell, D., 233-37
Campbell, H. A., 103
Campbell, H. F., 119
Campbell, J., 535
Campbell, M. T., 451
Campbell, P. A., 139
Campbell, R. C., 152
Campos, G. M., 134
Camu, F., 91
Camus, J., 36
Candela, L. R., 32
Candy, J. M., 554
Canellos, G. P., 101
Cannon, B., 590
Canterbury, J. M., 14
Cantor, A., 344, 347
Capen, C. C., 137
Capizzi, R. L., 103, 531, 532
Caranasos, G. J., 293, 356, 680
Carchman, R. A., 445, 453
Cardinal, J., 627, 632, 633
Cardinaux, F., 432
Care, A. D., 20, 77, 78
Carey, E. J., 398
Carey, R., 538
Carioli, V. J., 298
Carlini, E. A., 327
Carlisle, H. J., 343
Carlson, G. P., 93
Carlson, L. A., 269, 506
Carlson, L. D., 341, 342
Carlsson, A., 328, 413, 545, 551, 555
Carnaud, C., 281, 282, 288
Carne, S. J., 312
Carney, T., 201
Caro, C. M., 591
Caro, L. G., 33
Caro, M., 491
Caron, M. G., 575, 577, 581, 582, 585, 589, 591, 593, 594
Carone, F. A., 446, 448
Carpenter, C. C. J., 356, 358
Carpenter, D. O., 332
Carpenter, J., 535
Carpenter, S., 391, 392
Carr, A. A., 75
Carriere, S., 624
Carroll, P. T., 373, 378
Carson, R., 167, 168
Carswell, F., 205
Cartasegna, C., 205

688 AUTHOR INDEX

Carter, C. J. K., 100-2
Carter, M. R., 505
Carter, N. W., 17, 629
Carter, V. L., 85
Casati, C., 418
Casdorph, H. R., 506
Case, R. W., 189
Caso, A., 648, 660
Casper, A. G. T., 640
Castaneda, C., 653, 654, 658, 669
Castañeda, M., 442
Castle, J. D., 33
Castleden, C. M., 55, 59
Castro, J. A., 139
Catalona, W. J., 183
Catanzaro, F. J., 317
Catley, P. F., 152
Catt, K. H., 317
Cattan, A., 189
Caughey, W. S., 92
CAVAGNOL, R. M.,479-98
Cavalli, R. D., 200
Cavallito, C. J., 376
Cavanaugh, J., 550
Cavanaugh, J. H., 299
Cavanna, M., 99
Cavill, G., 491
Cedar, H., 99
Celesia, G. G., 370-73
Cerilli, J., 181
Chabner, B. A., 107
Chadwick, G. G., 169, 170
Chadwick, V. S., 16
Chakravarti, K. K., 119
Chakravorty, R. C., 183
Chambaut, A.-M., 578, 591
Chamberlain, A., 183
Chamberlain, D. A., 58
Chan, K., 54, 58
Chan, P-C., 444
Chan, Y. K., 189, 531
Chandler, D. W., 446, 449
Chandler, J. T., 262
Chandra, P., 453
Chang, C. C., 299, 396, 586
Chang, H. C., 425
Chang, K., 243
Chang, K-J., 579, 580, 582
Chang, M. M., 426, 430
Chang, T. M. S., 110
Changeux, J. P., 243
Chanh, P. H., 268
Chapman, J., 539, 549
Chapman, L. C., 71
Chapman, L. W., 68, 70-73
Chapman-Anderson, C., 252
Chapnic, B. M., 262
Chaput de Saintonge, D. M., 141
Charness, M. E., 581, 584, 588

Charreire, J., 288
Chase, L. R., 75-77, 446-48
Chase, T. N., 412-14, 613
Chasin, M., 331, 449, 453, 456, 458, 460, 591
Chason, J. L., 392
Chast, F., 329
Chatterjee, S. K., 444
Chattopadhyay, S. K., 444
Chau-Wong, M., 553
Chavaz, A., 53
Chavez de los Rios, J. M., 136
Chayoth, R., 443
Cheema, A. R., 187
Chen, T. F., 396
CHENEY, D. L., 369-86; 369-71, 373-80
Cheng, C. C., 121, 122
Cheng, C. Y., 505
Cheng, Y., 582
Cheng-Raude, D., 483
Chenoweth, M., 446, 448
Chenoweth, M. B., 86
Cheserak, W., 349
Cheung, D. K. K., 205
Cheung, W. Y., 445, 450-52
Chey, W. Y., 357
Chi, E. Y., 38
Chi, Y-M., 576
Chiariello, M., 444, 448
Chibata, I., 110
Chidsey, C., 315
Chidsey, C. A., 317-19
Ch'ien, L. T., 141
Chiesara, E., 50
Chignell, C. F., 361, 362, 565
Chikos, P. M., 84
Chin, P., 608
Chinn, C., 345
Chiong, R., 137
Chiou, W. L., 91
Chirito, E., 625, 630
Chisolm, J. J., 201-3, 205, 207
Chlopkiewicz, B., 531
Cho-Chung, Y. S., 453
Choi, L., 370, 374
Choi, R. L., 373-76
Choie, D. D., 208
Chong, E. D. S., 110
Chong, E. K. S., 271
Chong, G. C., 372
Chou, T., 300
Chretien, P. B., 181, 183
Chrisman, T. D., 450
Christ, D. D., 397
Christensen, C. N., 561
Christensen, J., 360, 361
Christensen, L. K., 297
Christensen, M., 294
Christensen, N. A., 139
Christiansen, C., 136

Christiansen, N. J. B., 51
Christiansen, R. O., 451
Christophe, J., 36
Christopher, N. L., 356
Christy, N. P., 511, 521
Chuang, S. T., 396
Chung, A., 360
Chung, E. K., 293
Chutkow, J. G., 72
Chytil, F., 512
Cinotti, G., 624
Ciosek, C. P. Jr., 455
Cirksena, W. J., 623
Citri, N., 110
Civinelli, J., 319
Claesson, L., 27
Claman, H. N., 516
Clapham, W. F., 634
Clapp, J. R., 68
Clare, R. A., 563, 569
Clark, B., 583
Clark, B. B., 141
Clark, C. G., 139
Clark, C. M., 446, 448
Clark, D. G., 85, 86
Clark, G. M., 318
Clark, I., 136
Clark, J., 201
Clark, J. F., 443, 451
Clark, J. K., 71
Clark, J. L., 32
Clark, K. E., 262
Clark, R. B., 331, 443, 451, 584, 587, 591, 594
Clark, W. G., 348
Clarkson, B., 103, 535
Clarkson, B. D., 103
Clarkson, T. W., 207
Claveria, L. E., 347
Clay, K., 453
Claybrook, D. L., 428
Clayman, S., 456
Clayton, B. E., 199
Clayton, G. A., 152
Clayton, J. W. Jr., 83, 84
Clegg, P. C., 266
Clemens, J. A., 612
Clement-Cormier, Y. C., 552
Clements, P. J., 186
Cleugh, J., 426
Cliffe, E. E., 248
Clifton, J. A., 357
Cline, M. J., 179, 182, 183, 187, 537
Clineschmidt, B. V., 612
Clody, D. E., 376, 458
Closse, A., 432
Cloutier, R. J., 608
Cluff, L. E., 293, 680
Coan, B. J., 505
Coates, V., 139

Coats, J. R., 172
Cobb, M. H., 248-50, 254
Coburn, J. W., 15, 17, 68-73, 75-78
Coceani, F., 269
Cochran, M., 16, 74
Cochrane, W. A., 141
Coe, F. L., 13, 14, 18
Coers, C., 396
Coffey, R. G., 443
Coffin, C. C., 170
Coffino, P., 448, 454, 464, 581, 584, 594
Coffman, P. Z., 327
Coggon, P., 126
Cohanim, M., 14, 71, 135
Cohen, B. H., 53, 57
Cohen, E. L., 371
Cohen, G. H., 282, 286, 288
Cohen, I. R., 288
Cohen, J. B., 243
Cohen, L., 444
Cohen, P., 187
Cohen, S., 586
COHEN, S. N.,561-73; 561, 564, 565
Cohn, C. K., 333
Cohn, D. V., 30, 77
Cohn, K., 295
Cohn, Z. A., 252
Colby, D., 170
Cole, L., 483
Cole, S., 152
Colebatch, J., 187
Colindres, R. E., 628
Collier, B., 37, 372
Collier, J. G., 264
Collins, P. R., 656, 664, 670
Collinsworth, K. A., 238
Colobert, L., 451
Colston, K. W., 135
Combs, G. F. Jr., 138
Comsa, J., 285
Conaway, H. H., 30
Condie, R. M., 109
Conen, P. E., 75
Conger, J. D., 634, 636
Conley, D. R., 360
Conn, H. O., 521
Connell, P. H., 550
Connett, R. J., 32
Conney, A. H., 297
Connor, T. B., 74, 75, 77
Conolly, M. E., 91
Conover, H., 72
Conrad, J. T., 397
Conroy, C. A., 370, 374, 375
Conroy, J., 539
Consolo, S., 372, 377
Constantino, R. T., 295
Cook, C. E., 118, 569

Cookson, D. U., 454
Coon, R. A., 92
Cooney, D. A., 98, 101, 110, 111
Cooper, B. R., 607, 612
Cooper, C. W., 77
Cooper, H. R., 139
Cooper, K. E., 342, 346
Cooper, L., 535
Cooper, M. J., 563, 569
Cooper, W. C., 208
Coore, H. G., 28, 35, 36
Cope, O., 72
Cope, O. B., 169
Copeland, D., 179, 182, 183
Copeland, E. M., 189, 538
Coper, H., 51
Copp, D. H., 29, 30
Coppolla, F. S., 183
Coraboeuf, E., 150
Corby, D. G., 294
Corcoran, J. W., 678
Cornelio, F., 390, 391
Cornwall, C. C., 208
Corrodi, H., 347
Corvino, B. G., 224-31, 234, 235, 237-39
Coscina, D. V., 610, 614
COSTA, E., 369-86; 299, 369, 370, 372-80, 412, 442, 450-52, 550, 554, 590
Costanzi, J., 532
Costanzi, J. J., 189, 288
Costanzo, L. S., 14
Costentin, J., 327, 332, 333
Cotten, M. deV., 679
Cotzias, G. C., 545
Coull, D. C., 299
Coulston, F., 199, 201
Counsell, R. E., 678
Coupland, R. E., 33
Court, W. A., 124, 129
Coverstone, M., 577, 581, 582
Cowan, F., 648, 649, 653, 654, 661
Cowan, G., 648, 649, 653, 654, 661
COX, B.,341-53; 332, 342, 347-49
Cox, J. W., 17, 20
Cox, P. J., 92
Coyle, J. T., 551, 593
Coyne, M. J., 360
Crabbe, J., 524
Craddock, C. G., 179
Craddock, P. R., 17
Craft, I., 134
Craig, L. C., 426
Cramer, H., 447, 448
Cramer, K., 201, 203, 207
Cramer, W., 31

Cranefield, P. F., 157
Cranston, W. I., 315, 345, 346
Crawford, M. A., 298
Crawford, T. B. B., 411, 412, 415, 426, 429
Crawshaw, L. I., 343, 346
Crayton, J. W., 442
Creehan, P., 447, 454
Creese, I., 552, 553
Crespí, G., 15
Creveling, C. R., 331, 590
Crispin-Smith, J., 376
Criss, W. E., 443, 448
Crofford, O. B., 456
Croll, G. A., 443, 453
Crone, H. D., 397
Cronholm, B., 418, 419
Crooks, J., 53, 55, 57
Crosby, D. G., 172, 174
Cross, B. A., 432
Crotty, J. J., 215
Crow, T. J., 547
Crowley, E. A., 312
Crowley, H. J., 458
Crowley, W. R., 614
Crowther, D., 535
Cruce, J. A. F., 610
Csaky, T. Z., 678
Csima, A., 75, 76, 78
Cuatrecasas, P., 243, 579, 580, 582
Cubeddu, X. L., 591, 594
Cucinell, S. A., 297
Cudihee, R., 295
Cumby, H. R., 348
Cumming, R. L. C., 205
Cummings, F., 183
Curran, P. F., 628
Currie, S., 397
Curry, D., 36, 37
Curtis, D. R., 380
Curutchet, H. P., 183
Curzon, G., 411, 412
Cushman, P. Jr., 521
Cytawa, J., 607
Czarnowska-Misztal, E., 135
Czyba, J. C., 139

D

D'Acosta, N., 139
Dahlquist, F. W., 243
Dailey, R. G. Jr., 124, 125, 129
Dalakos, T. G., 313
Dalderup, L. M., 136
Dale, D. C., 514
Dale, H. E., 388
Dale, H. H., 430, 575
Dalili, H., 235, 236
Dallman, P. R., 568, 569
Dalton, C., 458

Daly, J., 397, 402, 579
Daly, J. J., 183
Daly, J. W., 329, 331, 447, 576, 584, 587, 590-92
Dam, H., 137
Damato, A. N., 316
Daniel, M., 133, 134
Daniel, V., 448, 454, 464
Daniele, R. P., 179, 181
Danielli, J., 252
Danner, J., 248-50, 254
Danon, J. M., 391
Dao, T. L., 183
Da Prada, M., 28
Dardenne, M., 282, 284-87
Darling, M., 563, 569
Das, I., 446, 448
Dassonville, J., 90, 91
Data, J. L., 297
Datta, A., 443
Dauchot, P., 680
Daugharty, T. M., 635-37
Dauwalder, M., 33
David, D. S., 521
David, N. A., 320
David, O., 201
Davidoff, R. A., 427
Davidov, M., 315, 316
Davidson, A. R., 393
Davidson, G. M., 233, 238, 239
Davidson, J. M., 183
Davidson, L., 111, 545, 552, 553
Davies, B. N., 261, 263, 264, 266, 267
Davies, C., 299
Davies, D. S., 91, 563, 569, 678, 680
Davies, G. E., 455
Davies, J., 427, 430
Davies, J. A., 347
Davies, J. I., 455, 456
Davies, P. A., 263
Davis, B. B., 446
Davis, F. F., 110
Davis, H. A., 266
Davis, J. M., 299, 300, 550, 551
Davis, J. N., 411, 581-84, 588
Davis, N., 569
Davoren, P. R., 588
Dawes, P. H., 312
Dawson, R. M. C., 362
Day, A., 492
Day, G. M., 318
Day, M. D., 299
Dayton, P. G., 297, 563, 568, 569
Dean, H. J., 170
Dean, P. M., 29, 30, 39
Dearnaley, D. P., 262
Debeljuk, L., 432

DeBlanco, M., 17
Debons, A. F., 608
De Castro, C. R., 139
Decker, J. L., 520
Declercq, J. P., 123
DeConti, R. C., 185
Dedmon, R. E., 19
Deen, W. M., 637
Deetjen, P., 629, 630
de Fenos, O. M., 139
De Ferreyra, E. C., 139
de Freitas, A. S. W., 172, 174
DeGouyon, F., 75
DeGroat, W. C., 380
deGroot, W. J., 519
Deguchi, T., 590
DeHaan, R. M., 563
DeHaven, R. N., 369
deJong, R. H., 224-27, 236, 237, 239, 240
Dekirmenjian, H., 412, 419
de la Lande, I., 491, 492
de la Serna, J., 648, 653, 660, 662, 665
Delay, J., 654, 655, 661
Del Castillo, J., 656
Delea, C., 13, 17
Delea, C. S., 14, 136
Della Casa de Marcano, D. P., 126
Dellon, A. L., 181
DeLuca, H. F., 14, 17, 20, 133, 135-37
Delves, H. T., 199
DeMeyts, P., 243, 582, 587
Demos, J., 395
Deniker, P., 654, 655
Dennis, M. J., 429
Dennis, V. W., 624, 625, 640
De Oliveira, C. F., 183
de Qardener, H. E., 635
Derbes, V., 491
De Robertis, E., 31-33, 327, 358, 372
DeRoche, G. B., 591
De Rouffignac, C., 68, 69, 624
Derrer, E. C., 393, 394
de Sahagún, B., 648, 650-52, 660, 662, 664, 665, 669-71
Desalles, L., 578
Descarries, L., 613
Descoeudres, C., 640
Desgrez, P., 15
Desiderio, D., 432
Desnick, R. J., 108, 109, 111
Desser, P. C., 74
Dethlefsen, L. A., 530
DETTBARN, W.-D., 387-409; 390, 391, 394-402
Dettli, L. C., 51
Deutsch, E., 137
Deutsch, J., 243

DeVald, B., 183
De Vassal, F., 189
DeVellis, J., 591, 594
Devis, G., 29, 150
DeVita, V. T., 297
Devlin, J., 267
de Wardener, H. E., 634
Dewey, V. C., 140
De Wied, D., 425, 547
de Wolff, F. A., 141
Dews, P. B., 679
Dexter, R. N., 443, 448
Dhalla, N. S., 265, 442, 445, 457
Dhawan, B. N., 345
Diamond, J. M., 627
Diamond, S. S., 87
DIAZ, J. L.,647-75; 648, 651-54, 656, 658, 662-71
Diaz-Fierros, M., 512
Diaz Gomez, M. I., 139
Dickinson, G., 377
Dickson, L., 483
Didio, S. L., 200
Dietze, V. F., 50
DiFazio, C. A., 563, 567, 569
Digenis, P., 134
Digiovanni, J., 99
Diller, E. C., 17, 78
Dimich, A., 74
Dimitrov, N., 539
Diner, O., 32
Dingell, J. V., 590
Dingle, J. T., 133, 134
DIPALMA, J.R.,133-48; 139, 141
Dipeso, C. C., 648, 662
Diplock, A. T., 139
Dirks, J. H., 14, 67, 68, 70, 71, 623
DiSalle, E., 54, 57
DiScala, V. A., 71
Dismukes, K., 329-31, 590
Dismukes, R. K., 590
Dittmann, E. C., 90
Ditzion, B. P., 447, 448
Divac, I., 548
Dixit, K. S., 332
Dixon, J. E., 588
Dixon, M., 247, 248, 578
Dixon, R. H., 140
Dixon, W. M., 319
Dobbelstein, H., 389
Dobberstein, R. H., 658, 668
Dobbins, J. W., 359, 361
Dobkin de Ríos, M., 650-54, 669, 670
Dobson, A., 72
Dobson, J. G., 442
Doe, R. P., 71
Dohlwitz, A., 186
Dole, V. P., 243

Dolfini, E., 418
Doll, R., 316
DOLLERY, C.T.,311-23; 91, 299, 312, 314, 317, 318, 563, 569
Dolowy, W. C., 98, 99, 103, 104
Dominguez, J. H., 17
Dominitz, R., 35
Domino, E. F., 372, 376-78
DONE, A. K., 561-73; 215, 216, 221, 561
Donowitz, M., 355, 357, 359, 362
Dörfler, F., 158
Döring, H. J., 150-52, 154-57
Dorsey, D. J., 134
Doteuchi, M., 370, 371, 373, 376
Douglas, J. R., 267, 268
Douglas, W. W., 29-32, 34-38
Dousa, T. P., 446, 448
Dow, R. C., 412
Dowling, M., 103, 535
Dowling, R. H., 16, 359
Downing, D. T., 268
Downing, O. A., 271
Doyle, A. E., 317
Doyle, N. E., 288
Drach, G. W., 19
Drachman, D. B., 396, 397
Draffan, G. H., 91, 563, 569
Dragovich, J. A., 607
Dransfeld, H., 30
Dray, A., 427, 430
Dreifuss, F. E., 563, 564
Dreifuss, J. J., 29, 30, 32, 150, 269, 432
Dreisbach, R. H., 220
Drenick, E. J., 72
Dressler, D., 181
Drewinko, B., 532
Dreyer, D. A., 411
Drezner, M., 448
Dropp, J. J., 327
Dross, K., 369, 370, 373, 374
Drummond, G. I., 442, 452, 579
Drummond, J. C., 106
Drummond, M., 579
D'Snee, R., 199
Dua, P. P., 345
Duarte, C. G., 68, 71
Dube, W. J., 15
Dubnick, B., 140
Dubocovich, M. L., 268
Dubos, R., 97
Duce, B. R., 234, 235
Ducharme, D. W., 263
Duckert, F., 296
Duda, P., 269
Dudar, J. D., 372, 377

Dudel, J., 487
Dudrick, S. J., 183, 538
Duell, E. A., 447, 454
Duerr, A. C., 34
Duffield, J. C., 654
Duffy, E., 554
Duffy, M. J., 426, 430
Duggan, A. W., 380
Duhme, D. W., 294
Dujovne, C. A., 50, 505
Duke, E., 53, 55, 57
Dullum, C., 109
Dumitriu, C., 207
Dunbar, R. W., 233
Duncalf, D., 233, 238, 239
Duncan, T., 78
Duncan, W. A. M., 331
Dunham, E. W., 266
Dunlap, S. G., 537
Dunlop, D., 576
Dunn, A., 446, 448
Dunn, A. S., 444, 451
Dunn, M. J., 75, 76, 78
Dunn, T. F., 432
Dunne, J. F., 141
Dunnick, J., 578
Dunnick, J. K., 578
Dupont, J., 515
Duquesnoy, R. J., 443, 448, 453
Durant, C. J., 331
Durell, J., 419
Durr, J. C., 608
Dustan, H. P., 312, 315-17
Dworkind, J., 28, 35, 36
Dyball, R. E. J., 432, 433
Dyer, D. C., 261, 270
Dyer, R. G., 432, 433
Dyken, P., 563
Dyken, P. R., 563, 564

E

Eadie, M. J., 60
Eagan, R., 534
Eagle, H., 103
Eanes, E. D., 17
Earley, L. E., 358, 634-37
Earnest, D. L., 16
East, D. A., 13, 17
Eastwood, M. A., 360
Eaton, H. D., 134
Eaton, L. M., 396
Ebashi, E., 149
Eber, O., 428
Eberhardt, L. L., 168, 170, 171, 173
Eberstein, A., 388, 391
Ebert, M. H., 412
Ebner, F., 152
Eccles, J. C., 396, 425
Eccles, R. M., 396

Eccleston, D., 411, 412
Ecobichon, D. J., 568
Economou, S., 536
Edelman, I., 431
Edelstein, R., 189
Eder, M., 530, 534
Edery, H., 489, 490
Edminson, P. D., 329
Edstrom, A., 396
Edvinsson, L., 327
Edwards, B. A., 32
Edwards, B. R., 14
Edwards, D. J., 615
Edwards, J. M., 658, 668
Edwards, M. E., 32
Ehrenpreis, S., 271
Ehringer, H., 545, 552
Ehrnebo, M., 565
Eichler, O., 679
Eilber, F. R., 183, 189
Eilon, G., 136
Einhorn, L., 189, 533
Einhorn, V. F., 266
Eisen, A., 563, 564
Eisen, A. A., 392
Eisen, S. A., 442
Eisenberg, R. S., 389
Eisenberg, S., 499
Eisenstadt, W. A., 139
Eisner, M., 357
Ekengren, K., 133
Ekert, H., 187
Ekins, R. P., 448
Eknoyan, G., 71, 632
El-Ackad, T. M., 327
Elazar, Z., 483
Elde, R., 429, 432, 433
Eley, K. G., 271
Eliade, M., 654
Eliasson, M., 553, 554
Elkinton, J. R., 71
Ellinwood, E. H. Jr., 551
Elliott, H. W., 85, 86
Ellis, E. F., 569
Elmer, G. W., 99
Elmqvist, D., 396
El-Yousef, M. K., 299, 550
Emmerson, B. T., 201, 207
Endo, M., 149, 396
Enenkel, W., 152
Enero, M. A., 267
Engel, A. G., 396, 399, 401
Engel, R. R., 92
Engel, T. R., 239
Engel, W. K., 392-94
Engelbrecht, J. A., 264
Engelke, H., 55
Engert, R. F., 356
Engibous, D. L., 84
Engles, E., 487, 489
Engstedt, L., 186
Engstfeld, G., 156, 157

Enna, S. J., 553
Entman, M. L., 156, 442
Epling, C., 666
Epstein, A. N., 607, 609
Epstein, F. H., 78
Epstein, S. E., 442, 445, 457
Epstein, S. M., 443
Erb, W. H., 392
Erba, L., 205
Erez, M., 586
Erickson, C. K., 378
Erickson, R. W., 328
Ericsson, J. L. E., 624
Eriksson, L., 333
Erlij, D., 628
Ernst, A. M., 347
Ernst, P., 531, 532
Ernster, L., 137
Ervin, G. H., 612
Escalante, R., 661
Eskay, R. L., 432
Essex, H., 481
Estensen, R., 442
Estep, H., 75
Esther, L., 359
Estler, C.-J., 49
Eto, S., 151
Etschenberg, E., 90
Ettinger, B., 20
Eubanks, E. E., 614
Euler, U. S. von, 259, 263, 266, 268, 425, 430
Evan, I. M. A., 135
Evans, B. K., 610
Evans, D. P., 455
Evans, J. T., 189
Evans, J. V., 394, 396
Evanson, R. L., 67, 68, 70, 71
Even, E., 416
Everhart, W. H., 170
Ewald, R. W., 159
Ewe, K., 361
Ewton, M. F., 356
Ewy, G. A., 53, 58
Eyzaguirre, C., 388, 390

F

Fabre, J., 53
Fabricius, M., 159
Fabryka, E. F., 86
Facquet-Danis, J., 537
Fadiman, J., 667
Fahey, J. L., 179, 181, 188, 190
Faille, A., 531
Falch, D., 53, 294
Falchuk, K. H., 636
Falconer, J. D., 360
Fales, H., 491
Falk, G., 389, 391
Fallon, H. J., 505, 506
Faloon, W. W., 507, 508
Faloona, G. R., 357

Fambrough, D. M., 396, 397
Fan, W. C., 508
Fann, W. E., 49, 299
Faraci, R. P., 181
Farber, D. B., 447, 448
Farber, E., 538
Farber, M., 533
Farley, I. J., 550, 552
Farnebo, L. O., 263, 267
Farner, D., 62
Farnsworth, N. R., 121
Farquhar, M. G., 32, 33, 35
Farrell, P. M., 138
Farrer, D. N., 85
Fauci, A. S., 514
Fawcett, C. P., 37
Fawcett, D. W., 33
Fawcett, J. A., 419
Fawcett, P., 33, 34
Fayez, M. B. E., 655, 662
Fedak, S. A., 582, 585
Fedak, S. M., 582, 583, 585
Fee, W., 533
Feency, P. P., 250
Fefer, A., 188
Feger, J., 330
Feierstein, J. N., 190
Feinstein, H., 579
Feldberg, W., 344, 346, 349, 481, 482, 484
Feldman, E. B., 505
Feldman, J., 431
Feldman, P. E., 554
Feldstein, A. E., 346
Feldstein, M., 539
Felix, D., 432
Fell, H. B., 133, 134
Fellows, R., 432
Fencl, V., 425
Fenderson, O. C., 170
Feng, T. P., 396, 401
Fenichel, G., 390, 391
Fenichel, G. M., 396-402
Fenichel, J. A., 390
Feniuk, W., 270
Fennell, J., 483
Fenstermacher, J. D., 412
Fenton, J. J., 107
Ferguson, F. C., 37
Fernandez, L., 563, 564
Fernstrom, J. D., 614
Ferreira, S. H., 261, 266-68, 271
Ferrendelli, J. A., 450
Ferriero, D., 431
Ferris, R. M., 551
Fertel, R., 449-53, 458-62
Ficara, A. J., 446, 449
Fichman, M. P., 446, 448
Fiddler, M. B., 108, 109, 111
Fiehn, W., 388, 390
Field, J. B., 443
Field, M., 356-58

Fielding, S., 679
Figlin, R., 452, 458-61
Figulla, H.-R., 157, 158
Filburn, C., 360
Fillastre, J. P., 74
Fillion, G. M. B., 32
Finch, L., 332
Finck, A. D., 377
Findlay, J. A., 31
Fine, D., 319
Fine, L. G., 635
Fingerut, J., 357
Fingl, E., 355, 358
Fink, C. J., 36, 37
Fink, J., 37
Finkel, M. J., 137
Finkelstein, G., 357
Finkielman, S., 432
Finlayson, B., 12
Finnerty, F. A., 315-17
Fireman, P., 443
Firemark, H., 38
Firpo, J. J., 14
Fisch, C., 293
Fischbein, A., 206
Fischer, F., 482, 483
Fischer, G., 398, 400, 402
Fischer, G. H., 433
Fischer, J. C., 157
Fischer, L. J., 563, 566, 569
Fischer, R., 243, 530, 534
Fischer, S., 316
Fischer-Ferraro, C., 432
Fisher, A. E., 608
Fisher, G., 134
Fisher, J., 72
Fisher, J. C., 608
Fisher, J. W., 442
Fisher, L. A., 614
Fisher, L. J., 294
Fisher, V., 531
Fishlock, D. J., 357
Fishman, Y., 110
Fitzgerald, D. B., 117
Fitzgerald, R. J., 418
Fitzmaurice, M. A., 99, 101
Flaxman, B. A., 181
FLECKENSTEIN, A., 149-66; 150-52, 154-60
Fleckenstein, B., 150, 154, 157
Fleckenstein-Grün, G., 160
Fleisch, H., 20
Fleischer, N., 151
Fleischman, R., 103
Fleming, W. W., 396
Flesher, A. M., 139
Flessa, H., 531
Flink, E. B., 71, 74
Flores, S. E., 656, 665
Flower, R. J., 267-69
Flury, F., 481
Flynn, B., 532
Fodor, G., 658, 669, 670

Fog, R., 416, 417
Fogleman, D., 448
Foldes, F. F., 233, 238, 239, 376
Folk, B. P., 388, 390
Folkers, K., 433
Folkow, B., 313
Foltz, F. M., 134
Fong, H. H. S., 121
Foote, L. J., 99
Forbes, G. B., 199
Forbes, J. A., 315
Forbes, R. M., 203
Forcier, R., 534
Ford, S., 506
Fordtran, J. S., 356, 357
Forland, M., 15
Formal, S. B., 358
Forster, R. P., 68, 168, 172
Forte, L. R., 77
Forth, W., 359, 362
Foster, R. S., 343, 344
Foster, S. J., 591
Fothergill, L., 431
Fothergill, L. A., 431
Founier, C., 286
Fountas, P., 134
Fourcade, A., 188
Fournet, J. P., 75
Fowle, A. S. E., 294
Fowler, N. O., 300
Fox, F., 250
Fox, I. R., 142
Fox, J., 294
Fox, K. P., 393
Fox, Z., 563, 564
Frame, B., 134
Frame, M. H., 262, 264, 265, 268, 269
Francis, D. H., 455
Francis, J. E., 680
Franke, W. W., 37
Frankel, W. S., 239
Franklin, K. B. J., 610
Franklin, T. J., 591, 594
Franks, D. J., 451, 460
Franzen, D., 31
Franzén, S., 186
Fraser, D., 20, 75-78
Fraser, D. R., 135
Fraser, R., 72, 75
Fratantoni, J. C., 108
Fraysse, J., 445, 448
Frazer, A., 418
Frazier, P. D., 18
Freaney, R., 13, 75
Fredholm, B., 268, 269, 485
Fredholm, B. B., 262, 266, 268
Fredrickson, D. S., 499, 500, 504-6, 508
Free, C. A., 449, 453, 456, 458
Freed, J., 680

Freeman, B. W., 360, 361
Freeman, J. A., 390
Freeman, J. J., 373, 376
Freeman, J. T., 49
Freeman, S. E., 397
Frei, E. III, 100-2, 185, 187, 189, 530, 533-35
Freiberg, J. M., 313
Freireich, E. J., 183, 188, 189, 532-36
Freis, E. D., 319
French, J. E., 35
French, S. W., 590
Freund, H. J., 150-52, 154, 155, 157
Freund, J., 315
Frey, M., 156
Frey, T. S., 547
Freychet, P., 243
Friday, G. A., 443
Friedler, R. M., 75, 76, 78, 635, 640
Friedman, E., 378, 613
Friedman, M., 281, 282
Friedman, R. M., 453, 454
Friedman, S. A., 51
Friedman, W. F., 137
Friend, C., 188
Frier, H. I., 134
Frisk-Holmberg, M., 312
Fristedt, B. I., 201, 204
Fritz, R. R., 443, 444, 453, 462
Froesch, E. R., 448
Frohlich, E. D., 315, 317
Frohnert, P., 629
From, A., 608
Fromm, D., 356
Fromm, H., 16
Frömter, E., 625, 627, 629-31
Frontino, G., 50
Froscio, M., 444
Frost, P., 181
Fry, G. S., 648, 667
Fryer, C., 539
Fudenberg, H., 183
Fuhr, J. E., 454
Fujimori, H., 401
Fujita, T., 33
Fuller, R. W., 388, 609, 612
Fuller, T. J., 17
Fulton, C., 249-52
Furano, E., 486
Furchgott, R. F., 575, 576
Furlani, A., 99
Furnas, B., 533
Furst, P. T., 649, 653, 662, 663, 669
Furth, J., 539
Furth, J. J., 539
Furukawa, A., 397
Furukawa, H., 119
Furukawa, T., 397

Fuxe, K., 263, 347, 432, 433, 546, 608, 610
Fyro, B., 414, 421, 554

G

Gabbiani, G., 38
Gabreels, F. J. M., 563, 564
Gadd, R. E. A., 456
Gaddum, J. H., 425, 426, 429, 430
Gadea-Ciria, M., 369-72, 378, 379
Gaetano, G., 680
Gaffey, W. R., 208
Gage, F. H., 369
Gage, J. C., 199
Gage, P. W., 389
Gaginella, T. S., 360, 361, 363
Gagné, R. J. A., 14, 71
Gahrton, G., 186
Gakstatter, J. H., 169, 171
Gal, A. E., 98, 103
Gal, I., 134
Galand, G., 157, 158
Galante, J. G., 315
Galante, L. S., 135
Gale, C. C., 347
Gale, R. P., 181
Galeazzi, R. L., 298
Galindo, A., 332, 426
Gallagher, B. B., 141
Gallagher, J. C., 13
Gallina, A. M., 134
Gallo, D. G., 294
Galloway, D. B., 315
Galluzzi, N. J., 316
Galsky, A. G., 444
Gandolfi, A. J., 92
Ganellin, C. R., 331
Gang, M., 537
Ganong, W. F., 547
Gans, J. H., 505
Ganshorn, A., 565
Ganten, D., 432
Ganzer, U., 531
Gaoni, Y., 656, 668
Garabedian, M., 136
Garattini, S., 372, 377, 550, 554, 607, 612, 678
Garau, L., 370, 371, 376, 377
Garbarg, M., 325-30
Garber, B. T., 199
Garbers, D. L., 450
Garcia, D. A., 14, 135
García Jimenez, F., 656, 665
Gardiner, J. E., 372
Gardner, F. H., 442
Garelis, E., 411, 412
Garfield, C. F., 316
Gargouil, Y. M., 150, 157, 158
Garibay, K. A. M., 651, 671
Garnier, D., 150

Garrett, C., 158
Garrettson, L. K., 297, 563-65, 567, 569
Garver, D., 412
Garwood, F. A., 535
Gaschler, M., 448
Gaston, M. R., 110
Gaubatz, G. L., 332
Gaucher, S., 16
Gauld, E. N., 138
Gaumond, C., 109
Gauthier, M., 36, 37
Gavin, J. R., 243
Gavrilescu, N., 207
Gavrilovich, L., 315, 316
Gayton, R. J., 432
Gear, A. S., 315
Gee, T., 535
Gehan, E., 189
Gehan, E. A., 189
Geill, T., 137
Geissman, T. A., 127
Gelehrter, T. D., 297
Gencelly, R. E., 168
Genest, J., 432, 445, 448
Gent, J. P., 432
Gent, M., 305, 680
Gentleman, S., 249
Genton, E., 298, 305, 680
George, C. F., 314, 318
George, J., 432
George, S., 534-36
George, W. J., 264, 442, 450
Georgiev, V. S., 119
Gerald, M. C., 333
Geran, R. I., 117
Gerbode, F., 414, 417, 421
Gercovich, F., 536
Gerhardt, R. E., 298
Gericke, D., 453
Gerlach, J., 416, 417
Gerloczy, F., 139
Germain, G., 123
Gershoff, S. F., 19
Gershon, E., 135, 356, 358
Gershon, R. K., 182
Gershon, S., 378, 421, 550, 554
Gershwin, M. E., 286
Gertz, K. H., 634
Geschwind, I. I., 29, 30
Gessner, K., 625, 629, 630
Gessner, P. K., 346
Géy, K. F., 329
Gezenda, A. R., 169, 171
Gfeller, E., 325
Ghadimi, H., 106
Ghosh, P., 590
Giannella, R. A., 358
Giarman, N. J., 372, 376-78
Gibberd, F. B., 141
Gibson, E. S., 319, 320

Gibson, K. D., 205
Gibson, M. H., 530
Giebisch, G., 623, 626, 629, 631, 633, 636
Gifford, R. W., 311, 315
Gilberstadt, S., 17
Gilbert, J. B., 505
Gill, J. R., 640
Gillespie, E., 443, 455
Gillespie, J. S., 267
Gillette, J. R., 375
Gillette, P. C., 156
Gillingham, F. J., 415
Gilman, A. G., 451, 575, 577, 579-81, 584-87
Gilmore, C. J., 124, 129
Gilmore, E., 315, 317, 318
Gilmore, N., 266, 267
Gilmour, T. C., 200
Gingerich, R., 91
Ginn, D., 265
Ginn, H. E., 71
Ginsberg, N., 484
Giorgio, N. A., 243
Girard, A., 75, 77
Gitelman, H. J., 77
Gitter, S., 487, 489, 490
Gladtke, E., 563, 564
Glait, H., 190
Glancy, D. L., 445
Glaser, G. H., 397
Glass, D., 141
Glass, D. B., 442
Glauert, A. M., 133, 134
Glazko, A. J., 566
Gleason, M. N., 220
Gless, R. D., 119
Glew, R. H., 111
Glick, S. D., 348
Glickson, J. D., 243
Globerson, A., 283
Globus, D. L., 68
Glowinski, J., 329, 372, 373, 376, 546
Glueck, C. J., 506
Glynn, J. P., 110
Gnegy, M. E., 452
Godse, D. D., 614
Gohde, W., 532
Gokhale, S. D., 299
Golbey, R., 103
Gold, H. K., 445, 457
Gold, R. M., 608, 609
Goldberg, A., 205
Goldberg, A. I., 110
Goldberg, M., 14, 74, 640
Goldberg, M. E., 376
Goldberg, M. L., 443, 448
Goldberg, N. D., 442, 447, 450, 454
Goldberg, V. J., 680
Goldblatt, M. W., 259

Goldenberg, H., 449, 453, 456, 458
Goldfine, I. D., 243, 457
Goldin, A., 100
Goldin, H., 141
Goldman, A. S., 288
Goldman, D. E., 225, 228, 230, 232
Goldman, H. W., 613
Goldman, I. R., 152
Goldman, L. I., 181
Goldman, P. H., 579, 580
Goldman, R., 202
Goldsmith, R. S., 15
Goldstein, A., 282, 285, 577, 679
Goldstein, A. L., 282, 286-88
Goldstein, D. J., 432
Goldstein, E., 139
Goldstein, G., 283-86
Goldstein, L., 168, 172
Goldstein, M., 608, 610
Goldstein, R. B., 18
Goldstein, R. E., 445
Goldstein G., 284
Golenhofen, K., 158
Golub, S. H., 183
Gomez, M., 372, 378
Gómez-Acebo, J., 32
Gonda, A., 71
Gonick, H. C., 71
Gono, E., 201
Gonzalez, E., 628
Good, R. A., 183
Goode, D. J., 563, 564
Goodenow, J. S., 294
Goodgold, J., 388, 391
Goodhart, R. S., 133
Goodlet, I., 612
Goodman, D. S., 133, 134
Goodman, J., 568, 569
Goodman, J. M., 680
Goodman, M., 588
Goodman, R., 431
Goodwin, F. K., 411-13, 416, 418-22
Gopalakrishna, G., 376
Gorden, P., 243
Gordon, A., 243
Gordon, E., 411, 412
Gordon, E. K., 412-14, 419
Gordon, M., 679
Gordon, R., 555
Gordon, W. C, 186
Goren, E. N., 451, 452, 457
Gorgacz, E. J., 134
Görlitz, B. D., 152
Gorman, R. E., 442
Gorodetzky, C. W., 656, 665
Gorodischer, R., 569
Gorrod, J. W., 50
Gorshein, D., 442

Gorynia, I., 346
Gosch, F. C., 319
Gospodarowicz, D., 445, 448, 450
Gosselin, R. E., 220
Goth, A., 355, 358
Gottlieb, J. A., 189, 533
Gottlieb, T. B., 317-19
Gotto, A. M., 506
Gottschalk, C. W., 627-29, 640
Gouge, J. J., 36, 37
Gould, R. F., 174
Gould, R. G., 505
Goulding, R., 215
Gourlie, B., 532
Govindachari, T. R., 118
Goyer, R. A., 197, 199, 200, 203, 204, 206-8
Grabowska, M., 347
Grady, R. A., 123
Graham, D. T., 378
Graham, L. T. Jr., 427
Grahame-Smith, D. G., 443, 448
Grahmann, H., 55
Grandchamp, A., 628, 636
Graney, D., 361
Granger, P., 432
Granick, J. L., 205, 206
Granick, S., 205, 206
Grant, L. D., 607
Grant, P. T., 244
Grantham, S. J., 637, 639
Grau, J. D., 29, 30, 32, 150
Graudusius, R. T., 135
Graumann, W., 31
Gravenstein, J. S., 680
Gray, T. K., 357
Gray, R. W., 17, 135
Grayson, R., 215
Greeff, K., 30
Green, A., 534
Green, A. A., 187
Green, A. F., 300
Green, H., 328
Green, J. P., 325, 327
Green, M. D., 332, 341, 342, 348, 349
Green, R., 631, 633, 636
Greenberg, D., 546, 552
Greenberg, D. M., 104
Greenberg, J., 271
Greenberg, L. H., 442, 452, 457
Greenberg, N. H., 117
Greenberg, S., 264
Greenberger, N. J., 294
Greenblatt, D. J., 294
Greenblatt, M., 680
Greene, W. H., 187
Greengard, P., 224, 331, 442, 457, 461, 552, 587

Greenough, W. B. III, 356, 358
Greenspan, E. M., 678
Grega, G. J., 269
Gregoriadis, G., 109-11
Greider, M. H., 36
Greven, H. M., 425
Grewaal, D. S., 372
Grieco, H., 521
Griffey, M. A., 30
Griffin, T. B., 199, 201
Griffith, D., 17
Griffith, J. D., 550
Grill, V., 447
Grindey, G. B., 678
Gripe, K., 262, 268
Griswold, D. P., 530
Groblewski, G. E., 576
Grochowski, B. J., 109
Grodsky, G. M., 29, 31, 36, 37
Grollman, A., 62
Gross, L., 183
Gross, R., 530, 534
Gross, S. B., 200
Gross, S. R., 442
Grossman, M. I., 357
Grossman, S. P., 606
Groth, D., 535
Grove, J., 54, 57
Grower, M. F., 446, 449
Gruden, N., 199
Gruemer, H-D., 394
Grün, G., 150, 158-60
Grundy, S. M., 505
Grunfeld, Y., 487
Grün G., 150, 154
Gryglewski, R. J., 266
Grynderup, V., 427
Guay, G. F., 14
Guerra, F., 650, 651, 658, 666, 667, 671
Guha, A., 282, 285-87
Guichard, M., 537
Guidicelli, C., 19
Guidotti, A., 370, 371, 373, 376, 380
Guillemin, R., 29, 30, 432
Gulati, O. D., 299
Guldberg, H. C., 330, 411, 412, 415, 678
Gullbring, B., 186, 428
Gullikson, G. W., 360, 361
Gullino, P. M., 453
Gumpert, E. J. W., 411, 412
Gupta, M. L., 332
Gupta, S. K., 586
Gustafsson, L., 271
Gutenmann, W. H., 170, 171
Guterman, N., 479
Gutierrez-Hartman, A., 111
Gutman, A. B., 18
Gutmann, E., 396
Guton, A. C., 312, 316

Gutterman, J., 189
Gutterman, J. U., 182, 183, 185, 187-89
Guttler, R. B., 446, 448
Guyenet, P., 372, 373, 376
Guyenet, P. G., 372, 373
Guzmán, H. G., 660, 661
Gyory, A. Z., 630, 636

H

Ha, H., 426
Haanen, C., 535
Haas, H., 159
Haas, H. L., 329-33
Haas, T., 201
Haastert, H. P., 156-58
Haber, E., 579, 587, 588
Habermann, E., 482-85, 488, 489
Habibi, K., 199
Hackett, B. C., 319, 320
Haddox, M. K., 442, 447, 450, 454
Hadházy, P., 262, 270, 271
Haeger-Aronsen, B., 201, 203, 204
Haegermark, O., 485
Haeusler, G., 159
Haga, T., 373, 575, 585
Hagemann, R. F., 530
Hagler, L., 16
Hahn, F. E., 678
Hahn, G., 482
Hahn, M. A., 297
Hahn, R. A., 272
Hahn, T., 288
Hahn, T. J., 75, 76, 136
HAIT, W. N.,441-77; 444, 448, 451, 452, 459-62
Hakanson, R., 430
Hake, D., 531
Hakim, A. A., 358
Hales, C. N., 29-31, 36
Haley, T. J., 139
Halkin, H., 238, 294, 295
Hall, A. L., 130
Hall, G. H., 376
Hall, R. C., 134
Hall, T., 536
Hall, W. J., 266, 270, 271
Hall, Z. W., 590
Hallback, M., 313
Hallberg, L., 201
Hallick, R. B., 137
Halpern, B., 188, 189
Halprin, K. M., 447, 454
Halsall, T. G., 126
Halterman, R., 537
Haltiwanger, R. C., 124
Hamadah, K., 447-49
Hamashima, Y., 286, 287

Hambleton, J., 19
Hamburger, R. J., 624, 625, 640
Hamed, M. Y., 139
HAMELINK, J.L.,167-77; 170-72, 174
Hamer, J., 294
Hamet, P., 445, 448
Hamilton, H. E., 678
Hamilton, J. W., 30, 77
Hammes, G. G., 586
Hammond, D., 189
HAMMOND, P.B.,197-214; 200, 201, 205
Hammond, W. G., 13
Han, T., 111, 183
Hanahoe, T. H. P., 299
Handfield-Jones, R. P. C., 315
Handler, J. S., 456
Handley, S. L., 345-47
Handschumacher, R. E., 98, 101, 102, 109, 110
Handzel, Z. T., 288
Hancnson, I. B., 300
Hanieh, A., 415
Hanin, I., 370, 373-78
Hanna, S., 72, 75
Hanoune, J., 451, 458, 459, 578, 580, 591
Hanowell, E. G., 315, 316
Hansen, H., 482
Hansen, J., 316
Hansen, J. M., 51, 52, 56, 297
Hanson, J., 485
Hansson, L., 317
Harada, A., 331
Haranth, P. S. R. K., 376
HARDEN, T. K.,575-604; 577, 581, 583, 586, 588, 590-94
Hardesty, C. T., 101
Hardin, J. G. Jr., 521
Hardcastle, J. D., 361
Hardman, J. G., 442, 446, 450-52, 456, 459-61, 583, 640
Hardy, M. A., 286, 287
Hardy, W., 104
Hare, D., 629
Harington, M., 314
Harker, L. A., 305
Harley, J. D., 137
Haro, E. N., 508
Harper, D. T., 92
Harrah, M. D., 85, 86
Harrell, E. R., 447, 454
Harries, J. T., 359
Harris, A. J., 429
Harris, A. M., 84, 87-91
Harris, C. G. III, 458
Harris, D. J., 86
Harris, D. N., 449, 453, 456, 458, 460
Harris, E. J., 170

Harris, J., 179, 182, 183, 188, 356, 551
Harris, J. E., 184-86, 188
Harris, N. S., 288
Harris, R. S., 133
Harris, W. S., 86
Harrison, D. C., 295
Harrison, H. C., 19, 78
Harrison, H. E., 19, 78
Harrison, M. T., 75
Harrison, T., 72
Harry, J. D., 271
Hart, H., 19
HART, J. S., 529-43; 534-36, 538
Hart, R., 538
Hart, S. L., 361
Härtel, G., 158, 294
Hartenbower, D. L., 15, 75, 76, 78
Härtfelder, G., 159
Hartikainen, M., 158
Hartley, M. W., 207
Hartman, B. K., 584
Hartshorn, E. A., 677
Hartwell, J. L., 117-19
Harvey, A. M., 388
Harvey, D. R., 203
Harvey, R. F., 363
Harwood, J. P., 585
Hasan, A., 142
Hasan, J., 202, 203
Hashimoto, K., 159
Hashimoto, T., 428, 433
HASKELL, C.M.,179-85; 101, 179, 182, 183, 187, 189, 190
Hassing, G. S., 20
Hassler, R., 369
Hastings, C. W., 205
Hastreiter, A. R., 569
Hata, F., 36
Hathaway, P. W., 392
Hatt, A. M., 333
Hattan, B. A., 181
Haubrich, D. R., 375, 376
Hauser, D., 432, 581, 582, 586, 587
Hauser, R. L., 360, 361
Hauss, W., 532
Haussler, M., 14
Haux, P., 484, 485
Hava, M., 29, 31
Havard, C. W. H., 554
Havel, R. J., 499
Havener, W. H., 134
Haverman, R., 482
Hawk, M. H., 658
Hawker, C., 136
Hawkins, D. F., 563, 569
Hawkins, R. A., 370, 371, 373, 376
Hawthorne, J. N., 36

Hayase, K., 508
Hayase, S., 285
Hayat, M., 189
Hayduk, K., 432
Hayes, A., 534
Hayes, F., 535
Hayes, F. R., 170
Hayes, M. J., 54, 56, 60
Haynes, J., 297
Haynes, R. B., 319, 320
Hayslett, J. P., 636
Hayter, C. J., 634
Hayward, J. N., 345
Hazra, J., 271
Hazzard, W. R., 505
HEAGY, W.,243-58; 248-50, 254
Healy, K. M., 139
Heath, C., 298
Heaton, F. W., 68, 69, 71, 72, 75, 76, 78
Heaton, K. W., 363
Hebb, C., 376
Hecht, H. H., 317
Hechter, O., 578
Heddle, J. G., 141
Hedges, J. R., 359
HEDQVIST, P.,259-79; 261-71, 430
Hedwall, P. R., 262, 317
Heffelfinger, J. C., 297
Heffner, T. G., 608
Heffter, A., 649, 655, 662
Hegel, U., 627
Hegstrand, L. R., 331
Hegyi, T., 565
Hehl, U., 627
Heidland, A., 71
Heidrick, M. L., 442, 453, 454
Heikkinen, E. R., 447
Heim, R., 648-50, 652, 655, 660, 661
Hein, B., 154
Heinzerling, R. H., 139
Heizer, W. D., 355
Held, J., 550
Hellauer, H., 426
Helle, K., 32
Heller, A., 546
Hellman, B., 28, 36
Hellon, R., 344
Hellon, R. F., 345, 346
Hellström, I., 179, 181
Hellström, K. E., 179, 181
Hellstrom, L., 141
Helm, F., 189
Helrich, M., 92
Hemington, J. G., 446, 448
Hemminki, E., 680
Hemsworth, B. A., 370, 371, 373, 378, 380
Henderson, A., 356, 358

Henderson, C., 170
Henderson, D. A., 207
Henderson, G., 492
Henderson, H. F., 172
Hendrix, T. R., 355-57
Heninger, G. R., 414, 417, 421
Hennemann, H., 71
Henney, C. S., 181
Henriksen, O., 427
Henry, E., 183
Henry, J. L., 427, 429
Henry, P. D., 445, 457
Hensley, G. T., 357
Heppner, G., 183
Heppner, G. H., 185
Herberg, L. J., 610
Herberman, R. B., 183
Herbert, D., 456
Herbert, P. N., 500, 504-6, 508
Herbert, V., 142, 538
Herbst, A., 150, 154
Herding, J., 431
Herman, A., 271
Herman, A. G., 271
Herman, R. H., 16
Herman, R. L., 376
Herms, H. G., 678
Hermstein, N., 158
Hernández, F., 648, 650, 651, 660, 662, 664, 665, 669, 670
Hernandez, L., 617
Hernberg, S., 201-4
Herndon, C. N., 19
Herrán, J., 656, 665
Herrera-Acosta, J., 623, 634
Hersh, E., 189
Hersh, E. M., 182-89
Hersh, L. S., 111
Herz, W., 130
Hess, S. M., 331, 449, 453, 456, 458, 460, 591
Hession, C., 100
Hewick, D. S., 55, 62
Heyn, R. M., 189
Hibbert, S. R., 98
Hickie, R. A., 443, 453
Hickman, J., 109
Hickman, S., 103
Hicks, P. E., 332
Hicks, T., 357
Hiddemann, W., 532
Hierholzer, K., 629, 631, 636
Higgins, J. T., 358
Higgs, D. J., 138
Highman, B., 84, 85
Higson, J. E., 60
Hildebrand, E. M., 388
Hiley, C. R., 552, 586
Hill, A. V., 587
Hill, D. H., 186
Hill, H., 139

Hill, H. F., 347
Hill, J. M., 103
Hill, N., 103
Hill, R. C., 432
Hill, R. K., 658, 667
Hill, R. M., 567
Hillarp, N. aX8 Hiller, J. M., 431
Hillier, K., 267
Hills, A. G., 72
Hine, C. H., 85, 86, 200
Hines, J. D., 142
Hinley, J. B., 141
Hintz, H. P. J., 124, 125
Hippius, H., 325, 416
Hirohashi, M., 428, 433
Hirsch, A., 457
Hirsch, A. H., 451
Hirsch, J., 333
Hirsch, J. C., 327, 330
Hirschowitz, B. I., 451
Hirsh, J., 305, 680
Hirwe, A. S., 172
Hissa, R., 345, 346
Hitchcock, P., 139
Hittelman, K. J., 442
Hnik, P., 396
Ho, A. K. S., 590, 592
Ho, D. H. W., 100-2
Ho, H. C., 452
Ho, R. J., 591
Hobbs, D. H., 296
Hobe, R., 75
Hochella, N. J., 443, 448
Hodge, H. C., 220
Hodgins, D. S., 107
Hodgkin, A. L., 265, 389
Hodgkinson, A., 13-16, 19, 71
HOEBEL, B. G.,605-21; 606, 608-10, 612-17
Hoefer, J. A., 75
Hoeprich, P. D., 139
Hoffer, A., 656
Hoffer, B. J., 331, 332, 587
Hoffman, A. A., 19
Hoffman, B. F., 88, 293, 301
Hoffman, D. L., 20
Hoffmann, A., 456
Hoffmann, M., 456
Hoffmeister, F., 159
Hoffstein, S., 455
Hofmann, A., 649, 655, 656, 660, 665, 667, 669, 670
Hofmann, A. F., 16, 355, 357, 359
Hofmann, H., 482
Hofmann, W. W., 390
Hogben, C. A. M., 294
Hogberg, B., 485
Höglund, S., 186
Hohmann, B., 629
Hojer, B., 569

Hökfelt, T., 426, 428-30, 432, 433, 546, 608, 610
Hokin, L. E., 35
Hokkanen, E., 447
HOLCENBERG, J.S.,97-116; 98-101, 103-5, 109, 110
Holden, A. V., 169, 171
Holdstock, D., 486
Hole, D. R., 318
Holick, M. F., 135
Holker, B., 361
Holkstra, W. G., 138
Holland, J. G., 188
Holland, W., 75
Holland, W. W., 312
Hollenberg, M. D., 243, 581, 584
Hollenberg, N. K., 576, 586
Holley, K., 20
Hollifield, J., 312
Hollister, A. S., 612
Holloway, D. A., 51
Holm, G., 186
Holmes, B., 519
Holmes, E. C., 189
Holmes, J. C., 300
Holmgren, A., 186
Holmstedt, B., 357, 372
Holoye, P., 532
Holt, K., 20
Holtermann, O. A., 189
Holtzman, C. M., 508
Holtzman, E., 35
Holz, P., 140
Holzgreve, H., 635, 636
Holzman, N., 547
Homan, E. R., 110
Hommes, O. R., 141
Honour, A. J., 346
Hoobler, S. W., 299
Hook, E. B., 139
Hooper, J. A., 282, 286, 288
Hooper, K. C., 428
Hooper, W. D., 60
Hope, D. B., 32
Hopkins, C. R., 33
Hopkins, E. R., 32, 33, 35
Hopkins, H. A., 448
Hoppel, C., 563, 567, 569
Hori, T., 346
Horita, A., 346, 347
Horiuchi, K., 200
Horlick, L., 505
Horlick, L. L., 505
Horn, A. S., 611
Horning, M. G., 567
HORNYKIEWICZ, O.,545-59; 545, 550-54
Horovitz, Z. P., 458
Horowicz, P., 389
Horowitz, I. R., 356
Horrobin, D. F., 263

Horster, M., 624
Hörtnagl, H., 34
Hortobagyi, G., 189
Horton, C. L., 103
Horton, E. W., 266, 267, 269
Horton, L. J., 569
Horton, M. L., 84, 87-91
Horton, R., 73
Horton, R. W., 140
Horvath, C., 111
Horwitz, S. B., 119
Hoshi, M., 36, 37
Hoshiyama, M., 154
Hoskins, N. M., 680
Hosli, L., 329, 331, 332, 380
Hoszowska, A., 268
Houben, P. F. M., 141
Houck, J. C., 681
Houghton, G. W., 54, 57
Houssay, B. A., 29
Howald, W. N., 663
Howard, J. B., 563, 564
Howard, J. E., 19
Howard, J. L., 345, 412, 607
Howard, L., 264
Howard, M. R., 58, 294
Howe, E. S., 17
Howe, M. L., 287
Howell, R., 614
Howell, S. L., 33, 34, 36, 37
Hower, J., 201
Howie, V. M., 561
Hoyumpa, A., 55, 59, 60
Hrdina, P. D., 679
Hruban, Z., 134
Hsia, S. L., 447, 454
Hsiao, J. H., 91
Hsie, A. W., 453, 454
Hsu, P-Y., 443, 448, 453
Hsueh, W., 141
Huang, C. M., 33
Huang, M., 329, 331, 590, 592
Huang, N. N., 563
Huang, Y-C., 450
Hubbard, J. I., 265, 397
Huber, G. C., 623
Huber, W., 159
Hucho, F., 243
Hudak, W. J., 159
Hudgson, P., 393
Huet, P. M., 357, 363
Huffman, D. H., 294, 505
Hughes, J., 431
Hughes, L. E., 183
Hughes, M., 14
Huguenin, P., 534
Hui, W. H., 121
Hukovič, S., 427
Hullin, R. P., 448
Humbert, F., 628
Humphrey, D. C., 315
Humphrey, R., 532

Humphreys, M. H., 358, 637
Hunder, G. G., 525
Hunn, J. B., 172
Hunninghake, D. B., 505
Hunt, A. D., 140
Hunt, E. G., 168
Hunt, J. S., 189
Hunter, R., 141
Huong, T., 534
Huotari, R., 331, 332
Hurley, R. E., 316
Hursh, J. B., 198, 201
Hurwitz, A., 505
Huston, J. P., 613
Hutchins, M., 151
Hutchison, D. J., 105, 107
Hutter, O. F., 389
Hye, H. K. A., 325, 328
Hyman, A. L., 262, 264
Hymer, W. C., 28
Hynie, S., 445, 455

I

Ibrahim, M. Z. M., 327
Ice, R. D., 678
Ichord, R. N., 445
Ignarro, L. J., 442, 450, 455
Ihler, G. M., 111
Iizuka, Y., 428, 433
Ikehara, S., 286, 287
Ilfeld, D., 288
Illés, P., 263, 270, 271
Illner, P., 37
Imai, M., 624, 625, 627, 628,
  632, 634
Ingelfinger, F. J., 357
Inglis, A., 170
Inman, J. K., 206
Inoue, H., 72
Inouye, A., 426
Inscoe, J. K., 579
Insel, P., 581, 584, 594
Ireson, J. D., 299
Irion, E., 109
Iritani, C., 104
Irvine, R. E., 54, 57
Isaacs, H., 396
Isaia, J., 168
Isbell, H., 656, 665
Isenberg, H. D., 515
Iser, J. H., 359
Iseri, L. T., 680
Ishay, J., 483, 487, 489, 490
Ishida, A., 29, 35
Ishida, H., 36
Ishizuka, M., 455
Israel, L., 189
Ito, R., 298
Iucif, S., 134
Iven, H., 426
Iversen, L. L., 428, 679

Iversen, S., 551
Iversen, S. D., 679
Iwai, H., 457
Iyer, V., 390, 391
Izak, G., 188
Izbicki, R., 533
Izumi, F., 36

J

Jackson, C. E., 134
Jackson, I. M. D., 432
Jacob, E., 142
Jacob, H. S., 17
Jacob, J., 341, 346
Jacobowitz, D. M., 610
Jacobs, B. B., 181
Jacobs, B. L., 612-14
Jacobs, S., 582
JACOBSON, H. R.,623-46;
  624, 625
Jacoby, J. H., 613
Jagenburg, R., 203, 207
Jain, A., 507
Jakschik, B., 267, 268
Jalling, B., 563-65, 567, 569,
  570
James, S. L., 183
Jamieson, J. D., 33, 37
Jamison, R. L., 624
Jandl, J. H., 206
Janicki, R. H., 141
Janiger, O., 670
Janke, J., 152, 154-56
Janov, C., 515
Janowsky, D. S., 299, 447, 448,
  550
Jaques, R., 485, 486
Jard, S., 640
Jarett, L., 577, 581, 582, 587,
  588
Jasmin, G., 154
Jasper, H. H., 370-73
Játiva, M. C. D., 666
Javoy, F., 372
Jedrzejczyk, J., 397
Jeffcoate, S., 432, 433
Jefferson, J. W., 554
Jeffery, E. H., 139
Jell, R. M., 346
Jellinger, K., 545, 552
Jenden, D. J., 332, 370, 373-76,
  379
Jenkins, B. C., 451
Jenkins, L. J. Jr., 92
Jennekens, F. G. I., 133
Jenner, F. A., 448
Jenney, E. H., 140
Jennings, H. S., 244
Jensen, O. N., 141
Jensen, W. N., 206
Jentsch, J., 483

Jerina, D. M., 92
Jerks, J., 317
Jerrome, D. W., 35
Jesperson, S., 612
Jessell, T., 428, 429
Jessup, R., 428
Jewers, K., 117
Jhamandas, K., 377
Jodrey, L. H., 170
Johannessen, B., 75
Johansson, O., 429, 432, 433, 546, 608, 610
Johns, D. G., 107
Johnson, A. L., 319, 320
Johnson, A. O., 296
Johnson, B. F., 294
Johnson, C. B., 243
Johnson, D., 532
Johnson, D. G., 265
Johnson, D. W., 167, 168
Johnson, E. M., 267, 268
Johnson, G., 16
Johnson, G. A., 15
Johnson, G. L., 581, 583, 586, 591, 594
Johnson, G. S., 444, 445, 453, 454
Johnson, J., 356, 358
Johnson, J. M., 117
Johnson, M., 393
Johnson, R. A., 589
Johnson, W. L., 170
Johnson, W. P., 315
Johnsson, G., 317
Johnston, A. W., 299
Johnston, C. I., 317
Johnston, D., 532
Johnston, G. A. R., 380
Johnston, I. H., 380
Johnston, R., 391
Joiner, P. D., 262, 264
Jones, A. L., 33
Jones, C. W., 34
Jones, D. J., 446, 458
Jones, J. E., 74
Jones, R. A., 92
Jonsson, G., 610
Joo, P., 189
Jordan, D. A., 134
Jorgensen, T., 35
Jori, A., 54, 57, 418
Jose, D. G., 183, 187
Joselow, M., 205
Joselow, M. M., 207, 208
Joshua, H., 490
Josinovich, J. B., 446
Jowsey, J., 20, 75, 76, 78, 134
Joyce, J. W., 525
Jubert, A. V., 189
Juel-Jensen, B. E., 315
Julian, J. A., 512
Jung, R., 491

Junod, A., 35
Junstad, M., 265, 267, 268, 270
Jurgens, R., 137
Jusko, W. J., 563, 564, 567, 569
Juvancz, I., 139

K

Kacser, H., 327
Kadlec, O., 271
Kadowitz, P. J., 262-64, 270
Kaehny, W. D., 16
Kagan, B. M., 134
Kagedal, B., 312
Kahn, C. R., 243
Kahn, R. H., 442
Kahyo, H., 207
Kaiser, J., 158
Kakiuchi, S., 331, 452, 461, 590
Kakkar, V. V., 108
Kalbe, I., 50
Kalberer, E., 294
Kalbfleisch, J. M., 71
Kaley, G., 262
Kalisker, A., 590, 592
Kallberg, N., 567, 569
Kaller, H., 159
Kallistratos, G., 12
Kallman, B. J., 169
Kalman, S. M., 577
Kaluza, J., 347
Kamanabroo, D., 532
Kamberi, I. A., 29, 30
Kameyama, Y., 134
Kaminsky, N. I., 446
Kammermeier, H., 150-52, 154, 155, 157
Kampmann, J., 52, 56, 297
Kanazawa, I., 428, 429
Kandera, J., 431
Kanno, T., 29, 30
Kanof, P. D., 331
Kao, R. C. L, 203
Kapadia, G. G., 53, 58
Kapadia, G. J., 655, 662
Kapelner, S., 206, 563
Kapetansky, F., 134
Kaplan, H. R., 269
Kaplan, J. C., 451, 458, 459
Kaplan, J. M., 569
Kaplan, L., 667
Kaplan, N. O., 588
Kaplan, R., 13, 14
Kaplan, S. A., 455
Kaplan, S. L., 75, 77
Kaplinsky, E., 483, 490
Kapoor, I. P., 172
Kappas, A., 205, 206, 563, 678
Karaman, H., 136
Karch, F. E., 293

Karesoja, M., 295
Karim, A., 124
Karim, S. M. M., 264, 267
Karlberg, B. E., 312
Karlin, A., 243
Karmali, R., 263
Karnofsky, D., 103
Karnovsky, M. L., 425
Karon, M., 189
Karoum, F., 412
Karp, J., 539
Karpati, G., 391, 392, 394
Karpman, H., 152
Karppanen, H., 331, 332
Karsunky, K. P., 432
Kaser, O., 137
Kashgarian, M., 629, 636
Kashimoto, T., 36
Kasuya, M., 139
Katakkar, S., 189
Kataoka, K., 327, 369, 426
Kato, R., 50
Kattau, R. W., 388
Katz, B., 265, 398, 487
Katz, D. H., 287
Katz, F. H., 317-19
Katz, J., 234, 238
Kauffman, F. C., 391
Kauffman, R. E., 563, 564, 569
Kaufman, C. E., 71
Kaufman, J. W., 85, 86
Kaufmann, J. S., 299
Kaufmann, R., 156
Kaufmann, W., 104
Kavalach, A. G., 18
Kawakami, M., 432
Kawamura, S., 624, 625, 631
Kawashima, K., 453
Kayaalp, S. O., 269
Kaye, C. M., 55, 59
Kaye, G. I., 627
Keasling, H. H., 390
Keating, F. R. Jr., 523
Kebabian, J. W., 442, 457, 461, 552, 581, 582, 587, 590, 593
Kecskemeti, V., 266
Keenan, B. S., 99
Keenan, T. W., 33
Kehoe, R. A., 198-200
Keimowitz, R. I., 356, 636
Keist, R., 453
Kelemen, K., 266
Kellaway, C., 481, 482, 484
Keller, C., 454
Keller, R., 453
Keller, W. J., 667
Kellerth, J. O., 426, 428-30, 433
Kelley, P. R., 444, 448
Kello, D., 199
Kelly, P. J., 20
Kemp, J. A., 429, 430

Kemp, R. G., 443, 448, 453
Kenaga, E. E., 174
Kench, J. E., 207
Kendall, M. J., 54, 58
Kennedy, B., 539
Kennedy, G. L., 205
Kennedy, M. S., 347
Kephart, J. E., 33
Kerley, G. I., 123
Kermowitz, R. I., 635
Kerr, J. W., 443
Kerr, S. R., 172
Kerzner, B., 293
Kessler, J. A., 412
Kessler, R. H., 68
Kessner, D. M., 78
Keusch, G. T., 357
Kevern, N. R., 169
Kewitz, H., 369, 370, 373, 374
Key, B. J., 554
Khalil, S. A. H., 294
Khaliq, A., 189
Khalsa, M. S., 172
Khan, A., 103
Khankhanian, N., 189
Khanna, N. N., 563, 566, 569
Khoo, H. E., 199
Khoo, J. C., 442
Kiang, D., 539
Kibler, W. B., 396-400, 402
Kidder, G. W., 140
Kidman, A. D., 442
Kiesewetter, R., 57
Kiker, R., 519
Killander, A., 186
Killander, D., 186
Killmann, S. A., 529, 531, 532
Kim, D. K., 122
Kim, J. H., 103
Kim, U., 444
Kimberg, D. V., 135, 356-58
Kimura, H., 443, 448, 450
King, L. J., 92
King, M. L., 121
King, R. G., 72
Kinkel, A. W., 563, 564
Kinne, R., 636
Kinsey, M. D., 358
Kiorboe, E., 297
Kiosz, D., 565
Kipnis, D. M., 37, 442, 450
Kippen, I., 18, 19
Kirkegaard, L., 450
Kirklin, J. K., 140
Kirkpatrick, C. H., 454
Kirkpatrick, W. E., 343, 344
Kirpekar, S. M., 265
Kirshner, A. G., 32
Kirshner, N., 32, 34, 35
Kirwan, W. O., 360
Kiser, R., 519
Kitagawa, K., 429, 430

Kitchell, J. F., 172, 173
Kitto, G. B., 111
Kittredge, J. S., 244
Kiyomoto, A., 154, 159
Kizer, J. S., 432
Klachko, D. M., 388, 390
Klainer, E., 262
Klaus, W., 152
Kleeman, C. R., 68-73, 75-77
Klein, D. C., 451
Klein, E., 189
Klein, H. O., 530, 534
Klein, W. M., 668
Klein, E., 288
Klein Obbink, H. J., 134
Klenerova, V., 445
Klepzig, H., 152
Kleszynski, R. R., 74
Kligerman, M., 445, 448
Kligman, A. M., 134
Kline, K., 537
Klineberg, O., 653, 662
Klinenberg, J. R., 18, 19
Klipstein, F. A., 356
Klose, R. M., 623
Klotz, U., 55, 59, 60, 451
Knab, T., 670
Knaven, P. J. H., 141
Knelson, J. H., 199, 201
Knippers, R., 69
Knochel, J. P., 17
Knoll, J., 262, 263, 266, 270, 271
Knouss, R. F., 298
Knowles, F., 13, 20
Knowles, F. G. W., 433
Knox, A. E., 419
Knox, F. G., 636
Knox, G. V., 342, 343
Knudson, A. G. Jr., 133
Kobayashi, K., 134
Kobayashi, R. M., 329
Kobayashi, S., 33
Kobel, H., 649, 655, 660
Koblick, D. C., 138
Koch, C. E., 315
Koch, K. M., 636
Koch-Weser, J., 294, 296, 303, 317, 318
Kodama, T., 331
Kodicek, E., 135
Koehler, J. P., 392
Koening, H., 39
Koestner, A., 432
Kofman, S., 536
Kohlhardt, M., 150, 155-58
Kohn, A. J., 244
Kohner, E. M., 317
Koketsu, K., 265
Kokko, J. P., 624, 625, 627-34, 639
Kokubun, H., 159

Kolanowski, J., 524
Kolb, F. O., 20
Kolendorf, K., 51
Komiya, Y., 395
Komoda, Y., 124, 125
Komuro, K., 285
Konasewich, D. E., 174
Konings, A. W. T., 444
Konishi, S., 425-29
Kooh, S. W., 75
Kook, A. I., 283, 286
Koonce, J. F., 172, 173
Kopera, H., 426, 429
Kopin, I. J., 265, 329, 412, 679
Kopito, L., 202
Kopp, L. E., 446, 448
Koppel, M. H., 15
Korbut, R., 266
Koretz, S., 578
Koretz, S. H., 580
Korf, J., 413, 420
Korfmacher, S. D., 315
Kormendy, C., 49
Korn, S., 169, 171
Kornerup, H. J., 318
Kornetsky, C., 552-54
Kornfeld, S., 110
Korte, F., 680
Korus, R. A., 112
Koshland, D. E. Jr., 243
Koski, G., 425
Koslow, S., 375
Kosow, D. P., 108
Kosterlitz, H. W., 431
Kostial, K., 199, 200
Kostianovsky, M., 33
Kostis, J. B., 508
Kotani, M., 331
Kourides, I. A., 522
Kovacs, C. J., 448
Koysooko, R., 569
Koziorowska, J., 531
Kozyreff, V., 588
Krag, E., 357, 359
Kraicer, J., 29, 30, 37
Krakoff, I., 103
Krall, R., 200
Kramer, B., 199
Kramer, G. D., 446, 449
Kramer, S., 205
Kramer-Blankestijn, M., 513
Krans, H. M. J., 585, 588
Krantz, J. C. Jr., 90-92
Kranz, D., 50
Krasnegor, N. A., 679
Krasner, J., 565
Krasula, R. W., 569
Krauer, B., 563, 564, 569
Krause, H., 150, 155, 156, 158
Krauss, R. M., 500, 504-6, 508
Kredich, N. A., 99
Kreighbaum, W. E., 450, 451

Kreis, W., 100
Kreitner, D., 158
Kremer, W., 531
Kress, Y., 208
Kreusser, W. J., 640
Krikler, D., 152, 158
Krikler, D. M., 158
Krimsky, I., 608
Kripke, M. L., 181, 182
Krishna, G., 451, 455
Krishnamoorthy, M. S., 329, 330
Kristensen, M., 52, 56, 297
Kritchevsky, D., 502, 504, 680
Krivit, W., 109
Krivoy, W. A., 428
Krnjevic, K., 332, 426, 427, 429
Kroneberg, G., 152, 159
Krotkiewski, M., 513
Krueger, J., 425
Kruger, P. G., 327, 328
Kruk, Z. L., 347
Krulich, L., 37
Krumdieck, C. L., 141
Kruse, R., 136
Kuba, K., 397, 402
Kubic, V. L., 92
Kubikowski, P., 344, 346
Kuchel, O., 445, 448
Kudchodkar, B. J., 505
Kuehl, F. A. Jr., 442
Kuenzer, W., 565, 568
Kuffler, S., 487
Kuffler, S. W., 429, 590
Kuhar, M. J., 326, 327, 329, 330, 369, 372, 373, 375-80, 431
Kuhlmann, K., 51
Kuhn, E., 388, 390
Kuhn, W. L., 159
Kukovetz, W., 442, 457
Kukovetz, W. R., 456
Kulenkampff, H., 362
Kulshrestha, V. K., 333
Kunze, F. M., 200
Kunze, K., 395
Kunze, W., 57, 58
Kuo, J. F., 442, 457
Kuo, P. T., 508
Kuo, W-N., 442, 457
Kupchan, S. M., 119, 121, 124, 125, 127-30
Kupferberg, H. J., 563
Kupiecki, F. P., 446-48, 456
Kurland, L. T., 316
Kurokawa, K., 640
Kurz, H., 565
Kuschinsky, W., 636
Kusin, J. A., 134
Kutt, H., 297
Kvamme, E., 329

Kvetnansky, R., 679
Kwaan, H. C., 108
Kwiatowski, H., 325
Kwiecinski, H., 388, 390
Kwiterovich, P. O., 506
Kyle, G. C., 17
Kyle, L. H., 75

L

La Barre, W., 649
Labarthe, D. R., 316
Labella, F. S., 28
Labelle, E., 185
Labrie, F., 36, 37, 432, 433
Lacadie, J. A., 127-29
Lacaillade, C., 481
Lacefield, W. B., 388
Lacombe, M.-L., 580
Lacour, F., 188
Lacy, F. B., 624
Lacy, P. E., 32, 33, 36, 37
Lader, M. H., 679
Lader, S., 294
Ladinsky, H., 372, 377
Lagarde, A., 451
Lagercrantz, H., 271
Lagunoff, D., 38, 103
Lahav, M., 587
Lal, H., 679
Lal, S., 412
Lambert, E. H., 396, 399, 401
Lambert, L. A., 432
Lambert, M., 36
Lamberts, S. W. J., 513
Lamola, A. A., 205
La Montagne, A. E., 265
Lampart, C., 326-29, 348
Lampkin, B., 531
Lance, B. M., 181
Landa, J. F., 389, 391
Landahl, H., 36, 37
Landes, R. R., 19
Landis, D. H., 412
Landmark, K., 157
Lands, A. M., 576
Lands, W. E. M., 442
Landwehr, D. M., 623
Landy, M., 185
Lane, B. P., 134
Lane, M., 183
Lane, N., 627
Lang, E. P., 200
Lang, F. G., 454
Lang, M., 579
Langan, T. A., 157, 454
Langer, J., 481
Langer, S. Z., 267, 268
Langer, T., 500, 502, 503, 506
Langley, P. L., 388, 390
Langman, M. J. S., 54, 56, 60
Lanzotti, V., 538

Laparre, C., 534
Laragh, J. H., 312, 317
Larengood, R. W. Jr., 17
Large, B. J., 270, 299
Larkins, R. G., 135
LaRosa, J., 506
Larson, K. A., 122
Larsson, L. I., 327, 430
LaRusso, N. F., 355
Larvor, P., 75, 77
Lasagna, L., 50, 293
Lash, E. D., 100, 101
Laska, E. M., 316
LASKOWSKI, M. B.,387-409; 396-99, 401, 402
Lass, I., 489, 490
Lassen, N. A., 313
Lasser, M., 579
Lassiter, W. E., 627, 629, 640
Laster, L., 355
Laster, W. R., 530
Lastowecka, A., 29-32, 37
Latham, C. J., 606, 615
Latta, H., 202
Lau, J. R., 20
Lau, K., 14
Laudat, M-H., 580
Laurence, D. R., 299
Laursen, H., 52, 56
Lauwerys, R. R., 203-6
Laverty, R., 546, 547
Lavin, N., 455
Law, D. K., 183
Lawrence, E. C., 13, 14
Lawrence, W. Jr., 183
Lawson, A. A., 315
Lawson, N. L., 624, 625, 640
Lawton, R. L., 18
Lazarides, E., 38
Lazarini, W., 426, 429
Lazarow, A., 28
Lazarus, H., 106
Lazarus, S. S., 33, 34
LEAKE, C. D., 677-82;
LeBeux, Y. J., 38
Lebovitz, H. E., 448
Lech, J. J., 168
Ledilschke, B., 482
Lee, C. Y., 586
Lee, J. B., 264
Lee, K. S., 152
Lee, R. E., 198
Lee, S. C., 267
Lee, T., 553
Lee, T. C., 530
Leeman, S. E., 426, 430, 433
Leeming, J. T., 50
Leeper, R. D., 103
Lees, R. S., 499
Leeson, G. A., 140
LeFevre, H. F., 370

Lefkowitz, R. J., 575, 577, 579-85, 587-89, 591, 593, 594
Lefresne, P., 373, 376
LeGendre, G. R., 16
Le Grimellec, C., 68, 69, 624, 625
Legros, J. J., 32
Lehane, D. E., 183
Lehman, J. T., 251
Lehmann, H. E., 139
Lehmann, K., 55
Lehne, R., 451, 452, 460, 463
Lehninger, A. L., 97
Lehr, D., 613
Leibowitz, S. F., 333, 607, 610, 611
Leichtling, B. H., 591, 594
Leighton, J., 454
Leighton, M., 54, 57
Leikola, E., 51, 52, 56
Leishman, A. W. D., 299
Leitner, Z. A., 139
Lemaire, S., 36
Lemaire, W. J., 445
Lemann, J. Jr., 16, 17, 19, 71, 72
Lemay, A., 36, 37
Lembeck, F., 426, 428
Lemberger, L., 576, 679
Lempérière, T., 655, 661
Lenfant, J., 157, 158
LENHOFF, H. M., 243-58; 244, 246-54
Lennartz, K., 530, 534
Lennon, E. J., 16, 19, 71, 72
Lennon, V. A., 396
Lenon, H. L., 169, 170
Leonard, D. L., 207
Leonard, J. W., 315
Leonard, R. A., 442
Leong, L., 296
LeQuire, V., 390
Leray, F., 578, 591
Lergier, W., 430
Lerner, R. L., 505
Leshem, M. B., 606, 607, 612-15
Lesko, L., 578
Lesniak, M. A., 243
L'Estrange, J. L., 75
Leung, S., 85, 86
Levander, O. A., 138
Leveille, G. A., 508
Leventhal, B. G., 187, 537
Lever, J. D., 31
Levere, R. D., 205, 206
Levey, G. S., 442, 445, 457
Levi, J., 75-77
Levin, R. H., 185
Levin, R. M., 452, 458, 459, 461
Levin, S., 288

Levin, S. R., 31
Levine, L., 267
Levine, N., 287
Levine, R. R., 141, 295
Levine, S. G., 119
Levinsky, N. G., 635
Levinson, W., 457
Levintow, L., 104
Levitsky, S., 569
Levitzki, A., 577, 581, 582, 585, 586
Levy, B., 576
Levy, D., 138
Levy, G., 297, 563, 565, 566, 569
Levy, G. S., 445
Levy, J., 186, 442
Levy, M., 103
LEVY, R. I.,499-510; 499, 500, 502-6, 508
Lewis, J., 492
Lewis, J. A., 315
Lewis, J. C., 360, 361
Lewis, M., 108
Lewis, P. J., 317, 344, 345
Lewis, P. R., 369
Lewis, R. E., 159
Lewis, R. P., 294
Lewy, J. E., 628, 635, 636
Leyden, J. J., 134
Lheritier, J., 534
Li, T. H., 401
Liao, S., 578
Lichtenstein, L. M., 442, 443, 455
Lidbrink, P., 610
Liddell, D. E., 53, 57
Liddle, G. W., 446, 640
Lieb, A. J., 169
Lieber, C. S., 679
Liebow, C., 27
Lien, E. J., 678
Lifshitz, F., 78
Lifson, N., 358
Lilienthal, J. L. Jr., 388, 390
Lilis, R., 207
Lilius, H., 204
Lilly, L. F., 287
Lim, E. C., 507
Lim, T. W., 98, 103
Limacher, J. J., 331, 430
Limas, C. J., 319
Limbird, L., 582, 587
Limbird, L. E., 575, 582, 589
Lin, A. H., 578
Lin, J. C., 183
Lin, M. C., 585
Lin, T., 446, 448
Lin, Y. M., 450, 452
Linarelli, L. B., 640
Lincoln, T., 444
Lind, M., 563, 565, 566, 569

Lindall, A. W., 28
Lindeman, R. D., 71
Lindenbaum, J., 294
Lindgren, J.-E., 663
Lindholm, N., 513
Lindner, E., 158, 159, 425
Lindop, M. J., 54, 58, 60
Lindqvist, M., 413, 545
Lindquist, R. N., 678
Lindstedt, K. J., 244, 246, 250, 252
Lindstrom, J. M., 396
Lindup, W. E., 61
Lindvall, O., 546
Lineweaver, H., 247
Ling, N., 432
Ling, W. Y., 445
Lingard, J., 630
Lingard, J. M., 630
Lipat, G. A., 207, 208
Lipicky, R. J., 389
Lipinski, J. F., 325
Lippert, W., 139
Lippman, M. E., 512, 537
Lippmann, W., 457
Lipton, A., 103
Lipton, M. A., 412, 419
Lisk, D. J., 170, 171
Litchfield, M. H., 199
Little, S. A., 450
Littleton, G. K., 442
Litwack, G., 448, 454, 464
Litzow, J. R., 16, 19
Liu, Y. P., 109, 452
Livesley, B., 152
Livett, B. G., 32
Livingston, R., 103
LIVINGSTON, R. B., 529-43; 533-36, 538
Ljungdahl, A., 546
Llach, F., 75-77
Llorens-Cortes, C., 326, 328, 330, 333
Lloyd, H. H., 530
Lloyd, K. G., 369-72, 378, 379, 545, 552, 553
Lockhart, J. D., 561
Locklear, T. W., 356
Lockner, D., 186
Lockwood, T., 298
Lockwood, T. E., 668
Lodge, R., 315
Lodola, E., 49
Loeb, E., 103
Loeb, J. N., 522
Loeb, M., 251, 252
Loewi, O., 160
Logan, W. J., 679
Logsdon, P. S., 443
Lolley, R. N., 447, 448
LOMAX, P.,341-53; 332, 341-44, 348, 349

Lomo, T., 396, 397
Lonai, P., 286
Londos, C., 585
Long, A., 55, 58, 59
Long, E., 111
Long, G. J., 563, 567
Long, J. A., 33
Long, T. T., 19
Longmire, R., 179
Lonigro, A. J., 262
Loomis, W. F., 246, 248
Looney, W. B., 443, 448
Loos, M., 100
Lopes, R. A., 134
López, A., 661
López-Austin, A., 648, 650, 651
Lorand, L., 578
Lorber, S. H., 357
Lorden, J. F., 609, 610
Lorens, S. A., 612
Lorentz, W. B., 627, 628, 640
Losert, W., 456
Lossnitzer, K., 154
Loten, E. G., 451
Lotti, V. J., 344, 346
Loughnan, P. M., 563-65, 569
Louis, C. J., 443
Louis, W. J., 317
Love, A. H. G., 362
Lovejoy, F. H., 215
Lovell-Smith, C. J., 447, 448, 456
Lovely, P., 243
Lowbeer, T. S., 363
Lowitz, H. D., 624, 636
Lowndes, H. E., 398
Lowy, B., 648, 660
Lowy, P., 483
Lu, P. L., 101
Lu, P.-Y., 171
Lu, S. T., 119
Lucas, P. W., 75, 76
Luce, J., 532
Luchi, R. J., 298
Luckens, M. M., 215
Luckey, T. D., 284
Lucy, J. A., 38, 133, 134
Ludden, C. T., 299, 317
Luduena, F. P., 576
Ludueña, M. A., 38
Ludwig, F. L., 198
Ludwig, G. D., 17
Ludwig, J., 133
Luecke, R. W., 75
Luff, R. M., 345
Luft, R., 429, 432, 433
Lullin, M., 53, 58
Lullman, H., 391
Lumholtz, B., 52, 56, 297
Lumholtz, C., 649, 662, 663
Lunan, H. N., 680

Lundgren, G., 372
Lundgren, Y., 313
Lundholm, B., 376
Lung, E., 137
Lütold, B., 28
Lutz, M. D., 627, 632, 633
Lux, S. E., 500, 504-6, 508
Lynch, T. J., 445, 450
Lyons, M. M., 207, 208
Lytle, L. D., 614
Lytle, R. B., 401

M

MAAS, J. W.,411-24; 412, 419, 420
MacAuley, S. J., 135
Macchia, V., 444, 448
MacConnell, J., 491
MacDonald, M. M., 117
MacDougall, T. A., 656, 664
MacDowell, M. C., 623
Macek, K. J., 169, 171
MacEwen, J. D., 92
MacFadyen, B., 538
MacGregor, R. R., 77
Mache, K., 201
Machne, X., 224, 230
MacInnes, R. M., 636
MacIntosh, F. C., 370-72, 376, 396
MacIntosh, J. R., 628
Macintyre, E. H., 443
MacIntyre, I., 72, 75, 78, 135
Mackay, I. R., 183
Mackie, A. M., 244
Mackie, G. O., 250
MacKinney, A., 532
MacKinnon, J., 315
Mackler, B. F., 181
MacLean, P. D., 329, 332, 549
MacLellan, A., 103
MacManus, J., 75, 76, 78
MacManus, J. P., 451, 460
Macnab, R., 243
Maddaiah, V. T., 136
Maddox, G. L., 49
Maddux, G. W., 134
Madras, B. K., 614
Maesaka, J. K., 207, 208
Maetz, J., 168
Magnuson, J. J., 172, 173
Magnusson, T., 545
Maguire, M. E., 575, 577, 579-81, 584-87
Magyar, K., 262
Mahaffey, J., 75, 77
Maickel, R. P., 333
Maidhof, R., 71
Majchrowicz, E., 679
Majors, W. J., 201
Makman, M. H., 443, 445, 591

Malaise, E., 537
Malaisse, W. J., 29, 31, 150, 442
Malaisse-Lagae, F., 31, 38
Malamed, S., 34
Malani, F., 32
Malchoff, C. D., 580
Malcolm, D., 208
Malendin, H., 74
Malerczyk, V., 52, 55, 56, 565
Malik, K. U., 262, 264, 268
Malik, M. K. U., 554
Malmcrona, R., 317
Malmfors, T., 267
Malmo, R. A., 554
Maloof, F., 522
Mamrak, F., 331, 591
Manchanda, A. H., 117
Mandelli, M., 563, 564, 567
Mandel, W. J., 240
Mander, A. M., 183
Mandy, S. H., 447, 454
Mandy, W. J., 186
Manganiello, V., 455
Manganiello, V. C., 450
Mangos, J. A., 634
Manian, A. A., 552
Manji, P. M., 356
Manku, M. S., 263
Mann, C. V., 361
Mann, F., 481
Manninen, V., 294, 295
Manning, J., 206
Mansell, P., 536
Mansour, T. E., 249
Mantovani, A., 186
Many, N., 188
Mao, C. C., 379, 380
Marc, V., 412
March, B. E., 139
Marchand, N. W., 443, 453
Marchesi, V. T., 35
Marchetti, P., 372, 377
Marcilloux, J.-C., 609
Marco, G., 379
Marco, J., 512
Marconcini-Pepeu, I., 370, 371, 376, 377
Marcus, F. I., 53, 58
Marcus, R. J., 551
Margolis, F. L., 431
Margolis, S., 455
Margules, D. L., 607, 609, 610, 614
Marinetti, G. V., 578, 580
Mariscal, R. N., 250, 251
Mark, A. L., 262
Mark, G., 243
Markowitz, J., 481
Markowitz, R., 552-54
Marks, B. H., 432
Marks, J., 133, 138

Marks, N., 428
Markstein, R., 584
Markwardt, F., 456
Marley, E., 345
Marlowe, G. C., 568
Marquez-Julio, A., 432
Marsanico, R. G., 348
Marsden, C. A., 678
Marsh, J. M., 442, 445
Marshall, D. H., 12, 18
Marshall, G. J., 532
Marshall, G. R., 243, 248-50, 254, 268
Marshall, N. B., 168
Marshall, R. W., 12, 16, 18, 20
Marshall, V. F., 17
Martin, A. R., 397
Martin, B. R., 419, 585
Martin, G. E., 347
Martin, J. B., 432, 433
Martin, L. G., 75, 77
Martin, R. C., 189
Martin, S., 29, 30
Martin, T. J., 443
Martínez, M., 665, 668, 670, 671
Martinez-Maldonado, M., 71, 630
Martinez-Palomo, A., 628
Martino, J. A., 635
Martres, M. P., 326-31
Martt, J. M., 388
Maruyama, J., 530
Marver, H. S., 206
Marx, J. L., 179, 182, 188, 190
Mary, J. Y., 357, 363
Masbernard, A., 19
Mascher, D., 150, 157
Masek, K., 271
Maskrey, M., 342, 345
Masland, R. L., 401
Mason, D. T., 293, 301
Mason, H. L., 139
Massarelli, R., 370, 374
MASSRY, S.G.,67-82; 15, 17, 68-73, 75-78, 640
Masuda, T., 286, 287
Mathe58, 60
Mathias, A., 486
Mathieu, A., 624
Mathison, I. W., 293, 301
Matsuda, T., 36
Matsukado, Y., 331
Matsumoto, T., 455
Matsumura, K., 359
Matsuo, H., 432
Matsuo, N., 75, 77, 78
Mattern, J., 538
Matthew, H., 215, 300
Matthews, D. M., 141
Matthews, E. K., 28-30, 32, 39, 150

Matthews, H. L., 299
Matthews, R. H., 444
Matthysse, S., 546, 550, 551
Mattson, R. H., 141
Mattsson, H., 396
Matuchansky, C., 357, 363
Matuda, E., 650, 669, 670
Matz, L., 563
Mauck, H. P., 315
Maude, D. L., 630, 633
Mauer, A., 531, 534, 535
Mauer, L., 534
Maunsbach, A. B., 624
Mavligit, G. M., 182, 183, 185, 187-89
Maxfield, M. E., 86, 205
Maxwell, M. H., 202
Maxwell, R. A., 551
Mayer, C.-J., 158
Mayer, S. E., 360, 442, 583, 588
Mayfield, D. E., 239
Mayo, J. G., 530
Mayol, R. F., 451
Mazze, R. I., 233
Mazzullo, J. M., 293
McAfee, D. A., 442
McAllister, R. G., 312
McAuliff, J. P., 576
McBride, C., 189
McBride, C. E., 189
McBride, C. M., 189
McCall, D., 300
McCall, J. T., 19
McCann, S. M., 29, 30, 37
McClane, T. K., 419
McClure, D. J., 418
McColl, I., 361
McCollister, R. J., 71
McComas, A. J., 389, 397
McCormack, J. J., 294
McCormick, W., 480
McCoy, T. A., 103
McCracken, G. H. Jr., 563, 564, 569, 570
McCredie, K. B., 183, 188, 189
McCrory, W. W., 140
McCullough, J. L., 107
McDaniel, M. C., 282, 288
McDevitt, D., 312
McDonald, R. H., 299
McDonough, E., 183
McDougal, D. B. Jr., 450
McDowell, F., 297
McFadden, E. R. Jr., 519
McGeer, E. G., 372
McGeer, P. L., 372
McGiff, J. C., 262, 264, 268
McGill, D. B., 355
McGillion, F. B., 205
McGregor, G. A., 312
McGuffin, J. C., 612

McGuire, W. L., 536
McHenry, E. W., 141
McIndewar, I., 612
McIntosh, F. C., 376
McIntyre, A. R., 391
McIsaac, R. J., 269, 391
McKay, J., 123, 124
McKenna, T. J., 75
McKenzie, G. M., 551
McKinney, G. R., 449, 458
McKinney, W. M., 19
McKinnon, A. E., 172, 174
McLaughlin, J. L., 662, 663
McMahon, F. G., 677
McMahon, P. C., 315
McMillan, R., 179
McMillin, R. D., 530
McMullin, J. P., 13
McMurtry, R. J., 300
McNamee, M. G., 243
McNay, J. L., 318, 319
McNeill, J. H., 458
McNerney, J. M., 92
McNichol, G. P., 505
McNutt, N. S., 90
McPhail, A. T., 118, 126
McPherson, A., 269
McPherson, T. A., 189
McPhillips, J. J., 396
McWilliams, N., 531
Mead, J. F., 681
Mead, R., 480
Meadows, G. G., 99
Mechoulam, R., 656, 668
Medina, M., 325
Medina, M. A., 458
Meeter, E., 343, 344, 398, 400-2
Meffin, P., 238, 295, 563, 567
Megyesi, K., 243
Mehani, S., 198
Meier, J. P., 60
Meier, M., 317, 519
Meilman, E., 508, 515
Meinardi, H., 426
Meisel, J. L., 361
Meisler, J., 578
Meisner, M., 316
Meister, A., 103, 253, 254
Meister, S. G., 239
Mekhjian, H. S., 357, 359
Melam, H., 522
Melamed, E., 587
MELBY, J. C., 511-27; 513, 514, 517, 519, 523
Meldolesi, M. F., 444, 448
Meldrum, B. S., 140
Melekian, B., 75
Melin, J., 294, 295
Mellin, G., 204
Mellits, E. D., 207
Mellow, M. H., 294

Mellstedt, H., 186
Melmed, C., 392, 394
Melmon, K. L., 238, 293-95, 455, 581, 584, 594
Melnick, I., 19
Melon, J-M., 15
Melson, G. L., 446-48
Meltzer, M., 100
Menczel, J., 136
Mendell, J. R., 393, 394
Mendels, J., 418, 421
Mendelsohn, M. L., 529
Mendez, C., 157, 158
Mendlewicz, J., 681
Meng, K., 159
Menon, T., 589
Mercer, T. T., 198
Mergner, G. W., 90-92
Merrin, C., 183
Merritt, H. H., 388, 391
Merten, K., 55
Mertens, R. B., 360
Meshkinpour, H., 357
Messina, E. J., 262
Messing, R. B., 614
Messmer, W. M., 121
Metcalf, G., 344
Metcalf, R. L., 171, 172
Mettler, C. C., 548
Mettler, F. A., 547, 548
Meyer, J., 153
Meyer, J. L., 18, 19
Meyerhoff, B. G., 653, 662
Meyler, L., 140
Michaelson, D., 243
Michaelson, I. A., 327
Michaluk, J., 347
Michel, I. M., 449, 453, 456, 458
Michelakis, A. M., 208, 312
Mickelsen, O., 133, 135
Mickey, J., 582, 591, 593, 594
Mickey, J. V., 575, 582, 591, 593, 594
Mickiewicz, E., 190
Middleton, E., 443
Miele, E., 270
Mielke, B., 539
Mihich, E., 107
Miki, N., 36
Mikolajczak, K. L., 123, 124
Miledi, R., 265, 398, 590
Milgrom, H., 189
Millar, J. A., 205
Miller, A. A., 141
Miller, A. L., 296
Miller, D. D., 578
Miller, E. R., 75
Miller, J. G., 294
Miller, J. P., 451
Miller, R. E., 207
Miller, R. J., 552

Miller, R. P., 563, 566, 569
Miller, W. H., 442
Miller, Z., 445, 448
Milligan, J. W., 37
Mills, C. A., 139
Mills, I. H., 634
Mills, O. H., 134
Milman, H. A., 110
Milne, M. D., 294, 298
Milner, R. D. G., 29-31
Milosevic, M. P., 376
Mines, G. R., 151
Minor, L., 99
Minowada, J., 183
Minton, J. P., 444
Mintz, D. H., 446
Mircheff, A. K., 136
Mirkin, B. L., 561, 563, 567, 569, 678
Mironneau, J., 157, 158
Mirsky, A. F., 553
Misage, J. R., 299
Misantone, L. J., 609
Misiewicz, J. J., 357
Misu, Y., 265
Mitchard, M., 54, 58
Mitchell, A. A., 426
Mitchell, H., 483
Mitchell, I., 315
Mitchell, J. F., 370-72, 376, 377, 380
Mitchell, J. R., 299
Mitchell, M. S., 110, 181, 183, 185
Mitchell, T. G., 362
Mitchell, W. D., 360
Mitra, R. C., 356
Mittag, T. W., 373, 376
Mizel, S. B., 37, 38
Mizutani, A., 285
Mizutani, T., 285
Moawad, A., 261, 267
Modha, K., 16
Modigliani, R., 357
Moe, P. J., 186
Moelholm-Hansen, J., 297
Mogenson, G. J., 606, 609
Mogilner, B., 286
Mohs, J. M., 75, 77
Moir, A. T. B., 411, 412
Mok, H. Y. I., 359
Molinelli, E. A., 29
MOLINOFF, P. B.,575-604; 575, 577-81, 583, 584, 586-88, 590-94
Molloy, B. B., 609
Moloney, M., 13
Momcilovic, B., 200
Mommaerts, W. F. H. M., 578
Monahan, T. M., 443, 444, 453, 462
Monash, S., 235, 236

Moncada, S., 261, 268
Mondal, A., 356
Monier, J. F., 287
Monn, E., 451
Monnier, M., 333
Montague, W., 442
Montel, H., 267
Montes, L. F., 134
Montgomery, R. B., 610
Montgomery, R. G., 263
Montier, A. D., 265
Moody, T., 243
Mook, D. G., 608
Moore, D. C., 228, 233, 565
Moore, G. E., 576
Moore, J. F., 208
Moore, K. E., 551
Moore, M. M., 576, 592
Moore, M. R., 205
Moore, M. Z., 442
Moore, P. F., 456
Moore, R. A., 345
Moore, R. Y., 546
Mor, E., 136
Morales-Aguilera, A., 388-90
Moran, J. F., 586
Moran, N. C., 576
Moran, R. G., 678
Moreau, J. J., 656, 668
Morehead, R. M. Jr., 78
Morel, F., 68, 69, 630, 634
Moreland, T. A., 62
Morell, A. G., 109
Morgan, A., 90, 91
Morgan, B., 431
Morgan, B. A., 431
Morgan, D. B., 13
Morgan, J. M., 207
Morgan, J. P., 50
Morgan, P. H., 293, 301
Morgan, T., 634
Morganroth, J., 500
Mori, T., 110
Morii, H., 137
Morin, P., 534
Moritz, M., 357
Morley, J., 485
Morré, D. J., 33
MORRELLI, H.F.,293-309
Morrice, G., 134
Morris, F., 90
Morris, H. G., 591
Morris, H. P., 443, 448, 451
Morris, H. R., 431
Morris, J. A., 569
Morris, J. J., 298
Morris, M. E., 427, 429
Morris, V. C., 138
Morris, W. P., 591, 594
Morrison, R. C., 554
Morselli, P. L., 412, 563, 564, 567, 678

Morton, D. L., 179, 182, 183, 188, 189
Moses, A. M., 14
Mosko, S. S., 613
Moss, N., 68, 69
Moss, R. L., 432
Motais, R., 168
Motolinia, T. ca., 648, 660
Mott, M. G., 190
Mountain, C., 103, 534
Moutafis, C. D., 506
Moyer, J. H., 316
Mroczek, W. J., 315-17
Mrozek, K., 388-90
Mudge, G. J., 298
Muelder, A. H., 328
Mueller, P. K., 198
Muenter, M. D., 133, 134
Mukherjee, C., 575, 577, 581, 582, 589, 591, 593, 594
Mulas, M. L., 370, 371, 376, 377
Mulder, A. H., 243, 373
Muldowncy, Г. P., 13, 75
Mulhall, D., 426
Muller, C. W., 627
Muller, G., 52, 56
Muller, U., 52, 56
Mullikin, D., 582, 585, 591, 593, 594
Mullin, L. S., 86, 91
Muneyama, K., 451
Munkvad, I., 550
Munro, H. N., 614
Munro-Faure, A. D., 294
Munsat, T. L., 393
Munshower, J., 448
Munske, K., 456
Murad, F., 443, 446, 448, 450, 576
Murakami, N., 346
Murakami, U., 134
Murayama, Y., 634
Murphy, B. F., 138
Murphy, D. L., 393
Murphy, G., 545
Murphy, G. P., 111, 189
Murphy, J. V., 168
Murphy, P. G., 168
Murphy, S., 535
Murphy, W., 536, 538
Murray, A. W., 444
Murray, F. J., 297
Murray, J., 480
Muscatine, L., 250, 252
Muschek, L. D., 458
Musher, D., 17
Mustard, J. F., 305, 505
Mutch, L. M. M., 315
Myant, N. B., 506
Myers, B. D., 637
Myers, R. D., 342-47, 611, 614

Mylle, M., 629
Myllyla, V. V., 447

N

Nachmansohn, D., 679
Nagao, T., 159, 531
Nagao, Y., 124, 125
Nagasawa, J., 32, 34
Nagatomo, T., 388, 390
Nagode, L. A., 137
Nahmad, S., 653, 662
Nahmod, V. E., 432
Nahorski, S. R., 331, 581, 582
Naim, E., 579
Nair, K. G., 451
Nair, R. M. G., 432
Nakajima, H., 154, 159, 452
Nakamura, K., 345, 347
Nakamura, Y., 369
Nakao, K., 205
Nakata, Y., 428
Nakayama, K., 160
Nakayama, T., 346
Nakazato, Y., 38
Nance, D. M., 613
Nankin, H., 508
NARAGHI, M., 223-42;
Naranjo, C., 656
Naranjo, P., 653
Narimatsu, A., 157
Narod, M. E., 590
Nash, C. W., 298
Nashold, B. S. Jr., 411
Nassar, B. A., 263
Nation, R. L., 49, 55, 58, 59
Nauta, J. H., 549
Navar, L. G., 636
Nayler, W. G., 156
Neal, J. M., 663
Neal, M. J., 370, 371, 373, 378, 380
Needleman, P., 243, 267, 268, 680
Neel, H. B. III, 179, 181, 182, 188
Neelon, F. A., 448
Neely, W. B., 171, 172, 174
Neff, N. H., 370, 372, 432
Neidle, A., 431
Neims, A. H., 563-65, 569
Nell, G., 359, 362
Nelson, D., 492
Nelson, D. H., 73
Nelson, J. A., 535
Nelson, J. D., 563, 570
Nelson, S. R., 134
Nemoto, T., 183
Nenno, R., 140
Neptune, E. M., 362
Nesbakken, R., 75
Nesbit, M., 189

Nesbitt, J. A. III, 445, 448
Ness, P., 108
Nestorescu, B., 207
Neuberger, A., 205
Neufeld, A. H., 263, 268, 442
Neufeld, E. F., 98, 103
Neuman, M. W., 77
Neuman, R. E., 103
Neuman, W. S., 77
Neumann, K. H., 632
Neumann, W., 482-84
Neville, D. M., 243
Newbury, P. A., 55
Newcombe, D. S., 455
Newcombe, R. G., 183
Newman, E. V., 456
Newman, R. J., 136
Newman, T. M., 396, 401
Newmark, H., 133, 134
Newton, R., 20
Newton, R. W., 300
Ney, R. L., 443, 448
Ng, L. K. Y., 412
Ng, Y. L., 121
Ngai, S. H., 377
Niall, H. D., 426, 430, 433
Niaudet, P., 287
Nichol, C. A., 107
Nicholls, A., 141
Nicholson, P. A., 679
Nichool, R., 380
Nickander, R. C., 388
Nickerson, M., 576, 586
Nickerson, R., 534, 535
Nicklas, W. J., 38
Nicol, D. M., 103
Nicol, S. E., 442
Nicolas-Charles, P., 655, 661
Nicoll, R. A., 380, 425, 427, 429, 432, 433
Nicoloff, J. T., 446, 448
Nielsen, K. C., 327
Nielsen, R., 14
Nielsen, S. W., 134
Nielson, R., 14
Nieman, C., 134
Nies, A. S., 295, 297, 300
Nieto, D., 660, 661
Nikkanen, J., 201, 202, 204
Nikolsky, G. V., 168
Niles, A. M., 139
Nilsson, G., 426, 428-30, 432, 433
Nirenberg, M., 451, 584, 587
Nisbet, H. D., 152, 158
Nitowsky, H. M., 563
Nitz, R. E., 456
Nitze, H., 531
Nixon, P. F., 107
Nizze, J. A., 183
Noach, E. L., 141
Noble, D., 389

Noble, J., 300
Noda, H., 373
Noguchi, T., 138
Nolen, G. A., 134
Nonomura, Y., 396
Nordberg, A., 375, 377
Nordin, B. E. C., 12-15, 18, 74
Nordmann, J. J., 29, 32, 150, 432
Nordqvist, S. R., 538
Norman, A. W., 136
Normann, T., 75
Norris, A., 442
Norris, A. H., 53, 57
Norris, J. W., 141
Norris, R. M., 152, 158
Norstrom, R. J., 172, 174
North, K. A. K., 72
Novak, A., 490
Nowlin, J., 567
Nozaki, K., 198
Nüesch, E., 294
Nunes, W. T., 508
Nurminen, M., 202
Nusbaum, R. E., 200
Nussbaumer, J. C., 332, 333
Nybäck, H., 554
Nye, D., 171

O

Oakeley, H. F., 141
Oates, J. A., 299, 550
Oberdorf, A., 159
Oblath, R., 152
O'Brien, E. T., 315
O'Brien, P., 107
Ochwadt, B., 624, 636
O'Connell, T. X., 183
O'Connor, P., 13
O'Connor, R., 488, 492
O'Dea, R. F., 450
O'Donnell, S. R., 576
O'Donohoe, P., 13
O'Driscoll, K. F., 112
Oduah, M., 51
Oettgen, H. F., 100, 101, 103, 104
O'Fallon, W. M., 316
Ogilvie, R. I., 303, 563, 564
Ogin, G., 395
O'Hara, M., 579
Ohata, M., 13, 14, 20
Ohlsen, J. D., 530
Ohlsson, W. T. L., 201
Ohnuma, T., 112
Ohshima, M., 100
Oka, M., 36
Okamoto, M., 397
O'Keefe, D., 187
Oken, D. E., 633

Oki, T., 100
Ola'h, G. M., 660
Olander, R., 317
Old, L. J., 103, 104, 106
Oldham, R. K., 183
Oldham, S. B., 77
Olesen, J., 313
Olesen, O. V., 141
Olivari, A. J., 190
Oliver, C., 432
Oliver, I. T., 451
Oliver, J., 413, 623
Oliverio, V. T., 297
Olsen, W. A., 360, 361, 363
Olson, J. A., 134
Olson, R. E., 138
Olson, W. H., 390, 394-400, 402
Olsson, A. G., 506
Oltmans, G. A., 609, 610
Olton, D. S., 369
O'Malley, K., 53, 55, 57, 318, 319
Omdahl, J., 135
Omrod, A. N., 396
Onaya, T., 331
O'Neill, J. A., 395, 453
O'Neill, P., 270, 271
O'Neill, R. V., 172, 173
Ono, H., 159
Oomura, Y., 609
Opipari, M., 533
Oppenheim, J. J., 187
Opsahl, C. A., 610
Oram, S., 152
Orci, L., 35, 38, 628
O'Reilly, R. A., 295, 296
Orloff, J., 456, 625, 629, 631-34
Orma, A. L., 331, 332
Orö, L., 269, 506
O'Rourke, J., 22
Orr, E., 329, 333
Ortiz, J., 453, 454
Ortmann, R., 591, 594
Osborne, G. B., 624
Osmond, H., 656, 665
Ossorio, R. C., 179, 181, 188, 190
Otis, C. L., 446, 448
O'Toole, A. G., 450
O'Toole, C., 179, 181, 188
OTSUKA, M., 425-39; 396, 425-39
Ott, C. E., 636
Otten, J., 444, 445
Overhoff, H., 362
Overton, M., 454
Owen, M., 490
Owens, A. H. Jr., 186, 533, 535, 539
Owens, C. A., Jr., 137
Owman, C., 327

Oyama, V. I., 103
Oye, I., 576

P

Paakari, I., 331, 332
Paakari, P., 331, 332
Paasonen, M., 678
Paasonen, M. K., 429
Packham, M. A., 305
Padjen, A., 380
Paes, I. C., 508
Page, E. D., 263, 268
Page, I. H., 316
Pagel, H. D., 634
Pagliaro, L. A., 563
Paik, V. S., 449, 453, 456, 458
Paillard, F., 74
Pairault, J., 580
Paisley, J. W., 563, 564, 569, 570
Pak, C. Y. C., 11-14, 17, 18, 20, 78, 136, 446, 448
Palacois, J. M., 328
Palade, G. E., 27, 32, 33
Palkovits, M., 326, 333
Palm, C. R., 443
Palm, D., 140
Palmblad, J., 186
Palmer, D. S., 590
Palmer, G. C., 331, 458, 461, 590, 592
Palmer, J. S., 582
Palmer, K. H., 118
Palmeri, R., 137
Paloyan, E., 15
Pan, P., 451
Panagotacos, P. J., 138
Panczenko, B., 268
Panksepp, J., 608, 609, 613
Paoletti, R., 442
Pape, J., 317
Papeschi, R., 418
Papez, J. W., 549
Pappenheimer, J. R., 425
Paradise, R. R., 91
Paranjpe, M. S., 182
Pardi, G., 563, 564, 567
Pardue, W. O., 139
Pardy, R. L., 250
Parfitt, A. M., 15, 19, 71
Parikh, I., 579, 580
Paris, D. F., 169, 171
Parish, H., 480
Park, C. M., 183
Park, C. R., 243
Park, M. K., 261, 270
Parke, D. V., 92
Parker, C. W., 442, 443, 451, 454, 455
Parker, J. M., 394
Parker, K. L., 442

Parker, R., 492
Parkinson, C., 134
Parkinson, D. K., 75, 77, 78
Parks, L. C., 190
Parks, M. A., 450
Parks, R. E., 140
Parmley, W. W., 445, 448
Parodi, S., 99
Parrilla, R., 32
Parrot, R., 534
Parson, D. W., 72
Parson, F. M., 72
Parsons, J. A., 29, 30, 681
Parsons, M. E., 331
Parsons, R. L., 55, 59
Parsons, W. B., 139, 504, 506
Parsons, W. D., 563-65, 569
Passananti, G. T., 296
Pastan, I., 444, 445, 448, 453, 454
Pasternak, G. W., 431
Patch, K. R., 443
Paterson, A. H. G., 189
Paterson, J. W., 91
Patil, P. N., 272, 576, 578
Patlak, C. S., 412, 633
Paton, D. M., 679
Patsch, R., 563
Patterson, J. H., 563, 568, 569
Patterson, R., 522
Patterson, R. K., 198
Paudler, W. W., 123, 124
Pauk, G. L., 447, 448
Paul, A. G., 649, 662
Paul, B. B., 92
Paul, M. I., 447, 448
Paulet, G., 90, 91
Paulus, H. E., 186
Paunier, L., 75
Paustian, P. W., 262
Pavlovitch, H., 136
Pawlow, M., 208
Pawlson, L. G., 446
Payne, J. P., 297
Pazzagli, A., 376
Peacock, M., 12-15, 18, 20, 74
Pean, G., 75
Pearce, J. M. S., 392
Pearce, L. A., 328
Pearson, R. M., 318
Pearson, W., 536
Pease, C. N., 134
Peck, M., 492
Pedersen, E., 427
Pedersen, E. B., 318
Pederson, L., 167
Peery, C. V., 445
Peillon, F., 32
Peindaries, R., 346
Peiper, U., 159
Pelc, S., 396

Pelletier, G., 32, 36, 37, 432, 433
Penefsky, Z. J., 88
Penn, I., 181
Penn, P. E., 344
Penning, W., 206
Pennington, C. W., 662, 663, 667, 669
Pennington, R. J., 392
Pennington, S. N., 444
Penry, J. K., 563, 564
Pensuwan, S., 78
Pentchev, P. G., 98, 103
Pentikainen, P., 505
Peper, K., 150, 157
Pepeu, G., 370-72, 376-78
Percie-du-Sert, M., 537
Perel, J. M., 297
Perezamador, M. C., 656, 665
Perez-Gonzalez, M., 628
Peri, G., 357, 372, 377
Perkins, J. P., 331, 443, 449, 451, 575, 576, 578, 581, 583, 584, 586, 587, 590-94
Perkins, M. E., 576
Perlia, C., 536
Perlman, R., 457
Pernow, B., 426, 428-30, 433
Perrelet, A., 628
Perrenoud, M.-L., 578, 591
Perry, H. M. Jr., 317
Perry, H. O., 133
Perry, K. W., 612
Perry, S., 537
Perry, W. L. M., 415
Persson, B., 133
Persson, N. a., 271
Persson, T., 414
Pert, A., 333
Pert, C. B., 373, 431
Pert, C. D., 328
Pessayre, D., 357
Peter, J. B., 388, 390
Petersen, D. M., 49
Peterson, M. R., 548, 549
Peterson, R. G., 110
Petri, G., 372, 377
Petrie, A., 317
Petrie, J. C., 315
Petrovsky, D. D., 199
Petterson, U., 421
Petzold, G. L., 457, 461, 552
Pfeiffer, C. C., 140
Pfiffner, J. J., 428
Pfitzer, E. A., 200
Pflug, A. E., 54, 58, 60
Phebus, L., 614
Philips, F. S., 103
Phillips, B. J., 453
Phillips, J. H., 38
Phillips, M., 449, 453, 456, 458
Phillips, M. B., 458, 460
Phillips, R. A., 362

Phillips, S., 484
Phillips, S. F., 355-57, 359-61
Phillipson, O. T., 611
Phillis, J. W., 331, 332, 372, 427, 430
Picart, R., 33
Picatoste, F., 328
Pichard, A. L., 451, 458, 459
Pichot, P., 325, 655, 661
Pickering, B. T., 34
Pickleman, J. R., 15
Pickles, V. R., 266
Pictet, R., 34, 35
Piddington, S. K., 203
Piek, T., 487-89
Pierau, F. K., 427
Pierce, D. A., 444
Pierce, G. E., 183, 190
Pierce, H. I., 320
Pierce, N. F., 356
Piering, W. F., 71, 72
Pihl, E., 28, 36
Pike, M. C., 181
Pilar, G. R., 373, 378
Pilch, Y. H., 189
Pilkis, S. J., 243, 589
Pinaud, L., 395
Pinto, B., 15
Pinto, J. E. B., 31, 34
Piomelli, S., 205
Piotrowski, J., 200
Pipeleers, D. G., 37, 442
Pipeleers-Marichal, M. A., 37
Piper, P., 267
Pirch, J. H., 590
Pisano, J., 486, 487
Pisonic, M., 199
Pizarro, M. A., 524
Plattner, J. J., 119
Pleau, J. M., 284, 286, 287
Pledger, W. J., 451-53, 459, 460
Plescia, O. J., 453
Pless, J., 432
Pletscher, A., 28, 394, 411
Pletscher, R., 329
Plowman, T., 668
Pluchino, S., 590
Poch, G., 442, 456, 457
Podosin, R. L., 296
Pohl, S. L., 585, 588
Pohler, O., 20
Poirier, G., 36
Poisner, A. M., 29-32, 34-38
Polak, R. L., 371, 373, 376, 377
Poley, J. R., 355, 359
Polgar, P., 444, 448
Pollard, H., 325-30, 333
Pollard, T. D., 38
Pollock, B. H., 186
Polonovski, C., 75

Polonsky, J., 127, 128
Polson, J. B., 450
Pomare, E. W., 363
Pondron, G., 135
Popot, J. L., 243
Popovtzer, M. M., 15, 71
Portanova, R., 33, 34
Porter, C. C., 299
Porter, J. C., 432
Porter, J. W., 251
Porter, R. J., 563, 564
Posen, S., 102
Posner, J., 271
Post, A., 60
Post, R. M., 411-13, 416, 418, 420-22
Poste, G., 39
Postwood, R. M., 68
Potter, H., 181
Potter, L. T., 581
Potts, J. T. Jr., 426, 430, 433
Pouillart, P., 534
Poulos, B. K., 590, 593
Powell, C. E., 576
Powell, D., 426, 430, 433
Powell, E., 17, 20
Powell, J. A., 447, 454
Powell, N., 533
Powell, R., 49
Powell, R. C., 508
Powell, R. G., 123, 124
Powles, R., 189
Powley, T. L., 608-10
Prado, J., 486
Prager, M. D., 186
Prange, A. J. Jr., 412, 419
Prasad, A. S., 71
Prasad, K. M., 448, 453, 454
Prasad, K. N., 454
Pratt, R. F., 141
Prehn, R. T., 182
Prerovska, I., 201, 202
Prescott, L. F., 298
Preston, L. W., 315
Preuss, H. G., 141
Preuss, I., 55
Preusser, H. J., 398, 399
Pricam, C., 628
Price, K. S., 550, 552
Price, M. R., 179, 181
Prichard, B. N. C., 299, 300, 318
Prien, E. L., 18
Prien, E. L. Jr., 18, 71
Prien, E. L. Sr., 19
Prier, S., 74
Principi, N., 563, 564, 567
Prindle, K. H., 445, 457
Prinz, B., 201
Priola, D. V., 590
Prior, R. L., 189
Pritchard, D., 319

Prite, D., 505
Pritzl, P., 103
Procknal, J. A., 565
Promadhattavedi, V., 563
Proudfoot, A. T., 215
Prout, G. R. Jr., 183
Pruitt, A. W., 563, 568, 569
Prusiner, S., 99
Prusoff, W. H., 582
Prynn, R. B., 85
Przewlocka, B., 347
Puck, T. T., 453, 454
Pueschel, S. M., 202
Puglisi, L., 269
Pulczuk, N. C., 110
Puls, W., 159
Purdy, J. L., 454
Purvis, M. L., 19
Puschett, J. B., 640
Puszkin, S., 38
Putnam, R. W., 590
Pütter, J., 101
Puviani, R., 432, 433
Pyrah, L. N., 72

Q

Quadri, A., 54, 57
Quamme, C. A., 14
Quarfordt, S. H., 505
Quay, W. B., 329, 333
Quintao, E., 505
Quock, R. M., 346, 347

R

Rabinowitz, B., 445, 448
Rabinowitz, M., 578
Rabinowitz, M. B., 198, 199, 201
Rabson, A. S., 183
Racagni, G., 369-71, 373-79
Rachelefsky, G., 455
Rachelefsky, G. S., 455
Rachmilewitz, D., 361, 362
Radde, I. C., 75, 78
Raffauf, R. F., 658, 659, 666-68, 670, 671
Raftery, M. A., 243
Raich, P., 535
Raine, D. N., 202
Raisen, L., 18
Raisz, L. G., 78, 137
Raizner, A. E., 51
Rall, D., 530
Rall, T., 442
Rall, T. W., 331, 449, 576, 589-91
Ralston, A. J., 141
Ramadan, M. E., 104
Ramanathan, S., 445
Rambaud, J. C., 357, 363

Ramirez, A., 92
Ramirez, J., 659, 671
Ramming, K. P., 188, 189
Ramsey, T. A., 418
Ramussen, H., 136
Ramwell, P. W., 266, 270, 428, 680
Rand, M. J., 299, 300
Randall, P. K., 609, 610, 612, 614
Randic, M., 401
Randle, P. J., 35, 36, 457
Randrup, A., 550
Rane, A., 563, 564, 567-69, 678
Ranish, N. A., 390, 391
Rankin, J., 168
Rao, K. J., 14
Rao, K. S., 376
Rapoport, H., 119
Rapp, H. J., 188
Rasteger, A., 74
Rastogi, R. B., 679
Rathmayer, W., 487
Rautenberg, W., 345, 346
Rawlings, C. L., 360
Rawlins, F. A., 627, 628
Rawlins, M. D., 300, 344, 345
Ray, T. K., 578
Raymon, F., 239
Raymond, K., 294
Raymond, M. K., 444
Raynaud, C., 75
Re, R. N., 522
Read, A. E., 363
Rechsteiner de Vos, H., 136
Recker, R. R., 20
Rector, F. C., 356, 623, 625, 629, 630, 634
Rector, F. C. Jr., 71, 73, 632
Redding, T. W., 432
Reddy, C. R., 75, 76, 78
Reddy, V., 134
Redfern, P. H., 347
Redgrave, P. C., 344
Redmond, D. E. Jr., 412
Reed, A., 189
Reed, C. E., 454
Reed, R., 189
Reed, R. C., 182, 185, 187, 189
Reese, O. G. Jr., 19
Reeve, E. B., 15
Refsum, H., 157, 158
Regier, H. A., 172
Rehault, M. C., 326-29
Reich, E., 249
Reich, S., 296, 300
Reichard, G., 60
Reichelt, K. L., 329
Reichlin, S., 432
Reid, J. L., 299, 344, 345, 347, 680
Reid, W. D., 375

Reilly, J., 298
Reilly, M. A., 326, 329
Reimer, A. A., 250-52
Rein, A., 453
Reina, J. C., 199
Reinert, M., 481
Reinert, R. E., 168-70
Reinhardt, C. F., 86
Reiss, E., 14
Reissell, P., 295
Reitz, K., 483
Reizenstein, P., 186
Reko, B. P., 649-51, 658, 660, 661, 664-67
Reko, V. A., 656, 668
Remold-O'Donnell, E., 591
Renaud, L. P., 332, 432, 433
Rendell, M., 585
Rennels, E. G., 32
Rennick, B. R., 298
Renold, A. E., 35
Rentschler, R., 103, 534
Restivo, B., 319
Rethy, A., 588
Reuning, R. H., 294
Reuter, H., 30, 31, 150, 152, 157
Revuelta, A., 379, 452
Revuelta, A. V., 452
Rewerski, W., 344, 346
Reynolds, E. H., 141
Reynolds, F., 227, 228, 234
Reynolds, J. W., 563, 567, 569
Reynolds, W. A., 134
Rhodes, W., 648, 649, 653, 654, 661
Rhodin, J., 624
Rhyne, B. C., 197, 203, 204, 206
Ricanati, E. S., 71
Richardson, D. W., 315
Richardson, J. A., 295
Richens, A., 54, 57, 141
RICHEY, D.P., 49-65; 49, 50
RICHIE, D.M., 133-48
Richter, G. W., 208
Richter, H., 50
Rickenberg, H. V., 451
Rider, A. K., 506
Ridgway, E. C., 522
Riecker, G., 389
Riemer, J., 158
Rieselbach, R. E., 18
Rietra, P. J. G. M., 108, 109
Rifkin, D. B., 249
Rifkind, B. M., 500, 503, 505
Riggs, B. L., 20, 134
Riker, W. F. Jr., 397, 398, 401
Riley, V., 99, 101
Riley, W. D., 443
Ringer, S., 151
Rink, T. J., 31

Riska, N., 507
Ritchie, B., 224
Ritchie, J. M., 224
Ritter, S., 610
Ritts, R. E. Jr., 179, 181, 182, 188
Rivier, J., 432
Rivkin, I., 331, 591
Rivlin, R. S., 140
Rizek, J. E., 74
Robb-Smith, A. H. T., 35
Robens, J. F., 134
Robert, A., 270
Roberts, D. V., 396
Roberts, E., 104
ROBERTS, J., 97-116; 98-101, 103-7, 109, 110, 298, 401
Roberts, N., 431
Roberts, P. J., 243
Roberts, R. J., 563, 566, 569
Roberts, R. S., 319, 320
Roberts, S., 331
Roberts, W. C., 137
Robertson, C. R., 637
Robertson, P., 491
Robertson, W. G., 12, 13, 15, 18-20
Roberts-Thomson, I. C., 183
Robin, H., 137
Robins, R. K., 451
Robinson, B. F., 264
Robinson, D. S., 294
Robinson, E., 198
Robinson, G. A., 590
Robinson, R., 442
Robinson, R. R., 68
Robison, A., 445, 457
Robison, G. A., 331, 442, 449, 450, 454, 461, 576, 578, 583, 588
Roch, M., 370, 373-75
Rockel, A., 71
Rodbard, D., 582, 583, 585
Rodbell, M., 585, 588
Rodbro, P., 136
Roddie, I. C., 395
Rodensky, P. L., 293
Rodergas, E., 328
Rodgers, C. R., 169, 171
Rodgers, G. M., 442
Rodicio, J., 623, 634
Rodman, J. S., 77
Rodriguez, V., 183, 189
Rodriquez de Lores Arnaiz, G., 372
Roe, F. J. C., 140
Roe, T. F., 296
Roels, H. A., 203-6
Roels, O. A., 133, 138
Rogentine, G. N. Jr., 181
Rogers, J. C., 110
Rogers, K. J., 331

Rogers, M., 331
Rogers, N. L., 456
Rohde, R., 629
Roher, H. D., 446, 448
Röhl, D., 389
Roinel, N., 68, 69
Roitt, I. M., 455
Rojas, A. F., 190
Rolewicz, T. F., 563, 569
Roman, D., 512
Römer, D., 432
Romero, J. A., 581, 582, 590, 593
Rommelspacher, H., 369, 372, 378
Romsdahl, M., 532
Roncin, G., 90, 91
Ronnberg, A. L., 325, 327, 328
Ronnov-Jessen, V., 316
Roos, B-E., 414, 415, 418, 421, 555
Rosa, J., 284
Rose, C., 325-29, 348
Rose, G. A., 312
Rose, H. M., 117
Rose, L., 535
Rose, S. W., 563
Rosell, S., 266
Rosen, F., 107
Rosen, H., 51
Rosen, M. R., 293, 301
Rosen, O., 457
Rosen, O. M., 451, 452
Rosen, S., 624
Rosenblatt, S., 538
Rosenbluth, R. J., 98
Rosenbrook, W., 488
Rosenfeld, H. J., 106
Rosenfeld, S., 181
Rosenman, R. H., 315
Rosenoff, S., 539
Rosenqvist, U., 447
Rosenthal, G., 142
Rosenthal, J., 396, 397
Rosenthal, O., 72
Rosner, D., 189
Ross, E. J., 300
Ross, E. M., 575, 585
Ross, J. Jr., 445, 457, 588
Ross, M. J., 243
Rossen, R. D., 188
Rossier, J., 373, 376
Rossier, R., 566
Rossignol, S., 613
Rossner, S., 506
Rossoff, I. S., 677
Rostorfer, H. H., 141
Roth, J., 243, 457
Roth, J. A., 183
Roth, R., 12
Roth, R. H., 373
Rothberg, H., 140

Rothlin, R. P., 267
Rothman, P. E., 133
Rothman, S. S., 27
Rothschild, A., 484
Roti Roti, J. L., 530
Rotter, V., 283, 286
Rougier, O., 150
Rouiller, C., 35
Roumengous, M., 206
Rousseau, J. E., 134
Routtenberg, A., 547
Roventa, A., 207
Rowe, D. J. F., 136
Rowe, G., 390
Rowe, G. G., 297
Rowland, L. P., 394
Rowland, M., 238, 294, 295, 298
Rowland, N. E., 608, 615
Rowland, R. G., 446, 448
Rowlands, D. T. Jr., 179, 181
Roy, A. C., 455
Ruben, F. L., 186
Rubenstein, A. H., 32
Rubin, A., 679
Rubin, C. E., 359, 361
Rubin, R. P., 29, 30, 32, 149
Rubinstein, D., 92
Rubottom, G. M., 656
Rubulis, A., 507
Rudd, R. L., 168
Rude, R. K., 77
Rudel, R., 388-91
Rudland, P. S., 450
Rudman, D., 19
Rudo, F. G., 90-92
Rudy, T. A., 343-45
Rüegg, J. C., 158
Rufener, C., 35
Ruiter, M., 140
Ruiz, V., 536
Ruiz de Alarcón, H., 648, 660, 662, 665, 670
Rummel, W., 359, 362
Rumrich, G., 629-31, 633, 636
Runcie, J., 60
Rupak, D. M., 356
Rushforth, N. B., 250
Ruskin, B., 17, 136
Russell, J. C., 199, 201
Russell, J. T., 31, 150
Russell, R. G. G., 20
Russell, R. M., 134
Russell, T. R., 445, 448, 450, 451, 453
Russell, V., 591
Rutenburg, A. M., 444, 448
Rüther, E., 416
Rutledge, C. O., 590, 592
Rutstein, H. R., 85
Rutter, D. A., 109
Rutter, W. J., 34

Ryall, R. W., 426
Ryan, J., 589
Ryan, J. R., 507
Ryan, M. J., 262
Ryan, W. L., 442, 453, 454
Rymaszewska, T., 397

S

Saavedra, J. M., 326, 333
Sabatini, D. D., 33
Sachs, G., 451
Sachs, H., 33, 34
Sack, R. B., 358
Sack, R. L., 421, 422
Sackett, D. L., 319, 320
Sacks, G., 74
Sadoff, L., 190
Sadove, M. S., 519
Saelens, J. K., 370, 372-76
Safford, W. E., 650, 658, 669
Sagar, S., 108
Sagastume, E., 299
Sage, H. J., 32
Said, S., 357
Said, S. I., 357
Saito, K., 427, 429
Sakagami, M., 428, 433
Sakai, H., 288
Sakai, K. K., 432
Sakamoto, Y., 150
Sakmar, E., 294
Saks, B., 588
Sakuma, Y., 432
Salama, A. I., 376
Salassa, R. M., 523
Salen, G., 505
Salet, J., 75
Saller, C. F., 614
Salmon, J. H., 389
Salmon, S., 533
Salomon, J. C., 287
Salomon, Y., 585
Salvador, R. A., 576
Salway, J. G., 448
Salzmann, R., 271
Samaniego, S., 449, 453, 456, 458
Samaniego, S. G., 331, 591
Samanin, R., 612
Samiy, A. H. E., 68
Samli, M. H., 29, 30
Sampson, D., 111
Sampson, G. A., 448
Sampson, S. R., 29, 30
Samuel, P., 508
Samuels, M., 532
Samuelsson, B., 268
Sanborn, J. R., 171
Sanchez, N., 294
Sandler, G., 152
Sandstead, H. H., 208

Sanford, C. H., 442
Sanger, J. M., 38
Sanger, J. W., 38
Sannerstedt, R., 317
Sansone, F. M., 397
Sansur, M., 297
Santa, T., 396, 399, 401
Santhakumri, G., 333
Santhanam, P. S., 130
Santinoceto, L., 372, 377
Santos, G. W., 186
Sanwal, M., 28
Sanzenbacher, L. J., 13, 17
Sanz-Ibanez, J., 396
Sardi, A., 111
Sargent, T., 656
Sarmiento, L., 483
Sarna, G. P., 190
Sassa, S., 205, 206, 563
Satinoff, E., 344, 347
Sato, A., 331
Sato, H., 428, 432, 433
Sato, M., 159
Sato, P. T., 663
Sato, S., 563
Satoh, S., 272
Sattin, A., 447, 576, 591
Satyamurti, S., 396, 397
Sauberlich, H. E., 508
Sauer, J., 667
Sauer, R., 333
Saunders, D. R., 359, 361, 362
Sauviat, M. P., 150
Savard, K., 442
Saville, P. D., 20
Sawerthal, H., 484
Saxena, P. N., 347
Scales, A. H., 299
Scanlon, J., 201
Scarcia, V., 99
Scarpa, A., 156
Scatchard, G., 587
Schabel, F. M. Jr., 530
Schachter, M., 485, 486, 488-90
Schafer, J. A., 624, 625, 632, 633
Schaffer, J., 480
Schallek, W., 458
Schaller, K. H., 201
Schally, A. V., 432, 433
Schamroth, L., 158
Schanberg, S. M., 328
Scharp, C. R., 136
Scharrer, B., 425
Scharrer, E., 425
Schatz, M., 522
Schaumburg, H. H., 325
Schayer, R. W., 326, 328, 329
Schechter, B., 288
Scheel, D., 506
Scheel-Kruger, J., 612
Scheid, M. P., 284, 285

Scheinberg, I. H., 109
Schellenberg, D., 563
Schenk, E. A., 356
Schenk, R., 20
Schenkein, I., 101, 104
Schenken, L. L., 530
Schenker, S., 55, 59, 60
Schiavi, R. C., 181
Schiff, M., 181
Schiffer, L. M., 545
Schild, H., 425
Schildberg, F. W., 151, 152
Schildkraut, J. J., 419, 421
Schilkrut, R., 416
Schimpff, S. C., 187
Schlesinger, D. H., 284
Schlosser, L., 429
Schlossmann, K., 159
Schlumberger, J. R., 189
Schmer, G., 109, 110
Schmid, F., 105, 106, 110
Schmid, F. A., 100, 101, 104,
    105, 107
Schmid, P. G., 262
Schmidt, D. A., 75
Schmidt, E., 159
Schmidt, G. B., 519
Schmidt, K., 55
Schmidt, M. J., 331
Schmidt, R., 294
Schmidt, R. F., 397
Schmidt, S. Y., 447, 448
Schmidt-Gayk, H., 446, 448
Schmitt, G., 444
Schmitt, M. G., 357
Schneider, E. G., 636
Schneider, F. H., 32
Schneider, F. W., 451
Schneider, M., 189
Schneiderman, H. A., 250
Schnermann, J., 623
Schnur, J. A., 414
Schnure, F. W., 111
Schobben, F., 563, 564
Schoenfield, L., 360
Schönbaum, E., 341
Schonhofer, P. S., 451
Schöpf, J. A. L., 34
Schorah, C. J., 134
Schork, M. A., 454
Schramm, M., 579, 585
Schraven, E., 456
Schrecker, A. W., 117
Schrek, R., 104
Schrier, R. W., 15, 635-37
Schroder, C. H., 453
Schroder, J., 451
Schroder, J. M., 390
Schroeder, L. A., 390
Schroeder, W., 395
Schrogie, J. J., 296, 297
Schron, A., 30
Schubert, R. M., 129, 130

Schuberth, J., 370, 374, 375,
    377
Schuh, F. T., 391
Schulof, R. S., 282
Schultes, R. E., 649, 650, 652,
    656, 658, 660, 662, 665,
    667-70
Schultz, A. G., 119
Schultz, E. M., 680
Schultz, G., 456
Schultz, J., 331, 576, 590, 591
Schulz, R. A., 32, 34
Schumacher, A. M., 117
Schuman, J., 372, 373, 375, 376
Schumann, D., 658, 667
Schümann, H. J., 152
Schwab, J. H., 186-88
Schwabe, U., 458
Schwachman, H., 202
Schwarting, A. E., 658, 668
Schwartz, A., 156
Schwartz, C. J., 357
Schwartz, G. J., 565
SCHWARTZ, J.-C., 325-39;
    325-33, 348
Schwartz, J. H., 99
Schwartz, M. K., 100, 101,
    103, 104
Schwartz, R. S., 181, 182
Schwartz, S., 332, 426
Schwarzbeck, A., 159
Schwarzenberg, L., 189, 534
Schwertner, H. A., 678
Schwettmann, R. S., 73
Sclafani, A., 608
Scoggins, R., 530
Scoppa, P., 206
Scott, C. C., 140
Scott, C. W. Jr., 141
Scott, D., 72
Scott, H. R., 590
Scott, J. J., 205
Scott, M. L., 138
Scott, N. R., 345, 346
Scriabine, A., 317
Scribner, B. H., 298
Sealey, J. E., 317
Searle, C. E., 141
Sears, E. S, 427
Seashore, M. R., 397
Sebens, J. B., 413
Sebrell, W. H. Jr., 133
Secchi, G., 203, 205
Sedman, A. J., 294
Sedvall, G., 414, 421, 554
Seegmiller, J. E., 18
Seelig, M. S., 137
Seely, J. F., 71, 624-26, 629,
    630
Seeman, P., 553
Seferna, I., 271
Segaloff, A., 536
Segawa, T., 428

Seibert, G. B., 189
Seier, L., 139
Seifert, W., 450
Seiler, D., 388, 390
Seiler, K., 296
Seitelberger, F., 545, 552
Sekerke, H. J., 550
Sekowski, I., 508
Sela, M., 110
Selander, S., 201, 203
SELDIN, D. W.,623-46; 71,
    73, 624, 625, 629-32, 634
Seldin D. W., 623
Sellers, C. M., 376
Sellers, E. M., 296, 303
Sellinger, O. Z., 372, 378
Sellman, J. C., 623, 634
Selye, H., 300, 327, 393
Semenov, A., 481
Semmence, A. M., 315
Senesky, D., 640
Senft, G., 456
Senges, J., 388-91
Sensenbrenner, L. L., 186
Seraydarian, K., 578
Sereni, F., 563, 564, 567, 678
Sertel, H., 563, 569
Serum, J. W., 170, 171
Sethy, V. H., 372, 373
Sevilia, N., 581, 582, 585
Sewell, R., 535
Shafer, J. A., 632, 633
Shafer, S., 515
Shamma, M., 119
Shand, D. G., 295, 300, 312,
    563, 570
Shane, S. R., 74
Shank, R. P., 427
Shanks, R. G., 576
Shapiro, D., 98
Shapiro, L. J., 98, 103
Shapiro, S., 33, 34
Sharma, R. K., 443
Sharp, G. W. G., 579
Sharpe, D. M., 411, 412
Shaw, E., 249
Shaw, G. G., 332, 348
Shaw, J. E., 266, 270, 428
Shaw, J. W., 446, 448
Shaw, T. I., 265
Shaw, T. R. D., 294
Shaw, W. A., 75
Shear, M., 594
Sheard, M. H., 346
Sheeby, T. W., 141
Sheehan, J. D., 270, 271
Sheer, H., 356
Sheerin, H. E., 357
Sheffner, A. L., 394
Shein, H. M., 444, 448, 449,
    451, 452, 459-61
Sheiner, L. B., 294, 298
Shelanski, M. L., 37

Sheldon, D., 455
Shelley, W. B., 140
Shelp, W. D., 18
Shemin, D., 203
Shen, F., 14
Sheng, K. T., 563
Shepherd, A. M., 62
Shepherd, J. T., 395
Shepley, L., 206
Sheppard, H., 458
Sheps, S. G., 525
Sherman, G. P., 269
Sherman, K., 312
Sherrard, D., 14
Sherter, C., 300
Sherwin, R. P., 444, 451
Sherwood, L. M., 77
Shibata, S., 445
Shibusaki, S., 134
Shields, D. R., 396
Shields, R., 356
Shields, W., 103
Shifrin, S., 100, 109
Shiino, M., 32
Shills, M. E., 75, 78
Shimamoto, T., 457
Shimizu, H., 331
Shimizu, M., 285
Shinaberger, J. H., 15
Shipley, W., 539
Shipman, W., 483, 485
Shirai, M., 100
Shirger, A., 137
Shirkey, H., 561
Shkenderov, S., 484
Shock, N. W., 53, 57
Shoeman, D. W., 505, 563, 564
Shopsin, B., 421
Shore, N., 189
Shore, P. A., 294, 325, 344
Short, A. H., 54, 56, 60
Shoshkes, M., 137
Shoulson, I., 613
Shrager, M. W., 293
Shreeve, W. W., 36, 37
Shropshire, A. T., 263
Shtacher, G., 586
Shugart, H. H. Jr., 172, 173
Shulgin, A. T., 656
Shulman, M. G., 19
Shulman, R., 500, 504-6, 508
Shulman, R. S., 506
Shuman, D. A., 451
Shute, C. C. D., 369
Sica, R. E. P., 397
Sica, V., 579, 580
Siegel, C., 316
Siegel, F. L., 38
Siegel, J., 92
Siegel, R. K., 649, 656, 664, 670
Siekevitz, P., 27

Siersbaek-Nielsen, K., 51, 52, 56, 297
Sigel, C. W., 128, 129
Sigg, E. B., 554
Siggins, G. R., 331, 332, 587
Silbernagl, S., 630
Siletchnik, L. M., 93
Sillery, J., 359, 362
Silverman, L. M., 394
Silverman, R. W., 370, 374
Silverstein, M. J., 189
Silvis, S., 17
Sim, G. A., 118
Sim, J., 139
Simantov, R., 431
Simke, J. P., 370, 372-76
Simmonds, M. A., 345
Simmons, R. L., 206
Simon, C., 52, 55, 56, 565
Simon, E. J., 431
Simon, J., 373
Simon, J. R., 369, 373, 375-80
Simon, L. N., 451
Simon, M. L., 348
Simon, T. L., 108
Simonen, H., 295
Simonin, P., 53
Simonovic, I., 199
Simonsen, D. G., 104
Simpson, F. O., 311
Simpson, L. L., 265, 680
Simpson, W. T., 315
Simpson-Herren, L., 530
Sinclair, N., 485
Singer, A. L., 444, 451
Singer, F. R., 77
Singer, G., 610
Singer, R., 660, 661
Singh, B. N., 152, 158
Singh, J. N., 442
Singh, T., 539
Singhal, R. L., 679
Sinha, J. N., 332
Sinha, P. K., 448
Sinha, T., 446, 448
Sinichkin, A., 329
Sinnhuber, R. O., 169
Sinski, J., 491
Sitar, D. S., 563-65, 569
Sitka, U., 563
Sitt, R., 456
Sivakumar, B., 134
Six, K. M., 199
Sjo, O., 136
Sjoqvist, F., 297, 418, 419, 563, 565-67, 569
Sjöstrand, N., 266
Sjöstrom, R., 415, 418, 421
Skalko, R. G., 139
Skäberg, K-O., 186
Skea, J., 170
Skegg, D., 316
Skelton, C. L., 445

Skidmore, I. F., 451
Skillern, P. G., 134
Skinhoj, E., 313
Skinner, C., 299
Skipper, H., 536
Skipper, H. E., 530
Skjorten, F., 75
Skolnick, P., 331, 447, 584, 591
Skott, A., 555
Skovsted, L., 297
Skutelsky, E. H., 32, 33, 35
Skyberg, D., 75
Sky-Peck, H. H., 530, 536
Sladen, G. E., 359
Slangen, J. L., 607, 611
Slater, A., 38
Slater, F. D., 282
Slater, I. H., 576
Slater, J. H., 38
Slatopolsky, E., 77
Slikke, G. T. van der, 136
Sloan, H. R., 500, 504-6, 508
Slocumb, C. H., 521
Slorach, S. A., 32
Slotta, K., 484
Small, E., 649
Small, M., 283, 286-88
Smiesko, V., 442, 456
Smith, A. A., 448
Smith, A. D., 27-29, 32, 34, 35, 38
Smith, A. J., 299
Smith, A. L., 563, 564, 569, 570
Smith, A. N., 360
Smith, B. M., 331
Smith, C. L., 293
Smith, C. M., 370, 371, 380
Smith, C. R. Jr., 123, 124
Smith, D. F., 31
Smith, D. G., 86
Smith, D. H., 563, 564, 569, 570
Smith, E. R., 141
Smith, F. R., 133, 134
Smith, G. W. II, 17
Smith, H. D., 201
Smith, H. J., 152, 158
Smith, J. C., 376
Smith, J. W., 443, 454
Smith, L. H., 15, 16, 18-20
Smith, L. H. Jr., 15
Smith, M. J. V., 19
Smith, M. W., 426
Smith, P. E., 86
Smith, R. D., 607
Smith, R. E., 32, 33, 35
Smith, R. H., 75
Smith, R. I., 680
Smith, R. M., 124
Smith, R. P., 140, 220
Smith, R. T., 179, 181
Smith, S. E., 300

714   AUTHOR INDEX

Smith, T., 189
Smith, T. W., 58, 294, 431
Smith, W. J., 32, 35
Smith, W. M., 315, 316
Smith, W. O., 71
Smithee, G. A., 442
Smithells, R. W., 134
Smithies, A. R., 679
Smoake, J. A., 452
Smolen, P. M., 411
Snaith, R. P., 141
Sneden, A. T., 124, 125
Snee, R. D., 205
Sneyd, J. G. T., 447, 448, 451, 456
Snoddy, H. D., 388, 609
Snowman, A. M., 431
Snyder, P. D., 109
Snyder, R., 444, 448
Snyder, S. H., 243, 325-30, 348, 373, 376, 431, 546, 550-53, 577, 581-84, 587–88
Snyder, W., 13, 14
Snyderman, M., 189
Snyderman, R., 181, 581, 582
Sobel, A., 546
Sobel, A. E., 199
Sobel, B. E., 445, 457
Soda, D. M., 297, 563, 566, 569
Soda, K., 100
Söderlund, S., 636
Sodhi, H. S., 505
Soergel, K. H., 357
Soifer, D., 578
Sokal, J. E., 183, 189
Solé-Balcells, F., 15
Soler-Bechara, J., 133
Soll, A. H., 243
Solomon, A. K., 633
Solomon, H. M., 296, 297, 300
Solomon, N. A., 51
Soly, K., 239
Solymoss, B., 300
Somers, G., 29, 150
Somers, J. E., 388
Somers, K., 264
Somlyo, A. P., 158
Somlyo, A. V., 158, 442, 456
Sommerville, A. R., 448
Somogyi, G. T., 375
Somylo, A. P., 442, 456
Sondergaard, E., 137
Song, S-Y., 451
Sorby, D. L., 294
Sorensen, L. B., 207
Sorenson, R. L., 28
Soria-Herrera, C., 485
Sorimachi, M., 37, 38
Soscia, J. L., 133
Sourkes, T. L., 411, 412, 545
Sowton, E., 158

Soyka, L. F., 569
SPACIE, A.,167-77; 172
Spackman, D. H., 99, 101
Spanjer, W., 488
Spanner, S., 372, 374
Sparf, B., 370, 373-77
Sparks, F. C., 182, 183, 188, 189
Späth, E., 649, 655, 662
Spaziani, E., 677
Specht, W., 362
Spector, R. G., 141
Spector, S., 555
Speer, J. F., 189
Speight, T. M., 108
Speizer, F. E., 92
Spellacy, W. N., 445
Spencer, A. N., 250
Spiegel, A. M., 584, 585
Spiel, R., 152
Spielvogel, A., 136
Spiers, A. S. D., 105
Spierto, F. W., 77
Spillane, A., 13
Spink, W. W., 519
Spirt, N., 296, 300
Spittell, J. A. Jr., 137
Spitzer, A., 565, 636
Spjut, H. J., 444
Spooner, B. S., 38
Spoor, R. P., 37
Sporn, J. R., 578, 581, 583, 584, 587, 590, 592, 593
Sprague, J. M., 426
Sprague, R. G., 523
Sprangers, W. J. J. M., 141
Spratt, J. L., 158
Spratt, J. S. Jr., 444
Spreafico, F., 186
Sproles, A. C., 446, 449
Spurgeon, H. A., 590
Spurrell, R. A. J., 158
Srbova, J., 201
Srebro, B., 612
Srivastava, Y. P., 333
Stadler, H., 369-72, 378, 379
Stadler, J., 37
Stalling, D. L., 169, 171
Stamler, J., 319
Stamler, R., 319
Stamp, T. C. B., 136
Stanbury, S. W., 72
Stancel, G. M., 451
Stancer, H. C., 614
Standaert, F. G., 401
Stanton, E. S., 411
Starke, K., 267
Starkweather, D. K., 565
Starratt, A. N., 430
Starzl, T. E., 181
Statham, C. N., 168
Stauch, M., 154

Staverman, A. J., 631
Stavinoha, W. B., 458
Stavorski, J. M., 299
Stawarz, R. J., 590
Stawiski, M., 447, 454
Stawiski, M. A., 454
Steele, C. E., 139
Steele, G., 190
STEELE, T.H., 11-25; 17, 19
Steer, M. L., 577, 581, 582, 585, 586
Stefano, F. J. E., 267
Stefanovich, V., 455
Steffen, H., 28
Steg, A., 15
Stegaru, B., 159
Stein, D. H., 317
Stein, G., 58
Stein, H. B., 142
Stein, L., 610
Stein, M., 181
Steinberg, A. D., 286
Steinberg, D., 388, 442
Steinberg, S. A., 396
Steinborn, J. A., 370, 374
Steinbrunn, W., 295
Steiner, A., 508
Steiner, A. L., 450, 587
Steiner, D. F., 32
Steiner, G., 250
Steiner, M., 300
Steiner, P. M., 506
Steiness, E., 298
Stenberg, J., 317
Stenevi, U., 546
Stenson, R. E., 295
Stenson, W., 442
Stephens, D. S., 568
Stephenson, J. D., 345
Stermitz, F. R., 122
Stern, D., 37
Stern, L., 563, 566, 569
Stern, P., 427
Sterri, S., 329
Stevens, F. C., 452
Stevenson, I. H., 53, 55, 57, 62
Stewart, J. J., 360, 361, 363
Stewart, R. B., 293, 680
Stewart, T. H. M., 188
Stiles, M. H., 139
Stimson, W. H., 316
Stinus, L., 546
Stith, W. J., 107
Stjärne, L., 262, 263, 265-69
Stjernholm, R., 538
St.-Laurent, J., 421, 422
Stock, K., 451
Stockle, H., 629
Stocklein, P. B., 267, 268
Stockley, H. L., 271
Stockmann, V. A., 136
Stoepel, K., 159

Stöfen, D., 197
Stokes, J., 140
Stokes, J. W., 418
Stolbach, L., 183
Stoll, H. L. Jr., 189
Stoll, R. G., 294
Stolte, H., 629, 636
Stone, C. A., 299
Stone, L. J., 168, 169
Stone, N. J., 500, 504-6, 508
Stone, S., 152
Stoner, J., 450
Stopps, G. J., 205
Storm, D. R., 589
Storm-Mathisen, J., 327, 328, 330
Storr, J. M., 106
Stote, R. M., 15
Strada, S., 451, 460, 463
Strada, S. J., 450-53, 459, 460, 590, 592, 593
Stradlin, P., 319
Strand, L. J., 206
Strandberg, K., 266
Strandgaard, S., 313
Strandhoy, J. W., 636
Strange, P. G., 243
Strauch, M., 159
Straughan, D. W., 401
Straus, M., 534
Strauss, F. G. II, 15
Strauss, R. G., 141
STREBEL, L., 561-73
Streeten, D. H. P., 313
Streeto, J. M., 640
Stricker, E. M., 607-9, 614
Strisower, B., 505
Strisower, E. H., 505, 506
Strober, W., 181
Stromme, J. H., 75
Strong, C. G., 262
Strong, D. M., 286
Strong, J. M., 238, 239
Stroud, H. H., 140
Stroud, R. M., 243
Studer, R. O., 430
Stühlen, H. W., 153
Stuik, E. J., 203, 206
Stumpe, K. O., 624, 636
Stupp, Y., 188
Su, Y-F., 591, 594
Subramaniam, P. S., 130
Subramanian, N., 328
Subryan, V. L., 15
Suda, T., 136
Sudlow, M. F., 91
Sugasawa, T., 118
Sugerman, A. A., 139
Sugiyama, H., 243
Sugrue, M. F., 612
Suh, S. M., 75-78
Suhl, M., 421

Suhrland, G., 539
Suhrland, L. G., 185
Suijkerbuijk-Van Beek, M. M. A., 141
Suketa, Y., 206
Suki, W. N., 71, 73, 632
Sulakhe, P. V., 445, 457
Sulkes, A., 535, 536
Sullivan, T., 455
Sullivan, T. J., 442
Sulser, F., 461, 590, 611
Summers, W., 531
Sund, H., 243
Sundberg, D. K., 37
Sundler, F., 430
Sundwall, A., 370, 372, 374, 375, 377
Sung, C. P., 451
Surawicz, B., 300
Surber, E. W., 167
Suria, A., 380
Suszkiw, J. B., 373, 378
Sutherland, E. W., 442, 446, 449-51, 454, 456, 460, 576, 578, 583, 588, 589, 591
Suttie, J. W., 133
Sutton, R. A. L., 14
Suzuki, I., 285
Suzuki, S., 205
Suzuki, T., 205
Svenneb, G., 329
Svensson, T. H., 610
Svirbely, J. L., 84, 85
Swaine, D., 106
Swan, M., 75
Swanson, L. W., 584
Swash, M., 393
Swedberg, B., 186
Swedin, G., 266, 268, 269
Sweet, B., 505
Sweet, C. S., 262, 264
Swinny, B., 480
Swyryd, E. A., 505
Sy, W., 51
Szara, S., 655
Szechtman, H., 608
Szentivanyi, A., 454
Szerb, J. C., 370-72, 375-77
Szeto, J., 156

T

Taber, R. I., 347
Tadokoro, M., 636
Tager, J. M., 108, 109
Tagliabue, A., 186
Taira, N., 157, 272
Takabatake, Y., 33, 34
Takada, I., 200
Takagi, K., 586
Takagi, T., 397

TAKAHASHI, T., 425-39; 426-30
Takahasi, Y., 134
Takai, K., 100, 107
Takayanagi, I., 586
Takemori, A. E., 243
Takikawa, M., 609
Takizawa, S., 539
Täljedal, I. B., 28, 36, 457
Tallal, L., 103
Tallant, E. A., 445, 450
Tamao, F. A., 100, 101
Tamarkin, N. R., 412
Tamura, Z., 486, 586
Tanaka, Y., 135
Tang, A. H., 390
Tang, E., 104
Tang, F. L. M., 551
Tarazi, R. C., 312, 315-17
Targovnik, J. H., 77
Tasaki, T. K., 445
Tashjian, A. H. Jr., 75, 77, 78
Tasse, J. R., 397
Tassin, J. P., 547, 548
Tate, R., 575, 582, 591, 593, 594
Tate, S., 254
Tateson, J. E., 455
Tatra, G., 537
Tattersall, M., 539
Taussig, H. B., 137
Taylor, A. L., 446
Taylor, B. L., 243
Taylor, D. M., 141
Taylor, D. W., 319, 320
Taylor, E. L., 38
Taylor, G., 232
Taylor, G. J., 86
Taylor, G. S., 266
Taylor, H. L., 121, 125, 126
Taylor, K. M., 325-29, 348, 612
Taylor, P. T., 183
Taylor, R., 535
Taylor, R. E., 611
Taylor, S., 536
Taylor, S. A., 300
Taylor, W. A., 455
Taylor, W. J., 169, 171
Tchao, R., 454
Tebecis, A. K., 331, 332
Tedesco, J., 553
Teem, M. V., 359
Tegler, L., 312
Teien, A., 294
Teisinger, J., 201, 202
Teitelbaum, D. T., 215
Teitelbaum, P., 607, 608
Telford, I. R., 392
Tell, G. P. E., 579, 580
Teller, D. C., 100, 105, 109, 110

Tembe, V., 18
TEMPLE, A. R., 215-22; 215-17, 219, 221
Temple, R., 37
Temple, T. E., 208
Templeton, G., 17
Tengerdy, R. P., 139
Teo, T. S., 452
Teoh, P. C., 299
Tepper, L. B., 207
Terasaki, W. L., 451
Terenius, L., 431
Ter Haar, G. L., 197
Termini, B. S., 300
Terragno, N. A., 262
Terrill, J. B., 91
Teshima, Y., 452
Tha, S. J., 347
Thain, E., 486, 489, 490
Thaler, M. M., 568, 569
Thanassi, N. M., 455
Thesleff, S., 391, 396, 590
Thetford, B., 100-2
Thierry, A. M., 546
Thiesen, U., 55
Thirlwell, M., 533, 536, 538
Thoa, N. B., 265, 610
Thoenen, H., 345, 347
Thomas, C. W., 49
Thomas, D., 491, 492
Thomas, E., 15
Thomas, E. M., 134
Thomas, E. W., 443
Thomas, G. J., 124, 125
Thomas, J., 15, 563, 567
Thomas, L., 181
Thomas, L. J. Jr., 451
Thomas, M. L., 569
Thomas, P. H., 357, 360
Thomas, R., 488
Thomas, W. C. Jr., 19, 20
Thompson, D. D., 68
Thompson, E. A., 448
Thompson, E. B., 512, 537
Thompson, G. G., 205
Thompson, R. B., 71
Thompson, R. L., 548
Thompson, W. J., 450-52, 459, 460
Thomsen, J., 388
Thomson, P. D., 295
Thoren, P., 418
Thorn, G. W., 73
Thorn, N. A., 31, 32, 150
Thornburg, J. E., 551
Thornicroft, S. G., 152
Thornley, J. H., 296
Thorp, J. M., 505
Thorpe, S. R., 108, 109, 111
Thorsen, K., 416, 417
Threlfall, G., 141
Thresher, A. J., 445

Thurau, K., 624, 636
Thurm, R. H., 315, 316
Thurman, G. B., 282, 286, 288
Thyagarajan, B. S., 119
Thyrum, P. T., 298
Ticho, S., 319
Timmermans, H. A. T., 513
Ting, B. T., 30
Tinston, D. J., 85, 86
Tin-Wa, M., 121
Tisdale, M. J., 453
Tisher, C. C., 624, 628, 639
Tisman, G., 538
Tissot, R., 411
Tixier-Vidal, A., 33
Tobian, L., 262
Tobias, J., 539
Tobin, J. D., 53, 57
Tognoni, G., 563, 564, 567
Toivola, P., 347
Tola, S., 201, 202, 204, 205
Tolagen, K., 312
Tolchin, S. F., 186
Tomasi, V., 578, 588
Tomchick, R., 329
Tomita, M., 119
Tomkins, G. M., 448, 454, 464, 512
Torkelson, T. R., 84
Tormey, J. M., 627
Torrey, E. F., 548, 549
Tosa, T., 110
Toseland, P. A., 54, 57
Toskes, P., 75, 77
Totaro, J. A., 299
Toth, S., 300
Toulouse, P., 90, 91
Towers, R. P., 13
Townsend, J., 13, 14
Toyoda, T., 118
Toyokawa, K., 205
Tozer, T. N., 294
Trabucchi, M., 369-71, 373-79
Traeger, A., 57, 58
Trainin, N., 283, 286-88
Trechsel, U., 20
Tregear, G. W., 426, 430, 433
Trendelenburg, U., 578, 590
Treumann, F., 395
Trevisani, A., 588
Triem, S. C., 187
TRIFARÓ, J.M., 27-47; 28-32, 34-38
Triggle, D. J., 586
Triggs, E. J., 49, 55, 58, 59
Tripathi, O., 157, 158
Tripodi, D., 190
Trist, D. G., 455
Tritthart, H., 150, 152, 154, 156-58
Trochimowicz, H. J., 91
Trojanek, J., 121

Trojanowska, J., 200
Troll, W., 444
Troop, R. C., 318
Trottnow, D., 456
Troughton, V. A., 72
Trounce, J. R., 54, 57
Troutman, S. L., 624, 625, 632, 633
Troxler, F., 581, 582, 586, 587
Troy, J. L., 636
Trudinger, B. J., 563, 569
Trulson, M. E., 612-14
Trummel, C. L., 137
Trump, B. F., 624
Trygstad, C. W., 446, 448
Trzeciak, A., 430
Tschirdewahn, B., 152
Tschudy, D. P., 206
Tsuchiya, K., 207
Tsuzuki, O., 563, 566, 569
Tubiana, M., 537
Tucci, J. R., 446, 448
Tuck, D., 418, 419
Tucker, G. T., 54, 58, 60, 565
Tucker, S. G., 75
Tulloh, M., 534
Tune, B. M., 629
Tunell, R., 133
Tuomisto, J., 328, 678
Tuomisto, L., 328, 333
Turnberg, L. A., 356, 357
Turner, J. W., 415
Turpin, R. A., 72
Turtle, J. R., 442, 616
Tuttle, R. S., 62
Tweedale, M. G., 303
Twittenhoff, W. D., 159
Twose, P. A., 591, 594
Tyler, A., 442
Tyler, M., 491
Tymoczko, J. L., 578
Tyrer, J. H., 60
Tytgat, G. N., 361

U

Uchida, N., 118
Udén, A-M., 186
Udenfriend, S., 388, 486, 555
Udwadia, B. P., 299
Ugrai, E., 139
Uhlich, E., 629, 636
Uhlrecht, G., 158
Ulbricht, W., 388
Ullrey, D. E., 75
Ullrich, K. J., 629-31, 633, 636
Ulpian, C., 38
Umiel, T., 283, 286
Umphrey, J. E., 134
Umrath, K., 428
Ungerstedt, U., 546, 607, 609
Uphoff, D. E., 181

Urbanek, R., 565, 568
Urbina, M., 649, 650, 664, 665
Uren, J. R., 98, 106
Uretsky, N. J., 345
Urivetzky, M., 515
Urtasun, R., 539
Usdin, E., 612, 613, 679
Utiger, R. D., 432
Uttenthal, L. O., 32
Uvnäs, B., 32, 485
Uzunov, P., 449, 451, 452, 457-63

V

Vadlamudi, S., 100
Vale, W., 29, 30, 432
Valentin, H., 201
Valentine, M. D., 443
Valeri, V., 134
Valeriote, F., 530
Vallieres, J., 579
Valverde, I., 512
Van Arsdale, P. M., 585
Van Bekkum, D. W., 281, 282
van Benthem, R. M. J., 398, 400, 402
Van den Bergh, F. A. J. T. M., 108, 109
Van der Gugten, L., 611
van der Kleijn, E., 563, 564
Van Der Meer, C., 401
Vandlen, R., 243
Van Dyke, R. A., 92
Vane, J., 267
Vane, J. R., 261, 266-68, 271
Van Es, T., 110
Van Obberghen, E., 150
Van Praag, H. M., 413, 420
Van Rossum, J. M., 610
VanSanten, L., 17
Van Scott, E., 530
VAN STEE, E. W., 83-95; 84-91
Van Tienhoven, A., 345, 346
Van Valin, C., 169
Van Veelen, C. W. M., 133
Van Wijk, R., 453
Van Woert, M. H., 372, 545
Vapaatalo, H., 447
Varga, S., 300
Varma, R. N., 138
Varrady, P. D., 71
Vartia, K. O., 51, 52, 56
Vas, S. I., 453, 462
Vasilikiotis, G. S., 121
Vassanelli, P., 50
Vassort, G., 150
Vater, W., 159
Vatner, D., 581
Vaughan, E. D., 312, 317
Vaughan, G. L., 444

Vaughan, M., 450, 455
Vaughan Williams, E. M., 158
Vaz Ferreira, A., 31, 32
Veale, W. L., 342
Vecchi, A., 186
Veith, G. D., 174
Velasco, M., 318, 319
Vélez, T., 658, 665
Veltri, J. C., 216, 217, 221
Venter, J. C., 588
Venugopal, B., 284
Vera, J. C., 444, 448
Verdiere, M., 325-30
Verdiere-Sahuque, M., 329
Vere, D. W., 299
Verebely, K., 297
Vergnano, C., 205
Verhoust, P. J., 635
Verhulst, H. L., 215
Verlander, M. S., 588
Verma, A. K., 124, 125, 444
Vernikos-Danellis, J., 458
Vernot, E. H., 92
Verzar, F., 62
Vesell, E. S., 296, 565
Vest, M., 137
Vest, M. F., 566
Vestal, R. E., 53, 57
Vetulani, J., 590
Vick, J., 484, 485
Vidal, E., 90, 91
Viets, J., 262
Vignalou, J., 49
Vihko, V., 203
Vila-Porcile, E., 32
Vilhardt, H., 35
Viljoen, D., 205
Villablanca, J. R., 551
Villanueva, M., 512
Vincent, J., 75
Vincent, J. D., 432, 433
Vincenzi, F. F., 261, 270
Vine, W. H., 243
Virion, A., 331, 332
Viser, C., 519
Visser, B., 488
Viswanathan, N., 118
Viswanthan, C. T., 344
Vitaenzer, V., 678
Vitale, L. F., 207, 208
Viti, A., 269
Viveros, O. H., 32, 34
Vizi, E. S., 262, 263, 271
Voeller, K., 201
Vogel, J. R., 458
Vogelsang, A., 139
Vogler, W. R., 189, 531, 535
Vogt, M., 345, 429
Voisin, G. A., 182
Volk, B. W., 33, 34
Volkmann, R., 156, 158
Volm, M., 538

Volpe, B. T., 360
Von Bibra, E. F., 655, 656, 658
von Brücke, F. T., 554
von Henning, G. E., 159
Von Hungen, K., 331
von Oettingen, W. F., 84, 85
von Stedingk, M., 136
Voorhees, J. J., 447, 454
Vrelust, M.-T., 203

W

Wada, O., 205
Wada, T., 636
Waddell, W. J., 568
Wade, H. E., 105, 109
Wade, M. E., 185
Wadman, B., 186
Wagers, P. W., 680
Waggoner, J. G., 206
Wagman, J., 198
Wagner, H., 584
Wagner, H. R., 590
Wagner, J., 152
Wagner, J. G., 294
Wagner, O., 109
Wahl, M., 636
Wahlström, A., 431
Wain, H., 479
Wakabayashi, K., 29, 30
Walaszek, E. J., 328
Walczack, I. M., 112
Wald, A., 357
Waldeck, B., 545
Waldmann, T. A., 181, 355
Waldron, H. A., 197, 202, 203
Waldvogel, M., 448
Waley, S. G., 248
Walinder, J., 555
Walker, A. M., 623
Walker, C. M., 443, 453
Walker, J., 490
Walker, M. D., 678
Walker, M. M., 37
Walker, R. J., 429, 430
Walker, S. R., 91
Walker, T. M., 170
WALL, M. E., 117-32; 118, 119, 121, 125-27, 569
Wallace, J. E., 678
Wallace, K., 508
Wallace, S., 60
Wallach, S., 74
Waller, M. B., 347
Waller, S. L., 357
Wallick, E. T., 156
Wallis, D. I., 332
Walser, M., 68, 71, 75, 77, 78
Walsh, J. J., 316
Walsh, M., 90, 91
Walton, J. N., 392
Wan, S. H., 563, 564

Wanderling, J., 316
Wang, C., 369-71, 373-76, 378
Wang, C. T., 370, 374, 375
Wang, D. H., 138
Wang, F. L., 376
Wang, J. H., 452
Wang, P. F. L., 376
Wangeman, C. P., 658
WANI, M. C., 117-32; 118, 119, 121, 125-27
Wanitschke, R., 359, 362, 363
Wanstall, J., 492
Wara, D. W., 288
Ward, D. N., 432
Ward, I. L., 614
Wardell, W. M., 296
Ware, F. Jr., 391
Warnick, J. E., 397
Warren, B. T., 455
Warren, F. L., 658, 664
Warren, G. H., 678
Warren, W. A., 92
Warshauer, D., 139
Warshaw, A. L., 355
Warshaw, J. B., 579
Waser, P. G., 613
Wasserman, F., 293
Wasson, R. G., 648-56, 660, 661, 665, 666, 670
Wasson, V. P., 648-50, 660, 661
Watanabe, A. M., 156
Waters, K., 187
Waters, O., 13, 14
Watkin, D. M., 411, 412
Watlinger, C., 75
Watson, J. F., 68
Watson, M., 140
Waybrant, R. C., 170-72, 174
Wayss, K., 538
Webb, D., 453
Webb, D. R., 457
Webb, E. C., 248, 578
Webb, W. W., 505
Weber, G., 443, 448, 451
Weber, H. U., 138
Weber, K., 38
Weber, M., 243
Weber, W. W., 564, 565
Webster, G. D. Jr., 72
Webster, J., 78, 315
Webster, L. T., 239
Webster, P. D., 75
Webster, R. A., 141
Webster, R. G., 187
Webster, S. G. P., 50
Wecker, L., 396, 398-400, 402
Wedeen, R. P., 207, 208
Weder, H. G., 28
Weder, U., 160
Wedner, H. J., 442, 451
Weeks, J. R., 263
Weetall, H. H., 111

Wegman, D. H., 92
Wei, E., 199
Weihing, R. R., 38
Weil, J., 315
Weill, C. L., 243
Weily, H. S., 298
Weinberger, A., 18, 19
Weiner, B., 207, 208
Weiner, I. M., 14, 298
Weiner, J., 189
Weiner, R., 262
Weingartner, L., 563
Weinman, E. J., 632, 636
Weinryb, I., 449, 453, 456, 458
Weinshilboum, R., 265
Weinstock, M., 586
Weintraub, B. D., 522
Weintraub, M., 293
Weisbrode, S. E., 137
Weisbrodt, N. W., 360, 361
Weisenberg, R. C., 37
Weisleder, D., 123
WEISS, B., 441-77; 442, 444, 448-53, 455-63, 590, 592, 593, 680
Weiss, C. F., 297, 566
Weiss, C. M., 169, 171
Weiss, D. W., 188
Weiss, F. R., 141
Weiss, H. D., 678
Weiss, L., 313
Weiss, R., 156, 158
Weissbach, H., 329, 332
Weissman, G., 455, 515
Wekerle, H., 288
Welborn, W. S., 320
Welbundt, W., 629
Welch, A. D., 31
Weller, J., 451
Wellhoner, H., 483
Welling, L. W., 637, 639
Wells, J., 318, 319
Wells, J. N., 451, 452, 456, 459-61
Wells, S. A. Jr., 183
Wells, W. D. E., 54, 58
Wen, S. F., 67, 68, 70, 71
Wende, W., 153
Wennmalm, Å., 261, 262, 264-70
Wergedal, J. E., 17
Werkheiser, W. C., 678
Werko, L., 317
Werman, R., 425, 427
Werner, A. B., 612
Werner, R. J., 319
Wernick, G., 181
Wessels, J., 535
Wessels, N. K., 38
Wesson, L. G. Jr., 71
West, A. P., 550
Westby, G. R., 14
Westerlund, A., 317

Westfall, D. P., 396
Westfall, T. C., 262, 265
Weston, J. K., 566
Wettrell, G., 563-65, 568, 569
Wexler, I. B., 199
Whaley, W. G., 33
Whang, J., 530
Wheeler, G., 536-38
Wheeler, H. O., 360, 627
Wheeler, W., 533
Whitcomb, W. H., 442
White, A., 282, 285-87
White, B. G., 563, 564
White, C.
White, G., 316
White, J. M., 203
White, L. W., 505
White, N., 432, 433
White, P. T., 563, 564
White, R. J., 58
White, T., 326, 329, 332
White, W. F., 432
Whiteway, S. G., 170
Whitfield, F., 491
Whiting, B., 60
Whiting, M., 390, 391
Whitlock, R. T., 627
Whitney, J. E., 30
Whittaker, R. H., 250
Whittaker, V. P., 27, 426
Whittembury, G., 627, 628, 633
Whittingham, S., 183
Wick, T., 627
Wicks, W. D., 453
Wickson, R. D., 452
Wide, L., 186
Wiebelhaus, V. D., 451
Wieck, A. B., 201
Wieckowski, J., 397
Wiederholt, M., 629, 636
Wieland, T., 248
Wieneke, A. A., 390
Wiener, R., 515
Wiener, S. L., 515
Wiernik, P. H., 187
Wiesel, F.-A., 554
Wigton, R. S., 401
Wiklund, R. A., 577, 581, 584, 586, 587
Wilber, J. F., 37
Wilburn, R. L., 316, 319
Wilcox, W. R., 18
Wild, J., 134
Wile, A. G., 188
Wilk, S., 421
Wilkerson, C., 54, 58, 60
Wilkes, B., 186
Wilkinson, G. R., 55, 59, 60, 295, 297
Wilkinson, R., 13, 15
Willemot, J., 38
Willford, W. A., 168
Willi, H., 137

Williams, B. J., 590
Williams, D., 296
Williams, F. M., 53, 57, 91, 318, 563, 569
Williams, H. E., 15-17
Williams, H. L., 140
Williams, J. A., 28-30, 37
Williams, J. B., 75, 77
Williams, L. T., 575, 577, 581, 582, 587, 588
Williams, M. K., 202
Williams, R. B. Jr., 300
Williams, R. H., 450
Williamson, J. R., 156
Willingham, M., 454
Willis, G. L., 610
Willis, L. R., 636
Willis, P. W., 294
Willner, M., 137
Wills, H., 199, 201
Wills, M. R., 13
Wilson, A. E., 372, 377
Wilson, D. M., 15
Wilson, F., 187
Wilson, G. M., 680
Wilson, I. C., 419
Wilson, J. T., 561, 563, 564, 568-70, 678
Wilson, L., 37, 38
Wilson, M., 208
Wilson, M. H., 203, 207
Wilson, W. R., 264
Windhager, E. E., 626, 628, 633, 635, 636
Windorfer, A. Jr., 565, 568
Winegrad, S., 156
Winer, N., 388, 390
Wingate, D. L., 357, 359
Winkelman, A. C., 141
Winkelstein, A., 186
Winkle, R. A., 238
Winkler, H., 28, 32, 34, 35, 38
Winnacker, J. L., 77
Winokur, A., 432
Winsor, T., 152
Winston, F., 141
Winter, S. L., 139
Winzler, R. J., 252, 536
Wise, C. D., 610
Wise, W. D., 612
Wisenbau, T., 444
Wit, A. L., 157
Withrington, P. G., 261, 263, 264, 266, 267
Witkop, B., 479
Wittenborn, J. R., 140
Wittenmeier, K. W., 159
Witter, A., 425
Wittermann, E. R., 78
Witzke, F., 396
Wode-Helgodt, B., 414
Wodinsky, I., 537
Wohlfart, G., 391

Wolberg, W., 536
Wolcott, L., 388
Wold, F., 109
Wolf, G., 133
Wolf, H. H., 343, 345
Wolf, P., 329-33
WOLFE, B. B., 575-604; 577, 579-81, 583, 586, 588, 590-94
Wolfe, L. S., 269, 391
Wolff, D. J., 450-52, 459
Wolff, I. A., 123
Wolff, J., 37
Wolff, J. P., 183
Wolff, K., 482
Wolgin, D. L., 607
Wolstencroft, J. H., 432
Woltersdorf, O. W., 680
Wolthuis, O. L., 343, 398, 400, 402
Wong, E., 139
Wong, K., 553
Wong, N., 71
Wong, N. L. M., 14, 68
Wood, J. M., 151
Wood, P. L., 395
Woodard, C. J., 582, 583, 585
Woodin, A. M., 35, 390
Woodrow, M. L., 156
Woodruff, G. N., 429, 430
Woods, J. A., 101, 102
Woods, J. S., 111
Woods, J. W., 506
Woods, R. I., 262
Woodward, J. C., 75
Woodwell, G. M., 168, 169
Woolf, A. L., 394, 396
Woolfolk, D., 508
Wootton, I. D. P., 319
Wrenn, J. T., 38
Wrenn, S. M., 587, 588
Wright, F. S., 635
Wright, P. H., 91
Wright, R. K., 447, 454
Wright, T. L., 394, 395
Wriston, J. C. Jr., 98, 99
Wrong, O., 19
Wu, Y. J., 451, 452, 456, 459-61
Wunderlich, P., 636
Wurtman, R. J., 371, 614
Wyatt, R., 412
Wybran, J., 183
Wyllie, J. H., 266, 267
Wysenbeeck, H., 300

Y

Yablonski, M. E., 358
Yaffe, S. J., 565, 566, 569
Yajima, H., 429, 430
Yakir, Y., 283
Yaksh, T. L., 343, 344, 347, 370, 371, 376, 377, 380

Yamada, K. M., 38
Yamada, T., 331, 453, 454
Yamaguchi, I., 159
Yamaguchi, K., 118
Yamamoto, T., 36, 206
Yamamoto, Y., 100
Yamamura, H. I., 369-71, 373, 376, 377, 380, 546, 552
Yamane, T., 205
Yamashita, K., 154
Yamazaki, R., 452, 461
Yanagi, R., 569
Yanaihara, C., 428, 433
Yanaihara, N., 428, 433
Yang, H-Y. T., 432
Yang, M. G., 135
Yang, T. H., 121
Yang, T. J., 453, 454, 462
Yano, Y., 205
Yant, P. R., 172
Yao, L., 53, 58
Yarger, W. E., 627, 628
Yary, M. G., 133
Yates, C. M., 411
Yates, J. D., 294
Yatzidis, H., 134
Yawata, Y., 17
Yeager, D. W., 200
Yellin, T. O., 98, 99
Yendt, E. R., 14, 71, 135
Ygge, H., 563, 565, 566, 569
Yiengst, M. J., 71
Yokota, T., 397
Yokoyama, N., 119
York, D. H., 29, 30, 331, 332
Yorkston, N. J., 554
Yoshida, H., 36
Yoshioka, M., 586
Yosselson, S., 681
Young, A. B., 243, 328
Young, D. A., 36, 37
Young, J. A., 630
Young, L. B., 208
Young, R., 537, 539
Young, S. N., 412
Youngchaiyud, U., 183
Youngs, W. D., 170, 171
Yu, D. T. Y., 186
Yu, M. K., 394, 395
Yü, T-F., 18

Z

Zabriskie, J. B., 181
Zacest, R., 317, 318
Zacks, S. I., 396
Zajtchuk, R., 294
Zaki, S. A., 554
Zalin, R. J., 442
Zalman, A., 487
Zaltzman-Nirenberg, P., 555
Zanati, E., 107
Zanella, J., 576, 591

Zapf, J., 448
Zar, M. A., 263
Zatz, M., 581, 582, 590, 593
Zatz, M. M., 286
Zbar, B., 188
Zee-Cheng, K. Y., 121, 122
Zeitz, S., 522
Zellweger, H., 392
Zemlan, F. P., 613, 614
Zepernick, R., 236
Zetler, G., 426, 429
Zetterstrom, R., 137
Ziegler, F. D., 445
Ziegler, M. F., 128, 129

Zieher, L. M., 372
Zielhuis, R. L., 207
Zierler, K. L., 388, 390
Zierott, G., 55
Zighelboim, J., 179, 181, 188
Zigmond, M. J., 607-9
Zimmerly, V. A., 125
Zimmermann, B. G., 266
Zimmermann, P., 427
Zingg, R. M., 662, 669
Zipes, D. P., 157, 158
Zipori, D., 283, 286
Zirrolli, J. A., 579, 580

Zisblatt, M. A., 287
Zittoun, R., 537
Zivkovic, B., 412
Zsilla, G., 370, 373-75, 377,
    379, 380
Zull, J. E., 135
Zurier, R. B., 455, 515
Zur Nedden, G., 34
Zutaut, C. L., 75
Zweig, S. M., 637
Zwiebel, R., 629
Zwiren, G. T., 569
Zwisler, J., 249

SUBJECT INDEX

A

Absorption
  aging effects on, 50
  drug interactions affecting,
    294-95
  of lead
    from GI tract, 199
    from skin, 200
  reviews on, 678
Accumulation
  of chemicals by fish, 167-
    77
Acetaminophen
  pediatric aspects of, 563,
    566, 569
Acetazolamide
  on cyclic nucleotides, 456
  drug interactions with, 303
  and nephrolithiasis, 19
Acetohydroxamic acid
  in nephrolithiasis, 17
Acetylcephalotaxine
  antitumor studies of, 124
  structure of, 123
Acetylcholine (ACh)
  inhibition of synthesis of,
    372
  inhibiting drugs, 376
  measurement of brain turn-
    over of, 369-86
    actions of drugs on, 375-
      80
    conclusion, 380
    introduction, 369-70
    methods of, 370-75
  and myopathies, 396-98,
    400-2
  pediatric aspects of, 568
  postmortem changes in, 372-
    73
  and prostaglandins, 270-72
  receptors, 243
  release rates of
    measurement of, 371-72
  in thermoregulation, 342-44,
    349
  in venom, 488, 494
Acetylcholinesterase
  drugs acting on, 370, 376
2'-Acetylglaucarubinone
  antitumor activity of, 127
  structure of, 127
Acetylphenylhydrazine
  and β-adrenergic receptor,
    584-85
Acetylsalicylic acid
  aging pharmacokinetics of,
    61
  drug interactions with, 303

Acridine
  myopathies from, 388
ACTH
  suppression of secretion of,
    151
Actin
  in nonmuscle cells, 38
Actinia
  chemoreceptor of, 250-51
Actinomycin D
  on cancer immune response,
    184
  and vitamin K, 138
Activators
  external chemical
    classification of and func-
      tion in aquatic inverte-
      brates, 245
Actomyosin-like protein
  and hormone secretion, 38
Adenohypophysis
  mechanisms of hormone
    secretion in, 27, 33
Adenosine cyclic 3',5'mono-
    phosphate
  see Cyclic adenosine mono-
    phosphate
Adenosine monophosphate
    (AMP)
  as substance P blocker,
    427
Adenosine triphosphate (ATP)
  calcium sensitivity of, 151-
    52, 156
  in hormone release, 35-37,
    39
S-Adenosylmethionine
  to study β-adrenergic recep-
    tor, 579
Adenylate cyclase
  and β-adrenergic receptors,
    577-78, 581, 583-84,
    586-95
  and diseases, 442-50, 454,
    457-58
  dopamine-sensitive, 552
Adrenal cortical steroids
  on vitamin D, 135
Adrenal medulla
  hormone secretion mecha-
    nisms in, 27, 29-30, 32-
    33, 35, 37-38
Adrenal steroids
  and Mg excretion, 72-74
β-Adrenergic receptors
  see Receptors, β-adrenergic
Adrenergic systems
  on feeding control, 606-12
  local injections of drugs,
    606-7

neurochemical depletions,
    607-11
  perfusate collection, 611
  summary and conclusion,
    611-12
β-Adrenoceptor antagonists
  to identify receptor, 581-
    85
β-Adrenoceptor blockers
  aging pharmacokinetics of,
    59
  combination use in hyperten-
    sion, 315-16, 318-19
  in thermoregulation, 345
Adrenocortical atrophy
  and corticosteroids, 523
Adriamycin
  on cancer cell kinetics,
    533
  on cancer immune response,
    186
Aerosols
  lead
    toxicology of, 198-99
    metabolism of, 678
Age
  and lead disposition, 200
  pediatric pharmacokinetics,
    561-70
Aging
  effects of drugs on process
    of, 49
  pharmacokinetic consequences
    of, 49-65
    age-related changes in
      systems, 50-51
    changes in tissue respon-
      siveness, 61-62
    clinical studies, 51-59
    conclusion, 62
    introduction, 49
    plasma protein binding,
      59-61
Ailanthinone
  antitumor activity of, 127
  structure of, 127
Ajmaline
  cardiac effects of, 301
β-Alanyl-L-histidine
  see Carnosine
Alcohol (ethanol)
  and magnesium reabsorp-
    tion, 70-71
  see also Ethanol
Aldosteronism
  hypomagnesemia of, 72-73
Alkalinizing salts
  and nephrolithiasis, 19
Alkaloids
  anticancer drugs from plants,

118-24
benzophenanthridines, 121-22
camptothecin and related alkaloids, 118-19
cephalotaxus alkaloids, 123-24
dimeric benzylisoquinolines, 119-21
Alkylating agents
in cancer immune response, 184, 186
Allonitidine
antitumor activity of, 121
structure of, 122
Allopurinol
drug interactions with, 304
in treatment of uric acid calculi, 11, 18
Alloxan
aging pharmacokinetics of, 62
Alphrenolol
and β-adrenergic receptor, 584
Aluminum hydroxide antacids
and nephrolithiasis, 16-17
Ambenonium
myopathies from, 397
American Board of Medical Toxicology, 219
Amiloride
combination use of, 314
drug interactions with, 303
Amines
CNS metabolism of
drug effects on, 411-24
in thermoregulation, 341-49
9-Amino-acridinpropranolol
at β-adrenergic receptor, 587
p-Aminobenzoate
pediatric problems with, 566
γ-Aminobutyric acid (GABA)
on ACh turnover, 370, 379-80
p-Aminohippuric acid (PAH)
renal studies with, 6
γ-Aminoisobutyric acid
and myopathies, 394
Aminolevulinic acid dehydratase (ALAD)
lead sensitivity of, 203-6
Aminolevulinic acid synthetase (ALAS)
lead sensitivity of, 206
Aminophylline
in asthma, 455
Aminopyrine
aging pharmacokinetics of, 54, 57-58
para-Aminosalicylic acid (PAS)
compliance as problem in

dosage, 319
para-Aminosalicylic acid in vitamin C (PAS-C)
as hypolipidemic, 507-8
Amiodarone
cardaic effects of, 301
Amitriptyline
on CNS amine metabolism, 417-18, 420
discovery of, 9
Amobarbital
pediatric aspects of, 563
(+)-Amphetamine (AMPH)
on ACh turnover, 378
aging pharmacokinetics, 62
in control of feeding, 605-9, 611-12, 615-17
drug interactions with, 297, 299
psychosis from, 550-52, 554
in thermoregulation, 347
Ampicillin
aging pharmacokinetics, 55
pediatric aspects of, 563
Amprolium
renal transport characterization of, 5
Amylobarbitone
aging pharmacokinetics of, 54, 57
Anabolic steroids
drug interactions with, 304
Analgesia
see Pain relief, regional
Analgesics
aging pharmacokinetics, 58
reviews of, 579
Anaphylactic shock
from hymenoptera venom, 480
Anesthesia
on histamine in brain, 329
Anesthetic index, 240
Anesthetics
on ACh turnover, 377
Anesthetics, local
basic nature of, 227-28
molecular configuration of, 224-25
non-nitrogenous, 225
on sodium fluxes, 150
see also Pain relief, regional
Angiotensin II
as neurotransmitter, 432-33
Antacids
drug interactions with, 294
Anthopleura
chemoreceptor of, 250
Anthopleura elegantissima
chemoreceptors of, 249-50
Anthozoa

chemoreceptors of, 250-52
Antiallergy drugs
corticosteroids, 515-16, 519
Antiarrhythmics
arrthymias from, 293
interactions of, 301
on transmembrane action potential of heart, 301
Anticancer drugs
from plants, 117-32
Anticholinergics
on brain amine metabolism, 415
Anticholinesterases
and myopathies, 397
Anticoagulants
drug interactions with, 303-5
Antidepressants
and CNS amine metabolism, 417-20
review of, 679
tricyclic
on β-adrenergic receptor, 590
on CNS amine metabolism, 417-20
on cyclic nucleotides, 458-59
drug interactions with, 299-300
Antidiuretic hormone
histamine efffects on, 333
Antihistamines
drug interactions with, 300
Antihypertensives
combination use of, 311-20
interactions of, 302
Anti-inflammatory agents
aging pharmacokinetics of, 58
corticosteroids, 513-15
on cyclic nucleotides, 455
Antilymphocyte serum
on cancer immune response, 184
Antipolyvinylpyrrolidone
thymic factor on, 287
Antipsychotics
on ACh turnover, 379-80
on phosphodiesterase, 457-59
Antipyrine
aging pharmacokinetics of, 53, 57-58, 60
pediatric aspects of, 563
Antituberculosis drugs
drug interactions with, 297
Antitumor enzymes
criteria for, 99-100
Ant venom
characterization of, 490-92
Apamine

in bee venom, 483-84
Apatite
    and nephrolithiasis, 13, 16,
        18
Apis mellifera
    venom of, 481-85, 487, 492
Apomorphine
    on ACh turnover, 378-79
    structure of, 657
    on thermoregulation, 347-
        48
Aprindine
    cardiac effects of, 301
Arachidonic acid
    and prostaglandin biosynthe-
        sis, 260
Arecoline
    on ACh turnover, 375
Arginase
    in tumor chemotherapy,
        106
Aroclor
    fish accumulation of, 160
Artemsia absinthium
    psychopharmacology of,
        656
Arylaceticade
    on cyclic nucleotides, 355
Ascorbic acid (vitamin C)
    with para-aminosalicylic
        acid
        hypolipidemic activity of,
            507-8
    toxicity studies of, 141-42
    and urinary oxalate, 16, 19
Asparaginase
    bacterial and yeast sources
        of, 99
    on cancer cell kinetics, 532,
        534
    pharmacology and pharmaco-
        kinetics of, 100-3
    therapeutic usefulness of,
        103-12
    methods for improving,
        109-12
L-Asparaginase
    on cancer immune response,
        184, 186
Aspirin
    pediatric aspects of, 568
    on prostaglandin synthesis,
        267-68, 272
Asthma
    cyclic nucleotides in, 443,
        454-55
Atherosclerosis
    cyclic nucleotides in, 445,
        457
    and lipoproteins, 500
Atropine
    on ACh turnover, 371-72
    aging pharmacokinetics of,
        62
    local anesthetic effect of,
        233
    after myocardial ischemia,

680
Autoimmunity
    thymic control of, 287-88
Autologous rosettes
    thymic role in, 288
Autonomic neurotransmission
    prostaglandin mechanisms
        on, 259-79
    adrenergic neuroeffector
        junctions, 260-69
    cholinergic neuroeffector
        transmission, 270-72
    conclusions, 272
    ganglionic transmission,
        269-70
    introduction, 259-60
Azathioprine
    on cancer cell kinetics,
        533
Azidomorphine
    on ACh turnover, 377

B

Bacillus Calmette-Guerin
    (BCG)
    in cancer immunosuppres-
        sion, 187-89
    methanol-extracted residue,
        188
Backleak
    in proximal tubular reabsorp-
        tion, 628, 633-40
    diagram, 638
    passive, 633-40
Baclofen
    mechanism of action of,
        427
    substance P block by, 427
Bacterial enterotoxins
    laxative action of, 356
Barbital
    aging pharmacokinetics of,
        51, 60
Barbiturates
    on ACh turnover, 377
    aging pharmacokinetics, 56-
        57
    cardiodepressant activity
        of, 154
    drug interaction with, 304
    intoxication by, 680
Barium
    and hormone release, 29
B cells
    in cancer immunosuppres-
        sion, 180-81, 187
Beclomethasone dipropionate
    use and complications of,
        526
Bee
    venom of, 481-85
Bendroflumethiazide
    on cyclic nucleotides, 456
Benzoate Na
    pediatric aspects of, 566
Benzocaine

pain relief by, 233, 235
Benzodiazepines
    on phosphodiesterase, 458
Benzolamide
    drug interactions with,
        303
Benzophenanthridine alkaloids
    antitumor activity of, 121-
        22
    structures of, 122
Benzothiadiazine
    combination use of, 314-15
Benztropine
    on ACh turnover, 376
    on brain amine metabolism,
        415
Benzyl alcohol
    pain relief by, 225
Betamethasone
    clinical pharmacology of,
        511, 516-18
Bethanidine
    combination use in hyperten-
        sion, 318
    drug interactions with, 299,
        302
Beyer, Karl H. Jr.
    autobiographical chapter,
        1-10
Bicarbonate
    proximal tubular reabsorp-
        tion, 627, 629-33
Bile acids
    laxative action of, 359
Binding to surfaces
    and enzyme usefulness, 111-
        12
Biogenic amines
    CNS effects of psychophar-
        macologic drugs on, 411-
        24
    cyclic AMP on, 442
    and thyroid, 679
    in venoms, 493
Bisacodyl
    laxative action of, 359, 361-
        62
Bishydroxycoumarin
    drug interactions with, 295-
        97
Bleomycin
    on cancer cell kinetics, 532-
        33
β-Blockers
    see β-Adrenoceptor blockers
Blood
    cyclic nucleotides in, 442
    lead in (PbB), 199, 201-7,
        209
Blood pressure
    regulation of, 312-14
    review of drugs in, 680
    see also Hypertension
Boldine
    antitumor activity of, 121
    structure of, 120
Boloceroides

chemoreceptor of, 250-52
Bone marrow dependent lym-
    phocytes
    see B cells; Lymphocytes
Bone matrix
    lead disposition in, 200
Brain
    acetylcholine turnover in,
        369-86
    dopamine psychopharmacol-
        ogy, 545-56
    histaminergic mechanisms
        in, 325-39
        action on target systems,
            330-33
        conclusion, 333-34
        localization and metabolism,
            325-30
    tumor chemotherapy, 678
Bretylium
    cardiac effects of, 301
Bruceantarin
    antitumor studies of, 128
    structure of, 128
Bruceantin
    antitumor studies of, 128
    structure of, 128
Bruceantinol
    antitumor activity of, 128
    structure of, 128
Bruceolide esters
    antitumor studies of, 128
    structures of, 128
Brushite
    activity product for, 12
    and nephrolithiasis, 12-13,
        16-18, 20
Bulbocapnine
    antitumor activity of, 121
    structure of, 120
Bulk
    laxative effect of, 363
Bumetamide
    symposium on, 680
Bupivacaine
    pain relief by, 226-27, 238
    pediatric aspects of, 565
Burn treatment
    pharmacological aspects of,
        680
Butethamine
    pain relief mechanisms of,
        237
Butoxamine
    as β receptor antagonist,
        576
γ-Butyrolactone
    on ACh turnover, 377
Butyrophenones
    on cyclic nucleotides, 457
    dopamine antagonism by,
        552
    drug interactions with,
        299
Butyrylcholine
    pediatric aspects of,
        568

C

Cacaoquavitl
    psychopharmacology of,
        651-52, 671
Caffeine
    and calcium release, 31
    pediatric aspects of, 563-
        64, 567
    review of, 679
Calcitonin
    and magnesium excretion,
        70, 74-75, 78
    release mechanisms for,
        29-30
Calcium
    aging pharmacokinetics on,
        513
    corticosteroid effects on,
        513
    deficiency of
        and lead absorption, 199
        equilibrium in fluid and
            bone, 77-78
    on hydra feeding response,
        249
    and nephrolithiasis, 13-20
    and renal magnesium, 68-
        69, 73-78
    hypocalcemia of Mg deple-
        tion, 75-78
    specific pharmacology in
        myocardium, cardiac
        pacemakers, and vascu-
        lar smooth muscle, 149-
        66
    basic interaction in cardiac
        energy metabolism, 151-
        54
    biophysical membrane of
        drugs in myocardium,
        154-57
    inhibitors and promoters of
        Ca in vascular smooth
        muscle, 158-60
    introduction, 149-51
    pharmacological interven-
        tions in pacemaker acti-
        vity, 157-58
    summary, 160-61
    and vitamin D toxicity, 135-
        36
Calcium antagonists
    structures of, 153
Calcium disodium ethylenedi-
    aminetetraacetate (EDTA)
    on lead disposition, 201-2,
        205
Calcium ion
    in hormone secretion, 29-
        31, 35-37, 39
Calcium oxalate
    activity product of, 12, 15-
        16, 18
Calea zacatachichi
    psychopharmacology of,
        656

Calliactis
    chemoreceptor of, 250-51
Camptothicin
    anticancer use of, 118-19
    structure of, with analogues,
        118
Cancer
    cyclic nucleotides in, 443-
        44, 448-54
Cancer chemotherapy
    cell kinetics in, 529-43
        attempts at synchronization
            and recruitment, 530-34
        correlation of kinetic para-
            meters and clinical re-
            sponse, 534-38
        future directions, 538-39
        introduction, 529-30
    cyclic nucleotides in, 453-
        54
    immunologic aspects of, 179-
        95
        conclusions and future
            prospects, 190
        drug-induced immunosup-
            pression, 183-88
        immune response in cancer,
            179-83
        immunotherapy and chemo-
            immunotherapy, 188-90
        introduction, 179
        reviews of, 678
        risk-to-benefit ratio in,
            179
Cannabis indica
    psychopharmacology of,
        650
Cannabis sativa
    psychoactive drug from,
        649, 656
Carbachol
    in thermoregulation, 343
Carbamazepine
    drug interactions with, 297,
        304
    pediatric aspects of, 563
Carbenicillin
    pediatric use of, 563
β-Carboline
    structure of, 657
Carbonic anhydrase inhibitors
    drug interactions with, 303
Carbon tetrachloride
    vitamin E protection against,
        139
Carboxypeptidase G$_1$
    therapeutic use of,[1] 107
Carcinogens
    chemical
        exposure to, 680
Cardiac glycosides
    on cAMP, 457
    and Mg reabsorption,
        70
Cardiopep
    in venom, 485, 494
Cardiovascular diseases

cyclic nucleotides in, 445,
  456
Cardiovascular drug interactions, 293-309
  introduction, 293
  pharmacodynamic, 298-300
    amount/effect, 298
    at receptor site, 299-300
  pharmacokinetic, 294-98
    absorption, 294-95
    distribution, 295-97
    excretion, 298
    metabolism, 297-98
  specific drug types, 300-5
    antiarrhythmics, 301
    anticoagulants, 303-5
    antihypertensives, 302
    digitalis glycosides, 300-
      1
    diuretics, 303
Carinamide
  renal studies of, 6-7
Carnosine
  as neurotransmitter, 431
Castor oil
  laxative action of, 359-60
Catecholamines
  to assay β-adrenergic recep-
    tors, 578-81
  drug interactions with, 295,
    298
  mechanism of release of,
    32, 37
  in stress, 679
  in venom, 487
Catechol-o-methyltransferase
  (COMT)
  and β-adrenergic receptor,
    579
  review of, 678
Cecropia obtusifolia
  psychoactive drugs in,
    656
Cedronine
  antitumor studies of, 128
  structure of, 129
Cell division
  cyclic nucleotides in, 442
Cell kinetics
  in cancer therapy, 529-43
    attempts at synchronization
      and recruitment, 530-34
    correlation of kinetic para-
      meters and clinical re-
      sponse, 534-38
    future directions, 538-39
    introduction, 529-30
Cellulose phosphate
  and nephrolithiasis, 17
Central nervous system (CNS)
  amine metabolism in, 411-
    24
    antidepressants, 417-20
    antipsychotic drugs and
      human CNS amine metab-
      olism, 413-17
    introduction, 411-13

lithium, 421-22
  cyclic nucleotides in, 442
  stimulants of
    on ACh turnover, 380
Cephadrin
  pediatric aspects of, 565
Cephaloridin
  pediatric use of, 563
Cephalotaxine
  antitumor activity studies
    of, 124
  structure of, 123
Cephalotaxus alkaloids
  antitumor activity of, 123-
    24
  structures of, 123
Cephalothin
  pediatric aspects of, 563-
    64
Cephazolin
  pediatric aspects of,
    565
Ceramide trihexosidase
  therapeutic characteristics
    of, 103
Cerebral cortex
  β-adrenergic receptors of,
    392-93
Cerebrospinal fluid (CSF)
  biogenic amines in, 411-
    24
Chalones
  and cell growth, 681
Chelating agents
  on human lead disposition,
    201-2
Chelerythrine
  antitumor activity of, 122
  structure of, 122
Chemoreceptors
  aquatic invertebrate, 243-
    58
    chemical activation in
      lower organisms, 244
    classification of activators,
      245
    conclusions, 254
    evolutionary development
      of receptor proteins, 250-
      54
    introduction, 243-44
    mechanism of action of
      hydra glutathione recep-
      tor, 244-50
Chemotaxis
  bacterial, 243
  neutrophilic
    corticosteroid inhibition
      of, 514-15
Chemotherapy, cancer
  see Cancer chemotherapy
Children
  see Pediatric clinical phar-
    macology
Chloral hydrate
  drug interactions with, 296,
    304

Chloralose
  on ACh turnover, 377
Chloramphenicol
  drug interactions with, 297,
    304
  pediatric aspects of, 563-
    64, 566
Chlorcyclazine
  on thermoregulation,
    348
Chloride
  and myopathies, 389
  proximal tubular reabsorp-
    tion, 627, 630
Chlorimipramine
  on brain amine metabolism,
    418-19
p-Chloroamphetamine
  behavioral effects of,
    614
Chlorobromodifluoromethane
  (CBrClF₂)
  toxicology of, 84, 86-90
Chlorobromomethane (CH₂-
  ClBr)
  toxicology of, 84-85, 87-90,
    92
Chlorodifluoromethane
  (CHClF₂)
  toxicology of, 84, 93
Chlorohydrate
  on ACh turnover, 377
p-Chlorophenylalanine (PCPA)
  on feeding control, 612-15
  and myopathies, 394
β-(4-Chlorophenyl)-γ-amino-
  butyric acid
  see Baclofen
2,2-bis(p-Chlorophenyl)1-1,
  1-trichloroethane
  see DDT
Chloropractolol
  at β-adrenergic receptor,
    586
Chloroprocaine
  pain relief by, 238
Chlorothiazide
  combination use in hyperten-
    sion, 316
  historical story of, 7-8
Chlorpheniramine
  drug interactions with,
    299
Chlorpromazine
  on ACh turnover, 379
  on brain amines, 413-14
  and myopathies, 393
  on phosphodiesterase, 461-
    62
Chlorpyrifos
  fish accumulation of,
    171
Chlorthalidone
  combination use in hyperten-
    sion, 315
  on cyclic nucleotides,
    456

Cholecystokinin (CCK)
  laxative effect of, 357, 363
Cholera enterotoxin
  and laxative action, 356, 360
Cholesterol
  drugs affecting, 500-8
  and vitamin D, 136
Cholestyramine
  drug interactions with, 294, 304
  on lipoprotein catabolism, 504-6, 508
  and nephrolithiasis, 16
Choline
  brain uptake of
    assumptions about, 374
    sodium-dependent, 373, 378
Choline acetylase
  vitamin K inhibition of, 138
Choline acetyltransferase (CAT)
  drugs acting on, 370
Cholinergic neuroeffector transmission
  prostagladins on, 270-72
Cholinesterase (ChE)
  inhibition of
    chronic, 399-400
    and muscle fiber degeneration, 398
    reversible, 400-1
    and transmitter release, 397-98
    ultrastructural changes produced by, 399
Chromogranin A
  mechanism of release, 32
Chromonar
  on cyclic nucleotides, 456
Cimetidine
  on thermoregulation, 349
Circulating thymic factor bioassay
  biochemistry and isolation of, 284
Circulation
  regulation of by corticosteroids, 515
Clindamycin
  pediatric aspects of, 563-65
Clofibrate
  drug interactions with, 296, 304
  on lipoprotein production, 504-5, 508
Clonazepam
  pediatric aspects of, 563
Clonidine
  combination use in hypertension, 315, 319
  drug interactions with, 299, 302
  on histamine receptors,
    331-32
  in thermoregulation, 345
Clostridium sporogenes
  methioninase from, 100
Cloxacillin
  pediatric aspects of, 565
Clozapine
  on ACh turnover, 376, 379
  on brain amine metabolism, 416-17
  dopamine antagonism by, 552
Cnidarians
  as model for receptor studies, 244, 250
Cobalt
  and hormone release, 31
Cocaine
  on ACh turnover, 377
  pain relief by, 226, 231, 233, 235, 237, 239
Coffee
  review of, 679
Colchicine
  on hormone release, 36-37
  and myopathies, 397
Colestipol
  drug interactions with, 294
  as hypolipidemic, 507
Colistimethate
  pediatric aspects of, 563
Collagen
  and renal lithiasis, 17
Colonic cancer
  immune aspects of, 183
Colubrinol
  antitumor studies of, 125
  structure of, 125
Colubrinol acetate
  antitumor studies of, 125
  structure of, 125
Combination chemotherapy
  in cancer, 187-88
  in hyperlipoproteinemia, 508
  of hypertension, 311-23
  review of, 680
Compliance
  problems in hypertension therapy, 319-20
Compound 48/80
  and cAMP, 455
  on histamine release in brain, 328
  and venom peptides, 493-94
Computer
  methods for computation of absolute ion activities, 12
  Poisindex system, 219
  to study pharmacokinetics of aging, 59
Contraceptives
  oral
    see Oral contraceptives
Contractile proteins
  and hormone secretion mechanisms, 38
Convulvulaceae
  psychopharmacology of, 651, 656
Corals
  chemoreceptors of, 251
Cordylophora
  chemoreceptors of, 250, 252
Cornus striatum
  and schizophrenia, 547-48
Corticosteroids
  on cancer immune response, 184
  and nephrolithiasis, 17
Corticosteroids, systemic, 511-27
  action of, 511-16
    antiallergic and anti-immunologic, 515-16
    anti-inflammatory and antiallergic, 513-15
    biochemical and metabolic, 512-13
    regulation of circulation by, 515
  complications of therapy with, 521-26
    alternate-day regime, 525-26
    suppression of hypothalamic-pituitary-adrenal system, 523-25
    table of, 522
    topical and inhalant, 526
  modalities of therapy, 518
    chronic inhibition of ACTH, 521
    intensive short-term, 519-20
    low dose, chronic, palliative, 520-21
    prolonged, high dose suppressive, 520
    replacement, 518-19
  pharmacology of, 516-18
    relative anti-inflammatory potencies and half-lives, 517
    types, 516
Corticotroph
  and hormone release, 32
Cortisol
  clinical pharmacology of, 511-13, 516-19, 524
Corydine
  anticancer use of, 121
  structure of, 121
Corynebacterium parvum
  in cancer immunosuppression, 187-90
Coumarin
  drug interactions with, 296, 304
  from plants, 656

Creatine phosphokinase (CPK)
in myopathies, 392
Creatinine
aging effects on clearance
of, 51
Crysaora
chemoreceptors of, 251-52
Crystalloids
precipitation factors, 11-13
Curare
and myopathy, 400
Cushing's syndrome
Mg excretion in, 72
Cyclic adenosine monophosphate (cAMP)
biologic role of, 442
in disease, 442-64
table of, 443-47
histamine effect on, 331, 334
on hydra feeding response, 249
and laxatives, 356-57, 360-62
in proximal tubule, 627, 640
relationship of adrenergic receptors to formation of, 576, 584, 590-95
Cyclic guanosine monophosphate (cyclic GMP)
biologic role of, 442
in disease, 442-48, 450-51, 460, 464
table of, 443-47
Cyclic nucleotide phosphodiesterase
distribution, 450
endogenous activator of, 452-53
kinetic properties of, 451
multiple molecular forms, 451-52
substrate specificity, 451
Cyclic nucleotides
on hydra feeding response, 249
measurement as diagnostic aid, 448-49
review of disease role of, 680
as therapeutic agents, 441-77
biologic role, 442
development of drugs altering, 449-53
pathologic role of, 442-49
selective alteration of metabolism of, 458
summary, 464-65
therapeutic applications, 453-58
Cycloheximide
and β-adrenergic receptors, 593
and vitamin D, 136

Cyclophosphamide
on cancer cell kinetics, 533-34
on cancer immune response, 186
Cyclopropane
on ACh turnover, 377
Cysteine-degrading enzymes
therapeutic usefulness of, 106
Cystine-degrading enzymes
therapeutic usefulness of, 106
Cysteine-di-β-naphthylamide
substance P block by, 427
Cytochalasin B
and hormone secretion, 38
Cytochrome c
pediatric aspects of, 568
Cytochrome P450
lead effects on, 206
Cytosine arabinoside (ara-C)
on cancer cell kinetics, 530-31, 533, 535
on cancer immune response, 184-86

D

D-600
calcium antagonism by, 150, 153-55, 158
structure of, 153
Dactinomycin
and vitamin D, 135
Datura
psychopharmacology of, 650, 669-70
Datura stramonium
psychoactive drugs in, 649, 669
Daunomycin
on cancer immune response, 186
DDT
accumulation in fish, 167-72
Debrisoquin
drug interactions with, 299, 302
Defibrinating agents
enzymes as, 107-8
Dehydroailanthinone
antitumor activity of, 127
structure of, 127
Dehydrobruceantarin
antitumor activity, 128
structure of, 128
Dehydrobruceantin
antitumor activity of, 128
structure of, 128
Denervation
on β-adrenergic receptor-adenylate cyclase system, 589-90
Deoxycholic acid

laxative action of, 359
Deoxyharringtonine
antitumor activity of, 123
structure of, 123
Dependency
reviews of, 679
Depression
cyclic nucleotides in, 447
Designed discovery
Beyer's theory of, 7-8
Disipramine
on β-adrenergic receptor, 590
drug interactions with, 299
Desmethylimipramine (DMI)
on CNS amine metabolism, 419
and feeding control, 610
Desmosterol reductase
and myopathies, 388
Desoxycamptothecin
anticancer activity of, 118
Dexamethasone
clinical pharmacology of, 511, 516-18, 522-24, 526
on cyclic nucleotides, 455
Dextrothyroxine
see D-Thyroxine
Diabetes insipidus
cyclic nucleotides in, 446
Diabetes mellitus
cyclic nucleotides in, 446, 448
Diazepam
on ACh turnover, 380
aging pharmacokinetics, 55, 59-60
pediatric aspects of, 563-65, 567
20,25-Diazocholesterol (20,25-D)
myopathies induced by, 387-91
Diazoxide
combination use in hypertension, 316-17
on cyclic nucleotides, 456
drug interactions with, 296, 302, 304
pediatric aspects of, 563, 568
Dibenzopyran
structure of, 657
Dibromotetrafluoroethane (CBrF$_2$-CBrF$_2$)
toxicology of, 84
Dibromotrifluoroethane (CBrF$_2$-CHFBr)
toxicology of, 84
Dibucaine
pain relief by, 226
Dibutyryl cyclic AMP
in cancer chemotherapy, 453
proximal tubular reabsorption, 627, 640

Dichlorodifluoromethane
(CC1$_2$F$_2$)
toxicology of, 84, 86, 90-
92
2, 4-Dichlorophenoxyacetic
acid (2, 4-D)
myopathies induced by, 387-
91
Dichlorotetrafluoroethane
(CC1F$_2$-CC1F$_2$)
toxicology of, 84, 91
Dicloxacillin
pediatric aspects of, 565
Dieldrin
fish accumulation of, 169-
70
Diet
and Mg excretion, 71-72
in treatment of hyperlipoproteinemia, 501
Diethyldithiocarbamic acid
on thermoregulation, 347
O, O, -Diethyl-O(3, 5, 6-trichlo-
ro-2-pyridyl)phosphoro-
thioate
see Chlorpyrifos
Digitalis
and cholestyramine, 506
Digitalis glycosides
drug interactions with, 298,
300-1
Digitonin
on β-adrenergic receptor,
589
Digitoxin
drug interactions with, 296,
300
Digoxin
aging pharmacokinetics of,
53, 58-59
interactions with other drugs,
294-95, 298, 301
pediatric aspects of, 563-65,
568
Dihydroalprenolol (DHA)
and β-adrenergic receptors,
582-85, 587-89, 594
Dihydromorphine
and enkephalin, 431
Dihydrostreptomycin
aging pharmacokinetics of,
51-52, 56
2(R)-Dihydroxy-Y-(9-adenyl)-
butyric acid
on phosphodiesterase activity,
457
1, 2- or 1, 4-Dihydroxybenzene
on adrenergic receptors,
580
Dihydroxyl bile acids
laxative action of, 359-60
5, 6-Dihydroxytryptamine
(5, 6-DHT)
and control of feeding, 612
on thermoregulation, 347
5, 7-Dihydroxytryptamine
(5, 7-DHT)

and feeding control, 614
1, 25-Dihydroxyvitamin D
and nephrolithiasis, 20
Diisopropylfluorophosphate
(DFP)
and myopathy, 397-98, 400,
402
Diltiazem
calcium antagonism by, 154,
159
structure of, 153
Dimeric benzylisoquinolines
antitumor activity of, 119-
21
structures, 120
Dimethylquaternary propranolol
cardiac effects of, 301
N, N-Dimethyltryptamine
from plants, 655
Dinitrochlorobenzene (DNCB)
in studying cancer immunology, 183, 185
Dioctyl sodium sulfosuccinate
(DSS)
laxative action of, 362
Diperodon
pain relief by, 226
Dipropylacetate
pediatric aspects of, 563-
64
Dipyridamole
drug interactions with, 303
Disopyramide
drug interactions with, 301
Dissociation constant
determination of, 247
Disulfiram
drug interactions with, 297,
304
Diterpenoid triepoxides
antitumor studies of, 129
Diuretics
on cyclic nucleotides, 456
drug interactions with, 302-
3
in hypertension
case against routine use
of, 316-17
combination therapy, 314-
19
and magnesium excretion,
70-71
review of, 680
DNA synthesis
and cancer cell kinetics,
538-39
DOCA (Desoxycorticosterone
acetate)
and Mg excretion, 73-74
levo-DOPA
on ACh turnover, 378
aging pharmacokinetics of,
50
and pyridoxine, 140-41
and schizophrenia, 550,
554

Dopamine
on brain ACh turnover, 370,
372-73, 375, 378-79
receptor agonists, 378-
79
receptor blockers, 379
brain levels of
drug effects on, 411-22
feeding control, 607-8, 611-
12, 615
psychopharmacology of, 545-
59
brain DA and neuropathol-
ogy of behavior, 546-47
brain DA and schizophrenia,
550-55
conclusion, 555-56
introduction, 545-46
neuroanatomical substrates
of schizophrenia, 547-50
in thermoregulation, 347-
49
in venom, 487, 489
Dopamine-β-hydroxylase
and β-adrenergic receptors,
593
genetic aspects of, 681
release of, 32
Down's syndrome
cyclic nucleotides in, 446,
449
Doxepin
drug interactions with,
299
Doxycycline
aging pharmacokinetics, 55
pediatric aspects of, 563
Drug abuse
behavioral factors in, 679
Drug prescription
factors influencing, 681
Duchenne's muscular dystrophy
pharmacologic models of,
391-95, 403

E

Edrophonium
myopathies from, 397
EDTA
on β-adrenergic receptor,
249, 580
EHDP
see Ethane hydroxydiphos-
phonate
5, 8, 11, 14-Eicosatetrayonic
acid (ETA)
on prostaglandins, 268-69
Electrolytes
ionic requirements for
hormone release, 29-30
and laxative action, 355-63
Embryo
cyclic nucleotides in, 442
Endocrine diseases
cyclic nucleotides in, 446

Endocrine tissue
  mechanisms of hormone
    secretion by, 27-47
Endrin
  fish accumulation of, 171
Energy metabolism
  cardiac
    basic interactions of Ca
      and drugs in, 151-54
Energy requirements
  in hormone release, 35-36
Enkephalin
  as neurotransmitter, 431
Environment
  lead uptake from, 197-200
Environmental quality
  review of, 680
Enzyme abnormalites
  inherited
    and nephrolithiasis, 15
Enzyme deficiencies
  inherited
    replacement therapy for,
      108-9
Enzyme replacement therapy
  in genetic disease, 97
Enzymes
  in venoms, 493
Enzymes as drugs, 97-116
  concluding remarks, 112
  development of new enzymes,
    98-100
  characteristics of useful
    enzymes, 98-100
  sources, 98
  in vivo properties of thera-
    peutic enzymes, 100-9
  examples, 103-9
  pharmacology and pharma-
    cokinetics, 100-3
  methods for improvement of
    enzyme therapy, 109-12
    binding to surfaces, 111-
      12
    microcapsules, liposomes,
      and red blood cells, 110-
      11
    soluble chemical modifica-
      tion, 109-10
Enzyme specificity
  receptor role in, 253-54
Ephedrine
  drug interactions with, 297,
    299-300
  from plants, 668
Epilepsy
  cyclic nucleotides in, 447
Epinephrine (E)
  in asthma, 454
  drug interactions with, 299-
    300
  on feeding control, 612
  and local anesthetics, 236
  receptors, 575-95
  in venom, 487, 489
Ergot alkaloids
  in plants, 656

Ergotamine
  basic structure of, 657
Eritadenine
  on cyclic nucleotides, 457
Erythrina
  psychopharmacology of, 658,
    667
Erythrinane
  structure of, 657
Erythrocytes
  and enzyme therapy, 110-
    11
  lead effects on, 202-7
Eserine
  on acetylcholine release,
    371
Ethacrynic acid
  on cyclic nucleotides, 456
  discovery of, 8-9
  drug interactions with, 296,
    303-4
  and Mg excretion, 71
Ethane hydroxydiphosphonate
  (EHDP)
  on renal lithiasis, 20
Ethanol
  on ACh turnover, 378
  review of, 678-79
  and vitamin E, 138
  see also Alcohol
Ethchlorvynol
  drug interactions with,
    304
Ether
  on ACh turnover, 377
Ethosuximide
  pediatric aspects of, 563-
    64
Ethyl alcohol
  see Ethanol
Ethylenediaminetetraacetic
  acid
  see EDTA
1-Ethyl-4-(isopropylidenehydrazino)-1H-pyrazolo-
  (3,4-b)-pyridine-5-car-
  boxylic acid ethyl ester
  (SQ 20,009)
  on phosphodiesterase, 462-
    64
Ethylmorphine
  pain relief by, 226
Ethyl-parachlorophenoxyisobutyrate
  see Clofibrate
Evolutionary development
  of receptor proteins, 250-
    54
Excretion of drugs
  aging effects on, 51
  drug interactions affecting,
    298
  reviews on, 678
Exocytosis
  as hormone release mecha-
    nisms, 31-32
Extracellular fluid volume

and magnesium excretion,
  70-71
Eye disease
  cyclic nucleotides in, 447-
    48

F

Fabry disease
  therapy of, 109
Fagaronine
  antitumor activity of, 121
  structure of, 122
Fanconi's syndrome
  lead role in, 207
Feces
  laxative pharmacology, 355-
    67
Feeding control, 605-21
  amphetamine and adrenergic
    systems, 606-12
  fenfluramine and serotonergic
    systems, 612-15
  phenylpropanolamine and
    glucostatic systems, 615-
    17
  summary, 617
  terminology and abbrevia-
    tions, 606
Fendiline
  Ca antagonism by, 159
  structure of, 153
Fenfluramine (FEN)
  in control of feeding, 605-6,
    612-15
Fibrinolytics
  enzymes as, 107-8
Ficus
  psychoactive drugs from,
    656
Fire extinguishants
  toxicology of, 83-95
  acute, 84
  biotransformation, 91-93
  cardiac arrhythmias, 85-
    86
  cardiovascular pharmaco-
    dynamics, 86-90
  conclusions, 93
  general metabolism, 90-
    91
  introduction, 83-84
  neurological effects, 84-
    85
  uptake and distribution,
    91
Fish
  and chemical accumulation
    process, 167-77
  conclusion, 174
  fish growth and biomass
    dynamics, 172-74
  how fish acquire chemical
    residues, 168-71
  introduction, 167-68
  partition and kinetic mod-
    els, 171-72

unique aspects of problem, 168
Flufenic acid
  on cyclic nucleotides, 455
Fluoride
  and β-adrenergic receptor, 592
Fluoroalkanes
  toxicology of, 83-93
α-Fluorocortisol
  for aldosterone replacement, 518
5-Fluorouracil (5-FU)
  on cancer cell kinetics, 530-31
  on cancer immune response, 184-85, 189
Folic acid
  deficiency and tumor growth, 107
  toxicity of, 141
Free erythrocyte porphyrin (FEP)
  to study lead exposure, 205-6
Free radicals
  mechanisms of lipid damage and cell injury, 681
Fructose-6-diphosphatase
  and corticosteroid effects, 512
Furosemide
  combination use in hypertension, 316
  on cyclic nucleotides, 456
  drug interactions with, 302-3
  and Mg excretion, 71

G

Ganglionic transmission
  prostaglandins on, 269-70
Gastric cancer
  immune aspects of, 183
Gaucher disease
  therapy of, 109
Gentamycin
  pediatric aspects of, 563-64
Geriatric pharmacology
  pharmacokinetics, 49-65
Glaucarubinone
  antitumor activity of, 127
  structure of, 127
Glaucarubolone esters
  antitumor activity of, 127-28
  structure, 127
Glaucine
  antitumor activity of, 121
  structure of, 120
Glucagon
  and cyclic nucleotides, 457
  drug interactions with, 304
  laxative action of, 357

Glucocerebrosidase
  therapeutic usefulness of, 103
Glucocorticoids
  on β-adrenergic receptor, 592
  clinical pharacology of, 511-27
Glucose
  aging pharmacokinetics of, 50
  drug interactions with, 303
  and Mg excretion, 71
Glucose-6-phosphatase
  corticosteroid effects on, 512
Glucostasis
  and feeding control, 615-17
L-Glutamate
  and substance P, 427, 429
Glutamic-oxaloacetic transaminase (GOT)
  in myopathies, 392
Glutamic-pyruvic transaminase (GPT)
  in myopathies, 392
Glutaminase
  therapeutic uses of, 99, 103
Glutaminase-asparaginase
  therapeutic characteristics of, 102-5
  improvement of, 109-10
  usefulness, 104-5
γ-Glutamyl transpeptidase (GTP)
  specificity of, 254
Glutathione, reduced (GSH)
  receptors for in hydra, 243-50
  active GSH structure, 248-49
  cyclic nucleotides, 249
  determination of dissociation constant, 247
  determination in vivo of pH profile of receptor, 247-48
  evidence for GSH surface receptor, 246-47
  other factors, 249
  summary, 250
Glutethimide
  drug interactions with, 304
Glycerol
  drug interactions with, 303
  pain relief by, 225
Golgi apparatus
  functions of, 33
  as origin of secretory granules, 33-34
Gonadotroph
  and hormone release, 32, 35
Granule protein

mechanism of release of, 32
Granules
  and hormone secretion, 27-39
  origin and fate of granules, 33-35
  storage, 28
Griseofulvin
  drug interactions with, 304
Growth hormone
  and magnesium reabsorption, 70, 74
  suppression of secretion of, 151
Guanethidine
  combination use in hypertension, 318
  drug interactions with, 295, 297-99, 302
  and prostaglandins, 271
Guanidine
  and myopathies, 401
Guanine nucleotides
  on β-adrenergic receptors, 585
Guanosine cyclic 3',5'-monophosphate
  see Cyclic guanosine monophosphate
Guanylate cyclase
  in disease, 443-47, 450
5-Guanylimidodiphosphate (GMPPNP)
  on β-adrenergic receptor, 583, 585, 587, 594
Gut factor
  see Proctolin

H

Haliplanella
  chemoreceptor of, 250-52
Hallucinogens
  neurological aspects of, 679
Haloalkane propellants
  toxicology of, 83-95
  acute, 84
  biotransformation, 91-93
  cardiac arrhythmias, 85-86
  cardiovascular pharmacodynamics, 86-90
  conclusions, 93
  general metabolism, 90-91
  introduction, 83-84
  neurological effects, 84-85
  uptake and distribution, 91
Haloperidol
  on ACh turnover, 378-79
  on brain amines, 413-16
  dopamine antagonism by, 552-53

Halothane
  on ACh turnover, 377
  and glucose tolerance, 91
Harringtonine
  structure-activity of, 123
Heart
  arrhythmias
    haloalkane toxicology, 85-
    86
  cyclic nucleotides on, 442,
    445, 447
  diseases
    and vitamin D, 136
  energy metabolism
    basic interactions of Ca
    and drugs in, 151-54
    prostaglandins on, 261-62,
    269
    reviews of, 680
    specific calcium pharmacol-
    ogy in, 149-66
Heimia alkaloids
  psychopharmacology of, 656-
  58, 668
  structure, 657
Heme
  lead effects on, 202-7
Hemicholinium
  in myopathies, 400
Hemicholinium C-3 (HC-3)
  on ACh turnover, 372, 376
Hemoglobin
  lead effects on, 203-7
  schematic of, 204
Heparin
  mechanism of release of,
  32
1, 2, 3, 4, 10, 10-Hexachloro-6,
  7-epoxy-1, 4, 4a, 5, 6, 7, 8,
  8a-octahydro-1, 4-endo-
  endo-5, 8-dimethanonaph-
  thalene
  see Endrin
1, 2, 3, 4, 10, 10-Hexachloro-6,
  7-epoxy-1-4, 4a, 5, 6, 7, 8,
  8a-octahydro-1, 4-endo,
  exo-5, 8-dimethanonaph-
  thalene
  see Dieldrin
Hexamethonium
  on ACh turnover, 376
Hexobarbital
  aging pharmacokinetics of,
  51
Hexosamidase A
  therapeutic usefulness of,
  103
Hexylresorcinol
  pain relief by, 225
Histamine (HA)
  actions on brain target systems, 330-33
    cAMP, 331
    electrophysiological actions,
    331-32
    on vegetative functions and
    behaviors, 332-33

brain localization and
  metabolism of, 325-30
  anatomical disposition of
  histaminergic neuron
  pathways, 330
  biosynthesis, 326-27
  inactivation, 328-29
  occurrence and distribution, 325-26
  release, 328
  storage, 327-28
  turnover, 329-30
  mechanisms of release of,
  32, 37
  release of
    cyclic nucleotides on, 442,
    455
    in thermoregulation, 48-49
    in venom, 481-82, 484-86,
    488-89, 491-94
Histamine-N-methyltransferase
  in brain, 329
L-Histidine (L-his)
  in brain, 327
L-Histidine decarboxylase
  (HD)
  and histamine biosynthesis,
  326-27
Histidine-degrading enzyme
  in cancer chemotherapy,
  106
Hodgkin's disease
  immunologic defects with,
  183
  immunotherapy, 189
Holacanthone
  antitumor activity of, 127
  structure of, 127
Homeostasis
  and immune system in cancer, 182
Homeostatic thymus hormone
  description of, 284-85
Homograft
  thymic hormones in, 286-
  87
Homoharringtone
  antitumor activity of, 123
  structure of, 123
Homovanillic acid (HVA)
  and CNS DA metabolism,
  411-22
Honeybee
  venom of, 481-85
Hormones
  enteric
    and laxatives, 356
    secretion mechanisms, 27-
    47
    conclusion, 39
    effect of K ions on, 30-31
    exocytosis, 31-32
    introduction, 27
    ionic requirements for
    release, 29-30
    mechanisms of release,

35-39
    origin and fate of secre-
    tory granules, 33-35
    storage in granules, 28
    transmembrane potential
    of secretory cells, 28-
    29
Hornet
  venom of, 488-90
Hornet kinin
  characterization of, 489
Hyaluronidase
  in venom, 484, 489, 494
Hydra
  glutathione receptor of, 243-
  54
    active structure of gluta-
    thione, 248-49
    cyclic nucleotides, 249
    determination of dissocia-
    tion constant, 247
    determination in vivo of
    pH profile of receptor,
    247-48
    evidence for GSH surface
    receptor, 246-47
    evolutionary development
    of, 250-54
    other factors, 249
    summary, 250
Hydra attenuata
  chemoreceptors of, 248
Hydralazine
  combination use in hypertension, 316-19
  drug interactions with, 296,
  302
Hydra littoralis
  chemoreceptors of, 246-48
Hydrochlorothiazide
  combination use in hypertension, 318
Hydrocortisone
  on cyclic nucleotides, 455
6-Hydroxydopamine
  and β-adrenergic receptor,
  590, 592-93
  and feeding control, 605-6,
  608, 610-11, 615
  and myopathies, 394
  on thermoregulation, 345,
  347
Hydroxy fatty acids
  laxative action of, 360-
  61
5-Hydroxyindoleacetic acid
  (5-HIAA)
  to evaluate biogenic brain
  amines, 411-22
2(2-Hydroxy-3-isopropylamino-
  propoxy)iodobenzene
  on β-adrenergic receptors,
  586
5-Hydroxytryptamine (5-HT)
  on feeding control, 612-15
  on thermoregulation, 342,
  346-47, 349

see also Serotonin
5-Hydroxytryptophan
  on brain amine metabolism,
    420
Hydroxyurea
  on cancer cell kinetics, 530,
    532
Hydrozoa
  chemoreceptors of, 250-
    51
Hymenoptera venoms, 479-
    98
  ant, 490-92
  bee, 481-85
  clinical manifestations of
    envenomation, 480
  hornet venom, 488-90
  introduction, 479-80
  summary, 492-95
  wasp venom, 485-88
Hyperbilirubinemia
  drug problems in, 565
Hypercalcemia
  and tubular reabsorption of
    Mg, 70
Hypercalciuria
  and renal lithiasis, 13-15
Hypercholesterolemia
  drugs affecting, 500-8
Hyperoxaluria
  in nephrolithiasis, 15-16
Hyperparathyroidism
  cyclic nucleotides in, 446,
    448
  and nephrolithiasis, 13
Hypertension
  combination therapy of, 311-
    23
  conclusion, 320
  investigation of, 311-12
  practical problems, 319-
    20
  prediction of response,
    312
  rationale, 314-19
  regulatuon of blood pres-
    sure, 312-14
  cyclic nucleotides in, 445,
    448
Hyperthyroidism
  cyclic nucleotides in, 446,
    448
  and nephrolithiasis, 13
Hypertriglyceridemia
  drugs affecting, 500-8
Hyperuricosuria
  in nephrolithiasis, 18
Hypervitaminosis A
  description of, 133-34
Hypoglycemics
  on phosphodiesterase acti-
    vity, 457
Hypolipidemics, 499-510
  conclusion, 508
  drugs affecting lipoprotein
    catabolism, 505-7
  cholestyramine, 505-6

d-thyroxine, 506-7
drugs affecting lipoprotein
    production, 502-5
  clofibrate, 504-5
  nicotinic acid, 502-4
  introduction, 498-502
  other hypolipemics, 507-8
  colestipol, 507
  combined chemotherapy,
    508
  neomycin, 508
  PAS-C, 507-8
  β-sitosterol, 507
  review of, 680
  site of action of, 503
Hypothalamic releasing fac-
    tors
  as neurotransmitters, 432
Hypothalamus
  hormone secretion mecha-
    nisms in, 27, 33
Hypothyroidism
  cyclic nucleotides in, 305

I

Ifosfamide
  on cancer cell kinetics,
    532
Imipramine
  on CNS amine metabolism,
    418-20
  drug interactions with, 299
  myopathies from, 393-94
  on phosphodiesterase, 459
Immune response
  in cancer, 179-83
  diagram of, 180
  immune function in cancer
    patients, 182-83
Immunologic surveillance
  concept of, 181-82, 188
Immunology
  corticosteroids in, 515-16
Immunosuppression in cancer
  drug-induced, 183-88
  adriamycin, 186
  combination chemotherapy,
    187-88
  cyclophosphamide, 186
  cytosine arabinoside, 185-
    86
  daunomycin, 186
  5-fluorouracil, 185
  mercaptopurine, 185
  methotrexate, 185
  by microorganisms, 186-
    87
  stages in, 184
  vinca alkaloids, 186
Immunosuppressives
  mode of action of, 679
Immunotherapy
  in cancer, 188-90
  BCG, 189
  Corynebacterium parvum,
    189-90

levamisole, 190
Indoleacetic acid
  myopathies from, 388
Indoles
  from plants, 655
Indomethacin
  aging pharmacokinetics of,
    58
  drug interactions with, 296,
    303
  on prostaglandin, 268-69,
    271
Industrial toxicology
  lead, 202
Inhalation
  and fluoroalkane toxicology,
    83
Insulin
  receptors, 243
  release of
    cyclic nucleotides on, 442,
      457
    mechanisms of, 36-37
    specific blockers of, 150
Intermountain Regional Poi-
    son Control Center at
    University of Utah Medi-
    cal Center, 216, 221
Intestinal hyperoxaluria
  description of, 16
Intestine
  absorption of drugs in,
    678
  laxatives on, 355-67
Invertebrates, aquatic
  chemoreceptors of, 243-58
Iodohydroxybenzylpindolol
    (IHYP)
  on β-adrenergic receptor,
    582-85, 587, 591-92,
    595
Ion activities
  absolute
    computation of, 12
Ipomea violacea
  psychoactive drugs in, 650,
    652, 665
Iproveratril
  see Verapamil
Iron
  aging pharmacokinetics of,
    50
  and cholestyramine, 506
Islets of Langerhans
  hormone secretion mecha-
    nisms in, 27
Isobutylmethylxanthine
  on cyclic nucleotides, 456,
    462-63
Isocorydine
  antitumor activity of, 121
  structure of, 120
Isoharringtonine
  antitumor activity of, 123
  structure of, 123
Isoniazid
  drug interactions with, 297

and pyridoxine, 140
Isopropamide
  drug interactions with,
    299
Isoproterenol
  in asthma, 454
  drug interactions with, 299
  reversal of verapamil by,
    155, 157
  to study β-adrenergic recep-
    tors, 579-80, 585-88,
    590, 593-95
Isotopes
  to study brain ACh turnover,
    373-75

K

Kanamycin
  aging pharmacokinetics of,
    52
  pediatric aspects of, 563-
    64
K cells
  in cancer immunosuppres-
    sion, 181
Ketamine
  on ACh turnover, 377
Kidney
  drug interactions affecting,
    298
  lead effects on, 207-8
  lithiasis, 11-25
    conditions with increased
      urinary crystalloid con-
      stituents, 13-17
    disorders of nucleation
      induction, 17-19
    inhibitors of crystal forma-
      tion and growth, 19-20
    precipitation of crystalloids,
      11-13
  prostaglandins on, 267
  proximal tubular reabsorp-
    tion and regulation, 623-
    40
  renal handling of magnesium,
    67-75
    characteristics of tubular
      reabsorption of Mg, 67-
      69
    factors controlling urinary
      excretion, 70-75
    vasodilation, 71
  reviews of, 680
Kinins
  in hymenoptera venoms,
    486, 489

L

Lactic dehydrogenase (LDH)
  in myopathies, 392
Lanthanum
  and ion release, 31
  proximal tubular reabsorp-
    tion, 627

Laxatives, 355-67
  alteration of electrolyte
    movement, 356-58
  active ion secretion, 356-
    57
  mucosal damage, 358
  mucosal permeability, 357-
    58
  role of motility, 357
  conclusion, 363
  introduction, 355
  traditional classification of,
    358-63
    bulk, 363
    saline, 362-63
    stimulants, 359-62
    stool softeners, 362
Lead
  human exposure to, 197-
    214
    conclusion, 208-9
    disposition of lead, 200-2
    indices of, 205
    introduction, 197
    toxic effects vs exposure,
      202-8
    uptake from environment,
      197-200
Lead naphthenate
  toxicology of, 200
Lecithinase
  in venoms, 482
Leguminosae
  psychedelic drugs from,
    649, 651
Leonurus sibiricus
  psychopharmacology of,
    656, 666
Leukemia
  cell kinetics and therapy of,
    529-39
  immunologic defects in, 183,
    187, 189
  immunotherapy of, 187,
    189
  phosphodiesterase role in,
    462-64
  plants as source of drugs
    against, 117
Levamisole
  in cancer immunotherapy,
    188, 190
Lidocaine
  drug interactions with, 295,
    301
  pain relief by, 226, 232,
    236, 238
  pediatric aspects of, 563,
    565, 567
Limbic system
  and schizophrenia, 548-50
Lipoproteins
  classification according to
    mobility, 499
  drugs affecting, 499-508
    conclusion, 508
    drugs affecting catabolism,

    505-7
  drugs affecting production,
    502-5
  introduction, 498-502
  other drugs, 507-8
  metabolism of, 500-2
    normal, schematic, 501
    very low density, sche-
      matic, 500
    transport schematic, 503
    types of, 502
Liposomes
  in enzyme therapy, 110
Lithiasis, renal
  conditions with increased
    urinary crystalloid
    constituents, 13-17
  disorders of nucleation
    induction, 17-19
  inhibitors of crystal forma-
    tion and growth, 19-20
  precipitation of crystalloids,
    11-13
Lithium
  aging pharmacokinetics of,
    55
  on cancer cell kinetics,
    538
  and CNS amine metabolism,
    421-22
Liver
  β-adrenergic receptors in,
    591-92
Lophophora williamsii
  psychedelic drugs from,
    648, 650-51, 655, 662
Luteinizing hormone-releasing hormone (LHRH)
  in neurotransmission, 432
Lymecycline
  pediatric aspects of, 563-
    64
Lymphocytes
  role in cancer immunosup-
    pression, 180-81
Lymphocyte-stimulating hormones
  isolation and description of,
    284
Lymphomas
  immunologic defects in,
    183
Lysergic acid diethylamide
  (LSD-25)
  and substance P, 428
Lysolecithin
  in chromaffin granule mem-
    branes, 38-39
Lysosomal enzymes
  release of
    cyclic nucleotides on, 442
Lysosomal glycoprotein
  enzymes
  therapeutic characteristics
    of, 103
Lysosomal storage diseases
  therapy of, 108-9

Lysosomes
corticosteroid effects on, 514

M

Magnesium (Mg)
deficiency
and heart disorders, 680
and hormone release, 29, 31, 35
on hydra feeding response, 249
hypocalcemia of depletion, 75-78
renal handling of, 67-75
characteristics of renal tubular reabsorption of, 67-69
factors controlling urinary excretion, 70-75
Magnesium oxide
and nephrolithiasis, 19
Magnesium salts
laxative action of, 362-63
Mammotroph
and hormone release, 32, 35
Manganese
and hormone release, 31
Mania
cyclic nucleotides in, 447-49
Mannitol
drug interactions with, 303
and Mg excretion, 71
Marijuana
physiological disposition of, 679
ritual use of, 668
Mast cell degranulating peptide (MCD-peptide)
isolation and characterization of, 493-94
Mast cells
in brain, 327-28, 333
release mechanisms in, 32
Matrix substance A
in nephrolithiasis, 17
Maysenine
antitumor studies of, 125
structure of, 125
Maytanacine
antitumor studies of, 125
structure of, 125
Maytanbutine
antitumor activity of, 125
structure of, 125
Maytanprine
antitumor activity of, 125
structure, 125
Maytansine
antitumor studies of, 124-26
structure of, 125
Maytansine ethyl ether

antitumor studies of, 126
structure of, 125
Maytansinoids
antitumor studies of, 124-26
structures of, 125
Maytansinol
antitumor studies, 125
structure, 125
Maytanvaline
antitumor studies of, 125
structure of, 125
Mecamylamine
drug interactions with, 297 302
Meclofenamic acid
on prostaglandins, 268-69
Medial hypothalamus
and obesity, 606-9, 611, 614-15
Mefanamic acid
on cyclic nucleotides, 455
Melanotroph
and hormone release, 32-33
Melittin
characterization of, 483-84, 492
Membrane
effects
of drugs in myocardium, 154-57
fusion
and hormone release, 38-39
integrity
corticosteroid effect on, 514
transport
review of, 679
Meperidine
on ACh turnover, 377
aging pharmacokinetics of, 54, 58, 60
pain relief by, 225
Mepiperphenidol
early studies of, 6
Mepivacaine
pain relief by, 226, 234, 238
pediatric aspects of, 563, 567
Meprobamate
pain relief by, 225
Mepyramine
antihistaminic, 488
6-Mercaptopurine
on cancer immune response, 184-85
Mercurial diuretics
and Mg excretion, 71
Mercurials
cAMP on, 456
Mercury
fish accumulation of, 173
Mescaline

Mexican cultural aspects of, 655, 662
Metabolism of drugs
aging effects on, 50
drug interactions affecting, 297-98
reviews on, 678
Metaraminol
discovery of, 4
drug interactions with, 300
Methicillin
pediatric aspects of, 563
Methotrexate
on cancer cell kinetics, 531-35
in cancer chemotherapy, 103, 105, 107
on cancer immune response, 185
3-Methoxy-4-hydroxyphenethyleneglycol (MHPG)
and CNS NE metabolism, 411-12
3-Methoxy-4,5-methylenedioxyphenylisopropylamine
psychopharmacology of, 656, 663
Methoxyverapamil
and hormone release, 31
dl-O-Methyldauricine
antitumor activity of, 121
structure, 120
α-Methyldopa
on blood pressure, 302
combination use in hypertension, 315, 318-19
Methylene blue
and nephrolithiasis, 19-20
N-Methyl-isatin-β-semicarbazone
on phosphodiesterase, 547
α-Methylnorepinephrine
in temperature regulation, 345
Methylperidol
on brain amine metabolism, 415
Methylphenidate
drug interactions with, 297, 299
and schizophrenia, 550
Methylpinacolyloxyphosphoryl fluoride
see Soman
Methylprednisolone
clinical pharmacology of, 511, 516-18
and Mg excretion, 72
α-Methyl-p-tyrosine
and prostaglandins, 271
α-Methyltyrosine
with neuroleptics
antipsychotic effect of, 555
trans-2-Methyl-6-n-undecyl-

piperidine
in ant venom, 491, 494
Methylxanthines
on cyclic nucleotides, 460,
462, 464
Metiamide
on brain histamine, 332
Mexico
psychoactive plants of, 647-
75
Mexiletine
cardiac effects of, 301
Microbracon hebetor
venom of, 487-88
Microcapsules
in enzyme therapy, 110
Microcirculation
corticosteroids on, 514
Microtubules
in hormone release, 36-38
Minimine
in venom, 494
Minoxidil
on blood pressure, 302
combination use in hypertension, 317, 319
Mitogen
and MLC response, 286
Mixitl
identification and active
substances in, 648
Monoamine oxidase inhibitors
drug interactions with,
297
Monobromosalicyl alcohol
pain relief by, 225
Monocarboxylic acids
myopathies from, 388
Monosodium urate
in nephrolithiasis, 18-19
Moonshine whiskey
and lead poisoning, 207
Morphine
on ACh turnover, 377-78
Motility
role in fluid and electrolyte
movement, 357
Mucosa
damage, 358
permeability of, 357-58
Muscimol
on ACh turnover, 380
Muscle
cyclic nucleotides on, 442
smooth
prostaglandins on, 263
vascular smooth
specific Ca pharmacology
in, 149-51, 158-60
Muscular dystrophy,
Duchenne's
pharmacologic models of,
391-95, 403
ligation plus serotonin
model, 393-94
vascular model, 392-93
vasoactive amines, 394-95

Mushrooms
Mexican psychedelic drugs
from, 648-51, 653, 655
Myasthenia gravis
pharmacology of, 396-97
Myelin sheath
in pain relief, 230
Myocardial infarction
cyclic nucleotides in, 445,
448
Myocardium
specific calcium pharmacology in, 149-57
Myopathies, experimental,
387-401
conclusions, 403
general neuromuscular
diseases, 396-403
pharmacologically induced
myotonia, 387-91
pharmacologic models of
Duchenne's muscular
dystrophy, 391-95
Myosin
in nonmuscle cells, 38
Myotonia
pharmacologically induced,
387-91
by, 20, 25-diazocholesterol,
388-89
by 2, 4-dichlorophenoxy-
acetic acid, 388
membrane abnormalities,
389
relationship of nerve to
drug-induced myotonia,
390-91
similarities between human
and drug-induced myo-
tonias, 388
sites of drug action, 389-
90
Myotonia congenita
description of, 388
Myrmecia
venom of, 490-92, 494
Myrmecia forficata
venom of, 491
Myrmecia gulosa
venom of, 491, 494
Myrmecia pyriformis
venom of, 491-92, 494

N

Nacazul
psychopharmacology of,
650
Na$^+$, K$^+$ ATPase
and myopathies, 390
Nalidixic acid
drug interactions with,
303
Naloxone
and enkephalin, 431
Nanacatl
identification and active

substances in, 648
4-(1-Naphthylvinyl)pyridine
on ACh turnover, 376
Narcotic analgetics
on ACh turnover, 377-78
Narcotics
reviews of, 679
National Clearinghouse for
Poison Control Centers
on-line terminal to FDA
from, 220
Natriuretic factor
possibility of, 635
Neomycin
drug interactions with,
304
as hypolipidemic, 508
pediatric aspects of, 563
Neoplasia
antineoplastic agents from
plants, 117-32
alkaloids, 118-24
conclusions, 130
introduction, 117
nonalkaloids, 124-30
enzymic treatment of, 103-
7
deprivation of essential
amino acids, 106-7
deprivation of nonessential
amino acids, 103-6
by folate depletion, 107
and nephrolithiasis, 13
Neostigmine
and myopathies, 397, 401
Nephrolithiasis
pharmacology of, 11-20
Nerves
drugs acting on, reviews,
679
trophic function of, 396
Neurohypophysis
hormone secretion mecha-
nisms in, 27, 29-30, 32-
33, 35
Neurolemma
in pain relief, 230
Neuroleptics
and schizophrenia, 552-55
blockade of DA receptors,
553
blockade of DA-sensitive
adenylate cyclase, 552
blockade of synaptic re-
lease of DA, 553
mode of action of antipsychotics, 553-55
Neuromuscular disease, general
pharmacologic studies of,
396-403
acute cholinesterase inhibition and muscle fiber
degeneration, 398
cholinesterase inhibition
and transmitter release,
397-98

mechanisms for myopathy
development, 401-3
modification of myopathies,
400
muscle lesions during cholinesterase inhibition,
399-400
neural control of muscle
properties, 396-97
reactivation of phosphorylated ChE, 400
reversible ChE inhibition,
400-1
ultrastructural changes by
ChE inhibitors, 399
Neurophysins I and II
mechanisms of release of,
32
Neuropsychiatric diseases
cyclic nucleotides in, 447
Neurostenin
isolation of, 38
Neurotransmitters
peptide, 425-39
see also Peptide neuro-
transmitters
receptors, 243
Niacin
toxicity studies, 139-40
Nicotiana rustica
psychopharmacology of, 650,
656, 670
Nicotine
in ACh turnover, 376
Nicotinic acid
on lipoprotein production,
502-5, 508
Nifedipine
calcium antagonism by, 150,
153-54, 158-59
Nitidine chloride
antitumor activity of, 121-
22
structure of, 122
Nitrates
on blood pressure, 302
organic
surveys of, 680
Nitrites
and Ca antagonism, 159-
60
Nitroprusside
on blood pressure, 302
Nitrous oxide
on ACh turnover, 377
Norepinephrine (NE)
aging pharmacokinetics, 62
brain levels of
drug effects on, 411-22
and cyclic nucleotides, 457
drug interactions with, 299
and feeding control, 612
and local anesthetics, 236-
37
in myopathies, 393-94, 402
receptors, 575-604
release inhibition

by prostaglandin, 264-66,
271
on schizophrenia, 554-55
in thermoregulation, 344-
47, 349
in venom, 487, 489
Normetanephrine (NM)
drug effects on, 419
Nortriptyline
on CNS amine metabolism,
418-19
drug interactions with, 304
pediatric aspects of, 563,
566
on phosphodiesterase, 549
Nucleation induction
disorders of, 17-19
crystal nucleation by
organic matrix, 17
nucleation by heterologous
crystals, 17-19
Nuclei of brain
ACh turnover in, 369-80
Nucleotides
cyclic
see Cyclic nucleotides;
also specific ones
Nutrition
drug effects on, 681
Nymphea ampla
psychopharmacology of,
651, 669

O

Obesity
cyclic nucleotides in, 447,
456
pharmacology control of,
605-17
Octanoic acid
intestinal effects of, 360
Ololiuhqui
identification and active
substances in, 648-50,
652, 656-57, 665
structure of glucosides,
657
Oncogenesis
and immunologic status of
host, 181
Opiate receptor, 243
demonstration of, 431
Opipramol
on phosphodiesterase, 459
Oral contraceptives
drug interactions with,
304
and pyridoxine, 141
and vitamin A, 134
and vitamin E, 139
and vitamin metabolism,
678
Organophosphorus agents
and myopathies, 397-402
Osteoid
excess, 78

Osteoporosis
and vitamin D toxicity,
136
Oxacillin
pediatric aspects of, 563
Oxalate
and nephrolithiasis, 13, 15-
16
Oxotremorine
on ACh turnover, 375
in thermoregulation, 343,
349
Oxprenolol
combination use in hypertension, 318
Oxyphenbutazone
drug interactions with,
297
Oxyphenisatin
laxative action of, 359, 362
Oxytocin
blockers of, 150
mechanism of release of,
32, 34
as neurotransmitter, 432

P

Pacemakers
cardiac
specific calcium pharma-
cology in, 157-58
Pain relief, regional, 223-42
absorption rate, 233-34
absorption retardation by
vasoconstrictors, 236-
37
absorption from skin, 235-
36
basic nature of local anesthetics, 227-28
binding, 231-32
biotransformation, 237-38
cause of systemic reactions,
234-35
destruction in situ, 238-39
effect on metabolism, 231
esters and amides, 225-27
fiber size, 230-31
latent period, 232-33
lipid solubility and polar
association, 228
local vs systemic effects,
223-25
methods of testing, 240
molecular configuration of
local anesthetics, 224-
25
myelin sheath, 230
non-nitrogenous local anesthetics, 225
overlapping of actions, 233
penetration into nerve, 231
precautionary measure,
241
toxicity, 239
transmission of nerve

impulse, 229-30
Palythoa
  receptor of, 250-52
2-PAM
  see Pyridine-2-aldoxime
    methiodide
Pancreas
  hormone secretion mecha-
    nisms in, 27, 30, 32-38
Papaverine
  on cyclic nucleotides, 454,
    456, 459-60, 462
Paracetamol
  aging pharmacokinetics of,
    59
Paramethasone
  clinical pharmacology of,
    511, 516-18
Paraoxon
  myopathies from, 397-402
  pediatric aspects of, 578
Parasympatholytics
  on ACh turnover, 376
Parasympathomimetics
  on ACh turnover, 375-76
Parathyroid glands
  function of, 77
  hormone secretion mecha-
    nisms in, 27, 29
Parathyroid hormone (PTH)
  and magnesium excretion,
    70, 72, 75-77
  and nephrolithiasis, 13-14
  release mechanisms for,
    29-30
  and vitamin D, 135-36
Pargyline
  and myopathies, 394-95
Parkinson's disease
  dopamine in, 545
PAS-C (para-aminosalicylic
    acid in vitamin C)
  as hypolipidemic, 507-8
PCB (Polychlorobiphenyls)
  fish accumulation of, 171-
    73
Pediatric clinical pharmacol-
    ogy, 561-73
  clinical study approaches,
    565-70
    pharmacokinetics, 569
    quantitative studies of
      metabolism, table, 566-
      68
  introduction, 561-62
  postnatal pharmacokinetics,
    562-65
    apparent distribution vol-
      ume, 564-65
    developmental overview,
      562-65
    plasma concentration half-
      life, 562-64
    protein binding and meta-
      bolic processes, 565
  review of, 678
Penicillamine

in cystinuria, 11
  and pyridoxine, 141
D-Penicillamine (PCA)
  on lead disposition, 201-
    2
Penicillin
  aging pharmacokinetics of,
    51-52, 56
  compliance as problem in
    drug taking, 319
  pediatric aspects of, 563,
    565
Penicillin G
  aging pharmacokinetics of,
    51, 56, 60
Pennaria
  chemoreceptors of, 250
Pentobarbital
  on ACh turnover, 377-78
Pentolinium
  on blood pressure, 302
Pentylenetetrazol
  on ACh uptake, 380
Peptide hormones
  receptors of, 243
  reviews of, 681
Peptide neurotransmitters,
    425-39
  angiotensin II, 432-33
  carnosine, 431
  conclusion, 433
  enkephalin, 431-32
  hypothalamic releasing
    factors, 432
  neurophypophysial peptides,
    432
  proctolin, 430-31
  substance P, 425-30
Peptidergic neuron
  description of, 425
Perhexiline
  structure of, 153
Perinatal pharmacology
  symposium of, 678
Pethidine
  aging pharmacokinetics of,
    54, 58
Petit mal
  drugs used in, 680
Peyote
  psychopharmacological his-
    tory, 648-54, 662-64
Pharmacodynamics
  of drug interactions, 298-
    300
  amount/effect, 298
  receptor site, 299-300
Pharmacokinetics
  aging effects on, 49-65
    age-related changes in
      systems, 50-51
    changes in tissue respon-
      siveness, 61-62
    clinical studies, 51-59
    conclusion, 62
    introduction, 49
    plasma protein binding,

59-61
    drug interactions, 294-98
      absorption, 294-95
      distribution, 295-97
      excretion, 298
      metabolism, 297-98
    during postnatal human
      development, 562-65
Phenelzine
  on myopathies, 395
Phenethylamines
  in control of feeding, 605-
    17
  structural comparisons of
    monoamine neurotrans-
    mitters, 612
Phenobarbital
  aging pharmacokinetics of,
    54, 57
  drug interactions with, 294,
    297, 300
  pediatric aspects of, 563-
    65, 567
  and vitamin D, 136
Phenobarbituric acid
  aging pharmacokinetics of,
    60
Phenol
  anesthetic action of, 225
Phenolphthalein
  laxative action of, 362
Phenothiazines
  on brain amine metabolism,
    413-15
  on cyclic nucleotides, 457,
    461, 464
  dopamine antagonism by,
    552
  drug interactions with, 299-
    300
Phenoxybenzamine
  at β-adrenergic receptor,
    583
  drug interactions with, 299,
    302
  and myopathies, 393
Phenozelidine
  street use of, 679
Phentolamine
  at adrenergic receptor,
    583
  drug interactions with, 299,
    302
  on temperature regulation,
    345
Phenylacetate
  pediatric aspects of, 568
Phenylalanine ammonia-lyase
  therapeutic usefulness of,
    107
Phenylalanine mustard (L-PAM)
  on cancer cell kinetics,
    530
Phenylbutazone
  aging pharmacokinetics of,
    55, 57-61
  and cholestyramine, 506

drug interactions with, 297,
300, 303-4
pediatric aspects of, 563-
64
Phenylephrine
drug interactions with, 299
Phenylethylamine
from plants, 655
structure of, 657
Phenylhydrazine
and β-adrenergic receptor,
584
Phenylpropanolamine (PPA)
in control of feeding, 605-6
612, 615-17
drug interactions with, 299
Phenyramidol
drug interactions with, 297
Phenytoin
aging pharmacokinetics of,
54, 56-57, 60
drug interactions with, 296-
97, 300-1, 304
pediatric aspects of, 563-65,
567
and vitamin D, 136
Philanthus trangulum
venom of, 487-88
Phosphate
in nephrocalculi, 16-17,
20
Phosphodiesterase inhibitors
cyclic nucleotides
biologic role of, 442
development of drugs altering metabolism of, 449-
53
pathologic role of, 442-49
selective alteration of
metabolism of, 458
summary, 464-65
therapeutic use of, 453-
58
Phosphoenolpyruvate carboxykinase
corticosteroid effects on,
512
Phospholipase A (PLA)
in venom, 484, 489, 494
Phosphorylcholine
to lable brain choline, 374-
75
Physostigmine
on ACh turnover, 376
drug interactions with,
300
Picietl
psychopharmacology of, 650,
670
Picrotoxin
on ACh turnover, 380
Pilocarpine
on ACh turnover, 375
Pimozide
dopamine antagonism by,
552
in thermoregulation, 347

Pindolol
and β-adrenergic receptor,
584
Pineal organ
β-adrenergic receptors of,
593
Pipiltzintzintli
identification and active
substances in, 648, 650,
652, 668
Pituitary
peptide-like analgesic from,
679
Pituitary gland
hormone release mecha-
nisms of, 32, 36
Piule
psychopharmacology of,
651
Placenta
as enzyme source, 98, 108
Placental transfer of drugs
review of, 678
Plants
antineoplastic agents from,
117-32
sacred
Mexican, table of, 660-71
Plasma protein binding
aging effects on, 59-61
Plasminogen
therapeutic usefulness of,
108
Platelet aggregation
pharmacology of, 680-81
Pneumococcus
as source of therapeutic
enzymes, 98
Poisindex
description of, 219
Poison control centers, 215-
22
activities of, 220-21
information resources, 219-
20
introduction, 215-16
limitations and future needs,
221-22
regional: program description, 216-18
analytical capabilities,
217
communication and trans-
port, 218
information services, 217
treatment services, 217
staffing, 218-19
Polistes
venom of, 494
Polistes annularis
venom of, 486
Polistes apachus
venom of, 488
Polistes exclamanus
venom of, 486
Polistes fusicatus
venom of, 486

(Poly)dimethylsiloxane
in enzyme therapy, 112
(Poly)hydroxyethyl methacrylate
in enzyme therapy, 112
Polynucleosides
synthetic
in cancer immunotherapy,
188
Polypeptides
in venoms, 493
(Poly)N-vinyl pyrrolidone
and enzyme therapy, 112
Porphobilinogen (PBG)
lead effect on, 203
Potassium
depletion
and drug effects, 298
and hormone secretion, 28-
31, 37
on hydra feeding response,
249
and myopathies, 389
proximal tubular reabsorption, 627
Poyomatli
psychopharmacology of, 650-
51, 658-59, 671
Poyomaxochitl
psychopharmacology of, 651,
671
Practolol
at β-adrenergic receptor,
586
aging pharmacokinetics, 55,
59
Prazosin
combination use in hypertension, 317
Prednisolone
clinical pharmacology of,
511, 516-18, 520
Pregnancy
drug aspects of, 569
Prenylamine
Ca antagonism by, 153,
159
structure, 153
Prescription of drugs
factors influencing, 681
Prilocaine
pain relief by, 226, 234,
238
Primaquine
hemolysis from, 137
Probenecid
on brain amine metabolism,
412-13, 415-18, 420
Probenecid analogues
renal studies of, 6-7
Proboscidactyla
chemoreceptors of,
250
Procainamide
drug interactions with, 294,
298, 300-1
Procaine

pain relief by, 226-27, 232-
39
pediatric aspects of, 568
Procaine penicillin
aging pharmacokinetics of,
51
Proctolin
as neurotransmitter, 430-
31
Prolactin
on cancer cell kinetics,
539
Proline
receptor origin, 251-52
Propantheline
drug interactions with, 295
Propicillin
aging pharmacokinetics of,
52, 56
Propoxyphene
pediatric aspects of, 563
Propranolol
aging pharmacokinetics of,
55, 59
drug interactions with, 298-
302
in hypertension
combination use of, 312,
315, 318
and prostaglandins, 270
to study β-adrenergic receptors, 279-82, 586-88,
591
in thermoregulation, 345
Prostaglandins
on autonomic neurotrans-
mission, 259-79
adrenergic neuroeffector
junctions, 260-69
cholinergic neuroeffector
transmission, 270-72
conclusions, 272
ganglionic transmission,
269-70
introduction, 259-60
biosynthetic pathways of,
260
Prostaglandins
E_1
and β-adrenergic receptor,
584, 594-95
laxative action of, 357
E series
at adrenergic neuroeffector
junctions, 260-63, 265-66
F series
at adrenergic neuroeffector
junctions, 262-63, 266-67
in reproduction, 680
synthesis of
action of inhibitors of, 267-
69
Prostigmine sulfate
and myopathy, 400-1
Protein binding
in pediatric pharmacology,
565

Protoporphyrin IX (PROTO)
to study lead exposure,
205-6
Proximal tubule
reabsorption and its regulation, 623-46
diagram of backleak, 638
internephron heterogene-
ity, 625-26
intranephron heterogene-
ity, 624-25
introduction, 623
outward transport: active
and passive, 626-33
proximal tubule heterogeneity, 523-24
regulatory factors, 633-
40
Pseudohypoparathyroidism
cyclic nucleotides in, 447
Psilocybe sp.
Mexican sacred use of, 648,
650-53, 655, 660-61
Psilocybin
Mexican cultural uses of,
655, 661
Psoriasis
cyclic nucleotides in, 447,
454
Psychodysleptics
Mexican cultural uses of,
655-58
Psychopharmacology
genetic aspects of, 681
of Mexican plants, 647-75
basic structures, 657
botanical distribution and
identification, 649-52
conclusion, 659
history, 647-49
introduction, 647
psychopharmacology, 654-
59
table of, 660-71
uses and cultural roles of,
652-54
Psychoses
dopamine in, 545-46
Psychotherapeutic drugs
interactions of, 677
Psychotomimetics
on ACh turnover, 378
Psychotropics
on CNS amine metabolism,
411-24
symposium on, 679
Pulse injection
of isotopic ACh lab, 374-
75
Pulse-labeling methods
to study secretory mecha-
nisms, 33-34
Puromycin
on hormone release, 36
and vitamin D, 136
Push-pull cannula
to study brain ACh turnover,

369, 371-72
to study dopamine psycho-
pharmacology, 553
Puyomate
psychopharmacology of,
651
Pyrazolones
on cyclic nucleotides, 455
drug interactions with, 296
Pyridine-2-aldoxime methiodide (2-PAM)
and myopathy, 397, 400-1
Pyridinol
fish accumulation of, 171
Pyridoxal phosphate
enzymes which degrade,
99
Pyridoxine
deficiency
and tumor growth, 107
toxicity studies of, 140-41
drug interactions, 140-41
Pyrocatechol
on adrenergic receptor,
580
Pyrogen test
in steroid-treated patients,
524
Pyrophosphate
in nephrolithiasis, 20
Pyrrolizidine
psychopharmacology of,
658
structure of, 657

Q

Quantlapatzinzintli
psychopharmacology of,
665
Quassinoids
antitumor activity of, 126-
29
structures, 127-29
Quetzalpoyomaxochitl
psychopharmacology of,
651
Quinidine
drug interactions with, 294,
296-98, 300-1, 304
Quinolizidines
basic structures of, 657
psychopharmacology, 658,
667
Quinolones
on cyclic nucleotides, 455

R

Radiopharmaceuticals
organ-damaging, 678
Receptors
adrenergic
models of, 679
β-adrenergic, 575-604
and cAMP formation,
576

characterization of direct
binding assays for, 576-
78
classification of, 575-76
conclusion, 595
in vitro assays of, 578-87
in vitro properties of, 587-
89
regulation of, 589-95
chemoreceptors of aquatic
invertebrates, 243-58
dopamine
blockade of, 553
drug interactions at, 299-
300
Regional pain relief
see Pain relief, regional
Renal clearance techniques
Beyer's experience with,
5
Renin
diuretic manipulation of
levels of, 317
Reserpine
and breast cancer, 680
combination use in hypertension, 315-18
drug interactions with, 297,
299-300
on histamine release, 328
and myopathies, 394
Resorcinol
pain relief by, 225
Retinol-binding protein
description of, 133
Review of reviews, 677-82
Riboflavin
deficiency of
and tumor growth, 107
toxicity studies of, 140
Ricinoleic acid
laxative action of, 359-61
Rifampin
drug interactions with, 304
Rivea corymbosa
psychoactive drugs in, 650,
656, 665

S

Salicylalcohol
pain relief by, 225
Salicylamide
pediatric aspects of, 566,
569
Salicylates
aging pharmacokinetics, 60-
61
and corticosteroids, 521
drug interactions with, 294,
296, 303-4
pediatric aspects of, 563,
565-66
poisoning with, 680
Salicylic acid
aging pharmacokinetics of,
61

Saline
laxative action of, 362-63
Salvia divinorum
psychopharmacology of, 650,
652, 656, 666
Samaderin
antitumor studies of, 128
structure of, 129
Sanguinarine
antitumor activity of, 121-
22
structure of, 122
Sarcoidosis
and renal lithiasis, 13
Serin
and myopathy, 398
Sceliphron caementarium
venom of, 488
Schizophrenia
brain amine metabolism in,
416-17
dopamine in, 545-46
neuroanatomical substrates
of, 547-50
corpus striatum, 547-48
limbic system, 548-50
Scopolamine
in thermoregulation, 348
Scyphozoa
chemoreceptors of, 251
Secretin
laxative action of, 357
Selective phosphodiesterase
inhibitors, 441-77
biologic role of cyclic nucleotides, 442
development of drugs altering cyclic nucleotide
metabolism, 449-53
pathologic role of cyclic
nucleotides, 442-49
selective alteration of cyclic
nucleotide metabolism,
458
summary, 464-65
therapeutic use of, 453-58
Selenium
in glutathione peroxidase,
138
Senecio
psychopharmacology of, 658,
664-65
Serine dehydratase
isolation of, 106
Serotonin (5-HT)
brain effects of, 370
brain levels of
drug effects on, 411-22
in myopathies, 393-95
in venom, 488-89, 494
see also 5-Hydroxytrypt-
amine
Sex hormones
on cells and tissue transport, 677
Shock
corticosteroids in, 515, 519

Simaroubaceae
anticancer drugs from,
126
Sinicuiche
identification and active
substances in, 649
Siphonophores
chemoreceptors of, 251
β-Sitosterol
as hypolipidemic, 507
Skeleton
lead in, 200
Skin
lead absorption from, 200
Smooth muscle relaxants
and cyclic nucleotides,
456
Snake venom
therapeutic usefulness of,
108
Sodium
and Ca in cardiac pharma-
cology, 149-50
on hydra feeding response,
249
proximal tubular reabsorption, 627, 629
and renal Mg, 68, 70, 73-
74
Sodium ascorbate
on β-adrenergic receptors,
580
Sodium bicarbonate
in nephrolithiasis, 19
Sodium dichromoglycate
on asthma, 455
Sodium fluoride
and β-adrenergic receptor,
584
Sodium ion
and hormone secretion, 28,
30
Sodium metabisulfite
on β-adrenergic receptor,
580
Solenopsin A
in ant venom, 491
Solenopsis
venom of, 490-91, 494
Solenopsis saevissina
venom of, 490, 494
Soman (methylpinacolyloxyphosphoryl fluoride)
and myopathy, 398-99
Somatostatin
in neurotransmission, 432
Somatotroph
and hormone release, 32-
33, 35
Sophora secundiflora
psychoactive drugs from,
647
Spinal neurons
substance P on, 426-27
Spironolactone
combination use of, 314
drug interactions affecting,

298, 300-1, 303
Spleen
  prostaglandins on, 261,
    267
SQ 20009
  on phosphodiesterase, 462-
    64
SQ 20881
  on blood pressure, 302
Steroid pseudorheumatism
  description of, 521
Stimulus-secretion coupling
  explanation of, 29
Stool softeners
  pharmacology of, 362
Storage granules
  and hormone secretion,
    28
  see also Granules
Streptokinase
  therapeutic usefulness of,
    108
Streptomycin
  pediatric aspects of, 563
Striatum
  ACh turnover in, 369
Struvite
  and nephrolithiasis, 16
Strychnine
  on ACh turnover, 380
Substance P
  on brain ACh turnover, 370
  as neurotransmitter, 425-
    30
  antagonists, 427-28
  evidence for, 426-29
  inactivation of substance
    P, 428
  other possible functions,
    429-30
  in primary sensory neu-
    rons, 426
  release of substance P,
    428
  as sensory transmitter,
    428-29
  on spinal neurons, 426-27
  structure:activity, 428
Sulfadiazine
  aging pharmacokinetics of,
    60-61
Sulfadimethoxine
  drug interactions with, 296
Sulfalene
  pediatric aspects of, 563-
    64
Sulfamethizole
  aging pharmacokinetics of,
    59
  drug interactions with, 297
Sulfaphenazole
  drug interactions with, 296-
    97
Sulfinpyrazone
  drug interactions with, 296,
    303
Sulfisomidine

pediatric aspects of, 563-
    64
Sulfisoxazole
  pediatric aspects of, 563-
    64
Sulfonamides
  drug interactions with, 304
  pediatric aspects of, 565
Sulthiame
  drug interactions with,
    297
Sympathomimetics
  on thermoregulation, 342
Synergy
  of antihypertensives, 311
Syringaldehyde
  on β-adrenergic receptors,
    579
Syringic acid
  on β-adrenergic receptors,
    579

T

Tabun
  and myopathy, 398
Taenia coli
  Ca antagonizing drugs in,
    158
Tagetes lucida
  psychopharmacology of,
    652, 656
Taxane diterpenoids
  antitumor activity of, 126
  structure of, 126
Taxol
  antitumor activity of, 126
  structure of, 126
T cells
  in cancer immunosuppres-
    sion, 180-81, 187
  differentiation of, 282, 285
  importance of, 281
  induction of markers on
    precursors of, 285-86
Temperature regulation, 341-
    53
  acetylcholine, 342-44
  conclusion, 349
  dopamine, 347-48
  histamine, 348-49
  5-hydroxytryptamine, 346-
    47
  introduction, 341-42
  norepinephrine, 344-46
Teonanacatl
  psychoactivity of, 650, 652,
    660
Teratogens
  vitamin A, 134
Tetracaine
  pain relief by, 226, 233-35,
    238
2, 2', 4, 4'-Tetrachlorobiphenyl
  accumulation in fish, 171
Tetracycline
  aging pharmacokinetics of,

51-52, 56
  and hypolipidemics, 506
Tetraethyl lead
  toxicology of, 200
Tetrahydrocannabinol
  on ACh turnover, 378
Δ⁹-Tetrahydrocannabinol
  (THC)
  in Cannabis sativa
    regional variation in, 649,
      668
  structure of, 657
Tetrodotoxin (TTX)
  and hormone release, 31
  myocardial activity of, 157-
    58
  and myopathy, 397-98
  substance P block by, 427
Thalicarpine
  antitumor activity of, 119
  structure, 120
Thalidaisine
  antitumor activity of, 121
  structure of, 120
Theobroma cacao
  psychopharmacology of,
    651, 658, 671
Theophylline
  and calcium release, 31
  on cyclic nucleotides, 457-
    60
  pediatric aspects of, 563-
    65
Therapeutic orphan
  pediatric pharmacology,
    561
Thermoregulation
  see Temperature regulation
Thiamin
  toxicity studies of, 139
Thiazides
  combination use in hyperten-
    sion, 317-18
  drug interactions affecting,
    298, 302-3
  and hypolipidemics, 506
  in nephrolithiasis, 14-15,
    18
Thioguanine
  on cell kinetics, 535
Thiopental
  aging pharmacokinetics of,
    61
Thioridazine
  on brain amine metabolism,
    415-16
  dopamine antagonism by,
    552
Thiothixene
  drug interaction with,
    299
Thomas J. Fleming Poison
    Information Service, 216
Thromboxanes (TX)
  biosynthetic pathways of,
    260
Thymic hormones, 281-91

biological activities, 285-88

clinical activities, 288-89

introduction, 281-82

one or several, 285

preparation, assay, and biochemistry of thymic factors, 282-85

Thymic humoral factor (THF) on antibody responses, 287

bioassay, biochemistry, and isolation of, 282-83

clinical uses of, 288-89

Thymic hypocalcemic factors description of, 285

Thymidine $_3$ tritiated (^{3}HTdR) to study cancer cell kinetics, 529

Thympopoietins I and II bioassay, biochemistry, and isolation of, 283-84

Thymosin antitumor response of, 287

bioassay, biochemistry, and isolation of, 282

clinical uses of, 288

Thymus hormones of, 281-91

Thymus dependent lymphocytes see Lymphocytes; T cells

Thyrocalcitonin laxative action of, 357

Thyroid and biogenic amines, 679

Thyroid drugs drug interactions with, 304

Thyroid gland mechanisms of hormone secretion in, 27, 29

Thyroid hormone and magnesium reabsorption, 70, 74

Thyroid stimulating hormone suppression of secretion of, 151

Thyrotroph and hormone release, 32, 35

Thyrotropin-releasing hormone (TRH) in neurotransmission, 432

D-Thyroxine drug interactions with, 304

on plasma lipids, 506-7

Ticrynafen uricosuric potency of, 19

Tienilic acid uricosuric potency of, 19

Tlapatl identification and active substances in, 648, 650

Tlitlitzen psychopharmacology of, 652

Tobramycin pediatric aspects of, 563

α-Tocopherol see Vitamin E

Tolbutamide drug interactions with, 296, 304

pediatric aspects of, 563, 568

Toloatzin psychopharmacology of, 650, 652

Toxicology exposure of humans to lead, 197-214

poison control centers, 215-22

reviews of, 680

Transmembrane electrolyte movements fast channel-slow channel, 150, 159

Transmembrane potential in secretory cells, 28-29

Triamcinolone clinical pharmacology of, 511, 516-18

Triamterene combination use of, 314

drug interactions with, 303

Trichlorofluoromethane (CCl_3F) toxicology of, 84, 90-92

3, 5, 6-Trichloropyridinol in fish, 170

Trichlorotrifluoroethane ($CCl_2F\text{-}CClF_2$) toxicology of, 84, 91

Triclofos drug interactions with, 304

Tricyclic antidepressants see Antideppressants, tricyclic

Trifluoperazine on phosphodiesterase, 458-61

Trifluorobromomethane ($CBrF_3$) toxicology of, 84-91

α, α, α-Trifluoro-2, 6-dinitro-N, N-dipropyl-p-toluidine (Trifluralin) fish accumulation of, 172

Trihexyphenidyl on brain ACh turnover, 376

Trimethaphan camphor sulfonate on substance P, 427

Trimethopham drug interactions with, 302

Tripdiolide antitumor activity of, 129

structure of, 129

Tripelennamine in pain relief, 233

Triptolides antitumor studies of, 129-30

structures of, 129

Tropane psychopharmacology, 658, 669

structure of, 657

Tryptamine structure of, 657

Tryptophanase therapeutic potential of, 99-100

Tubularia chemoreceptors of, 250

Tumor-cell labeling index to predict clinical response, 530, 534-38

Tumors cell kinetics, 529-39

Turbicoryn psychopharmacology of, 656

Turnera diffusa psychopharmacology of, 659, 671

Tyramine drug interactions with, 297

Tyrosine isomers chemoreceptors for, 252-53

Tzinzintlapatl identification and active substances in, 648, 650

U

Undulatone antitumor activity of, 127

Urea drug interactions with, 303

and Mg excretion, 71

Uric acid in kidney stones, 18

Urine conditions with increased crystalloid constituents, 13-17

factors controlling excretion of Mg in, 70-75

changes in filtered load, 70

changes in tubular reabsorption, 70-75

Urokinase therapeutic usefulness of, 108

Uterus Ca antagonizing drugs in, 158

V

Vanilylmandelic acid (VMA) drug effects on, 419

Vascular beds

prostaglandins on, 262, 269
Vasoconstrictors
  and local anesthetics, 236-37
Vasodilators
  combination use in hypertension, 317-18
Vasopressin
  blockers of, 150
  mechanism of release of, 32, 34
  as neurotransmitter, 432
Vein, portal
  calcium-antagonizing drugs in, 158
Venoms
  hymenoptera, 479-98
  ant, 490-92
  bee, 481-85
  clinical manifestations of, 480
  hornet, 488-90
  introduction, 479-80
  summary, 492-95
  wasp, 485-88
Ventral bundle
  and feeding control, 606, 609
Ventriculolumbar gradients
  for brain amines, 412
Verapamil
  Ca antagonism by, 150-51, 153-59
  cardiac effects of, 301
  structure of, 153
Veratrum alkaloids
  myopathies from, 388
Vespa crabo
  venom of, 488-89, 494
Vespa orientalis
  venom of, 489-90, 494
Vespa vulgaris
  venom of, 486, 494
Vespula arenario
  venom of, 488
Vespula pennsylvanica
  venom of, 488
Viminol R$_2$

on ACh turnover, 377
Vinblastine
  on cancer cell kinetics, 532-33
  on hormone release, 36
  and myopathy, 397
Vinca alkaloids
  on cancer cell kinetics, 530
  on cancer immune response, 184, 186
Vincristine
  on cancer cell kinetics, 530-31, 533-34
Vitamin A
  interaction with vitamin E, 134
  toxicity of, 133-34
  teratogenic, 134
Vitamin B-12
  and ascorbic acid, 142
Vitamin D
  Ca antagonists effect on, 154
  corticosteroid effects on, 513
  toxicity, 134-37
  calcium role in, 135
  drugs affecting, 136
  parathyroid hormones, 135
Vitamin E
  interaction with A, 134
  toxicity of, 138-39
Vitamin K
  drug interactions with, 304-5
  toxicity of, 137-38
Vitamins
  metabolism of
  oral contraceptive effects on, 678
Vitamin toxicity, 133-48
  conclusions, 142
  fat-soluble vitamins, 133-39
  water-soluble vitamins, 139-42

W

Warfarin
  aging pharmacokinetics, 62
  drug interactions with, 294, 296
  and hypolipidemics, 506-7
Wasp
  venom of, 485-88
Wasp kinin
  characterization of, 486
Water
  histamine effects on, 333
Waterhouse-Friderichsen syndrome
  corticosteroids in, 519
Water transport
  and laxatives, 355-63
Weed killers
  myopathies from, 388

X

Xanthine
  psychopharmacology of, 658-59, 671
  structure of, 657
X irradiation
  in cancer immune response, 184
X-ray contrast media
  design of, 678
Xylocaine
  see Lidocaine
Xylose
  aging pharmacokinetics, 50

Y

Yahutli
  psychopharmacology of, 652

Z

Zoanthus
  chemoreceptor of, 250-51
Zymogen granules
  ATP-induced release from, 36

CUMULATIVE INDEXES

CONTRIBUTING AUTHORS VOLUMES 13-17

A

Adriani, J., 17:223-42
Allen, J. L., 14:47-55
Anichkov, S. V., 15:1-10
Aranda, J. V., 16:427-45
Austen, K. F., 15:177-89
Azarnoff, D. L., 16:53-66

B

Bach, J.-F., 17:281-91
Back, K. C., 17:83-95
Bapna, J. S., 14:115-26
Barbeau, A., 14:91-113
Baumgarten, H. G., 16:101-11
Bender, A. D., 17:49-65
Bevan, J. A., 13:269-85
Beyer, K. H. Jr., 14:355-64; 17:1-10
Bignami, G., 16:329-66
Binder, H. J., 17:355-67
Björklund, A., 16:101-11
Brater, D. C., 17:293-309
Brodie, B. B., 14:271-88
Burks, T. F., 16:15-31

C

Calabresi, P., 16:367-79
Carter, S. K., 14:157-83
Cavagnol, R. M., 17:479-98
Changeux, J.-P., 15:83-103
Chase, T. N., 13:181-97
Chasseaud, L. F., 14:35-46
Cheney, D. L., 17:369-86
Cho, A. K., 13:371-90
Christensen, J., 15:243-58
Clineschmidt, B. V., 16:113-23
Clouet, D. H., 15:49-71
Cohen, J. B., 15:83-103
Cohen, S. N., 17:561-73
Coleman, J. E., 15:221-42
Colquhoun, D., 15:307-25
Costa, E., 14:491-511; 17:369-86
Cox, B., 17:341-53

D

Dandiya, P. C., 14:115-26
DeFeudis, F. V., 15:105-30
de Jong, W., 14:389-412

Dettbarn, W.-D., 17:387-409
deWied, D., 14:389-412
Díaz, J. L., 17:647-75
DiPalma, J. R., 17:133-48
Dollery, C. T., 17:311-23
Done, A. K., 17:561-73
Drill, V. A., 15:367-85
Dungworth, D. L., 16:381-99

E

Eknoyan, G., 13:91-106

F

Fairshter, R. D., 16:465-86
Fanelli, G. M. Jr., 14:355-64
Fassett, D. W., 15:425-35
Ferreira, S. H., 14:57-73
Fishbein, L., 14:139-56
Fleckenstein, A., 17:149-66
Forsham, P. H., 15:351-66
Freund, G., 13:217-27
Frost, D. V., 15:259-84

G

Genest, J., 16:287-308
Gillespie, J. R., 16:465-86
Gillette, J. R., 14:271-88
Goldstein, E., 16:447-63
Gosselin, R. E., 16:189-99
Green, J. P., 14:319-42
Grob, D., 16:215-29
Gross, F., 13:57-90
Guthrie, G. P. Jr., 16:287-308

H

Habermann, E. R., 14:1-8
Hackney, J. D., 16:465-86
Hait, W. N., 17:441-77
Hamelink, J. L., 17:167-77
Hammond, P. B., 17:197-214
Harden, T. K., 17:575-604
Hart, J. S., 17:529-43
Haskell, C. M., 17:179-95
Havel, R. J., 13:287-308
Heagy, W., 17:243-58

Hedqvist, P., 17:259-79
Heppner, G. H., 16:367-79
Hoebel, B. G., 17:605-21
Holcenberg, J. S., 17:97-116
Hornykiewicz, O., 17:545-59
Hubbard, J. I., 13:199-216
Huffman, D. H., 16:53-66
Hunn, J. B., 14:47-55
Hyman, A. L., 15:285-306

I

Iwatsubo, K., 15:49-71

J

Jacobson, H. R., 16:201-14; 17:623-46
Jenden, D. J., 13:371-90
Jöchle, W., 13:33-55
Johnson, C. L., 14:319-42
Joiner, P. D., 15:285-306
Jordan, G. W., 15:157-75; 16:447-63
Juchau, M. R., 14:219-38

K

Kadowitz, P. J., 15:285-306
Kaliner, M., 15:177-89
Kane, J. P., 13:287-308
Kang, S., 14:319-42
Karam, J. H., 15:351-66
Kehoe, J. S., 16:245-68
Kelley, W. N., 15:327-50
Knoll, J., 16:487-502
Kokko, J. P., 16:201-14
Kosterlitz, H. W., 15:29-47
Kuchel, O., 16:287-308

L

Laskowski, M. B., 17:387-409
Leach, R. M. Jr., 14:289-303
Leake, C. D., 13:455-63; 14:521-29; 15:465-72; 16:1-14, 503-10; 17:677-82
Legator, M., 15:387-408
Lenhoff, H. M., 17:243-58
Levy, R. I., 17:499-510
Lish, P. M., 15:259-84
Livingston, R. B., 17:529-43

Lomax, P., 17:341-53
Loughnan, P. M., 16:427-45

M

Maas, J. W., 17:411-24
MacKenzie, M. R., 16:447-63
Magazanik, L. G., 16:161-75
Maibach, H., 16:401-11
Manning, M., 13:5-17
Marder, E., 16:245-68
Maren, T. H., 16:309-27
Marshall, J. M., 13:19-32
Martinez-Maldonado, M., 13:91-106
Massry, S. G., 17:67-82
Matin, S. B., 15:351-66
McGaugh, J. L., 13:229-41
Meek, J. L., 14:491-511
Melby, J. C., 17:511-27
Merigan, T. C., 15:157-75
Minneman, K. P., 16:33-51
Mitchell, J. R., 14:271-88
Möhring, J., 13:57-90
Molinoff, P. B., 17:575-604
Molitch, M. E., 14:413-34
Morrelli, H. F., 17:293-309
Mueller, W. J., 14:289-303
Murphy, D. L., 13:181-97

N

Naraghi, M., 17:223-42
Natochin, Yu. V., 14:75-90
Needleman, P., 16:81-93
Neims, A. H., 16:427-45
Nelson, K. W., 16:95-100

O

Odell, W. D., 14:413-34
Ogilvie, R. I., 15:131-55
Oldendorf, W. H., 14:239-48
Osebold, J. W., 16:447-63
Oswald, I., 13:243-52
Otsuka, M., 17:425-39

P

Paoletti, R., 15:73-81
Park, C. R., 14:365-88
Paton, W. D. M., 15:191-220

Paulus, H. E., 13:107-25
Phalen, R. F., 16:381-99
Pilkis, S. J., 14:365-88
Pinto, S. S., 16:95-100
Plaa, G. L., 16:125-41
Porte, D. Jr., 16:269-85
Posternak, T., 14:23-33

Q

Quastel, D. M. J., 13:199-216

R

Radomski, J. L., 14:127-37
Raffel, S., 13:1-4
Richey, D. P., 17:49-65
Ritchie, D. M., 17:133-48
Roberts, J., 17:97-116
Rozman, R. S., 13:127-52

S

Samson, F. E., 16:143-59
Sastry, B. V. R., 13:253-67
Sasyniuk, B. I., 15:131-55
Sawyer, W. H., 13:5-17
Schildkraut, J. J., 13:427-54
Schoental, R., 14:185-204
Schou, M., 16:231-43
Schwartz, J.-C., 17:325-39
Schwartz, L. W., 16:381-99
Scriabine, A., 16:113-23
Seldin, D. W., 17:623-46
Simpson, L. L., 14:305-17
Sirtori, C. Jr., 15:73-81
Slavik, M., 14:157-83
Smith, D. E., 14:513-20
Smith, P. H., 16:269-85
Smith, R. P., 16:189-99
Smythies, J. R., 14:9-21
Spacie, A., 17:167-77
Spano, P. F., 15:73-81
Spector, S., 13:359-70
Stannard, J. N., 13:325-57
Steele, T. H., 17:11-25
Stewart, G. T., 13:309-24
Stewart, R. D., 15:409-23
Strebel, L., 17:561-73
Su, C., 13:269-85
Suki, W. N., 13:91-106

Sweet, C. S., 16:113-23

T

Takahashi, T., 17:425-39
Taylor, T., 14:35-46
Temple, A. R., 17:215-22
Thoenen, H., 13:169-80
Thrupp, L. D., 14:435-67
Tilles, J. G., 14:469-89
Tranzer, J. P., 13:169-80
Trifaro, J. M., 17:27-47
Tyler, W. S., 16:381-99

V

Valdecasas, F. G., 15:453-63
Vane, J. R., 14:57-73
Van Stee, E. W., 16:67-78; 17:83-95
Vesell, E. S., 14:249-70

W

Waddell, W. J., 13:153-68
Wall, M. E., 17:117-32
Wani, M. C., 17:117-32
Warner, M., 16:427-45
Waterfield, A. A., 15:29-47
Watson, J. T., 13:391-407
Weihe, W. H., 13:409-25
Weiss, B., 17:441-77
Weiss, G. B., 14:343-54
Wesson, D. R., 14:513-20
Whitehouse, M. W., 13:107-25
Wilkinson, G. R., 15:11-27
Wilson, A. F., 16:465-86
Wilson, J. G., 14:205-17
Winters, W. D., 16:413-26
Witschi, H., 16:125-41
Wogan, G. N., 15:437-51
Wolfe, B. B., 17:575-604
Wurtman, R. J., 16:33-51

Y

Yaffe, S. J., 14:219-38

Z

Zbinden, G., 16:177-88
Zimmering, S., 15:387-408

CHAPTER TITLES VOLUMES 13 - 17

PREFATORY CHAPTERS
Windsor Cooper Cutting (1907-1972)   S. Raffel   13:1-4
Rudolf Buchheim and the Beginning of a Phar-
macology as a Science   E. R. Habermann   14:1-8
How I Became a Pharmacologist   S. V. Anichkov   15:1-10
How I Am   C. D. Leake   16:1-14
A Career or Two   K. H. Beyer Jr.   17:1-10
ALLERGY AND DRUG SENSITIVITY
Allergy to Penicillin and Related Antibiotics:
Antigenic and Immunochemical Mechanism   G. T. Stewart   13:309-24
Immunologic Release of Chemical Mediators
from Human Tissues   M. Kaliner, K. F. Austen   15:177-89
Cutaneous Pharmacology and Toxicology   H. Maibach   16:401-11
ANESTHETICS, ANALGESICS, AND ANTIINFLAMMATORY AGENTS
Nonsteroid Anti-Inflammatory Agents   H. E. Paulus, M. W. White-
                                                      house   13:107-25
New Aspects of the Mode of Action of Non-
steroid Anti-Inflammatory Drugs   S. H. Ferreira, J. R. Vane   14:57-73
Mechanisms of Tolerance to and Dependence
on Narcotic Analgesic Drugs   D. H. Clouet, K. Iwatsubo   15:49-71
Effects of Drugs on the Electrical Activity of
the Brain: Anesthetics   W. D. Winters   16:413-26
The Pharmacologic Principles of Regional
Pain Relief   J. Adriani, M. Naraghi   17:223-42
ANTIMICROBIAL, ANTIVIRAL, AND ANTIPARASITIC CHEMOTHERAPY
Chemotherapy of Malaria   R. S. Rozman   13:127-52
Newer Cephalosporins and "Expanded-Spectrum"
Penicillins   L. D. Thrupp   14:435-67
Antiviral Agents   J. G. Tilles   14:469-89
Enchancement of Host Defense Mechanisms by
Pharmacological Agents   G. W. Jordan, T. C. Merigan   15:157-75
AUTONOMIC PHARMACOLOGY
The Pharmacology of 6-Hydroxydopamine   H. Thoenen, J. P. Tranzer   13:169-80
Micropharmacology of Vertebrate Neuromus-
cular Transmission   J. I. Hubbard, D. M. J. Quastel 13:199-216
The Use of Neuropoisons in the Study of Cholin-
ergic Transmission   L. L. Simpson   14:305-17
Physiological and Pharmacological Roles of
Prostaglandins   P. J. Kadowitz, P. D. Joiner,
                                                      A. L. Hyman   15:285-306
Basic Mechanisms of Prostaglandin Action on
Autonomic Neurotransmission   P. Hedqvist   17:259-79
BEHAVIORAL AND PSYCHOPHARMACOLOGY
Chronic Central Nervous System Toxicity of
Alcohol   G. Freund   13:217-27
Drug Facilitation of Learning and Memory   J. L. McGaugh   13:229-41
Neuropharmacology of the Affective Disorders   J. J. Schildkraut   13:427-54
Drugs of Abuse 1973: Trends and Developments   D. E. Smith, D. R. Wesson   14:513-20
Pharmacology of Marijuana   W. D. M. Paton   15:191-220
Behavioral Pharmacology and Toxicology   G. Bignami   16:329-66
Psychopharmacological Implications of
Dopamine and Dopamine Antagonists: A
Critical Evaluation of Current Evidence   O. Hornykiewicz   17:545-59
Pharmacologic Control of Feeding   B. G. Hoebel   17:605-21
CANCER CHEMOTHERAPY AND IMMUNOPHARMACOLOGY
Chemotherapy of Cancer   S. K. Carter, M. Slavik   14:157-83
Selective Suppression of Humoral Immunity by
Antineoplastic Drugs   G. H. Heppner, P. Calabresi   16:367-79
Immunologic Aspects of Cancer Chemotherapy   C. M. Haskell   17:179-95
Thymic Hormones: Biochemistry, and

Biological and Clinical Activities | J.-F. Bach | 17:281-91
The Clinical Applications of Cell Kinetics in Cancer Therapy | R. B. Livingston, J. S. Hart | 17:529-43
CARDIOVASCULAR PHARMACOLOGY
Drugs and Lipid Metabolism | R. J. Havel, J. P. Kane | 13:287-308
Antiarrhythmic Drugs: Electrophysiological and Pharmacokinetic Considerations | B. I. Sasyniuk, R. I. Ogilvie | 15:131-55
Central Noradrenergic Control of Blood Pressure | A. Scriabine, B. V. Clineschmidt, C. S. Sweet | 16:113-23
Evaluation of Thrombogenic Effects of Drugs | G. Zbinden | 16:177-88
Renin and the Therapy of Hypertension | G. P. Guthrie Jr., J. Genest, O. Kuchel | 16:287-308
Pharmacological Basis for Combination Therapy of Hypertension | C. T. Dollery | 17:311-23
The Effect of Hypolipidemic Drugs on Plasma Lipoproteins | R. I. Levy | 17:499-510
CLINICAL TOXICOLOGY AND DRUG INTERACTIONS
Current Concepts About the Treatment of Selected Poisonings: Nitrate, Cyanide, Sulfide, Barium, and Quinidine | R. P. Smith, R. E. Gosselin | 16:189-99
Vitamin Toxicity | J. R. DiPalma, D. M. Ritchie | 17:133-48
Poison Control Centers: Prospects and Capabilities | A. R. Temple | 17:215-22
Cardiovascular Drug Interactions | D. C. Brater, H. F. Morrelli | 17:293-309
COMPARATIVE PHARMACOLOGY
Uric Acid in Nonhuman Primates with Special Reference to its Renal Transport | G. M. Fanelli Jr., K. H. Beyer Jr. | 14:355-64
Fish and Chemicals: The Process of Accumulation | J. L. Hamelink, A. Spacie | 17:167-77
Aquatic Invertebrates: Model Systems for Study of Receptor Activation and Evolution of Receptor Proteins | H. M. Lenhoff, W. Heagy | 17:243-58
ELECTROLYES AND MINERAL METABOLISM
Pharmacology and Toxicology of Lithium | M. Schou | 16:231-43
Pharmacology of Magnesium | S. G. Massry | 17:67-82
Proximal Tubular Reabsorption and Its Regulation | H. R. Jacobson, D. W. Seldin | 17:623-46
ENDOCRINE PHARMACOLOGY
Mechanism of Action of Insulin | S. J. Pilkis, C. R. Park | 14:365-88
Drug Effects and Hypothalamic-Anterior Pituitary Function | D. de Wied, W. de Jong | 14:389-412
Antidiabetic Drugs After the University Group Diabetes Program (UGDP) | J. H. Karam, S. B. Matin, P. H. Forsham | 15:351-66
The Pharmacology of the Pineal Gland | K. P. Minneman, R. J. Wurtman | 16:35-51
Neuropharmacology of the Pancreatic Islets | P. H. Smith, D. Porte Jr. | 16:269-85
Clinical Pharmacology of Systemic Corticosteroids | J. C. Melby | 17:511-27
ENVIRONMENTAL AND INDUSTRIAL PHARMACOLOGY AND TOXICOLOGY
Toxicology of Radionuclides | J. N. Stannard | 13:325-57
The Effect of Temperature on the Action of Drugs | W. H. Weihe | 13:409-25
Toxicology of Food Colors | J. L. Radomski | 14:127-37
Toxicity of Chlorinated Biphenyls | L. Fishbein | 14:139-56
Effects of Chemicals on Egg Shell Formation | W. J. Mueller, R. M. Leach Jr. | 14:289-303
Selenium in Biology | D. V. Frost, P. M. Lish | 15:259-84
Genetic Toxicology | M. Legator, S. Zimmering | 15:387-408
The Effect of Carbon Monoxide on Humans | R. D. Stewart | 15:409-23
Cadmium: Biological Effects and Occurrence in the Environment | D. W. Fassett | 15:425-35
Mycotoxins | G. N. Wogan | 15:437-51
Toxicology of Inhalation Anesthetics and Metabolites | E. W. Van Stee | 16:67-79

Arsenic Toxicology and Industrial Exposure | S. S. Pinto, K. W. Nelson | 16:95-100
Chemicals, Drugs, and Lipid Peroxidation | G. L. Plaa, H. Witschi | 16:125-41
Morphological Methods for Evaluation of
Pulmonary Toxicity in Animals | D. L. Dungworth, R. F. Phalen,
L. W. Schwartz, W. S. Tyler | 16:381-99
Methods for Evaluating the Toxicological Effects
Gaseous and Particulate Contaminants on
Pulmonary Microbial Defense Systems | E. Goldstein, G. W. Jordan,
J. W. Osebold, M. R. Mac-
Kenzie | 16:447-63
Evaluation of Abnormal Lung Functions | A. F. Wilson, R. D. Fairshter,
J. R. Gillespie, J. Hackney | 16:465-86
Toxicology of Haloalkane Propellants and Fire
Extinguishants | K. C. Back, E. W. Van Stee | 17:83-95
Exposure of Humans to Lead | P. B. Hammond | 17:197-214
GASTROINTESTINAL PHARMACOLOGY
Pharmacology of the Esophageal Motor Func-
tion | J. Christensen | 15:243-58
Gastrointestinal Pharmacology | T. F. Burks | 16:15-31
Pharmacology of Laxatives | H. J. Binder | 17:355-67
HISTORY AND HIGHLIGHTS OF PHARMACOLOGY
Pharmacological Research in India | P. C. Dandiya, J. S. Bapna | 14:115-26
History and Highlights of Spanish Pharmacology | F. G. Valdecasas | 15:453-63
History and Highlights of Pharmacology in
Hungary | J. Knoll | 16:487-502
Ethnopharmacology of Sacred Psychoactive
Plants Used by the Indians of Mexico | J. L. Diaz | 17:647-75
MECHANISMS OF ACTION OF DRUGS AND CHEMICALS
Stereoisomerism and Drug Action in the Nervous
System | B. V. Rama Sastry | 13:253-67
Cyclic AMP and Cyclic GMP | T. Posternak | 14:23-33
Biochemical Mechanisms of Drug Toxicity | J. R. Gillette, J. R. Mitchell,
B. B. Brodie | 14:271-88
Application of Quantum Chemistry to Drugs
and Their Interactions | J. P. Green, C. L. Johnson,
S. Kang | 14:319-42
The Cholinergic Receptor Protein in Its Mem-
brane Environment | J. B. Cohen, J.-P. Changeux | 15:83-103
Chemical Reactions of Sulfonamides with Car-
bonic Anhydrase | J. E. Coleman | 15:221-42
Common Mechanisms of Hormone Secretion | J. M. Trifaró | 17:27-47
In Vitro Study of β-Adrenergic Receptors | B. B. Wolfe, T. K. Harden,
P. B. Molinoff | 17:575-604
METABOLIC FATE OF DRUGS AND CHEMICALS
Clinical Relevance of Drugs Affecting Trypto-
phan Transport | R. Paoletti, C. Sirtori Jr.,
P. F. Spano | 15:73-81
Developmental Aspects of the Hepatic Cyto-
chrome P450 Monooxygenase System | A. H. Neims, M. Warner, P.
M. Loughnan, J. V. Aranda | 16:427-45
Pharmacokinetic Consequences of Aging | D. P. Richey, A. D. Bender | 17:49-65
MISCELLANEOUS
Enzymes as Drugs | J. S. Holcenberg, J. Roberts | 17:97-116
NEUROMUSCULAR PHARMACOLOGY
Use of Drugs in Myopathies | D. Grob | 16:215-29
The Pharmacology of Experimental Myopathies | M. B. Laskowski, W.-D. Dett-
barn | 17:387-409
NEUROPHARMACOLOGY AND NEUROCHEMISTRY
Serotonin and Central Nervous System Function | T. N. Chase, D. L. Murphy | 13:181-97
Drug Research and Human Sleep | I. Oswald | 13:243-52
Drugs Affecting Movement Disorders | A. Barbeau | 14:91-113
Regulation of Biosynthesis of Catecholamines
and Serotonin in the CNS | E. Costa, J. L. Meek | 14:491-511
Amino Acids as Central Neurotransmitters | F. V. DeFeudis | 15:105-30
Mechanisms of Drug Action at the Voluntary
Muscle Endplate | D. Colquhoun | 15:307-25
Neurotoxic Indoleamines and Monoamine

Neurons	H. G. Baumgarten, A. Bjork-lund	16:101-11
Pharmacology of Drugs that Affect Intracellar Movement	F. E. Samson	16:143-59
Functional Properties of Postjunction Membrane	L. G. Magazanik	16:161-75
Identification and Effects of Neural Transmitters in Invertebrates	J. S. Kehoe, E. Marder	16:245-68
Pharmacologic Control of Temperature Regulation	B. Cox, P. Lomax	17:341-53
Pharmacologic Implications of Brain Acetylcholine Turnover Measures in Rat Brain Nuclei	D. L. Cheney, E. Costa	17:369-86
The Effects of Psychopharmacological Agents on Central Nervous System Amine Metabolism in Man	J. W. Maas	17:411-24
Putative Peptide Neurotransmitters	M. Otsuka, T. Takahashi	17:425-39
PERINATAL PHARMACOLOGY		
Factors Determining the Teratogenicity of Drugs	J. G. Wilson	14:205-17
Perinatal Pharmacology	S. J. Yaffe, M. R. Juchau	14:219-38
Pediatric Clinical Pharmacology and the "Therapeutic Orphan"	A. K. Done, S. N. Cohen, L. Strebel	17:561-73
PHARMACOKINETICS, DRUG ABSORPTION, AND EXCRETION		
Bioavailability of Drugs from Formulations After Oral Administration	L. F. Chasseaud, T. Taylor	14:35-46
Movement of Drugs Across the Gills of Fishes	J. B. Hunn, J. L. Allen	14:47-55
Carcinogenicity as Related to Age	R. Schoental	14:185-204
Blood-Brain Barrier Permeability to Drugs	W. H. Oldendorf	14:239-48
Relationship Between Drug Distribution and Therapeutic Effects in Man	E. S. Vesell	14:249-70
Pharmacokinetics of Drug Disposition: Hemodynamic Considerations	G. R. Wilkinson	15:11-27
Therapeutic Implications of Bioavailability	D. L. Azarnoff, D. H. Huffman	16:53-66
PHARMACOLOGICALLY ACTIVE NATURAL SUBSTANCES		
Antineoplastic Agents From Plants	M. E. Wall, M. C. Wani	17:117-32
Histaminergic Mechanisms in Brain	J.-C. Schwartz	17:325-39
The Pharmacological Effects of Hymenoptera Venoms	R. M. Cavagnol	17:479-98
RENAL PHARMACOLOGY		
Renal Pharmacology, with Special Emphasis on Aldosterone and Angiotensin	F. Gross, J. Möhring	13:57-90
Tubular Sites and Mechanisms of Diuretic Action	W. N. Suki, G. Eknoyan, M. Martinez-Maldonado	13:91-106
Renal Pharmacology: Comparative, Developmental, and Cellular Aspects	Yu. V. Natochin	14:75-90
Effects of Drugs on Uric Acid in Man	W. N. Kelley	15:327-50
Diuretics: Sites and Mechanisms of Action	H. R. Jacobson, J. P. Kokko	16:201-14
The Pharmacology of Renal Lithiasis	T. H. Steele	17:11-25
REPRODUCTION AND FERTILITY		
Corticosteroid-Induced Parturition in Domestic Animals	W. Jöchle	13:33-55
The Pharmacology of Contraceptive Agents	W. D. Odell, M. E. Molitch	14:413-34
Oral Contraceptives: Relation to Mammary Cancer, Benign Breast Lesions, and Cervical Cancer	V. A. Drill	15:367-85
REVIEW OF REVIEWS		
Review of Reviews	C. D. Leake	13:455-63
		14:521-29
		15:465-72
		16:503-10
		17:677-82
SMOOTH MUSCLE PHARMACOLOGY		
Effects of Catecholamines on the Smooth Muscle of the Female Reproductive Tract	J. M. Marshall	13:19-32

Sympathetic Mechanisms in Blood Vessels:
Nerve and Muscle Relationships   J. A. Bevan, C. Su   13:269-85
Cellular Pharmacology of Lanthanum   G. B. Weiss   14:343-54
Organic Nitrate Metabolism   P. Needleman   16:81-93
Specific Pharmacology of Calcium in Myocardi-
um, Cardiac Pacemakers, and Vascular Smooth
Muscle   A. Fleckenstein   17:149-66
STRUCTURE-ACTIVITY RELATIONSHIPS AND MEDICINAL CHEMISTRY
Synthetic Analogs of Oxytocin and the Vasopres-
sins   W. H. Sawyer, M. Manning   13:5-17
Relationships Between the Chemical Structure
and Biological Activity of Convulsants   J. R. Smythies   14:9-21
In Vitro Models in the Study of Structure-
Activity Relationships of Narcotic Analgesics   H. W. Kosterlitz, A. A. Water-
                                                      field   15:29-47
Relations Between Structure and Biological
Activity of Sulfonamides   T. H. Maren   16:309-27
Selective Cyclic Nucleotide Phosphodiesterase
Inhibitors as Potential Therapeutic Agents   B. Weiss, W. N. Hait   17:441-77
TECHNIQUES
Radioimmunoassay   S. Spector   13:359-70
Applications of Integrated Gas Chromatography/
Mass Spectrometry in Pharmacology and Toxi-
cology   D. J. Jenden, A. K. Cho   13:371-90
Application of New Analytical Techniques to
Pharmacology   J. T. Watson   13:391-407